SYNOPSIS OF

PEDIATRICS

To
The health and happiness of children everywhere
and to all who help them achieve these goals.

"Present knowledge is not half utilized;
present knowledge is not half of future knowledge."
William G. Lennox, M.D.

SYNOPSIS OF
PEDIATRICS

Editor

JAMES G. HUGHES, B.A., M.D.

Emeritus Professor of Pediatrics, University of Tennessee Center for the Health Sciences, and formerly Chairman of the Department of Pediatrics;
Director, Center for Children in Crisis, Le Bonheur Children's Medical Center;
formerly Medical Director, Le Bonheur Children's Hospital,
Memphis, Tennessee; Brigadier General, Army of the United States (Ret.)

Associate Editor

JOHN F. GRIFFITH, B.A., M.D.

Professor and Chairman, Department of Pediatrics, and Professor of Neurology,
University of Tennessee Center for the Health Sciences;
Medical Director, Le Bonheur Children's Medical Center

With the collaboration of 50 present or past faculty members of the University of Tennessee Center for the Health Sciences and 3 guest contributors

SIXTH EDITION

with **191** *illustrations*

The C. V. Mosby Company

ST. LOUIS • TORONTO • PRINCETON 1984

MOSBY

A TRADITION OF PUBLISHING EXCELLENCE

Assistant editor: Terry Van Schaik, Sandy Gilfillan
Editing supervisor: Lin Dempsey
Manuscript editor: Diane Ackerman
Book design: Staff
Cover design: Nancy Steinmeyer
Production: Judy Bamert, Margaret B. Bridenbaugh, Ginny Douglas

SIXTH EDITION

Printed in the United States of America

The C.V. Mosby Company
11830 Westline Industrial Drive, St. Louis, Missouri 63146

Library of Congress Cataloging in Publication Data

Main entry under title:

Synopsis of pediatrics.

Includes bibliographical references and index.
I. Pediatrics. I. Hughes, James G. (James Gilliam), 1910-
II. Griffith, John F., 1934-
[DNLM: 1. Pediatrics.
WS 100 S993]
RJ45.S96 1984 618.92 83-26705
ISBN 0-8016-2310-3

GW/VH/VH 9 8 7 6 5 4 3 01/C/027

Contributors*

ROBERT G. ALLEN, M.D.†

Clinical Professor of Surgery

COURTNEY L. ANTHONY, Jr., M.D.

Associate Professor of Pediatrics; Chief, Division of Pediatric Cardiology

FREDERICK F. BARRETT, M.D.

Professor of Pediatrics; Chief, Division of Pediatric Infectious Diseases, Director, Infectious Disease Service, Le Bonheur Children's Medical Center

TULIO E. BERTORINI, M.D.

Associate Professor Neurology; Department of Neurology

DENNIS D. BLACK, M.D.

Instructor, Department of Pediatrics; Division of Pediatric Gastroenterology

MICHAEL BOND, M.S.

Third Year Dermatology Resident

R. E. BROWN, B.S., M.D.

Director of Laboratories, Ft. Worth and Cook Children's Hospitals, Ft. Worth, Texas; Formerly Associate Professor of Pathology and Pediatrics and Director of Laboratories, Le Bonheur Children's Medical Center

C. HAL BRUNT, B.A., M.D.

Clinical Associate Professor of Psychiatry; Medical Director, Lakeside Hospital, Memphis, Tennessee

GEORGE A. BURGHEN, M.D.

Associate Professor of Pediatrics; Chief, Section of Pediatric Endocrinology/Metabolism

ALVRO M. CAMACHO, M.D.

Clinical Professor of Pediatrics

LAWRENCE T. CH'IEN, M.D.

Director of Child Neurology, T.C. Thompson Children's Hospital, Chattanooga, Tennessee; formerly Associate Professor of Pediatrics and Neurology; Director, Neurology/Psychology Division, St. Jude Children's Research Hospital, Memphis, Tennessee

LLOYD. V. CRAWFORD, Jr., M.D.

Clinical Professor of Pediatrics; Chief, Section of Pediatric Allergy

JAMES N. ETTELDORF, Ph.D., M.D.

Emeritus Professor of Pediatrics; Member, Division of Pediatric Endocrinology/Metabolism

SANDOR FELDMAN, M.D.

Associate Professor of Pediatrics; Associate Member, Division of Pediatric Infectious Diseases; Director, General Pediatric Service, St. Jude Children's Research Hospital, Memphis, Tennessee

JOSEPH NEWTON FISHER, Jr., B.A., M.D.

Associate Professor of Medicine and Pediatrics; Co-Assistant Director of Clinical Research Center

PHILIP GEORGE, B.A., M.D.

Professor of Pediatrics; Chief, Division of Pediatric Pulmonary Medicine

*Except when specified otherwise, contributors are from the faculty of the University of Tennessee Center for the Health Sciences, Memphis, Tennessee.
†Deceased.

MARVIN I. GOTTLIEB, B.S., Ph.D., M.D.

Director, Institute for Child Development, Hackensack Medical Center; Professor of Pediatrics, University of Medicine and Dentistry of New Jersey, Formerly Professor of Pediatrics and Director of Clinic for Exceptional Children, Le Bonheur Children's Medical Center

JOHN F. GRIFFITH, B.A., M.D.

Professor and Chairman, Department of Pediatrics; Professor of Neurology; Medical Director, Le Bonheur Children's Medical Center

CHARLES W. GROSS, M.D.

Otolaryngologist, Le Bonheur Children's Medical Center; Formerly Chairman, Department of Otolaryngology

HENRY G. HERROD, B.S., M.S., M.D.

Associate Professor of Pediatrics; Chief, Division of Pediatric Immunology

ROGER L. HIATT, B.S., M.D.

Professor and Chairman, Department of Ophthalmology

JAMES G. HUGHES, B.A., M.D.

Emeritus Professor of Pediatrics; Director, Center for Children in Crisis, Le Bonheur Children's Medical Center

WALTER T. HUGHES, Jr., M.D.

Professor of Pediatrics; Chief, Infectious Diseases Division, St. Jude Children's Research Hospital, Memphis, Tennessee

JOHN A. HUNTER, Jr., A.B., M.A., Ph.D.

Assistant Professor, Department of Psychiatry and Behavioral Sciences, Eastern Virginia Medical School, Norfolk, Virginia; Director, Family Sexual Trauma Program and Director of Adolescent Unit at the Community Mental Health Center and Psychiatric Institute, Norfolk, Virginia; Formerly Clinical Instructor, Department of Psychiatry University of Tennessee Center for the Health Sciences

GERALD R. JERKINS, M.D.

Assistant Professor of Urology; Instructor, Department of Pediatrics

PAUL KING, M.S., M.D.

Clinical Assistant Professor of Psychiatry; Medical Director, Adolescent Services, Lakeside Hospital, Memphis, Tennessee

RONALD H. KIRKLAND, M.D.

Otolaryngologist, Le Bonheur Children's Medical Center

SHELDON B. KORONES, B.S., M.D.

Professor of Pediatrics and Obstetrics/Gynecology; Director, Newborn Center

SHEON LYNCH, M.T. (ASCP)

Supervisor of Chemistry, Le Bonheur Children's Medical Center Laboratory

JOSÉ MARÍN-GARCIÁ, M.D.

Associate Professor of Pediatrics; Member, Division of Pediatric Cardiology

ALVIN M. MAUER, B.A., M.D.

Professor of Medicine and Pediatrics; Chief, Medical Hematology/Oncology; Director, Cancer Program, University of Tennessee Center for the Health Sciences; Formerly Director, St. Jude Children's Research Hospital, Memphis, Tennessee

H. NORMAN NOE, M.D.

Associate Professor of Urology; Assistant Professor of Pediatrics

DAVID M. ORENSTEIN, M.D.

Assistant Professor of Pediatrics; Member, Division of Pulmonary Medicine; Director, Cystic Fibrosis Center, Le Bonheur Children's Medical Center

SUSAN R. ORENSTEIN, M.D.

Instructor, Department of Pediatrics, Division of Pediatric Gastroenterology

ROBERT S. PINALS, M.D.

Professor of Medicine; Director, Division of Connective Tissue Disease; Chief, Section of Rheumatology

FREDERICK P. RIVARA, M.D., M.P.H.

Associate Professor of Pediatrics and Community Medicine; Associate Director, Ambulatory Pediatrics, Le Bonheur Children's Medical Center

E. WILLIAM ROSENBERG, M.D.

Professor and Chief, Division of Dermatology, Department of Medicine

SHANE ROY III, B.S., M.D.

Professor of Pediatrics; Member, Section of Pediatric Nephrology

JERRY L. SHENEP, M.D.

Instructor of Pediatrics; Assistant Member, Division of Infectious Diseases, St. Jude Children's Research Hospital, Memphis, Tennessee

ROBERT B. SKINNER, Jr., M.D.

Instructor, Division of Dermatology, Department of Medicine

F. BRUDER STAPLETON, M.D.

Associate Professor of Pediatrics; Chief, Section of Pediatric Nephrology

MARCUS J. STEWART, B.S., M.S., M.D.

Clinical Professor of Orthopedic Surgery; Chief, Division of Orthopedics, Kennedy Veterans Administration Hospital, Memphis, Tennessee

GREGORY L. STIDHAM, M.D.

Associate Professor of Pediatrics and Anesthesiology; Chief, Critical Care Division; Director, Intensive Care Unit, Le Bonheur Children's Medical Center

ROBERT L. SUMMITT, M.S., M.D.

Professor of Pediatrics, Anatomy and Child Development; Dean, College of Medicine

DONALD ALAN TAYLOR, M.D.

Clinical Assistant Professor of Pediatrics and Neurology

HERSHEL P. WALL, B.S., M.D.

Professor of Pediatrics; Associate Dean of Admissions and Student Affairs; Chief, Division of Ambulatory Pediatrics; Acting Director, Clinic for Exceptional Children, Le Bonheur Children's Medical Center

JEWELL C. WARD, M.D., Ph.D.

Assistant Professor of Pediatrics and Biochemistry; Chief, Inborn Errors of Metabolism Laboratory; Member, Division of Pediatric Genetics

ABBY LOIS WASSERMAN, M.D.

Assistant Professor of Pediatrics; Director, Division of Psychiatry and Psychology, St. Jude Children's Research Hospital, Memphis, Tennessee

DAVID F. WESTENKIRCHNER, M.D.

Assistant Professor of Pediatrics; Associate Director, Intensive Care Unit, Le Bonheur Children's Medical Center

PETER F. WHITINGTON, B.A., M.D.

Associate Professor of Pediatrics; Chief, Division of Pediatric Gastroenterology, University of Tennessee

GENE L. WHITINGTON, M.D.

Associate Professor of Pediatrics; Member, Division of Pediatric Gastroenterology

EARLE L. WRENN, Jr., B.A., M.D.

Clinical Associate Professor of Surgery and Pediatrics

PETER W. ZINKUS, B.A., M.A., Ph.D.

Assistant Professor of Pediatrics; Pediatric Psychologist, Clinic for Exceptional Children, Le Bonheur Children's Medical Center

---

NOTE: Throughout this textbook, unless the sense of the sentence specifically requires appropriate sex designation, use of the words *he, his,* and *him* invariably also mean *she, hers,* and *her*. Terms such as *he/she* are linguistic monstrosities that distract the reader, and vividness of expression often suffers when plural forms substitute for the singular to avoid sex connotation.

Preface to Sixth Edition

Rapid progress in the biomedical sciences and increasing emphasis on the biosocial aspects of pediatrics have greatly improved our depth of understanding of disease processes and their treatment, and have widened the scope of pediatric practice to include many aspects of childhood not formerly considered inherently a part of this specialty.

Particularly because of vigorous research in the numerous pediatric subspecialties, new knowledge has been gained concerning many organic entities. This has led to markedly improved therapy. The amazing proliferation of technologic advances for precise study of disease processes, as well as for treatment, enable the physician to be far more effective in the prevention, diagnosis, and treatment of a wide variety of diseases.

Concomitantly, there is now laudable emphasis on developmental and learning disabilities, child psychology and child psychiatry, family maladjustment, child abuse and neglect, foster care, adoptions, and a variety of other factors that may affect the child adversely.

Because of this rapid progress, medical textbooks require frequent revision—every 4 years in the case of this text. The sixth edition of the *Synopsis of Pediatrics* seeks to bring up to date topics included in previous editions and to add new material as indicated.

Extensive changes have been made in the present edition. Five new chapters have been added: Pediatric Intensive Care, Pediatric Urology, Pediatric Dermatology, Pediatric Otolaryngology, and Laboratory Values–The Pediatric Range. Eight existing chapters have been completely rewritten by new authors: Mental Retardation, Nutrition and Nutritional Disturbances, Fluid and Electrolyte Homeostasis, Injuries and Poisonings in Childhood, The Digestive System, Arthritis in Childhood, Inborn Errors of Metabolism, and Cystic Fibrosis. The remaining 25 chapters have been revised as indicated. References to pertinent medical literature, appearing at the end of each chapter to encourage the reader to study more deeply the material covered in this somewhat abbreviated textbook, have been expanded.

The central purpose of the book remains the same: to cover the major portion of the broad field of pediatrics in a clear, straight-forward manner with emphasis on a practical approach to diagnosis and treatment, as well as proper attention to basic mechanisms of disease. It is not intended to be a complete, detailed textbook.

The popularity of this book leads us to believe that it fills a useful purpose in affording a rapid and clearcut introduction to this specialty, and that it contains sufficient material to guide the student and physician in the diagnosis and management of the great majority of conditions seen in pediatric practice.

It is now 21 years since the *Synopsis of Pediatrics* first appeared in print. And it is time to begin shifting responsibility for its editorship. Therefore Dr. John F. Griffith, Chairman of the Department of Pediatrics of the University of Tennessee Center for the Health Sciences and Medical Director of the Le Bonheur Children's Medical Center, has kindly and ably joined me as Associate Editor in preparation of this sixth edition. On the next go-round he will be Editor, and perhaps I shall be around to serve happily in an editorial consultative capacity.

Since this is the last time I shall be writing a preface for this textbook, I should like to take this opportunity to thank all contributors, past and present, for their valued participation in the various editions of the *Synopsis of Pediatrics*. And thanks also to their patient secretaries, who typed and retyped the many manuscripts, being often required to decifer calligraphy as baffling as that of the Rosetta stone. Finally, appreciation is expressed to The C.V. Mosby Company for its professional excellence and unfailing graciousness.

We recognize that this text is not really a synopsis in the usual sense of the term. But it was born in 1963 and christened with its present title as one of a series of synopses published by The C.V. Mosby Company. Like a child, it has grown and developed through the years, and we have been reluctant to cause it to have the failure-to-thrive syndrome. Therefore we have nourished it to its present status.

We now send our offspring into the wide world of medical readership and trust it will merit a kindly reception. We hope it will continue to prove useful in encouraging knowledge of, and interest in, the fascinating field of pediatrics.

James G. Hughes

Preface to First Edition

The pace of modern medicine is so rapid and the fields of the various specialties so broad that even the most devoted physician finds it difficult to keep abreast of progress. Even the specialist has difficulty mastering his specialty.

Harassed by the demands of a crowded curiculum, the medical student is often confused. He is confronted either with texts that are lengthy and detailed or with compendia and manuals that give useful information but which, because of their brevity, cannot cover basic fundamentals.

The busy physician, shouldering the load of a heavy practice, must also, at times, read as he runs. Although he often yearns for the leisurely hours to pursue his topics of interest, it becomes increasingly difficult to find them. Books and journals are legion, but his time is limited.

The intern and the resident perhaps have somewhat more time to read and are in close contact with the teaching staff. However, they, too, can profit from presentations that condense and crystallize important medical information.

With these thoughts in mind, we have prepared this *Synopsis of Pediatrics* in the hope that it will make accurate information more easily available. It does not, of course, pretend to rival the excellent pediatric reference texts that are indispensable to this specialty. Nor does it seek to present something about everything. Indeed, many things have been left out intentionally. However, the reader will note the strong orientation toward explanation of the fundamental mechanisms of disease in an effort to bridge the gap between basic science and clinical pediatrics. Only in this way can a full appreciation of disease be obtained and logical therapy applied. Unless medicine be scientific, we had best stop speaking of medical science.

Of course, there would not be so many textbooks if anyone had solved the riddle of combining brevity and clarity with a proper degree of comprehensiveness. The degree to which these qualities can be joined is the challenge of medical writing. We do not presume to have solved this problem. Perhaps it can never be solved since condensation and simplification are double dangers. We recognize that it is a somewhat hypertrophied synopsis, but since the child is our subject, we had to let it grow.

A new method of medical illustration, evolved recently by the writer, is used here for the first time. It consists of organ, arrow, and label overlays superimposed upon the picture of a child. These prefabricated items afford considerable flexibility in making teaching slides or illustrations.

I wish to thank the various contributors for the material they submitted and particularly acknowledge their indulgence in many instances in permitting me to make changes in manner of presentation and literary style. Although twenty voices cannot be alike, there is, at least, a harmony.

I would also like to express the appreciation of our group to the various publishers, editors, and authors who so generously permitted reproduction of material from their publications. We are also grateful to the secretaries of the department who toiled diligently to type the text.

James G. Hughes

Contents

1 The Scope of Pediatrics

Pediatrics is the study of growth and development of the child from the genetic background and moment of conception through adolescence, and the science and art of the prevention, diagnosis, and treatment of the diseases of children from birth through adolescence, whether these disturbances be physical, mental, or emotional. It is a profound concern with, and an abiding interest in, everything that contributes to the final product—a healthy adult ready to take his place in life.

Pediatrics is the knowledge of genetics, for this governs the seed. It is the knowledge of the events of prenatal life, for this is the soil in which the seed grows. It is the knowledge of the newborn, the infant, and the young child, for this is the early growth period. And it is the continued scientific and empathetic supervision of the child until he achieves maturity.

The single most characteristic feature of pediatrics is that it deals with the growth and development of the child, comprising all those changes in size and form and in complexity of function that constitute growing up. It is this fact that distinguishes it as a specialty—one of the broadest and one of the most interesting.

Physicians dealing with children must be continually aware, for example, of the differences in physiologic maturity of newborn and young infants as compared to the older infant and younger child and to an even greater extent the older child or adolescent. There are differences for these various age levels in (1) functioning of various organ systems, (2) degree of immunity to diseases, (3) response to the effects of disease, (4) drug dosages and tolerance to drugs, (5) mental and motor ability, and (6) pattern of emotional response.

Thus pediatrics encompasses a fascinating and almost endless variation that distinguishes it from other specialties that focus only on certain systems or regions of the body or that are related entirely to adults, who are more or less of similar size and maturity of functions. These differences between children and adults have been summed up in the statement, "The child is *not* a little man."

GENETICS

The pediatrician must maintain a lively interest in genetics. Although the mechanisms of heredity are working long before the pediatrician sees the newborn child, he is the first to observe deviations occasioned by defective genes. Thus congenital malformations fall within the province of the pediatrician, who may call on various specialists to help in the management of such children.

Heredity also determines those subtle enzymatic abnormalities known as inborn errors of metabolism. These, too, are usually first detected by the pediatrician, who must know how to diagnose them and how to treat those susceptible to clinical management.

Finally, a sound knowledge of heredity is important in regard to the effects it has on general growth and development—knowledge that may explain body build, facial appearance, intellectual level, and many other facets of the child.

Interest in genetics has quickened by virtue of remarkable discoveries regarding chromosomes. Determining true sex through study of the chromatin pattern of cells has afforded a practical application of genetics. Most of all, however, photographing chromosomes, arranging them in pairs, and thereby demonstrating alterations in chromosomal patterns that account for certain clinical conditions have stimulated a tremendous interest in genetics. Furthermore, an increasing number of genetically transmitted diseases can now be diagnosed in utero by technologic procedures. To what extent these explorations toward the earliest beginnings of life will someday afford a better understanding and possible control of various diseases constitutes an exciting challenge.

PRENATAL EVENTS

It is said that the Chinese reckon a child to be 1 year of age at birth. Of course, it is not a year, but the major portion of a year of intrauterine growth and development that precedes the birth of the baby. If heredity and intrauterine environment are normal, a normal baby may be born. However, just as heredity may determine abnormality, so also may adverse prenatal influences.

Some adverse prenatal factors that may distort intrauterine growth and development to cause death, deformity, premature delivery, or subsequent disability are (1) poor prenatal supervision, (2) maternal malnutrition, (3) acute or chronic maternal diseases (systemic or specifically affecting the reproductive organs), (4) maternal infections that permit organisms to cross the placenta and infect the unborn child (usually viral agents such as that of rubella; less often bacterial or protozoal agents), (5) faulty implantation and hormonal imbalance, often leading to threatened abortion or miscarriage, (6) pelvic irradiation, (7) deleterious effects of certain drugs or toxic substances such as excessive alcoholic intake or excessive smoking during pregnancy, and (8) rarely, trauma.

Knowledge of such factors is of great aid in evaluation of the sick newborn infant or the child who later shows evidence of brain damage that may have occurred from adverse prenatal influences. Furthermore, if such factors act within the early months of gestation, growth and development may be so distorted that the resulting abnormalities may closely mock or even be clinically indistinguishable from genetically determined malformations.

LABOR AND DELIVERY

Since the baby may be profoundly affected by the vicissitudes of labor and delivery, knowledge of what transpired as the child was born is of great significance. Proper interpretation necessitates that the pediatrician know as many of the circumstances as possible, including the following:

1. Whether any one or combinations of the above high-risk factors occurred
2. Whether the baby was born in the home, in the hospital, or en route to the hospital
3. The mother's condition (fever, foul vaginal discharge, etc.)
4. Whether she is primiparous or multiparous
5. Type of delivery (spontaneous, induced, or operative—including cesarean section or use of forceps)
6. Fetal presentation
7. Duration of the stages of labor
8. Relative intensity of labor
9. Whether cephalopelvic disproportion existed
10. Time interval between rupture of the membranes (spontaneous or induced) and birth of the baby
11. Drugs used for analgesia or anesthesia, doses, routes of administration, and timing with respect to delivery
12. Whether labor was induced and managed by an intravenous oxytocic agent
13. Whether any untoward event occurred such as maternal hemorrhage or severe hypotension
14. The infant's birth weight, gestational age, and condition at the moment of birth, including Apgar rating
15. Whether resuscitation was required and, if so, methods employed
16. Condition of the baby when sent from the delivery room to the nursery

It is apparent that teamwork between the obstetrician, in recording pertinent information, and the pediatrician, in interpreting this information, is of great importance.

NEWBORN PERIOD

Patterned by genes, nurtured in the womb, and launched by labor and delivery, the infant now enters the newborn period. So rapid are the adaptive adjustments to extrauterine existence that the pediatrician needs to have a thorough knowledge of the newborn infant's anatomy, physiology, and behavior. Because the handicaps of low birth weight infants are even greater, they require special knowledge.

To watch life begin here in the outer world is one of the real fascinations of pediatrics. Although events usually proceed normally, many threats exist, including congenital malformations perhaps incompatible with life or for which immediate operation is necessary. Birth damage is also usually first observed in the newborn period, but may not become apparent for months or even years. Infections rank high on the list of dangers, and their prevention and treatment are of the utmost importance.

Other special problems include (1) initial resuscitation, (2) maintenance of respiration, (3) affording oxygen in proper concentrations, (4) special feeding methods for premature and sick infants, (5) particular care with respect to fluid and electrolyte therapy, (6) careful regulation of drug dosage because organ immaturity handicaps detoxification and excretion, (7) conditions causing anemia or hyperbilirubinemia, and (8) vomiting, diarrhea, and surgical conditions of the alimentary tract. These are only a few examples of the many problems often posed in care of the newborn infant.

When one considers that most childhood deaths occur during the newborn period or during the first year of life, one can understand why pediatrics is increasingly concerned with research into the causes and treatment of many threatening conditions that appear at these times.

INFANCY PERIOD

After the newborn period, usually defined as the first month of life, the baby enters the period termed infancy, comprising the first 2 years of life. This is an era of extremely rapid growth and development physically, mentally, and emotionally. The details of this development are described in Chapter 2. Organ systems mature rapidly, and the relative instability of homeostasis in the newborn period gives way to a more secure status—the infant has better control of his various physiologic and biochemical functions. Physical growth proceeds at a remarkable rate. The child's birth weight may double by about 5 months of age and triple by about 1 year of age. Length increases rapidly, and the various parts of the body grow in size and form according to predetermined patterns. The infant also gains increasing neuromotor ability, passing through well-defined and orderly stages of achievement.

Paralleling physical growth and development is the amazing rapidity with which the normal baby learns. By 2 years of age he can speak short sentences, knows much about the home and family, and demonstrates a lively interest in exploring the environment. These first 2 years are also of cardinal importance in the emotional life of the child. They constitute formative years in the development of his personality; much of what it will be later is determined even at this early time.

From a preventive viewpoint the physician plays an important role throughout this period. Through serial health examinations frequently in the first year and somewhat less often during the second year, the adequacy of physical growth is checked with the use of growth charts. Simple tests are applied to determine whether development is progressing satisfactorily in the motor, language, adaptive, and personal-social fields. The physician affords parents opportunities to discuss the behavior of the child and gives advice on the numerous problems of management that concern parents, thus seeking to foster good attitudes and a healthy emotional environment to encourage psychologic security and stability. He seeks to detect behavior problems at their incipiency so that corrective action can be taken before they reach major magnitude. At such examinations the nutritional status of the child is surveyed and advice is given concerning the diet. The physician also performs a complete physical examination to detect conditions not previously noted so that early treatment may be instituted.

Immunization against certain preventable infectious diseases is also included in these supervisory health conferences. Thus the infant is immunized against diphtheria, pertussis, tetanus, measles, rubella, poliomyelitis, and mumps.

Counseling in prevention of accidents, a leading cause of death, is an important part of the health supervisory visits. Much of pediatric practice is concerned with health supervision, immunization, and other preventive aspects, including evaluation of the adequacy of growth and development. The remainder consists of the diagnosis and management of a wide variety of diseases that affect various organs or systems and range from the relatively simple and common conditions to those of great severity.

PRESCHOOL PERIOD

The preschool period follows the same general trends established in the period of infancy. Physical growth is proceeding at a somewhat slower pace, mental development is progressing steadily, and emotional patterns are becoming more fixed. Supervisory health visits are now made somewhat less often and are similar to those described for the period of infancy. Normal children are usually well established on a satisfactory diet by this time (although they may not eat enough to satisfy their parents), immunizations have progressed into the booster phase, and problems of emotional origin are increasing in frequency.

Personality development. In the period of infancy the environment of the child is restricted chiefly to the home. Other than members of the family, the child's contacts are limited. He is a fledgling not yet ready to fly. In the preschool period he leaves the nest and enters a new world: the neighborhood, the shopping center, the Sunday school, and perhaps the nursery and kindergarten. He meets many new people, young and old, and is called on to make an increasing number of personality adjustments. If he has been reared properly in infancy and guided wisely during the preschool period, he will socialize rapidly, gain more and more self-confidence, and adjust well in an increasingly complex world. If his lot has been otherwise, he may fail to adjust, becoming one of the many children with emotional problems. Furthermore, he may be so poorly prepared to enter school that he either totally fails to accept it or becomes greatly disturbed by it. For these reasons and others discussed elsewhere (Chapter 4), behavior problems are common in the preschool period.

Common infectious diseases. Increasing contacts with people also mean increasing contacts with germs. Preschool children are ready prey for the currently unpreventable common contagious diseases. This age group also has a relatively high incidence of infections of the respiratory and gastrointestinal tracts as compared to other age groups. In these early battles with bacteria and viruses, immunity to many of them is achieved so that later in childhood the incidence of contagious diseases and respiratory and gastrointestinal tract illness diminishes.

Accidents. Only the indiscriminating infant excels the preschool child in capacity to invite accidents. Most accidents involving infants occur in the home, but those involving the adventurous preschool child occur outside the home to an increasing degree. The frequency of traffic accidents involving this age group rises as the years pass. It is a shocking fact that in the United States accidents are the leading cause of death of children from 1 to 14 years of age—small wonder that pediatricians and many other groups are so interested in accident prevention.

Malformations and malignant conditions. Advances in prevention of disease and improvements in therapy have changed the face of pediatric practice. Diseases formerly common, threatening, and often fatal now occur far less often. Thus diphtheria is a rarity, deaths from diarrheal disorders are greatly diminished, and death from respiratory tract infection occurs less frequently. As in leaving the mountains one notes the foothills, congenital malformations and malignant conditions, no longer overshadowed by the massive incidence of common disease, now evoke more interest. Congenital malformations and malignant conditions are among the top four causes of death of children from 1 to 14 years of age.

In pediatrics, interest centers on three major facets of the malformation problem: the genetic aspect, the etiologic role of adverse prenatal influences, and the remarkable advances in pediatric surgery and rehabilitative procedures. The identification of abnormal chromosome patterns in several syndromes of defective development has introduced a new era in which the etiology of many other malformations is being elucidated. Early detection of inborn errors of metabolism, and in several instances their successful management, is a great advance in the care of certain afflicted infants. Although scientists now see, as through a glass darkly, little prospect for prophylaxis of genetically determined anomalies, advances in knowledge of genetics may lead to as yet unforeseen opportunities to modify or control human development.

The residual defects of damage from adverse prenatal factors may become apparent in the newborn period or later on, depending on severity of the insult, timing in relation to gestation, and structures altered. This type of damage expresses itself clinically in two chief ways: malformations, perhaps indistinguishable from those genetically determined, and brain damage. Such anomalies of development are of a wide variety and pose many problems in diagnosis and management.

Increasing interest in malignant conditions of childhood stems partly from the fact that cancer, including leukemia, is one of the chief causes of death of children in the United States but is primarily a result of improved and more widely available diagnostic and therapeutic methods. As with cancer in other age groups, there is a premium on early diagnosis. Hence, during all health examinations, pediatricians should be alert to the possibility of a malignant condition when a mass is detected, when the hematologic picture is suggestive, or when other indicative evidence is present.

Therapeutic advances have been achieved by greatly improved pediatric surgical techniques that permit formidable operations to be performed with relative safety and by the availability of a rapidly enlarging armamentarium of anticancer drugs of increasing effectiveness.

Syndromes of brain damage. Syndromes resulting from brain damage are noted frequently in young children and present many medical, social, economic, and educational problems. Residual defects of brain damage express themselves clinically in one of, or a combination of, four major entities: (1) neuromotor defect (cerebral palsy), (2) epilepsy, (3) mental retardation, and (4) brain damage behavior syndrome. To these major manifestations may be added visual-perceptual-motor disabilities, handicaps of speech and hearing, and various learning disabilities (see Chapter 3). Because of the variety and frequency of clinical manifestations caused by brain damage, pediatricians are often involved in complex diagnostic and therapeutic problems related to these conditions. Among other things they need to have knowledge of and fully utilize various consultants and community facilities in the comprehensive management of the problems of these unfortunate children.

Many other problems in the preschool period might be considered, but from the discussions given it is apparent that during these early years the scope of pediatrics is exceptionally broad.

SCHOOL PERIOD

The school years are generally the healthiest. Having passed through the potential danger period of the early years and having met and conquered a variety of pathogenic agents, to some of which immunity has been established, schoolchildren are relatively free of disease. They continue to have their share of respiratory tract infections but usually handle them well. Certain diseases to which they were formerly not so susceptible may now appear, such as rheumatic fever, a disease far more common among children of school age than among others.

Residual defects previously incurred are still present. The child must learn to live with them and to adapt to them as well as he can, seeking to participate as fully as possible in those activities commensurate with his clinical condition. Parents, too, must often make profound adjustments to the child's disability. Obviously, the psychologic repercussions of being handicapped have an increased opportunity to prey on the child's mind. He sees other children more active on the playground and in after-school activities. Later, as an adolescent, the social disadvantages of being handicapped may bring many a lonely moment.

The principal psychologic difficulties of the school years, however, come at the time of entry into school and in the first few years afterward, when so many adjustments must be made. The overprotected child who was practically a prince in his home now belongs to the masses. The socially shy child who stayed too much within his shell is now cast into the crowd. The child who was blessed with affection and warmth within the home is now taught in a large class by a busy teacher who, despite inherent kindness, does not have time to be parent to all. The child whose intellectual level is not up to that of the class repeatedly trips on the barriers of lessons that are easily hurdled by others. The child who has never been treated roughly is spoken to abruptly, sees another child punished in class, or in other ways derives an opinion that school is a hostile place and he had best be home.

The inner tensions thus occasioned erupt in psychosomatic manifestations of great variety. The child may become nervous, fearful, or insecure, pleading not to be sent back to school and being most willing to forfeit his academic career. When words fail to achieve his desires, he speaks in another language—the language of the organ systems. His chief spokesman is his stomach, so easily upset. Recurrent vague abdominal pain plagues the child, the parents, and sometimes the puzzled physician. It is noted that the syndrome is peculiar: the pain appears in morning hours as the time for school approaches, or strikes in the midst of difficult lessons, or elects to visit the child in the evenings when the parents, in their laudable desire to help with studies, put on the pressure to achieve. Vomiting often follows the pain. If the child is 6 years old, he may have that common syndrome—never so called in scientific literature but noted by all physicians to the young—September vomiting. It is an epidemic of upset stomachs, limited almost exclusively to first-grade children, which appears chiefly just before the dreaded trip to school and is rapidly cured by the child's being permitted to remain at home.

Many problems center on academic difficulties. The most common derive from the fact that the child simply does not have the intellectual ability to keep pace with his peers. Many a child well-schooled in social graces—polite, well-mannered, and well-spoken—is really dull-normal in intellect. Parents may be shocked at the idea that the child who appears so smart is really not. Only careful comprehensive psychologic testing will reveal the true facts; it should be done in every instance of school failure. Other causes for academic difficulties are lack of motivation to learn because of emotional problems in the home or elsewhere, cultural deprivation, poor hearing, impaired vision, run-down general physical condition, and special handicaps to learning, chief of which is specific reading disability (dyslexia).

THE PEDIATRICIAN AS THE CHILD'S ADVOCATE

The pediatrician's role is that of advocate for the child, not merely in the field of prevention and treatment of disease but also in every aspect of the child's life that affects normal growth and development—physically, mentally, psychologically, and socially. The constant objective is to so protect and rear the child that he becomes a healthy, happy, well-adjusted, independently functioning adult well-equipped to make a maximum contribution to society. Thus the proper pediatrician—the "complete pediatrician"—has an enormous interest in and concern for the familial, social, educational, environmental, legal, and moral milieu in which the child grows and develops. Adverse circumstances in any of these areas may thwart the child's achievement of his personal maximal potential for growth and development in the broadest, most comprehensive sense.

As a group, pediatricians are the most dynamic, properly aggressive, and strongly organized of all the medical specialties in mounting and pursuing programs for the health and welfare of children. These objectives are achieved by the unusual strength and effectiveness of our national pediatric societies, especially the American Academy of Pediatrics—some 20,000 strong in the United States and growing rapidly at the state and national levels.

The major pediatric organizations have established a Council of Pediatric Societies that has been instrumental in fostering national legislation for improvement of the health care of children. Expert panels of pediatricians frequently advise Congress concerning proposed legislation in the child health field. Numerous committees of pediatric experts focus continually on various aspects of child health care, conduct analyses, and promote national and state programs. Constant efforts are made to extend good health care to all children by means of adequate organization of private practice groups, support of Medicaid and other health programs for children, and proper medical insurance coverage.

As advocate for the child, the pediatrician is often called on by public and civic groups and by the mass media to discuss various aspects of child health. Thus the pediatrician becomes a spokesman for the child and capitalizes on these opportunities to expand and improve the public's knowledge of what constitutes good health services for children.

ACADEMIC AND RESEARCH ACTIVITIES

The physician entering pediatric training may cultivate an interest in research and may wish to train further in one of the many fields that follow the lines of the pediatric subspecialties (cardiology, hematology, endocrinology, metabolism, allergy, neurology, genetics, psychiatry, public health pediatrics, diseases of newborn infants, pathology, infectious diseases, etc.). Of all the specialties, pediatrics has one of the most vigorous, varied, and interesting research programs. Other physicians completing pediatric training may wish to remain within the academic ranks, where they find rich opportunities for teaching and research. In the atmosphere of a university or medical center there are the rewards of constant association with those who are working out new solutions to old problems, breaking down barriers of ignorance, and teaching the students and house staff who will be the physicians of the future.

James G. Hughes

2 Growth and Development

Growth and development represent a continuous interaction of biologic processes that are initiated at conception and terminate at death. The integrity and the quality of these processes are influenced by a myriad of variables, including genetic, physiologic, biochemical, psychologic, and socioeconomic factors. Physicians are uniquely responsible for safe-guarding and enhancing growth and development. The traditional medical role focuses on preventing, detecting, and treating the noxious influences that can impair these biologic processes. Among physicians the challenge is particularly demanding for the pediatrician, inasmuch as most of growth and development is completed during the first few years of life. Professionals providing health care for children must be aware of the various genetic, nutritional, hormonal, emotional, and economic impediments (among others) that can severely disturb the milieu for normal growth and development. Failure to recognize antecedent high-risk factors and signals that herald disturbed patterns of growth and development may result in serious and permanent disabling sequelae. Students of pediatrics, regardless of their level of training, should be familiar with the complex processes that constitute growth and development.

Conceptually, growth and development are often used synonymously, or at least to imply a symbiotic relationship. *Growth* implies a physical change, usually resulting from either an increase in cell number or cell size. *Development* suggests a change or modification in capacity to function; for example, the enhancement of a skill. Two additional processes, maturation and learning, are intimately associated with growth and development. *Maturation* is a biologic process of progressive change leading to utilizations—a sophistication of growth and development that ultimately permits function by the organism (or cell). *Learning* is basically a permanent alteration of behavior that results from experience. Learning in part depends on a satisfactory end product of the maturational process. A child is unable to walk until the necessary cellular growth is complete in the various locomotive organs (muscles, bones, and nerves) and maturation and integration of the participating systems is completed. The child cannot learn to walk unless the neuromusculoskeletal systems are capable of working as a unit. It is obvious that biologic functions can be seriously impaired if adverse influences disrupt the growth-development-maturation-learning complex. The four biologic processes are intimately related and often mutually dependent. The sophistication of physical, mental, cognitive, emotional, and social abilities of an individual are all components of normal growth and development.

The pediatrician actively participates in providing an optimum environment that will ensure proper growth and development for his patients. To appreciate deviations from the normal, it is assumed that the professional is well versed in the acceptable range of normal values. The normal parameters of maturation vary among individuals and within each chronologic age bracket. The physician, as well as all health professionals concerned with growth and development, must be familiar with the range of variabilities and norms. For example, the age-related norms for language, motor skills, and sexual maturation must be appreciated as they apply to a particular child and within the framework of a developmental sequence.

The *periods of growth,* which are common to all normal individuals, have been categorized into four major sequential groups: (1) a relatively rapid growth during infancy with a gradual deceleration until about the fourth year of life, (2) a slow but uniform period of growth until puberty, (3) a prominent adolescent growth spurt, and (4) a relatively gradual decrease in the rate of growth until completion of maturity. The general sequential pattern is consistently recognized both for height and weight. Many of the internal organ systems, such as the respiratory, circulatory, digestive, and excretory systems, follow a similar pattern. However, all the organ systems do not follow this general format; for example, lymphoid tissue, nervous system, head circumference, and thyroid gland have unique developmental patterns. Lymphoid tissue grows rapidly during childhood but decreases in mass size at the onset of puberty. The growth of the nervous system is also an exception to the general rule of linear growth. The unique characteristics of nerve tissue, such as lack of neuronal replication, evoke particular modifications of traditional growth patterns. Head circumference increases rapidly after birth, but this growth is of short duration. A sharp decrease in rate of increase in head size is noted until about 10 years of age. Similarly, the thyroid gland manifests a unique pattern of growth. Growth is constant from birth to maturity, without the characteristic rapid acceleration during infancy and preadolescence.

Cellular growth can be related to three phases of activity: (1) hyperplasia, (2) hyperplasia and hypertrophy, and (3) hypertrophy (Fig. 2-1). *Hyperplasia* implies an increase in the number of cells in an organ, whereas *hypertrophy* suggests an increase in bulk as a result of increased cell size. Most organs pass through these three stages, a process that depends on the slowing and subsequent cessation of deoxyribonucleic acid (DNA) replication (Fiser and Hill, 1977). Analysis of DNA content serves as a measure of cell number in a tissue or organ. The amount of DNA increases linearly during the prenatal period, decelerates slightly after birth, and reaches a maximum at age 8 to 12 months. Accumulation of protein within the cell continues

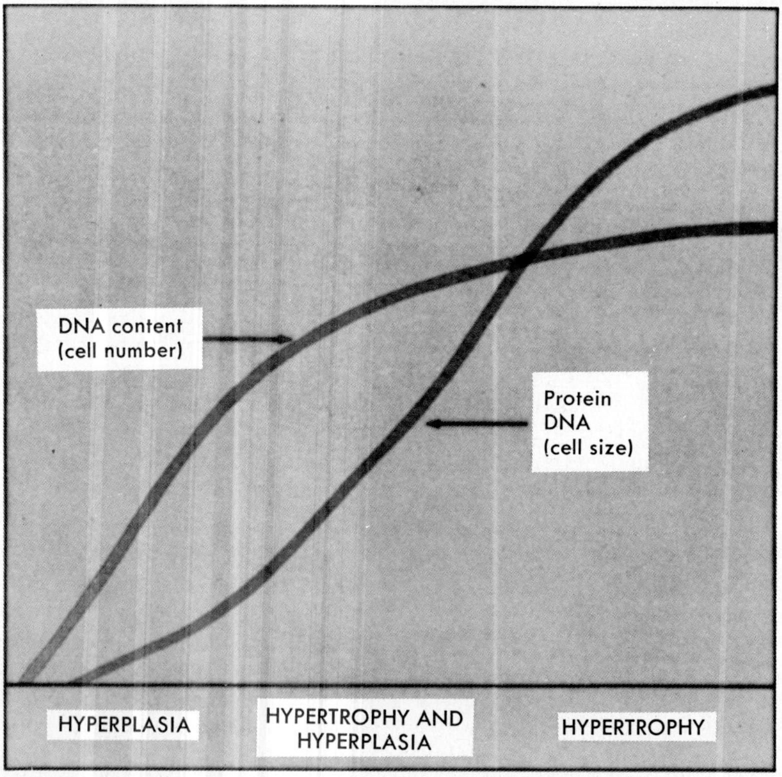

Fig. 2-1. Three phases of cellular growth. In any organ, cell replication precedes increase in cell size.

after DNA replication ceases. Initially, organ growth results from active mitosis, with an increase in cell numbers. Later, growth results from hypertrophy of existing cells. This concept is significant in understanding the mechanisms of either growth-retarding or growth-promoting influences on various tissues.

FACTORS INFLUENCING GROWTH AND DEVELOPMENT

Growth and development can be modified by a myriad of exogenous and endogenous influences, working independently or in combination with one another. Several of these factors will be reviewed briefly.

Heredity. Hereditary characteristics depend on the action of genes or the combined actions of several genes. Each individual inherits a large assortment of these basic units. Genes are formed from DNA and consist of two helical chains of alternate sugar (deoxyribose) and phosphate, which are linked with purine and pyrimidine bases. The purines (adenine and guanine) and the pyrimidines (cystosine, uracil, and thymine) project from the sugars and are joined by hydrogen bonds.

It has been estimated that humans may have as many as 50,000 genes. The developmental potentials of a person are couched in the gene complement, established at fertilization. Each gene exerts an influence on the developing embryo and fetus and sets a template for future growth of the child. Potentials for growth and development are determined by the interplay of inherited genes. Genetic expression can be modified by a variety of environmental factors. In essence, genetic constitution may prognosticate the potentials and format of growth and development, but these patterns can be modified by various exogenous influences.

Prenatal environment. Faulty development and malformations may result from harmful elements in the embryonal and fetal environment. During the interval from fertilization to delivery of the newborn, the growing organism may be insulted by a myriad of exogenous factors. Injuries incurred during the embryonic period (gestational age from conception to 12 weeks) may cause an arrest of development and serious malformations. Regardless of etiology, exogenous insults during embryonic life may interfere with the normal processes of organogenesis. On the other hand, during the period of fetal development (gestational age 12 to 40 weeks) intrauterine injuries or insults have an effect similar to that incurred during postnatal life. Regardless of the type of offending influence or the time during gestational life that the injury occurs, the developing organism may be compromised by depression or deviations of normal growth and developmental patterns. Examples of exogenous prenatal factors that can severely impair growth and development include the following:

1. Maternal infections
   a. Rubella
   b. Cytomegalic inclusion disease
   c. Syphilis
   d. Toxoplasmosis
2. Maternal endocrine disorders
   a. Diabetes mellitus
   b. Hypothyroidism
3. Maternal nutritional disorders
4. Genetic disorders
   a. Isoimmunization disorders
   b. Metabolic disorders (e.g., PKU)
   c. Skeletal anomalies (e.g., achondroplasia)
   d. Chromosomal abnormalities (e.g., Down syndrome)
5. Maternal chemical-toxin exposure
   a. Hallucinogens
   b. Sedatives
   c. Thalidomide
   d. Aspirin
   e. Phenytoin, or diphenylhydantoin
   f. Alcohol
   g. Excessive smoking
6. Maternal radiation exposure
7. Maternal-fetal abnormalities
   a. Abnormal fetal positions
   b. Abnormalities of the placenta
   c. Abnormalities of the cord
   d. Abnormalities of labor
   e. Trauma at delivery

Postnatal environment. After delivery a variety of environmental conditions may adversely modify genetic potentials for growth and development. Depressed socioeconomic conditions have been associated with retardation of growth in some children as a result of (1) poor nutrition, (2) increased incidence of acute and chronic illness, (3) inadequate medical supervision and care, (4) crowded and inefficient housing and sanitation, and (5) nonsupportive psychologic inputs. Studies reveal that newborns whose families are poor tend to be smaller than infants born in higher economic classes, (Lippman and Owen, 1977). Children from moderate-to-high income families are taller, heavier, and more advanced in skeletal and dental maturity. Apparently these variations are independent of ethnic and racial grouping. In addition to the suppressant effects of socioeconomic deprivation, the considerations must also focus on differences in maternal age, quality of prenatal care, family size, and spacing of pregnancies. Also, the quality of "mothering" within the first 3 years of life may be a very influential factor affecting growth and development.

Sex. The influence of sex on patterns of growth and development is readily apparent. Girls are usually slightly shorter than boys at all ages until adolescence. During the period from approximately 11 to 14 years of age, girls may be taller than boys. During the adolescent growth spurt, boys grow more rapidly and surpass their female counterparts. Girls generally weigh less than boys, reflecting anatomic differences and possible dietary influences. It is recognized that there is a differential sex timetable. Girls usually develop (mature) approximately 2 to 2½ years earlier than boys. However, it should be noted that at full maturity boys are usually 6 inches taller than girls. In essence, it takes boys approximately 3 years longer than girls to complete adolescent growth, but at the end of this period final growth of the male surpasses that of the female. On the other hand, it appears that at all ages boys have more advanced muscular development.

Endocrine system. Numerous hormone-producing organs have been linked directly and indirectly with growth and development: pituitary gland, thyroid gland, gonads, pancreas, adrenal glands, and others. The *pituitary gland* is probably one of the most important of the endocrine organs that regulate growth and development. *Growth hormone* apparently functions by stimulating DNA synthesis and cell multiplication. This hormone has a major influence on increasing cell numbers during the period from late infancy to adulthood. Growth hormone (1) stimulates the transport of amino acids across cell membranes and promotes the synthesis of protein, (2) promotes cartilage growth, (3) increases total fatty acid catabolism and mobilizes free fatty acids, and (4) increases the metabolism of carbohydrates.

The *thyroid gland* is probably second in importance only to the pituitary gland in regulating growth and development. Whereas thyroid hormone greatly influences fetal and neonatal growth, the growth hormone of the pituitary gland exerts less of an effect during this period. *Thyroid hormone* is actively secreted by the fetal gland. Absence of thyroid hormone during fetal life can adversely affect brain growth, causing microcephaly, as a result of diminished cell size and cell numbers. Ultimately, retarded behavioral development will be observed. During late fetal life and early infancy, thyroid-hormone deficiency appears to interfere with cell multiplication; in later life its deficiency influences cell size. Thyroid hormone acts as a catalyst that increases oxidative processes of the tissues, increasing the activity of the respiratory enzymes. Thyroid hormone (1) promotes body growth and development, (2) enhances skeletal growth and development, (3) promotes sexual maturation, (4) influences mental development, (5) increases metabolic rate, and (6) is associated with cutaneous texture, including hair growth.

The *gonads* are apparently activated during puberty, as reflected by increased secretion of androgens, estrogens, and their metabolites. *Testosterone* (1) increases protein formation (as an interaction with insulin); (2) increases the formation of cholesterol, triglycerides, and free fatty acids; (3) enhances muscular development; (4) promotes bone maturation and epiphyseal closure; and (5) increases sexual maturation, as evidenced by enlargement of the scrotum, penis, prostate, and by spermatogenesis. *Estrogens* (1) stimulate linear growth, with acceleration of skeletal maturation and fusion of the epiphyses (at puberty); (2) stimulate growth and differentiation of the genitalia and secondary sex characteristics; and (3) effect a decrease in serum cholesterol and triglycerides.

Insulin from the *pancreas* complements the action of growth hormone, promoting the accumulation of protein within the cell. In addition, insulin enhances the building of protein from amino acids in the absence of glucose.

The *adrenal glands* are important to growth and development. The adrenal cortex produces hormones that are important in the control of (1) water and electrolyte balance (aldosterone), (2) carbohydrate-protein balance (corticoids), and (3) masculinization and nitrogen retention (androgens). Direct influence on growth depends on the relative amounts of the antagonistic

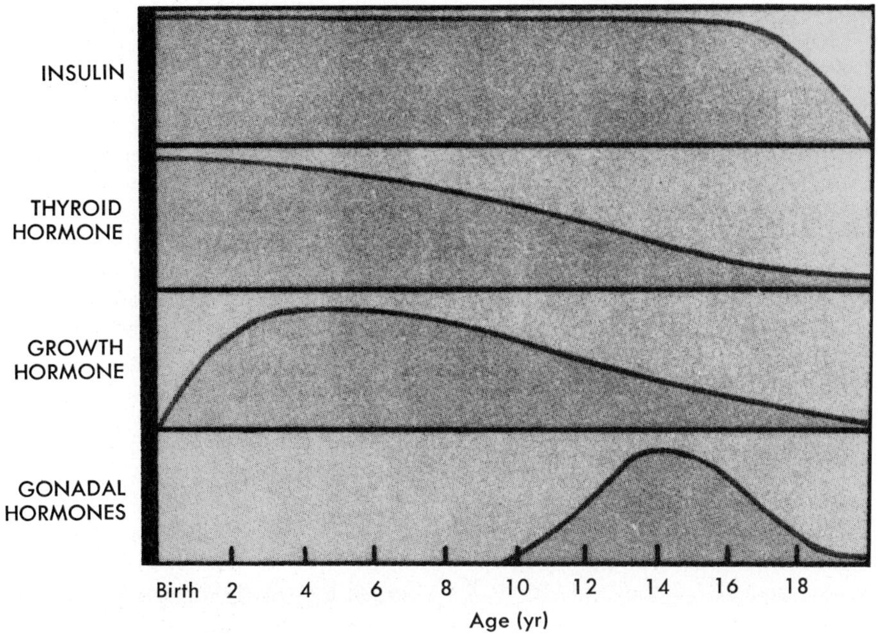

Fig. 2-2. Hormones influencing growth during childhood.

corticoids and androgens secreted. The androgens have a marked influence on skeletal maturation and various aspects of secondary sexual development.

It must be stressed that hormones do not work in isolation. The major hormones are in balance and work in concert to promote normal growth and development (Fig. 2-2).

Nutrition. Abnormalities of nutrition may directly influence cell division and cell growth and thereby modify total growth and development. One of the earliest signs of malnutrition is the failure to gain weight despite a relatively normal increment in height. There are many diverse causes of inadequate nutrition, which extend from uterine life through adulthood, including placental dysfunctions, chronic illness and disease, inadequate dietary intake, maternal neglect, and others. Caloric deficiency during the active phase of cellular hyperplasia may be responsible for smaller cell size, diminished organ size, and depressed total body growth. Malnutrition during the active phases of organogenesis, growth, and development may cause irreversible damage and suppression.

Although malnutrition is often used synonymously with "starvation," overfeeding is also a very serious health hazard. Overfeeding during the critical periods of growth and development may have a detrimental influence on stature. Excess caloric intake can increase the number of cells in organs, influence adipose depots, and result in obesity.

Disease. Chronic disease states, regardless of etiology, can cause growth failure in the infant or toddler. Cystic fibrosis, renal disorders, intestinal malabsorption, and infectious diseases are examples of disorders critically affecting growth and development. During periods of remission, or on correction of the offending influence, the rate of growth may be accelerated (i.e., "catch-up growth"). As normal channels of growth are approached the rate may return to normal, but when growth failure has been severe and prolonged the child may never regain his normal growth potential. Also, repeated adverse disease influences can interfere with statural growth, resulting in delayed bone maturation, extension of the growth period, and ultimate diminution of potential growth. It should be recognized that motor, language, cognitive, and psychosocial development may also be depressed by chronic diseases. The time of insult is as significant as the duration. Disease states occurring in infants and young children may more seriously affect growth and development than if the same disorders occur in older children.

OBJECTIVE MEASUREMENTS OF PHYSICAL GROWTH

Physical growth may be assessed by a variety of parameters: (1) weight, (2) height, (3) head circumference, (4) anthropometry, (5) growth charts, (6) osseous development, (7) dental development, (8) developmental patterns, and (9) physical motor development. It is most important that standardized techniques and instruments be employed in performing these measurements. The value and validity of the assessment may depend on the accuracy and skill of the assessor.

Weight. The "average" newborn weighs between 2.5 kg and 4.6 kg at birth; the median is 3.27 kg for boys and 3.23 kg for girls. Infants weighing less than 2.5 kg at birth are classified as *low birth weight infants*. Approximately 10% of the weight may be lost during the first 3 or 4 days after birth. This physiologic weight loss represents a loss of excessive extracellular fluid and meconium, in addition to relative lack of food and fluid intake. Most infants regain this lost weight and approximate their birth weight within 10 days. During early infancy the weight gain is approximately 20 g/24 hr, decreasing to 15 g/24 hr during the second 6 months of life. Birth weight is usually doubled between 4 and 6 months of age and tripled by 1 year. The "average" child in the second year of life gains 2.5 kg and thereafter gains 2 kg every year for the next 3 years. During the steady growth period in childhood the child gains about 3 kg a year until the adolescent growth spurt.

Height. Among newborns, height varies between 45 cm and 55 cm, with a median of 50.5 cm for boys and 49.9 cm for girls. Length in-

A

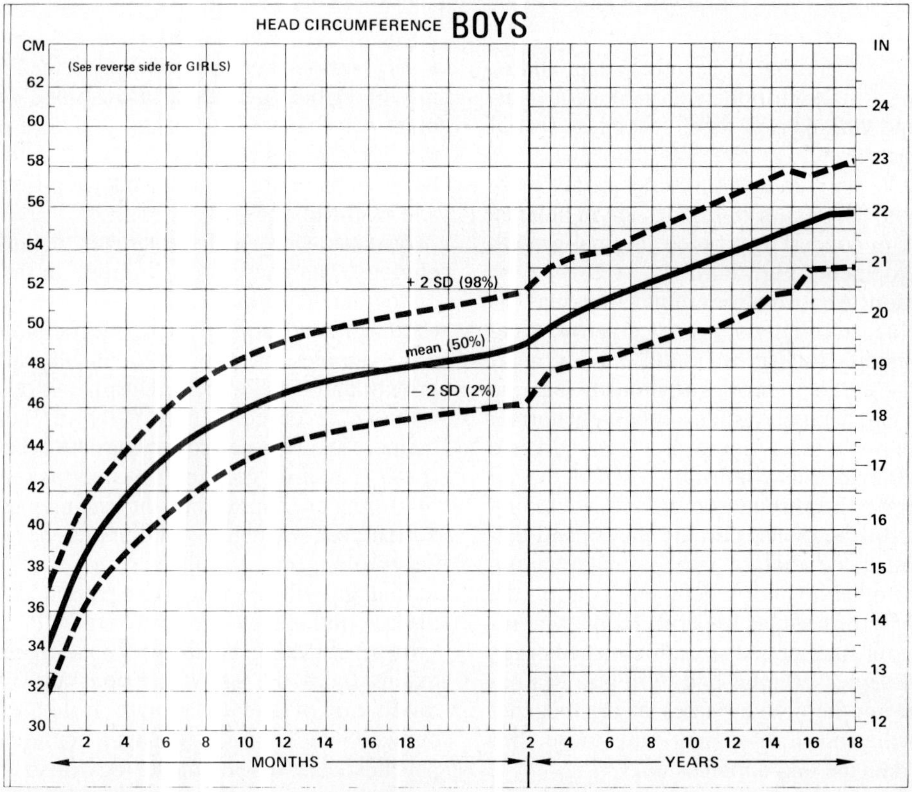

Fig. 2-3. Head circumference. **A,** Boys. **B,** Girls. (From Nellhaus, G.: Pediatrics **41:**106, 1968. Copyright © Academy of Pediatrics, 1968.)

creases by about 50% during the first year of life. In the second year of life the child grows about 12 cm in length and about 7 cm a year between 3 and 5 years of age. During early school years, height gain is steady at about 6 cm a year until the adolescent growth spurt.

Head circumference. During infancy, head circumference is usually a reliable indicator of brain growth. During the first 6 months of life the cellular DNA content of the brain increases and then reaches a plateau. Head circumference follows this pattern. Brain growth after 6 months can be attributed to a continuing increase in weight, protein, and ribonucleic acid (RNA) content in each cell (hypertrophy). Children with severe malnutrition have a diminution in total brain weight, protein, RNA, and DNA, with a proportional delay in increase of head circumference.

At birth, head circumference measures approximately 34 to 35 cm, and increases by approximately 10 cm during the first year. Subsequently the rate of gain decreases, and growth is 1.25 cm a year from age 5 until maturity. A head circumference growth chart, from birth to adulthood, is illustrated in Fig. 2-3.

The posterior fontanel usually closes by the sixth week of life. The anterior fontanel is open for a longer period, closing between the ninth and eighteenth months. A slight separation of the bones of the skull may be noted at birth, but most sutures close by the end of the sixth month.

Anthropometry. Anthropometry refers to the measurement of skinfold thickness. Approximately 50% of body fat is present in the subcutaneous tissue layers, and a correlation exists between fat content and skin thickness. Measurements with skinfold calipers are believed to reflect accurately the relative fat deposition. It has been proposed that anthropometry is *the* most valid assessment of physical growth, body composition, and general nutritional status.

Text continued on p. 22.

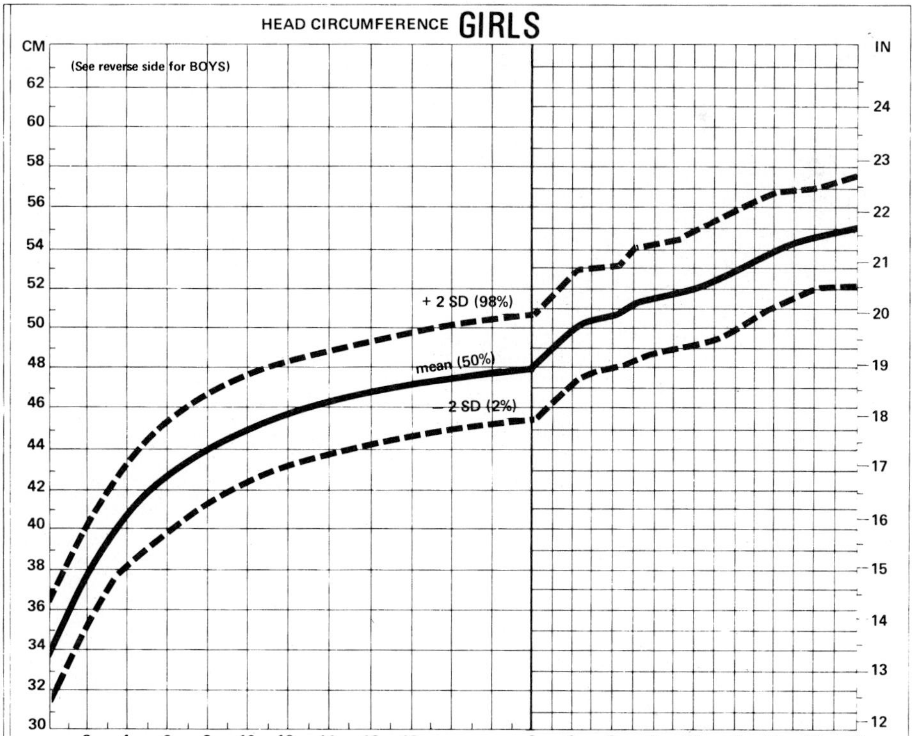

B

Fig. 2-3, cont'd. For legend see opposite page.

A

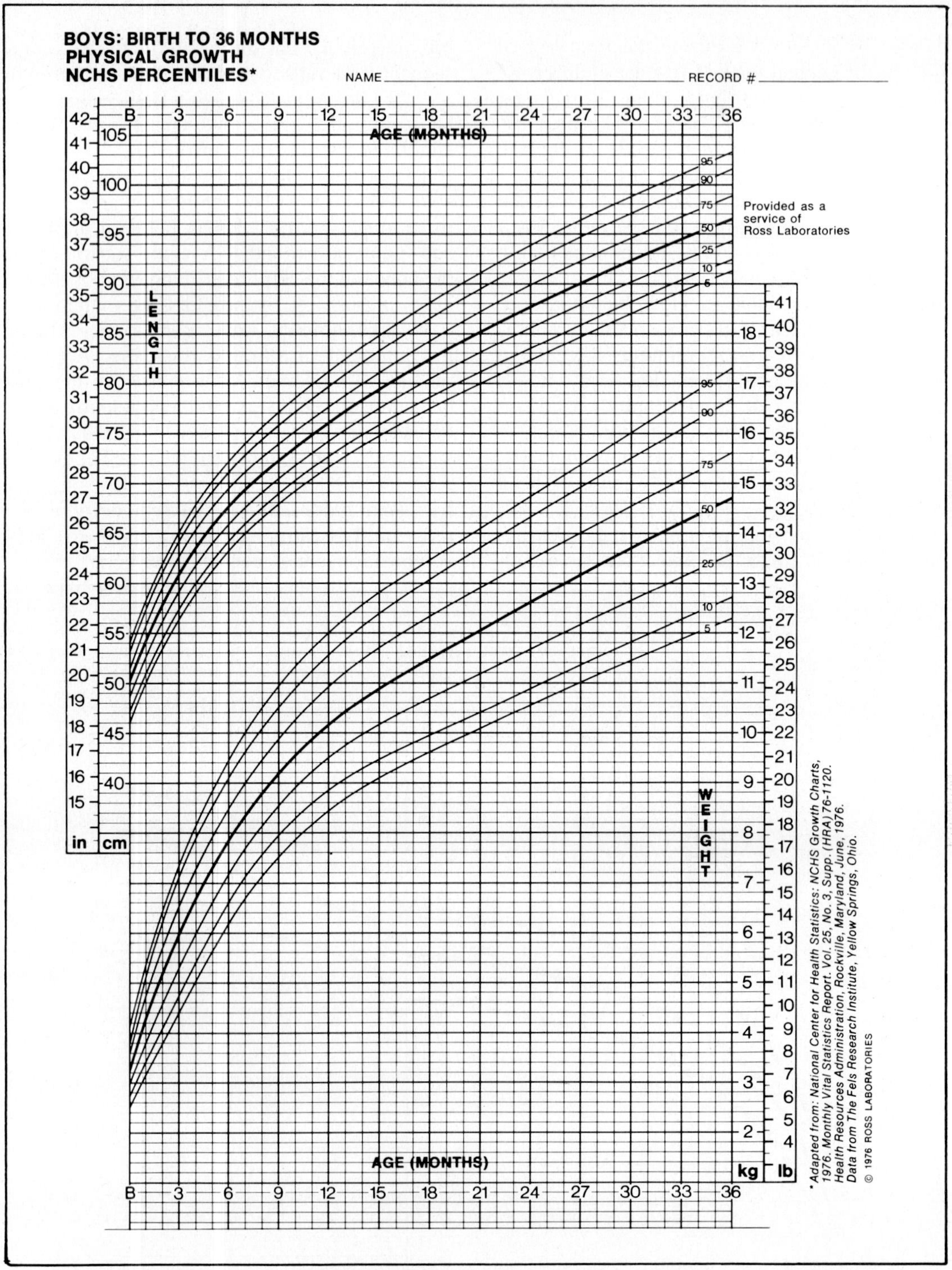

Fig. 2-4. Physical growth, NCHS percentiles. **A,** Boys: birth to 36 months. **B,** Girls: birth to 36 months. (Modified from National Center for Health Statistics: NCHS growth charts, 1976; Monthly vital statistics report, vol. 25, no. 3, supp. [HRA] 76-1120, Health Resources Administration, Rockville, Md., June, 1976; Data from The Fels Research Institute, Yellow Springs, Ohio. Published by Ross Laboratories, Columbus, Ohio, 1976.)

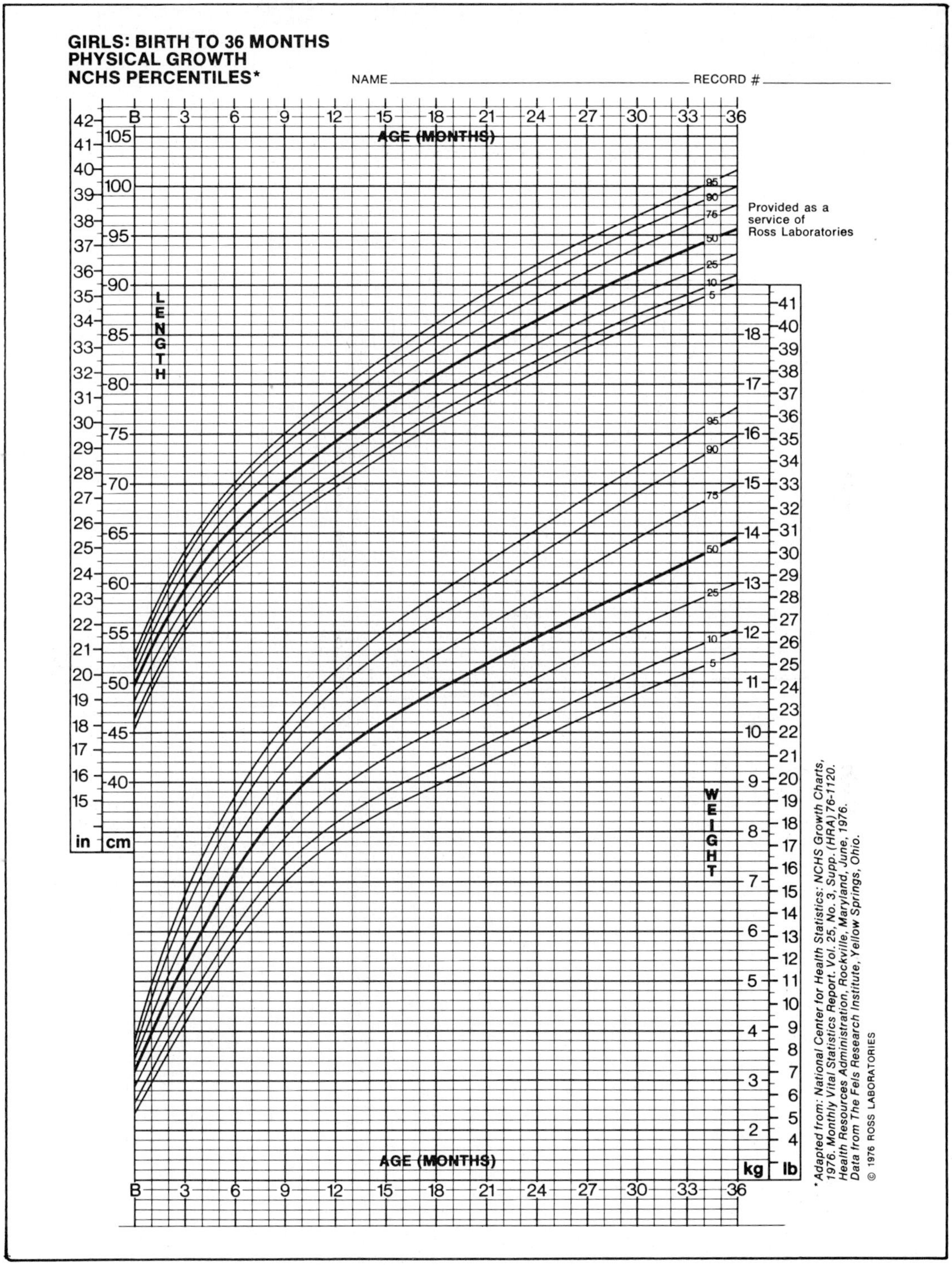

B

Fig. 2-4, cont'd. For legend see opposite page.

A

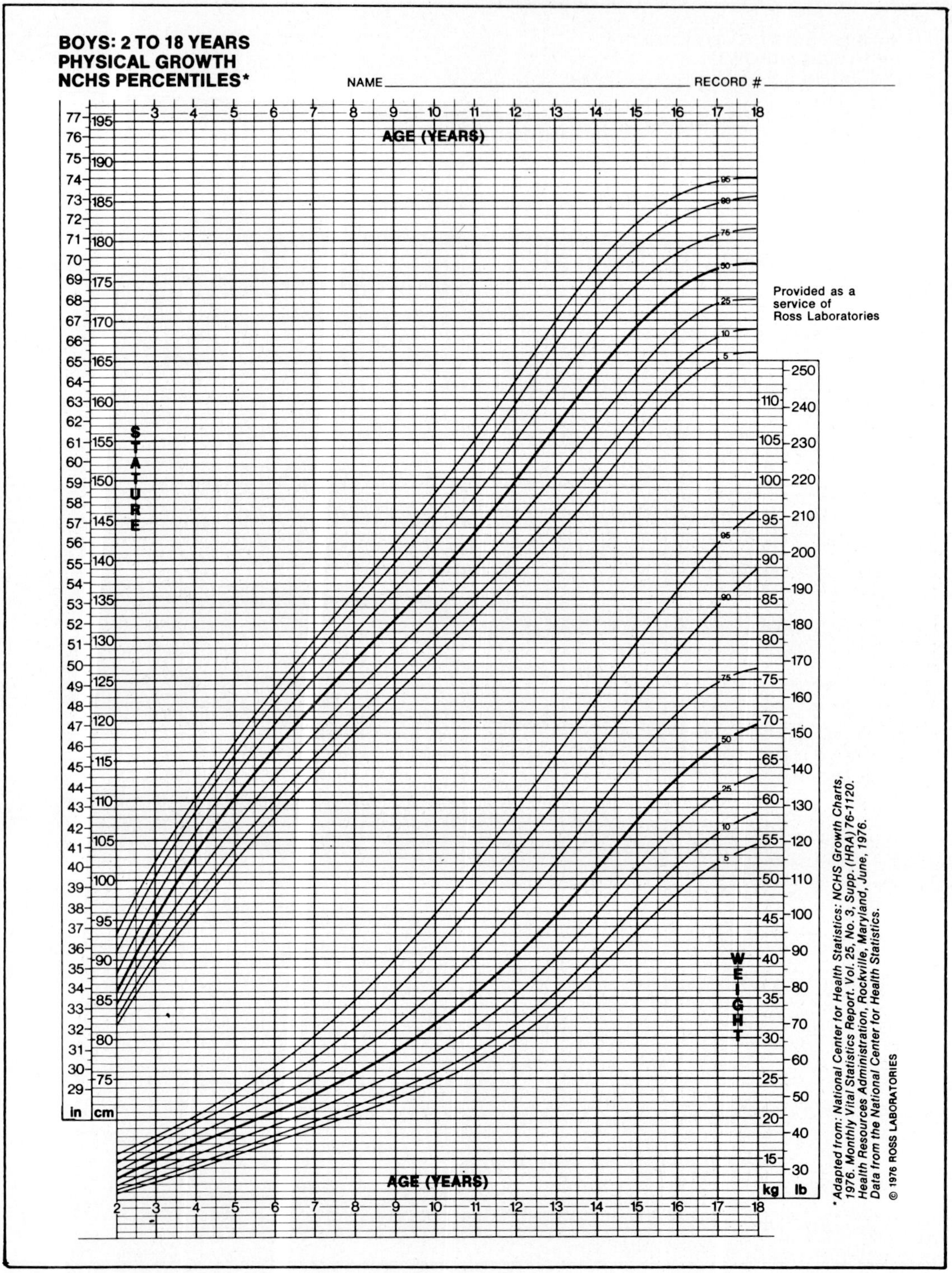

Fig. 2-5. Physical growth, NCHS percentiles. **A,** Boys: 2 to 18 years. **B,** Girls: 2 to 18 years. (Modified from National Center for Health Statistics: NCHS growth charts, 1976; Monthly vital statistics report, vol. 25, no. 3, supp. [HRA] 76-1120, Health Resources Administration, Rockville, Md., June, 1976; Data from the National Center for Health Statistics. Published by Ross Laboratories, Columbus, Ohio, 1976.)

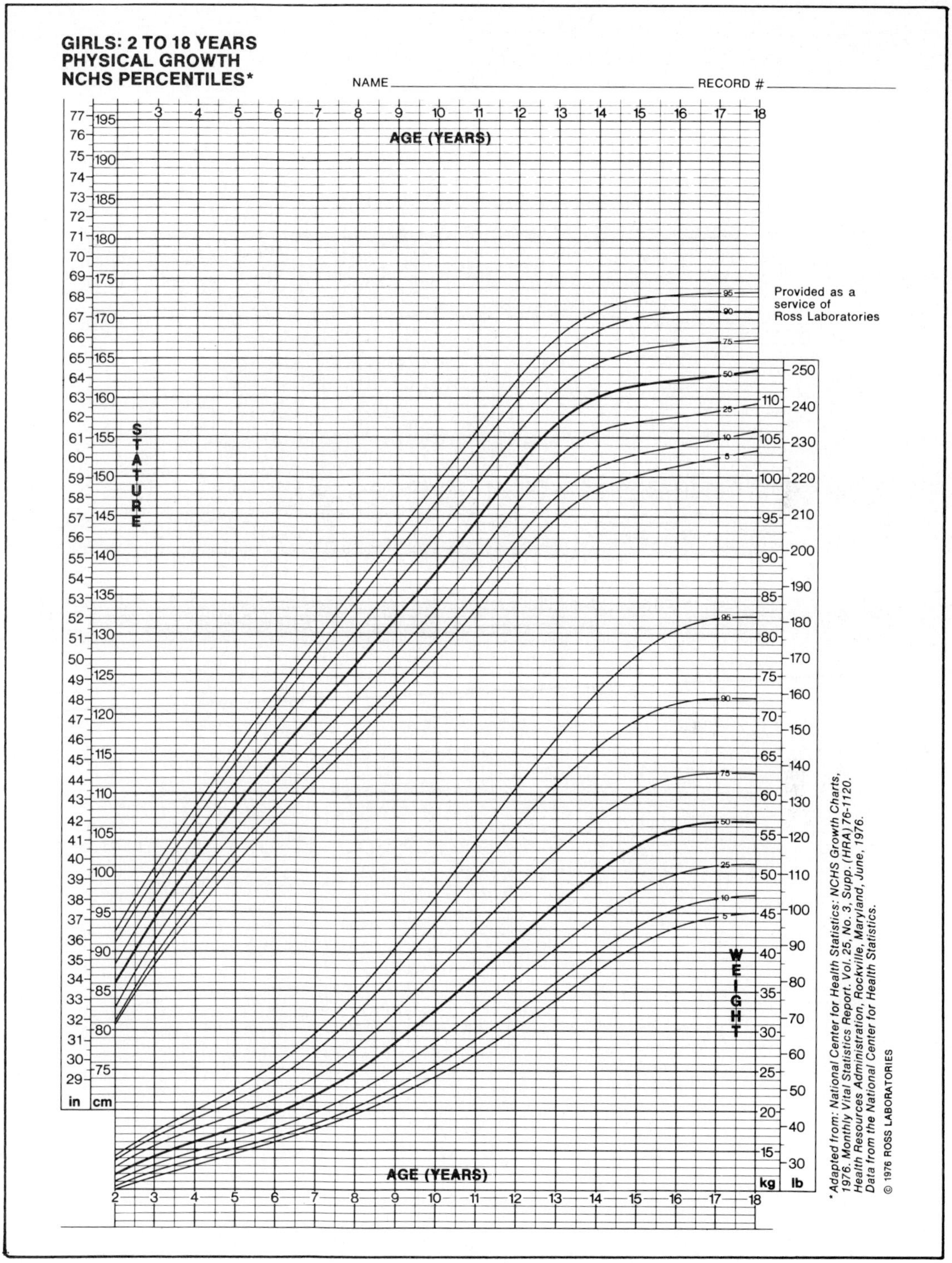

B

Fig. 2-5, cont'd. For legend see opposite page.

A

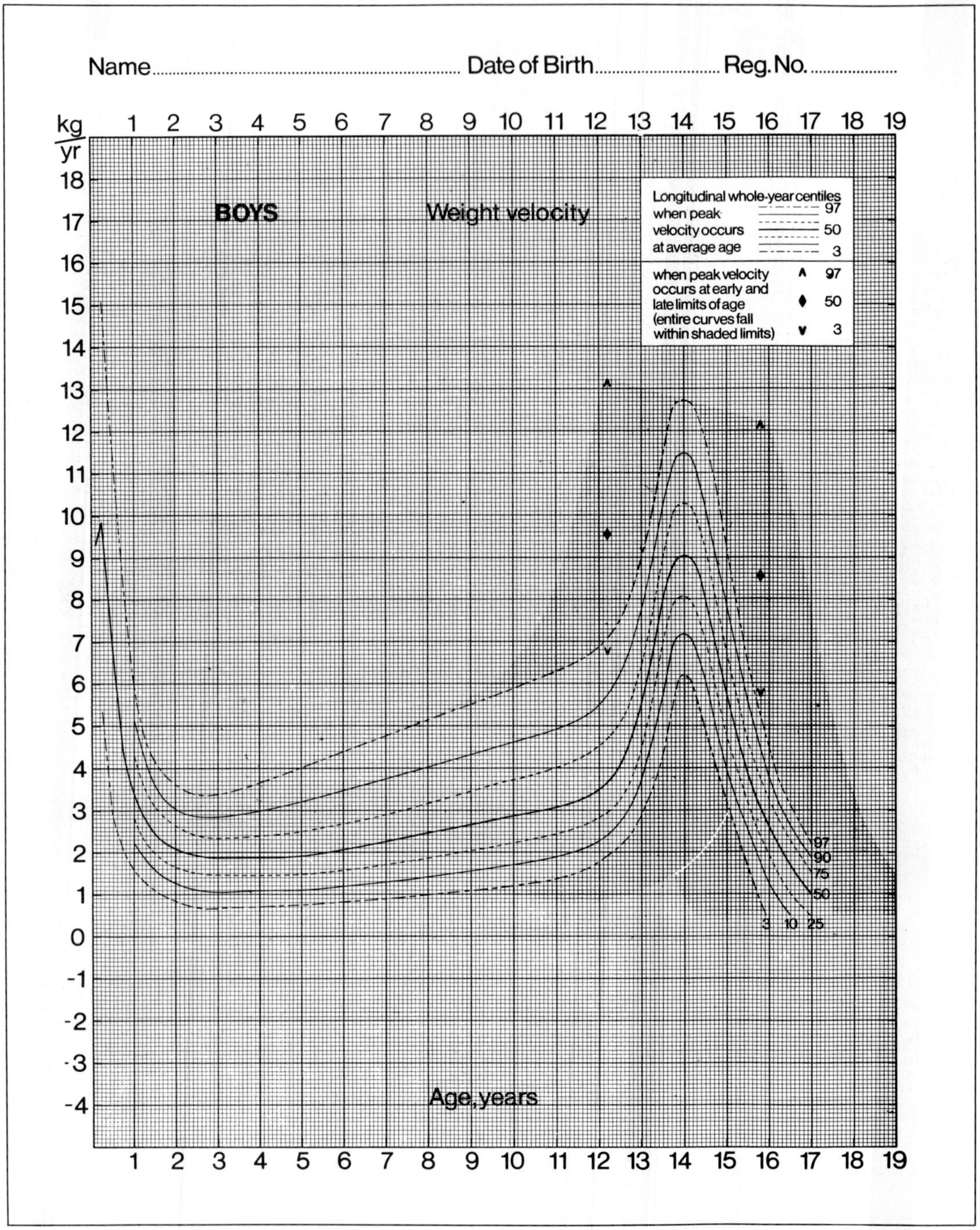

Fig. 2-6. A, Boys: weight velocity. **B,** Boys: height velocity. (Chart prepared by J.M. Tanner and R.H. Whitehouse, University of London Institute of Child Health for The Hospital for Sick Children, London; courtesy Creaseys, Ltd., Castlemead Publications, Hertford, England.)

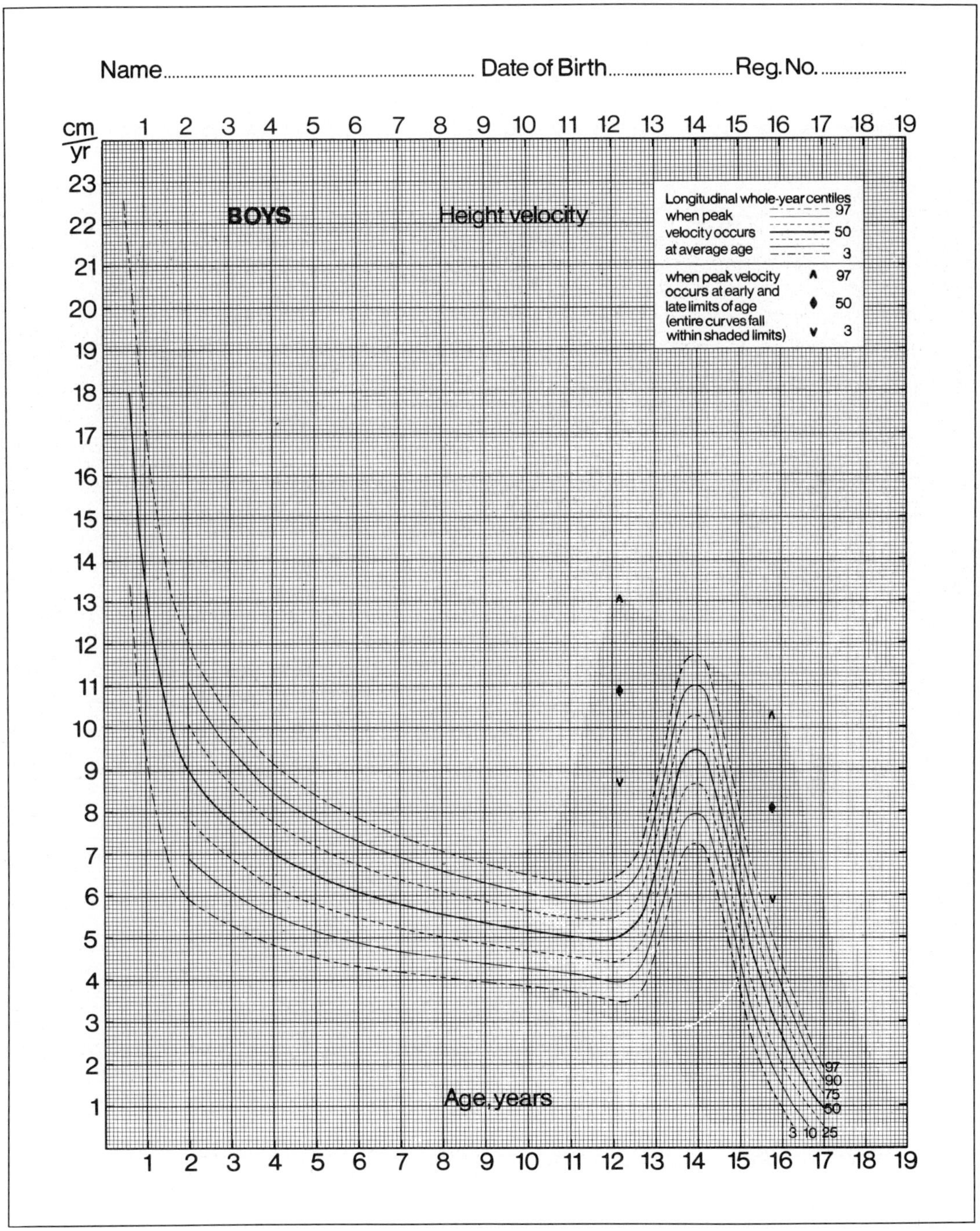

B

Fig. 2-6, cont'd. For legend see opposite page.

A

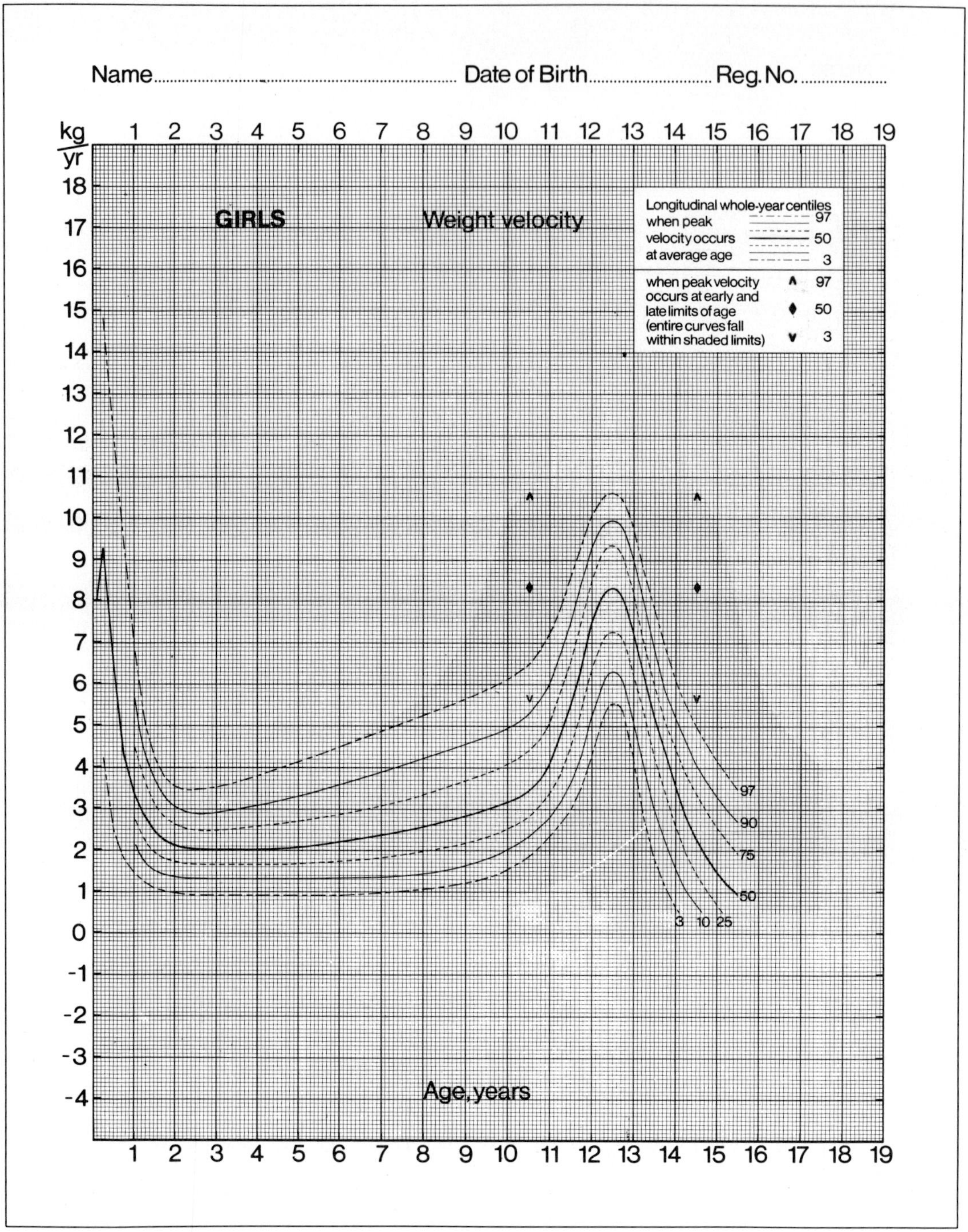

Fig. 2-7. A, Girls: weight velocity. **B,** Girls: height velocity. (Chart prepared by J.M. Tanner and R.H. Whitehouse, University of London Institute of Child Health for The Hospital for Sick Children, London; courtesy Creaseys, Ltd., Castlemead Publications, Hertford, England.)

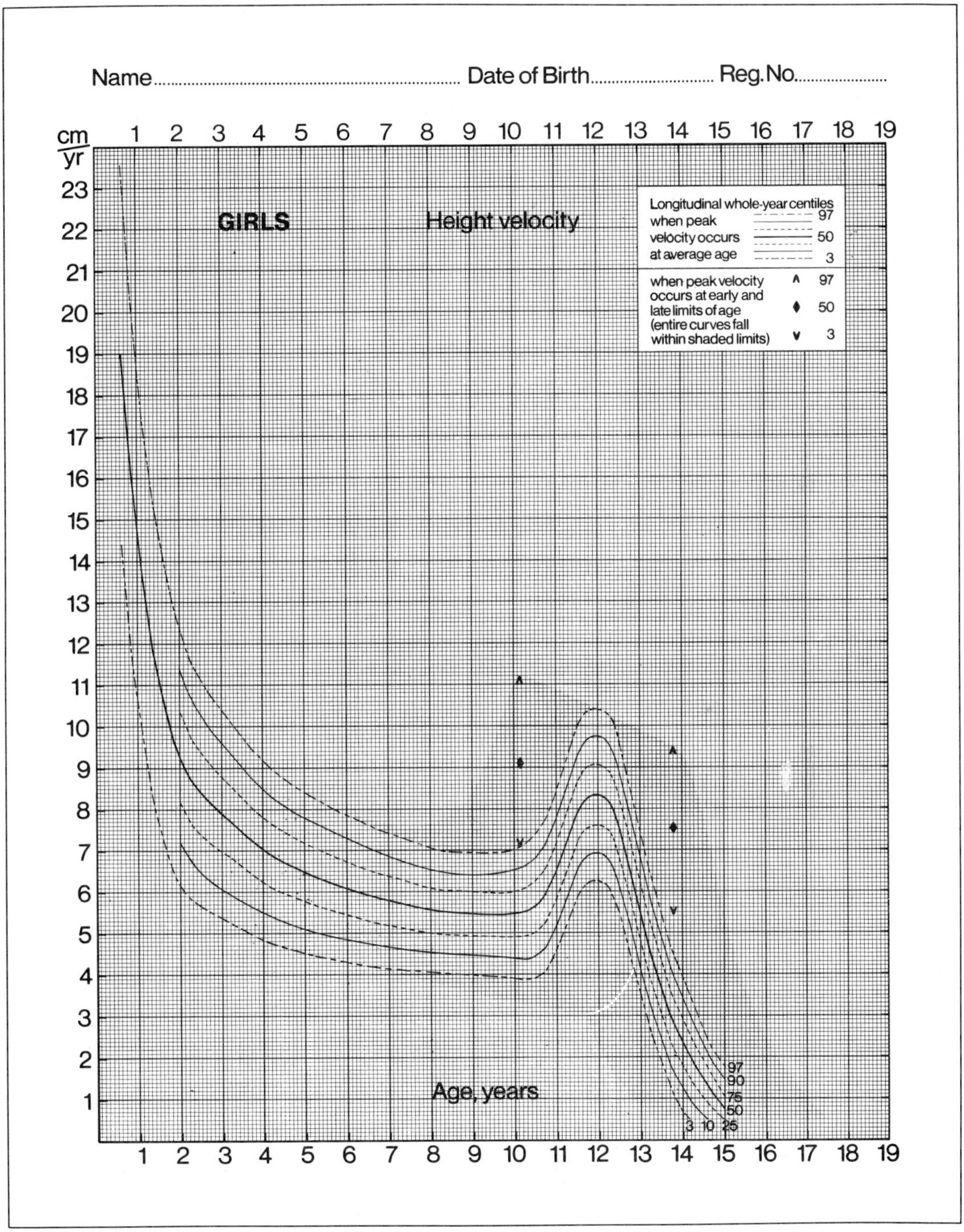

B

Fig. 2-7, cont'd. For legend see opposite page.

However, these measurements are relatively complex, time consuming, and more subject to error than weight and height. Consequently they are used less frequently in assessing physical growth. The most common sites of measurements are the triceps and subscapular regions (Tanner and Whitehouse, 1967).

Growth charts. The use of growth charts for assessing weight, height, and rate of growth is valuable and practical. With these charts the child's progress can be plotted and compared to the range of normal. The growth chart is a presentation of normal growth in terms of curves plotted along percentile levels. After serial measurements the evaluator can quickly visualize whether or not a normal growth pattern has been obtained or a deviation has occurred. *Distance curves* provide information on the height and weight at each age and are regular smooth curves without individual peaks. They are most valuable when the child is seen only once and no estimation of developmental age is available. The National Center for Health Statistics (NCHS) has prepared *percentile distance curves* to more accurately assess the physical growth of children in the United States. Seven percentiles are available for two age groups: birth to 36 months and 2 to 18 years (Figs. 2-4 and 2-5).

The distance curve is inadequate when information is needed about change over time in weight or length. The true growth pattern is reflected in the *velocity curve*, which is derived from measurements at regular intervals from the distance curve. For example, a child may fall below the third percentile on a distance curve, whereas the child's rate of gain over time may actually be within normal limits. Children do *not* have as strong a tendency to remain in the same percentile positions on velocity curves as they do on distance curves. There is a pattern of moving from outer percentile positions toward more central positions. During adolescence the "typical" distance curves are misleading because the percentile ranges of growth vary remarkably. If the child matures early, he moves to a higher percentile before dropping back to his preadolescent percentile. Conversely, if a child matures late, he moves to a lower percentile before regaining at maturity his preadolescent percentile.

Velocity charts for boys' and girls' height and weight gains from birth to adulthood are illustrated in Figs. 2-6 and 2-7. From birth through 2 years the weight velocity decline is more rapid than at any other time. The growth rate decelerates but steadily increases from 3 years until puberty. During the adolescent growth spurt there is rapid acceleration of growth for the first time in postnatal life. Peak velocity occurs at the middle of puberty, after which there is rapid deceleration until growth ceases.

Height velocity in boys is greater than in girls at birth but becomes equal in both sexes at about 7 months of age. From 7 months to 4 years the rate of height gain is greater in girls, becoming equal again until adolescence, at which time boys surpass girls. A boy's weight velocity is also greater than a girl's at birth, but is equal by 8 months. Boys gradually drop below girls in weight until adolescence, when boys become heavier. Weight velocity is affected more by exogenous factors than is height velocity (Tanner et al., 1966).

Bone development. Bone age is the average osseous development for children at a given chronologic age. It is a valuable index of physiologic maturity.

At birth the following five ossification centers are present in 90% of infants born at term: (1) distal end of the femur, (2) proximal end of the tibia, (3) talus, (4) calcaneus, and (5) cuboid. The first ossification centers to appear at 5 to 6 months of age are the capitate and hamate of the wrist. Ossification occurs from secondary centers of cartilage and follows a definite pattern until maturity. Variations do occur that are within the range of normal. Girls, as a rule, have a more advanced bone age than boys. Once the epiphyses have fused, further bone growth can no longer occur.

Bone development can be determined by radiographs, comparing the subject with a standard set of films representing children of a comparable age. The ossification centers that should be present at ages up to 5 years are outlined in Table 2-1. In children up to 6 years of age the wrist is the most reliable area from which to determine bone age.

Assessment of sexual maturation. Childhood sexual maturation culminates in puberty. These pubescent changes mark the beginning of adolescence, which involves not only physical changes but also psychologic factors. The crit-

Table 2-1. Normal bone development

Age (yr)	Joint examined (x-ray film)	New ossification centers present
Birth	Knee (lat.)	Distal femoral and proximal tibial epiphyses
	Ankle (lat.)	Talus, calcaneus, cuboid
1	Wrist (AP)	Capitate, hamate, distal epiphysis of radius
	Shoulder (AP)	Epiphysis of head of humerus
	Hip (AP)	Epiphysis of head of femur
	Ankle (lat.)	External cuneiform, distal tibial epiphysis
2	Shoulder (AP)	Greater tuberosity of humerus
	Elbow (AP)	Capitellum of humerus
	Ankle (lat.)	Distal epiphysis of fibula
3	Wrist (AP)	Triquetrum (triangularis) epiphyses of phalanges and metacarpals
	Ankle (AP)	Internal cuneiform, metatarsal epiphyses
4	Wrist (AP)	Lunate
	Hip (AP)	Epiphysis of great trochanter
	Knee (lat.)	Proximal epiphysis of fibula
	Ankle (lat.)	Middle cuneiform, navicular
5	Wrist (AP)	Trapezium (multangulum majus), navicular (scaphoid)
	Elbow (AP)	Proximal epiphysis of radius
	Knee (lat.)	Patella

Modified from Holt, L.E., Jr., et al.: Pediatrics, ed. 13, New York, 1962, Appleton-Century-Crofts.

ical period of adolescence with all its implications for a healthy and well-adjusted adulthood will not be discussed in this chapter. However, as part of objective measurements of physical growth, the Tanner Sexual Developmental Stages are briefly reviewed in the outline below.

Boys: genital development (Fig. 2-8)

Stage 1 Preadolescent. Testes, scrotum, and penis are about the same size and proportion as in early childhood.

Stage 2 Scrotum and testes are enlarged. Skin on scrotum is reddened and changed in texture. Little or no enlargement of penis is present at this stage.

Stage 3 Penis is slightly enlarged, which occurs at first mainly in length. Testes and scrotum are further enlarged.

Stage 4 Increased size of penis with growth in breadth and development of glans is present. Testes and scrotum larger; scrotal skin darker more than in earlier stage.

Stage 5 Genitalia adult in size and shape.

Girls: breast development (Fig. 2-9)

Stage 1 Preadolescence. Elevation of papilla only.

Stage 2 Breast bud stage. Elevation of breast and papilla as small mound. Enlargement of areola diameter.

Stage 3 Further enlargement and elevation of breast and areola with no separation of their contours.

Stage 4 Projection of areola and papilla to form a secondary mound above the level of the breast.

Stage 5 Mature stage. Projection of papilla only caused by recession of the areola to the general contour of the breast.

Both sexes: pubic hair (Fig. 2-10 for girls)

Stage 1 Preadolescent. The vellus over the pubes is not further developed than that over the abdominal wall; that is, no pubic hair.

Stage 2 Sparse growth of long, slightly pigmented downy hair, straight or curled, chiefly at the base of the penis or along labia.

Stage 3 Considerably darker, coarser, and more curled. The hair spreads sparsely over the junction of the pubes.

Stage 4 Hair now adult in type, but area covered is still considerably smaller than in the adult. No spread to the medial surface of the thighs.

Stage 5 Adult in quantity and type with distribution of the horizontal (or classically "feminine") pattern. Spread to medial surface of thighs but not up linea alba or elsewhere above the base of the inverse triangle (spread up linea alba occurs late and is rated Stage 6).

Dentition. Eruption of the deciduous teeth in infants usually begins at about 6 months of age. Dental eruption is characterized by wide variations in terms of the rapidity and pattern of eruption. Some infants are born with teeth; in others the first tooth may not appear until the infant is approaching 1 year of age. Normal children usually erupt 20 deciduous teeth by the age of 3 years. The general order of eruption and age at eruption and shedding are illustrated in Table 2-2. Although the first permanent tooth

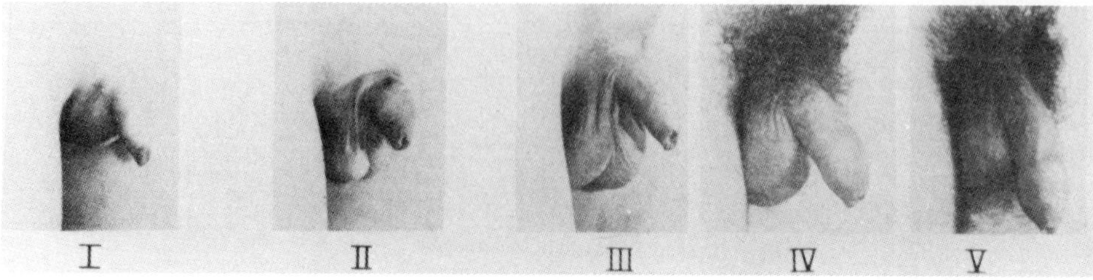

Fig. 2-8. Genital development in boys. *Stage I,* Prepubertal; *stage II,* enlargement of testes, appearance of scrotal reddening, and increase in scrotal rugations; *stage III,* increase in length and to a lesser extent breadth of penis, with further growth of testes; *stage IV,* further increase in size of penis and testes and darkening of scrotal skin; *stage V,* adult.

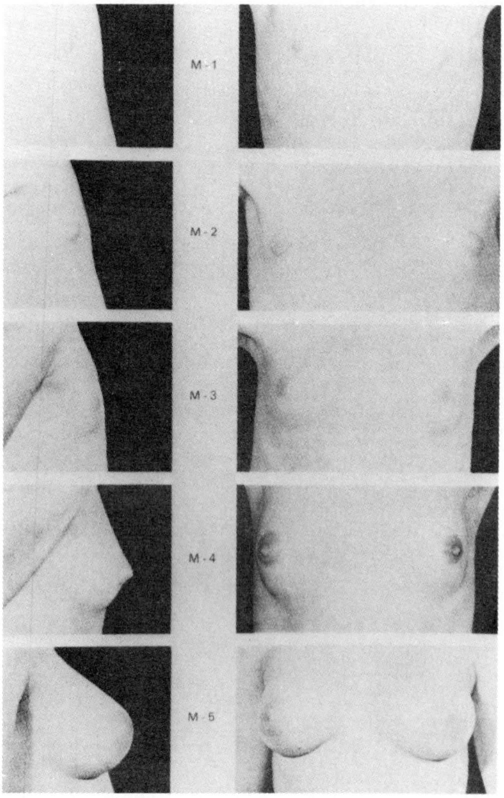

Fig. 2-9. Breast development in girls. *Stage I,* Prepubertal; *stage II,* budding; *stage III,* appearance of small adult breast; *stage IV,* areola and papilla form a secondary mound; *stage V,* adult.

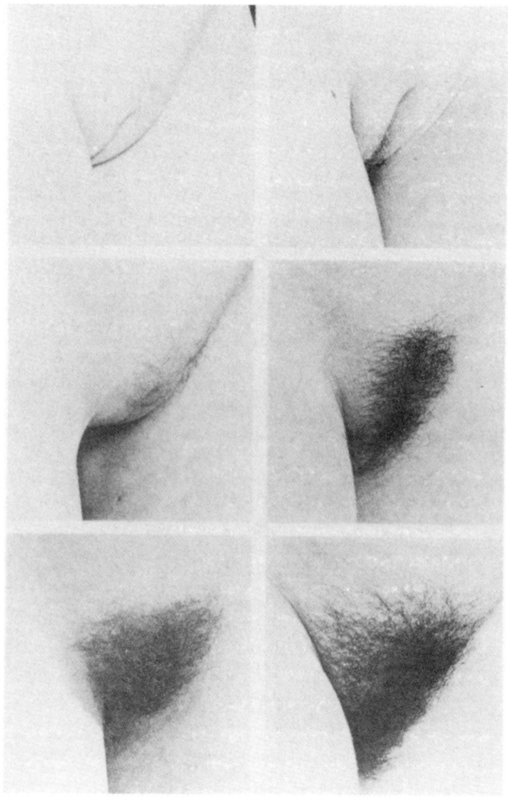

Fig. 2-10. Stages of appearance of pubic and labial hair in girls. *Stage I,* Prepubertal; *stage V,* adult.

usually does not erupt until 6 years of age, children should receive regular dental examinations beginning at 3 years of age. The patterns of shedding the deciduous teeth and eruption of the permanent teeth can also be used as an index of maturation. The patterns are outlined in Tables 2-2 and 2-3.

Developmental patterns. Development progresses in a cephalocaudal direction and is an indication of nervous system maturity. There is a characteristic sequence of appearance of the developmental achievements, with a recognized range of normal variation. The time of acquisition of the major developmental achievements from birth to 9 years of age can be divided into five main areas: (1) gross motor, (2) fine motor, (3) adaptive, (4) language, and (5) personal-social (Table 2-4).

Physical motor development. Physical growth and psychomotor development is greatest during the first 3 years. Children attain a state of *readiness* before proceeding to develop new motor skills. Both sexes are generally equal in their skills at this time. During the preschool period, physical development begins to taper, and distinctions become apparent between boys and girls. Reaction times become quicker and more efficient, especially eye-hand coordination and manual dexterity skills. There is increasing agility, especially in the lower extremities. Boys become better than girls in jumping, climbing, and ball throwing, whereas girls are better in such skills as hopping and bicycling. Some of these differentials in development may be related to the fact that after 4 years of age 75% of the total body weight is caused by muscle development. Girls have larger muscle cells than boys, but they do not exhibit superior strength because boys have more muscle cells than girls (about 3:2 ratio).

During midchildhood, motor development continues at a relatively slow rate. Even though muscle growth is extremely rapid during this time, muscle function is still relatively immature. The child is usually awkward and inefficient in motor movement. The child may exhibit frequent changes in tempo, revealing an inability to sit still for long periods of time. During this developmental period large muscle movement and coordination are being perfected. Fine

Table 2-2. Normal pattern of eruption and shedding of deciduous teeth

Teeth	Eruption (age in mo)		Shedding (age in yr)	
	Lower	Upper	Lower	Upper
Central incisors (4)	6	7½	6	7½
Lateral incisors (4)	7	9	7	8
First molars (4)	12	14	9½	11½
Canines (cuspids) (4)	16	18	10	10½
Second molars (4)	20	24	11	10½
Incisors	Range, ±2 months		Range, ±6 months	
Molars	Range, ±4 months			

Table 2-3. Normal pattern of eruption of permanent teeth

Permanent teeth	Lower (age in yr)	Upper (age in yr)
First molars (6 yr molars) (4)	6-7	6-7
Central incisors (4)	6-7	7-9
Lateral incisors (4)	7-8	8-9
Bicuspids (first and second premolars) (8)	9-11	10-12
Canines (eye teeth) (4)	10-12	10-12
Second molars (12 yr molars) (4)	12-13	12-13
Third molars (wisdom teeth) (4)	17-22	17-22

Table 2-4. Age of acquisition of major developmental achievements

Area	Achievement
4 weeks	
Motor	
Gross	Asymmetric tonic neck reflex positions predominate
	Head sags forward in sitting
Fine	Hands fisted
	Hands clench on contact
Adaptive	Regards object in line of vision only
	Follows to midline
	Drops toy immediately
Language	Vague indirect regard (receptive)
	Small throaty noises (expressive)
Personal-social	Stares indefinitely at surroundings
	Regards observer's face and diminishes activity
16 weeks	
Motor	
Gross	Symmetric postures predominate
	Head steady in sitting
	Head lifted 90° when prone on forearms
Fine	Hands engage
	Scratches and clutches
Adaptive	Eyes follow slowly moving object well
	Arms activate on sight of dangling toy
	Regards toy in hand and takes to mouth
	Regard goes from hand to object when sitting
Language	Laughs aloud
	Excites and breathes heavily
Personal-social	Spontaneous social smile
	Hand play with mutual fingering
	Pulls garment over face
	Anticipates food on sight
28 weeks	
Motor	
Gross	Sits briefly leaning forward on hands
	Supports large fraction of weight in standing
	Bounces actively in supported standing
Fine	Has radial palmar grasp of toy
	Rakes at small pellet with whole hand
Adaptive	One-hand approach and grasp of toy
	Bangs and shakes rattle
	Transfers toy from one hand to other
Language	Vocalizes "m-m-m" when crying
	Talks to toys
Personal-social	Takes feet to mouth
	Reaches for and pats mirror image
40 weeks	
Motor	
Gross	Sits steady indefinitely
	Creeps and pulls to feet at rail
Fine	Crude release of toy
	Plucks pellet easily with thumb and index finger
Adaptive	Matches 2 objects in hands
	Index finger approach
	Spontaneously rings bell
Language	Says "Mama" and "Dada" with meaning
	One other "word"
Personal-social	Waves "bye-bye" and does pat-a-cakes (or other nursery trick)
	Feeds self cracker and holds own bottle
12 months	
Motor	
Gross	Walks with 1 hand held
	Stands momentarily alone
Fine	Neat pincer grasp of pellet
Adaptive	Tries to build tower of 2 cubes
	Releases cube in cup (after demonstration)
	Serial play with objects
Language	Two words besides mama and dada
	Gives toy on request or gesture
Personal-social	Offers toy to image in mirror
	Cooperates in dressing
15 months	
Motor	
Gross	Toddles independently
	Creeps upstairs
Fine	Puts pellet into bottle
Adaptive	Builds tower of 2 cubes
	Puts 6 cubes in and out of cup
	Incipient imitation of stroke
Language	Jargons
	Four to six words, including names
	Pats pictures in book
Personal-social	Says "thank you" or equivalent
	Points or vocalizes wants
	Indicates wet pants
	Throws objects in play or refusal
18 months	
Motor	
Gross	Walks, seldom falling
	Seats self in small chair and climbs into adult chair
	Hurls ball in standing position

Table 2-4. Age of acquisition of major developmental achievements—cont'd

Age	Domain	Achievement
18 months—cont'd	Fine	Turns pages of book 2 or 3 at once
	Adaptive	Builds tower of 3 or 4 cubes
		Imitates stroke with a crayon and scribbles spontaneously
		Dumps pellet from bottle
	Language	Ten words
		Looks selectively at pictures and identifies 1
		Names ball and carries out 2 directions ("on the table," "to mother")
	Personal-social	Pulls toy on string
		Carries and hugs doll
		Feeds self in part, with spilling
2 years	Motor	
	Gross	Runs well, no falling
		Walks up and down stairs alone
		Kicks large ball on request
	Fine	Turns pages of book singly
	Adaptive	Builds tower of 6 or 7 cubes
		Aligns cubes for train
		Imitates vertical and circular strokes
	Language	Uses pronouns
		Three-word sentences; jargon discarded
		Carries out 4 directions with ball ("on the table," "on the chair," "to mother," "to me")
	Personal-social	Verbalizes toilet needs consistently
		Pulls on simple garment
		Inhibits turning of spoon in feeding
		Plays with domestic mimicry
3 years	Motor	
	Gross	Alternates feet going upstairs
		Jumps from bottom step
		Rides tricycle, using pedals
	Fine	Holds crayon with fingers
	Adaptive	Builds tower of 9 or 10 cubes
		Imitates 3-cube bridge
		Names own drawing
		Copies circle and imitates cross
	Language	Uses plurals
		Gives action in picture book
		Gives sex and full name
		Obeys 2 prepositional commands ("on," "under")
3 years—cont'd	Personal-social	Feeds self well
		Puts on shoes and unbuttons buttons
		Knows a few rhymes or songs
		Understands taking turns
4 years	Motor	Walks downstairs alternating feet
		Does broad jump
		Throws ball overhand
	Adaptive	Draws man with 2 parts
		Copies cross
		Counts 3 objects with correct pointing
		Imitates 5-cube bridge
	Language	Names 1 or more colors correctly
		Obeys 5 prepositional commands ("on," "under," "in back," "in front," "beside")
	Personal-social	Washes and dries face and hands; brushes teeth
		Distinguishes front from back of clothes
		Laces shoes
		Goes on errands outside of home
5 years	Motor	Skips, alternating feet
		Stands on 1 foot more than 8 seconds
	Adaptive	Builds 2 steps with cubes
		Draws unmistakable man with body, head, etc.
		Copies triangle
		Counts 10 objects correctly
	Language	Knows 4 colors
		Names penny, nickel, dime
		Descriptive comment on pictures
		Carries out 3 directions
	Personal-social	Dresses and undresses without assistance
		Asks meaning of words
		Prints a few letters
6 years	Motor	Advanced throwing
		Stands on each foot alternately, eyes closed
	Adaptive	Builds 3 steps with blocks
		Draws man with neck, hands, and clothes
		Adds and subtracts within 5
		Copies diamond
	Language	Uses Stanford-Binet items (vocabulary)
	Personal-social	Ties shoelaces
		Differentiates morning and afternoon
		Knows right from left
		Counts to 30

motor skills are gradually improving by trial and error. The child increases his competency levels and thereby increases self-confidence and self-esteem.

SPEECH AND LANGUAGE DEVELOPMENT

Language is a communication system that includes oral, written, and gestural modalities. Four systems contribute to the development of acceptable vocabulary, phrases, and sentences in both oral and written communication: *phonology* (sound features), *semantics* (meaning), *syntax* (word order), and *morphology* (rule system). Speech is oral communication—the act of verbal expression.

Language influences all modes of intellectual and social adaptation (motor, cognitive, or personal-social) and critically affects growth and learning. The integration of language with behavior is a gradual process often exhibiting wide ranges of variation. However, most children follow a general pattern of development in the acquisition of communicative skills. It is recognized that age alone is not the sole criterion for assessing language development; other influences must be considered.

Language development involves two major modalities: comprehension and expression. The development of communicative skills depends on the ability of children to perceive and analyze the language in their environment. The child must perceive words to understand them. Expression, in turn, depends on adequate comprehension. The processes are ongoing, involving continued listening experiences, development of concepts for everyday living, use of language to influence others in the environment, and preparation for their education. Adequate language skill involves mastering *vocabulary* (semantics), *sentence structure* (syntax), and a *rule system* (morphology).

The birth cry is the infant's initial speech utterance. Although it has no particular language meaning, it heralds the beginning of communication. It can be regarded as a prelinguistic stage that ultimately leads to the child's understanding and use of words. Babies begin to vocalize early in life, and they find pleasure in producing and listening to sounds. The characteristic vocalization during the first 9 months is *babbling,* which is a mixture of vowel and consonant sounds that become speechlike. This is followed by *echolalia,* when the baby begins to match the sounds of others. At this time the child is perceiving auditory signals and repeating them without attaching significant meaning. At 9 months of age the babbling becomes *jargon,* or meaningful verbalization, which employs a variety of sounds. At approximately 1 year of age the child begins to pair action with words. At this time the child should be able to follow one-part, simple commands. In addition, the child is expected to recognize pictures, which he may not be able to name. After 1 year of age most infants produce meaningful speech. *Words* are usually spoken beginning between the ages of 9 and 12 months.

Development in *sound acquisition* spans a continuum from simple to compound. Sounds requiring gross articulation movement *(p, b, m)* are among the first to be acquired. Sounds that require fine motor coordination of the articulators may not be uttered until the child is older. The sounds *s, j,* and *r* and blends such as *sw, bl,* and *tr* appear later in the developmental stages of articulatory acquisition.

Single words normally continue to develop gradually between 12 and 18 months of age. Two- and three-word *sentences* are noted by 18 to 20 months of age. Sentence usage represents the true beginning of language. A 2-year-old acquires words, whereas a 3-year-old uses them. Between 18 months and 3 years, sentence length increases, and children begin to learn grammatical essentials. During the preschool years the variety of sentence structure increases, and the sophistication of speech improves through the use of verb tenses, more complex sentence structure, and speech sounds. Between the ages of 3 and 6 years, persistent questioning related to language, interests, and the environment is at a peak. After the preschool years the child's major interests involve surroundings. Speech is used primarily for communicating with others—*socialized speech*.

Parents are often apprehensive about their child's language development. It is the role of health providers to familiarize parents with this developmental process. Parents and professionals should recognize signs indicative of possible hearing loss in young children and should be aware that impaired auditory acuity can cause (1) delays in speech development, (2) inappropriate response to auditory stimuli, (3) inadequate discrimination of sounds and speech, (4) frequent requests for repetition of conversation, and (5) articulation errors. Parents are influential in the development of the child's speech and language. A preschooler's time is spent primarily with his parents, and activities are usually family oriented.

Guidelines (Lillywhite, 1962) for referring children for professional speech and language assessment include the following:

1. A child who is not talking by 2 years of age
2. Speech that is unintelligible after age 3
3. Sounds more than 1 year late in appearance, according to developmental sequence
4. Omissions of initial consonants after age 3
5. A child who uses predominantly vowel sounds in speech
6. No sentence usage by age 3
7. Obvious faulty sentence structure by age 5
8. A child who is embarrassed by his speech at any age
9. A child who is noticeably nonfluent after age 5
10. Pitch inappropriate to age and sex
11. Abnormal rhythm, rate, and inflection after age 5

PSYCHOSOCIAL AND PERSONALITY DEVELOPMENT (see also Chapter 4)

The child is expected to respond and adapt to the demands of society with increasing sophistication. The timetables for psychosocial and personality development are not clearly defined. A myriad of factors may enhance or depress the rates of psychosocial maturity. Some espouse the concept that personality development results primarily from predetermined genetic processes. Others postulate that environmental experiences are the most critical factors in determining personality traits. The two theoretical positions are commonly referred to as the *nature-nurture controversy*. Most developmental theorists hypothesize that personality is shaped by the interplay of temperament and environment.

Three category classifications of temperament in children have been identified. The *"easy" child* is adaptable, has regular sleeping and eating schedules, is cheerful, learns rules quickly, and adjusts well to school. The *"difficult" child* withdraws from new stimuli, has irregular body functions and habits, has negative moods and frequent temper tantrums, and adapts poorly to school and new situations. The *"slow-to-warm-up" child* has low activity levels and low-intensity reactions, withdraws from stimuli, and rejects changes.

These general temperament characteristics may prevail throughout childhood and influence the psychosocial development stages of the child. Health providers must appreciate these influences to counsel parents adequately regarding adjustments to the major developmental stages (infancy, toddler, preschool, and school-age).

Infant. The most important psychologic milestone during infancy is the establishment of *trust*. The infant must learn to trust the environment and the caregiver to fulfill basic needs such as food, shelter, elimination, and sensory input. Infancy is a "taking in and taking hold" period. Sensory stimulation is provided, and basic needs are met through oral experimentation: sucking, burping, spitting, biting, and cooing.

During the first 6 months of life the infant participates in a symbiotic relationship with the mother. Between the sixth and ninth month, an ego and self-awareness develop. The infant realizes that he is separate from mother. He begins to respond to others with gestures and verbalizations. With the realization that mother is separate from others, he begins to experience awareness of strangers and anxiety about them.

At about 8 months the infant begins to demonstrate the cognitive milestone of object permanence. He begins to realize that objects may exist even when out of sight. The awareness is established that his mother still exists when she leaves his visual field. During the latter part of the first year, the infant begins to experience separation anxieties, becoming distressed when loved ones leave him. He resists sleep and cries when his parents leave for the evening. Peekaboo and other hiding games may help the infant to cope with separation anxieties. With a close maternal-infant attachment during the first year of life, trust and security develop, allowing the infant healthy beginnings of ego development and personality. If trust and security do not develop, the infant becomes fearful and rejecting of others, and future development is hindered.

Toddler. The most important psychosocial achievement of the toddler is the development of autonomy, or independence. With newfound motor skills the toddler learns to explore and venture out on his own. He develops an awareness that he can in part exert control over his environment. The toddler learns to "let go of" his mother, toys, and body functions. In his search for independence the toddler frequently tries short periods of separation from his mother but looks for reassurances of her presence. If trust and security have not been established at an earlier age, autonomy will fail to develop. The child with faulty autonomy traits will be clinging and dependent.

The toddler reveals some self-control during this period. He begins to understand the meaning of "no" and "yes." He often becomes obstinate and angry as he experiments with independence. At one moment the toddler displays a temper tantrum, and at the next he is trying to please his parents. At this time, children who are rejected by their parents stop trying to win love. They search for pleasures elsewhere, and this often results in behavior problems. Parents must also set limits for behavior, using consistent disciplining techniques. They should allow for sufficient development of independence during toddlerhood. Substitutions should be provided for anger and temper tantrums.

Children engage in solitary play during the toddler period because of immature socialization skills. The toddler may be very imaginative, creating make-believe friends. He may express fears of storms, dogs, and the dark.

Toilet training is probably one of the major concerns of parents at this time. Before experimenting with toilet training, parents should be aware of the readiness signs. The maturity required for toilet-training includes (1) sufficient vocabulary to express toileting needs, (2) awareness that voiding or a bowel movement has occurred, and (3) the necessary fine and gross motor skills to permit the mechanical aspects of toileting.

Preschooler. The developmental task of the preschooler is achieving *initiative*. Initiative is a basis for the preschooler's future sense of ambition and purpose. He begins to initiate attachments to others outside his nuclear family members. Although the concept of empathy is still difficult for the preschooler to grasp, at 4 to 5 years of age he is able to initiate shared play with other children. Gradually he learns to cooperate with playmates. During this period the preschooler overcomes strong attachments to the parent of the opposite sex and begins to identify with the parent and friends of the same sex.

Sibling rivalry, fears, and autocratic behaviors are sometimes troubling to parents during this time. If a baby is born, the preschooler may become jealous and for the first time realizes that he must share his parents' love. He often regresses to previous behavior patterns, such as thumb-sucking, bed-wetting, or temper tantrums, but if given love and understanding, he finally accepts the new sibling. He realizes that a parent's love can be shared.

Children of this age continue to have vivid imaginations. Frequently, nightmares and fears of the dark, death, imaginary creatures, and physical injury are worrisome concerns. These fears are very real to the child and cannot be ignored. The peak age for the development of autoerotic behavior is from 3 to 4 years and is part of the child's self-discovery process. This is a normal phenomenon and should be treated with a matter-of-fact attitude by the parents.

The preschooler is curious and demanding. He often becomes angry to the point that temper tantrums seen in toddlers may reemerge. Temper outbursts may result from a desire to prove independence. Attention, even in the form of punishment, may reinforce the undesirable behavior. Appropriate punishment such as withdrawal of privileges, toys, etc. may be used. Praise, attention, and love should always be given when the child exhibits a desired behavior. In most cases, consistency and time will help eliminate an undesirable behavior.

School-age child. Industry, ambition, and self-worth are the most important developing values during the middle years of childhood. If these concepts are to develop adequately, children must experience successes both at home and at school. Repeated failures engender rejection from peers, teachers, and parents, resulting in a negative self-concept. Parents can help increase their child's self-confidence by being honest, providing opportunities for creativity, helping him succeed in activities, and providing positive reinforcement.

The school-age child ventures forth to form

deeper relationships with children of the same age and sex. However, the family still represents the major form of security. The school-age child is less egocentric and more empathetic. He is able to share thoughts with others, resulting in increased cooperation and collaboration with peers. There are newfound participations in organized groups and activities. Groups and clubs formed by the school-age child have rules, ceremonies, oaths, and other structures comparable to society's rules. Membership is exclusive in these groups, and rules must be followed to gain acceptance and approval. Peer groups help to provide the child with a practical knowledge of social structure, leadership, justice, injustice, and loyalties. These groups also become a way of socialization to gain support and reassurance and to "escape from parents." Values of the group may become more important than those of the parents. By the age of 8 to 9 years, the transfer of affiliation and loyalty to the peer group may be established.

Parents become distressed when their child loses his affectionate nature and becomes a "stranger" to the family. They are appalled at the odd mannerisms, language, and silence that their child may exhibit. During this period, parents may be tempted to become their child's "pal" to win back his approval. It is important that parents continue their adult roles. Children still require the parental role model to help them in time of need and to provide support, comfort, and guidance.

Children begin to learn differences between ideal and real situations, which leads to disparity and disillusionment. This is apparent in attitudes toward parents, who were once perceived as being incapable of doing wrong. Without the realization that parents can make mistakes, children become disillusioned and may temporarily reject them. By the age of 9 years, children usually learn to accept the fact that their parents can, and do, make mistakes.

School-age children learn to help themselves. They learn to love! They learn to understand the concepts of past and future. Fears are often associated with school, social relationships, and economic difficulties. The child may be very curious, seeking the reasons behind how and why things work.

Moral development should also occur during this period. Rules of right and wrong are first learned from parents at about 8 to 9 years. However, they may not be understood or appreciated. By the age of 9 or 10, children become aware of the meanings and purposes of rules, which they eventually begin to respect.

Children who have not mastered previous stages of development will experience some forms of emotional instability. Those who lack

Table 2-5. Screening tools and tests

Test	Ages	Description
Neonatal Behavioral Assessment Scale (Brazelton)	First few days of life	Behavioral assessment scale and psychologic scale for newborn; tests for neurologic adequacy, behavioral states of consciousness, and ability to quiet when stimulated; training required for accuracy
Neonatal Perception Inventory (Broussard and Hartner)	Birth to 4 wk	Evaluates mother's perception of an average baby and her own baby
Caldwell Home Inventory	Birth to 3 yr	Home observation to assess following areas: (1) emotional and verbal responsitivity to mother, (2) avoidance of restriction and punishment, (3) organization of environment, (4) provision of appropriate play materials, (5) maternal involvement with child, and (6) opportunities for variety in daily routine
The Washington Guide to Promoting Development in the Young Child	1 to 52 mo	Assesses developmental tasks of feeding, sleeping, playing, language, discipline, toileting, and dressing; suggested activities presented to enhance growth and development in each area
Denver Developmental Screening Test	Birth to 6 yr	Assesses four parameters of development: (1) personal-social, (2) fine motor adaptation, (3) language, (4) gross motor; very easily administered
The Developmental Profile (Alpern and Boll)	Birth to preadolescence	Screens development in physical, self-help, social, academic, and communication areas

love and the capacity to love often have behavior problems, with higher incidences of stealing and lying. During this stage of development, parents need to set rules and limitations on behavior (and to provide the rationale for them). The school-age child should be handled with understanding but also with firmness. The child should be allowed to voice his viewpoints!

• • •

The pediatrician is in a strategic position to monitor and assess language and psychosocial development, as well as physical growth and development (Table 2-5). Routine evaluations should be made in an effort to prevent or detect developmental problems at the earliest possible stage. The physician is in an excellent position to counsel parents and children and to assist them through normal development and the minor problems that occur during each stage.

Hershel P. Wall
Marvin I. Gottlieb

REFERENCES

Fiser, R.N., and Hill, D.E.: Chronic disease and short stature, Postgrad. Med. **62:**103, 1977.

Lillywhite, H.: Doctor's manual of speech disorders, J.A.M.A. **167:**850, 1962.

Lippman, G., and Owen, G.: Nutritional status of infants and young children: USA, Pediatr. Clin. North Am. **24:**211, 1977.

Tanner, J.M., and Whitehouse, R.N.: Standards for subcutaneous fat in British children: percentiles for thickness of skinfolds over triceps and below scapula, Br. Med. J. **1:**446, 1967.

Tanner, J.M., et al.: Standards from birth to maturity for height, weight, height velocity, weight velocity: British children 1965, part I, Arch. Dis. Child. **41:**454-471; part II, 613-635, 1966.

SELECTED READINGS

Cheek, D.B., et al.: Human growth: body composition, cell growth, energy and intelligence, Philadelphia, 1968, Lea & Febiger.

Erikson, E.H.: Childhood and society, New York, 1963, W. W. Norton & Co. Inc.

Faulkner, F., editor: Human development, Philadelphia, 1966, W.B. Saunders Co.

Hatten, J.T., and Hatten, P.W.: Natural language, Tucson, 1974, Communication Skill Builders, Inc.

Hoffman, M.L.: Personality and social development, Ann. Rev. Psychol. **28:**295, 1977.

Hopper, R., and Naremore, R.C.: A practical introduction to communication development, New York, 1973, Harper & Row, Publishers.

Illingworth, R.S.: The normal child: some problems of the first five years and their treatment, London, 1968, J & A Churchill, Ltd.

Johnston, R.B., and Magrab, P.R., editors: Developmental disorders: assessment, treatment, education, Baltimore, 1976, University Park Press.

Knoblock, H., and Pasamanick, B.: Gesell and Amatruda's developmental diagnosis: the evaluation and management of normal and abnormal neuropsychologic development in infancy and early childhood, New York, 1974, Harper & Row, Publishers.

Lowry, G.H.: Growth and development of children, Chicago, 1973, Year Book Medical Publishers, Inc.

Tanner, J.: Growth at adolescence, ed. 2, Oxford, 1962, Blackwell Scientific Publications, Ltd.

3 Educational Health and Development: The Learning-disabled Child

During the past decade *developmental-behavioral pediatrics* has become established as a major medical specialty, serving the needs of children and their families with a variety of biosocial and educational problems. A primary responsibility of pediatric medicine is to *improve the quality of life for all children,* including those whose psychologic, educational, and social potentials are compromised by chronic handicapping conditions. The following chapters review the genetic imbalances, infectious diseases, metabolic disorders, degenerative processes, and other noxious conditions that can disrupt and impair normal growth and development. The "traditional" role for physicians relates to diagnosing, treating, and preventing these acute disorders and emergency situations. Comprehensive health care for children, however, implies a much broader spectrum of pathologic disorders that may seriously jeopardize the child's future, including mental retardation, learning disabilities, communication handicaps, behavior and emotional disorders, maturational delays, neuromotor dysfunctions, and other chronic handicapping conditions.

During the past 2 decades the primary care physician has been mandated an important role in safeguarding and enhancing the child's development in all areas, including emotional, psychologic, educational, and social growth (American Academy of Pediatrics, 1977). To accommodate these changing demands and priorities in primary care pediatrics, modifications are necessary in the didactic and clinical content of training programs for medical students (Gottlieb and Zinkus, 1980) and pediatric residents (Wolraich, 1980). In addition, continuing education programs for physicians in practice must provide opportunities to review and discuss the impact of chronic handicapping disorders on the child, the family, the educational system, and the community (American Academy of Pediatrics, 1980).

The physician, as an active participant in multiple disciplines, is frequently called on to manage complex educational and psychosocial problems. To fulfill this commitment, an expanded gestalt of the child is essential; a profile that is only constructed by interdisciplinary assessment. Interdisciplinary (team) intervention is synonymous with developmental-behavioral pediatrics. In association with professionals from various disciplines, the primary-care physician can contribute to formulating an in-depth description of the child and his total environment. The construction of this profile is a continuing process, ideally initiated as early as possible in the life of the child and family. Early intervention is the key to preventing many of the devastating chronic sequelae of developmental disabilities and behavior disorders.

Developmental-behavioral pediatrics is concerned with the prevention and early remediation of chronic handicapping disorders of childhood. The specialty is dedicated to improving the quality of life for all children in the broadest context of human development. Pediatricians have increasingly assumed the role of advocate for the *learning-disabled child.* Perhaps this growing concern is nurtured by a sensitivity for the intimate relationship between general health, neurologic function, academic achievement, self-esteem, and social adaptation. Physicians are cognizant of the numerous adverse influences that can disturb the delicate balance between the nervous system, learning skills, and psychosocial development. The physician must share in the responsibility of ensuring that *all* children receive an optimal learning experience consistent with their emotional and intellectual capacities. The American Academy of Pediatrics (1973a and b) advocates active medical participation in the early identification of children with learning disabilities.

Scientific advances that limit life-threatening situations, improved delivery of health services, and changing social attitudes contribute to a reorganization of pediatric priorities. Developmental disabilities and behavioral disorders have emerged as special interest areas in pediatric medicine. Within this broad constellation of disorders, learning disabilities is the one issue that has probably received most attention. The alarming incidence of impaired learning, coupled with the potential for severe psychosocial complications, has generated intense public, professional, and legislative concern. Federal legislation (Public Law 94-142) mandates free public education for all handicapped children with disturbed learning who require special education resources. The legal and social implications of learning problems have dictated a more active participation by physicians, calling on them to blend their expertise with that of others in the diagnostic and therapeutic process (American Academy of Pediatrics, 1978). For many practicing pediatricians, however, the learning-disabled child represents a previously unexplored area of study and a clinical challenge.

This chapter presents an overview of several critical issues in educational health and development. We attempt to define specific roles for the pediatrician, encouraging an active medical intervention for the learning-disabled child. Although this chapter focuses primarily on the child with impaired learning skills, it will hopefully serve to stimulate a more global interest in the general field of developmental and behavioral pediatrics.

HISTORICAL BACKGROUND

The historical ledger does not reveal an abundance of entries recording the contributions of medicine on behalf of children with educational disabilities. Paradoxically, the initial impetus for professional concern was apparently spawned by the pioneer efforts of physicians (Goldberg and Schiffman, 1972). In 1877 Kussmaul, a German physician, described an aphasic loss of the ability to read despite adequate speech, vision, and intellect. He introduced the term *word-blindness* to depict this disability. In 1896 W. Pringle Morgan, an ophthalmologist, is credited with providing the first definitive analysis of a specific reading disability in a report in the *British Medical Journal* (Thompson, 1966). He described an intelligent child who experienced difficulty in learning to read and suggested the descriptive label *congenital word-blindness*. James Hinshelwood, also an ophthalmologist, contributed articles in 1895 to *Lancet* on word-blindness and visual memory, reporting that the problem was not caused by an oculomotor dysfunction. He suggested that the disturbance was the result of cerebral cortex agenesis, specifically localized to the angular gyrus. Following these historic observations, the medical literature contained sporadic reports periodically reflecting the physician's interest in learning disabilities, particularly in disorders of reading. Apert in 1924 and Potzl in the same year introduced the concept that children with reading disabilities were manifesting a maturational or developmental delay rather than an anatomic lesion in the central nervous system. In 1925 Samuel Orton defined several neurologic deficits that appeared to be associated with reading disabilities, calling attention to an apparent association with confused laterality, reversals, left-handedness (or ambidexterity), and mirror-writing. The term *strephosymbolia* was formulated to characterize the disorder. In almost a quarter of a century of research Orton demonstrated that children with specific language disabilities were capable of being educated, thereby avoiding academic underachievement and emotional reactions (Thompson, 1966).

In the early 1920s the concept of a "brain damage behavioral syndrome" was recognized as a complication of acute attacks of epidemic encephalitis lethargica. Within a decade a group of children was described as "organically driven" with erratic attention spans, presumably as a consequence of a brain stem dysfunction. Alfred Strauss, a neuropsychiatrist, and coworkers (Strauss and Lehtinen, 1947) recognized "brain-injured children" who exhibited hyperactivity, impulsivity, distractibility, and perseveration. Subsequently, these children were found to have educational delays apparently resulting from perceptual disturbances and "subtle" neurologic abnormalities. Special education was recommended to assist children having academic difficulties as a result of perceptual deficits. The concept of brain-injured children became an increasingly popular etiologic classification but unfortunately was linked synonymously with all disorders of learning.

It is apparent that before 1940 physicians were primarily concerned with acute problems that threatened the physical health of the child. Following the publications of Erikson, Gesell, Freud, Ilg, and others, disorders of behavior, personality, and learning became significant topics in child health care. The rapidly growing interest in developmental and behavioral pediatrics reflected the combined concerns of parents and professionals. Quite dramatically, medical interest appeared to experience a metamorphosis from passive neglect to active intervention.

In the early 1960s the first federal conferences were organized to share interests in the learning-disabled child. In 1964 parents organized a national group, the Association for Children with Learning Disabilities. Physicians have been summoned with increasing frequency to share their expertise in the care of learning-impaired children. Overall there has been a positive and energetic response to this call by pediatricians and pediatric neurologists (Schain, 1977). Medical interest in learning disorders is reflected by various activities. The American Academy of Pediatrics has included learning disabilities as part of its continuing education program. The topic is a suggested area for study in recertification, and medical schools have included these issues in the didactic curriculum for students. Clinical experiences in developmental disabilities are provided for residents in pediatric training. Fellowships have been designed, and numerous articles, chapters, and books are authored by physicians (Schain, 1977; Kinsbourne and Caplan, 1979; Gottlieb, 1979; Gottlieb et al., 1979; Levine, et al., 1980a; Levine, et al., 1980b; Levine et al., 1981).

Historically, the clinical profile of children with impaired learning was, in part, fashioned by legislative policies. In 1963 a government committee redefined the child with minimal brain dysfunction (Clements, 1966). The designation *minimal brain dysfunction* had previously been used synonymously with learning disability. In the same year Congress passed Public Law 88-164, which designated funds for special education training. Several years later the category of learning disabilities was removed from that of crippled and health-impaired children and was established as a division under the United States Office of Education. Funds became available when Congress enacted the Learning Disabilities Act as Title VI-G of the Elementary and Secondary Education Act of 1970. Several revisions of terminology have transpired. The most recent modification was enacted in the Special Education for All Handicapped Children Act of 1975 (Public Law 94-142). In the overall historical perspective of pediatric research, learning disabilities has been a relatively unexplored area.

CLASSIFICATION AND TERMINOLOGY

A learning disorder can obviously interfere with academic achievement, temporarily or permanently, but may also deleteriously influence emotional and social development. Learning disabilities in their broadest context include a potpourri of organic and functional disorders that result in poor school performance. A general etiologic grouping would include a spectrum of chronic handicapping conditions of childhood, such as mental retardation, physical handicaps, economic and cultural deprivation, central nervous system processing dysfunctions, maturational delays, prolonged somatic illnesses, unrealistic parental expectations, emotional and behavioral disorders, and ineffectual educational management. The design of these classification systems is dependent on a variety of concepts, including neurologic, educational, psychologic, psycholinguistic, and other discipline-oriented models.

Disorders of learning represent a heterogeneous group of clinical entities. Academic underachievement results from the interaction of multiple neurologic and behavioral factors that depress overall performance. Children with learning disabilities have been characterized from various professional viewpoints reflecting interest in etiology, symptomatology, and therapeutic responsiveness. Consequently an array of labels have been generated: hyperkinetic syndrome, minimal brain dysfunction, perceptually handicapped, dyslexia, visual-motor disability, specific reading disability, slow learner, lazy, and poorly motivated. The assigned label may reflect the area of expertise (or bias) of the professional evaluating the child (Warren, 1978). The range and numbers of descriptive terms attest to the fact that these children do *not* have characteristics definable as a syndrome.

A satisfactory functional organization of learning disorders has not been formulated because of semantics, tunnel-vision approaches, poorly defined basic mechanisms, and the diversity of concepts of etiology and therapy. One classification segregates disorders of learning into four major categories: (1) psychogenic, (2) neurogenic, (3) developmental language disabled, and (4) environmental (de Hirsch, 1974). The first category, *psychogenic* learning disabilities, includes children with psychotic disturbances as well as children with nonpsychotic disorders such as phobic reactions, motivational difficulties, passive attitudes, and compulsive and "fantasy-ridden" states. Children in the second group, with *neurogenic* learning disabilities, are classically considered to have brain injuries ranging from mild to severe. Included in this category are children with cerebral palsy, convulsive equivalents, seizures, and obvious neurologic deficits. Associated neurobehavioral signs may include irritability, hyperactivity or hypoactivity, short attention span, confusion in left-right orientation, and visual-motor incoordination. The third group, *dyslexic* children, have disorders in using printed and written forms of language. Although these children have adequate intellectual abilities, opportunities for learning, intact emotional development, and normal neurologic examinations, they demonstrate reading disabilities categorized under the general scope of developmental language disorders. The fourth category, learning disorders related to *environmental deprivation,* includes children whose academic achievement is limited by detrimental by-products of a depressed environment. The noxious elements include malnutrition, substandard medical and dental care, disturbed family relationships, inadequate housing, and socioeconomic deprivation. Educational readiness may be endangered as a consequence of motivational depression, poorly developed educational attitudes, lack of challenging and organized preschool stimulation, and a variety of undetected organic handicaps.

The various definitions of learning disabilities generally exclude children whose academic underachievement is a result of a neurologic deficit, disturbed emotionality, or environmental deprivation. Original federal legislation (Public Law 91-230, sect. 602-15, April 13, 1970) defined learning disabilities for funding purposes and was restated in the Special Education for All Handicapped Children Act of 1975 (Public Law 94-142):

> Children with special learning disabilities exhibit a disorder in one or more of the basic psychologic processes involved in understanding or in using spoken or written language. These may be manifested in disorders of listening, thinking, talking, reading, writing, spelling or arithmetic. They include conditions which have been referred to as perceptual handicaps, brain injury, minimal brain dysfunction, dyslexia, developmental aphasia, etc. They do not include learning problems which are due primarily to visual, hearing, or motor handicaps, to mental retardation, emotional disturbance, or to environmental disadvantage.

The Council for Exceptional Children (Bateman and Schiefelbusch, 1969) proposed the following definition:

> A child with learning disabilities is one with adequate mental ability, sensory processes and emotional stability who has specific deficits in perceptual, integrative or expressive processes which severely impair learning efficiency. This includes children who have central nervous system dysfunction which is expressed primarily in impaired learning efficiency.

It has been emphasized that *relevance* is the key for selecting a definition of learning disorder (Gallagher, 1966). One definition to satisfy all disciplines would be almost impossible to formulate. Although the definition may have a specific significance for the user, it can be confusing or controversial for other professionals.

INCIDENCE

Statistical analyses that attempt to precisely define the population of academic underachievers by specific etiology are extremely difficult to compile. Learning disorders are not reportable entities; underdiagnoses and overdiagnoses are common, and confused semantics have contributed to a statistical dilemma.

A relatively large proportion of schoolchildren have been identified with learning disorders and reading problems. Estimates vary from 10% to 20%, involving approximately 5 to 10 million children. It has been conservatively calculated that in the United States approximately 15% of schoolchildren exhibit developmental lags in their education (Goldberg and Schiffman, 1972; Walzer and Richmond, 1973). However, only 2 million schoolchildren are enrolled in special education programs for handicapping conditions of all types (American Academy of Pediatrics, 1972).

Regardless of the statistical survey that is considered to be most accurate, the minimal estimate indicates that an alarmingly large segment of the pediatric population faces educational jeopardy. The problem of learning disabilities, by any standard of measurement, appears to be of epidemic proportions and constitutes a national crisis.

ETIOLOGY

The medically oriented concept of the epidemiology of learning disabilities implies a central nervous system dysfunction. The neuropsychologic concept suggests that high-risk factors encountered during the prenatal, perinatal, or postnatal periods presumably alter neuronal function and capacities or cause maturational delays. Neurologic insults incurred during early life presumably may be manifested years later by impaired learning ability and specific defects in cognitive skills. A medically based etiologic classification is limited in scope but has particular value for physicians by (1) indicating needed areas for strengthening preventive medicine, (2) defining a population of children considered at risk, and (3) identifying children who require careful monitoring during the preschool period. A myriad of factors have been suggested as the etiologic basis for learning disorders:

- Prenatal and perinatal factors
  - Genetic constitution
  - Low birth weight for gestational age
  - Prematurity
  - Complicated labor and delivery
  - Gestational bleeding
  - Maternal infections
  - Maternal metabolic disorders
  - Maternal malnutrition
  - Maternal drug abuse
  - Trauma
- Fetal malnutrition
- Neonatal factors
  - Cyanotic episodes
  - Convulsions
  - Subdural hematoma
  - Malnutrition
  - Kernicterus
  - Septicemia
- Postnatal factors
  - Organic handicaps
  - Severe dehydration
  - Meningitis
  - Encephalitis
  - Severe head injury
  - Ingestion of toxins
  - Chronic somatic illness
  - Malnutrition
  - Economic and cultural deprivation

It is readily apparent that the list contains the essential elements of a high-risk classification. The final common pathway of the conditions cited is a disruption in the homeostasis of the central nervous system, resulting in disturbances in cognitive abilities. The implication is that learning disabilities basically represent a neurologic dysfunction. However, the concept is too limiting an approach and fails to recognize equally significant causes.

A more ''global'' etiologic classification (Walzer and Richmond, 1973) follows; it stresses the interaction of a variety of factors influencing psychosocial adaptation:

- Biologic factors
  - Intrinsic neural organization
    - Cognition, perception, attention
  - Motor disorders
  - Sensory disorders
    - Visual, auditory, kinesthetic
  - Language pathways
  - Seizures
  - Somatic handicaps
  - Vigor
- Psychologic factors
  - Sensory deprivation
  - Infant-maternal interaction
    - Insufficiency, distortion, discontinuity
  - Perception (psychologic)
  - Adaptational patterns
  - Cognitive capacities
  - Anxiety
  - Self-concept
  - Personality development
- Sociocultural factors
  - Child-rearing patterns
  - Economic level
  - Housing
  - Nutrition
  - Urban-rural locale
  - Subculture
  - Minority group
  - Prejudice
  - Educational facilities
  - Employment opportunities
  - Medical services
  - Social services
  - Educational expectations
  - Teacher expectations

Learning disabilities may be envisioned as a product of the interaction of psychoeducational, sociocultural, and neurobiologic factors. The active interplay between the three categories contributes to molding a developmental, educational, and social profile of the child, adolescent, and ultimately the adult.

SPECIFIC LEARNING DISABILITIES: AN OVERVIEW

Disorders of learning have been roughly segregated into two broad categories of specific and nonspecific disabilities. However, the final outcome may be the same for both groups: academic underachievement, poor self-concept, and eventually impaired social adjustment.

The term *specific learning disabilities* generally includes dyslexia, visual and auditory processing disturbances (perceptual disorders), dysgraphia, dyscalculia, and attention deficit disorder. It is important to note that learning difficulties may occur as a result of varying combinations of these disorders more often than existing as deficits in isolation. The definition excludes academic underachievement caused by mental retardation, emotional disturbances, impaired peripheral sense organs, or environmental disadvantage; the latter are *nonspecific* causes.

Dyslexia. Since the first use of the word *dyslexia* by the German ophthalmologist Berlin in 1887, volumes of descriptions have been assembled in an attempt to delineate the child with a reading disability. The range of interpretations of dyslexia has included a general categorization of learning disability, behavioral reactions, and a specific type of reading disability. Dyslexia has been defined more precisely as a reading disorder caused by an inability to associate auditory input and vocalizations with graphic symbols (White et al., 1973). The dyslexic reader has been characterized as exhibiting associated deficits such as letter and word reversals, poor spelling skills, poor handwriting, and minor neurologic signs.

Slow readers generally are divided into two categories: (1) primary dyslexia (developmental dyslexia) associated with normal intelligence and absence of an obvious cause of the reading disability and (2) secondary dyslexia, a reading disorder caused by an obvious difficulty such as brain injury or environmental disadvantage. It has been estimated that in the United States approximately 10% of all children are handicapped by a reading disability; perhaps 25% or more of this group have developmental dyslexia.

A general classification of reading retardation (a significant discrepancy between the actual reading level and level expected based on mental age) has been organized; it is a classification based on etiology (Rabinovitch, 1968):

Primary reading retardation (developmental dyslexia): A disorder in which the "capacity to learn to read is impaired without definite brain damage suggested in the history or on neurologic examination." The disability is characterized by difficulty in processing letters and words as symbols, apparently resulting from "a disturbed pattern of neurologic organization." The concept implies an endogenous etiology.

Reading retardation secondary to brain injury: A disorder associated with documented neurologic deficits and other aphasic difficulties. Evidence of brain injury is revealed in the history (e.g., encephalitis, head injury).

Reading retardation secondary to exogenous factors: Implies that the child has the potential for achieving a reading level commensurate with age and intelligence, but potential is compromised by anxiety, depression, other emotional factors, inadequate schooling . . . and other exogenous influences.

Evidence supporting the concept of a specific developmental dyslexia includes the specific nature of reading errors, familial and male sex incidences, absence of perceptual deficits and serious brain injury, lack of obvious emotional disturbances, and failure to read despite conventional teaching in the face of average or above-average intelligence.

Dyslexia is most likely associated with specific deficits in one or more aspects of linguistic functioning or verbal processing. However, a clearly defined etiologic base has not been established. The proposed origins for developmental dyslexia have included (1) maturational lags (lags in specific cortical association areas cause a delay in acquiring developmental skills), (2) impaired cerebral dominance (poor lateralization to the left hemisphere of language representation), (3) biochemical abnormalities (higher monoamine oxidase and thyroxine levels), and (4) neuroanatomic abnormalities and dysfunctions (Long and Murray, 1982). These postulates represent preliminary research probes that require more extensive analysis, investigation, and replication.

Visual processing dysfunctions. Visual perceptual ability encompasses the processes of receiving, integrating, and interpreting visual stimuli. Children with intact visual acuity but impaired central nervous system processing abilities may be educationally disadvantaged. Impaired central nervous system processing can interfere with (1) discriminating details composing an object; (2) blocking out unimportant visual stimuli, permitting an appreciation of dominant visual clues; (3) combining several visual clues into groups, thereby deriving a meaning from the total visual impression; (4) classifying an object into a previously organized visual category; and (5) comparing a visual hypothesis with an actual object as it is perceived and visually transmitted to the nervous system (Chalfant and Scheffelin, 1969).

Visual processing skills appear to develop in a sequential pattern from birth to approximately 6 years of age. However, a range of normal biologic variation is anticipated. Maturational lags or dysfunctions can disrupt proper use of visual inputs and are reflected as disturbed learning experiences. During the learning process, disturbances in the processing of visual stimuli in the cerebral cortex disrupt three major functions: (1) spatial orientation and relationships, (2) visual discrimination, and (3) object recognition.

Dysfunctions in spatial orientation are observed educationally as confused laterality (left-right discrimination), reversals and rotations of letters and numbers, and poor depth perception. Children with visual perceptual deficits often exhibit difficulty in copying and matching geometric designs, copying letters and numbers, dressing and buttoning, reading, and organizing directions. Visual discrimination may relate to size, shape, sequence, rate of presentation, duration, and numbers of stimuli presented. Academic confusion may result from impaired visual discrimination skills. The child may exhibit difficulty with figure-ground differentiation; the more complex the background material, the more difficult it will be to correctly identify the dominant visual clue. Similarly, the child may be unable to recognize an object unless all the visual clues are presented (visual closure). Literally, the child experiences a *visual agnosia,* although recognition may be achieved through tactile sensation. The inability to synthesize, or blend, visual stimuli into a meaningful whole or to recognize missing components of an incomplete visual presentation causes deficits in learning. Visual processing deficiencies may compromise a child's academic progress by interfering with his reading abilities—a *visual dyslexia.*

It is readily apparent that a child will require intact visual processing skills to adjust successfully in complex academic and social environments. Children with deficits in visual-motor coordination, left-right orientation, visual memory, spatial orientation, visual closure, visual distraction, and discrimination and attention, singly or in combinations, are at risk educationally and socially.

Auditory processing dysfunctions. Auditory perceptual maturity is probably completed by approximately 7 years of age, recognizing a biologic range of variation. Maturational lags and auditory processing dysfunctions, similar to visual processing deficits, can adversely influence academic performance. Indeed, auditory processing disturbances appear to be a major cause of impaired learning by markedly interfering with reading abilities (Rampp, 1972).

The child with an auditory processing disability may reveal weaknesses in auditory attention, auditory memory, auditory sequencing, sound discrimination, auditory synthesis (blending), auditory closure, and auditory temporal relationships. Attending to auditory stimuli may be extremely difficult for a child who is unable to interpret such stimuli in a meaningful way. Despite intact auditory acuity, the child may be unable to discriminate between similar sounds. Anatomically the auditory processing disturbances probably represent a temporal lobe dysfunction. Deficits in the ability to analyze and synthesize speech sounds creates a formidable task for the child when he is expected to master the traditional phonetic approach to reading. Reading disturbances resulting from underlying auditory processing deficits have been described as an *auditory dyslexia.*

Disturbances in auditory serial memory are commonly associated with academic difficulties such as reciting the alphabet; naming the days of the week, the months, and the seasons; and remembering addresses and telephone numbers. Children with this deficit function poorly when challenged with a multiple series of directions. At times the child may appear to be responding inappropriately to verbal commands, reflecting the inability to correctly interpret the auditory stimuli.

Children with either visual or auditory processing deficiencies appear to have lower thresholds for distraction. Frequently they experience great difficulty sorting out unimportant stimuli and are literally distracted and confused by all stimuli. Weaknesses in processing skills are often associated with behavioral disturbances. The children are often singled out for their behavioral "disabilities," including easy distractibility, short attention span, poor motivation, daydreaming, and academic disinterest. However, the basic fault is not one of emotions and attitude; rather, it is a manifestation of central nervous system processing disturbances and a resultant impairment of learning skills.

It is of medical interest to speculate on a relationship between impaired peripheral sense organ function and a subsequent central processing deficiency. For example, intermittent hearing losses associated with chronic otitis media may be linked to inadequate stimulation of the central nervous system, which is ultimately recognized as delayed communicative skills (Sak and Ruben, 1982) and auditory perceptual disturbances. The suggested interaction stresses the need for concerted medical attention long after the otitis media and hearing problems have been corrected. The residue may be an auditory processing deficiency and a learning disability (Zinkus and Gottlieb, 1978a and b; Zinkus et al., 1978; Gottlieb, 1979; Gottlieb et al., 1979).

Auditory-visual integration dysfunctions. The ability to associate, or match, auditory and visual stimuli forms the basis for language development and ultimately the development of reading skills (Geschwind, 1965). Auditory-visual integration dysfunctions are frequently found in learning-disabled children and probably form the basis of more severe learning problems. During the early school years the child with auditory-visual integration deficits experiences difficulty in learning the letters of the alphabet. He often misnames letters, despite the considerable amount of time teachers and parents devote to his learning this task. Later, dyslexic-type reading patterns emerge, suggesting that a deficit in auditory-visual integration probably forms the basis of many dyslexic disturbances. Reading skills may be poor, and tasks such as spelling from dictation also prove to be extremely difficult. The auditory input of the dictated word becomes distorted at the cortical level, and the resulting written word seldom resembles the correct spelling. The association between phoneme and grapheme is markedly disturbed, and bizarre configurations of letters are common. Distortions in letter arrangements occur even with words previously learned.

The etiology of auditory-visual integration disturbances is poorly understood. Lesions in the temporal-parietal area of the dominant hemisphere, especially in the region of the angular gyrus, have been implicated (Geschwind, 1965). However, learning-disabled children with auditory-visual integration deficits seldom exhibit discrete abnormalities on electroencephalograms (EEGs) or other standard neurologic tests.

Dysgraphia. The inability to produce the written symbols of a language is the primary feature of dysgraphia. The disorder is typically a manifestation of disturbed language function as evidenced in graphic expression (writing). Dysgraphia in isolation is a rare occurrence among learning-disabled children. Frequently, writing (penmanship) is impaired, but this deficit results from visual or auditory processing disorders (or both), visual-motor coordination problems, or deficits in auditory-visual integration. The differential diagnosis of impaired graphic skills involves evaluation of the full range of perceptual skills.

Dyscalculia. The inability to execute arithmetic operations at a level commensurate with the child's intellectual ability may be evidence of dyscalculia. Dyscalculia is seldom observed in isolation. More often the child has perceptual deficits that disrupt the ability to accurately perform arithmetic problems. For example, a child with visual-spatial orientation problems will have extreme difficulty correctly aligning the columns of figures in a simple arithmetic problem, leading to subsequent computation errors. Dyscalculia, or faulty arithmetic skills, is recognized, but the basis for the difficulty stems from visual processing disorders. Failure to perform adequately in arithmetic is frequently observed in association with similar inabilities to function adequately in reading or spelling.

Attention deficit disorder (ADD). A variety of terms have been used interchangeably to describe the child with an ADD, including *minimal brain dysfunction, hyperkinetic syndrome, clumsy child syndrome, perceptually handicapped,* and *hyperkinetic reaction of childhood.* ADD, as characterized in the *Diagnostic and Statistical Manual of Mental Disorders* (DSM-III), is associated primarily with developmentally inappropriate attention and impulsivity. Two subtypes have been delineated: Add with hyperactivity and ADD without hyperactivity. The former, as diagnostically defined in the DSM-III (1980), includes:

A. Inattention (at least 3 of the following):
   1. often fails to finish things he or she starts
   2. often doesn't seem to listen
   3. easily distracted
   4. has difficulty concentrating on schoolwork or other tasks requiring sustained attention
   5. has difficulty sticking to play activity
B. Impulsivity (at least 3 of the following):
   1. often acts before thinking
   2. shifts excessively from one activity to another
   3. has difficulty organizing work (not due to cognitive impairment)
   4. needs a lot of supervision
   5. frequently calls out in class
   6. has difficulty awaiting turn in games or group situations
C. Hyperactivity (at least 2 of the following):
   1. runs about or climbs on things excessively
   2. has difficulty sitting still or fidgets excessively
   3. has difficulty staying seated
   4. moves about excessively during sleep
   5. is always "on the go" or acts as if "driven by a motor"
D. Onset before the age of seven
E. Duration of at least six months
F. Not due to Schizophrenia, Affective Disorder, or Severe or Profound Mental Retardation

ADD (formerly *minimal brain dysfunction*) as a diagnostic entity has been debated by physicians, and two divergent concepts have emerged. One group suggests that ADD is a syndrome (Haller, 1975; Shaywitz et al., 1978); the other claims it is a myth (Schmitt, 1975). The "believers" perceive the child with ADD as having a complex of learning difficulties and behavioral problems despite average or above-average intelligence. The incidence has been variously reported at 5% to 10% of school-age children, with a marked male preponderance estimated as high as 6 to 1. The etiologic factors are assumed to be various prenatal, perinatal, and postnatal cerebral insults—the so-called high-risk factors—such as anoxia, infections, and traumas. These injuries presumably do *not* cause gross neurologic disturbances (seizures, paralyses, etc.) but do cause more subtle dysfunctions in the central nervous system. The cardinal manifestations of ADD include an array of neurologic, learning, and behavioral signs and symptoms: hyperactivity, short attention span, distractibility, impulsivity, emotional lability, specific learning deficits (perceptual problems), poor self-concept, and "soft" neurologic signs. The soft, or equivocal, neurologic signs include general coordination deficits, transient strabismus, dysdiadochokinesia, excessive synkinesis, poor finger coordination, confused laterality, inability to perform tandem gait, tremors, hyperreflexia, and articulation deficits. Therapeutic intervention for children with ADD may involve a combined approach, including special education, counseling, and medication.

"Nonbelievers" suggest that ADD was established by using invalid criteria. They regard the soft neurologic signs as indications of neurologic immaturity, transient in nature, rather than a consequence of injury. No pathognomonic neurologic sign has been identified with ADD, psychologic examinations do not reveal characteristic patterns, and EEG changes are nonspecific. The syndrome status is similarly questioned because of the alleged high incidence and sex distribution, which has not been confirmed in some communities and countries. In addition, it is well known that children with major central nervous system disease do not typically exhibit the symptoms attributed to ADD. Finally, pathologic evidence is lacking from postmortem studies, which fail to reveal any brain damage in patients assumed to have ADD. It is argued that more harm can be caused by the label than is commonly recognized, paralyzing school systems, frightening parents, and stigmatizing the children. The nonbelievers advocate eliminating ADD as a medical entity.

Special considerations. Within the broad framework of learning disorders, several unique issues deserve mention. These particular difficulties and situations, although not categorized as specific learning disabilities, can profoundly influence educational progress and psychosocial productivity. Early detection and intervention, however, may be associated with a favorable prognosis. The need for some medical participation is apparent.

Children with overt *organic handicaps* (blindness, deafness, mental retardation, or cerebral palsy) will require some special education programming and considerations. Ideally modifications in the classroom environment will focus on meeting individual and realistic goals for the child's progress, providing opportunities for enhancing learning potentials. One must establish priorities when designing a program for the child with multiple handicaps. Periodic reassessments may be valuable in redesigning the educational prescription.

Similarly, children with *behavioral and emo-*

tional disorders will require special educational adjustments in their school program. The severity of their problem may determine the need for placement in a self-contained program. The curriculum design may include behavior modification approaches as well as the adjunct use of medications. Active medical supervision of drugs is essential in the coordinated educational program, and monitoring will require active dialogue between teacher, parent, and physician. The unique problems of the autistic child will necessitate special education interventions (Morgan, 1981).

Gifted and talented children are similarly deserving of special mention. The "gift" of superior intelligence or an outstanding talent (music, mathematics, leadership, etc.) will often demand adaptations of the traditional educational environment to enhance these skills. There is a need to provide special assistance without engendering elitism or disrupting normal peer interactions. Consideration of the type of educational program should be couched within the framework of the child's physical, social, and educational levels of development. Acceleration and grouping may not be the ideal approaches to prevention of academic boredom. The physician should be able to contribute a meaningful component in providing a profile of child and family as it relates to the construction of an educational program (Freeman, 1979; Adamson, 1982; Gottlieb and Williams, 1982).

There are various other topics of interest relating to learning disabilities: the learning-disabled adolescent (Kinsbourne and Swanson, 1980; Daniel, 1981), the learning-disabled juvenile delinquent (Gottlieb and Zinkus, 1981), available resources in higher education, career counseling, and counseling for poor self-concept. These issues similarly require intervention from the primary care physician.

EMOTIONAL SEQUELAE OF LEARNING DISORDERS

The child in educational jeopardy has a marked disadvantage in a society that places an extremely high value on achievement, rewarding individuals who are successful and ignoring or punishing those who are unsuccessful. Children who deviate from "normal" pathways of academic achievement and progress usually create concern, anxiety, and stress for parents, teachers, and those who are attempting to help the child reach his full potential.

Problems in learning often occur at critical points in a child's development. During the interval from 5 through 9 years, children initiate attempts at independent functioning and definition of the self (identity). The developmental changes formulate the basic structure of their future personality. Considerable emotional damage can be precipitated by protracted periods of anxiety and stress emanating from a tense or disappointing classroom experience.

Parental responses to the underachieving child are often unrealistic and harsh, expressing their feelings of guilt and disappointment in the form of anger and hostility. The child in educational jeopardy experiences a continual atmosphere of anxiety and frustration both at home and at school. As a result, the learning-disabled child may present characteristic behavioral features at the time of the evaluation. The child often enters the examining room with his eyes and head down, realizing that once again he is expected to perform for someone who will reveal his lack of ability. He frequently exhibits defensive behaviors, attempting to excuse what he anticipates to be a poor performance. The child becomes increasingly frustrated with his inability to successfully perform a task, exhibiting aggressiveness toward the examiner in the form of resistance, poor cooperation, lack of attention, or a flippant attitude. These defensive maneuvers are relatively uncommon in the normal, well-adjusted child who is performing adequately in school. Lack of success experiences generates additional emotional stress, which compounds the difficulties engendered by the specific learning disability. The child anticipates difficulty in almost every situation and becomes emotionally paralyzed with fear of failure and expected rejection. Because school attendance is mandatory and the child cannot leave physically, he compensates by withdrawing psychologically, daydreaming and thinking more pleasant thoughts of enjoyable times. He avoids what he regards to be aversive stimuli: the teacher, the blackboard, and classmates. Occasionally the child with learning disabilities will manifest psychosomatic complaints and symptoms of school phobia or school aversion. If the academic environment remains uncomfortable, the child may participate in school truancy or, in some instances, school vandalism.

The hyperkinetic child is of special concern because overactivity is a very disturbing and disrupting classroom behavior for teacher and peers. It is a constant source of tension for all concerned. Unfortunately, it has been erroneously assumed that hyperkinetic behavior is associated only with attention deficit disorder. This is not true; in addition to organic origins, hyperactivity may be associated with anxiety, tension, and frustration. Situational hyperactivity may be induced by an emotional state (a pressured situation), which is sometimes overlooked in haste to define an organic etiology. The child who reacts aggressively to the teacher frequently craves attention, gaining recognition by acting-out behaviors. It is ego saving for the learning-disabled child to blame and feel angry

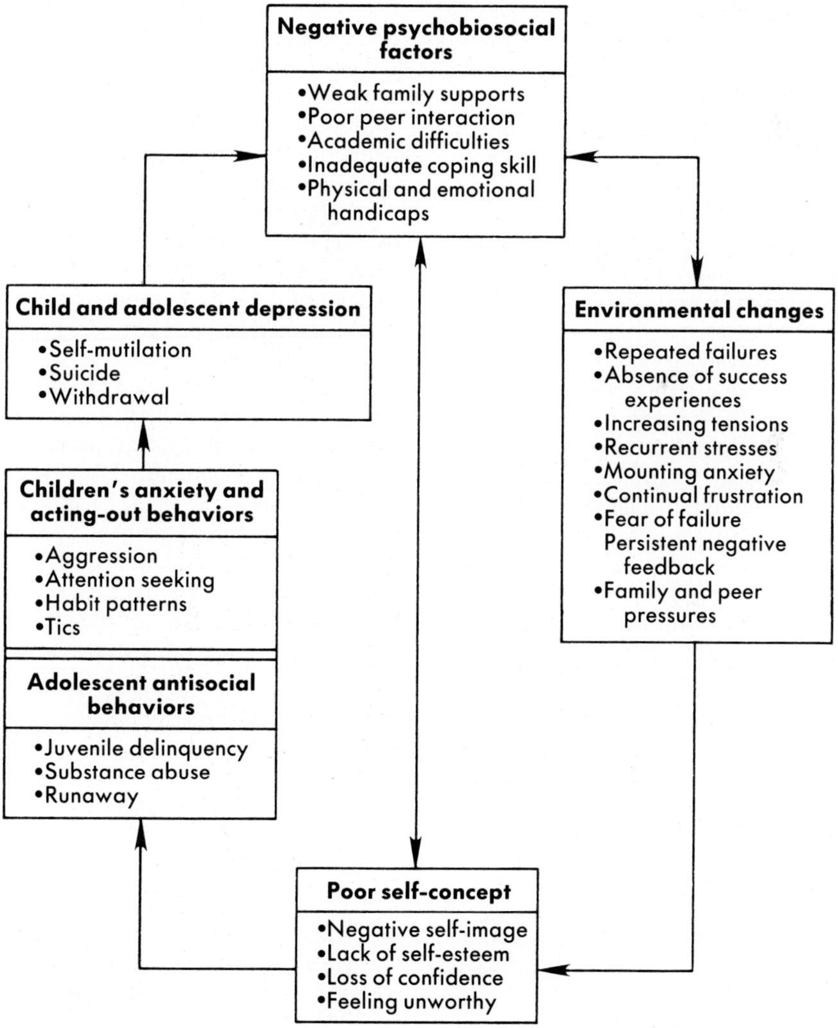

Fig. 3-1. Schema of cyclic, self-perpetuating nature of poor self-concept in children and adolescents.

toward the teacher, rather than to accept personal responsibility for failure. Frequently the emotional components of the learning disability represent a more serious threat than does the specific learning disorder per se (Fig. 3-1).

A complex relationship exists between the physical, cognitive, and emotional components of a child's development. The learning-disabled child experiences numerous obstacles that prevent a healthy interaction between these factors. The bottom line of repeated frustrations, anxieties, and negative reenforcements is a loss of self-esteem and a lack of self-confidence (Gottlieb and Williams, 1982; Shaw et al., 1982). The disrupted balance can ultimately result in disturbed behaviors in the classroom, as previously discussed. Eventually the effects of poor self-concept extend beyond the school environment to involve behaviors at home. Chronic feelings of worthlessness, lack of confidence, and depression, if untreated, may result in serious adolescent and adult personality disorders. An undiagnosed and untreated learning disability may be an important precursor for aberrant behavior such as juvenile delinquency (Fig. 3-1).

Numerous investigations have revealed that an overwhelming percentage of youthful offenders are severely retarded in reading; the reading disabilities are not caused by antisocial and rebellious attitudes that reduce the "teachability" of the youthful offender, but by underlying specific learning disabilities (Zinkus and Gottlieb, 1978a). Perceptual handicaps are found in a large percentage of youthful offenders and can cause poor academic skills. The severity of the reading disability has been directly related to the seriousness of the perceptual deficits, confirming a relationship between learning disorders and delinquent behavior (Zinkus and Gottlieb, 1978b). Many juvenile delinquents present a history in which there are prominent characteristics of the attention deficit disorder (hyperactivity, short attention span, poor impulse control, and distractibility).

Health care professionals must be aware of the long-term sequelae of learning disabilities, which, if left untreated, may culminate in severe behavioral disturbances. The child who is continually frustrated may attack the system that causes his discomfort, that is, the school and society in general. Early diagnosis and treatment, beginning with the child's physician, is of primary significance in preventing these emotional and behavioral complications.

DIAGNOSIS: THE PHYSICIAN'S CONTRIBUTION

Although learning disabilities are fundamentally educational problems, there are important roles for physicians in diagnosis and management through early detection, physical examination, neurologic assessment, judicious referrals to other professionals, coordination of multidisciplinary efforts, medication management, family counseling, consulting with school personnel, and patient advocacy (Golden, 1982).

There are no pathognomonic signs to characterize children with learning disabilities. Resolution of the differential diagnosis usually requires the combined efforts of selected professionals, including the physician, psychologist, language specialist, special and general educators, and other members of the health service team. Interdisciplinary cooperation is required to define the multiple problems of the learning-disabled child, as well as to delineate his various strengths.

Despite criticism from some professionals (including physicians), the complex nature of disorders of learning has prompted increased physician involvement. Past medical apathy may have been the result of little or no formal training in this area, the time-consuming nature of the problem, and the lack of assignment of a specific role on the interdisciplinary team.

Nevertheless, a role for the physician is mandated by several unique circumstances:

- Physicians are the first professionals to relate to children, defining a responsibility in early detection of developmental disabilities.
- Physicians are usually the first professionals to be contacted by anxious parents, defining a role in counseling.
- Physicians have a particular expertise in medical and neurologic skills, defining a role in resolving the differential diagnosis.
- Physicians are solely responsible for prescribing and monitoring medications, defining a role in therapy management.
- Physicians frequently consult with other professionals, defining a role in coordinating the interdisciplinary team.
- Physicians usually have longer contact with the child and family, defining a role in monitoring and follow-up services.

- Physicians are respected by the families they serve, defining a role in preventing intervention by untried or fraudulent approaches.
- Physicians have training in neurologic disorders and child development, defining a research role in learning disorders.

The broad scope of interdisciplinary communication and interaction necessitates that physicians keep current in their medical readings and that psychoeducational literature be added to their self-improvement programs. The physician must expand his vocabulary to understand and appreciate the contributions of an interdisciplinary effort. A former president of the American Academy of Pediatrics suggested that "perhaps sociology should be a prerequisite for studying medicine, as are physics and chemistry today" (Thompson, 1974).

At the turn of the century a physician's involvement with schools was primarily to consult on methods of controlling outbreaks of infectious diseases. Today the pediatrician and family physician are being called on with increasing frequency to become advocates for children with a variety of school-encountered learning difficulties (Table 3-1). Parents and teachers are aware of the need for medical evaluation when a child is suspected of having a learning disorder, particularly when there are evidences that impaired learning stems from organic or emotional deficits. In addition, the physician is often expected to offer counsel to parents and professionals regarding the relative values of diagnostic and therapeutic programs. The concept of a training program in "educational pediatrics" as a subspecialty of pediatrics has been considered (Menkes, 1972). The school physician would assume the role of a specialist in educational disorders, working closely with parents, teachers, and associated professionals.

The format of the medical evaluation, when examining a child with a suspected learning disorder, can be designed to follow patterns used in solving traditional pediatric problems.

Comprehensive history. The initial comprehensive history is one of the most important facets of the total assessment procedure. Careful questioning about past medical events may reveal evidence of high-risk conditions that relate to the child's current educational difficulties. Details regarding gestation, labor, delivery, neonatal period, and early infancy may provide meaningful etiologic clues. Analysis of the maturational sequence, including comparisons with siblings' rate of development, may reveal evidences of neurologic lags. Details of progress in speech, motor, and social skills are retraced. The medical account is complemented with detailed social, behavioral, educational, and family histories. The accumulation of historical data, in essence, outlines a profile of the child, as recalled by the parents and involved professionals.

The history also includes information obtained from the child. Communicative children often provide meaningful insights about the difficulties they experience and their reactions to these problems.

Additional data should be obtained from other involved professional sources. Teachers are usually most cooperative in sharing their observations of a child's academic achievements and behavioral characteristics; contact by telephone or written report is essential for a meaningful evaluation. Records of previous examinations, school achievement, and medical information should be reviewed and analyzed.

General and neurologic examinations. A child with a suspected disorder of learning requires a thorough physical examination, including screening of visual acuity by use of a Snellen chart and auditory acuity with a pure tone audiometer. The more sophisticated visual screeners and impedance audiometry are encouraged as part of routine office use. It is the physician's responsibility to detect and treat remedial impedances to good educational health, for example, poor vision, impaired hearing, dental disorders, anemia, and other acute and chronic medical problems. The need for a thorough and comprehensive physical examination cannot be stressed too emphatically. In a review by the American Academy of Pediatrics (1972) the following was reported:

> About 3% of children in the early school years have some kind of hearing defect (rarely sufficient to be handicapping), about 25% have distant vision less than 20/20 Snellen (almost all correctable with glasses), about 1% are considered to have major speech disorders (most of which are correctable or improve spontaneously), about 10% to 20% are considered to have a reading disorder, 3% are considered mentally retarded (most are educable), and approximately 1% are epileptic (most are controlled).

Table 3-1. Differential diagnosis of disturbed educational development

	Specific learning disability	Mental retardation	Organic handicap (e.g., hearing loss)
History of high-risk factors	Possible relation to complications of pregnancy and delivery	Possible relation to complications of labor and delivery; genetic faults	May have history of infections or trauma (e.g., chronic otitis media)
Developmental milestones	May exhibit isolated developmental delays (e.g., speech or motor coordination)	Delays may be noted in all areas of development	Usually normal; developmental delay may be isolated (e.g., delayed speech)
Physical examination	Usually normal	Usually normal findings as related to specific syndromes (e.g., Down syndrome)	Abnormality may be apparent on examination (e.g., scarred tympanic membrane)
Neurologic examination	Usually normal; may detect soft, or subtle, neurologic signs	Varies with extent of central nervous system damage	Abnormality of affected organ
EEG	Usually normal	Varies from normal to abnormal	Usually normal
Teachers' observations	Puzzling; may perform well in some areas academically and socially	Child unable to compete at grade level or with children of same age	Academically functions well in uninvolved areas; peer rapport good
School achievement	Depressed in affected areas and gradually spreads	Depressed for age; functions better in Special Education Program	Depressed in areas that require use of affected sensory skill
Psychologic evaluation	Some normal performances and some areas depressed	Usually depressed in all areas	Depressed in areas requiring use of affected modality
Parents' observations	Usually no problems except for school difficulty; does well with friends	Usually no family disruption; plays with younger children	Functions well in uninvolved areas
General remarks	May have no problems until starting school; preschool identification encouraged; may have superimposed behavioral disorder	Suspicions may be aroused in preschool period because of developmental delays or dull affect	Occasionally exhibits associated behavioral difficulties; deficits a medical challenge

Complete neurologic examination is an essential component of the medical evaluation. The child is examined for evidences of nervous system dysfunction (Table 3-2). The learning-disabled child does not usually exhibit gross abnormalities of the nervous system. Neurobehavioral characteristics frequently associated with learning disorders include hyperactivity (occasionally hypoactivity), short attention span, impulsivity, emotional lability, perceptual-motor impairments, coordination deficits, disorders of memory and thinking, communication disorders, and an array of "subtle" neurologic signs (Page and Grossman, 1973). There are no specific neurologic or behavioral examinations to delineate adequacy of nervous system function as related to learning abilities. However, the association of abnormal neurologic signs (variously labeled as soft, equivocal, or subtle) with behavioral characteristics common to learning disabilities and ADD is considered valuable in the differential diagnosis by some (Table 3-3). Grossman (1978) states that soft neurologic signs is an ambiguous term, de-

Cause			
Somatic illness	**Psychosis**	**Behavioral disorders**	**Socioeconomic (cultural) deprivation**
Usually none	Usually none	Usually none	Usually none; possible history of poor prenatal care
Usually normal; occasionally development irregular	Usually normal	Usually normal	Usually normal
Depends on specific type of somatic disorder (e.g., cardiac, renal, etc.)	Usually normal	Usually normal	Usually normal
Usually normal unless a problem of nervous system	Usually normal or minor abnormalities	Usually normal	Usually normal
Usually normal; question of some abnormalities	Usually normal	Usually normal	Usually normal
Change in performance related to onset of illness	Bizarre responses; may be withdrawn and unresponsive	Attention-seeking behaviors; may annoy classmates; acting-out behavior; islands of good behavior	May be characterized as "poorly motivated"
Poor performances during periods of illness; otherwise normal achievement	Erratic but usually very poor	Varies; can and frequently does do well	Generally performance poor when in competitive academic atmosphere
May be depressed as result of illness	Bizarre responses, possibly with islands of normal function	Good results if child cooperates	Generally depressed; can reflect cultural bias of test items
No difficulty except for illness	Disturbed parent-child relationships; siblings, peer, and social relationships are poor	Better on a 1 to 1 basis; occasional parent-child disturbances	Functions well in own cultural environment; friends with similar circumstance
Family aware of acute or chronic nature of illness	Preschool behavior may be obviously that of a disturbed child	Behavioral disorder may have onset with start of school or exaggerated when school begins	Evidences of socioeconomic depression; functions well at home and with neighborhood peers; slow in school

fining no clear association with specific central nervous system function. The soft signs may be normal at a younger age but regarded as a dysfunction at an older age.

Special laboratory procedures. Results of the history, as well as the physical and neurologic examinations, may prompt further laboratory investigation. Although there are no specific medical laboratory tests associated with learning disabilities, information gathered from EEGs, skull radiographs, and blood chemistries may be valuable in defining other neurologic disorders.

The EEG is of limited value in the diagnostic evaluation of the child with a specific learning disability. However, the EEG is an important diagnostic tool in children with suspected convulsive disorders, neurologic findings suggestive of a focal lesion, suspected progressive neurologic deterioration, unexplained outbursts of abnormal behaviors, a question of absence seizures being confused with daydreaming or "loss of contact," and a history that suggests a convulsive equivalent.

Skull radiographs are rarely of value in as-

Table 3-2. Neurologic signs that may be associated with disorders of learning

Sign	Test	Area of nervous system
Choreiform movements	Outstretched arm and fingers	Basal ganglia
Excessive synkinesis	Thumb-to-finger approximation	Parietal lobe
Fine motor incoordination	Dressing and buttoning	Cerebellum
Dysdiadochokinesia	Hand pronation-supination	Cerebellum
Graphesthesia	Letter tracing on skin	Parietal lobe
Dysmetria	Finger-nose test	Cerebellum
Simultagnosia	Simultaneous touch	Parietal lobe
Visual-motor incoordination	Bender-Gestalt test Slosson drawing test	Temporal lobe Occipital lobe
Gait disturbance	Heel-and-toe walking Hopping and skipping Tandem gait	Cerebellum Basal ganglia
Stereognosis	Touch-and-tell test	Parietal lobe
Abnormal ocular movements	Following moving objects	Frontal lobe Occipital lobe Brain stem
Tightness of muscle groups	Examination of muscle groups	Motor areas
Asymmetric deep tendon reflexes	Examination of reflex activity	Upper motor neurons
Confused laterality	Identification of right and left and crossing over	Parietal lobe
Articulation defects	Repeating words	Temporal lobe Frontal lobe (Broca area)

Table 3-3. Neurobehavioral characteristics that may be associated with attention deficit disorder and learning disorders

Characteristic	General remarks
Hyperkinesis	May be evidenced during infancy as restlessness and poor sleep habits; older children exhibit activity without purpose, disinhibited behavior; activity level increases under stress; may be outgrown during teenage years
Short attention span	Inability to perform tasks that require concentration; low threshold for auditory or visual stimuli; distracted easily; ''flitting'' of attention
Distractibility	Capable of concentration in quiet environments but easily interrupted; forced responsiveness to visual and auditory stimuli
Emotional lability	Mood swings; emotionally labile; overreaction to minimal situations; volatile
Frustration	Low threshold for temper; temper tantrums, outbursts, and aggressive behavior
Impulsivity	Actions may be considered inappropriate; talks out and acts out but does not think out
Poor social adaptation	Socially immature; may act silly, clownlike, or inappropriately
Concrete thinking	Concretism; problem increases as educational tasks become more abstract
Communicative disorders	Delay in speech development; articulation errors
Behavioral disorders	Feelings of insecurity, rejection, anxiety; evidences of attention-seeking behavior; lack of self-confidence; poor self-concept
Anxiety reactions	Nervousness, fear reactions, tics, phobias, aggressive behavior
Depressive reactions	Feelings of worthlessness, apathy, hostility; aggressive behavior; sleep and eating disturbances; pervasive sadness

sessing the child with a learning disability and are reserved for children in whom the examiner suspects problems such as intracranial masses, vascular abnormalities, or neurocutaneous syndromes.

Urine amino acid assays, chromosomal studies, and complex metabolic surveys are usually reserved for patients with suspected mental retardation or specifically related syndromes. These laboratory examinations are not part of the routine evaluation of children with learning disorders.

Laboratory procedures such as urine analysis and hemoglobin determination are usually part of the basic pediatric examination.

Developmental screening. Jean Piaget pioneered the concept that the young child is capable of learning from the beginning of infancy, stressing that the first 2 years of life are the important building blocks for subsequent cognitive development (Maier, 1969). Modifications that enrich the milieu would improve a preschooler's learning capabilities, suggesting that goal-oriented, stimulating play materials and environments would enhance the potentials of the developing nervous system.

One of the primary objectives in screening preschool children is to determine whether performance and behavior are within the range of normal developmental variation. Occasionally the assessment provides information about social maturation and readiness for participation in nursery and kindergarten experiences. The prerequisites for adaptation to preschool programs presumes an ability to (1) interact and play well with other children, (2) follow simple commands, (3) conform to simple rules of behavior, (4) feed and dress with a minimum of supervision, (5) remain separated from parents for prolonged periods during the day, and (6) be motivated for a preschool experience. Early identification programs attempt to find the child at risk and initiate therapeutic preschool experiences. Physicians have been challenged with the responsibility of administering preschool developmental screening inventories, as well as traditional health analyses, because of their unique position of being the first professionals to serve children (Hass and Scovell, 1977). In addition, physicians have the opportunity to monitor a child's development from birth over an extended period and during this interval may intervene to enhance readiness for the formal learning experience.

Although the screening of preschool children for possible educational weaknesses is encouraged, caution must be exercised, inasmuch as no single testing instrument can specifically identify a learning disability. However, detection of developmental delays should prompt a more formal evaluation by a multidisciplinary team. A variety of assessment measures are available for evaluating the maturational level of preschool children. Five popular developmental screening inventories were compared on relevant technical and practical criteria (Thorpe and Werner, 1974). Although valid criticisms have been proposed, the testing instruments can provide a descriptive developmental profile of the preschool child. The inventories evaluated included the (1) Denver Developmental Screening Test, (2) Head Start Developmental Screening Test and Behavior Rating Scale, (3) Cooperative Preschool Inventory, (4) School Readiness Survey, and (5) Thorpe Developmental Inventory. The five screening tests were designed to assess a child's developmental status before and after initiating special education and health programs. The limitations are based on the fact that norms are not universally applicable; much depends on the expertise of the examiner and the data analyzer. Screening tests are not infallible but serve as good triage inventories to evaluate strengths and weaknesses.

One of the more popular screening inventories used in appraising the developmental abilities of children from birth to 6 years of age is the Denver Developmental Screening Test (DDST). The screening also finds application in evaluating functional levels of children older than 6 years whose abilities fall in the preschool range. The DDST is based on the standardized appraisal of developmental skills in four areas: (1) gross motor, (2) fine motor–adaptive, (3) language, and (4) personal-social. The DDST should not be misconstrued as a test to measure intelligence. However, the screening can reveal delays in these several areas of development and thus single out the developmentally delayed preschooler for more extensive evaluation. The test is readily administered in an office setting and can be effectively administered by office personnel. The DDST may be used as a "developmental growth chart," in much the same way

A

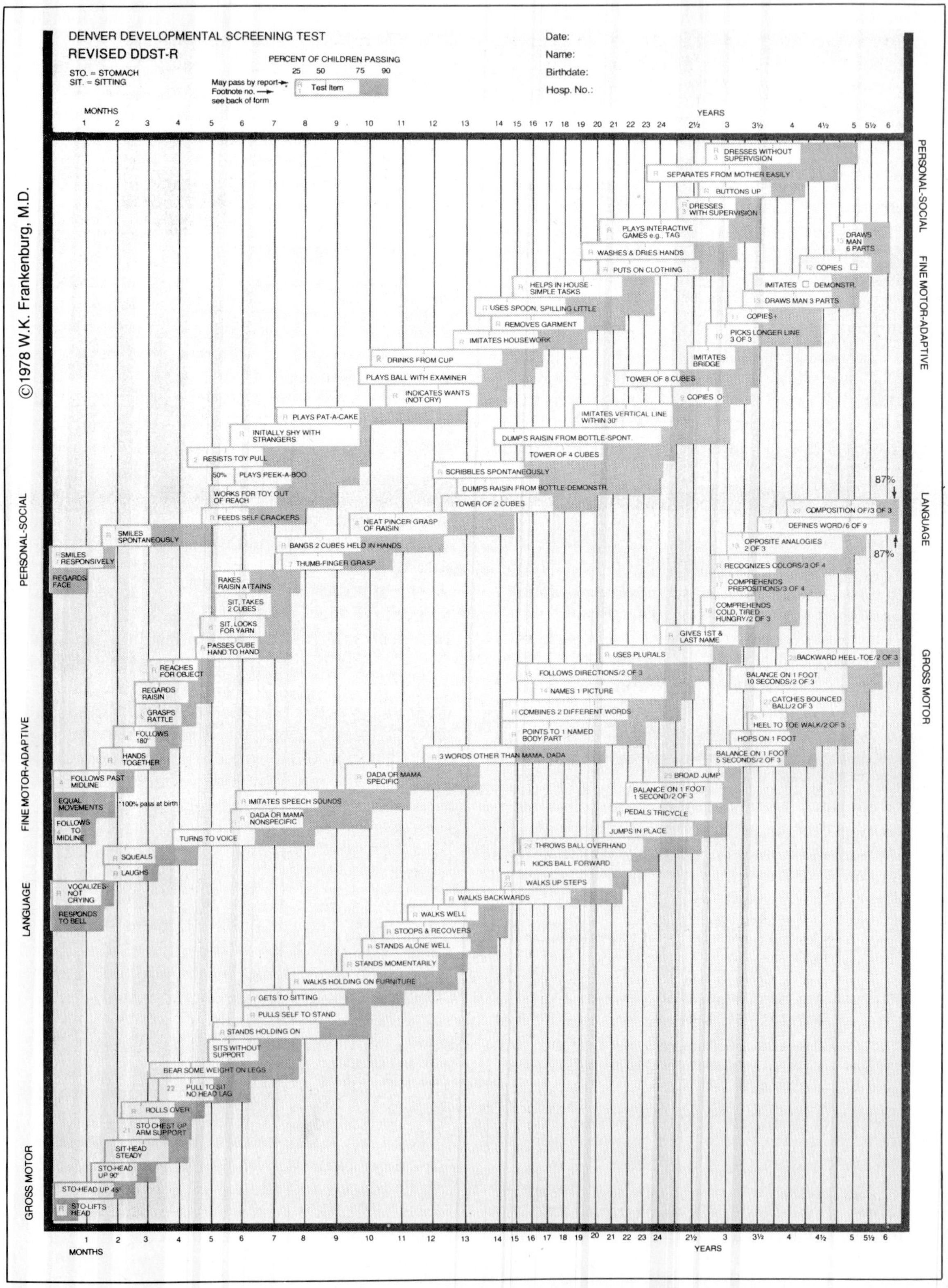

Fig. 3-2. A, DDST scoring sheet.

DATE

NAME

DIRECTIONS — BIRTHDATE

HOSP. NO.

1. Try to get child to smile by smiling, talking or waving to him. Do not touch him.
2. When child is playing with toy, pull it away from him. Pass if he resists.
3. Child does not have to be able to tie shoes or button in the back.
4. Move yarn slowly in an arc from one side to the other, about 6" above child's face. Pass if eyes follow 90° to midline. (Past midline; 180°)
5. Pass if child grasps rattle when it is touched to the backs or tips of fingers.
6. Pass if child continues to look where yarn disappeared or tries to see where it went. Yarn should be dropped quickly from sight from tester's hand without arm movement.
7. Pass if child picks up raisin with any part of thumb and a finger.
8. Pass if child picks up raisin with the ends of thumb and index finger using an over hand approach.

9. Pass any enclosed form. Fail continuous round motions.
10. Which line is longer? (Not bigger.) Turn paper upside down and repeat. (3/3 or 5/6)
11. Pass any crossing lines.
12. Have child copy first. If failed, demonstrate

When giving items 9, 11 and 12, do not name the forms. Do not demonstrate 9 and 11.

13. When scoring, each pair (2 arms, 2 legs, etc.) counts as one part.
14. Point to picture and have child name it. (No credit is given for sounds only.)

B

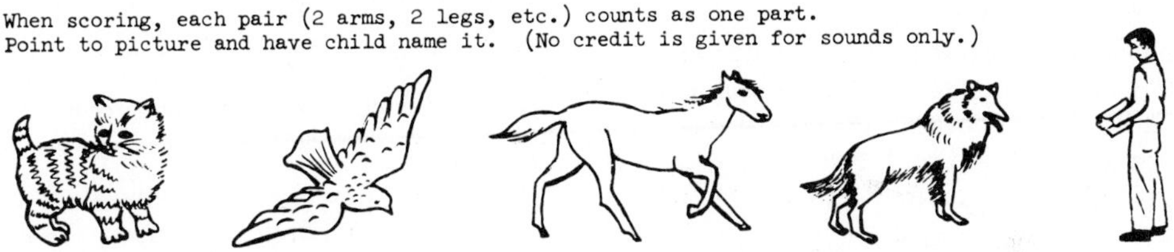

15. Tell child to: Give block to Mommie; put block on table; put block on floor. Pass 2 of 3. (Do not help child by pointing, moving head or eyes.)
16. Ask child: What do you do when you are cold? ..hungry? ..tired? Pass 2 of 3.
17. Tell child to: Put block <u>on</u> table; <u>under</u> table; <u>in front</u> of chair, <u>behind</u> chair. Pass 3 of 4. (Do not help child by pointing, moving head or eyes.)
18. Ask child: If fire is hot, ice is ?; Mother is a woman, Dad is a ?; a horse is big, a mouse is ?. Pass 2 of 3.
19. Ask child: What is a ball? ..lake? ..desk? ..house? ..banana? ..curtain? ..ceiling? ..hedge? ..pavement? Pass if defined in terms of use, shape, what it is made of or general category (such as banana is fruit, not just yellow). Pass 6 of 9.
20. Ask child: What is a spoon made of? ..a shoe made of? ..a door made of? (No other objects may be substituted.) Pass 3 of 3.
21. When placed on stomach, child lifts chest off table with support of forearms and/or hands.
22. When child is on back, grasp his hands and pull him to sitting. Pass if head does not hang back.
23. Child may use wall or rail only, not person. May not crawl.
24. Child must throw ball overhand 3 feet to within arm's reach of tester.
25. Child must perform standing broad jump over width of test sheet. (8-1/2 inches)
26. Tell child to walk forward, heel within 1 inch of toe. Tester may demonstrate. Child must walk 4 consecutive steps, 2 out of 3 trials.
27. Bounce ball to child who should stand 3 feet away from tester. Child must catch ball with hands, not arms, 2 out of 3 trials.
28. Tell child to walk backward, toe within 1 inch of heel. Tester may demonstrate. Child must walk 4 consecutive steps, 2 out of 3 trials.

<u>DATE AND BEHAVIORAL OBSERVATIONS</u> (how child feels at time of test, relation to tester, attention span, verbal behavior, self-confidence, etc,):

Fig. 3-2, cont'd. B, DDST direction sheet.

as the traditional plotting of the child's height and weight, when administered periodically as part of the pediatric examination (Fig. 3-2).

General abilities screening. Screening of educational readiness by physicians need not be limited to preschool children. Children of school age suspected of specific learning disabilities, as evidenced by poor academic performances and behavior disorders, are frequently referred initially to physicians for evaluation. In many instances diagnostic testing had been previously performed by a psychologist, educator, or other allied health professional. The medical and neurologic examination may reveal no major deficits, but this does not preclude further medical investigation. Physicians are urged to perform their own educational screening inventories—a triage that can consist of a collection of test items of the physician's design. If administered as part of an annual examination, these screening tests may direct attention to an impending educational problem. It must be emphasized that results of a screening examination are *not* to be interpreted as an estimation of intelligence or a formal evaluation of scholastic achievement. A standardized psychologic or educational test must be administered by a professional trained in administration, scoring, and interpretation.

A collection of evaluation items can be assembled to assess a wider range of learned skills such as reading, spelling, arithmetic, and writing, as well as visual and auditory processing skills. The objective of the examination is to demonstrate the presence and possible severity of a child's perceptual, educational, or behavioral disability. The screening is not intended to elicit a definitive diagnosis of a specific learning disability. Caution must be exercised in designing a screening test, avoiding duplication of test materials (which would invalidate standardized examinations). A screening examination has been employed at the University of Tennessee Center for the Health Sciences/Le Bonheur Children's Medical Center (Thompson and Gottlieb, 1973).

The means of assessing the child's academic and perceptual skills may be a potpourri of the physican's own design. The screening test for school age children used at the University of Tennessee Center for the Health Sciences, Clinic for Exceptional Children, utilizes both verbal and performance tests, freely adaptable to children of various ages and stages of development. The test contains oral questions concerning elementary factual information such as compositions of familiar objects, names of the days of the week, and identification of well known historical figures (e.g., Who discovered America?). Verbal questions formulated to test the child's judgment and reasoning abilities (What would you do if you cut your finger? What is the best thing that ever happened to you? If you had one wish, what would it be?) often give valuable insights concerning the child's power of abstraction. Responses to questioning of this nature give the examiner impressions of a child's level of social adaptation and occasionally provide clues to psychopathology.

Performance tasks may be designed that do not require the use of pencil and paper. For example, a child can be asked to select a specific item from an assortment of letters and numbers. Similarly, recognition of deleted letters from an incomplete alphabet sequence may be presented as a task that does not require graphic expression.

Perceptual and academic exercises requiring visual motor coordination and pencil skills can be utilized. The reproduction of geometrical designs, patterned after the Bender-Visual-Motor Gestalt Test, may reveal errors of angulation, rotation, perseveration, and loss of the gestalt, information which suggests weaknesses of visual perception and visual-motor coordination. Other tests of visual-motor integration include tracing the path of an imaginary automobile over a maze-like road or supplying missing parts for an incomplete human figure drawing.

The modality of auditory perception may be screened by determining the child's ability to: (1) follow multiple serial commands, (2) repeat sequences of letters, (3) demonstrate phonetic discrimination, and (4) perceive the content and format of directions and questions.

The physician may gain insights about a child's basic skills in reading, spelling, arithmetic, and perceptual development by offering age and grade level skill test items.

It is stressed once again that medical screening measures usually serve to indicate gross learning deficits and general areas of academic weakness. They are *not* intended to provide definitive diagnostic labels or prescriptive educational programs. Probably one of the most significant values of the screening inventory is to assist in a more efficient referral to various allied health professionals, for example, psychologist, speech pathologist, or special educator. The examination does not eliminate the need for interdisciplinary evaluation but makes referral selection more precise and meaningful.

Interdisciplinary interaction. The resolution of the differential diagnosis and the design of an effective therapeutic program for a child with a learning disorder depends on a meaningful multidisciplinary effort. Each member of the interdisciplinary team contributes his specialty-related expertise, to be incorporated into a cumulative profile of the child's strengths and weaknesses. Physicians are expected to contribute their particular expertise and are often solicited to serve as the team coordinator. The team coordinator synthesizes accrued data and amalgamates individual professional evaluations into a meaningful composite. Physicians assuming this role must have an appreciation of the standardized testing procedures and the implications of performance results. The parents, concerned professionals, and agencies are in turn familiarized with the diagnostic findings as collectively expressed by the interdisciplinary effort. Regardless of the physician's total involvement, he should be aware of the contributions afforded by other allied health professionals in the diagnostic procedure.

The clinical psychologist provides essential information relating to the child's level of intellectual function and potential, visual and auditory processing skills, academic achievement, and behavioral and emotional profiles (Table 3-4). The psychologist attempts to define discrepancies between intellectual function and academic achievement, searching for factors that have created this paradox. In addition, psychologic evaluation provides useful data for

Table 3-4. Examinations used in the differential diagnosis of learning disorders

Name	Test age range	General remarks
Intelligence and readiness tests		
Stanford-Binet Intelligence Scale	2 yr to adulthood	Test of general intellectual development that predominantly tests verbal intelligence Series of subtests grouped into age levels measuring comprehension, abstract reasoning, concept formation, and visual-perceptual skills
Wechsler Intelligence Scale for Children (WISC)	5 to 15 yr	Excellent test of general intellectual ability; may reflect some cultural bias Full-scale IQ reflects overall intellectual level Verbal IQ indicates intellectual ability related to verbal skills such as comprehension, abstract reasoning, vocabulary, memory, and arithmetic; subtests are sensitive to auditory perceptual and language deficits Performance IQ indicates intellectual ability related to nonverbal skills such as visual sequencing, visual-spatial relationships and visual-motor coordination; subtests are sensitive to deficits in visual-perceptual skills Difficulty with certain subtests may reflect presence of a learning disability
Wechsler Intelligence Scale for Children—Revised (WISC—R)	6 to 16 yr	1974 Revision of the WISC; reduces cultural bias of WISC
Peabody Picture Vocabulary Test (PPVT)	2 to 18 yr	Test that essentially measures receptive language and ability to recognize pictures; raw scores converted into mental ages and standard score IQ Test may reflect a cultural bias
Slosson Intelligence Test for Children and Adults (SIT)	2 yr to adulthood	Screening test based on Gesell Scales and Stanford-Binet scale that provides a verbally oriented evaluation
Vineland Social Maturity Scale	Infancy to 25 yr	Developmental schedule concerned with child's ability to look after his needs, function independently, and take responsibility; items grouped into age levels Social age (SA) and social quotient (SQ) can be completed from the scale
Columbia Mental Maturity Scale	3 to 12 yr	Nonverbal test that measures mental age and IQ Developed for use with cerebral-palsied children; child responds by pointing or nodding; test therefore has usefulness with handicapped persons
First Grade Screening Test	Late kindergarten or early first grade	Test that screens potential first grade student for readiness of first grade experience May identify child who will need special assistance
Raven's Colored Progressive Matrices	4½ to 11½ yr	Nonverbal test of general intelligence May provide information regarding perceptual accuracy, reasoning ability, and visual discrimination

In part modified from Warren, S.A.: Psychological evaluation for the mentally retarded, Pediatr. Clin. North Am. **15:**943, 1968; and The pediatrician and the child with mental retardation, Evanston, Ill., 1971, American Academy of Pediatrics.

Continued.

Table 3-4. Examinations used in the differential diagnosis of learning disorders—cont'd

Name	Test age range	General remarks
Perceptual development		
Wechsler Intelligence Scale for Children—Revised	6 to 16 yr	Subtests can be used to measure the full range of auditory and visual perceptual skills as well as to provide intelligence levels
Slosson Drawing Coordination Test	1 through 12 yr	Test of visual-motor coordination and spatial perception
Bender-Visual-Motor Gestalt Test	5 yr to adulthood	Test of visual-motor coordination and spatial orientation Sensitive to perceptual disorganization resulting from brain damage and emotional disturbances Patterns copied are checked for angulations, distortions, rotations, perseveration, fragmentation, organization
Illinois Test of Psycholinguistic Abilities (ITPA)	2½ to 9½ yr	Test evaluates auditory and visual perceptual skills levels expressed in age; assesses 9 psycholinguistic abilities reported as a language age
Visual Retention Test (Benton)	8 yr to adulthood	Tests visual motor skills, spatial perception, and visual memory Emotional disturbance may impair performance
Frostig Developmental Test of Visual Perception	Preschool ages	Screening examination for visual perceptual skills
Speech and language development		
McDonald Deep Screening Articulation Test	3 yr to adulthood	Rapid method of evaluating a child's articulation of several commonly misarticulated consonants
Triota Screening Test	2 yr to adulthood	Computerized test that screens for articulation, language, and listening skills Normalizes data
Wepman Auditory Discrimination Test	3½ yr to adulthood	Screening examination for ability to discriminate minimal acoustic differences
Achievement and reading tests		
Wide Range Achievement Test Metropolitan Achievement Test Stanford Achievement Test Gray Oral Reading Test	School-age children	Widely used test in school systems that compares child's academic achievement with that of other children of same age and grade level Significant discrepancies may indicate learning disability
Emotional development		
Thematic-Apperception-Test (T-A-T)	Adolescents and adults	Person interprets individual and social situations pictured on cards and projects self into scenes he interprets, revealing possible emotional conflicts
Children's-Apperception-Test (C-A-T)	3 to 10 yr	Adaptation of T-A-T for younger children that comprises series of animal picture cards aimed at problems of early childhood; child projects experiences and problems into card interpretations
Rorschach Ink Blot Test	Adolescents and adults	Individual reports what he sees in the various ink blots and projects needs, anxieties, and conflicts
Draw-A-Person Test (DAP)	3 to 13 yr	Test measures IQ on ability to draw person with details; provides insights as to self-concept and is information-gathering device for insights into a child's feelings
Sentence Completion Test	School-age children	Disorganization may reflect perceptual problems

the educator designing a remedial program. Monitoring a child's progress may be a mutual undertaking of psychologist and teacher. Professionals trained in the area of communicative disorders—speech pathologists and audiologists—are often required to lend their professional skills in the diagnostic and therapeutic process. It is frequently necessary to employ sophisticated techniques for assessing auditory acuity (free field audiometry or electroacoustic impedance audiometry), language development, and auditory processing abilities. Special and general educators monitor the child's educational progress, processing skills, and behavioral reactions. A battery of educational, perceptual, and behavioral inventories can be administered individually or in group settings. Social workers and pediatric nurse practitioners are involved in the diagnostic procedure, using home and school visits, parent and teacher interviews, and developmental and behavioral screenings. The composition of the diagnostic team is usually determined by the nature and severity of the child's problem and the individual needs of the child and family. No single routine pattern of professional intervention is recommended.

THERAPY: THE PHYSICIAN'S ROLE

It has been emphasized that learning disorders are complex problems that often contain elements of emotional, behavioral, social, perceptual, and academic disturbances. Regardless of the professional contributing to the diagnosis, it is ultimately the teacher who is called on to instruct the child. The teacher, either a general or a special educator, assumes the responsibility of getting the educational job done. The interdisciplinary effort is of great value in defining the child's relative strengths and assists the teacher in designing the remedial program.

There are four basic approaches (Hewett, 1973) that are used to assist the child with special education needs: (1) the *psychotherapeutic approach,* which is basically concerned with the child's motivations, attitudes, family relationships, and psychologic difficulties; (2) the *neurologic approach,* which defines the child's educational lags in terms of dysfunctions of the nervous system (visual and auditory perceptual deficits, eye-hand incoordination, and other manifestations of impaired neurologic circuitry); (3) the *academic approach,* which relates to the child's academic achievement in mastering educational challenges (reading, writing, and arithmetic); and (4) the *behavioral approach,* from which the teacher attempts to define the child's functional ability in school, (i.e., what behaviors may be interfering with efficient functioning). It is obvious that no single approach is meaningful in isolation and that all four are intimately associated and enjoy a symbiotic relationship.

Although rehabilitation is primarily an educational process, the physician has a vital function in providing several inputs into the total therapeutic program. Frequently the pediatrician or family physician is responsible for (1) counseling, (2) monitoring continued health care, and (3) if necessary, directing a medication program.

Counseling. The physician is often responsible for counseling with teachers, sharing the findings of the interdisciplinary team, but he does not dictate the educational approach. Periodic communication with teachers is encouraged, including a review of the child's educational progress and effects of behavioral modifications.

A professional relationship should be maintained with the parents. As a rule, children with disorders of learning have parents who are in need of some type of counseling and support. Parents are vulnerable because they want to "make it better for our kids than we had it"—a philosophy deeply rooted in the desire that their children achieve higher levels of education than they were able to attain. A threat to this dictum creates parental anxieties, feelings of guilt, and an atmosphere of confusion. The physician is often the most instrumental professional in providing counseling to help parents adjust to the problems of a learning-disabled child (Todd and Gottlieb, 1976).

Counseling, or in-depth explanations, are usually provided only for the parents of a learning-disabled child. However, it is frequently the child who would benefit most from some form of professional communication. The contact can be made directly by a physician, teacher, or psychologist or indirectly through the parents. Regardless of the method of communication, the child may be provided some insights into the nature of his difficulties. It is not unusual for learning-disabled children to harbor a host of anxieties, feelings of insecurity and rejection, fears of being retarded, and a variety of misconceptions about their lack of ability. Lack of success experiences, unrealistic teacher and parent pressures, inability to express anger and frustrations, and disrupted sibling and peer relationships all contribute to the child's poor motivation and decreasing confidence. Frequently, children with disorders of learning exhibit evidences of poor self-concept and refer to themselves as "dumb and stupid." Siblings and peers may taunt the child, characterizing him as "queer," "retarded," "lame," or "weird." Unfortunately, uninformed and insensitive adults may hide similar feelings. It may be necessary for the physician to intervene, serving as the child's advocate, to provide counseling for parents, teachers, and child. The child's educational career, personality, and social adjustments are at risk. Effective counseling may require multiple family contacts and, at times, group meetings. Needless to say, in a busy medical practice adequate time may not be available for this type of intervention. It is important, however, that the physician make provisions with other professionals for counseling services as they are needed. Regardless of the source of paramedical assistance offered, the parents anticipate continued physician interest and direction. In contrast to school personnel, whose relationship usually changes on a yearly basis, the physician is expected to provide a constant and stable role on the interdisciplinary team over an extended period of time.

One aspect of parental counseling deserves special mention. Frequently, parents contact their physician to seek advice about new and often untried tutorial programs, teaching aids, medications, and special classes or schools claiming to offer new hopes for the learning-disabled child. The physician may be required to differentiate between quality and quackery. If unfamiliar with these programs, the physician should seek professional consultation for his own clarification. Parents often feel frustrated and guilt ridden, falling prey to gimmicks and unprofessional shortcuts to resolve their child's educational difficulties. The physician may be the stabilizing factor, preventing parents from acting impulsively in selecting methods for helping their child.

Effective counseling requires an appreciation of the controversial intervention strategies that have been recommended for the learning-disabled child (Silver, 1975). Physicians have a particular obligation to become knowledgeable about the variety of controversial approaches to managing the child with learning disabilities. The psychosocial and financial traumas experienced by affected families render them vulnerable to the "quick cure" advocates. The primary care physician is mandated the responsibility of becoming familiar with "old approaches" and recent advances, learning to recognize when science is weak in supporting a recommended management approach (Gottlieb, 1979; Brown, 1982). Controversy should not necessarily imply "wrong," "harmful," "worthless," "chicanery," or any other totally negative connotation. In most instances *controversial* suggests "poorly documented," "uncontrolled experiment," and "hypothesis based solely on several case history reports." The validity of a controversial claim can only be resolved in the crucible of sophisticated research that adheres to the principles of the scientific method. The effective counselor cannot give carte blanche approval or completely dismiss the queries of anxious and vulnerable parents of learning-disabled children.

A variety of discordant issues that deserve brief mention have erupted regarding diagnostic and therapeutic approaches to children with impaired learning. The issue of the *self-contained classroom versus mainstreaming special education programs* has generated concern because of the stigmatizing effect of educational isolation. However, the feasibility of instructing children with special needs in a regular classroom setting has provoked debate. The controversy is exaggerated by a myriad of social, legal, moral, and financial implications as well as the basic dilemma in the desired method of achieving educational goals. The *academic versus perceptual training* paradox is similarly unresolved. The argument centers on the issue of whether the time spent on a one-to-one basis with a learning-disabled child is more efficiently used by teaching academics or by attempting to improve perceptual skills. Advocates of each program present evidence to support their claims. The issue of *psychostimulant drugs versus behavior modification programs* for hyperactive children has also been a topic of medical debate. Drugs may not get at the basic pathology involved but are in some instances an effective adjunct in a program for the hyperactive learning-disabled child. The abuse of drug therapy has caused strong opposition to drug use in general. It has been argued that psychologic behavior modification is the best approach to the child with hyperkinesis. The problem is not an all-or-none issue, and valid indications exist for both (or combined) forms of therapy. The concepts of *neurologic retraining, optometric exercises,* and *orthomolecular medicine* have likewise provoked professional concern. Incompletely documented experiments have resulted in strong statements of caution by various professional associations. The value of patterning exercises has been criticized because of the lack of supporting evidence and inherent strains placed on the family constellation. The association between certain ocular deficits as a cause of academic deficiency has been similarly challenged. The use of megavitamins as a nutritional approach to learning disorders has likewise been debated. The claim that synthetic flavors and colors (food additives) are factors in hyperkinesis and learning disabilities is currently an issue of research investigation. The American Academy of Pediatrics has recommended nonparticipation in these programs or reservation of approval until further documentation is obtained.

Controversy in diagnostic and therapeutic management of learning disabilities suggests the following: (1) parents of learning-disabled children are extremely anxious and vulnerable, (2) parents desire rapid cures for the child's problem, (3) established programs are not always successful, (4) parents may not receive proper counseling regarding their child's problem or acceptable therapeutic interventions, and (5) in the interest of patient and public protection, physicians must be knowledgeable concerning community resources and controversial interventions.

Chemotherapy. Therapists assisting learning-disabled children frequently recognize that several problems must be resolved simultaneously: academic deficiencies and behavioral disturbances, including hyperactivity, short attention span, distractibility, impulsivity, and disturbed peer relationships. A common solicitation of the physician working with educationally handicapped children is a request for medications for the hyperactive child. Methylphenidate and possibly the other psychostimulant medications may affect attention processes in hyperactive children. However, they may not affect the higher cortical processes required to ensure long-term academic gains (Adams, 1982).

The term *hyperactive* has occasionally been used interchangeably with *learning disabled*. However, physicians should recognize that hyperkinesis has no single cause. Hyperactivity has been associated with a variety of origins: (1) genetic or familial causes; (2) certain drugs; (3) medical disorders such as hyperthyroidism; (4) neurologic problems, for example, cerebral palsy or lead intoxication; (5) environmental conditions in which controls are lacking; (6) emotional disturbances; (7) developmental delays; and (8) situational disorders such as a pressured educational setting. No one medication is expected to resolve *all* these difficulties. The judicious use of drugs in assisting the learning-disabled child is a medical challenge (Gottlieb, 1975). Dextroamphetamine and methylphenidate are popular adjuncts to assisting the learning-disabled child. A variety of other drugs have been tried but appear to be less effective, including phenytoin (Diphenylhydantoin), imipramine, diphenhydramine, chlorpromazine, thioridazine, and primidone. Paradoxically, it has been observed that the barbiturates may exaggerate symptoms of hyperactivity.

The majority of children referred to as hyperactive are probably not organically "driven." Many exhibit behavioral difficulties that are precipitated by uncomfortable learning situations such as pressured school and home environments. Amid the confusion of what constitutes hyperactivity and the besieging requests from parents and teachers, a variety of medications have been instituted empirically, often with little or no beneficial effect. After thorough diagnostic evaluation, the physician should carefully select and monitor the psychopharmacologic agent selected for use.

Careful monitoring is necessary to establish the adequate dosage of the psychotropic drugs; their use requires careful medical supervision (Schain, 1972). *Methylphenidate hydrochloride (Ritalin)* is not recommended for children under 6 years of age. The drug is usually started with an initial dose of 5 mg/24 hr orally (before breakfast and lunch). Gradual increments of 5 to 10 mg weekly are titered; the average dose is 15 mg/24 hr, and daily dosage above 60 mg is not recommended. *Dextroamphetamine sulfate (Dexedrine)* is not recommended for children under 3 years of age. Children 3 to 5 years old are usually started with 2.5 mg/24 hr orally, with increments titered at 2.5 mg at weekly intervals. For children 6 years of age and older, therapy can be initiated with 5 mg/24 hr, and gradual increments of 5 mg at weekly intervals are titered. The drug can be divided into morning and noon doses. The average daily dose is 10 mg/24 hr, and the maximal dose is 30 mg/24 hr. *Pemoline (Cylert)* is a central nervous system stimulant but is structurally dissimilar to methylphenidate and the amphetamines. It is administered as a single oral dose each morning; the recommended starting dose is 37.5 mg/24 hr. The dosage can be titered by increments of 18.75 mg at weekly intervals; the effective daily dose ranges from 56.25 to 75 mg, and the maximum recommended dose is 112.5 mg/24 hr. Pemoline is not recommended for children under 6 years of age.

Once a drug program has been established, it is usually maintained during the school year. Medications may be discontinued during the intervals when the child is not attending school. The need for continued medication may be observed during these "rest periods." Undesirable side effects, including insomnia, anorexia, weight loss, gastrointestinal disturbances, growth suppression, and personality changes may require reduction of dosage or discontinuation of the drug. It has been debated that the prolonged administration of these drugs may be related to a general suppression of growth in height and weight.

Drug selection and administration may be more efficiently regulated with the use of rating scales. Medications should be discontinued, after appropriate dosage adjustments, if they fail to achieve the desired goals of behavior modification at home and at school as well as improved academic attention. However, it must be stressed that psychotropic drugs do not make children learn. Drugs should be regarded as a useful adjunct for educational rehabilitation and behavioral modification. Medications are *not* a substitute for specific rehabilitative programs.

SUMMARY

The physician has a unique and vital role in the care of learning-disabled children. Medical intervention and expertise is essential in the diagnostic and therapeutic management of these problems. Accumulated knowledge of high-risk factors during pregnancy, infancy, and early childhood suggests an additional role for pediatricians in research directed toward prevention of learning disorders.

Pediatricians have an opportunity to serve children almost from birth, defining a responsibility for early identification of developmental weaknesses in preschool children. Federal legislation mandating free public education for *all* handicapped children adds further to the obligations of physicians to become actively involved with the learning-disabled child. Changing social attitudes and values have been an additional stimulus for medical involvement.

The physician's commitment to a child's *educational health and development* is multifaceted, including (1) early screening and identification of developmental disabilities in preschool children; (2) medical management of organic disorders interfering with educational progress; (3) prescribing and monitoring psychopharmacologic agents used as an adjunct in therapy; (4) coordination of efforts of an interdisciplinary team; (5) counseling of parents, professionals, and child; (6) knowledge of community resources, enabling meaningful referral for diagnostic and therapeutic services; (7) coordination of follow-up services; (8) recognition of controversial issues for meaningful service to child and family; (9) initiation of research in prevention, diagnosis, and management; and (10) serving as an advocate for the child.

A child's educational health and development is a major factor influencing psychosocial development. Aberrant adolescent behaviors and loss of adult productivity may relate directly to adverse learning environments. The physician must assume the responsibility for enhancing educational development and thereby affording each child a better opportunity for a quality-oriented life.

Marvin I. Gottlieb
Peter W. Zinkus

REFERENCES

Adams, W.: Effect of methylphenidate on thought processing time in children, J. Dev. Behav. Pediatr. **3:**133, 1982.

Adamson, W.C.: The gifted child: a psychodynamic profile, J. Dev. Behav. Pediatr. **3:**170, 1982.

American Academy of Pediatrics: School health: a guide for physicians, Evanston, Ill., 1972, The Academy.

American Academy of Pediatrics Council on Child Health: Statement: children with learning disabilities, Evanston, Ill., 1973a, The Academy.

American Academy of Pediatrics Council on Child Health: Statement: early identification of children with learning disabilities—the preschool child, Evanston, Ill., 1973b, The Academy.

American Academy of Pediatrics: Recertification: a plan for practicing physicians, News and Comments **28:**1, 1977.

American Academy of Pediatrics: PL 94-142: appropriate education for each handicapped child, News and Comments **29:**1, 1978.

American Academy of Pediatrics: New directions in care for the handicapped child (An AAP–sponsored in-service training course for primary care physicians), Evanston, Ill., 1980, The Academy.

Bateman, B.L., and Schiefelbusch, R.L.: Minimal brain dysfunction. Public Health Pub. No. 2015, sect. II, p. 7, Washington, D.C., 1969, National Project on Learning Disabilities in Children, Phase two.

Brown, G.W.: A loss of nerve, J. Dev. Behav. Pediatr. **3:**88, 1982.

Chalfant, J.C., and Scheffelin, M.A.: Central processing dysfunctions in children: a review of research, National Institute of Neurological Diseases and Blindness Monograph No. 9, Washington, D.C, 1969, U.S. Department of Health, Education, and Welfare.

Clements, S.D.: Minimal brain dysfunction in children, National Institute of Neurological Diseases and Blindness Monograph No. 3, Public Health Services Pub. No. 1415, Washington, D.C., 1966, U.S. Department of Health, Education, and Welfare.

Daniel, W.A., Jr.: Adolescence, adolescents, and learning disorders, J. Dev. Behav. Pediatr. **2:**105, 1981.

de Hirsch, K.: Learning disabilities: an overview, Bull. N.Y. Acad. Med. **50:**459, 1974.

Diagnostic and Statistical Manual of Mental Disorders, ed. 3, Washington, D.C., 1980, The American Psychiatric Association.

Freeman, J.: Gifted children, Baltimore, 1979, University Park Press.

Gallagher, J.J.: Children with developmental imbalances: a psychoeducational definition. In Cruickshank, W.M., editor: The teacher of brain injured children, Syracuse, N.Y., 1966, Syracuse University Press.

Geschwind, N.: Disconnexion syndromes in animals and man, Brain **88:**585, 1965.

Goldberg, H.K., and Schiffman, G.B.: Dyslexia: problems of reading disabilities, New York, 1972, Grune & Stratton, Inc.

Golden, G.S.: Evaluation of the child with school failure: determining learning disabilities. In Frankenburg, W.K.: Children are different, behavioral development, Monograph No. 3, 1982, Ross Laboratories Publications.

Gottlieb, M.I.: Pills: pros and cons of medications for school problems, Acta Symbolica **6:**35, 1975.

Gottlieb, M.I.: The learning-disabled child: controversial issues revisited. In Gottlieb, M.I., Zinkus, P.W. and Bradford, L.J., editors: Current issues in developmental pediatrics: the learning-disabled child, New York, 1979, Grune & Stratton, Inc.

Gottlieb, M.I., and Williams, J.E.: Self-concept. In Plaisted, M., editor: Feelings and their medical significance, Ross Laboratories **24:**23, 1982.

Gottlieb, M.I., and Zinkus, P.W.: A medical student curriculum on the needs of exceptional children. In Guralnick, M.J., and Richardson, H.B., Jr., editors: Pediatric education and the needs of exceptional children, Baltimore, 1980, University Park Press.

Gottlieb, M.I., and Zinkus, P.W.: Reflections: the learning-disabled youthful offender, J. Dev. Behav. Pediatr. **2:**1, 1981.

Gottlieb, M.I., et al.: Chronic middle ear disease and auditory perceptual deficits, Clin. Pediatr. **18:**725, 1979.

Grossman, H.J.: Neurologic assessment and management of learning disorders, Pediatr. Ann. **7:**63, 1978.

Haller, J.S.: Minimal brain dysfunction syndrome, Am. J. Dis. Child. **129:**1319, 1975.

Hass, G., and Scovell, M.: A guide to administration, diagnosis, and treatment for the early and periodic screening, diagnosis, and treatment program (EPSDT) under Medicaid, Washington, D.C., 1977, U.S. Department of Health, Education, and Welfare and American Academy of Pediatrics, p. 54.

Hewett, F.M.: Strategies of special education, Pediatr. Clin. North Am. **20:**695, 1973.

Kinsbourne, M., and Caplan, P.J.: Children's learning and attention problems, Boston, 1979, Little, Brown & Co.

Kinsbourne, M., and Swanson, J.W.: Anticipatory guidance for classroom conduct and learning problems, J. Dev. Behav. Pediatr. **3:**112, 1980.

Levine, M.D., et al.: A pediatric approach to learning disorders, New York, 1980a, John Wiley & Sons, Inc.

Levine, M.D., et al.: The pediatric examination of educational readiness: validation of an extended observation procedure, Pediatrics **66:**341, 1980b.

Levine, M.D., et al.: Developmental output failure: a study of low productivity in school-aged children, Pediatrics **67:**18, 1981.

Long, R.L., and Murray, M.E.: Neurophysiologic aspects of developmental dyslexia (review), J. Dev. Behav. Pediatr. **3:**2, 1982.

Maier, H.W.: Three theories of child development: the contributions of Erik H. Erikson, Jean Piaget, and Robert R. Sears, and their applications, New York, 1969, Harper & Row, Publishers, Inc.

Menkes, J.H.: A new role for the school physician, Pediatrics **49:**803, 1972.

Morgan, S.B.: The unreachable child: an introduction to early childhood autism, Memphis, 1981, Memphis State University Press.

Page, E., and Grossman, H.J.: Neurological appraisal in learning disorders, Pediatr. Clin. North Am. **20:**599, 1973.

Rabinovitch, R.D.: Reading problems in children: definitions and classifications. In Keeney, A.H., and Keeney, V.T., editors: Dyslexia: diagnosis and treatment of reading disorders, St. Louis, 1968, The C.V. Mosby Co.

Rampp, D.L.: The behavioral characteristics of children exhibiting auditory processing disturbances, Proceedings of First Memphis State University Symposium on Auditory Processing and Learning Disabilities, Memphis, 1972, Memphis State University Press.

Sak, R.J., and Ruben, R.J.: Effects of recurrent middle ear effusion in preschool years on language and learning, J. Dev. Behav. Pediatr. **3:**7, 1982.

Schain, R.J.: Neurology of childhood learning disorders, ed. 2, Baltimore, 1972, The Williams & Wilkins Co.

Schain, R.J.: Learning disabilities: a medical responsibility? In Gottlieb, M.I., and Bradford, L.J., editors: Learning disabilities: an audio journal for continuing education, New York, 1977, Grune & Stratton, Inc.

Schmitt, B.D.: The minimal brain dysfunction myth, Am. J. Dis. Child. **129:**1313, 1975.

Shaw, L., et al.: Developmental double jeopardy: a study of clumsiness and self-esteem in children with learning problems, J. Dev. Behav. Pediatr. **3:**191, 1982.

Shaywitz, S.E., et al.: The biochemical basis of minimal brain dysfunction, J. Pediatr. **92:**179, 1978.

Silver, L.D.: Acceptable and controversial approaches to treating the child with learning disabilities, Pediatrics **55:**406, 1975.

Strauss, A., and Lehtinen, L.: Psychopathology and education of the brain injured child, New York, 1947, Grune & Stratton, Inc.

Thompson, H.C.: Contributions of medicine to the quality of life for children. In Brown, L.E., editor: Quality of life, Acton, Mass., 1974, Publishing Sciences Group, Inc.

Thompson, L.J.: Reading disability: developmental dyslexia, Springfield, Ill., 1966, Charles C Thomas, Publisher.

Thompson, R.C., and Gottlieb, M.I.: Educational jeopardy, an interdisciplinary problem: the physician's contribution, Acta Symbolica **4:**46, 1973.

Thorpe, H.S., and Werner, E.M.: Developmental screening of preschool children: a critical review of inventories used in health and educational programs, Pediatrics **53:**362, 1974.

Todd, M., and Gottlieb, M.I.: Interdisciplinary counselling in a medical setting. In Webster, E.J., editor: Professional approaches with parents of handicapped children, Springfield, Ill., 1976, Charles C Thomas, Publisher.

Walzer, S., and Richmond, J.B.: The epidemiology of learning disorders, Pediatr. Clin. North Am. **20:**549, 1973.

Warren, S.A.: Problems encountered with learning difficulties, Pediatr. Ann. **7:**12, 1978.

White, C.S., et al.: Dyslexia: is the term of value? Acta Symbolica **4:**6, 1973.

Wolraich, M.: A one-month rotation in developmental disabilities. In Guralnick, M.J., and Richardson, H.B., Jr., editors: Pediatric education and the needs of exceptional children, Baltimore, 1980, University Park Press.

Zinkus, P.W., and Gottlieb, M.I.: Disorders of learning and delinquent youth: an overview. In Gottlieb, M.I., and Bradford, L.J., editors: Learning disabilities an audio journal for continuing education, vol. II, New York, 1978a, Grune & Stratton, Inc.

Zinkus, P.W., and Gottlieb, M.I.: Learning disabilities and juvenile delinquency, Clin. Pediatr. **17:**775, 1978b.

Zinkus, P.W., et al.: Developmental and psychoeducational sequelae of chronic otitis media, Am. J. Dis. Child. **132:**1100, 1978.

4 Child Psychology and Psychiatry

Viewpoint of a general pediatrician

The fundamental objective of pediatrics is to guide children safely and happily through childhood so that they will become healthy, well-adjusted, normal young adults. Thus the pediatrician is concerned with keeping the well child well and with comprehensive consideration of the child as a whole so that physical, mental, and emotional growth and development will achieve their maximal potential. Much of pediatric practice is concerned with such supervision of the relatively normal child. The remainder is devoted largely to the diagnosis and treatment of a wide variety of illnesses, most of which are of a temporary nature.

Unfortunately, there is often undue preoccupation with organic illness, and insufficient attention is paid to the prevention, diagnosis, and treatment of disorders of emotional origin that arise in pediatric practice. Indeed, many physicians manifest little or no interest in such matters.

Fortunately, this situation is changing. The incidence of organic illnesses has decreased through improvements in nutrition, housing, sanitation, immunization, health education, and serial health supervision of the growing child. Furthermore, better control of many of these diseases has been achieved by chemotherapeutic agents and antibiotics, improved supportive measures such as fluid and electrolyte therapy, and wider dispersion of diagnostic and treatment facilities that bring modern medicine to more of the people. The organic illnesses will, of course, be with us always, and they will forever constitute an important part of pediatric practice, although they now occur less frequently and are easier to manage. Meanwhile, chronically handicapping conditions, including emotional disorders of childhood, loom larger in importance than they did in times past.

Actually, there is no such thing as a purely organic illness or a purely emotional disorder. One does not become sick in the flesh or in the spirit alone. Every organic illness is invariably associated with some degree of psychic disturbance, not only of the child himself but also of his parents and others to whom he is dear. Similarly, every emotional disorder is to some degree accompanied by a disturbance in body function, ranging from the trivial and inconsequential to psychosomatic manifestations of such intensity as to mock organic entities.

One may visualize illness, then, as a spectrum in which the almost purely organic conditions are at one end and the almost purely psychic conditions are at the other, with all possible combinations and variations between. One of these factors ordinarily predominates, but there is always a combination. It often takes a perceptive physician to determine the extent to which each participates.

Unless the physician dealing with children bears these concepts constantly in mind, he will not be able to provide truly comprehensive care to his pediatric patients. Furthermore, unless he realizes the frequency of so-called psychosomatic complaints in children and how closely they mock organic disease, he may become lost in a diagnostic maze when confronted with the nervous child who has functional headache, inexplicable abdominal pain, recurrent vomiting, obsessive obesity, or a wide variety of other overt manifestations of psychic tensions.

A physician for children needs to know how the personality of the child develops normally, factors that influence that development, how deviations from normal can be prevented through anticipatory counseling, the role that psychic factors play in organic illness, and how to diagnose and treat at least the more common emotional problems of children. Knowledge of personality development and factors that influence it is essential to understand the child and to interpret the child to the parents in response to their many questions about his behavior. Anticipatory counseling in preventive mental hygiene is necessary to avoid circumstances and attitudes that foster childhood behavior problems; it should be part and parcel of the pediatric supervision of every child. Reasons have already been expressed regarding the need to evaluate the psychic veneer that overlays all organic illness.

The physician need not be expected to manage successfully all established behavior problems he encounters in practice, but at least he should be interested in them and should be able to treat the simpler ones. He may rightfully wish to send patients having behavior problems of mild degree, and certainly those of severe degree, to a psychiatrist, preferably a pediatric psychiatrist if one is available. However, he cannot send all patients having behavior problems to psychiatrists because there are not enough psychiatrists to see more than a small fraction of all the children who have such problems. Unless he manages the simpler cases, the children will receive no attention whatsoever and their psychic disturbances may become ingrained, chronic, more complex, and decidedly more difficult to eradicate.

The physician who is actively interested in childhood behavior problems will find many rewards, including the knowledge that the quality of his supervision may mean the difference between a happily adjusted child who grows up to be a normal adolescent and adult and one who becomes increasingly maladjusted. Furthermore, he will gain many interesting and fascinating insights into the lives of people. And surely people are at least as interesting as the diseases they bear.

EMOTIONAL DEVELOPMENT (see also Chapter 2)

The personality of the child depends to a great extent on genetic endowment, but it is molded primarily by environmental circumstances. In the latter category are included the multiplicity of factors that impinge on the personality of the child as he passes through the various developmental stages of infancy and childhood.

Physical, mental, and emotional growth and development proceed simultaneously and are intimately related. As the child grows in size, his mental capacity also increases, and his emotional processes become increasingly complex. Thus the newborn infant is not only physically and mentally immature but also his emotional reactions are at an instinctive level. His world is a narrow one, encompassed perhaps by the confines of a single room and the presence of a limited number of people. With few exceptions he is oblivious to environment, although he cries from hunger and discomfort and is obviously in need of affection. As physical development and increasing mental capacity permit him to enlarge his sphere of interest, more and more psychic influences subtly mold him, and one sees the growth of habits and the formation of attitudes toward persons and things.

Although personality and basic attitudes are well established at an early age, they are continually subject to modifications and refinements governed by subsequent experience. Thus like Tennyson's Ulysses we are indeed a part of all that we have met.

Just as Shakespeare described the seven ages of man, psychiatrists and psychologists have divided personality development into sequential stages, beginning in earliest infancy and extending through childhood and adolescence. However, it must be remembered that there are no precise demarcations and that one stage blends almost imperceptibly into the next. This gradually unfolding personality development parallels, and indeed depends on and is intimately related to, physical and mental growth.

Schopenhauer is said to have defined the initial cry of the newborn baby as an expression of rage at entering a hostile world. Although such pessimism may be unwarranted, the halcyon days of intrauterine life are indeed a far cry from the tumult of the outer world. At any rate, the newborn infant does express discomfort in no uncertain terms by much crying from hunger, wet diapers, and handling by attendants and parents.

During the newborn period and for the first few months the infant is thought to be functioning at an instinctive level, his guiding objectives being to satisfy raw, basic drives for animal comfort. During this period he is growing rapidly, physically and mentally, and is gaining an increasing degree of neuromotor control. He is beginning to take more notice of his surroundings and is becoming more capable of exploring his limited environment. He learns to follow objects briefly with his eyes and to hold an object placed in his hand. He may smile if stimulated to do so.

Through the countless repetitions of feeding, bathing, changing diapers and clothing, and so on, the young infant comes to know his mother or the mother substitute at about 3 months of age. He may stop crying at her approach, thus indicating he realizes that his need of the moment is about to be satisfied by her. This is construed to be the earliest evidence that he is now aware of himself and that he is different from others and the world around him. The infant now becomes increasingly aware of and attached to his mother, who is the central person in his life (alas, only later, as a rule, does the child become attached to his father). She represents to him security, gratification of needs, and relief from discomfort. The degree to which the mother is oriented toward the infant affects greatly the quality of this relationship. If her feelings and attitudes are those of acceptance and affection, the child will blossom in the warmth of her love. If she is fearful of her ability to manage the infant, does not accept him fully, or even rejects him psychologically, her uncertainty will be transmitted to him and will be reflected in the way he reacts.

Thus the basic foundations of psychologic security are being laid down in these first 12 to 18 months. The attitudes the infant will exhibit later on in his relationships to others are now crystallizing. Although subject to subsequent modification, it is thought that patterns for interpersonal relationships established at this early age carry into later childhood and even adulthood.

The infant who is so unfortunate as to lack the warm affection of his mother or one who is for a prolonged period in a hospital or institution where not enough mothering of infants exists may suffer the emotional deprivation of regimentation. He may become apathetic, listless, and anorexic, may sleep poorly, and may even fail to develop at a normal rate (pseudoretardation). It is believed that sometimes lasting emotional scarring ensues, possibly revealing itself years later as inability to establish warm relationships with others or even as lack of interest in others.

Throughout the period of infancy the child's rapidly developing physical and mental powers drive him to explore his environment to an increasing and almost ceaseless degree, thus widening his horizons. Details of these developmental achievements are discussed on pp. 25 to 28. Of high importance for personality development are his contacts with those about him, leading him into more and more complex interpersonal relationships.

By the end of infancy and the beginning of early childhood he is walking well, his language is improving rapidly, and his self-concept is sharpening. By now he clearly feels he is a distinct person and is beginning to socialize to a much greater degree.

Throughout these early years the child is developing a mind of his own. He learns to say "yes" and "no" but at first sometimes confuses their meaning. He is becoming much more independent and even rebellious at the many necessary restrictions placed on his raw drives. His curiosity is boundless as he views, approaches, touches, grasps, handles, and explores whatever he finds of interest, frequently putting objects into his mouth to discover what they are like. This is the period when household accidents and poisonings are more likely to occur. The pediatrician should emphasize this particular point to the parents of the young child so that they may take necessary preventive measures to avoid these catastrophes.

By age 18 to 24 months children have established the concept of whether they are boys or girls. Experience indicates that when there has been confusion regarding true sex and the child is "assigned" to the wrong sex, the child assumes the psychologic orientation of the assigned sex rather than that of the true sex. For example, a truly female child with the adrenogenital syndrome may be mistakenly reared as a boy until proper studies reveal that the child is actually a girl. If the assigned sex is now changed and attempts are made to change the sexual orientation of the child (change to manner of dress of the newly assigned sex, toys, play habits, and so on), confusion may arise in the mind of the child, initiating considerable insecurity and tension.

Although there is much more that could be said regarding the development of the personality of the child, the foregoing brief sketch and subsequent comments in this chapter indicate the chief forces during the early years. The patterns of the child's inner life are now laid down in great part. The stage is set for the play that follows—the subsequent reactions of the child to the world and the people about him constitute the various acts, leading to a happy ending or perhaps a tragedy.

Although there are many angles from which one might view the development of the personality of the child, it is helpful to think of the roles played by such factors as (1) whether the child obtains gratification of his basic emotional needs; (2) the attitudes of parents and other adults toward him; (3) the psychic environment of the home; (4) his relationships to other children, not only his siblings but also his associates in the neighborhood, at school, and later in the community at large; (5) the effects of organic illness on his personality; (6) whether brain damage has altered his behavior; (7) his mental development; and (8) whether he has a learning disability. In the evaluation of problems of emotional origin, careful consideration should be given to these governing factors in the life of the child.

BASIC EMOTIONAL NEEDS

Although in the attempt to categorize the basic emotional needs of children there are differences in emphasis and expression, there is rather general agreement. These needs may be listed as follows: (1) love and affection, (2) security, (3) acceptance as an individual, (4) self-respect, (5) achievement, (6) recognition, (7) independence, and (8) authority.

Love and affection. The most important emotional need of the child is to be loved by his parents and to know that whatever happens he is sure of their love. Without it he may become insecure and tense, exhibit nervous habits, take refuge in functional complaints, be openly or secretly jealous of more favored siblings, overcompensate by explosive aggressiveness, or nurse his wounds in secret resentment and smouldering hostility. He may be so emotionally blighted that he is forever incapable of forming warm attachments and friendships, growing up to be a cold and distant adult.

Parents ordinarily do not need anyone to tell them to love their children. The perpetuation of the human race rests on the probability that they will. Loving is as important as being loved. It is as much a need of the parent as it is of the child. It is not largesse—a gift that is given because it seems appropriate to give a gift. Like the quality of mercy, it is not strained. Thus in the usual circumstances of the fortunately normal home the parents surround their children with the warmth of affection. Without a shred of pedantic preparation they adopt the informality that is so appealing to children—the little games, the kind words, the loving glances, the stories that are read, the songs that are sung. They are not above a romp or a tussle—the sophisticated equivalent of the she-wolf playing with her cubs.

However, there are some unfortunate parents who were reared in unhappy circumstances and whose personalities were never permitted to bloom. Although the variations on the theme are endless, these are essentially the ones who never became adjusted to the warmth of the world. They love their children, but they do not have the knack of showing it. They give formal protestations of devotion, but they do not know that children grade parents by actions and attitudes, not words. Frequently they cannot understand why they do not get along with their children better when they do everything for the children and tell them that they love them. Cast in a somewhat formal mold, they cannot unbend from austerity. Frequently the child interprets this to mean a lack of love. On the other hand, one or both parents may have been abused or neglected as children, and so have been impaired in their ability to love and to tramsmit that love to their children.

In the evaluation of behavior problems in children the physician must observe constantly for evidence as to whether the child is really receiving the affection that children so normally crave, whether he is in reality rejected, or whether he feels unloved because his parents cannot transmit their love to him—indeed, may keep it tightly locked from him, as from others.

An almost certain clue that the parent does not have the normal, spontaneous warmth of feeling toward the child is the undue insistence on reading material to understand the child's development. When parents continually request information regarding child rearing, and particularly when they seek authoritative approval and explanation of even the simplest things, it is evidence that they are grossly uncertain as to their roles as parents. It usually means that they are either afraid of the child and all the implications and responsibilities his presence occasions or that they secretly wish they did not have him. These comments are not directed toward well-balanced, intelligent, but inexperienced parents who want to learn more about the child and his development. It is not the desire for further knowledge that is questioned but the reasons why the desire is so intense.

The child needs not only the love of his parents but also the love of others in the home. He requires discipline, of course, and he is not always permitted to do what he wants to do, but back of it all he needs to feel a sense of belonging, of being wanted and accepted. As he passes through childhood the friendship and affection of companions will play increasingly important roles in his personality development. And, as all adults know, the need to be loved is a never-ending one.

Security. As the young child grows up in his increasingly complex world, there arise many threats to his sense of security. Perhaps the first of these are the animal threats of hunger, coldness, and discomforts of all kinds. Later, in usual circumstances the threats are of a psychologic nature and fundamentally involve whether he obtains gratification of his basic emotional needs. The child with his raw drives runs headlong into all the restraining influences of family and community that seek to civilize and make him into a conforming member of the family and society. He is constantly being told what he can and cannot do, he is finding out what he can and cannot have, and he is forming opinions as to whether he is liked or disliked. Buffeted by these experiences, he has many opportunities for feelings of uncertainty and insecurity. Later, as an adolescent, looking out over the broad ocean of adulthood, he experiences the trepidation of those who sail the unknown. And for the rest of his life, if he is normal, there will be at least some insecurity—the normal uncertainty that all will forever go well.

Almost every behavior problem of any degree of importance is associated with an element of insecurity. The evidence may be obvious in a child's tenseness and nervousness, or it may be camouflaged by aggressive overcompensation. Sometimes it is a secret sorrow that the child hides within himself.

So numerous are the factors that may breed insecurity that they can be only briefly discussed here. Except for those areas of the world in which merely to survive is an achievement, perhaps the most frequent cause of insecurity in children is marital discord. The strength of the home is the child's island of security in his insecure world. It is the fortress to which he retires when things go badly for him outside the home. His parents are the authoritative figures to whom he looks for guidance, advice, solace, and encouragement. They set the emotional tone of the home, and he reacts to the way they act and behave. When children see their parents at odds, bickering, quarreling, separating, or obtaining a divorce, their sense of security is threatened to its very foundations, as though the troops observed the uncertainty and mutual hostility of their commanders.

Clever parents seek to hide their discord, but children know their parents so thoroughly—their actions, their manner of speaking and of looking, and their moods—that this seldom is successful. Even if the parents were capable of quarreling without the children knowing it, they are not the same parents after the quarrel as they were before: they have been changed by it, and their unhappiness is often expressed in undue leniency based on the thought that at least the child should be happy in this wretched home, or in undue strictness resulting from short temper. Management of the child is unsteady, and as the horse knows the nervous rider, the child feels the change.

Threatening illness of a parent or loved one also poses a threat to security, although properly prepared children may accept the inevitable. Death of a parent, especially for the young child, is often followed by insecurity.

Many other causes of insecurity exist. Rejection of children or failure to accept them warmly is a frequent cause. Sibling rivalry is often the reason. Social ineptitude that prevents the establishment of firm friendships is common. Physical handicaps of all sorts may make children insecure, ranging from truly severe handicaps that prevent full participation in the activities of other children to those of minor significance. From the child's point of view, security depends greatly on personal appearance. Obesity, a scrawny figure, skin blemishes such as acne or even freckles, the shape of the nose, and a thousand other things loom large in importance to the child. Lack of skill in sports or in social graces, academic difficulties in school, a somewhat cold and aloof teacher, excessive teasing at home or school, and a long list of other factors each may play a part. There is also the insecurity of transplantation—the frequent changes in residence from one location to another that require the child to adapt to a new home, neighborhood, school, and community. Just as shrubs and flowers would never take root if transplanted too frequently, the frequently transplanted child may encounter difficulties in adjustment that manifest themselves as insecurity. However, some children take such changes as easily and happily as migratory birds, especially if in the new location the same old pattern of living exists, as is often true of the children of military personnel who change from one post to another.

Sometimes the child is deeply concerned about his health. In the chronically ill child there is a real basis for this feeling, making it all the more important for the physician to help the child and his parents face the illness and the future bravely and intelligently. In every chronic illness, especially those that will leave residual defect, it is the duty of the physician to inventory not only the incapacities of the child but also his remaining strengths and potentialities and to help plan a program to give confidence and happiness to the child within the framework of his handicap. (See pp. 75-79.)

Sometimes, however, the child is not really organically ill but merely thinks he is, and he thinks it so hard that it almost becomes a reality. Thus the physician sees a child with some of the symptoms of heart disease whose heart is strictly normal, one who has abdominal pain but a perfect set of viscera, or one with some other paradoxical condition. The child may be unwittingly copying the symptoms of another—someone with the real disease whose manifestations his symptoms mock. In other instances the child is merely using his symptoms to gain an objective—to stay home from school, to have a parent remain by his side, and so on. When the diagnostic studies fail to elucidate the answer and bewilderment continues as to what is really wrong with this child, the pattern of neurotic illness becomes ingrained. The concern the parents and even the physician show toward the child and his "illness" may engender considerable insecurity.

From these remarks it is clear that a search for factors causing insecurity is indicated in the workup of every child with a major behavior problem, that numerous causes for insecurity exist, and that many of them may be difficult to determine.

Acceptance as an individual. Because children differ physically, mentally, and emotionally, it is important to avoid attempts to channel rigidly their activities, interests, and ambitions. They should be accepted for what they are, rather than be cast into roles for which they are not adapted. Most parents find little difficulty in accepting the child for what he is; the mere fact that they have a child is to them a bountiful blessing. They usually soon discover that they do not have a perfect one, but they easily allow for minor imperfections. There are always some things about the child that they might wish to see improved, and they may seek a change without upsetting the child. They may stimulate the child to do better in this or that way, but they do not exert too much pressure. Handled properly, the child may be channeled into better behavior and new interests and may receive enormous benefit from the friendly counsel of wise parents.

On the other hand are parents who fail to accept the child for what he is, either rejecting him in one way or another or seeking to overhaul him to fit their own ideas. The child without musical talent drearily plunks the piano to satisfy his parents but hates the idea and may begin to hate them too; the clumsy boy without good coordination is forced into competitive sports only to suffer the indignities of repeated failures; the mediocre student is spurred on, only to stumble on the academic heights for which he was never intended; and the shy, sweet-natured child of creative ability is swept into the maelstrom of ceaseless social activity in order that he may be a part of the "right group." The inevitable disappointments that arise when he is defeated in these campaigns planned by his parents have severe effects on the child. Failure to achieve goals set by parents breeds defeatism and frequently leads to secret hostility and resentment. The docile child may work his heart out to satisfy his parents, knowing that at least his perseverance may win approval. The strong-willed child more often makes his dissatisfactions known, sometimes in explosive scenes of rebellion. The parents may then be startled to find that the child resents what in their opinion is so good for him.

Although in individual cases the reasons for failure to accept the child for what he is may be obscure, in others it is perfectly clear. Often the parents are trying to afford opportunities to the child that were denied them in some way when they were children—a laudable motive, but impracticable in the particular instance. If they never attended college, they may be intent on the child's doing so, although he may not have the necessary intellectual ability. Perhaps opportunities for music lessons were not afforded them; therefore they wish to make sure that their child does not lack in this respect. And so it goes—the parents seeking their own reincarnation through the lives of their children.

All too often it is not the desire to afford the child an opportunity that was denied to them in childhood but rather the need to win vicarious victories through the achievements of the child. When the child excels, it is as though the parents excelled. In a sense the child is pitted against the world so that the parents may taste sweet victory.

As in most things, this situation of parents living through the lives of their children is a matter of degree. It is, of course, normal to wish to afford to children whatever one thinks is for their benefit, and it is only natural that parents who remember keenly the defects of their childhood wish to make it better for their child. And pride in the accomplishments of one's children is certainly normal and universal. It is only when these attitudes get out of bounds that they cause trouble.

Self-respect. The child needs to feel his worth and his adequacy to meet his problems, achieve success, and have this success recognized. Anything that instills ideas of inferiority disturbs him greatly and may lead to a defeatist attitude, an inferiority complex, timidity, and seclusiveness in an effort to avoid his problems. He may, on the other hand, resort to aggressive behavior to compensate for his feelings of inferiority.

In the management of behavior problems in childhood the physician often finds that situations have occurred that tend to destroy the child's self-respect. High on the list are the all too frequent invidious comparisons parents and relatives make between brothers and sisters. The child's bad behavior is compared minutely to a sibling's good behavior, and the bad behavior becomes all the worse. Not only has he been criticized by his parents, perhaps justifiably so, but he has also been set against a sibling, who now becomes the shining light of virtuosity and approval. The child feels inferior, and the flame of sibling rivalry burns bright. Perhaps the children bring home their report cards, which are then brought forth during the dinner hour for minute scrutiny, comparison, approval, or damning, and the comments crackle. One child wins the honors, the next does moderately well, but the third, who has done poorly, may be criticized severely.

Perhaps in the schoolroom a child answers a question improperly, writes poorly, or in other ways does not achieve the desired level of performance. The teacher, harassed by the burdens of a large class and having little time for diplomacy, may openly state or infer by her attitude that the child is a dunce. The inherently clumsy child may be teased and jeered at on the playground because of lack of ability.

All these wounds to sense of pride and self-respect take their toll on the child and play important roles as causes of behavior problems. If all who deal with children would only remember that they, too, have feelings and sensibilities and should be handled with the same consideration one would wish for one's self, there would be fewer whose spirits have been crushed by harsh criticism, ridicule, and all the other things that poison self-respect. One should never forget the implications of the statement "Inasmuch as ye have done it unto one of the least of these."

Achievement. The maturing capacities of the growing child must find their outlet in achievement. The child learns to sit, to stand, to walk, to run, to ride a tricycle and then a bicycle, and later to drive a car. He is dynamic, active, questing, adventurous. He is not, like so many adults, merely maintaining his status quo. But his drive to achieve is often thwarted. Because of parental overprotection, he may be prohibited from joining his playmates in activities that are really safe but are considered by his parents to be hazardous. He is not permitted to climb trees, to ride a bicycle on the quiet neighborhood street, or to be out in a cold wind—a wind that is bound to bear on its breath the seeds of sickness. Parental precautions surround him like a stockade. The meek child may accept these restraints because he has learned to obey his parents. The more independent child resorts to arguments, pleadings, and scenes of high indignation, and by his vehemence may win the right to take part in normal activities. Regardless of the pattern of reaction, the net result is an injury to parent-child relationships.

In other instances the thwarting of achievement is a matter of parental convenience rather than overprotection. It is often so much easier to do things for the child than to bother with the learning period that enables him to do them for himself. Thus parents feed, dress, and bathe children long past the time when they could accomplish these things for themselves. They solve the child's school problems to make his studies easier. They manage the child's schedule with such efficiency that the smooth routine of the overly organized home is seldom upset. Things get done—and quickly—because the parents are seeing that they get done. However, the child is not learning to achieve any goals but is merely being led through life with a ring in his nose.

Recognition. As far as young children are concerned, virtue is seldom its own reward. They need recognition of their achievements and the approval of parents and playmates. Yet many a parent shows little interest in the child's activities and accomplishments. Perhaps the parents have become unduly absorbed in the management of the home, in their business affairs, and in their social life. In one way or another they may not be noticing the child as much as he needs to be noticed. Some parents are on the go so much that they really have little time with the child. Often the members of the family have such full schedules of activities that the home is really nothing but a launching pad, or like a restaurant a place to eat, or like a hotel a place to sleep. The child may be afforded all the necessities of life and may realize that back of it all his parents really love him, but he so seldom feels the pat of approval that there is an emptiness in his life.

In the evaluation of behavior problems it is interesting to note how frequently parents devote almost all their time with the child directing his activities, telling him to do this or that, not to do other things, criticizing him for breaking the house rules, and marshaling him up and down throughout the day to such an extent that he never feels the glow of their approval. The parents are often well-motivated in behaving in this manner. The harrassed mother, perhaps overburdened with work or household chores, or the mother who makes large chores out of little ones, may be so intent on keeping a perfect home that she places law and order and neatness above all else. The father, seeking to give his family a higher standard of living, drives on and on in his business activities, spends longer and longer hours making more and more money, and comes home late for dinner worn out, seeking peace and quiet and an early bed. Too often he has little time for his children, who may be asleep anyway before he arrives. Household duties, social life, business effort—whatever it is, the child is being neglected. A child is his parents' most important business. If this business is neglected, there is bound to be a bankruptcy of affection.

Independence. As the child grows, his maturing powers permit him to be increasingly the master of his fate. Under the guidance of his parents and others he learns to make more and more decisions, to become self-reliant, and in effect is trained to take his place as an adult capable of guiding his destiny. Wise parents, realizing their responsibility to equip the growing child to become a psychologically mature adult, foster the gradual development of independence, although at the same time maintaining the steady discipline and kindly authority that are necessary to prevent liberty from becoming license.

However, some parents do not permit the child to develop his independence. For many a parent, emancipating a child is a psychologic struggle. They wish to perpetuate his babyhood, are pleased that his childhood lisping persists longer than it should, and in countless other ways treat him as a baby when he is a child, and as a child when he is fully grown. And so the parents, seeing themselves grow older, cling to each golden moment of the childhood years. The poor child, never knowing independence, meekly forfeits it; never knowing freedom, never yearns for it; and grows in size but not in spirit, becoming all too often the weak, indecisive, incompetent adult who must turn to others for every decision and lean on them for the support he was trained to expect. Fortunately, a spirited child cannot be tamed so easily and, like a lively colt, breaks out of the corral of parental oversupervision into a wider world in which he can range more freely.

The acquisition of independence is sometimes blighted not by parental overprotection but by parental autocracy. The domineering parent who treasures authority, permits no one to challenge his word, and rules the home with an iron hand may see to it that independence does not rear its ugly head, just as a general quells the mutterings of his troops. There will be only one big bull in the pasture. But because like breeds like, he may have sired others of equally fiery spirit. In such homes the tensions run high, and the horns of the parent are all too often locked with those of the children. At first the child seldom wins, receiving many a psychic wound along the way, but finally, usually as an older adolescent well-trained on the family battlefield, he emerges with some degree of freedom and a greater measure of real independence.

Authority. Without the stabilizing influence of a certain measure of authority mixed with affection, the child will flounder emotionally. He needs to know the rules of the home, the neighborhood, the school, and the community. He can learn these things only by training and experience, and the training requires the steady but firm guidance of his parents.

The central purpose of discipline and authority is to prepare the child to accept the restrictions on behavior that he will encounter all through life. In this complex world a certain degree of conformity is mandatory, at least as one's actions affect others. The parents are not disciplining the child so that they may win the immediate contest; they are training him so that he will not go trampling through the world. Better to let him have his tears now, when there are parents to give comfort, than to let him go forth from the home to fall prey to his own arrogance and lack of self-control.

Unfortunately, many parents, like King Lear, forfeit their authority to their children. In some instances the parents are basically weak themselves and psychologically incapable of leadership. In other circumstances the pattern of the home life is so chaotic that no chain of command really exists. The parents may have failed to establish their positions of authority because they are never around enough to make their influence felt, perhaps placing more stock in business and social life than in seeing that their own house is in order. In other instances naïve parents do not know the difference between cordial relationships with their children, although still maintaining control, and excessive informality that makes them almost one with the children. It is as if the officers had stripped themselves of their insignia and joined the ranks. Finally, parents sometimes fail to exercise a proper degree of authority because they are basically uncertain in their approach to their children and fear that to act may distort in some way the child's personality.

Regardless of the cause, the result is often disastrous. The child may become impudent, arrogant, and demanding and may grow up to be a person who fails utterly to accept restraints and authority. From such backgrounds come many so-called juvenile delinquents. Although their delinquency is not to be condoned, it cries out to be understood, and it was their parents who were initially the delinquent ones—delinquent in not having taught the child to accept the restraints of the world.

Although it is never easy to rear a child, sensible parents establish fair rules for the home and then see that they are followed. They do not set up such a complicated system of rules that it is almost impossible for an active child to conform. And they do not believe that the child has committed an unpardonable sin if he is guilty of a minor infraction. They realize that people do better when led than when driven, and so they set good examples of behavior themselves. Through all the administration of discipline and authority they let their real affection for the child be evident. Using the principle of the conditioned reflex, perhaps without knowing it, they are so consistent in the application of penalties for bad behavior that the child becomes conditioned to good behavior. They praise the child for being good and withhold praise for being bad. They send him instantly from the room when he misbehaves, realizing that social ostracism, even at an early age and for only brief periods, is the most effective of punishments for the young child. They set no time limit for the punishment because they are observant enough to see that the small child does not wear a wristwatch and cannot tell time. The child is told to come back when he feels that he can behave properly. When he does return (perhaps in an incredibly short time), he is not reminded again and again of his poor behavior. Instead, he is warmly accepted to show that good behavior brings happy times and bad behavior brings unhappiness. The key to all this is, of course, consistency and the fact that the punishment so quickly follows the "crime."

Although parents need not feel terribly guilty for giving their children an occasional "good hard spanking" (it is noted that this phrase is used only by adults), observant parents soon see that the "good" spanking does little good. It usually creates far more problems than it solves, despite the unjustified perpetuation of the erroneous dictum, "Spare the rod and spoil the child." Beating on children is hardly the way to teach kindness, and losing one's temper is scarcely the way to foster self-control. Furthermore, it is a terribly unimaginative approach for an adult, who should be able to outthink a child and to steer him to better behavior by way of his mind instead of his gluteus maximus. When parents repeatedly spank their children, there is something wrong with the parents and perhaps with the child. In any event, such actions finally make the child more resentful of his parents, more fearful of them, and more distant toward them.

Other methods to maintain a proper degree of control in the home may be used, such as withdrawal of certain privileges for a limited period. For a younger child the greatest catastrophe that could occur is a temporary ban on viewing television. For a young teenager, temporary denial of the use of the family telephone, interpreted by him to be a virtual excommunication from the outer world, is a major disaster. Later on, forbidding the use of the family car for a day or two, prohibiting dating for a weekend, or other meaningful but not harsh punishments may prove effective.

If parents spent more time stimulating children to want to behave and showed their approval of good behavior more frequently and openly, the end result would be far better.

PARENTAL ATTITUDES

The chief parental attitudes to investigate are whether they truly love the child, whether they actually reject him, whether they overprotect him, and whether they unduly dominate him. Although these factors have been discussed to some extent in preceding pages, further comments seem indicated.

Love. Love and affection for the child are the most important parental attitudes. Most parents easily demonstrate their affection for the child in countless ways that he understands and accepts, but some parents find this difficult to do. They feel uncomfortable in meeting the child at his level of interest. Encouraging such parents to express their affection more openly may result in improvement of a behavior problem. However, in many instances the pattern of formality is too ingrained to change.

Rejection. Causes for rejection are many, including (1) immaturity of young parents, who find themselves incapable of easily assuming the obligation of parenthood; (2) an undesired pregnancy when the parents are economically insecure; (3) use of pregnancy to patch a broken romance in the thought that the advent of the child will call for cessation of hostilities; (4) the child's presence as an interference with the mother's career; (5) the child not being of the desired sex or not meeting expectations physically, intellectually, or emotionally; (6) sometimes the fact that the child is chronically handicapped or deformed; and (7) scientific detachment, whereby the mother or father prefers psychologic dissection to parental affection, viewing the child as an interesting biologic experiment warranting constant analysis of attitudes and actions.

Actually, parents seldom wholly accept or completely reject a child. Fortunately, acceptance ordinarily dominates, but any child is at least occasionally a problem. The most considerate and affectionate parent finds it difficult to suppress transient feelings of rejection when the child tracks muddy footprints indoors, breaks treasured objects, or in other ways creates a scene. On the other hand, the most rejected of children may experience warm moments of acceptance, but they are only as the winter sun, quickly hidden by clouds.

Rejection is more often concealed and less often openly expressed. Because it is abnormal not to love one's flesh and blood, guilt feelings arise, and parents may seek to assuage their consciences by overcompensation. In lieu of love and affection they shower the child with material comforts, request meticulous medical supervision, encourage eating to the point of causing obesity, and in other ways unconsciously seek to hide their abnormal emotions from the eyes of the world.

Overprotection. In their normal desire to spare their child the vicissitudes of life, some parents overprotect him. They pick him up and walk him about whenever he cries; they feed, dress, and bathe him long past the time when he could do these things himself; they select only the nicest, most malleable playmates; they overemphasize medical supervision, they urge food to stave off illness and thereby produce obesity; they do the homework for the schoolchild; and in countless other ways they lay a carpet of flowers along life's thorny paths. Such children often emerge as submissive, indecisive, incompetent adolescents at the mercy of a world that treats them with intolerable impartiality.

Some overprotected children become docile and submissive, are agreeable to all parental desires, are shy and seclusive, fit poorly into groups, or may be channeled into hypochondriasis. Others run roughshod over their parents (who never exercise firm authority), become impolite and even impudent, and are domineering, aggressive, and increasingly insistent in their demands.

Domination. Another factor meriting consideration is parental domination and overambition. There is an uncrowned king in many a home. Imposition of autocratic discipline, insistence on perfect performance, and planning more for the child than the child can achieve may give rise to tension, insecurity, and feelings of inferiority and failure. Children may react with complaints of fatigability, headache, abdominal pain, or vomiting. Dawdling and delay may become prominent features of behavior—the childhood equivalent of a slowdown strike. Other children resent domination and become rebellious. As the child grows older, open conflict may occur, and the child's vehemence may gain him freedom from oppression.

Fortunately, most parents know the wisdom of dominating their children just enough to civilize them and to give them the stability that goes with a measure of parental authority. Most parents are so pleased with their children that they do not spend too much time or effort erecting lofty ambitions for them. After all, the saving grace of the world is that there are so many normal people in it.

OTHER FACTORS WITHIN AND OUTSIDE THE HOME

Relationships to others in the home. The evaluation should also include determination of relationships in the home between the child and adults other than the parents and the child's relationships with siblings. With regard to other adults the same information is sought as is obtained about the parents. Sibling rivalry is natural in some degree but frequently becomes excessive. It is fostered by invidious comparisons between children, favoring one child more than another, and in other ways accentuating the competition for affection of parents that is normal with all children.

Other factors in the home. Many other factors in the home also affect the adjustment of the child. One may list them as space for play and other activities, economic status, social status, social attitudes of parents, family educational standards, illness of parents, broken homes, and the way in which discipline and punishment are meted out.

Factors outside the home. The principal factor outside the home is often the school. One seeks to know the relationship between the child and his teachers, how he performs in his work, and how he gets along with his schoolmates in and out of the classroom. The relationship of the child to his peers and associates in the neighborhood and community also deserves study.

PHYSICIAN'S INITIAL CONTACT WITH THE PROBLEM

In his approach to behavior problems a physician either actively searches or passively waits. If he is properly oriented and alert to the psychologic aspects of children, he may note early deviations from normal in his contacts with the child in the office or the home and may tactfully afford an opportunity for the parents to mention the problem. This is the preferable approach because it often permits early consideration of the problem before it has become more serious. Thus when the physician observes that the child clings to the mother unduly, exhibits great shyness, sucks his thumb during much of the visit, or in other ways openly demonstrates a tendency to a beginning problem, he may diplomatically inquire whether the child often acts in this way and whether it has been a concern to the parents. This should be expressed in an understanding and sympathetic manner, without a trace of criticism. If managed properly, many a parent will feel that the physician is truly interested in the child and will express the problem more fully, leading to subsequent management of it. This is the questing approach—the active searching out of the problem. Of course it can be overdone, and it can give rise to undue concern on the part of the parent if the approach is not tactful. But it is just the opportunity many parents need to bring themselves to discuss openly something that they have already felt to be wrong. One must remember that many parents are inherently shy and reserved, that some have never thought of mentioning minor behavior problems to their physician, and that others have not really recognized the actions of the child as showing a deviation from preferred behavior.

Too often the physician never concerns himself with a behavior problem until the parents themselves openly request help. By then many a problem has achieved major significance, and the golden opportunity to erase it has passed. This passive waiting for parental complaint explains much of the failure of preventive mental hygiene.

SCOPE OF EVALUATION

The basic information desired is the child's mental status, whether his emotional needs are being met, the attitudes of his parents, the parent-child relationships, the relationships between the child and other adults in the home, his relationship to siblings, and how he gets along in the neighborhood, the school, and the community at large. One must also determine whether organic illness is present and, if so, to what extent it is affecting the adjustment of the child. Furthermore, certain tests, mentioned later, may be of much importance in obtaining a comprehensive evaluation.

One of the commonest errors is to peck at the problem in piecemeal fashion. Bed-wetting is treated as an isolated event, destructiveness is managed superficially, and temper tantrums are handled by temporary maneuvering. There is undue fixation on the immediate aspect of the problem but insufficient consideration for the underlying reasons. The approach is thus a probing patrol action rather than a full advance. This road leads only to frustration because the problem is being treated rather than the child. Analyzing and managing abnormalities of behavior without full evaluation is like treating organic illness without a complete history and physical examination. One should remember that the overt action of the child, the external expression of the behavior problem, merely represents the outcropping of internal disturbance. What may appear to be identical abnormalities of behavior in two children often arise from different causes and require different treatment.

ARRANGING THE FIRST CONFERENCE

Perhaps the commonest error in approaching behavior problems is failure to plan properly. Too often, when it is suddenly discovered in the rush of practice that one of the children has a behavior problem, the physician is tempted to evaluate the situation superficially. This can lead only to inadequate therapy based on insufficient information.

When it is apparent that there is a behavior problem of more than minor proportions, the physician should immediately suggest a reappointment for the specific purpose of considering it fully. Parents quickly sense the value of special consideration—indeed, they often hunger for an opportunity to pour out their problem.

Depending on the complexity of the problem, more than one conference with the parents and with the child may be required. Subsequent conferences are also arranged by specific appointment so that the physician is not harassed by the ordinary demands of practice.

CIRCUMSTANCES OF THE CONFERENCE

Whether to have both parents present at the first interview or to have conferences with them separately depends on the nature of the problem. If the physician has advance information that the parents are at odds, it is usually profitable to hold separate conferences with them, at least at first. If an acceptable degree of harmony prevails, there is great advantage in obtaining at the beginning the opinion of both parents. Separate interviews are held later. Too often the father is left out completely on the basis that he is too busy at work. This is a mistake because one needs to learn the father's attitudes toward the problem and the family, and the physician also wants the father to gain an understanding of what is wrong so that he may be able to help the child more intelligently.

Suitable privacy and freedom from distracting interruptions should be afforded. The physician cannot bob in and out of a conference room and expect to elicit confidence and cooperation. It is better to guarantee 20 to 30 minutes of privacy and solve the problem in a series of conferences than to prolong an interview to the point at which it becomes impossible to fend off other duties of practice. In fact, there are positive benefits in working up a problem through a series of short conferences. Parents often need time to think about what was said in the first conference and to make up their minds concerning how far they want to bare their souls to this particular physician. It is common experience for them to withhold delicate information until the third or fourth conference. Also, suggestions that the physician has made when a slight change in management is clearly indicated may be bearing fruit and stimulating confidence.

Two chief objectives of such conferences are to evaluate the problem accurately and to win the cooperation of the parents and the child. The first ingredients for success are genuine interest and real sympathy for the problem and the people involved.

The physician should remember that, when first interviewed, parents are often nervous, uncertain, and apprehensive or defensive and feel inadequate, guilty, or confused. An important essential is to put them at their ease. One should especially avoid an attitude of criticism or condemnation. We are physicians, not judges. A friendly, objective manner is best.

It often helps to tell the parents early in the first interview that their problem, although important, is not highly unusual but is common to many families. The knowledge that others face the same problem and that the physician has often dealt with similar situations is reassuring.

Without interrupting the parents unduly, it is helpful to insert a casual remark from time to time, such as "I can see how you must have been disturbed by that" or "I can appreciate how you thought that was a wise thing to do." The physician should show no surprise at whatever is said. If he has been practicing many years, few things will surprise him anyway.

The capacity to be a good listener is all-important. The skilled physician gives his patients and parents medical "attention" in the literal sense of the word. Although they often pour out their problem in a disconnected fashion that lacks the orderly sequence of an intern's history, he understands that this is normal and that getting it off the chest or telling all helps clear many tensions. It is quite like a religious confession.

Note taking is reduced to a minimum, since fast and furious scribbling interferes with the flow and continuity of the parent's story.

The first conference with the parents may be thought of as consisting of three parts: (1) the initial statement in which they describe the problem as they see it, (2) questions by the physician to bring out in greater detail matters that the parents have mentioned, and (3) completion of the history by questions covering aspects not previously discussed.

In general, the physician should be careful not to interrupt the initial story if at all possible. One is studying these parents, just as they are evaluating him, and much can be learned about them by the manner in which they present the case. Only if endless rambling ensues should the physician venture an occasional remark to get the story back on the subject.

When the parents have come to the end of their remarks, the physician asks questions that elicit more information on phases of the problem that the parents have already mentioned. When, as is usual, several aspects of behavior have been brought up, he selects the one that is psychologically least traumatic to the parents and begins with it, then considers the next least disturbing, and so on. Thus step by step the material is considered in an ascending order of severity. In the early stages mutual understanding is being established between the physician and the parents, and by his approach they become more willing to give full information concerning the more disturbing features of the problem.

After everything the parents have voluntarily mentioned has been considered, the physician then obtains in this and succeeding conferences the necessary information to round out the total evaluation of the child, parental attitudes, parent-child relationships, and other matters affecting the emotional life of the child.

The physician should be careful not to go too far in the first interview. Questions involving intimate details of the lives of the parents and their relationships to one another should be avoided unless the parents themselves bring them up or unless there is a clear opening for their introduction. If the problem is not a simple one requiring only a minor degree of guidance, additional interviews will be needed anyway, and the physician should give the parents an opportunity to think things over before going on. If the right approach has been made in the first conference, the parents will talk together and agree that the physician is trying to be helpful and has a personal interest in their problem. It is often amazing to see what additional information will then be given in the second conference. The initial story may be completely changed. The very heart of the problem may be revealed.

In obtaining the psychiatric history, the physician should avoid the step-by-step application of an outline. Of course a mental outline is used, but parents often resent steady interrogation. The same information can be obtained more informally and pieced together.

EXAMINATION OF THE CHILD

The medical history of the child may be taken in the child's presence, since he is accustomed to having the physician ask the parents questions while he is in the room. After the history and the physical examination he can amuse himself in the waiting room or elsewhere while the physician talks in private with the parents. In some instances, especially in dealing with older children, it may be better to interview the parents without the child for the first conference on the behavior problem.

The physical examination should be done with special thoroughness. Parents frequently ascribe abnormal behavior to physical disease. The "thorough examination" is helpful to convince the physician of the absence of an organic condition that would explain the problem but most of all to give the parents the same assurance. A superficial survey and a hasty statement that the child "seems all right" may completely destroy confidence.

When minor physical abnormalities are encountered, only experience will indicate whether they account for all or any part of the behavior problem. Such minor abnormalities should be corrected, if possible, but their etiologic role should be played down, or the parents will subsequently be disappointed when improvement of the physical condition does not lead to improvement of the behavior problem.

Once having examined the child carefully, it is important not to reexamine him repeatedly. This may give the impression to the parents and to the child that perhaps there is some doubt in the physician's mind and that there is a possibility that some organic condition may actually be the cause of the trouble. These lingering doubts may be difficult to dispel.

TESTS AND LABORATORY PROCEDURES

A routine urinalysis and complete blood cell count should be performed, and additional tests may be indicated by material brought out in the history and examination. The purpose should be to request only the minimal number of laboratory tests. In certain instances, however, the parents will not be content unless some special test is performed, such as obtaining a chest radiograph. In such circumstances it is part of the therapy to obtain the test. The opposite approach obtains when the physician orders a large number of tests without adequate reason, merely in the hope of "turning up something." This may lead to frightening experiences for the child and undue expense for the parents.

Clinical psychologic evaluation should be obtained if the child is having difficulty in school, if there are other apsects of the case that suggest impaired mentality, and especially if the problem is obscure. In practice the majority of children with behavior problems do not require psychologic evaluation.

If a child appears to pay little attention to his parents' requests or does poor work in school, it is wise to evaluate hearing ability by means of an audiogram. If he holds books close to his eyes, complains of discomfort of his eyes, or has difficulty seeing what is on the blackboard, his visual acuity should be determined. If he experiences unusual difficulty in reading or writing, the possibility of a specific reading disability should be explored.

CONFERENCES WITH THE CHILD

Conferences with the child often help determine the nature of the disturbance and establish the proper rapport for subsequent solution of the problem. The level at which the conference is pitched is all-important. The approach must be carefully related to the child's age and intelligence or the physician will be too advanced for one child and will insult the intelligence of another. Children are sometimes resentful toward anyone who pries into their thoughts and feelings and may show a bristling defensiveness. A patronizing attitude is especially to be avoided, as is lecturing or condemning the child. Sometimes it is better at first to say nothing to the child concerning his problem but to talk casually of school or sports or of his other activities, thus remaining the one adult who does not seem to peep into his soul. Careful maneuvering may later result in much information from the child as he grows friendly and trusts the physician more.

CONFERENCES WITH TEACHERS AND OTHERS

Because the school plays an important part in the child's emotional life, a conference or at least a telephone conversation with the teacher may be helpful. The physician should also ask the teacher to send a brief letter describing how the child impresses her in his academic work and behavior. Teachers almost invariably cooperate in this, and much valuable information may be gained. One should remember that, as a group, schoolteachers help solve more problems than they create and logically resent any implication that they may have contributed to the child's disturbance.

Sometimes it is advisable to talk with other adults who live in the home or who have frequent contact with the family, such as grandparents or an aunt.

GENERAL APPROACH TO THERAPY

Granted that a complete evaluation has been made, the physician should correct simultaneously, if possible, all deviations from normal behavior. Attempting to solve all the overt problems at once is often helpful because they usually arise from similar fundamental causes. Thus if the child has temper tantrums, a feeding problem, and enuresis, it is usually advisable to approach all the problems together rather than in piecemeal fashion. In other instances it may be better to work first with one simple aspect of a complicated problem.

Sudden changes in management may be less effective than more gradual alteration. Sometimes a child, particularly an older one, becomes wary when a complete reversal of methods of management is accomplished suddenly. Announcements that "things are going to be better" are less effective than quietly making them so.

Suggestions for improvements in management should be practical and applicable in the particular situation. For example, there is little advantage in stressing the need for more room for the children when it is apparent that financial limitations prevent more spacious quarters. When parents are unable to provide what the physician has declared necessary, they are put into an unhappy position that may accentuate their own difficulties.

THE EMOTIONAL IMPACT OF CHRONIC DISEASE

All organic diseases have a psychologic impact on the child and his family, varying from minimal emotional tensions during transient and relatively insignificant illness to potentially severe and lasting psychologic effects in chronic disease. Physicians and other members of the health team should keep this concept continually in mind and give appropriate attention to the psychologic overlay that invariably accompanies organic disease, at the same time properly diagnosing and treating the organic disturbance.

The following discussion concerns how physicians and others may so manage the child with chronic disease and his family that emotional problems may be minimized. The emphasis is on understanding the type of child and family with which one is dealing, analysis of the emotional impact on child and family, and preventive and therapeutic actions that may be taken. A systematic approach that has been found to be practical and useful is presented.

One may conceive of six major factors as having important influence on the degree to which emotional disturbances accompany chronic disease: (1) nature of the chronic disease or handicap, (2) age of the child at onset of disease, (3) parental attitudes and emotional balance, (4) emotional adjustment of the child at the onset of the disease, (5) threats to the basic emotional needs of the child, and (6) availability of special facilities and programs.

Nature of the chronic disease or handicap. Chronic diseases and handicaps range from those that are minimal to those that are severe, even life-threatening. Therefore, the physician needs to ask himself the following questions: (1) Is the diagnosis accurate? (2) What is the prognosis? (3) Is the condition disfiguring? (4) Will it greatly restrict the activities of the child and his participation in school and social contacts with his age group? (5) Is there a treatment that gives hope to success? (6) Is excellent treatment easily available to this particular child? (7) How will the cost of treatment be borne?

Accuracy of diagnosis. An accurate diagnosis, early established, does much to emotionally stabilize the parents and the child who is old enough to appreciate medical uncertainty. Nothing exceeds fear of the unknown in creating anxiety and tensions. Therefore, diagnostic measures should be planned intelligently, executed promptly, and should be so well-coordinated that the result is known as soon as possible. A poorly planned, piecemeal diagnostic approach may be completely upsetting. Unfortunately, all chronic diseases are not easily diagnosed. When there continues to be doubt, appropriate consultants are called in, and the fact that they *are* called in is, in itself, a stabilizing factor. . . .

A physician should request a consultant under the following circumstances: (1) when he does not know what he is dealing with and needs another opinion; (2) when he *does* know the diagnosis, but the treatment is out of his field; (3) whenever he makes the accurate diagnosis of a chronic disease of major importance or a disease with an invariably fatal outcome; and (4) when the family is anxious because of uncertainties in diagnosis or treatment and is about to request a consultant.

In the case of major chronic disease or uniformly fatal disease, parents invariably feel better when a second physician has also certified the diagnosis and approved the treatment.

Requesting a consultant when one senses that the parents are about to suggest one is not done to save face. It is done for the child's sake—specifically, to permit the suggestion of a consultant who could really be of help.

Once an accurate diagnosis is established, one is able to analyze the other items regarding the nature of the disease or handicap.

Prognosis. Chronic diseases range from those that are easily controlled to those that may become progressive, or may eventually cause death. Armed with the right diagnosis, the physician is, of course, able to predict the probable outcome of the illness, at least in general terms. Nevertheless, in view of unpredictable variations in certain chronic diseases (rheumatoid arthritis, for example), determining the outlook is often far from exact. The best that can be done in most instances is to adopt an optimistic attitude and to emphasize that the child may well fall into the group that makes good progress.

Is the disease or handicap disfiguring? It makes a great difference whether the disease or handicap is disfiguring—whether it is visible or invisible. One might even say whether it is audible, as in children with severe cleft palate who may never speak perfectly despite skillful operations. If the defect is disfiguring, it will have a more profound emotional impact on the child and parents than if it is invisible, as in diabetes. It will also be essential to correct the disfiguring defect surgically, where this can be done, and as early as possible in order to lessen the period of maladjustment of the child and the parents.

Restriction of activities. The degree to which a chronic disease or handicap restricts a child's activities has great bearing on his emotional, social, and intellectual growth and development. At one end of the spectrum are bedridden invalids and at the other those whose chronic disease or handicap interferes only slightly with their activities.

If the child's activities must be greatly restricted, special attention should be given to affording contacts with other children, within the limits of his clinical condition. Thus, his friends should be encouraged to visit him in the hospital or home, and as close a contact as possible should be maintained with his social world.

Does treatment give hope to success? The parents and the child old enough to understand will be much comforted, and therefore better adjusted, if there is a treatment that offers hope of success. Diabetes, with all its difficulties, may be well controlled. Epilepsy may be perfectly controlled. The child with celiac disease may blossom under proper treatment. Not so the child with severe scoliosis, advanced renal insufficiency, sickle cell disease, and a host of other permanently difficult problems.

Is excellent treatment easily available for this child? Unfortunately, not all children have excellent treatment facilities easily available. There are innumerable children in our nation who are geographically remote from medical centers. This includes those who must cross the asphalt jungles of metropolitan complexes to reach medical facilities. They are remote in the sense of the time and effort necessary to attend special clinics for the chronically ill or handicapped. Fortunately, much effort is being made to reduce these geographic and temporal barriers to good medical care. The psychologic burdens of the child and his parents will obviously be reduced if good longitudinal care is easily available.

The cost of treatment. Chronic diseases and long-term handicaps are notably expensive. Federal, state, and city medical programs for children are often available, and voluntary health agencies and medical insurance include more and more of the nation's population. Yet these programs do not always cover the entire cost of care, and family finances often suffer.

Age of the child at onset of disease. The age of a child at the onset of a chronic disease or physical defect strongly influences the degree of emotional impact. The simplest example is the very young infant who is, of course, psychologically oblivious to the fact that his illness or defect makes him different from others. However, an infant less than 6 months of age may react to hospitalization with what has been called a "global" reaction—alterations in patterns of feeding, sleeping, and elimination. In the second half of the first year, he may react to prolonged hospitalization by what has been termed "stranger anxiety" and "separation anxiety."

The child 1 to 3 years of age may also have anxiety based on separation and on fear of hospital strangers, and may show regressive behavior. Under the emotional impact of regimentation and hospitalization, he may become detached, withdrawn, fail to eat well, and may even become permanently blighted emotionally if lack of sensory stimulation and warm affection lasts too long.

As the child grows older and his self-image becomes better established, he begins to react to disease and hospitalization not only with separation anxiety, but many fears—fears of painful procedures and fears in regard to harm to his body. Deeper anxieties now flood his mind—the thwarting of achievement goals, worry over loss of independence, concern over future occupation, fear that he will not be accepted socially, and damage to his self-image. Small wonder he so often becomes withdrawn, embittered, and reacts with aggressive overcompensation.

Parental attitudes and emotional balance. Adjustment of parents and, in turn, the child depends to a great extent on parental attitudes and the degree of emotional balance of the parents prior to the onset of the child's illness.

Thus, one is especially interested in evaluating whether the parents have the normal love and affection for the child, whether they actually reject him, whether they are overprotective, or whether they are domineering. We need to know whether they can give him the warmth of love and affection that every child deserves and the chronically ill child specifically requires.

Every parent initially rejects the diagnosis of a chronic disease in his child. This is a normal, impulsive flight from the truth, through self-protective denial of the diagnosis. Once the diagnosis has been accepted, the child himself may be rejected, although the converse is usually true: afflicted children usually call forth great parental love and sympathy. Nevertheless, there are undoubtedly secret moments of rejection. But these transitory rejection thoughts, born of the burden of the disease and the dashed hopes of the parents, are usually quickly overcome by the much greater love for the child. However, when parents catch themselves thinking this way, they have deep guilt feelings.

Indeed, parents invariably have guilt feelings when the diagnosis of a deformity, chronic illness, or a fatal disease is made. The physician should always recognize this fact and attempt to relieve the parents of false thoughts that they contributed to the child's condition. It is amazing how gratified parents are for this open approach, and how obviously relieved they are for the absolution of their presumed sin.

Overprotectiveness is another parental attitude that needs evaluation. It may have been present before the onset of the chronic disease, and it understandably flourishes during the management of the condition. There is ordinarily a surge of sympathy for any afflicted person, most of all one's own child. This is so normal and so therapeutic for the parents that it is often difficult to hold in check. But, if it is overdone, it will harm the child's adjustment to his handicap. He may feed on overprotectiveness, demand more and more attention, resign from doing even the simplest things for himself or others, and become insistent and even domineering and tyrannical.

Overprotectiveness may also impair treatment. Having given in to the child on so many fronts, parents may also give in on strict adherence to the home treatment schedule.

Pity often accompanies overprotectiveness. Pity is, of course, invariably and understandably present. However, the parents should not openly pity the child. He will then begin to pity himself, and this will defeat efforts to encourage him to accept his situation bravely and make the most of his remaining capacities.

Though fortunately in the minority, one does encounter self-willed, domineering parents—often with strong feelings of rejection—who make it all the more difficult for the child to adjust to his illness. They sometimes give the physician a rough time: questioning the diagnosis, debating the treatment, concentrating on the minutiae of home treatment, holding the child to a superstrict schedule, and expecting a Spartan bravery with little consolation.

We also need to know something of the personal relationships between the parents. Marital discord may have been present all along, but the burden of a chronically ill child often accentuates it. Parents may blame each other for the child's illness. One may accept the diagnosis and the other may not. They may debate the treatment and whether the physician is capable. Their families may pit them against each other. One may want to shop for an optimistic diagnosis and the other may not. Disagreements centering about the chronically ill child may also lead to divorce. . . .

For the above reasons, it is important once the diagnosis is established to have a series of gentle but frank talks with the parents, not only about the many other things mentioned above, but also about how the chronic illness conceivably might impair their marriage.

They should be encouraged to maintain their normal business and social life insofar as possible; if they can get away from the child at times, their strength to carry on may be renewed.

When their families insist on them showing the physician newspaper clippings or magazine articles concerning miraculous cures or a uniformly successful treatment, the physician should not act in a condescending manner. He should accept the article and write the author, asking him to send an early reply. Almost invariably, the author writes back that he was misquoted and really has nothing new. When these letters are shown to the parents, pressure on the physician is diminished and he stands in the proper position of having been quite willing to pursue any conceivably hopeful lead.

The physician should identify other individuals in the family circle who are close to the parents and the child and who therefore exercise an influence on how the parents adapt to the illness, and who play prominent roles in the family dynamics.

With the knowledge of the parents, the physician should properly orient these influential relatives concerning the nature of the disease, what they can do to help minimize emotional impact, and how they can best help the parents. They should be so well informed that they understand the situation as well as the parents. They should be particularly cautioned against blaming one or both parents for the child's illness, and they should be told that the physician has strongly recommended that the parents continue to be as active as possible in their usual activities outside the home.

Emotional adjustment of the child at the onset of the disease. Just as the parents react to the child's disease against the background of their prior emotional adjustment, so does the child respond from his own emotional baseline. A happy, secure, sociable, sufficiently independent, achieving child who feels warmly accepted by parents, siblings, and associates is, of course, best prepared to weather the emotional storms of a chronic disease or handicap. An unhappy, insecure, overly dependent, socially inept child without a strong self-image, and who already feels unloved, is the least prepared.

One of the physician's chief responsibilities is to determine what sort of a child he is dealing with from the standpoint of emotional balance. Having determined this, the physician can plan more intelligently for the care of the child.

Threats to the basic emotional needs of the child. One might list the basic emotional needs of children (and of adults) as follows: (1) love and affection; (2) security; (3) acceptance as an individual; (4) self-respect; (5) achievement; (6) recognition; (7) independence; and (8) authority or discipline. Knowing how these basic needs are threatened by a chronic disease or handicap helps the physician in his efforts to minimize the emotional impact.

Love and affection. The child may feel that he is being punished or deserted by his parents when he is hospitalized and has to undergo extensive and sometimes painful tests. He may feel guilty and rejected. Now that he has a chronic illness or a handicap, he may feel himself to be a burden on the family and that they will now prefer his brothers and sisters.

Security. The chronically ill child has a multitude of threats to his security. Among them are fear of the unknown when the diagnosis is in doubt; fear of the known when the diagnosis is certain; fear of being abandoned; fear of pain; fear of death; worries about the destruction of his self-image; anxiety about possible mutilation, as from operations; long thoughts about his future (social acceptability, vocation, marriage); and, high on the list, concern that he is different from his fellows.

Acceptance as an individual. A feeling of being accepted for what he is is a basic emotional need of every child. But now the illness has changed him. He is different, feels the difference, and knows that others know he is different. He magnifies the importance of this and he may well imagine that, since he has changed, his parents and his friends may no longer accept him as they once did. . . .

The parents, too, have to adjust to the changed child. Perhaps their expectations for him are now thwarted, or blighted. His appearance may have been permanently changed for the worse, as when severe facial burns are suffered. Perhaps he has nephrosis and is taking corticosteroids that in a high dosage can change him into a fat caricature of the beautiful child they formerly had. A 6-year-old child in our city screamed and wanted to "go to God" when she saw her steroid-bloated face for the first time in a mirror. How casually we talk of "moon facies" but seldom tell the child that his appearance will be changed while the dosage is high. Why do we not take photographs of his face before therapy is begun so that we can remind him that his appearance will return to that of the photograph when the drug dosage is decreased or treatment discontinued?

Self-respect. The chronically ill child, or the child with a severe handicap, may suffer a loss of self-respect. He may think the disease is a punishment for his wickedness, or for his hostile thoughts toward his parents, or a personal weakness. His inability now to achieve his goals may weaken his self-respect. His changed body image and self-concept may make him feel inadequate.

Achievement. The maturing capacities of the growing child must find their outlet in achievement. But achievement may be blocked by the chronic disease or handicap. The athletic boy can no longer excel in sports. The popular girl may not even be able to attend social events. The sense of success in life is gone, and the child lies in bed or sits in restriction amidst his broken dreams. Of all the bitter pills to swallow, the worse may be this thwarting of dynamic achievement. . . .

The physician should take not only the usual negative inventory—what is wrong with the child—but also a positive inventory—what potentialities remain. Unfortunately, too many physicians are content if they pin down the diagnosis in all its details and ramifications, satisfied that they have catalogued all the defects. Too few carefully evaluate the remaining capacities of the child and specifically seek to develop his strong points.

As an example, a 12-year-old boy had severe rheumatic carditis, with aortic regurgitation and mitral insufficiency of such a degree as to permit him to walk only a block or two slowly. Formerly a fine athlete, now he could not compete. He refused to ride to school in the family car, preferring to go on his own, however slowly. Participation in social activities was greatly limited.

The physician arranged for him to be trained by a radio-television repairman, and soon the boy was the idol of his group because of his ability to repair radio and television sets. The town photographer then accepted him for special instruction. He learned rapidly, set up his own darkroom, and began developing prints for his friends. His father interested him in collecting stamps. His continued sense of achievement helped immeasurably to maintain his emotional adjustment and he remained, as he was before his illness, one of the most secure and popular boys in his town.

On the other hand, a 14-year-old girl with mild rheumatoid arthritis was converted into a confirmed hypochondriac by an overly protective mother and a doting aunt. They sympathized too openly over her most minor complaints, waited on her hand and foot, encouraged her to remain at home in bed when resumption of activity had been advised, and in other ways adopted an overly lenient attitude toward the prescribed home management. She retired from the world—dropped out of school, drifted away from her friends and soon did not want them to visit her, lost ambition to achieve, and accepted the role of martyr to an illness that was never more than mild and by no means incapacitating.

We should remember that we are not only responsible for the prevention of disease where that is possible, and the prompt diagnosis and adequate treatment of it when it does occur, but also for comprehensive rehabilitation of those who are left with residual impairment. Rehabilitation means much more than improvement in the mere physical aspects of the disease. It also means detailed attention to the emotional impact, and a positive approach in order to minimize the impact.

Recognition. All children need recognition of their achievements and approval of their parents and associates. Yet in many instances there is such a concentration on the chronic disease itself that only the disease is recognized—the child is important only because he has the problem. The child should know that others realize the impact of the illness on him, and sympathize, but that they also notice his good qualities and approve of him and the way he bravely faces his handicap. He needs to feel that he amounts to something, even though he is ill or handicapped.

Independence. Chronic illness or handicap thwarts to a variable degree the acquisition of independence. Indeed, the illness often requires the child to be dependent on others at the very time he most needs a greater degree of independence.

Small wonder that many children who become chronically diseased or handicapped go through a period of denial of the diagnosis and reject the idea that they will have to suffer limitations, have to depend more on others. Small wonder also that they often overcompensate with a rebellious attitude—sometimes a virtual defiance of the disease and its treatment—and a hostility to all connected with it—parents, physicians, and nurses.

Authority or discipline. In the complex and sometimes chaotic world of the child, there is a vital need for the steady exercise of kindly yet firm parental discipline and authority. When the child is ill, there is a great tendency to diminish, or even to abandon, authority and discipline. The ordinary, sensible rules and restrictions break down. This road leads to tyranny by the child, who takes over the family in a domineering manner, using his illness as a lever to get what he wants.

The physician should encourage parents to maintain a sensible degree of authority and discipline. Even the chronically ill child must learn to accept the restrictions on behavior that the civilized world demands of its inhabitants. Of what avail is it to rehabilitate him physically if he then emerges as a headstrong, self-willed, impetuous person?

Special facilities and programs. Space does not permit consideration of all the ways in which the environment can be arranged to improve the outlook for the chronically ill child—improved hospital construction, motel-hospital arrangements, rooming in for parents, playroom, recreational programs, hospital teaching programs, homebound instruction, special education, medical foster homes, and parent group discussions. But it is clearly apparent that the objective of minimizing the emotional impact of chronic diseases can best be achieved when proper facilities, programs, and personnel well-experienced in the management of such children are available. . . .

• • •

Viewed in the above manner, the management of a child with a chronic disease or handicap becomes intellectually challenging, exciting, and personally rewarding.*

James G. Hughes

Psychiatric aspects of childhood

The pediatrician is often the first professional to whom the parents go when either they or the school has some question about the behavior or emotional development of their child. In the case of the preschool child the child's physician may be the person who actually detects some deviation from normal psychosocial or behavior development. The child's primary care physician may feel comfortable in handling personally these types of problems or may feel that referral to or consultation with a child psychiatrist is in order.

The optimal situation for the patient is to have the pediatrician and the child psychiatrist working together with open communication and mutual respect. The pediatrician can contact the child psychiatrist either before or after recommending consultation to the family, but he must make sure that both the family and the psychiatrist are fully aware of the referral. The family has to know that a psychiatrist has been asked to become involved, whether the child is an outpatient or an inpatient. Moreover, the better prepared the family and the patient are regarding the referral for psychiatric services, the more likely they will see the referral in a positive light.

On first seeing the patient and the family, the child psychiatrist will do a complete psychiatric evaluation to arrive at a diagnostic impression and to decide on the type of treatment to recommend. The evaluative process involves: (1) history taking from both parents and child, (2) observation of child alone and with parents (or whole family if other members of the family are present), (3) physical examination as necessary, (4) laboratory studies if necessary, (5) psychologic testing if indicated, and (6) information from outside sources (referring physician, school, social service agencies, courts, etc.).

Depending on the psychiatrist's preference, the history taking can be done with the parents and child together, separately, or a combination of both. One must first clarify what the family sees as the problem and what they hope will be accomplished by seeing the psychiatrist. Besides the presenting problem, the history should include the child's development from the time of conception up to the present day. The family history is important, for it can indicate not only illnesses in other family members but also how the family functions as a unit. It is important to assess the role of the child in his family and social environment.

The assessment of the child in his family is augmented by the observation of the child with his family. One may see the child as the intermediary between two parents who are at odds with one another. The child may be the scape-

---

*From Hughes, J.G.: Emotional impact of chronic disease, Jacobi Award Address (given before the A.M.A. Section of Pediatrics 1975), Am. J. Dis. Child. **130:**1200, Nov., 1976, Copyright 1976, American Medical Association.

goat for family problems in general. A handicapped or chronically ill sibling may be diverting a lot of the family's emotional resources to his care, whereas the identified patient's symptoms may be a cry for much-needed attention. Also, a family interview acknowledges that the patient's problems are actually the whole family's problems and that the whole family has to work together to overcome these difficulties.

The next phase of the evaluation is the interview with the child alone. Done by a trained psychiatrist, the psychiatric interview with children has been shown to have a high degree of reliability and validity (Rutter and Graham, 1968). How the interview of the child is conducted depends on the age of the child. The younger the child, the more play is involved; the older the child, the more verbal exchange is used. Regardless of the method, the psychiatrist will try to elicit strengths and assets as well as maladaptive aspects of development. During the time with the child the psychiatrist will observe the mental status of the child as well as his physical attributes. Mental status includes interactions with the examiner, self-confidence, mood, memory, sociability, self-expression, understanding, attention span, distractibility, verbalization, intelligence, orientation, thought processes, activity, coping mechanisms, use of fantasy, and formation of conscience and self-concept. Physically, the psychiatrist will notice any congenital anomalies or neurologic disturbances. Various tasks may be given to screen for learning disabilities, distractibility, and attention span (Silver, 1976) because many children with learning disabilities develop emotional problems secondary to frustrations and failures in school. If the psychiatrist believes that further physical workup is necessary, this will be discussed with the referring physician, and if another consultation is indicated (i.e., neurologic, surgical, etc.) they both should agree on it.

During the evaluation the psychiatrist may formulate questions that can only be answered by specific educational, psychologic, speech and language, or biologic tests. After discussing these tests with the parents, the psychiatrist makes the appropriate referral. After the results of the assessments are received, the psychiatrist discusses the treatment program with the child and the parents in light of this information. After a treatment program is decided on, which may or may not involve psychotherapy, the psychiatrist contacts the persons to be involved with the treatment/educational program and the referring physician to share the results of the psychiatric evaluation and plans for treatment. Because the primary physician will have continued contact with the patient and the family, it is imperative that he knows what the treatment plans are to make sure that the family follows through with them or, if not, the reasons why. Treatment modalities that are commonly used are outlined by Campbell and Shapiro (1975):

1. Treatment of the child
   a. Educational and remedial techniques
   b. Socialization groups
   c. Operant conditioning techniques
   d. Individual psychotherapy (play and interview therapy)
   e. Psychoanalytic techniques
   f. Other psychotherapies
   g. Residential milieu treatment
   h. Group therapies
2. Treatment of the parent
   a. Counseling
   b. Mirroring and identification with trained professionals
   c. Individual psychotherapy
3. Treatment of the family

In summary, Simmons (1974) outlines the topics to be considered in a diagnostic evaluation:

1. Presenting problem
2. Family description
3. Family history
4. Sociocultural issues
5. Birth, development, and medical history
6. Peer relationships and activities
7. Previous and present school experience
8. Educational, psychologic, and biologic studies
9. Other professional evaluations
10. Mental status
11. Diagnostic formulation
12. Diagnostic impression
13. Recommendations

Diagnostic formulation and assessment do not end with the initial evaluation but are ongoing processes interwoven with the treatment program.

DIAGNOSTIC CLASSIFICATION

The third edition of the *Diagnostic and Statistical Manual of Mental Disorders* (DSM-III) of the American Psychiatric Association was published in 1980. (Work is already in progress on DSM-IV.) The diagnostic scheme presented in DSM-III is multiaxial. Each person is described in terms of 5 axes:

I. Clinical syndromes
II. Specific developmental disorders (the learning disabilities)
III. Physical disorders and conditions
IV. Severity of psychosocial stressors
V. Highest level of adaptive functioning past year

Most of the categories are primarily descriptive, with no implications regarding known etiology, prognosis, and treatment. In DSM-III there is no assumption that each mental disorder is a discrete entity. Although all persons described as having the same mental disorder show at least the defining features of the disorder, they may well differ in other important ways that may affect clinical management and outcome. The purpose of DSM-III is to provide clearer descriptions of diagnostic categories to enable clinicians and researchers to diagnose, treat, study, and communicate about the various disorders with specific criteria in mind.

Listed below is an abbreviated outline of Axis I disorders from the DSM-III. Selected disorders are considered in detail in the discussion that follows.

- I. Disorders usually first evident in infancy, childhood, or adolescence
  - A. Mental retardation
  - B. Attention deficit disorder
    - 1. With hyperactivity
    - 2. Without hyperactivity
  - C. Conduct disorder
    - 1. Undersocialized or socialized
    - 2. Aggressive or nonaggressive
  - D. Anxiety disorders of childhood or adolescence
    - 1. Separation anxiety disorder (including school phobia)
    - 2. Avoidant disorder of childhood or adolescence
    - 3. Overanxious disorder
  - E. Other disorders of infancy, childhood, or adolescence
    - 1. Reactive attachment disorder of infancy
    - 2. Schizoid disorder of childhood or adolescence
    - 3. Elective mutism
    - 4. Oppositional disorder
    - 5. Identity disorder
  - F. Eating disorders
    - 1. Anorexia nervosa
    - 2. Bulimia
    - 3. Pica
    - 4. Rumination disorder of infancy
    - 5. Atypical eating disorders
  - G. Stereotyped movement disorders
    - 1. Transient tic disorder
    - 2. Chronic motor tic disorder
    - 3. Tourette's disorder
    - 4. Atypical stereotyped movement disorder
  - H. Other disorders with physical manifestations
    - 1. Stuttering
    - 2. Functional enuresis
    - 3. Functional encopresis
    - 4. Sleepwalking disorder
    - 5. Sleep terror disorder
  - I. Pervasive developmental disorders
    - 1. Infantile autism
    - 2. Childhood onset pervasive developmental disorder
    - 3. Atypical pervasive developmental disorder
- II. Substance use disorders
  - A. Drugs
  - B. Alcohol
- III. Schizophrenic disorders
- IV. Paranoid disorders
- V. Psychotic disorders not elsewhere classified
  - A. Schizophreniform disorder
  - B. Brief reactive psychosis
  - C. Schizoaffective disorder
  - D. Atypical psychosis
- VI. Affective disorders
  - A. Major affective disorders
    - 1. Bipolar disorder
      - a. Manic
      - b. Depressed
      - c. Mixed
    - 2. Major depression
  - B. Other specific affective disorders
    - 1. Cyclothymic disorder
    - 2. Dysthymic disorder (or depressive neurosis)
- VII. Anxiety disorders
  - A. Phobic disorders
  - B. Anxiety states
  - C. Post-traumatic stress disorder
- VIII. Somatoform disorders
  - A. Somatization disorder
  - B. Conversion disorder
  - C. Psychogenic pain disorder
  - D. Hypochondriasis
  - E. Atypical somatoform disorder
- IX. Dissociative disorders
  - A. Psychogenic amnesia
  - B. Psychogenic fugue
  - C. Multiple personality
  - D. Depersonalization disorder
  - E. Atypical dissociative disorder
- X. Psychosexual disorders
  - A. Gender identity disorders
  - B. Paraphilias
  - C. Other psychosexual disorders (including ego-dystonic homosexuality)
- XI. Factitious disorders
- XII. Disorders of impulse control not elsewhere classified
- XIII. Adjustment disorders
- XIV. Psychologic factors affecting physical condition

XV. Conditions not attributable to a mental disorder that are a focus of attention or treatment
   A. Malingering
   B. Borderline intellectual functioning
   C. Childhood or adolescent antisocial behavior
   D. Academic problem
   E. Uncomplicated bereavement
   F. Noncompliance with medical treatment
   G. Parent-child problem
   H. Other specified family circumstances
   I. Other interpersonal problem

ATTENTION DEFICIT DISORDER (see also pp. 40 and 41)

The essential features of attention deficit disorder are developmentally inappropriate short attention span and impulsivity. Along with these behaviors, poor concentration and distractibility are usually present. Previously this disorder has been referred to by a variety of names, including hyperkinetic syndrome, hyperactive child syndrome, minimal brain dysfunction, minor cerebral dysfunction, etc. DSM-III uses *attention deficit disorder* (ADD) because attention difficulties are the central and sustaining feature of those children, adolescents, and adults plagued with this disorder. Excessive motor activity (hyperactivity) may or may not be present. If present, hyperactivity tends to be haphazard, poorly organized, and not goal directed.The hyperactive youngster may also become normally active in adolescence even though the underlying attention difficulties persist.

In school, attentional difficulties and impulsivity are evidenced by the child's not staying with tasks and having difficulty organizing and completing work. The work is sloppy and is performed in an impulsive fashion. Group situations are particularly difficult for the child, and attentional difficulties are exaggerated in the classroom, where sustained attention is expected. At home, attentional problems are shown by failure to follow through on parental requests and instructions and by inability to stick to activities, including play, for periods of time appropriate for the child's age. Typically, symptoms of this disorder in any given child vary with the situation and the time. It is the rare child who displays signs of the disorder in all settings, or even in the same setting at all times. The child with ADD is least likely to show his symptomatology in the one-to-one setting of the physician's office.

Associated features vary according to age and may include negativism, bossiness, stubbornness, antisocial behavior, obstinance, bullying, increased mood lability, low frustration tolerance, temper outbursts, low self-esteem, depression, and lack of response to discipline. Often these children have learning disabilities with which one must deal. In addition, "soft" neurologic signs, perceptual-motor dysfunctions, and EEG abnormalities may be present. Academic difficulties are common. Social functioning may be impaired as well. This is a common disorder, with estimates of 3% to 10% of prepubertal children manifesting it. Boys are 5 to 10 times more likely to have the disorder than girls, although girls are more likely to have ADD without hyperactivity. ADD appears to run in some families, with a significant percentage of the parents having had ADD as children and being psychiatrically disturbed as adults (Cantwell, 1972).

Normal overactivity as seen in some children must be differentiated from the haphazard, poorly organized quality in the hyperactive child with this syndrome. Children from disorganized, chaotic, or inadequate home situations may have difficulties in sustaining attention and goal-directed behavior. In such cases it may be difficult, if not impossible, to determine if the disorganized behavior is a result of the chaotic environment, the child's innate psychopathology, or a combination of both. Anxiety disorders may influence attention and motor activity, but a source for the anxiety can usually be found on evaluation. Moreover, as anxiety is reduced, attention and motor activity improve, whereas with ADD symptoms are unrelated to emotional conflict.

Central nervous system stimulants are the current drugs of choice in children with ADD, with or without hyperactivity (Table 4-1). Improvement in behavior occurs in 67% to 75% treated with the stimulants. Worsening can be expected in 5% to 10% (Cantwell, 1977). Satterfield et al. (1974) believe that the stimulants help to restore the central nervous system to a more normal state in which the child can be in control of screening out sensory input and controlling motor responses while permitting a wider range of behavioral patterns. The most common drugs of this category used are dextroamphetamine, methylphenidate, and pemoline. Caf-

Table 4-1. Examples of psychotropic medication for children (2 to 12 years of age)

Name	Indications	Clinical effects	Side effects	Suggested oral dosage range (mg/24 hr)
Neuroleptics (antipsychotics)				
Chlorpromazine (Thorazine)	Psychoses Mental retardation with behavior problems Acute anxiety states	Antipsychotic effects: reduced aggression, activity, excitability, and tics	Extrapyramidal symptoms, dystonic reactions,* dry mouth, drowsiness, seizures, hypersensitive reactions, and restlessness	10-200
Haloperidol (Haldol)	Psychoses Stereotyped movement disorders (Tourette)			0.5-6 (.05 mg/kg/day-0.15 mg/kg/day)
Tricyclics (antidepressants)				
Imipramine (Tofranil)	Depression Nocturnal enuresis School refusal Hyperkinesis	Reduces symptoms of depression and anxiety	Constipation, dry mouth, drowsiness, sweating, ECG findings, and hallucinations	25-100 (3 mg/kg/day)
Amitriptyline (Elavil)	Depression School refusal	Reduces symptoms of depression		25-100
Desipramine (Norpramine)	Depression	Reduces symptoms of depression		25-100
Stimulants				
Dextroamphetamine (Dexedrine)	Attention deficit disorder	Improved concentration and attention; reduced activity	Insomnia, appetite loss, irritability, and stomachaches	5-40
Methylphenidate (Ritalin)	Attention deficit disorder			5-60
Pemoline (Cylert)	Attention deficit disorder			37.5-112.5
Miscellaneous				
Diazepam (Valium)	Somnambulism, pavor nocturnus (night terrors)	Reduces symptoms	Drowsiness, fatigue, ataxia	1-10 h.s.
Diphenhydramine (Benadryl)	Anxiety, insomnia, and acute dystonic* reactions caused by neuroleptics		Dry mouth, hallucinations, and skin rash	25-300 (5 mg/kg/day)
Lithium carbonate	Manic episodes Severe aggression	Controls manic-depressive illness; reduces certain aggressive symptoms	Fine hand tremor, polyuria, mild thirst, nausea, and toxic signs: diarrhea, vomiting, drowsiness, muscular weakness, and incoordination	450-1800 (plasma levels of 0.6 to 1.2 mEq/L)

*For acute dystonic reactions caused by neuroleptics, use diphenhydramine, 25 to 50 mg intramuscularly.

feine has been recommended as a substitute for the psychostimulants (Schnackenberg, 1973), but in controlled, double-blind studies caffeine was not significantly better than placebo in controlling the behavioral manifestations of ADD (Garfinkel et al., 1975; Arnold et al., 1978). Methylphenidate and dextroamphetamine are not significantly different from each other in their ability to control the symptomatology of ADD. Moreover, if one of these medications is not efficacious, the other should be tried because in the Arnold et al. study (1978), a child had almost as good a chance (60%) of responding well to the second of these two stimulants after the first one failed as did another child of responding to the first drug tried (65%). Failure to respond to either drug did not seem to substantially reduce the chance of benefit with the other medication. Pemoline is a longer-acting medication than the other two stimulants and appears to work equally as well (Cantwell, 1977), although long-term clinical trials have not been completed. In deciding on dosage, the goal is to prescribe the smallest dose necessary to get the desired response. A peak enhancement of learning in hyperactive children was found to be at a lower dose than the peak improvement of social behavior (Weiss and Hechtman, 1979). Therefore it is important to target the symptoms one is going to treat before initiating medication. Anorexia, insomnia, headaches, stomachache, nausea, tearfulness, and pallor are common side effects with all the stimulants. Safer and Allen (1975) found that methylphenidate may cause growth inhibition that may persist as long as the medication is given, with possibly a compensatory growth spurt when the medication is stopped. Cantwell (1977) has seen several children who developed mild to moderate depressive episodes in the course of treatment with the short-acting stimulants. These episodes required the cessation or reduction of dosage of stimulant and the use of imipramine to alleviate the depression. No addiction or dependency has been reported with the use of the stimulants for ADD or hyperactivity.

There are some reports that imipramine is effective in 40% to 85% of children with ADD, but after 2 to 3 months the behavior deteriorates again (Cantwell, 1977). The Food and Drug Administration has not approved imipramine for routine use in ADD at this time.

Phenothiazines may be indicated and are more effective than stimulants for certain children. They are not, however, the drugs of first choice. Their potential toxicity is greater than the stimulants and their efficacy is not as well-documented (Cantwell, 1977).

Besides the use of medication in these children, any or all of the intervention approaches discussed below may be necessary for a given child. Individual psychotherapy for the child is indicated for the treatment of the secondary emotional symptoms of depression, low self-esteem, anxiety, and poor peer relationships. Behavior modification is useful in controlling some of the poor classroom and home behavior. Children with significant learning disabilities require specific educational management based on a thorough psychoeducational assessment. Most importantly, the successful management of the child with ADD requires the involvement of his entire family. The family, along with the child, has to be taught the nature and phenomenology of the syndrome. Blame and guilt must be dissipated. The child's environment should be structured so that there are regular daily routines and firm limits on his behavior. Situations known to cause difficulty, overstimulation, and excessive fatigue are to be avoided. The siblings can also be encouraged to act as surrogate therapists, helping the child with ADD gain new skills, increase desirable behavior, and decrease maladaptive behavior. There is no hard scientific evidence to support megavitamin therapy, elimination diets, or hypoglycemic diets as beneficial in the treatment of ADD.

As adolescents, even though the hyperactivity decreases, these children continue to be distractible, emotionally immature, and unable to maintain goals. Failures in school subjects are common, as is juvenile delinquency. However, by adulthood most of these persons have gained control of their impulsiveness and do not commit further delinquent acts (American Academy of Pediatrics Committee on School Health, 1981). The level of functioning as an adult varies with severity of the impairment, which is strongly affected by the home and school environment.

CONDUCT DISORDERS

The essential feature of the conduct disorders as outlined in DSM-III is a repetitive and persistent pattern of conduct in which either the basic rights of others or major age-appropriate societal norms or rules are violated. The behavior is more serious than the ordinary mischief and pranks of children and adolescents. Four attributes designated in DSM-III compose the subtypes: undersocialized, socialized, aggressive, and nonaggressive.

Undersocialized types are characterized by a failure to establish a normal degree of affection, empathy, or bond with others. Appropriate feelings of guilt or remorse are usually absent. The socialized types do show social attachment to others (i.e., gangs), but may be callous and lack guilt when those outside their group are made to suffer.

Aggressive types demonstrate repetitive and persistent patterns of aggressive conduct in which the rights of others are violated by either physical violence against persons or thefts outside the home involving confrontation with a victim. Nonaggressive types are characterized by an absence of conduct in which other people are confronted.

Difficulties at home, at school, and in the community are common, as are smoking, drinking, substance abuse, and precocious sexual activity. Self-esteem is usually poor, although an image of toughness is portrayed. Poor frustration tolerance, irritability, temper outbursts, and recklessness are often present. The child usually blames others for difficulties and does not feel responsible for problems. The child also usually feels unfairly treated and mistrustful of others. Academic performance is usually poor. Attention deficit disorders may or may not be present. The child "gives" only when there is an immediate advantage and does things with the question of "What is in it for me?" Manipulative behavior is common. The person may be sorry when caught in an antisocial act but not sorry for the act itself.

It is thought that parental rejection, inconsistent management with harsh discipline, early institutional living, frequent shifting of parental figures, and being an illegitimate, only child are predisposing factors to the development of the undersocialized type. Predisposing factors for the socialized type include large family size, association with a delinquent subgroup, and an absent father (through divorce, separation, or alcohol abuse). Conduct disorders are more common in children with parents who have antisocial personality disorders or abuse alcohol.

Children or adolescents exhibiting conduct disorders need a thorough evaluation by a child psychiatrist. Other psychiatric illnesses must first be ruled out; then a comprehensive treatment program should be instituted. The earlier these children are identified, the easier they are to treat. Severe forms tend to become chronic, qualifying for the adult diagnosis of antisocial personality disorder, a situation to be avoided if possible. The family's functioning with emotional stability, appropriate child-rearing techniques, and a strong personal commitment on the part of the parental figures are important factors in preventing or eliminating conduct disorders.

ANXIETY DISORDERS

For the child and adolescent age group three subclasses are included in the DSM-III in which anxiety is the predominant characteristic: separation anxiety disorder, avoidant disorder, and overanxious disorder.

In separation anxiety disorder the child manifests excessive anxiety on separation from major attachment figures (mother, grandparent, etc.) or from home or other familiar surroundings. These children may refuse to visit or sleep over at a friend's home, go to camp, or even go to school. In the entity of school phobia the key issue is a separation anxiety between the mother (or less commonly, the father) and the child who are bound tightly in a hostile dependency relationship. These children may refuse to stay alone even in their own bedrooms. They may insist on staying close to the parent, following the parent wherever she may go. Physical complaints are common when separation is anticipated or occurs. When separated from their parents, these children worry about accidents occurring to their parents or to themselves. Concerns about dying are common, as are fears of robbers and kidnappers. These children often have difficulty falling asleep, and nightmares, especially with the theme of separation, may be a recurring problem.

Children with separation anxiety tend to come from caring families that are closely knit. It occurs equally in boys and girls. Usually, the disorder occurs after a specific incident in the child's life, usually a death, an illness, or a move. Through the use of psychotherapy the child and the family are able to come to grips with the underlying concerns manifesting themselves as anxiety.

In the avoidant disorder, the child or adolescent avoids contact with strangers, resulting in problems with social functioning in peer relationships. Yet in the home and with other people the child knows, the relationships are warm and satisfying. These children desire affection and acceptance; their major problem area is meeting new people.

Children suffering from the overanxious disorder worry about most things, especially future events, past behavior, competence in a variety of areas, and things in general. Worries about what other people think are constantly bothering them. These children demand a lot of reassurance about their variety of worries. They are markedly self-conscious and embarrass easily, are usually tense, and cannot relax. Somatic complaints are frequent. This disorder appears more commonly in eldest children, small families, upper socioeconomic groups, and in families in which there is a concern about performance, regardless of the child's level of performance.

DISORDERS WITH PHYSICAL MANIFESTATIONS

Enuresis and encopresis are fairly frequent behavior problems brought to the attention of the physician. Enuresis is the discharge of urine and encopresis is the discharge of feces in places not considered proper for elimination. There are both primary and secondary enuresis and encopresis. Primary enuresis or encopresis refers to a child who has never gained bladder or bowel control either during the day (diurnal) or at night (nocturnal); secondary enuresis or encopresis occurs in a child who had control for a period of time (4 to 6 months) and then started wetting or soiling again.

Enuresis

McLaine (1979) writes that the incidence of enuresis is about 19% of children between the ages of 4 and 5 years and decreases with increasing age (8% at age 8 and 5% at age 10). About 1% to 2% of adolescents remain enuretic. Enuresis is seen more often in boys and in children with a positive family history. Enuresis is primary in about 75% of cases. About 80% of enuretic children have nocturnal enuresis alone, 5% have diurnal enuresis alone, and 15% have both nocturnal and diurnal enuresis. About 15% of enuretic children also have encopresis, whereas about 25% of the children with encopresis also have enuresis. According to Leventhal (1981), secondary enuresis occurs commonly in school-age children; 5% to 20% of children who were dry at age 5 years relapse before age 11 years. Diurnal enuresis, especially if it is secondary, is considered a more serious problem than nocturnal enuresis, and physical as well as psychologic factors should be considered.

After all organic causes for the enuresis have been eliminated, the question of treatment arises. Major treatment methods include behavior modification, bladder training, medication, and counseling. Regardless of the treatment regimen, the child must want to stop wetting and want to take an active interest in the treatment.

Behavior modification can involve either positive or negative reinforcement; the former is usually more successful. Putting a star or stickers on the calendar to signify nights when the bed is kept dry is very encouraging to children.

In another approach to behavior modification, an alarm awakens the child who wets the bed. The initial aim of this treatment is to awaken the child as soon as urination begins; the ultimate goal is to have the child awaken before voiding. The alarm system works best in children over 7 years of age and probably should not be used in children under 5 years.

Bladder training or stretching is a way of increasing the functional capacity of the bladder. The child is told to drink as much as possible during the day and to hold his urine for increasing lengths of time, up to a maximum of 30 to 40 minutes. Once a day the child should hold his urine as long as possible, and the voided urine should be measured. With bladder capacities above 240 to 360 ml, bed-wetting may stop.

Imipramine hydrochloride (1 to 3 mg/kg one-half hour before bedtime) has been shown to be effective in helping children stop bed-wetting (McLain, 1979). Its mechanism of action is unknown, although there has been much speculation. The major drawback to this approach is that when the imipramine is discontinued a large percentage of children start wetting again. The side effects are mostly caused by the

Table 4-2. Treatment protocol for encopresis

Treatment phase	Treatment program	Comments
Initial counseling	1. Education and "demystification" of the problem 2. Removal of blame 3. Establishment and explanation of treatment plan	Include drawings, review of colonic function, shared observation of x-rays; emphasize need for intestinal "muscle-building"
Initial catharsis Inpatient	1. High normal saline enemas (750 ml bid) 3 to 7 days 2. Biscodyl (Dulcolax) suppositories bid, 3 to 7 days 3. Use of bathroom for 15 minutes each meal	Patient admitted when: 1. retention is very severe 2. home compliance likely to be poor 3. parents prefer admission 4. parental administration of enemas is inadvisable psychologically
At home	1. For moderate to severe retention, 3 or 4 cycles as follows: a. Day 1. Hypophosphate enemas (Fleet's adult) twice b. Day 2. Biscodyl (Dulcolax) suppositories twice c. Day 3. Biscodyl (Dulcolax) tablet once 2. For mild retention, senna or danthron; one tablet daily for 1 to 2 weeks.	1. Dosages or frequency may need alteration if child experiences excessive discomfort 2. Admission should be considered if there is inadequate yield
	Follow-up abdominal X-ray to confirm adequate catharsis	
Maintenance	1. Child sits on toilet twice a day at same times each day for 10 minutes each time 2. Light mineral oil (at least 2 tablespoons) twice a day usually for at least 4 to 6 months 3. Multiple vitamins, 2 a day, between mineral oil doses 4. High roughage diet, usually bran cereal 5. In severe cases use of an oral laxative (senna or danthrone) for 2 to 3 weeks, then alternate days for 1 month (given between mineral oil doses)	1. A kitchen timer may be helpful 2. A chart with stars for sitting may be good for children under 7 3. Bathroom reading encouraged 4. Mineral oil may be put in juice or Coke or any other medium 5. Vitamins to compensate for alleged problems with absorption secondary to mineral oil 6. Diet should be applied, but not to the point of coercion
Follow-up	1. Visits every 4 to 10 weeks, depending on severity, need for support, compliance, and associated symptoms 2. Telephone availability to adjust doses when needed 3. In case of relapse: a. check compliance b. use of oral laxative (e.g., Senokot) for 1 to 2 weeks c. adjust dosage of mineral oil 4. Counseling and/or referral for associated psychosocial and developmental issues	1. Duration of treatment program may be as long as 2 to 3 years or as short as 6 months 2. Signs of relapse: a. excessive oil leakage b. large caliber stools c. abdominal pain d. decreased frequency of defecation e. soiling 3. Physician should spend time alone with the child 4. In cases slow to respond, physician should sustain optimism: persistence cures almost all cases (eventually)

Modified from Levine, M.D.: Pediatr. Rev. **2**:285, 1981.
All dosages and frequencies are for an average-sized 7-year-old child. Appropriate adjustments should be made for smaller and larger patients.

drug's anticholinergic properties: irritability, dry mouth, sleep disturbances, constipation, tachycardia, orthostatic hypotension, urinary retention, and blurred vision.

Counseling is usually done in conjunction with the above-mentioned treatments by the treating physician. If serious psychopathology is suspected, referral to an appropriate person for evaluation and therapy is indicated.

Encopresis (see also p. 350)

The incidence of encopresis is approximately 1.5%, with a male-to-female ratio of 6:1 (Bellman, 1966). Encopresis may or may not be associated with constipation. If constipation is present, prolonged retention of stool leads to impaction, rectal distention, loss of bowel tone, and finally, functional megacolon. The large amount of stool in the rectum produces a partially dilated anal sphincter with subsequent overflow soiling (intermittent leakage of liquid stool and mucus flowing around the impaction).

Evaluation involves a complete history, including psychosocial factors and physical examination. When the incontinence is clearly deliberate, antisocial and other psychopathologic features are common. Smearing the feces may be deliberate and has to be differentiated from the accidental smearing that takes place as the child tries to hide feces passed involuntarily.

Treatment includes emptying the colon of any retained stool, keeping the stools soft, and training the child in regular bowel habits. In encopresis in which stools of normal caliber are passed without evidence of constipation, a behavioral approach is recommended, such as using the star chart for positive reinforcement. In the case of chronic impaction with stool withholding and overflow soiling, many different approaches have been used in dealing with this problem of emptying the bowel and keeping it empty while the child learns proper bowel habits. Levine (1982) outlines an effective treatment protocol for this type of encopresis, in Table 4-2. Encopresis has a fairly high relapse rate. If significant resistance is met in the child or family regarding treatment, or if psychosocial problems appear to be at the root of the encopresis, referral to a psychiatrist is in order (Table 4-2).

SLEEP DISORDERS

Sleep disturbances such as nocturnal enuresis, nightmares, night terrors, sleepwalking, and sleeptalking begin in the preschool years. Excluding nightmares, these conditions are classified as non-REM (NREM) dyssomnias and are associated with emergence from Stage 3-4 NREM sleep. A child may experience two or more of these disorders at different times. Often there is a positive family history. The disorders are paroxysmal, characterized by nonresponsiveness to the environment. The child's actions appear automatic, and retrograde amnesia is present for the episode (Guilleminault and Anders, 1976).

Night terrors (pavor nocturnus) and nightmares must be differentiated, as their treatment and course differ. Table 4-3 compares these two phenomena on several variables.

In night terrors the child abruptly sits up with a panicky scream, is inconsolable, and cannot be awakened. There is increased autonomic discharge, with tachycardia and tachypnea. These episodes, which can last for 1 to 20 minutes, disturb the parents more than the child,

Table 4-3. Comparison of nightmares and night terrors

	Nightmares	Night terrors
Stage of sleep	REM	Stage 3-4 NREM
Amount of anxiety	+ +	+ + +
Amount of autonomic discharge	+	+ + +
Amount of motility	+	+ + +
Amount of vocalization	±	+ + +
Amnesia	No	Yes
Ability to be awakened	Easy	Difficult
Person most disturbed by the episode	Child	Parent(s)

Modified from Wasserman, A.: Common behavioral disorders of childhood. In Gottlieb, M., editor: Concise textbook of developmental pediatrics, New York, Medical Examination Publishing Co., Inc. (in press).

who doesn't remember anything the following morning. The DSM-III points out that episodes of sleep terror are more likely if the person is fatigued, has experienced a stress, or has taken a bedtime dose of a tricyclic antidepressant or neuroleptic.

Essential features of sleepwalking are repeated episodes of arising from bed during sleep and walking about for several minutes to half an hour. Guilleminault and Anders (1976) estimate that 15% of all children between the ages of 5 and 12 years have walked in their sleep at least once. Sleeptalking may occur during sleepwalking, but the speech is usually a mumble and makes little sense. Parents need to protect the child from hurting himself. Purposeful walking and speech during sleep time, unlike the NREM syndromes discussed above, suggest psychologic disorders, and a more intensive evaluation is in order.

PERVASIVE DEVELOPMENTAL DISORDERS

The DSM-III gives the characteristics of pervasive developmental disorders as *distortions* in the development of multiple basic psychologic functions that are involved in the development of social skills and language, such as attention, perception, reality testing, and motor movement. Many basic areas of psychologic development are affected at the same time and to a severe degree. The qualitative abnormalities that these children display are not normal for any stage of development. Included under this heading are infantile autism, childhood onset pervasive developmental disorder, and the atypical pervasive developmental disorder.

The diagnostic criteria for infantile autism, as outlined in DSM-III, are onset before 30 months of age; pervasive lack of responsiveness to other people (autism); gross deficits in language development; if speech is present, peculiar speech patterns such as immediate and delayed echolalia, metaphoric language, pronominal reversal; bizarre responses to various aspects of the environment (e.g., resistance to change, peculiar interest in or attachments to animate or inanimate objects). Delusions, hallucinations, loosening of associations, and incoherence, which occur in schizophrenia, do not occur in infantile autism.

Other aspects of autism include disturbances in responses to sensory stimuli (hyperreactivity or hyporeactivity); disturbances in the capacity to relate appropriately to people, objects, or events; resistance to learning or practicing a new activity; stereotyped movements; unusual fears; difficulties in feeding and sleeping; temper tantrums; and self-abuse. Autism is associated with lower intelligence; three fourths of autistic children have an IQ less than 70 (Stewart and Gath, 1978).

In evaluation there will be minimal eye contact, little or no evidence of meaningful play, and a history of lack of cuddliness. Cooperative play and friendships do not exist. As the child gets older, some attachment to significant people may develop, but will be of a superficial, immature quality. The physical appearance of the child is often normal, with relatively intact gross motor abilities. Development of unusual "scatter skills" is common—islands of normality with isolated, nonfunctional skills such as memory for insignificant past events or reading words without comprehension. Mood is often labile. The child may lack appreciation for dangerous situations (heights, fire, motor vehicles, etc.). Lack of speech development by 5 years of age indicates a poor prognosis.

Autism is rare (2 to 4 cases per 10,000). It is three times more common in boys than in girls. Predisposing factors include maternal rubella, phenylketonuria, encephalitis, meningitis, and tuberous sclerosis. Family dynamics and parental personality structures do not seem to affect the development of autism. However, siblings have an increased risk (2%) of being autistic (Stewart and Gath, 1978).

In mental retardation there are often behavior abnormalities similar to those seen in infantile autism (autistic-like); however, the full syndrome is not present. The mentally retarded child shows flat developmental delays in all areas related to intellectual functioning and slow gradual progress to a plateau. These children will demonstrate responses to sensory inputs, people, and objects appropriate to their level of intellectual function. In infantile autism, uneven, fragmented intellectual development is present. The autistic youngster does much better on manipulative or visual-spatial skills and recent memory than on verbal skills, especially those requiring logical or abstract thinking.

Specific language disabilities must be ruled out because such children may show autistic-like behaviors. There are two major subtypes of the developmental dysphasias: receptive type (difficulty in comprehending oral language) and expressive type (difficulty in expressing verbal language). However, these children show evidence of an "inner language" with gesturing and imitations to communicate. No disturbance in relatedness or in response to sensory inputs is present.

Heller disease (infantile dementia) needs to be distinguished from autism. Here the child has normal development for the first 2 years of life. At a specific time of onset a progressively downhill course starts, with motor restlessness and loss of speech at about 4 to 5 years old. The EEG is abnormal and there is an increase in plasma and spinal fluid lipids.

Painstaking behavior treatments do seem to improve self-help and social skills in autistic children. The brighter children also gain in language development and formal education through use of behavior methods. Psychotropic medications have been tried, but no one drug seems to help the overall disability of autism.

Some autistic children eventually are able to lead independent lives, with only minimal signs of the essential features of the disorder but still show social awkwardness and ineptness. In general, one sixth make an adequate social adjustment and are able to hold a regular job by adulthood, one sixth make a fair adjustment, and the remainder are severely handicapped and unable to lead independent lives. IQ and the development of language skills are the major factors related to long-term adaptation.

The diagnostic criteria for childhood onset pervasive developmental disorder includes: (1) gross and sustained impairment in social relationships, (2) onset of the full syndrome after 30 months of age but before 12 years of age, (3) absence of delusions, hallucinations, incoherence, or marked loosening of associations, and (4) at least three of the following: (a) sudden excessive anxiety, (b) constricted or inappropriate affect, (c) resistance to change in the environment, (d) oddities of motor movement, (e) abnormalities of speech, (f) hypersensitivity or hyposensitivity to sensory stimuli, and (g) self-mutilation.

The disturbance in social relations may include lack of appropriate affective responsivity, inappropriate clinging, asociality, lack of empathy, and lack of peer relationships. These disturbances prevail over time. Bizarre ideas and fantasies, often of a morbid nature, are common. Some children may become preoccupied with a given object. Childhood onset pervasive developmental disorder is more common in males than females. Although the prognosis is guarded, it is probably better than in infantile autism.

The diagnosis of an atypical subtype of pervasive developmental disorders is reserved for children with developmental distortions in basic psychologic functions resulting in problems with social skills and language who cannot be classified as having either autism or childhood onset developmental disorders.

SCHIZOPHRENIA

The onset of schizophrenic disorders is usually during adolescence or early adulthood. Generally, onset is insidious, with a decline in school performance as disordered thinking appears. Language may become incoherent in form, and the content of thought may become delusional. Various types of delusions may be present, including thoughts of being controlled by others or by outside forces, ideas of reference in which unrelated events are given personal significance, and the belief that others can hear one's thoughts. Hallucinations are the main disturbances in perception. Auditory hallucinations are more common, but tactile and somatic hallucinations are occasionally present. If visual, gustatory, or olfactory hallucinations occur, the question of an identifiable intracranial process or toxic reaction should be examined.

The expressed or observed emotion (affect) is blunted or inappropriate. For example, the patient may laugh or smile while describing how he is being persecuted. He may become preoccupied and withdrawn, with serious disturbances in interpersonal relationships. Premorbid personality disorders may be evident and are often described as paranoid, introverted, or borderline. After the initial episode the symptoms may subside, but a complete return to the premorbid personality is unlikely. The illness is chronic and recurrent but can be helped significantly with psychiatric treatment, including medication and a supportive life-style. The physician must be especially supportive to the parent who suffers from schizophrenia and other major mental disorders to provide a protective influence for the vulnerable children.

Schizophrenia occurs in all parts of the world in about 1% of the population and is equally common in men and women. Genetic factors are important in that the disorder has a higher prevalence in biologically related family members. However, nongenetic factors are noted to be important, as indicated by the relatively low concordance rate, even in monozygotic twins.

TOXIC PSYCHOSIS

Disorientation to time, person, and place with loss of recent memory, along with visual hallucinations, are hallmarks of a toxic psychosis. Hallucinations of a toxic condition tend to be self-orienting. The patient may refer to the hospital as his home and to the nurse as a relative. A central feature is a disturbance of the ability to sustain attention even to such activities as watching television. Onset is sudden and may be related to trauma, illness, fever, or drug ingestion. A history should always be obtained from a relative or close acquaintance. The patient may be agitated, hyperalert, or hypoalert and may show increased or decreased motor activity and signs of autonomic arousal such as dilated pupils, flushed face, sweating, elevated systolic blood pressure, and tachycardia. Symptoms tend to be fluctuating rather than fixed, with cognitive impairment more marked at night or in the dark, and communication more lucid in the morning. The duration of a toxic psychosis is brief, averaging one week.

Drug screening tests of blood and urine, plus a careful physical examination, may reveal the cause if drug abuse has occurred. Involuntary movements, especially coarse tremors, are the most common neurologic signs. Difficulty in naming objects and impaired writing ability may be present. A normal EEG helps to rule out toxic psychosis, in conjunction with information gathered from the history, physical examination, and mental status. If toxic psychosis is present or highly suspected, no medication should be given. Physical restraints are in order if the patient is agitated and will not respond to talking with a person who is constantly at his side.

NONTOXIC PSYCHOSES

If a child has psychotic agitation and a toxic etiology has been ruled out, then chemical restraint is preferable. Chlorpromazine (Thorazine) may be given intramuscularly—1 mg/kg to a total of 50 mg. Precautions to avoid orthostatic hypotension should be taken by having the patient remain horizontal and by having the blood pressure and other vital signs carefully monitored. Oral antipsychotic medication may be started concomitantly. Many antipsychotic medications are available; they are also known as neuroleptics, or major tranquilizers.

In all children with a psychosis, medication is symptomatic treatment. The target symptoms in the pervasive developmental disorders are the self-injurious, overly aggressive, and ritualistic self-stimulating behaviors and stereotyped movements that interfere with learning and socialization. Those children who are withdrawn and without speech need stimulation, not sedation, to aid learning. Haloperidol is another widely used and effective medication in patients with a psychotic disorder. Table 4-1 summarizes the use of psychotropic medication. Dosage should be started at low levels and gradually increased in divided doses. Chlorpromazine has more sedative-hypnotic qualities than does haloperidol, which is somewhat more stimulating. Dextroamphetamine and methylphenidate are contraindicated in psychotic children. In older children, antipsychotic medication is aimed at decreasing hallucinations and delusions and in helping to integrate thinking so that learning may progress.

Medication is only one part of a multimodality treatment program that includes day and hospital programs in which special education has a central role. Behavioral management techniques are both helpful and supportive. Family therapy may be exploratory or supportive, and supportive individual psychotherapy should be offered.

AFFECTIVE DISORDERS

The essential feature of affective disorders is a disturbance of mood. The illness involves either a manic episode or a depressive episode, or both, and is often cyclic. Affective disorders (manic-depressive disorders) may reach psychotic proportions in the manic phase or depressive phase (although most depressions are not that severe). However, the disorders may initially occur as primarily manic or depressive, rather than cyclic. These disorders have been rarely described in younger children but have been increasingly diagnosed in adolescents. In this chapter, depression will be described separately from manic and manic-depressive episodes.

Manic episodes

Episodes of mania are characterized by euphoria and expansiveness, increased psychomotor activity, irritability and aggressiveness, distractibility, flight of ideas, and loss of sleep. Hypersexuality and use of bizarre clothing may be symptoms. The features of schizophrenic thought disorder are absent. The groups of symptoms appear as a complex of behaviors occurring with increasing frequency after puberty, and may or may not reach psychotic proportions. Mania is rarely identified before puberty. However, it has been suggested that the specific behaviors of explosive anger and hostility, poor attention span and distractibility, lying, stealing, fire-setting, and extreme recurrent mood swings in younger children are the equivalent of mania and respond to lithium carbonate as in older patients (DeLong, 1978). Symptoms in the form of shifting emotional states, unusual tension and anxiety, hyperactivity, irritability, inflated self-esteem, and decreased need for sleep have been reported before puberty and suggest a predisposition to manic-depressive disease.

A positive family history of manic-depressive illness should alert the clinician to evaluate the child carefully. It is likely that manic episodes have been misdiagnosed as hyperactivity because of the apparent difficulty in differentiating the disorders. Case reports of adolescents who subsequently develop manic-depressive illness have revealed earlier diagnoses of hyperactivity or hyperkinesis. Ongoing clinical studies will be helpful in identifying the disorder and studying family histories and the response to medication.

Lithium carbonate is widely known to be effective in the treatment of certain manic-depressive disorders in adults, and has been shown to be useful in treating children and adolescents (Annell, 1969; Feinstein and Wolpert, 1973). Studies using lithium in the treatment of children with ADD with hyperactivity have not demonstrated effectiveness (Greenhill, *et al,* 1973). It is important to note that blood lithium levels and thyroid and renal function need regular monitoring when lithium is prescribed. Antipsychotic medication may be added if the mania reaches psychotic proportions.

Campbell and Shapiro (1975) outline a recommended treatment schedule for use of lithium in children over age 3. The starting dose is 450 mg/24 hrs, with weekly increases of 250 to 300 mg until a therapeutic response is reached or to a maximum of 1800 mg/24 hrs. Plasma levels of lithium are maintained within the range of 0.6 to 1.2 mEq/l. Specific laboratory studies before and during lithium maintenance include complete blood count, hematocrit, urinalysis, blood urea nitrogen (BUN), thyroxin iodine level, free-thyroxin level, and electrocardiogram (ECG).

Depressive episodes

Depression is defined as a low mood accompanied by feelings of sadness, despair, and unhappiness. It is a universally experienced, normal feeling state, as seen in a grief reaction. As a diagnosis or component of illness, depression will have the clinical manifestations of a dysphoric mood with the appearance of sadness, loss of interest, irritability, and self-deprecatory ideation, including feelings of worthlessness, guilt, and suicidal thoughts. Agitated aggressive behavior may be present along with sleep disturbance, change in attitude toward school, lowered school performance, and diminished socialization. Somatic complaints of pain are frequently present, as well as a loss of usual energy and a change in appetite, with recent weight loss or gain. In prepubertal children, separation anxiety may develop and be seen in the clinging of the child to the parent, school avoidance, and fears that the parents or child will die. Negativistic or antisocial behavior may be present. Antisocial presentation is more frequent in boys and in older children. Adolescents with depressed feelings may be restless, irritable, uncooperative, aggressive, sulky, withdrawn, and have feelings of wanting to leave home. Inattention to personal appearance, difficulties in school, and instances of alcohol or drug use are common. It is widely thought that of the adolescents who abuse drugs about one third are depressed, one third are experimenting, and one third have character disorders.

Following is a diagnostic classification of depressive syndromes in childhood and adolescence, organized according to developmental stage, beginning with infancy:

- Infancy
  - Anaclitic depression or reactive attachment disorder of infancy
- Childhood
  - Acute depressive reaction
  - Chronic depression
  - Masked depression
- Adolescence
  - Primary depression
    - Unipolar (no episode of mania)
    - Bipolar (manic-depressive, at least one episode of mania)
  - Secondary depression
  - Atypical depression

Depression in infancy. Anaclitic (a leaning on) depression or reactive attachment disorder of infancy is a severe reaction to maternal and stimulation deprivation that was first described by Spitz (1946). He observed that mature, healthy babies who were separated from their mothers in the second half of the first year of life and did not have adequate stimulation became apprehensive with frequent crying and insomnia. They began to refuse food, resulting in weight loss or failure to gain. The babies became withdrawn and fixed to the center of the bed, with staring and lack of smiling. Similar clinical pictures have been reported in monkey infants who were systematically submitted to similar early traumatic events. The infants progressed through the stages of protest, despair, and detachment. Questions remain about the complete reversibility of such a severe state as detachment, and the development of later psychopathology. Although it is rare to see this disorder in the severe form today, some cases of "failure to thrive" are similar. The clinician should be alert to identifying the characteristics because they may be missed early on. Treatment is to stop the pathologic process and provide supplemental caregiving.

Acute depressive reactions in childhood. Acute depressive reactions in children frequently follow a stressful and traumatic life event. However, because it frequently goes unrecognized, delays in referral for medical care may be 2 or 3 months after the onset of the depression. The child usually has a history of normal adjustment; the family has only mild psychopathology and no history of depressive illness.

Chronic depression in childhood. Chronic depression indicates the child has had previous episodes of depression and a marginal premorbid adjustment. Often one parent will have recurrent depressive illness and the child will have had early life separation experiences with loss of significant people. In children under age 6, a depressed mood may have to be inferred from a persistently sad facial expression.

Masked depression in childhood. Masked depression may appear in the course of depressive illness in childhood. Many clinicians object to the concept of acting-out behavior masking depression and insist that true depression is present but not observed. In the history the clinician may identify depressive symptoms, especially the appearance of sadness, which may have become pervasive. Subsequently, hyperactivity, aggressive behavior, and even delinquency may develop. Hypochondriasis and psychosomatic illness are common in these children. Diagnosis of masked depression may be made by observing or identifying by history a periodic purely depressive picture and using projective testing techniques. This clinical entity should always be considered in the differential diagnosis of hyperkinesis or ADD. Accurate diagnosis of depression will lead to more effective use of proper medication and psychiatric counseling.

Primary unipolar and bipolar depression. Primary depression in adolescence has been described in two forms. Unipolar depression refers to single or recurrent episodes of depression with no episodes of mania. The onset of unipolar depression tends to be earlier, and the persons affected have a higher premorbid emotional instability. The bipolar (manic-depressive) patient will have had at least one episode of mania. This condition is associated with a history of depression in female family members. Genetically, bipolar illness has been shown to be X-linked on the Xga locus. Thus a mother may pass it on to a son or daughter, whereas a father may pass it on only to his daughters. The distinction between unipolar and bipolar depression is essential because the use of specific medication follows from the diagnosis. Lithium carbonate is specifically useful in bipolar illness, primarily the manic phase, but has not been shown to be substantially beneficial in unipolar depression.

Secondary depression. Secondary depression has the same signs and symptoms as does primary depression but is superimposed on a serious physical illness or a preexisting psychiatric illness (nondepressive).

Atypical depression. Atypical depression of adolescence has an earlier onset, a less remitting chronicity, and premorbid psychiatric difficulties. More irritability and interpersonal discord is present. On long-term follow-up, clinical reports reveal that many of this atypical group develop severe personality disorders and major mental illnesses. However, no definitive systematic studies have been done.

Diagnosis and treatment. In considering a differential diagnosis for depressive syndromes in childhood and adolescence, the clinician should always take a careful three-generational family history. As pointed out by Akiskal and McKinney (1975), major depressive disorders result from the interaction and integration of several factors, including physiologic stressors, genetic predisposition, psychosocial stressors, and developmental predisposition. Biochemical studies have demonstrated a decrease in brain catecholamines (norepinephrine) and indoleamines (serotonin) in depression.

A diagnostic aid in determining depression is the Dexamethasone Suppression Test (DST). The overnight DST was developed originally as a screening test for patients with Cushing disease. When hypersecretion of cortisol was identified also in patients with severe depression, the DST was studied in this population as well. Many reports have confirmed that patients with depression have abnormal DST results (Carroll et al., 1981).

The recommended protocol for the DST in psychiatric practice calls for oral administration of 1 mg dexamethasone in tablet form at 11 PM for postpubertal patients and ½ mg for prepubertal patients. The next day, blood samples for plasma cortisol are drawn at 4 PM and 11 PM. An elevated plasma cortisol concentration in either blood sample signifies an abnormal or positive test result. The criterion plasma cortisol concentration is 5 μg/dl with good radioimmunoassays.

With this procedure the sensitivity of the DST for depression (true-positive rate) is about 65% and the specificity (true-negative rate) is about 95%. Based on these results, an abnormal DST result will carry a high diagnostic confidence (predictive value) for depression. However, a negative test result will not rule out the diagnosis of depression.

The medications most successful in treatment are the tricyclic antidepressants (Table 4-1). Their action is thought to inhibit the reuptake of such neurotransmitters as norepinephrine and thus to increase available norepinephrine at the neuroreceptor site. Studies revealing these findings have been largely in adults. Currently, research is under way with adolescents and children.

Treatment for depression involves multiple modalities, including varying degrees of individual, family, and group psychotherapy and active socioenvironmental therapy on an outpatient or inpatient basis, as indicated. The pediatrician or family physician has an essential role to play in the prevention, early identification, prompt referral for consultation, ongoing management, and follow-up of these disorders. Treatment failure at all ages often results in suicide attempts and death.

SUICIDE (see also p. 110)

Suicide is one of the leading causes of death among young people. All suicide thoughts and attempts should be regarded as expressions of unhappiness and viewed as a cry for help. Peak ages for suicide are in the late teenage years and after age 45 years. Girls attempt suicide more often than boys, but boys are three times as successful in accomplishing suicide. In the under-12 age group, the most frequently chosen method in successful suicides is hanging by boys and drug overdose by girls. Above age 12, the method of choice by boys and girls is to use firearms. Children and adolescents who have a chronic physical or mental illness are at high risk. Family history of suicide and depression, as well as family problems and pressures, should alert the clinician to the seriousness of the attempt and the potential for further attempts. A frequent precipitating event is a family crisis, in which parents or school will show an overly rigid response to antisocial behavior common to adolescent development. Many successful suicides occur in those who are highly competitive in academics and find frustration or failure unacceptable. Social isolation is ominous. Return to school with a normal attendance pattern is a predictor of good outcome.

To evaluate a suicide attempt or suicide potential, the following procedures should be helpful:

I. In a suicide attempt, take a brief history and do a full physical examination to confirm the complaint and to evaluate the physical status of the patient. Begin management for coma, psychosis, delirium, drug ingestion, or trauma when indicated.

II. If the patient needs no physical management or necessary measures have been completed, evaluate for necessity of psychiatric admission (with or without a psychiatric consultation).

   A. Evaluation of a suicide attempt usually requires presence of both parents. All family members should be interviewed together and separately. Any person currently involved in the patient's care should be contacted. Also, if recent events are not clear, friends or other family members may have to be contacted. Social service will be helpful in facilitating this part of the evaluation.

   B. The following basic information should be gathered, in most cases by the physician from the family and the patient. This will take approximately 30 minutes.

      1. Inquire about any present or previous care for physical, emotional, or social problems. What is the current relationship to any helping person and how well did the family cooperate? Characterize previous suicide plans or attempts.
      2. Find the exact method and time of an attempt. Inquire about a suicide note, communication with anyone, exact location of the attempt, chance of being found, and the patient's knowledge of the lethality of the method.
      3. Evaluate the patient's motivation. Specifically, does the patient have a wish to die? If so, what are the reasons and what are the expectations after death for self and loved ones? If the patient did not wish to die, what are the expectations from an attempt? Has there been a recent loss, especially the death of a family member? Has there been the anniversary of a past loss? Has there been a recent loss of a boyfriend or girlfriend or sibling (to school or army, etc.)? Is there illness in the family? Is the patient pregnant or afraid of being pregnant?
      4. Evaluate the mental status of the patient. Observe agitation or motor retardation. Note affect, especially anxiety, about the attempt and the extent of depression. Any evidence of psychosis is ominous. Note the presence of psychotic or illogical thoughts, especially paranoia. To help rule out mild delirium, observe the state of consciousness. Is there restlessness, disorientation, memory loss, agitation, fearfulness, hallucinations, or affective lability?
      5. Evaluate the resources available to the child outside the hospital. Note in general how the family responds. Are they ambivalent about the child? Does the family wish to be rid of the child? Does anger or concern predominate? Are they willing to seek help? Are they aware of the seriousness of the situation? Is there family history of suicide, divorce, or mental illness? Are there current marital problems?
      6. Evaluate internal resources of the patient. Find out about performance at school. Note any delinquent behavior or arrest. Record previous mental health services. Inquire whether there are any close friends. Social isolation is the most reliable single differentiation between successful and attempted suicides. Note the parent's attitude toward the family. Characterize any recent personality change.

III. Determine need for consultation with a child psychiatrist.

ANOREXIA NERVOSA
(see also pp. 107 to 108)

Cases of anorexia nervosa appear to be increasing. In 1976, Crisp et al. found anorexia nervosa in 1% of 16- to 18-year-old female British students. In addition to increased incidence, increased awareness of this syndrome has also played a role in bringing more of these cases to treatment. Maloney and Klykylo (1983) believe that anorexia nervosa appears to be reaching epidemic proportions in upper socioeconomic-level girls. The analogue to anorexia in the upper socioeconomic boys may be "obligatory running" (Yates et al., 1983).

Essential features of anorexia nervosa as outlined in DSM-III are intense fear of becoming obese, disturbance of body image, significant weight loss, refusal to maintain a minimal normal body weight, and amenorrhea. The usual age of onset is early to late adolescence. Anorectic children under age 12 and over age 18 at time of onset tend to be atypical in symptomatology; they also carry a more serious prognosis.

Anorexia is a misnomer because the girls are usually preoccupied with thoughts of food and are denying their hunger. They willingly refuse to eat in "a pursuit of thinness," "weight phobia," or "fear of fatness." The typical patient is a white, middle-to-upper-class female (10% are male) who has a history of being overweight, started dieting, but was unable to stop losing even when her normal weight was attained. The typical anorectic patient is preoccupied with physical exercise and will push herself beyond the usual limits of endurance. The main types of anorexia nervosa are related to the age of the patient, as follows: (1) anorectic patients who diet and abstain from food, age 10 to 14 years; (2) anorectic patients who binge and vomit, age 19 to 30 years; and (3) anorectic patients who abstain from food for a period, then binge, then either vomit or abstain from food again, age 15 to 18 years.

Besides the amenorrhea caused by anorexia, approximately 25% of the patients develop amenorrhea before the weight loss occurs (Vande Wiele, 1977). Other symptoms include constipation, often with complaints of abdominal pain, disturbed sleep, cold intolerance with disturbance of shivering, syncope, agitation or lethargy, sensitivity to noise, and vomiting. Physical findings comprise the following: cachexia, dry or scaly skin, increased lanugo-like body hair, bradycardia, hypotension, hypercarotenemic skin, peripheral edema, hypothermia, acrocyanosis, petechiae, and hair loss. Laboratory findings include decreased thyroid function test values, abnormalities in cortisol and growth hormone secretion, decreased gonadotropins, hypercarotenemia, other evidence of hypothalamic dysfunction, elevation of blood urea nitrogen, abnormal glucose tolerance test, leukopenia (with or without anemia), abnormal ECG, and hypoplastic bone marrow. Some other problems seen in anorexia nervosa are gastric ulcers (Kline, 1979), sucrose sensitivity (Lacey et al., 1977), and the superior mesenteric artery syndrome (Sours and Vorhaus, 1981). Psychologic problems such as fatigue, depression, apathy, and withdrawal, in addition to cognitive disturbances, occur secondary to the starvation itself. A number of investigators suggest that depression is an integral part of this disorder (Bruch, 1973; Crisp, 1977).

Treatment of anorexia nervosa is multidimensional. The patient's failing physiologic functions must be supported. If the weight loss is 25% or more of the premorbid weight, hospitalization is usually indicated. Electrolyte imbalance needs to be corrected. Nutritional balance must be restored and sufficient weight gain must be generated to allow for independent function. Tube feeding or parenteral hyperalimentation may be necessary if the girl continues to refuse to eat.

Most workers in the field of anorexia nervosa use a combination of nutritional supplementation, behavior modification, and supportive and insight-oriented psychotherapy. Psychologic support and reorganization of pathologic behavior patterns are necessary so that nutritional and psychosocial adjustments are maintained even after weight gain has stabilized and psychotherapy is no longer necessary. Therapy can be done either as an inpatient or as an outpatient. Usually there is a combination of inpatient and outpatient work because therapy continues after hospitalization to make sure the advances made during the hospitalization continue.

Besides individual psychotherapy, group therapy, family therapy, and work with the parents (either as a couple or as individuals) are methods that have proved to be very effective. Psychotropic drugs are sometimes employed, although most anorectic patients will refuse to take drugs. The drugs used include antidepressants, chlorpromazine, diphenylhydantoin, and some experimental drugs. Electroconvulsive therapy, insulin shock, and leukotomy have been used with varying degrees of success.

The typical features of the families of anorectic children, as outlined by Minuchin et al. (1978), are as follows: mothers—perfectionistic, at odds with themselves in terms of achievement and competence; fathers—seductive, sometimes withdrawn, aloof from the family; family organization—built around fragility, hurt, and pain from failure and disappointment, seeks perfection and relies heavily on maintaining external appearances as a means of hiding weaknesses and maintaining an appealing front. Rules for the family are established and rigorously followed. Emotions are not to be expressed, and aggression is suppressed and hidden. Any transgression results in disgust and tension.

Drossman et al. (1979) outline the psychologic, behavioral, and perceptual features seen in anorexia nervosa. Psychologically, there is no predominant psychiatric diagnosis. Features of depression, anxiety, and obsessional thoughts may exist. There is lowered self-esteem and social anxiety. Average intelligence is present but overachievement and perfectionism exist. A number of workers, however, feel that anorexia nervosa is a primary affective disorder (Barcai, 1977; Cantwell et al., 1977; Moore, 1977; Winokur et al., 1980). They feel that the eating disorder is a variant of unipolar (depressive) or bipolar (manic and depressive) affective disorders. Symptoms pointing towards this view include hyperactivity, early morning awakening, racing thoughts, speaking under pressure, apparent euphoria, and spells of depression with guilt and self-reproach. Cantwell (1977) and Winokur (1980) note an increased incidence of affective disturbances in parents and siblings of anorectic patients close to the incidence of primary affective disorders in family studies of probands with primary affective pathology.

Behavior symptomatology includes preoccupation with food, willful semistarvation, hyperactivity, and decreased sexual interest. However, the girls maintain their personal appearance. A number of those suffering from anorexia nervosa vomit and purge to help lose weight. Some also start binge eating (bulimia).

Perceptual problems are exemplified by the disturbed body image, in which there is an overestimation of the size of the face and torso. The misperception of bodily sensations is shown by the distorted hunger awareness and the denial of fatigue. There is also a sense of ineffectiveness, with a poorly developed sense of autonomy and a feeling of being controlled by the environment rather than being in control of it.

Regardless of treatment method, 25% to 50% of anorectic patients have severe symptoms or remain unchanged at follow-up. Weight restoration immediately after treatment does not correlate with long-term outcome. Morbidity of anorexia nervosa includes recurrent episodes of weight loss, frequent hospitalizations, depression, persistent amenorrhea, infertility, and bulimia with or without vomiting. Psychosocial difficulties that may remain for anorectic patients, even after they are of normal weight, include peer and parental relationships, psychosexual adjustment, social isolation, and feelings of powerlessness in social relationships.

Overall mortality rates are about 6% (range 0% to 21.5%). Life-threatening states include inanition (35% to 40% below usual body weight or 25% to 30% if weight loss has occurred in less than 3 months), cardiac arrhythmias (with and without electrolyte imbalances), state of listlessness, significant metabolic stress (i.e., infection), superior mesenteric artery syndrome, and severe depression (resulting in suicide).

Two review articles of outcome data are summarized in Table 4-4. The article by Hsu (1980) reviews 16 studies, all in English. The studies had to have 15 subjects and a mean duration of follow-up longer than 2 years. The diagnostic criteria had to be clearly stated. Schwartz and Thompson's (1981) article includes 12 studies done since 1964. Their studies had to have sample sizes larger than 25 subjects and an average follow-up of more than 2 years. The authors of the studies they reviewed had to attempt to compile data in a systematic, statistical way rather than by impressions or in a case-by-case fashion. These articles illustrate the large variability of outcome among these patients.

BULIMIA

Bulimia is a syndrome whose major component is episodic binge eating. Usually the patient binges on high-caloric, sweet foods that are rapidly consumed. These binges are usually terminated by self-induced vomiting, sleep, abdominal pain, or social interruption (usually the food is eaten secretly). Although such binges may be pleasurable, guilt, self-criticism, and a depressed mood follow. The bulimic patient may or may not have had anorexia nervosa previously.

Bulimic patients do differ in a number of ways from restricting or fasting patients (Garfinkel et al., 1980; Casper et al., 1980). Bulimic persons experience a strong appetite, are more extroverted and sexually involved, feel more irritated and restless when hungry (fasting patients cherish hunger feelings and derive a sense of mastery from them), feel more psychic distress, experience more guilt and anxiety, have more somatic complaints, are sensitive in interpersonal relations, and don't sleep as well. The craving for food can be induced by frustration, tension, and boredom. They are of an older age than the fasting patients and are seen by others as more depressed, worried, and discouraged. Bulimic persons also show other signs of problems with impulse control, such as alcohol and drug abuse, kleptomania, self-mutilation, and even suicide attempts. There is also significantly more maternal obesity among bulimic patients compared to restricting patients.

The usual course is chronic over a period of years. The binging may alternate with fasting

Table 4-4. Comparison of review articles by Hsu (1980) and Schwartz and Thompson (1981) regarding outcome of patients with anorexia nervosa

	Hsu	**Schwartz and Thompson**
Nutritional outcome at follow-up	41%-81% Normal weight 15%-25% Weight was persistently below 75% of average 2%-7% Overweight by 15% or more	50% Of those alive had completely recovered 31% Experienced some improvement (some were obese) 19% Did not change significantly
Eating behavior at follow-up	33% Eating normally 50% Still consciously and purposely avoiding high-caloric foods 14%-50% had bulimia 10%-28% had vomiting Common: Laxative abuse Anxiety when eating with others	No mention made
Menstrual outcome at follow-up	33%-75% Menstruating Common: Menstrual irregularity Weight increase and improvements in mental attitude preceded return of menstruation Some patients of normal weight were still amenorrheic	No mention made
Psychiatric outcome at follow-up	63%-100% Continue to have morbid attitude toward weight and shape 44%-46% Diagnosed as definite or probable affective disorder Depressive symptoms common 24%-45% Admitted social phobia 13%-44% Had obsessive compulsive features Sociopathic behavior has been reported	46% Anorectic patients remain highly symptomatic in areas not related to food or weight (may be low estimate; only extreme symptoms were mentioned)
Psychosocial outcome at follow-up	High proportion in full-time employment Social anxiety common 20% Unable to differentiate themselves emotionally from the family (most still anorectic) 50% Of those with financial independence and living away still felt unable to resolve intense hostile dependent feelings in the family	Anorectic patients are able to work, even up to death from illness (quality of work not reported)
Psychosexual outcome at follow-up	20% Of patients clearly abnormal in attitude and behavior in sexual matters Sexual frigidity and fear of pregnancy was not rare, even among those who married	55% married or "kept company" Even those who married showed poor personal and sexual adjustment

or normal eating. Electrolyte imbalance and dehydration can occur. Parotid swelling (Levin et al., 1980) and loss of dental enamel (Hurst et al., 1977) secondary to acidic vomitus is not uncommon.

Although there is no definite form of treatment for bulimia, most women improve with psychotherapy. The therapist must be alert to any depression in the bulimic patient because suicide is the most common cause of death in this disorder (Crisp, 1982).

CONVERSION DISORDER (HYSTERIA)

Conversion disorder or *hysteria* (a word coined by Hippocrates) has interested physicians for 4000 years who have had the problem differentiating "real" versus "imagined" and "organic" versus "functional." The simplistic view of separating the brain and the body continues in the minds of many clinicians.

Since early times, when the disorder was associated with a convulsive condition said to occur in widows and spinsters, conversion disorder has most commonly been thought of as associated with the hysterical personality, or what is now called histrionic personality disorder. Both conversion symptoms and the histrionic personality are seen in girls and women more often than boys. The personality type is described as suggestible, overdramatic, flamboyant, immature, dependent, and manipulative.

The diagnostic criteria for conversion disorder according to DSM-III are as follows:

A. The predominant disturbance is a loss of or alteration in physical functioning, suggesting a physical disorder.
B. Psychologic factors are judged to be etiologically involved in the symptom, as evidenced by either:
   1. A temporal relationship between an environmental stimulus that is apparently related to psychologic conflict or need and the initiation or exacerbation of the symptom.
   2. The symptom enables the person to avoid some activity that is noxious to her.
   3. The symptom enables the person to get support from the environment that otherwise might not be forthcoming.
C. Determination that the symptom is *not* under voluntary control.
D. Failure to explain the symptom by a known physical disorder after appropriate investigation.

If the symptoms are limited to pain alone, they are grouped in the category of psychogenic pain disorder, in which pain dominates the clinical picture. Disturbances in sexual functioning are considered outside of this category.

Typical symptoms of conversion disorder include blindness, which shows constricted tubular peripheral visual fields that are pathognomonic of hysterical amblyopia, conversion syncope, convulsive-like phenomena, intense weakness, coordination disturbance, paralysis, vomiting, aphonia, akinesia, dyskinesia, paresthesias, anesthesia, hyperventilation, and others. Rarely, conversion symptoms may involve the autonomic or endocrine system. Conversion symptoms are rare in adults in the modern western world as compared to other cultures, but more frequent in children who are more marginal in their thinking as a function of their stage of development.

The clinical picture in children is most often multisymptomatic (immobilized fingers, enuresis, back pain). The duration of illness is frequently several months or a year before hospitalization. The "classical" pseudoneurologic symptoms are prominent. Disabling life stresses occur in most cases. Absence of a history of life stresses with resulting symptoms would make questionable the diagnosis of conversion disorder. Cases will predominantly be those of adolescent or preadolescent girls who show many characteristics of the histrionic personality and a calm mental attitude of "la belle indifference." When occurring in boys, more passive personalities are noted, with submission to parental expectations.

In childhood, incidence is about equal among girls and boys. Peak ages are 9 to 10 years and 13 to 14 years, but it does occur in preschoolers.

Preschoolers are suggestible, labile in emotional reactions, more likely to express feelings in somatic terms rather than in words, and are more concrete in concepts about body function. A frequently reported symptom in a preschooler is a paralyzed arm that occurs after the child has been punished for aggressive behavior. Reality testing is usually intact, with no marked personality disorganization. Prognosis with treatment is generally good. Absence of serious pathology in parents is more favorable for outcome. In longitudinal studies, 40% of children who developed histrionic or sociopathic personalities as adults had some conversion symptoms before age 8. Thus there may be some link emerging between conversion symptoms and antisocial or delinquent behaviors. Yet many of these children grow up to be obsessional personalities who are over-controlled in their behavior.

This diagnosis should never be made solely on the basis of ruling out organic disease. When conversion disorder is suspected, one should search for positive criteria such as:

The symptom occurs in a psychologically uncomfortable situation, and often acts as some sort of solution or escape from the situation. A sexual seduction, a demand for performance, or a traumatic event may be reported.

The symptom accrues some sort of secondary gain in a more long-term fashion (e.g., increased care from the family, justification for failure, avoidance of school, or another unpleasant expectation).

There should be some evidence of poor psychological adjustment; that is, school adjustment, peer adjustment, family adjustment, depression, or anxiety. Sometimes poor adjustment manifests itself as the "too perfect" child.

There are various psychologic reasons to choose a particular symptom. There is often some significant identification; that is, the patient knew someone who had or whom he thought had had a similar symptom, or the patient has had a similar symptom in the context of a previous physical illness. The symptom may be the paralysis of an organ involved in a forbidden wish (the arm in a wish to punch, or the eye in a wish to see). The symptom may be the same as the suffering wished on someone else.

Child psychiatric consultation need only be made on *emergency* basis if admission to the hospital for psychiatric reasons is thought necessary. Admission to the hospital is best avoided when the diagnosis of conversion reaction is suspected. One careful physical examination is better than several examinations, so as not to reinforce the symptomatology. Necessary diagnostic procedures should be performed, if at all possible, as an outpatient. If admission for diagnostic procedures is necessary, psychiatric evaluation should be postponed until the patient is in the hospital. Extra unnecessary diagnostic procedures should never be done to "prove" to the patient or family that the problem is not physical, for a paradoxical effect is often seen, even when the results of the tests are negative. Moreover, tests often come back with ambiguous results.

Admission for psychiatric reasons may be considered necessary if the symptom is incapacitating and does not improve with firmness and reassurance, or if the family seems incapable or unwilling to take care of the child at home. In this case, the primary care physician should contact the child psychiatrist with the family's knowledge. This is an excellent example of how pediatrics and child psychiatry working together can be of benefit to the incapacitated child.

*Abby L. Wasserman**
C. Hal Brunt

---

*Dr. Wassermann's contribution to this chapter was partially supported by Grant 5 T01 14866 from the National Institute of Mental Health.

REFERENCES

Akiskal, H.S., and McKinney, W.T., Jr.: Overview of recent research in depression, Arch. Gen. Psychiatry **32:**285, 1975.

American Academy of Pediatrics Committee on School Health: School health: a guide for health professionals, 1981, Evanston, Ill., 1981, The Academy.

Annell, A.L.: Lithium in the treatment of children and adolescents, Acta Psychiatr. Scand. **207**(suppl.):19, 1969.

Arnold, L.E., et al.: Methylphenidate vs. dextroamphetamine vs. caffeine in minimal brain dysfunction, Arch. Gen. Psychiatry **35:**463, 1978.

Barcai, A.: Lithium in adult anorexia nervosa, Acta Psychiatr. Scand. **55:**97-101, 1977.

Bellman, M.: Studies on encopresis, Acta Pediatr. Scand. **170**(suppl.):1, 1966.

Bruch, H.: Eating disorders: obesity, anorexia nervosa, and the person within, New York, 1973, Basic Books, Inc., Publishers.

Campbell, M., and Shapiro, T.: Therapy of psychiatric disorders of childhood. In Shader, R.I., editor: Manual of psychiatric therapeutics, Boston, 1975, Little, Brown & Co.

Cantwell, D.P.: Psychiatric illness in families of hyperactive children, Arch. Gen. Psychiatry **27:**414, 1972.

Cantwell, P.D., et al.: Anorexia nervosa—an affective disorder? Arch. Gen. Psychiatry **34:**1087-1093, 1977.

Cantwell, D.P.: Psychopharmacologic treatment of the minimal brain dysfunction syndrome. In Weiner, J.M., editor: Psychopharmacology in childhood and adolescence, New York, 1977, Basic Books, Inc., Publishers.

Carroll, B.J., et al.: A specific laboratory test for the diagnosis of melancholia: standardization, validation and clinical utility, Arch. Gen. Psychiatry **38:**15-22, 1981.

Casper, R.C., et al.: Bulimia: its incidence and clinical importance in patients with anorexia nervosa, Arch. Gen. Psychiatry **37:**1030-1035, 1980.

Crisp, A.H., et al.: How common is anorexia nervosa? A prevalence study, Br. J. Psychiatry **128:**549-554, 1976.

Crisp, A.H.: The differential diagnosis of anorexia nervosa, Proc. R. Soc. Med. **70:**686-688, 1977.

Crisp, A.H.: Anorexia nervosa at normal body weight: the abnormal normal weight control syndrome, Int. J. Psychiatry Med. **11:**203-233, 1982.

Delong, G.R.: Lithium carbonate treatment of select behavior disorders in children suggesting manic-depressive illness, J. Pediatr. **93:**689, 1978.

Drossman, D.A., et al.: Anorexia nervosa, Gastroenterology **77:**1115-1131, 1979.

Feinstein, S.C., and Wolpert, E.A.: Juvenile manic-depressive illness: clinical and therapeutic considerations, J. Am. Acad. Child Psychiatry **12:**123, 1973.

Garfinkel, B.D., et al.: Methylphenidate and caffeine in the treatment of children with minimal brain dysfunction, Am. J. Psychiatry **132:**723, 1975.

Garfinkel, et al.: The hetrogeneity of anorexia nervosa: bulimia as a distinct subgroup, Arch. Gen. Psychiatry **37:**1036-1040, 1980.

Greenhill, L.L., et al.: Lithium carbonate in the treatment of hyperactive children, Arch. Gen. Psychiatry **28:**636, 1973.

Guilleminault, C., and Anders, T.F.: Sleep disorders in children, Adv. Pediatrics **22:**151-174, 1976.

Hsu, L.K.G.: Outcome of anorexia nervosa, a review of the literature (1954-1978), Arch. Gen. Psychiatry **37:**1041-1046, 1980.

Hurst, P.S., et al.: Teeth, vomiting, and diet: a study of dental characteristics of seventeen anorexia nervosa patients, Postgrad. Med. J. **53:**298-305, 1977.

Kline, C.L.: Anorexia nervosa: death from complications of ruptured gastric ulcer, Canad. J. Psychiatry **24:**153-156, 1979.

Lacey, J.A., Stanley, P.A., Crutchfield, M., and Crisp, A.H.: Surose sensitivity in anorexia nervosa, J. Psychosom. Res. **21:**17-21, 1977.

Leventhal, J.M.: Enuresis. In Gabel, S., editor: Behavioral problems in childhood, New York, 1981, Grune & Stratton, Inc.

Levin, P.A., et al.: Benign parotid enlargement in bulimia, Ann. Intern. Med. **93:**827-829, 1980.

Levine, M.D.: The schoolchild with encopresis, Pediatr. Rev. **2:**285, 1981.

Levine, M.D.: Encopresis: its potentiation, evaluation, and alleviation, Pediatr. Clin. North Am. **29:**315-330, 1982.

Maloney, M.J., and Klykylo, W.M.: An overview of anorexia nervosa, bulimia, and obesity in children and adolescents, J. Am. Child Psychiatry **22:**99-107, 1983.

McLain, L.G.: Childhood enuresis. In Gluck, L., editor: Current problems in pediatrics, Chicago, 1979, Year Book Medical Publishers Inc.

Minuchin, S., et al.: Psychosomatic families: anorexia nervosa in context, Cambridge, Mass., 1978, Harvard University Press.

Moore, D.C.: Amitriptyline therapy in anorexia nervosa, Am. J. Psychiatry **134:**1303-1304, 1977.

Rutter, M., and Graham, P.: The reliability and validity of the psychiatric assessment of the child. I. Interview with the child, Br. J. Psychiatry **114:**563, 1968.

Safer, D., and Allen, R.: Side effects from long-term use of stimulants in children, Int. J. Ment. Health **4:**105, 1975.

Satterfield, J.M., et al.: Pathophysiology of the hyperactive child syndrome, Arch. Gen. Psychiatry **31:**839, 1974.

Schnackenberg, R.C.: Caffeine as a substitute for schedule II stimulants in hyperkinetic children, Am. J. Psychiatry **130:**796, 1973.

Schwartz, D.M., and Thompson, M.G.: Do anorectics get well? Current research and future needs, Am. J. Psychiatry **138:**319-323, 1981.

Silver, L.B.: The playroom diagnostic evaluation of children with neurologically based learning disabilities, J. Am. Acad. Child Psychiatry **15:**240, 1976.

Simmons, J.E.: Psychiatric examination of children, Philadelphia, 1974, Lea & Febiger.

Sours, J.A., and Vorhaus, L.J.: Superior mesentric artery syndrome in anorexia nervosa: a case report, Am. J. Psychiatry **138:**519-520, 1981.

Spitz, R.A., and Wolf, K.M.: Anaclitic depression. II. An inquiry into the genesis of psychiatric conditions in early childhood, Psychoanal. Study Child **2:**313, 1946.

Stewart, M.A., and Gath, A.: Psychological disorders of children, a handbook for primary care physicians, Baltimore, 1978, The Williams & Wilkins Co.

Task Force on Nomenclature and Statistics of the American Psychiatric Association: Diagnostic and Statistical Manual of Mental Disorders, ed. 3, Washington D.C., 1980, The Association.

Vande Wiele, R.L.: Anorexia nervosa and the hypothalamus, Hosp. Pract. **12:**45-50, 1977.

Weiss, G., and Hechtmann, L.: The hyperactive child syndrome, Science **205:**1348, 1979.

Winokur, A., et al.: Primary affective disorder in relatives of patients with anorexia nervosa, Am. J. Psychiatry **137:**695-698, 1980.

Yates, A., et al.: Running—an analogue of anorexia? N. Engl. J. Med. **308:**251-255, 1983.

SELECTED READINGS

Berlin, I.N.: Bibliography of child psychiatry, New York, 1976, Human Sciences Press.

Chess, S., and Thomas, A., editors: Annual progress in child psychiatry and child development, New York, Brunner/Mazel, Inc.

Freedman, A.M., et al.: Comprehensive textbook of psychiatry, ed. 3, Philadelphia, 1980, The Williams & Wilkins Co.

Journal of the American Academy of Child Psychiatry (bimonthly), Baltimore, The Williams & Wilkins Co.

Lewis, M.: Clinical aspects of child development, ed. 2, Philadelphia, 1981, Lea & Febiger.

Noshpitz, J.D.: Basic handbook of child psychiatry, New York, 1979, Basic Books, Inc., Publishers.

Rutter, M., and Hersov, L.: Child psychiatry, London, 1977, Blackwell Scientific Publications, Ltd.

Stewart, M.A., and Gath, A.: Psychological disorders of children—a handbook for primary care physicians, Baltimore, 1978, The Williams & Wilkins Co.

5 Adolescence

The term *adolescence* evokes a variety of mental images. Some will recall their teen years with pleasure, time perhaps having blurred the memory of the more difficult episodes. Others will wish to forget the trauma of "growing up" and the emotional turmoil surrounding the discovery of sexuality, rebellion from parental authority, conformity to peer pressures, and many other issues that bubble to the surface at this time of life. A universally accepted definition of adolescence is difficult to find, but it is perhaps best considered as that period extending from the beginning of secondary sexual development until physical maturity has been achieved. Clearly, this is a broad definition that will take in many preteens and may include some persons in their early twenties. Hand in hand with sexual maturation, physical growth characteristically makes a final rapid surge at this period, and, as noted already, these changes are accompanied by emotional development that hopefully will prepare the boy or girl for a responsible role in "adult" society.

In this chapter we can only attempt to provide a few vignettes concerning adolescence. For more extensive coverage the reader is referred to the texts by Daniel (1977) or Shen (1980) or to the other references (Committee on Adolescence, 1968; Erikson, 1963).

In addition to a description of normal physical and emotional growth and development, we would like to focus on a few problems that are seen with particular frequency at this age or that require insight into the evolving psychology of the adolescent for optimal management. These are nutritional disturbances, drug abuse, suicide, and reaction to chronic illness.

APPROACH TO THE ADOLESCENT

Many physicians, whether their training has been in pediatrics, internal medicine, or other disciplines, are uncomfortable when dealing with the adolescent patient. The adolescent, in turn, is often ill-at-ease in the pediatrician's office, surrounded by infants and children, or in the office of the internist or generalist, where all the patients may appear to the teenager to be ancient (i.e., over 30). Thus the physician who wishes to see adolescent patients will be well advised to limit his practice exclusively to this age group (a risky financial venture in most localities for the physician in full-time private practice) or to try to arrange to see all his adolescent patients on the same day so that they will not have to share the waiting room with younger or older age groups.

Although it is important to obtain a history from parents whenever possible, this is generally best accomplished before the adolescent's visit, either over the telephone or person-to-person. Because the first appointment for an adolescent is almost always made by the parent, perhaps at the urging of school officials or others, it is essential to discover *before* the visit, if at all possible, why the patient is being referred and what is expected of the physician. The adolescent should be told that any information shared with his doctor is confidential and that none of it will be divulged (without his permission) to parents or anyone else. The only exception to this is information that might pose a serious threat to the life or health of the patient were it not shared with a responsible family member. Even then, this should almost always be done with the teenage patient's foreknowledge.

Perhaps the most important clue to success in dealing with adolescents is to treat them with the dignity and respect that any thoughtful physician would afford an adult patient. This requires that the patient be seen alone without parents or other adults in the room at the time of the interview, that questions and answers be clearly stated without resorting to medical terms or jargon, and that the physician retain a neutral attitude. The physician who becomes judgmental or speaks in a condescending or excessively authoritarian manner will have little success with the adolescent; on the other hand, neither will the physician who attempts in dress or speech to adopt the life-style of his teenage patients.

Most adolescents have such little memory for the details usually sought by physicians in a conventional history form that a meticulous review of systems with the patient will generally bring forth little information. In fact, it is fair to say that the teenager who can recite in great detail his medical history and symptomatology is probably neurotic. It is important, however, to discover what is bothering the adolescent patient and what his symptoms mean to him. A teenage boy without benefit of any sex education at home or in the schools may be greatly disturbed by nocturnal emissions. A teenage girl (and perhaps her parents as well) may be enormously apprehensive at unilateral appearance of breast development, not realizing that this is a normal variation. Adolescents of either sex may have somatic complaints such as headache or abdominal pain, which a careful history and physical examination might reveal as more likely caused by emotional distress than by organic illness.

Physical examination should be approached matter-of-factly and performed in a systematic fashion, with adequate explanation given to special procedures. A pelvic examination performed by the male physician should always be done with a nurse in attendance and with great gentleness to allay fear and avoid discomfort. Despite apparent nonchalance, adolescents are curious about their own health and bodies and will appreciate assurance as to the normality of the examination. That curiosity can also serve as reason for a return visit, when it seems indicated, by a statement such as, "Let's get a blood count and urinalysis and have you come back next Tuesday to see me so we can discuss the results." By the second visit the teenager may feel sufficiently relaxed to "open up" and discuss matters he was unwilling to bring up at the first encounter.

In summary, to be successful in caring for adolescents, the physician must be patient, sympathetic, and unhurried and not easily offended, outwardly judgmental, or critical. Although time consuming and at times enormously frustrating, the rewards are worth the price.

PHYSICAL GROWTH AND DEVELOPMENT (see also Chapter 2)

Acceleration of linear growth and sequential development of secondary sexual characteristics are expected coincident changes during adolescence. When growth is delayed or sexual maturation seems slow or inadequate, the physician may be consulted. It is important therefore that those caring for adolescents be aware of the normal progression of maturation and able to recognize when there are significant deviations from what would be anticipated for an individual at a particular age.

Much of the data on variation in the timing and pattern of pubertal changes in both sexes derives from the careful studies of Marshall and Tanner (1969 and 1970), who have followed over 400 boys and girls in Great Britain longitudinally for more than 20 years. Tanner's standards of genital development in boys, breast development in girls, and pubic hair maturation in both sexes are well known and widely available and will not be repeated here. Table 5-1 indicates the usual sequence of sexual maturation in boys and girls. The important thing to note is the rather wide range of normal for the appearance of secondary sexual characteristics in both sexes. Unfortunately, many physicians fail to perform an adequate examination of the genitals and as a result are unsure of themselves when attempting to distinguish normal from abnormal development. Measurements of height, weight, and estimates of genital maturation should be made routinely and growth data plotted.*

A decline in the rate of linear growth in early adolescence will often be detected only if the data are plotted on a growth chart. Such a finding should always be of concern and should prompt investigation to uncover the cause. While such a fall in linear growth may be secondary only to a physiologic delay in sexual maturation, other causes must be kept in mind.

*Standard growth charts are available from the National Center for Health Statistics, Health Resources Administration, Hyattsville, Md. 20782.

Table 5-1. Sequence of events at puberty

Girls		Boys	
Event	**Average age* (range)**	**Event**	**Average age* (range)**
Height spurt	10.5 (9.5-14.5)	Growth of testes	11.5 (9.5-13.5)
Enlargement of areola and budding of breast	11 (8-13.5)	Pubic hair	12.3 (9.5-15)
Pubic hair	11 (8-14)	Growth of penis, prostate, and seminal vesicles	12.5 (11.5-14.5)
Development of breast, pigmentation of areola, axillary hair, and uterine enlargement	13 (10-16)	Height spurt	12.5 (10.5-16)
Menarche	13† (10-16.5)	Axillary and facial hair, subareolar breast tissue	14 (12-17)
Ovulation	14 (11-18)	Full growth of penis and voice change	15 (13.5-16.5)
		Full growth of testes and maturation of spermatogenesis	16 (14.5-18)

Modified from Marshall, W.A., and Tanner, J.M.: Variations in the pattern of pubertal changes in girls, Arch. Dis. Child. **44:**291, 1969 and Marshall, W.A., and Tanner, J.M.: Variations in the pattern of pubertal changes in boys, Arch. Dis. Child. **45:**13, 1970.

*Age of onset (years) unless otherwise indicated.

†Mean age of menarche in North American girls is approximately 12.6 (Root, 1973).

These include acquired hypothyroidism, Cushing syndrome, and hypopituitarism secondary to tumors or other causes or to gastrointestinal disorders such as Crohn disease. In general, endocrine disorders presenting as growth failure in adolescence are associated with weight that is appropriate for, or in excess for, height, whereas adolescents with gastrointestinal disorders and growth failure generally are underweight. For a detailed discussion of the endocrine aspects of pubertal development, the reader is referred to Root's (1973) excellent review.

EMOTIONAL CHANGES IN ADOLESCENCE (see also Chapter 4)

The emotional changes of puberty appear to parallel the physical changes. In the early teens young people are comparing their secondary sexual changes with those of others, and body changes become an important preoccupation in this age group. The development of breasts in the young girl and body hair and genital development in the young boy bring with them the prospect of future adult sexual functioning. Additional pubescent changes include a surge of both aggressive and sexual feelings, which must be dealt with by the teenager and used for further growth. Control over these emotions becomes a major task, and a number of adolescent conflicts arise from difficulties in this area. Table 5-2 lists general stages of adolescence.

Attaining independence from parents is a necessary and central task of adolescence. The decrease of parental influence, however, is coupled with anxiety over the loss of a sense of support. The latency-aged child nearly always takes his parents' views for granted. The teenager, on the other hand, may feel confused and isolated without an understanding of the possible etiology of these emotions. As a result, the young person will often turn to other significant adults (i.e., teachers, employers, coaches, etc.) for a new supportive relationship.

The movement toward independence can also be seen as a recreation of an earlier stage of development. The toddler period is noted for the achievement of motor control, coupled with the child's new ability to walk away from parents. Erikson (1963) calls this "autonomy vs. shame and self-doubt." Others have written extensively about the *separation-individuation phase* of child development, which begins at about 18 months. The child begins to believe that he has an identity that is separate from that of his mother. The method by which this stage is handled by the mother is vitally important. If the move toward autonomy is not supported, the child may feel a sense of abandonment; independence brings with it the loss of mother's support. As the adolescent strives toward a separation from parents, these old issues again resurge, and feelings of despair, loneliness, and abandonment

Table 5-2. Stages of adolescence

Early	Mid	Late
Rapid physical growth	Usually at peak of struggle with parents for independence	Usually more stable and has established satisfactory independence
Beginning to move away from influence of family and to that of peer group	Peer group usually has replaced parents' influence on behavior standards	Relates well to members of opposite sex and is able to love and be loved
Great concern with body image, particularly in relation to other members of same sex	Desire to be attractive is less related to body image than to opinion of opposite sex	Dating partner may have supplanted parents and peers as primary influence
Often spends much time in abstract thought about self	Thoughts more outward directed and adolescent more involved with world around him	Thoughts center around possibilities of careers, education, life-styles, marriage, etc.

Modified from Daniel, W.A.: Adolescents in health and disease, St. Louis, 1977, The C.V. Mosby Co.

may be rekindled. The young person may guard against these feelings by not truly achieving the necessary independence. Behavioral problems may result from the adolescent's attempt to seek relief from anxiety in the form of impulsive behavior. Action becomes a method of avoiding painful problems and, at the same time, may serve to keep the young person in a dependent position, since unacceptable behavior invites adult countermeasures and the placing of limits.

Adolescents with problems in this area handle separation poorly. Going away to school or breaking up with a boyfriend or girlfriend brings feelings of panic. This sometimes results in an abandonment type of depression, which the young person will handle with impulsive action. It is not unusual in the emergency room to see a teenage girl who has overdosed with a drug after breaking up with her boyfriend. The feelings of abandonment are acute and are dealt with in a self-destructive fashion.

In normal adolescent development the achievement of peer group relationships becomes important. The peer group provides a sense of belonging, which, as family ties weaken, becomes a new attachment and support. The peer group often reflects the values of one teenager. Conformity to a peer group involves adapting certain sets of behaviors and values. These values may be growth promoting in areas such as sports or arts and reflect the group's interest. Likewise, a group may reflect antisocial types of attitudes such as those manifested by delinquent gangs or drug abusers.

Adolescence is a time for sexual experimentation. Especially in early adolescence, mutual masturbation and other homosexual encounters are common among boys and girls. This should not be construed as necessarily correlating with homosexuality in later years. These homosexual contacts merely reflect a time of experimentation with new feelings and a new drive. Fixed patterns of behavior come later.

Shortly after the successful attainment of a group identity comes the struggle of dealing with members of the opposite sex. Peer group conversations pertaining to sexual matters are often quite frank. Dealing with feelings of sexual drive, attaining some social sophistication, and relating to members of one's own peer group in regard to sexual matters all become areas of concern for the teenager. As noted for contacts with members of the same sex at an early age, heterosexual contacts in the beginning most often represent experimentation rather than a true feeling. Popular terms such as *crush,* and *puppy love,* are descriptive of this period. The onset of a true heterosexual relationship does not come about until the end of adolescence or even later. Again, the achievement of a relative separation from parental ties and the realization of a degree of autonomy are necessary prerequisites.

NUTRITION

Iron deficiency

A number of surveys have indicated that adolescents are at risk for iron deficiency, but the reported prevalence rate has varied considerably, depending on the criteria for diagnosis. In one survey of adolescents 12 to 17 years old, 15.5% of boys but only 2.4% of girls had hematocrits below the acceptable lower limits of normal (40% for boys and 36% for girls). The fact that boys had a higher incidence of iron deficiency than girls, though surprising at first encounter, is consistent with the observation that increases in blood volume and muscle mass associated with growth at puberty are considerably greater in boys than in girls, and consequently the requirement for iron is higher. Girls with heavy menstrual loss of blood are at particular risk for iron-deficiency anemia, however, as are pregnant adolescent girls who frequently have little, if any, iron stores on which to draw. The recommended daily allowance (RDA) for iron during adolescence is 18 mg, and many available surveys indicate that both boys and girls during this period rarely achieve the RDA for iron in their diet (Food and Nutrition Board, 1976).

Obesity

Excessive accumulation of body fat is perhaps the commonest form of "metabolic abnormality" seen in affluent societies. Accurate estimates of the incidence in adolescents are not available, but even casual observation suffices to document obesity as a significant problem in Western culture.

Obesity is best considered as a syndrome rather than a specific entity. Certainly there are many factors that may contribute to the excessive accumulation of adipose tissue, including (1) heredity, (2) inactivity, (3) overeating, (4) endocrine-metabolic disorders, and (5) psychologic problems.

Heredity. The separation of genetic from environmental influences is difficult, but the occurrence of obesity in some inbred strains of animals and studies of human twins reared apart strongly support the concept of a primary genetic cause of adiposity. Furthermore, anthropometric types tend to predict which individuals may become obese, the ectomorph rarely developing a significant weight problem.

Inactivity. A number of studies have provided data linking obesity to inactivity. Bullen, using a time lapse photographic technique, studied adolescent girls at camp and noted that the obese were inactive 70% of the time compared to the nonobese, who were inactive only 20% of the time, even though both groups were involved in the same "active" sports of volleyball, swimming, and tennis (Bullen et al., 1964).

Overeating. Although it seems axiomatic that one must eat excessively to become obese, the actual amount of food consumed by some moderately overweight adolescents may be less than that of their normal-weight peers. The key to this apparent mystery is most likely activity, as just noted. Several studies have suggested that overfeeding in infancy may lead to obesity in the older child and by inference in the adult, since approximately 80% of obese youngsters remain overweight as adults.

Endocrine-metabolic disorders. Despite a folklore shared by physicians and laity alike that attributes obesity to a "glandular problem," demonstrable metabolic disorders are seldom encountered as a cause of excessive weight. Nevertheless, one must be alert to the possibility of Cushing syndrome, acquired hypothyroidism, or even more rarely a hypothalamic lesion when confronted with an obese teenager, especially if the weight gain is of recent origin and there is evidence of a decline in the rate of linear growth.

Psychologic problems. During adolescence, achieving a change in eating habits is very difficult. The damage to a teenager's self-concept is already present and possibly irreparable. There are feelings of loneliness, rejection, and low self-esteem. Eating may be the only means of satisfaction for the obese teenager, and it becomes an effective way of dealing with stress and anxiety. It also becomes a method of emotionally remaining a child and avoiding the stresses of a peer group, sexuality, and independence. If the adolescent has been obese as a child he already has to face his teenage years with deficiencies in establishing patterns of self-control and mastery. The obese young person seems to react to psychologic cues rather than to physiologic ones. For example, obese individuals tend to eat when food is in sight, the aroma of food is present, or the clock says it is mealtime, rather than because they are hungry. The obese youngster often eats because of boredom, which in turn may be the result of his exclusion from sports or social acceptance by his obesity—a vicious cycle.

The results of treatment for obesity are poor, the primary problem with the obese adolescent being compliance. The achievement of a permanent modification of eating patterns is most important and, at the same time, the most difficult task. The simplest way, of course, is to follow a low-calorie, nutritionally balanced diet, but lasting results are obtained only when the diet becomes a part of the person's eating behavior, rather than an interim measure. Though it sounds simple, this is most difficult to achieve. Frustration with minimal weight loss after much psychologic anguish causes many to discontinue the diet. Other obese young people tend to gravitate toward fad diets: high-fat, low-fat, and high-protein diets, as well as water diets, grapefruit diets, rice diets, and finally starvation. Again, because of the failure of real behavioral change, the weight is usually regained.

Self-help groups such as Weight Watchers and T.O.P.S. have achieved fair results with adults. The groups can provide intensive support and reinforce greatly the goals that the physician is trying to achieve. If the program is made up entirely of adults, however, most adolescents will stop attending.

Medication has little, if any, role in the treatment of obesity. Amphetamines do suppress appetite but are accompanied by side effects and possible physical dependence. Also, tolerance to the anorectic effect develops rapidly, usually in about 2 weeks. Other types of "medicines," such as thyroid preparations given to patients without thyroid problems, human chorionic gonadotropin (HCG), and diuretics in the absence of a physiologic problem are potentially dangerous and of dubious benefit.

Since it appears that psychologic factors play such as important role, one might believe that psychiatric treatment would be beneficial, but as already stated, the results have usually been poor. Recently there is some evidence that behavior modification techniques might be helpful. Many of the methods serve to keep the dieter constantly aware of the problem. Keeping a food diary, thinking before eating, putting the fork down after each mouthful, and chewing completely are examples. Other aids include shopping or cooking only on a full stomach, sticking to a strict shopping list, and keeping the serving dishes off the table so that it is more difficult to get seconds. The results with these techniques appear to offer some promise (Stunkard et al., 1972).

Anorexia nervosa (see also pp. 95 to 97)

Anorexia nervosa is a syndrome with a usual onset at puberty or postpuberty. Most anorectic patients are female and have experienced a weight loss of 25% or more. Other characteristic symptoms include amenorrhea, constipation, preoccupation with food, abdominal pain, and intolerance to cold. Patients are generally hyperactive despite their emaciated appearance, behavior that is quite the opposite of what a physician would expect in someone who is starving. There may be self-induced vomiting as well as abuse of laxatives. There is a distortion in body image perception in which the anorectic person believes she is overweight even though she may be remarkably emaciated. Most patients will deny anorexia, or lack of hunger, saying simply that they do not wish to eat. On physical examination they appear as gaunt, skeletal beings who characteristically insist that there is nothing seriously wrong with them. Usually they exhibit hypotension, bradycardia, hypothermia, and dry skin with abundant lanugo-type hair. Dependent edema is often present, especially in the patient who is beginning to gain weight with refeeding.

An endocrine disorder, especially hypothyroidism or hypopituitarism, is often suspected. Indeed, a number of endocrine laboratory tests may be abnormal, including low plasma gonadotropins, absent circadian rhythm in plasma cortisol, low 17-ketosteroids and 17-hydroxycorticoids, low basal metabolic rate, and borderline or low plasma thyroid function tests, especially serum triiodothyronine. Paradoxically, an exaggerated response to adrenocorticotropic hormone or metyrapone may occur. Because of the constellation of physical findings and laboratory abnormalities, some have proposed that anorexia nervosa is a primary hypothalamic disorder affecting the satiety center and various releasing hormones. The best evidence to date, however, indicates that the hormonal changes are secondary to inanition and that they are reversible by refeeding and restoration of normal body weight.

A major contributor to knowledge about the psychologic factors in anorexia is Bruch (1973). She suggests that the rejection of food is seen as a defensive attempt to maintain a sense of identity and separateness from mother. Often mother and food are equated, and the child has not distinguished between them in the phase of separation-individuation with the development of a sense of autonomy. Starvation gives the young girl a sense of control and identity. As a result she is able to "win" a struggle for independence from her mother.

It is important for the physician to be able to identify a potential anorectic patient among the many normal adolescents who are dieting. The patient with anorexia will give the impression that she is dieting without an effort and that the dieting is not an ordeal, sacrifice, or battle. The anorectic patient will insist that there is no reason to eat because she does not see herself as thin.

The treatment approaches are quite varied. Hospitalization is certainly indicated when the situation is life-threatening. Most patients are strongly resistant to treatment and will thwart the best efforts of the physician and the hospital staff. They must be observed for self-induced vomiting after meals, searched for hidden laxatives, and stopped from engaging in excessive exercise such as running in the halls. The anorectic person often will drink a large amount of water before weighing time. Some have even concealed weights in their hair or within body cavities in an attempt to feign weight gain.

Behavior modification techniques have frequently been used because they are simple and most patients respond (Stunkard et al., 1972). Some believe, however, that the rapid changes and coerciveness of the treatment may have some adverse effects. Others use a regimen of bed confinement, forced feeding, and psychotropic medication. The most commonly used classes of drugs are phenothiazines and tricyclic antidepressants. Tube feeding is sometimes used, but carries a risk of overhydration, as well as allowing the patient to remain in a passive attitude concerning her condition. Some consider a modification of the family constellation as the primary intervention once the patient is no longer in medical danger. A family pattern that appears to be overprotective and enmeshed encourages dependence and inhibits self-reliance. Treatment of the family attempts to effect the adolescent's achievement of independence.

Bulimia (see also pp. 97 to 98)

Bulimia is another eating condition common in the teenage group that is characterized by episodes of binge eating followed by the teenager's guilt over loss of control. They sometimes appear similar to anorectic patients because they attempt to control weight by dieting, vomiting, and using laxatives. They eat by gorging—often sweet, high-caloric items—after which they diet and often fast. The mood is frequently one of depression and remorse after the binge eating episode.

SUBSTANCE ABUSE

It is difficult to have a clear idea of the degree of drug and alcohol abuse in the teenage population. Certainly the abuse problem is extensive, and drug use directly or indirectly plays a role in many referrals to juvenile court. In the regular use of a drug an alteration of mood, or "high," is sought. The user may be psychologically dependent, using drugs or alcohol to alleviate anxiety. If the person is experiencing withdrawal symptoms, he is showing drug dependence that can be defined as an addiction. Habituation is a craving for euphoria before the development of physical dependence.

Marijuana is derived from the plant *Cannabis sativa,* and the active ingredient is called tetrahydrocannabinol (THC). The potency of the drug appears to depend on the climate in which it is grown and the portion of the plant used, the leaves (called "grass") being less potent than the resin ("hash"). Marijuana from Mexico ("Acapulco gold") or Colombia ("Colombian gold") is usually more potent than that grown in the United States.

When marijuana is smoked, an effect is produced that lasts about 2 to 4 hours. The drug is a mild hallucinogen, causing some enhancement of visual and auditory perception. The person may believe that he is engaging in meaningful conversation when in fact he is speaking gibberish. Time becomes distorted, and an uncaring and dreamy attitude becomes apparent. The effects of marijuana may be quite unpredictable and often may depend on the social context in which it is being used.

Experimental and occasional social use of marijuana is common among teenagers. The drug-dependent adolescent will spend a great portion of his time "high," using marijuana to avoid the stresses of school and of interpersonal relationships. The nature of the peer group will often change as a result of adopting a life-style that assigns less importance to social norms.

LSD, also called "acid," is one of the most potent mind-altering substances. The LSD "trip" lasts for several hours, and there appear to be vivid visual hallucinations and impairment of ego functions. For this reason it was previously thought that there was a relationship between the LSD reaction and schizophrenia. However, further research did not bear this out.

Other hallucinogens are psilocybin and mescaline. Psilocybin is the active drug from a type of Mexican mushroom used originally by the Aztecs. Mescaline is the active ingredient of peyote. These produce alterations in perceptual and sensory experiences that are usually pleasant. At times the "trip" is unpleasant, however, with feelings of terror and frightening visual images. Usually these can be managed by placing the individual in a quiet, dimly lit room with the physician or a friend talking to him in a reassuring manner until he gets back in touch with reality.

Another drug was made originally for veterinarians as an immobilizing agent for subhuman primates. The active substance is phencyclidine (PCP), and it is the parent substance of the anesthetic ketamine. The drug is known as PCP, "angel dust," and "crystal." Because of its unpleasant side effects, it is often misrepresented as LSD or THC by drug pushers. The PCP experience is often marked by anxiety and psychotic thought disorder. Rarely are there visual hallucinations, which helps to distinguish the PCP experience from that produced by LSD. Body image distortions, such as elongation of limbs and contraction or expansion in body size, usually occur. PCP produces psychotic symptoms such as thought blocking and disorganized thinking. Physiologic signs include vertigo, diaphoresis, nausea, and vomiting. Large doses may result in myoclonic convulsions and coma. Nystagmus is common, as is hypertension.

PCP intoxication is becoming a frequent diagnosis in emergency rooms. Placing the patient in a dark room to cut down stimulation is very helpful. Diazepam may be used for myoclonus. If a neuroleptic is needed, haloperidol should be used because phenothiazines may produce significant hypotension.

There are several other drugs that are abused to produce a perceptual experience. Anticholinergic drugs, or atropine itself, may be used to produce a toxic psychosis. Methaqualone (Quaalude), a sedative-hypnotic drug, is said to produce tingling sensations and perceptual alterations. Young teenagers often sniff glue, aerosols, gasoline, and most recently the typewriter eraser product Liquid Paper. Cardiovascular drugs that cause vasodilation have also been abused by teenagers.

The amphetamines, known as "speed," have long been abused. They may be taken orally (diet pills) or intravenously ("speeding") and produce a feeling of euphoria and sleeplessness. The drugs have long been used by students and truck drivers to stay awake. After large doses a paranoid psychosis may result. The withdrawal symptoms are usually quite unpleasant and have been called "crashing."

Cocaine is also a stimulant drug, but the effects seem to come faster and last a much shorter time. Cocaine is usually inhaled ("snorted") or injected intravenously. A combination of cocaine and heroin is called a "speedball." There do not appear to be acute side effects of cocaine use, but long-term users often have severely injured the nasal septum from repeated inhalation.

Heroin addiction presents an entirely different problem in that the patient may have to be hospitalized for withdrawal. Although detoxification may be achieved on an outpatient basis if the young person is sufficiently motivated, hospitalization is usually necessary. Methadone substitution is the procedure of choice at present, the dose depending on the amount of heroin used. After the appearance of withdrawal symptoms, an initial dose of 10 mg methadone can be given orally. If the patient becomes drowsy, subsequent doses are decreased. No more than 15 to 20 mg twice a day is necessary. Once a stabilization dose is achieved, the dose can be reduced by 5 mg/24 hr with complete withdrawal within 10 days.

The abuse of alcohol is becoming a major health hazard among our youth. Immature teenagers tend to drink like alcoholic persons—until intoxicated or sick or until all alcohol is gone. This pattern of drinking leads to the development of alcohol-dependence patterns in only a few months. The attitude of society worsens the problem, with the view of alcohol as a "social lubricant" rather than as a potentially dangerous drug. Adults not aware of the danger of adolescent alcohol dependence often do not consider it a problem until the alcoholism has fully developed.

SUICIDE (see also pp. 94 and 95)

Adolescent suicide is now the second leading cause of death among young people, accidents being first. This is only a partial picture, however, since 5 to 20 serious threats or attempts are made for every successful suicide. Boys outnumber girls in successful suicides, but the ratio of attempts is about 3:1 girls to boys. Protestants have the highest rate among religious groups and Catholics the lowest. Girls tend to take pills or slit their wrists, whereas boys often will either hang or shoot themselves. Attempters are generally younger in age than those who complete the act.

The verbal and nonverbal expressions of suicide are frequently seen as a cry for help. This appears to be more characteristic of the adolescent than the adult. Often there has been a smouldering family situation with sporadically occurring conflicts. Episodes of crying spells, running away, impulsive physical action, and perhaps minor suicide gestures often precede the actual attempt. Quite often the attempt is manipulative in nature, directed against parents by children who believe that they have lost their parents' love. This loss may be real or only fantasized (Morrison and Collier, 1969). When parents fail to attentively listen to a young person's dreams and aspirations or, worse yet, belittle them, an impasse is created in which the young person may feel that he is unable to find a solution. He then must acquiesce to his parents' wishes or alternatively choose a course that he believes may anger his family. A feeling of hopelessness may occur in which suicide is often considered the only "solution."

Tension in the home is an important factor leading to attempted suicide. One marriage in three ends in divorce, which is often bitter, the children becoming pawns used by the parents for their own needs. It is not at all surprising, therefore, that the vast majority of young suicide attempters come from broken or from disturbed homes. When families are often in conflict, with constant quarreling or with one parent alcoholic or institutionalized, the resultant anger in the young person may be handled either by running away or by suicide.

There are a number of *risk factors* that give valuable clues to a possible adolescent suicide and must not be overlooked. The first is an absence of a significant personal relationship. A young person who has lost a *significant other* in a love relationship or has lost a parent is at risk. The use of drugs and alcohol is a second factor, often being an inappropriate way of dealing with problems. If this should fail, then suicide may be seen as the method of choice to deal with a situation. A young person who shows a marked behavior change with his peers or at school may be severely depressed. Loss of appetite, neglect of schoolwork, rejection of good friends, and a lack of interest in personal appearance are ominous signs. Finally, family communication problems are a crucial sign and have been referred to previously.

The role of the physician can be of extreme importance. It is interesting to note that many depressed youngsters have recently seen a physician for a somatic complaint before making the suicide attempt. The important thing is to listen for clues of an emotional problem and refrain from being judgmental. A number of times this is enough to diffuse the stress adequately. An actual suicide attempt should *always* be followed by a psychiatric consultation. Teenagers too often are sent home from the emergency room after the medical danger is past. The reason for the attempt must be explored, either individually or in family sessions, to rectify a dangerous pattern of behavior.

COPING WITH CHRONIC ILLNESS (see also pp. 75 to 79)

As emphasized already, adolescents need to know that they are "normal," and they may become greatly concerned over illness and any attendant changes in life-style that they perceive as setting them apart from their peers. What happens to the adolescent when confronted with a chronic or potentially debilitating condition or illness? Many factors will shape his response, but the most important perhaps is his premorbid adjustment. Illness, after all, does not occur in a vacuum. The child has already had achievements and strengths, as well as weaknesses and prior failures, and his past record of coping with the latter will in all likelihood predict his ability to deal with a more serious and threatening situation. The psychologic meaning of illness to the adolescent is of great importance in determining his response and will usually depend on age. For the *early adolescent,* management of serious illness is often extremely difficult because of the real or imagined threat it poses to body image. If serious illness occurs before the adolescent has matured from an idealized body image concept to a real one, there is danger that normal psychologic development will fail to occur. Separation from the peer group and confinement because of illness may cause great difficulty in coping. The *midadolescent* usually has problems in contending with illness that center around the issues of independence from parents or other adults, acceptance by peer groups, and sexuality. Illness in the *older adolescent,* on the other hand, more often brings problems in relationships with boyfriend or girlfriend or one's choice of vocational-educational goals. At this stage, illness usually is only slightly related to body image, independence, or ability to function sexually.

Every adolescent suffering from a chronic disease will have given himself some explanation for his condition, and these answers will generally make better sense to him than the learned and sometimes incomprehensible explanation given by his physician. One must find out what the adolescent thinks about the cause and meaning of his illness. Only after that has been aired and discussed is he likely to hear and comprehend the physician's information.

In the paragraphs that follow, diabetes mellitus has been used as an example of a chronic illness with which an adolescent must learn to cope. However, with only slight changes many other conditions, ranging from sickle cell disease to seizure disorders, could be substituted in these discussions.

Living with a chronic illness such as diabetes inevitably results in some psychic side effects (Ack, 1974). Among the commonest and most likely to be debilitating are those involved with (1) dependency, (2) activity-passivity, (3) self-concept, and *environmental* factors that include (4) family, (5) school, (6) social life, and (7) sports.

Dependency. Throughout childhood, and especially in adolescence, the child struggles to emancipate himself from the control of adults. Just as he is beginning to accomplish that goal, diabetes occurs and some of this independence must be surrendered. Under such pressure some will regress, shrug their shoulders, and in effect say, "You take over. You give my injections, test my urine, make my doctor appointments, and I will be an obedient, quiet, docile child again." For others, dependency is so distasteful that they may behave in erratic and perhaps dangerous and self-destructive ways to try and prove themselves independent—not only from adult domination but also from the restrictions imposed by the disease. In the diabetic adolescent this may mean "fudging" of urine tests for sugar, ignoring dietary advice, or, worse still, deliberate avoidance of insulin injections with resulting ketoacidosis.

Activity-passivity. Activity is the natural way that children react to their environment, and enforced passivity is resisted by children at all ages. The adolescent who has had diabetes mellitus for any length of time often lives with a great deal of anxiety about the disease, fearing insulin reactions, diabetic acidosis, and coma, as well as the long-term complications of the disease, which he increasingly comes to know and fear. If activity is curtailed by poor control and frequent reactions or by misguided parents or physicians who attempt to "protect him" by prohibiting participation in sports and other activities, the adolescent's anxiety is all the more increased.

Self-concept. The view we hold of ourselves is one of the major determinants of our behavior and the level of adjustment we achieve. For the adolescent to be ill in a society that emphasizes physical development and beauty is to be "different," and to be different is often interpreted as being in some way "inferior." All people, but young people in particular, need social interaction to achieve a proper perspective about themselves. However, if such interaction tends to magnify the adolescent's feeling of being different and increases anxiety, the usual response will be to withdraw. Not infrequently we see teenagers with diabetes mellitus who have withdrawn from their peer group rather than explain why they cannot have an ice cream sundae after school or why they must be at home on time for dinner rather than stay out with the gang an extra hour. Most adolescents have a terrible dread of being different and interpret such difference from their peers as a sign of failure.

Family. Appreciation of a number of other

factors that might be considered environmental are of importance in helping the adolescent cope with his condition. The first of these is the family. The family's reactions to an adolescent with chronic illness obviously are quite important. Are they supportive, overprotective, or indifferent? The impact of diabetes on the emotional health of the family must also be considered in caring for the adolescent. To live with someone who has diabetes is to live under chronic stress. If the family structure is shaky to begin with, the occurrence of diabetes in one of the children may exaggerate preexisting difficulties. The appearance of diabetes in one family member will to some extent change the life-style of the entire family. For example, vacation plans may need to be altered so that the family stays near a medical facility, eating habits of the family may change to accommodate the diabetic individual's need for meals at regular times, and so on. Although various changes may individually be small, when added together they exact a toll.

School. Teachers are often fearful of a child with a chronic illness, and their fears and misconceptions need to be allayed by the physician or other health care specialists. In the case of diabetes, teachers should know about insulin reactions and the need for prompt treatment with sugar, the necessity of regular mealtimes, and, on the other hand, the importance of not singling out the adolescent and making him feel different.

Social. The adolescent with diabetes should be encouraged to establish normal peer relationships and not be ashamed to acknowledge to his friends that he has diabetes. Most of them will be understanding and appreciative of this shared knowledge, as well as supportive both emotionally and in a practical way (e.g., recognizing insulin reactions) if they are sufficiently acquainted with the situation.

Sports. Coaches and parents alike tend to be overprotective of youngsters with diabetes. Unless the physician intercedes for them strongly, these adolescents are likely to spend most of their time "on the bench," rather than on the playing field. It should be pointed out to all concerned that many professional athletes have diabetes and are able to manage very well indeed.

THE MEDIA

By high school graduation, the average American child has watched 15,000 hours of television and approximately 350,000 commercials. Much of the programming is a potential mental health hazard to young people (Rothenberg, 1983). The American Academy of Pediatrics (1978) has issued a position paper recommending an increased awareness of viewing habits and making assessments of the potential influence on youth.

Another major influence is today's rock music and the movies. Themes of violence, hate, and drug use are reflected in much of the music. Society appears to tolerate movie scenes that show people smoking marijuana, heavy social drinking on television shows, and lyrics of songs such as "Sweet Leaf" and "Cocaine." Beer commercials portray an image of recreation and beer going together. Parents may take a firm position against drug use, but television, the movies, radio, and some music stars give a different impression.

• • •

In summary, to be successful in providing quality medical care to an adolescent, the physician must be not only competent in understanding the pathophysiology of diseases that affect adolescents but must also be aware of and concerned with the psychologic factors that affect the young person and his family.

Joseph N. Fisher
Paul King

REFERENCES

Ack, M.: Psychological problems in long-standing insulin-dependent diabetic patients, Kidney Int. **1**(suppl.):141, 1974.

American Academy of Pediatrics: Policy statement, Forty-eighth Annual Meeting, Chicago, 1978, The Academy.

Bruch, H.: Eating disorders, New York, 1973, Basic Books, Inc., Publisher.

Bullen, B.A., et al.: Physical activity of obese and non-obese adolescent girls appraised by motion picture sampling, Am. J. Clin. Nutr. **14:**211, 1964.

Committee on Adolescence: Normal adolescence; its dynamics and impact, Report No. 68, Group Adv. Psychiatry **6:**751, 1968.

Daniel, W.A.: Adolescents in health and disease, St. Louis, 1977, The C.V. Mosby Co.

Erikson, E.H.: Childhood and society, ed. 2, New York, 1963, W. Wolarton & Co.

Food and Nutrition Board: Iron nurture in adolescence, Pub. No. (HSA) 77-5100, Washington, D.C., 1976, Department of Health, Education, and Welfare.

Marshall, W.A., and Tanner, J.M.: Variations in the pattern of pubertal changes in girls, Arch. Dis. Child. **44:**291, 1969.

Marshall, W.A., and Tanner, J.M.: Variations in the pattern of pubertal changes in boys, Arch. Dis. Child. **45:**13, 1970.

Morrison, G.C., and Collier, J.G.: Family treatment approaches to suicidal children and adolescents, J. Am. Acad. Child Psychiatry **8:**140, 1969.

Root, A.W.: Endocrinology of puberty, J. Pediatr. **83:**1, 1973.

Rothenberg, M.B.: The role of television in shaping the attitudes of children, J. Am. Acad. Child Psychiatry **22:**86-87, 1983.

Shen, T.J.Y.: The clinical practice of adolescent medicine, New York, 1980, Appleton-Century-Crofts.

Stunkard, A., et al.: New therapies for the eating disorders: behavior modification of obesity and anorexia nervosa, Arch. Gen. Psychiatry **26:**391, 1972.

6 Mental Retardation

Disorders of higher cerebral function involving intellect and adaptive behavior are often grouped under the heading of *mental retardation* or *mental deficiency. Mental retardation* is the most frequently applied and widely accepted term for this type of developmental disorder. The most commonly used definition of mental retardation is that of the American Association on Mental Deficiency: "Mental retardation refers to significantly subaverage general intellectual functioning existing concurrently with deficits in adaptive behavior, and manifested during the developmental period." *Significantly subaverage* refers to intelligence scores more than two standard deviations below the mean, as compared to the normal population (intelligence quotient [IQ] less than or equal to 70 on most tests). However, mental retardation is not defined by IQ score only—adaptive behavior must also be deficient. Mental retardation should be distinguished from derangements of higher cerebral function that are acquired in later life, including *dementia*. Dementia is loss of memory and other intellectual processes caused by progressive brain degeneration. Many of the conditions that cause mental retardation in childhood may also cause progressive loss of developmental milestones and intellect, that is, dementia. They are discussed in more detail in Chapter 23, Inborn Errors of Metabolism, and Chapter 29, Diseases of the Nervous System.

Mental retardation is a symptom of higher brain dysfunction involving the cerebrum (primarily the cortical association areas), resulting in repeated recognizable deviation from normal function. It is not a specific diagnosis but rather is a sign of underlying functional disturbance that can have many causes. After thorough evaluation, a specific pathologic process may or may not be identified. Nonetheless, every attempt should be made to understand pathogenesis and determine etiology when possible.

Mental retardation often coexists with other developmental handicaps, including abnormalities of motor development (cerebral palsy) and special sensory development (hearing or vision). Because of the unavoidable stigma associated with a diagnosis of mental retardation, the diagnosis should *only be made* when it is reasonably certain that there are no other physical, sensory, psychologic, learning, or environmental problems to account for the deficiency. If reasonable diagnostic certainty is not present, it is far better to describe a person's performance level and avoid labels.

Mental retardation is the single largest neurologic problem in society today. Approximately 3% of the population of the United States (6,900,000 persons) may be considered mentally retarded. Of the total number, 10%, or approximately 690,000 persons, are sufficiently handicapped to make them incapable of independent living. The *incidence* (number of cases per given time period) of many conditions that cause mental retardation has decreased, owing to better genetic counseling, prenatal diagnosis, and improvement in general medical care. However, the life expectancy of many mentally retarded persons has increased because of improved medical care and better general living conditions for the handicapped. Thus the average *prevalence* (number of cases at a given time) of mental retardation has remained relatively static. Because of the modern trend away from institutionalization, the total number of persons living in public residential facilities has declined steadily over the last decade. Nonetheless, the severity of affliction and the cost of care of institutionalized persons is increasing. In 1982 there were approximately 120,000 persons in state or public institutions in the United States at a cost of over 3.7 billion dollars. This figure does not include severely mentally retarded persons in home care or private institutions. It also does not include an accounting of the cost of financial aid, public housing, and loss in productivity related to the care of these persons at home or in private institutions.

INTELLIGENCE TESTING

It may be very difficult to distinguish the mentally retarded child from the child with other developmental problems, especially at an early age. Children with static encephalopathy from motor system injury (cerebral palsy) that is acquired perinatally may have coexisting mental retardation. However, such a child may have voluntary motor, involuntary movement, or speech disorders of such magnitude that reasonable assessment of intelligence cannot be made by conventional means. Thus the separation of intellectual or cognitive function from other brain function (motor or sensory) is dependent on the testing modality. Age and degree of central nervous system maturation are also important considerations. By necessity, in the first 12 to 18 months of life, scales of development heavily weigh motor and special sense development, which are intimately associated with myelination of the central nervous system. During the second year of life the normal child begins to acquire language, and developmental measurements must include speech and language assessment. The skills of the 2-year-old child with impaired hearing and resultant faulty speech and language or of the 2-year-old child with dysarthria because of motor system injury will be underestimated if pure language scales are used. In the third year of life and later, use of symbolic language and thought replaces concrete, object–oriented, thinking. By 4 to 6 years of age most children are ready to take more conventional tests of intelligence involving expressive and receptive language, abstract reasoning, and accumulated experience.

Formal evaluation of development in the first 2 years of life is greatly reliant on basic sensory, motor, and language skills. Commonly used measures include the Cattell Infant Intelligence Scale and the Bayley Scales for Infant Development. After this early period, measurement of cognitive ability becomes more complex and less dependent on simple developmental milestone achievement. Pioneers in the field of intellectual evaluation recognized this complexity but desired a simple representation of intelligence level for ease of expression and comparison. Alfred Binet introduced the concept of *mental age* (MA) to indicate average achievement level for any chronologic age (CA). In 1916, Terman derived the IQ from the ratio of MA/CA multiplied by 100. Although introduced over 60 years ago, the IQ score remains the most universally applied measure of intelligence. Popular instruments for IQ assessment in widespread use include the Stanford-Binet Intelligence Scale, the Wechsler Intelligence Scale for Children-Revised (WISC-R), Wechsler Preschool and Primary Scale of Intelligence (WPPSI), and the Wechsler Adult Intelligence Scale (WAIS).

These currently used tests of intellectual ability actually use *derivation IQ* rather than the simpler *ratio IQ* described above. (The term *IQ*, as commonly used today, refers to derivation IQ.) Derivation IQ is computed using standardized tables in which reference population IQ scores have been converted to a normal distribution with a mean of 100 and equal standard deviation values for every age. For the Stanford-Binet one standard deviation is 16, whereas with the Wechsler scales one standard deviation is 15. A person's actual test scores are converted to IQ values using such tables. Derivation IQ scores are more stable across different age groups and thus more easily comparable. In addition, individual percentile rank may be obtained from the derivation IQ.

CLASSIFICATION

Many classification systems are applied to mentally retarded individuals. Each primarily reflects the major interest of the group using the system (medical, social, educational, or economic). However, no entirely satisfactory classification system exists for mental retardation. Because division by severity of involvement is the cornerstone of most classifications, it follows that division by IQ score, however controversial, is a common basis for classification (Table 6-1). Using this classification criterion, persons who fall more than two standard deviations below the mean are considered to be mentally retarded. Severity of mental retardation is based on the number of standard deviations past this two standard deviation mark.

Persons with IQ scores between 70 and 80 are sometimes referred to as *borderline mentally*

Table 6-1. Classification of mental retardation as a function of IQ score

A.A.M.D.* level	Standard deviations below mean	Stanford-Binet IQ (SD = 16)	Wechsler IQ (SD = 15)
Mild	2-3	52-67	55-69
Moderate	3-4	36-51	40-54
Severe	4-5	20-35	25-39
Profound	>5	≤19	≤24

Modified from Grossman, H.J., editor: Manual on terminology and classification in mental retardation, Washington, D.C., 1973, American Association on Mental Deficiency.
*American Association on Mental Deficiency.

Table 6-2. Functional classification of mental retardation

AAMD* level	Educational level	Functional level	Social-medical level
Mild	Educable	Independent	Subcultural
Moderate	Trainable		
Severe	Dependent	Dependent	Pathologic
Profound			

*American Association on Mental Deficiency

retarded. This is a controversial category and the term should probably be avoided.

Grouping by IQ number or number of standard deviations from the mean may not be useful for all purposes, and other more descriptive groupings may be used (Table 6-2). Generally, these can be considered *functional classification systems* and include consideration of educational and vocational potential and suitability for independent living. The educable retarded generally fall in the mildly affected group, and differ from persons of normal intellect mainly in cognitive ability. The trainable group may be taught self-help and employment skills and often are capable of independent living. They correspond to the moderately retarded group. The dependently retarded, although perhaps capable of many self-help skills, usually cannot live independently and often are institutionalized.

A particularly useful classification system, first proposed by Lewis in 1933, is based on whether the variation present could be considered normal or abnormal (pathologic). The first, or normal variation group consists of mildly to moderately retarded persons who occupy the lower extreme of the normal distribution curve—the opposite of superior or genius. This is variously termed the *subcultural, familial-cultural,* or *physiologic* group. Members are difficult to characterize, as the group blends imperceptibly into the normal population. It is the largest group, accounting for 90% of all mentally retarded persons. In addition, most familial cases fall in this group. Definite etiologic diagnosis is usually not possible. Persons may be delayed in all developmental areas from an early age or have relatively normal motor development. Significant cognitive disability may not be discovered until school age. Major morphologic abnormalities are usually not present and only school performance level may distinguish them from their more normal counterparts. The subcultural group is medically as well as socially and economically important because of its size, family clustering, and increased incidence of chronic disease when compared to the normal population. A disproportionately large number of these persons are from lower socioeconomic classes, suggesting that poor living conditions, at least in part, may be an etiologic factor. Because this group is a normal expression of individual intelligence variation within the population, it can be considered an index of the mental vitality of society as a whole. Interestingly, the number of persons in this mildly to moderately retarded group tends to diminish with age. This is a result of finishing school, where identification usually takes place, and joining the labor force, where they may function independently in their daily lives.

Table 6-3. Comparison of subcultural and pathologic groups of mental retardation

	Subcultural	Pathologic
Number of retarded citizens represented	90%	10%
I.Q. Level–A.A.M.D.*	Mild	Moderate to profound
Physical appearance	Usually normal	Often abnormal
Associated neurologic signs	Rare	Common
Etiologic diagnosis	Rare	Common
Parents/siblings	Abnormal (Similar)	Usually normal
Socioeconomic class	Cluster in lower groups	Distribution similar in all classes
Institutionalization	Rare	Common

Modified from Lewis, E.O.: Types of mental deficiency and their social significance, J. Ment. Sci. **79:**298, 1933.
*American Association on Mental Deficiency

The second group of mentally retarded persons may be considered the abnormal variation or *pathologic* group, as most cases are caused by definite organic lesion or abnormality. Common causes include chromosome abnormalities, other genetic or metabolic factors, birth trauma, and major developmental abnormalities of the nervous system. Most members are severely to profoundly retarded, although some may be only moderately affected. They are more evenly distributed with regard to socioeconomic class than the subcultural group. Physical abnormalities and dysmorphic features as well as infertility are common in this group. There is a high incidence of other neurologic problems, including seizures and cerebral palsy. They require high-level care and are often institutionalized. Most importantly, after appropriate evaluation, the etiology is usually apparent in this group. For comparison of the subcultural and pathologic groups, see Table 6-3.

PATHOPHYSIOLOGY

An understanding of normal nervous system development is required to understand the pathophysiology of mental retardation. Embryologic development of the central nervous system may be conveniently divided into early and late phases. The *early phase* consists of *dorsal induction* (neural tube formation) and *ventral induction* (forebrain and face differentiation.) It is largely complete by the end of the sixth week of gestation. During this important phase there is progressive increase in complexity of the rostral neural tube, resulting in the formation of the primordia of the cerebral hemispheres, ventricles, and brain stem. Abnormalities of this phase of development often lead to early spontaneous abortion or are not compatible with survival after birth. Survivors, although often mentally retarded, are usually considered as suffering from genetic or chromosome disorders or neural tube defects, based on the morphologic abnormalities present at birth. Toxins, ionizing radiation, intrauterine infection, and metabolic and genetic diseases all have been implicated as causes of abnormality in the early phase of brain development. These factors may also adversely influence events during any of the later developmental phases.

Insults to the central nervous system occurring during the *later phase* of fetal development are important determinants of mental retardation. This coincides with a particularly vulnerable period of brain development and may result in significant functional derangement unaccompanied by obvious morphologic abnormality. Major events during this phase include neuron proliferation, migration, organization, and myelination.

By the conclusion of the sixth week of gestation, the primitive nervous system has already undergone complex growth and differentiation rostrally. Primitive nerve cells lying in the periventricular zones of the paired telencephalic hemispheres begin the stage of *neuronal proliferation,* which peaks in the second to fourth month of gestation. Abnormalities involving this stage of rapid cell division include both microcephaly and macrocephaly, resulting from inhibition or stimulation of cell differentiation. Microcephaly may be familial or may be associated with chromosomal abnormalities. Intrauterine infections as well as teratogens such as ionizing radiation or alcohol are also associated with microcephaly. Macrocephaly may also be familial or may be seen in neurocutaneous syndromes including tuberous sclerosis and neurofibromatosis. Not all patients with microcephaly or macrocephaly are mentally retarded.

Between 3 and 6 months of gestation, neurons migrate in orderly sequence from their origin in the periventricular zones to take their place in the cerebral cortex. At the conclusion of *neuron migration* (20 to 24 weeks of fetal life), the cortex has its full adult complement of 16 to 22 billion neurons. Abnormalities of this stage of development include agenesis of portions of the cerebral walls (schizencephaly), decreased number of gyri (lissencephaly), broad gyri and abnormal cortical lamination (pachygyria), polymicrogyria, and neuronal heterotopias. Infants born prematurely during this period are at risk of having hypoxic-ischemic injury or periventricular-intraventricular hemorrhage. This may lead to significant cognitive disorder in surviving patients.

Growth of axons and dendrites and synaptic formation continue from late gestation through the first few years of life. Abnormalities of synaptic and dendritic development have been demonstrated in the brains of mentally retarded persons. However, many abnormalities in this stage of *neuron organization* are beyond the resolution of traditional neuropathologic techniques. In some patients with significant mental retardation, neither gross nor microscopic alterations may be seen. Because of its duration, postnatal as well as prenatal factors can affect neuron organization. Neonatal asphyxia with hypoxic-ischemic encephalopathy, a major cause of both mental retardation and cerebral palsy, probably affects neuron interconnection formation at this stage of development.

Myelination begins during fetal development, but the majority of myelination occurs in the first and second years of life. The primary clinical manifestation is the rapid development of major motor milestones during infancy. Later in development, myelination of major association areas of the brain is associated with the development of abstract thought processes and experiential learning. When myelin formation is affected by the leukodystrophies, metabolic disorders, infection, hypoxemia, infarction, or

Table 6-4. Major etiologic categories of pathologic mental retardation

Major etiologic category	Principal diagnostic clues	Specific examples with associated symptoms or signs
Chromosome abnormality	Association of certain physical findings suggests diagnosis, which must be confirmed by karyotyping	Down syndrome: hypotonia, upslanting palpebral fissures, flat facial profile, simian crease Trisomy 13: holoprosencephaly, cleft lip or palate, seizures, polydactyly
Syndromes without chromosome abnormality	Diagnosis depends on identification of constellation of characteristic features	de Lange syndrome: synophrys, thin downturning lips, micromelia, short stature Prader-Willi syndrome: hypotonia, obesity, small hands and feet, hypogonadotropic hypogonadism Rubenstein-Taybi syndrome: broad thumbs and toes
Congenital infection	Neonatal: hepatosplenomegaly, petechiae, seizures, intrauterine growth retardation, chorioretinitis Later: intracranial calcification, microcephaly, hydrocephalus, chorioretinitis, cataracts, hearing deficit	Rubella: hearing loss, cataract, cardiac defects Cytomegalovirus: hepatosplenomegaly, petechiae, thrombocytopenia, seizures, periventricular calcification Toxoplasmosis: chorioretinitis, hydrocephalus, intracranial calcification Herpes simplex: vesicular rash, meningoencephalitis
Inborn errors of metabolism and storage diseases (with known enzymatic abnormality)	Seizures (early), ataxia (late), peculiar odor, hepatosplenomegaly, metabolic acidosis, neurologic or developmental deterioration, large head, macular cherry red spot	Phenylketonuria: blond hair, blue eyes, eczema, musty odor Galactosemia: cataract, hepatosplenomegaly Mucopolysaccharidoses: skeletal abnormalities, coarse features, corneal clouding Lesch-Nyhan syndrome: self-mutilation, choreoathetoses Tay-Sachs disease: macular cherry red spot

trauma, cognitive skills are usually impaired.

Brain development and function potentially can be adversely affected in a number of ways at any of these major developmental stages. However, the deleterious effects of a teratogen may vary depending on when the exposure occurs during development. Thus exposure to ionizing radiation during the first trimester may lead to microcephaly and severe mental retardation, whereas similar exposure later in development may cause no measurable injury. There may also be important response variables among individuals. Some children of mothers who drink excessive amounts of alcohol during pregnancy develop the fetal alcohol syndrome, whereas others do not. Similarly, a small number of patients with untreated phenylketonuria develop normal intelligence, whereas most have severe mental retardation and other neurologic abnormalities. Finally, there is evidence to support the claim that central nervous system injuries are reversible. For example, although fetal, neonatal, and infantile undernutrition may lead to mental retardation, some of the brain dysfunction may be reversible even after prolonged relative starvation. In summary, an understanding of mental retardation must include knowledge of brain development from several perspectives, including relative vulnerability to injury at various developmental stages, individual variability, and relative recovery potential. In general, the earlier the insult to the nervous system, the more severe the outcome.

ETIOLOGY

Any process that can affect the developing nervous system may lead to mental retardation. Most are more fully discussed elsewhere in this book. Table 6-4 lists the major etiologic classes of mental retardation with some key physical findings and diagnostic clues. More complete lists of conditions causing mental retardation can be found in any of the general references at the end of the chapter.

EVALUATION

Once a child is suspected of being mentally retarded, a careful evaluation should be undertaken to answer the following questions:

1. What is the current level of function? (confirmation and quantitation)
2. What is the nature of the problem? (pathogenesis)
3. Why is the problem present? (etiology)

Table 6-4. Major etiologic categories of pathologic mental retardation—cont'd

Major etiologic category	Principal diagnostic clues	Specific examples with associated symptoms or signs
Neurodegenerative disease (without known enzymatic abnormality)	Hallmark is loss of or failure to obtain developmental milestones. Certain features or signs suggest diagnosis	Neuronal ceroid lipofuscinosis: retinal degeneration, blindness, seizures Alexander disease, Canavan disease: large head Pelizaeus-Merzbacher disease: nystagmus
Toxic and endocrine disorders	Diagnosis may be suspected by physical appearance but must be confirmed by history of exposure or appropriate diagnostic tests	Fetal alcohol syndrome: prenatal growth deficiency, short palpebral fissures, microcephaly, hypoplastic philtrum Creatinism (neonatal hypothyroidism): prolonged neonatal jaundice, large posterior fontanel, umbilical hernia, hypoactivity
Neurocutaneous syndromes	Depigmented macules, café au lait spots, adenoma sebaceum, facial hemangioma	Tuberous sclerosis: depigmented macules, adenoma sebaceum, intracranial calcification Neurofibromatosis: café au lait spots, neurofibromas, cutaneous lipomas
Perinatal problems	History of traumatic birth, meconium staining, prematurity, low Apgar scores, asphyxia	Periventricular-intraventricular hemorrhage: sudden or saltatory deterioration in a premature neonate with seizures, fall in hematocrit, lethargy, bulging fontanel (confirmed by CT or ultrasound scanning) Perinatal asphyxia with hypoxic-ischemic encephalopathy: seizures, hypoactivity, jitters, irritability, hypotonicity or hypertonicity

4. Are there environmental risk factors that may be modified to affect outcome?
5. Are treatable, preventable or familial conditions present, necessitating genetic counseling?
6. Are other explanations present? (child neglect, abuse or deprivation, chronic disease, special sense abnormality, learning disability, psychosis, or autism)
7. What is the best currently available approach to help the patient achieve his full human potential?

History and physical examination. A carefully obtained, thorough history is of primary importance. The age of onset of problems or the age at which concern was first expressed should be noted. It is important to determine if the problem is static (slow or no milestone advancement) or progressive (loss of milestones). Progressive problems often are caused by metabolic or degenerative disease. A history of difficulty during pregnancy, labor, or delivery may be the only information available to substantiate a specific etiologic diagnosis. Prenatal factors indicating high risk include teenage pregnancy, poor prenatal care, alcohol, cigarette or other drug consumption, poor maternal nutrition, maternal illness (rubella, herpes, toxoplasmosis), and maternal systemic illness including epilepsy, diabetes, and toxemia. High-risk perinatal factors include prematurity, postmaturity, small size for gestational age, precipitous birth, low Apgar scores, and asphyxia. The birth process itself may be associated with trauma to the brain. Once born, the neonate is at risk for asphyxia, with resulting hypoxic-ischemic encephalopathy or infection (viral or bacterial). The premature infant is particularly susceptible to hemorrhage in the periventricular areas with resultant destruction of neurons and potential neurons. Each infant at high risk should have a thorough neurologic examination in the neonatal period and comprehensive developmental follow-up examinations. Early identification of developmental delay is important because some children can be helped by remedial therapy before they enter preschool or kindergarten.

A complete family history should be taken to determine whether other siblings are similarly affected. Inquiry should be made about early or unexplained infant death, epilepsy, cerebral palsy, or other neurologic or psychiatric disease. The possibility of consanguinity should be explored. The *environmental-socioeconomic history* should include age, parents' marital status, educational status, and source of income of the family. The *developmental history* should include gross motor, fine motor, and language milestones as well as personal and social adaptive skills.

The physical examination should be tailored to the age and developmental capabilities of the patient. In all cases height, weight, and head circumference should be measured and plotted on standard growth charts. The general physical examination should determine if any acute or chronic medical problems or physical abnormalities are present that might affect development. The physical features specific for certain mental retardation syndromes are quite varied; for a partial list see Table 6-4.

The neurologic examination should include a description of the current level of development. Transillumination of the skull should be performed, and the size and position of the fontanels and sutures should be noted. This information may be particularly significant when correlated with serial measurement of head circumference. When specific neurologic abnormalities are present (i.e., hemiparesis, macrocephaly, or seizures), mental retardation is frequently an associated feature.

Diagnostic studies. Several screening procedures are employed to further identify, quantitate, and confirm abnormalities suspected from the history and physical examination. Useful screening tests for general development in the infant and younger child include the Denver Developmental Screening Test and the Lexington Developmental Scale. The acquisition of speech and language is an important part of early childhood development and should be quantitated. Several instruments are available for this, including the Peabody Picture Vocabulary Test.

The special senses of vision and hearing should likewise be evaluated. One can measure vision using pictures of common objects (Allen cards) or an *E* chart in the younger child. The standard Snellen chart is used for older children, and visual response to objects of decreasing size is useful in evaluation of infants. For the younger child, hearing is best evaluated by quantitation of behavioral response to a sound source. A great deal of experience, however, is necessary for proper interpretation of sound field audiometry. Standard audiometry with quantitation of number of correct responses is used in older children who are cooperative. Newer visual and auditory evoked potential measurements are now available to evaluate the functional integrity of the visual and auditory pathways, even in the uncooperative or very young patient. These screening procedures and tests of special sense development should be considered logical extensions of the physical examination.

Time-consuming, expensive, or potentially dangerous tests are to be avoided when there is little chance the results will affect therapy. However, even the most expensive diagnostic procedure is relatively cost effective when compared to a lifetime of dependent living or loss of employment potential. Most diagnostic efforts will be directed toward the pathologic group, the lower 10% of mentally retarded persons. However, every reasonable attempt should be made to establish the etiologic diagnosis in *all cases* of mental retardation. In the case of a mildly retarded person this might involve only the time and expense of sending for birth records or the mother's prenatal records. In a severely retarded person with normal parents it is justifiable to include chromosome analysis and metabolic screening in the evaluation. Other well-accepted indications for metabolic evaluation include: two or more affected members in the same family, infantile and especially neonatal seizures, recurrent episodes of altered consciousness, and the presence of other associated neurologic signs or symptoms. Commonly used metabolic tests are discussed in Chapter 23.

Several specific neurodiagnostic tests are widely available and may aid in etiologic diagnosis when *selectively* applied. They are of greatest value in the investigation of severely retarded persons. The yield is further increased when specific or focal abnormalities are found on neurologic examination. In certain cases they may be applied to the larger subcultural group to help determine etiology or to answer specific questions about brain structure or function. For example, routine skull radiographs allow indirect quantitation of cerebral volume and provide detail of skull shape and maturation. Premature closure of one or more of the cranial sutures (craniosynostosis) may occur in isolation or in association with other craniofacial abnormalities, as in Crouzon, Apert, or Pfeiffer syndromes. Intracranial calcifications may be seen in cases of congenital infection (toxoplasmosis or cytomegalovirus) or in tuberous sclerosis.

Computed tomography is currently the best commercially available method to evaluate central nervous system anatomy. New generation scanners give excellent detail of brain parenchyma, including differentiation between gray and white matter. Conditions that affect gray matter may be associated with unusually prominent cerebral sulci or may have no obvious CT abnormality. Abnormally lucent white matter may be seen in the leukodystrophies. CT is especially useful for the evaluation of suspected hydrocephalus or porencephaly.

The EEG is a means to monitor cortical electrical activity that allows evaluation of brain wave maturational patterns as well as paroxysmal events (seizures). Certain patterns, such as hypsarrhythmia or the slow spike-wave pattern of Lennox and Gastaut, suggest poor developmental or intellectual outcome.

Other specific neurodiagnostic tests may be occasionally valuable in the diagnosis of mental retardation. The peripheral nerve conduction velocity is usually slow in a number of rare conditions associated with mental retardation, such as metachromatic leukodystrophy, Krabbe disease, spinocerebellar degenerations, and hereditary peripheral neuropathies. The electromyogram (EMG) is useful in distinguishing between neurogenic and myogenic weakness but usually does not help establish etiologic diagnosis in mental retardation. However, some persons with myotonic muscular dystrophy are mentally retarded, and the EMG demonstration of myotonia helps confirm this diagnosis.

Psychometric testing. Psychometric testing should be performed when the patient is old enough or advanced enough to cooperate. In many cases it is only through this specific testing that mild or moderate mental retardation can be separated from learning disabilities or motivational problems. Emphasis should be placed on identifying strengths as well as weaknesses of each person with a view to recommending appropriate educational placement or vocational training. Severely retarded persons can benefit from the proper learning experience.

Diagnosis. Mentally retarded persons should first be given a descriptive diagnosis that emphasizes current level of function. Classification into a subgroup is often possible as part of the descriptive diagnosis. Specific etiologic diagnosis and level of certainty of diagnosis should be provided if possible.

EXAMPLE:

Descriptive diagnosis. Eight-year-old moderately mentally retarded, Stanford Binet IQ 50. Patient follows instructions well, no behavioral problems, functionally independent at home

Etiologic diagnosis. Down syndrome, confirmed karyotype, Trisomy 21.

Descriptive diagnosis. Six-year-old, profoundly mentally retarded. Static encephalopathy manifested by spastic quadriparesis, seizure disorder, and absence of communication skills.

Etiologic diagnosis. Perinatal asphyxia with hypoxic-ischemic encephalopathy, 5-minute Apgar 1 (heart rate only).

The well-being of severely and profoundly mentally retarded persons is largely dependent on the care and resources of the family and community. The physician, educator, psychologist, physical and occupational therapist, speech pathologist, and social worker are important resources for both. At a young age most severely and profoundly mentally retarded persons can be taken care of at home, provided specialized support is available. Although many communities have appropriate preschool and school programs, the emotional and financial commitment to the family can be enormous. Seemingly minimal problems such as transportation to school can be quite difficult to overcome, especially for working parents. Occasionally, residential school placement is desirable to give the child proper nutritional, emotional, and educational support for optimal growth.

The physician should assume many of the professional responsibilities related to the care of this group of retarded persons. These may include (1) conducting the initial medical evaluation to include an etiologic diagnosis if possible; (2) continuing medical care to prevent complications; (3) providing information to the family and other professionals concerning diagnosis, prognosis, and medical treatment; (4) helping to ensure that proper educational and other professional services are available to the patient and optimally used to enhance best quality of life; (5) providing emotional support for the family and patient; and (6) counseling the family about institutionalization when appropriate.

Mildly and moderately retarded persons differ from the general population primarily in cognitive ability. Often they are from underprivileged social and economic backgrounds. Children with relatively normal intelligence but with a severe learning disability may be difficult to separate from this group. They represent the largest group of mentally retarded citizens and pose a great challenge to society. The physician should attempt to make an etiologic diagnosis in these patients even though it is more difficult than with the more severely affected group of patients. The psychometric process helps to identify relative *strengths* as well as weaknesses and to encourage proper educational placement and support. Defining relative strengths helps to engender a sense of self-esteem and assists in the design of educational programs and employment. The importance of early intervention cannot be overemphasized. With proper support, most members of this group can be gainfully employed. They need minimal, if any, living supervision. As they blend into the labor force, their numbers seem to diminish with advancing age.

• • •

In summary, variations exist within the subdivisions of mental retardation. Mildly retarded persons may be unrecognized because many are employed and can live independently. Mild to moderately retarded persons with disorders of the special senses or with severe motor handicap may not be capable of independent living for a number of reasons. More severely affected persons usually remain dependent but can learn and grow from experience and should be afforded the opportunity for personal advancement. The medical approach to mentally retarded children should be individualized, as with any other medical or neurologic problem. There are few areas in medicine in which the physician can hope to have as great an impact on the quality of life for the individual patient.

Donald A. Taylor

SELECTED READINGS

Adams, R.D., and Lyon, G.: Neurology of hereditary metabolic diseases of children, New York, 1982, McGraw-Hill Book Co.

Adams, R.D., and Victor, M.: Principles of neurology, New York, 1981, McGraw-Hill Book Co.

Allen, H.A.: Testing of visual acuity in preschool children: norms, variables, and a new picture test, Pediatrics **19:**1093, 1957.

American Medical Association Conference on Mental Retardation: Mental Retardation: a handbook for the primary physician, JAMA **191:**183, 1965.

Barlow, C.F.: Mental retardation and related disorders, Philadelphia, 1978, F.A. Davis Co.

Carter, C.H., editor: Medical aspects of mental retardation, Springfield, Ill., 1978, Charles C Thomas, Publisher.

Conley, R.W.: The economics of mental retardation, Baltimore, 1973, Johns Hopkins University Press.

Crome, L., and Stern, J.: Pathology of mental retardation, Baltimore, 1972, The Williams & Wilkins Co.

Dodge, P.R., and Porter, P.: Demonstration of intracranial pathology by transillumination, Arch. Neurol. **5:**594, 1961.

Dodge, P.R., et al.: Nutrition and the developing nervous system, St. Louis, 1975, The C.V. Mosby Co.

Friede, R.L.: Developmental neuropathology, New York, 1975, Springer-Verlag New York, Inc.

Grossman, H.J., editor: Manual on terminology and classification in mental retardation, Washington, D.C., 1973, American Association on Mental Deficiency.

Huttenlocher, P.R.: Dendritic development in neocortex of children with mental defect and infantile spasms, Neurology **24:**203, 1974.

Huttenlocher, P.R.: Synaptic and dendritic development and mental defect. In Buchwald, N.A., and Brazier, M.A.B., editors: Brain mechanisms in mental retardation, New York, 1975, Academic Press, Inc.

Illingworth, R.S.: The development of the infant and young child, Edinburgh, 1975, Churchill Livingstone.

Lewis, E.O.: Types of mental deficiency and their social significance, J. Ment. Sci. **79:**298, 1933.

Menkes, J.H.: Textbook of child neurology, Philadelphia, 1980, Lea & Febiger.

Menolascino, F.J., and Egger, M.L.: Medical dimensions of mental retardation, Lincoln, 1978, University of Nebraska Press.

Panel on Developmental Neurological Disorders: Technical document to the National Advisory Neurological and Communicative Disorders and Stroke Council, NIH Pub. No. 79-1919, Bethesda, Md., 1979, National Institute of Health.

Purpura, D.P.: Dendritic spine "dysgenesis" and mental retardation, Science **186:**1126, 1974.

Purpura, D.P.: Normal and aberrant neuronal development in the cerebral cortex of human fetus and young infant. In Buchwald, N.A., and Brazier, M.A.B., editors: Brain mechanisms in mental retardation, New York, 1975, Academic Press, Inc.

Purpura, D.P., and Reaser, G.P., editors: Methodological approaches to the study of brain maturation and its abnormalities, Baltimore, 1974, University Park Press.

Rapin, I.: Children with brain dysfunction, New York, 1982, Raven Press.

Robinson, N.M., and Robinson, H.B.: The mentally retarded child, New York, 1976, McGraw-Hill Book Co.

Scheerenberger, R.C.: Public residential services for the mentally retarded, 1982, National Association of Superintendents of Public Residential Facilities for the Mentally Retarded, 1982.

Smith, D.W.: Recognizable patterns of human malformation, Philadelphia, 1982, W.B. Saunders Co.

Towbin, A.: Mental retardation due to germinal matrix infarction, Science **164:**156, 1969.

Volpe, J.J.: Neurology of the newborn, Philadelphia, 1981, W.B. Saunders Co.

7 Autosomal Abnormalities

The chromosome constitution *(karyotype)* of the normal human somatic cell consists of 44 *autosomes* and 2 *sex chromosomes*. The chromosomes occur in pairs: 22 pairs of autosomes and the sex pair, one member of each pair having been donated by the germ cell of each parent of the person. For a schematic representation of gametogenesis showing reduction of the chromosome number from the diploid number 46 to the haploid number 23 and restoration of the diploid number by fertilization, see p. 603.

A second application of the term *karyotype* refers to the *photographic* representation of the human chromosomes arranged in pairs or groups in order of descending size, according to the position of the constricted area *(centromere)* that joins the two *chromatids* of any metaphase chromosome, and more recently according to certain morphologic characteristics produced by specific staining techniques. Chromosomes whose centromeres are equidistant from the ends of the chromatids are designated *metacentric,* those whose centromeres are very near one end of the chromatids are designated *acrocentric,* and those with intermediately placed centromeres are designated *submetacentric*. In the human being a satellite (a small mass of chromatin separated from the main body of the chromosome by a narrow stalk) is attached to the short arm of each acrocentric chromosome (except the Y chromosome), although these are not always visible in the microscope.

Until approximately 14 years ago, available routine techniques allowed identification of only a few pairs of human chromosomes—numbers 1, 2, 3, 16, Y, and usually 17 and 18. Pairs 13, 14, and 15 and the late-replicating X chromosome could be identified by *autoradiography,* a rather cumbersome and time-consuming procedure. Within the past 14 years a number of new techniques have been developed that have not only permitted specific identification of each chromosome but also have led to new insights into chromosome structure and behavior and to detailed definition of structural chromosome abnormalities. Two techniques now used routinely are the so-called *G-banding* procedures, which use Giemsa staining of pretreated chromosomes, and the *Q-banding* procedure, which involves the analysis of chromosomes stained with quinacrine and examined with the fluorescent microscope. The banding patterns produced by these techniques were described in the report of the 1971 Paris Conference on Standardization in Human Cytogenetics, and updated and supplemented in 1975, 1978, and 1981 with information on new techniques and the knowledge gained therefrom. Significant technical advances have occurred since the first reports on chromosome banding in the early 1970s. Original *banding maps* (Fig. 7-1) were based on the analysis of condensed metaphase chromosomes. Techniques that allow the study of early metaphase, prometaphase, and prophase chromosomes have been developed. Studies of such high-resolution banded chromosomes have led to refinements in banding maps, with division of metaphase bands into multiple subbands. This has led to the identification of small deletions and duplications not previously discernible and to more accurate assignment of breakpoints in structural chromosome rearrangements. Techniques for the hybridization of human cells with cells from other species have allowed the mapping of specific genes to specific chromosomes, even to specific bands of those chromosomes. New knowledge regarding chromosome behavior in genetically determined diseases inherited in straightforward Mendelian fashion, and in response to environmental mutagens, has emanated from the use of techniques to demonstrate exchange of chromosome material between sister chromatids of replicated chromosomes. The demonstration of *fragile sites* within chromo-

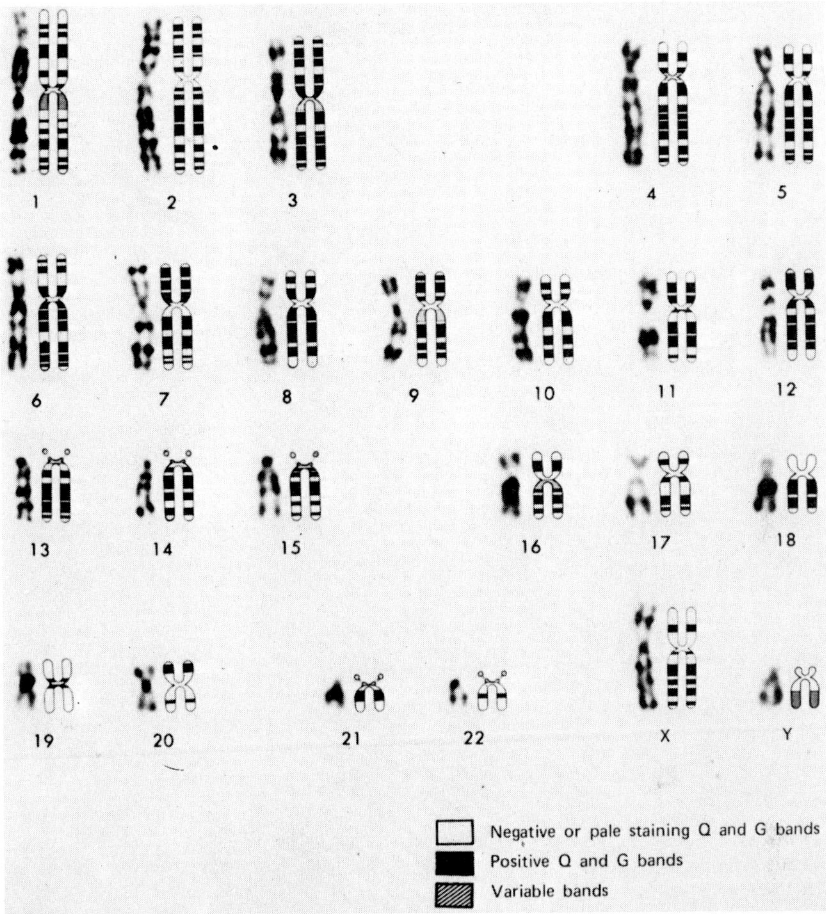

Fig. 7-1. Human karyotype demonstrating schematically the banding pattern (G-banding) of each chromosome in the right-hand member of each pair and photographically the banding pattern in Giemsa-stained chromosomes in the left-hand member of each pair. Q-banding patterns are in general similar, but because they are demonstrated by fluorescence microscopy, bands that are dark in G-banded chromosomes are bright in Q-banded chromosomes, and vice versa. (Courtesy A.T. Therapel, Memphis.)

somes has generated excitement regarding such conditions as X-linked mental retardation and has opened new avenues for research into the pathogenesis of genetic disease. Various combinations of the above techniques are now also providing opportunities for further investigation into the etiology and pathogenesis of diseases heretofore of unknown cause, including cancer.

Karyotypes in this chapter will, in general, depict chromosomes stained by the G-banding technique, the Q-banding technique, or both. Fig. 7-1 illustrates the characteristic banding pattern diagrammatically on the right for each chromosome and photographically from an actual stained cell on the left. An example of a normal female banded metaphase karyotype is shown in Fig. 7-2, and that of a normal male is shown in Fig. 7-3.

Since the inception of techniques for human chromosome analysis 28 years ago, it has become obvious that chromosome abnormalities account for significant human morbidity and mortality. In at least 7% of all human pregnancies the conceptus bears an abnormality in the number or the structure of the chromosomes. It has been estimated that 90% of these abnor-

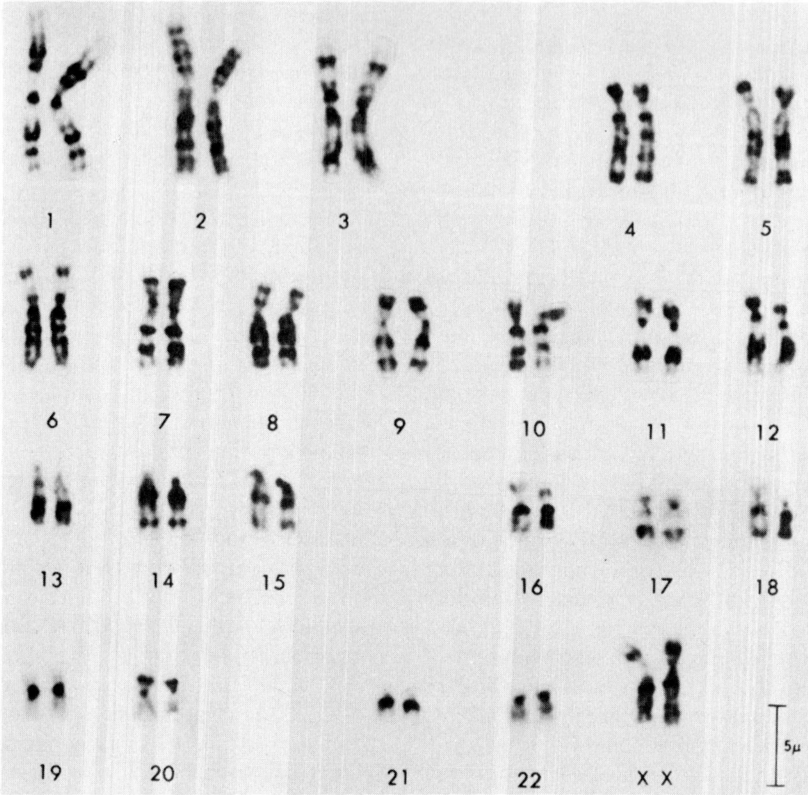

Fig. 7-2. Normal G-banded female karyotype, designated 46,XX. Pairs 1, 2, and 3 comprise group A; pairs 4 and 5, group B; pairs 6 through 12 and the X chromosome, group C; pairs 13 through 15, group D; pairs 16 through 18, group E; pairs 19 and 20, group F; pairs 21 and 22, group G.

malities result in aberrant development, but only about 10% of the developmentally abnormal conceptions produce liveborn infants. The other 90% terminate in spontaneous abortion. Further estimates indicate that approximately 50% of the products of recognizable spontaneous abortion have a chromosome abnormality. *At least* 1 in 200 liveborn infants harbors an *unbalanced* chromosome abnormality, one that involves a gain or loss in net chromosomal material. Approximately one half of these involve the autosomes; the other half discussed in Chapter 22 concern the sex chromosomes. Approximately 1 in 500 persons in the normal population harbors a balanced chromosome rearrangement without obvious clinically detectable effects. Minor variations in the karyotype, the significance of which is yet to be determined, may occur in as much as 20% of the general population. The incidence of significant chromosome abnormalities in certain selected subpopulations is striking. Sex chromatin positive males are almost six times as common in mentally defective populations as the 1 in 1000 general population figure, the highest frequency being in the high-grade mentally defective population. At least 4% of children with multiple congenital anomalies have a chromosome abnormality, and the incidence of recognizable chromosome aberrations in clinically unclassifiable mentally retarded children with three or more congenital anomalies is approximately 10%.

Since the discovery of autosomal trisomy in Down syndrome in 1959, a number of clinical syndromes have been attributed to chromosome aberrations. Those involving the sex chromosomes are reviewed briefly in the discussion of sex differentiation and development (pp. 615 to

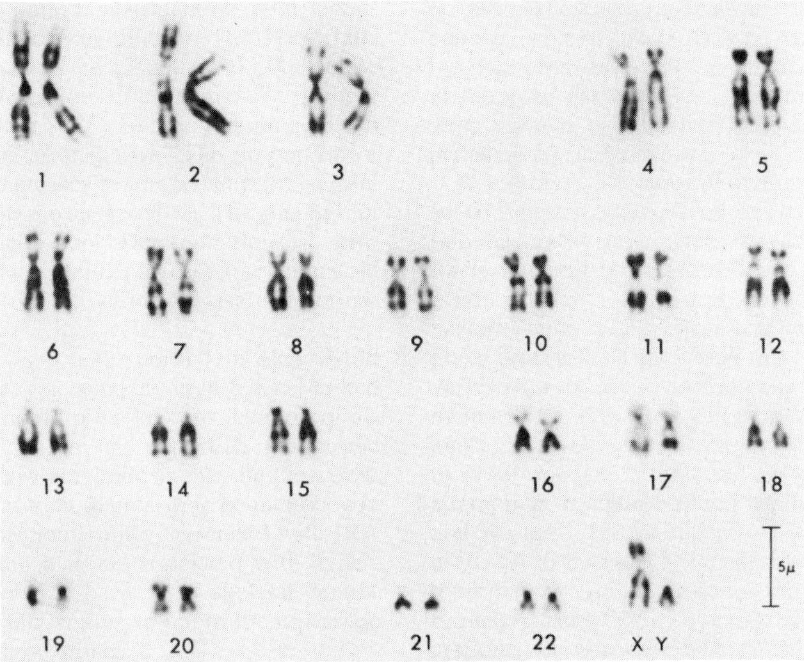

Fig. 7-3. Normal male karyotype, G-banded, designated 46,XY. Note the characteristic Y chromosome.

629). Only abnormalities of the autosomes will be discussed here.

TRISOMY

Trisomy is probably the most frequently encountered autosomal abnormality. Trisomy for a given chromosome occurs when that chromosome is present in triplicate instead of in the normally encountered pair (disomy). Trisomy is usually the result of chromosomal *nondisjunction* in meiosis. The total somatic chromosome number is *47* instead of *46*. Three *autosomal trisomy syndromes*—Down syndrome (trisomy 21), trisomy 18, and trisomy 13—have been well defined. For a number of years, and since the advent of chromosome banding techniques, others have been delineated (e.g., trisomy 8).

Down syndrome. Down syndrome was the first condition found to be caused by autosomal trisomy. In 1959 Lejeune and colleagues found that cells from patients with Down syndrome contained 47 chromosomes and that an extra small acrocentric (G group) chromosome was present. They designated this chromosome abnormality *trisomy 21,* a term that was widely accepted, although it was difficult to differentiate the two pairs of chromosomes in the G group by older techniques. The advent of banding techniques has allowed the identification of the chromosome that is trisomic in Down syndrome as the smaller of the two pairs in the G group. Nevertheless, because of the prior use of the term *trisomy 21,* the involved chromosome was designated number 21. The karyotype of a male with trisomy 21 and Down syndrome is shown in Fig. 7-4. Meiotic nondisjunction leading to trisomy 21 is shown in Fig. 7-5.

Down syndrome is not rare; the incidence is approximately 1 in 800 live births. It occurs in all racial groups and in all areas of the world. A definite correlation exists between the incidence of Down syndrome and advanced maternal age (Fig. 7-6); approximately 20% of the mothers of children with this condition are 35 years of age or older at the time of the birth of their affected offspring. Table 7-1 shows the single year maternal age correlation with the incidence of trisomy 21 from ages 20 to 49. The table reveals the sharp increase in risk after a maternal age of 35 years.

The application of chromosome-banding tech-

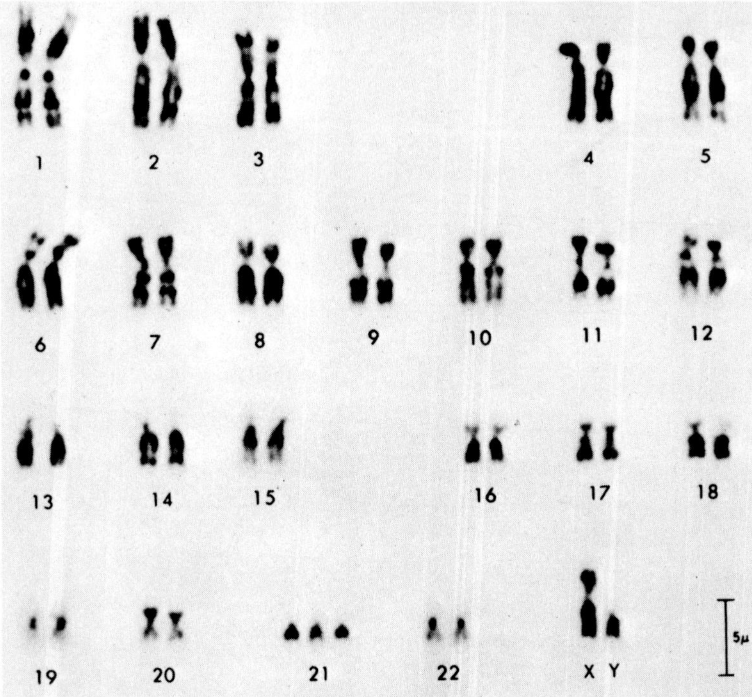

Fig. 7-4. G-banded karyotype of male with trisomy 21: 47,XY, +21. The G group chromosome in triplicate, number 21, has a banding pattern that allows it to be distinguished clearly from number 22. (From Summitt, R.L.: Pediatr. Ann. **2**:40, 1973.)

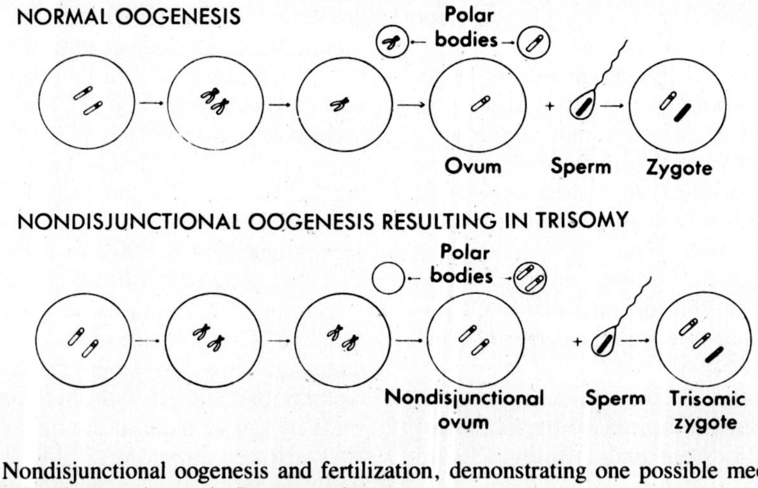

Fig. 7-5. Nondisjunctional oogenesis and fertilization, demonstrating one possible mechanism of misdivision leading to trisomy in Down syndrome.

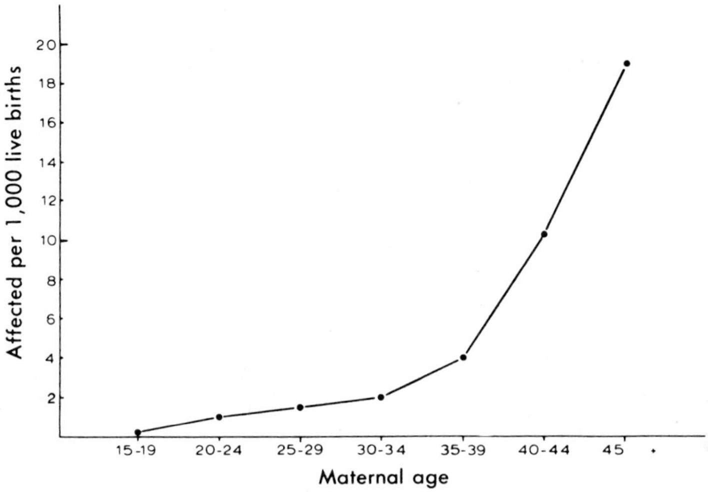

Fig. 7-6. General frequency of Down syndrome relative to maternal age. (Data from Carter, C.O., and Evans, K.A.: Lancet **2:**785, 1961.)

Table 7-1. Estimated rates of Down syndrome

Maternal age (years)*	Trisomy 21 estimated rate	All chromosome abnormalities estimated rate	Maternal age (years)	Trisomy 21 estimated rate	All chromosome abnormalities estimated rate
<15	1/1000	1/435	32	1/715	1/333
15	1/1000	1/435	33	1/625	1/295
16	1/1110	1/455	34	1/500	1/244
17	1/1250	1/475	35	1/385	1/196
18	1/1430	1/500	36	1/294	1/159
19	1/1666	1/525	37	1/227	1/128
20	1/1666	1/525	38	1/175	1/103
21	1/1666	1/525	39	1/137	1/83
22	1/1666	1/525	40	1/106	1/66
23	1/1430	1/500	41	1/82	1/52
24	1/1250	1/475	42	1/67	1/42
25	1/1250	1/475	43	1/50	1/33
26	1/1110	1/455	44	1/38	1/26
27	1/1000	1/435	45	1/30	1/21
28	1/1000	1/435	46	1/23	1/16
29	1/910	1/400	47	1/18	1/13
30	1/910	1/400	48	1/14	1/10
31	1/830	1/370	49	1/11	1/7

From Hook, E.B., and Cross, P.K., Am. J. Hum. Genet. **31:**136A, 1979, and Hook, E.B., et al.: Am. J. Hum. Genet., **34:**128A, 1983.

*Age at last birthday at delivery.

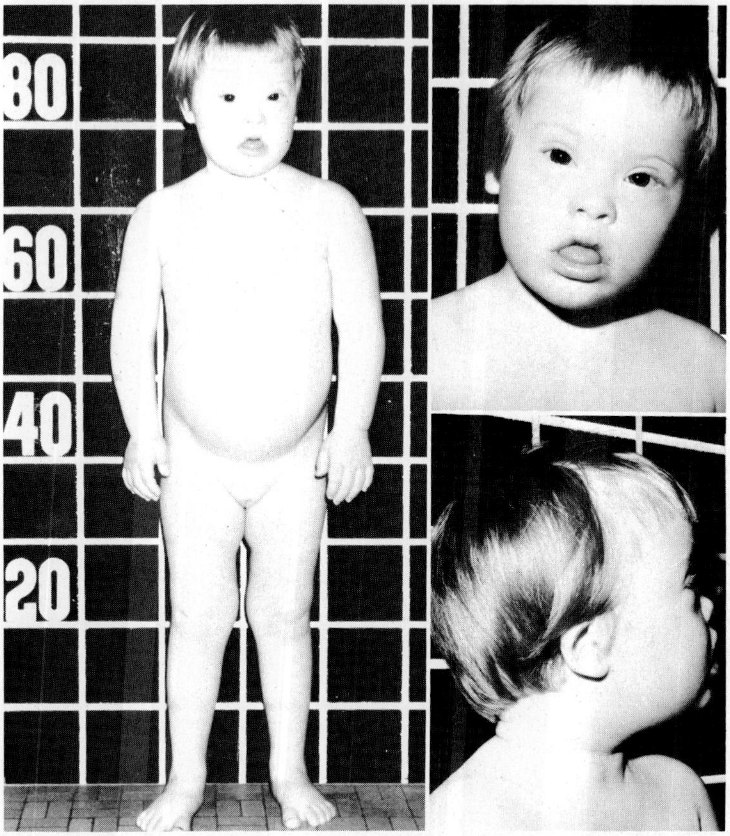

Fig. 7-7. Three-year-old girl with Down syndrome.

niques has made it possible to determine in a number of instances whether the extra chromosome 21 in a patient with Down syndrome is derived from the mother or the father. Despite the long-known correlation between the incidence of Down syndrome and advancing maternal age, in fully 30% of the cases studied, the extra chromosome was derived from the *father*. A number of recent studies have addressed the possibility of a correlation between advancing paternal age, independent of maternal age, and the incidence of Down syndrome. Although results have not been consistent, critical analysis of available data reveals *no* convincing correlation between advancing paternal age and incidence of Down syndrome. Overall, the error in cell division that leads to trisomy 21 in the offspring occurs most often in the first meiotic division in oogenesis in the mother (Fig. 7-5), as revealed by banding studies on parental origin.

Down syndrome is almost invariably associated with *significant* mental retardation, as are most conditions involving *any gain or loss* of total autosomal mass. A child with the typical clinical phenotype of Down syndrome is shown in Fig. 7-7. Because diagnosis can almost always be made clinically, chromosome analysis is used for laboratory confirmation and, more importantly, to identify the unusual *mosaic* or *translocation* karyotype that might indicate heritable Down syndrome and that will be mentioned later. Diagnosis is not based on the presence of (nor is it excluded by the absence of) any one or two phenotypic abnormalities of Down syndrome; rather, it is based on the *total* clinical phenotype of the patient. The abnormalities commonly encountered by the clinician are summarized in Table 7-2. Patients suffering from Down syndrome may succumb to heart disease; they are highly susceptible to respiratory infections.

Table 7-2. Anomalies of Down syndrome

Area	Common (50% or more of patients)	Less than 50% of patients
General	Hypotonia; shortness of stature	
Central nervous system	Mental deficiency, IQ = 25 to 50	Seizures
Cranium	Relatively flat occiput	
Eyes	Oblique palpebral fissures; inner epicanthic folds; speckling of iris (Brushfield spots); short and sparse eyelashes	Strabismus Nystagmus Cataract
Ears	Small; overlapping upper helices; attached lobules	Low set
Nose	Flat nasal bridge; small nose	
Mouth	Hypoplasia of maxilla ± narrow palate; protruding tongue ± fissuring	
Mandible	Micrognathia	
Neck	Broad and/or short in appearance	Laxity of skin
Hands	Short hands and fingers; clinodactyly of fifth finger; simian crease pattern; dermal—distal palmar axial triradius, high frequency of ulnar loops on digits	Single crease, fifth finger
Feet	Gap and/or plantar furrow, first and second toes; hallucal loop distal (small) or arch tibial pattern	
Thorax		Funnel or pigeon chest
Abdomen	Diastasis recti	Umbilical hernia
Genitals	Male—small penis	Cryptorchidism
Radiographic findings	Hypoplasia of second phalanx of fifth finger	Decreased acetabular, iliac angles
Cardiac		Atrial septum primum defect; ventricular septal defect; tetralogy of Fallot
Intestine		Duodenal atresia; tracheoesophageal fistula

Modified from Smith, D.W.: Autosomal abnormalities, Am. J. Obstet. Gynecol. **90:**1055, 1964.

Once a diagnosis of Down syndrome is made (and it can usually be made in the newborn period), the parents must be counseled regarding the meaning of the diagnosis and must be informed of the risk of recurrence. In general, once a couple has had an infant with Down syndrome, the risk that they will have a second affected offspring is low (approximately 1%). This fact should be encouraging to prospective parents. However, the risk in a given case cannot be accurately estimated without chromosome analysis, since Down syndrome is sometimes the result of chromosome *translocation*. In such cases the long arm of the extra chromosome 21 is attached to another chromosome, most commonly the long arm of a D or another G group chromosome. Such translocations involving entire arms of two acrocentric chromosomes are termed *Robertsonian translocations*. In a patient with 21-D translocation Down syndrome the karyotype includes 46 chromosomes, with only 4 chromosomes in the G group and only 5 normal chromosomes in the D group instead of the normal 6 chromosomes, but with an extra C-like chromosome that is the result of fusion of a number 21 and a D chromosome (Fig. 7-8) and that is designated t(Dq21q) according to the 1971 Paris Conference on Standardization in Human Cytogenetics. Banding techniques have allowed identification of the D chromosomes involved in Dq21q translocations as number 14 or 15, and only rarely number 13. Approximately 3.5% of all cases of trisomy 21 syndrome are the translocation variety. Of these, 44% involve chromosome 21 and a D chromosome, and 56% involve number 21 and another G chromosome. Translocation Down syndrome may occur as a sporadic event or may be inherited from a so-called *translocation heterozygote*. In such a heterozygous parent the karyotype includes 45 chromosomes with only 3 chromosomes in the G group, 5 chromosomes in the D group, and the C-like t(Dq21q) fusion chromosome. The parent whose karyotype is shown in Fig. 7-9, although her cells contain only 45 chromosomes, is phenotypically normal because the only chromosome mass lacking is the short arms of the two fused chromosomes and

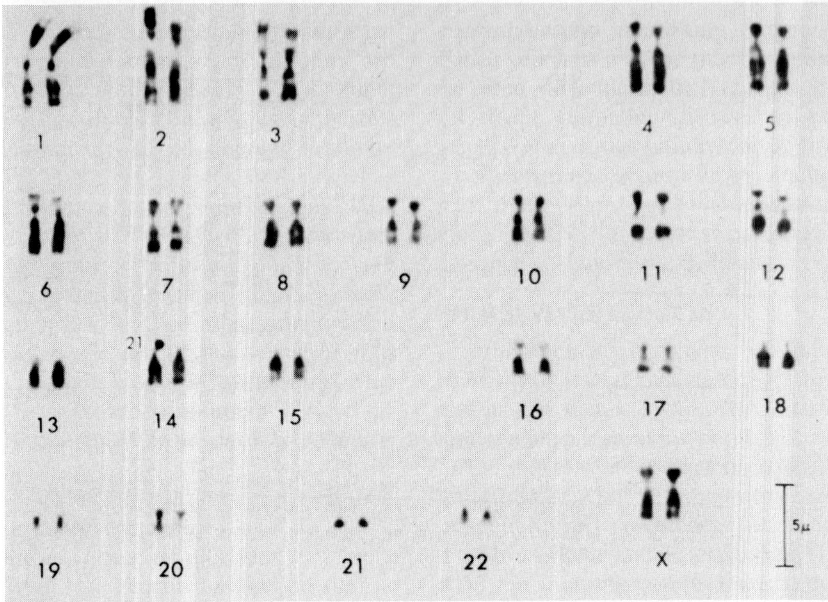

Fig. 7-8. G-banded karyotype of female with Down syndrome caused by a 21-14 translocation, designated 46,XX,-14, + t(14q21q). Note that the short arm of one chromosome 14 is longer than that of any other D group chromosome because the long arm of chromosome 21 is attached thereto. Thus the karyotype demonstrates trisomy 21.

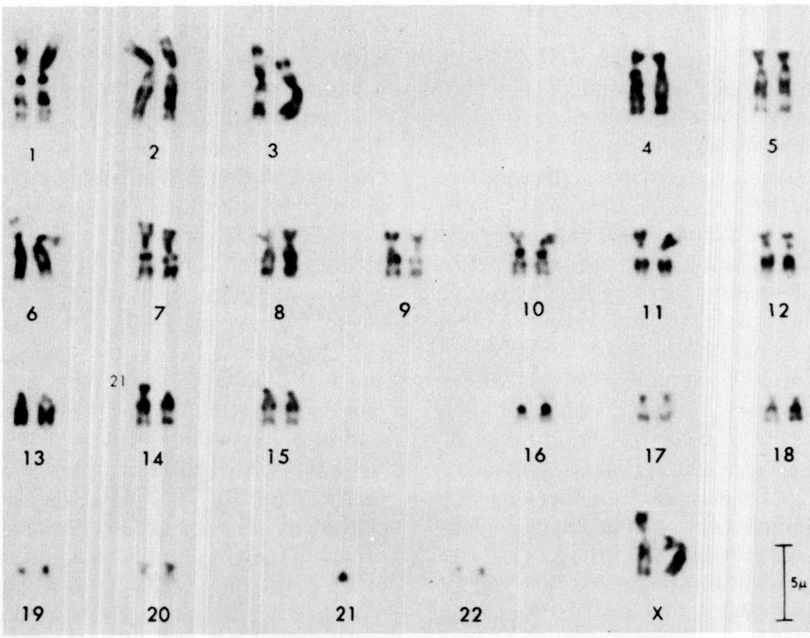

Fig. 7-9. G-banded karyotype of phenotypically normal female carrier of 14-21 translocation, designated 45,XX,-14,-21, + t(14q21q). Although the total chromosome number is 45, with only one apparent chromosome 21, the second chromosome 21 is attached to number 14.

because the absence of short arms of two acrocentric chromosomes involved in a Robertsonian translocation produces no deleterious effects.

Such an abnormality may be transmitted in normal persons through multiple generations of a family. Approximately 9% of children with Down syndrome born to mothers younger than 30 years of age suffer from the condition because of translocation; about one fourth of this group have inherited the condition. Thus the chances of finding an inherited translocation if one analyzes the chromosomes of a patient with Down syndrome born to a mother younger than 30 years of age are about 1 in 40. In contrast, only about 1 out of 300 children with Down syndrome are born to mothers 30 years of age or older from an inherited translocation. Translocation Down syndrome bears no correlation with advancing maternal age.

In contrast to the low risk of recurrence in those instances resulting from meiotic nondisjunction, the risk of an offspring with Down syndrome being born to a *mother* who is heterozygous for a 21-D translocation is relatively high. Observations have not borne out the theoretical risk of 1 in 3 that any offspring will be affected, 1 in 3 that any will (like the mother) be a heterozygous carrier of the translocation, and 1 in 3 that any will be phenotypically and karyotypically normal. With proper correction for bias of ascertainment the risk of an affected offspring to a heterozygous carrier mother, if that mother was ascertained through a person with Down syndrome because of an unbalanced 21-D translocation, is about 10% with any pregnancy. The likelihood of an offspring who is a phenotypically normal heterozygote (like the mother) for the same translocation is about 50%, and that of a normal offspring with a normal karyotype is about 40%. On the other hand, the probability of an affected offspring is less than 5% if the *father,* ascertained through an affected family member, is the heterozygous carrier of the translocation. If *either* parent is a carrier of a 21-21 translocation, all liveborn offspring *will be affected.* If the mother carries a 21-22 translocation, the risk of an affected offspring with any pregnancy is about 7%, although data are few. In the case in which karyotypically normal parents have previously had a liveborn or stillborn infant with 47, +21 Down syndrome, or have had an abortion with trisomy 21, we have counseled that the recurrence risk is in the previously mentioned 1% range. Hook and others have recommended the use of a recurrence risk of 1% *added to* the maternal age-related risk.

Trisomy 18. In 1960, trisomy 18 was described simultaneously by Patau and associates and by Edwards and associates. It apparently occurs much less frequently than Down syndrome; the most accurate figure available is 1 in 8000 live births. The condition has been seen more commonly in females than in males. A positive correlation with advanced maternal age is apparent in this condition, which is also assumed to be the result of meiotic nondisjunction.

The infant with trisomy 18 (Fig. 7-10) is typically small at birth, even when born at term, and fails to thrive from the outset. Most patients die within the first few months of life. The anomalies commonly seen with the syndrome are summarized in Table 7-3. The diagnosis of trisomy 18 syndrome, like that of Down syndrome, can usually be made on the basis of the *total* clinical phenotype.

The karyotype of a patient with trisomy 18 includes 47 chromosomes (Fig. 7-11), with an extra chromosome 18. The extra chromosome 18 may rarely be attached (translocated) to another chromosome.

Trisomy 13. Patau and associates first described trisomy 13 in 1960. Since then, many occurrences have been reported. The frequency is approximately 1 in 20,000 live births. The commonly encountered anomalies in this condition are summarized in Table 7-4, and the typical appearance of the patient is shown in Fig. 7-12. The phenotype in this syndrome is more variable than that in either Down syndrome or trisomy 18 syndrome. The karyotype typical of an affected infant is illustrated in Fig. 7-13. Other less common chromosome abnormalities, such as 13-D translocation, are encountered as a cause of trisomy 13.

Other trisomies. The routine use of chromosome-banding techniques in most laboratories over the past 8 years has led to the delineation of trisomy syndromes other than the three that have been known for 2 decades. The best evidence for the existence of a clinical syndrome attributable to trisomy of a whole chromosome is available for trisomy 8, trisomy 9, and tri-

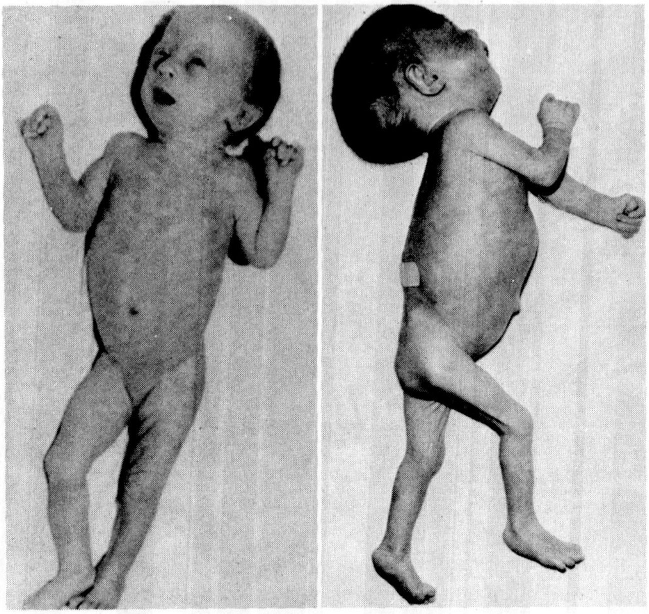

Fig. 7-10. Female infant with trisomy 18 syndrome.

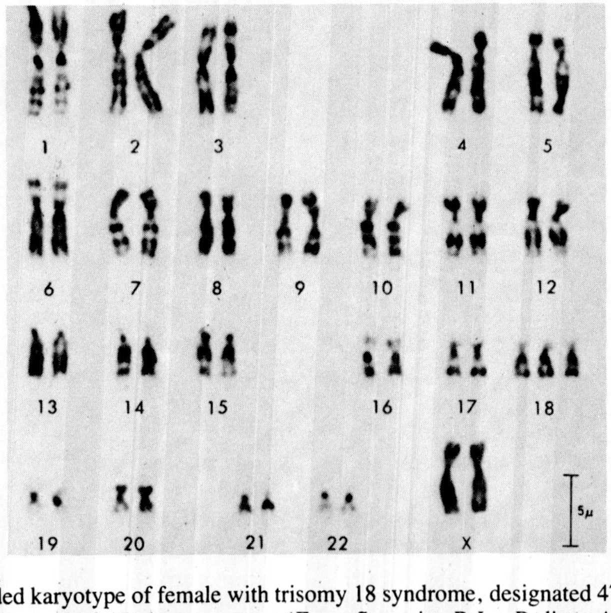

Fig. 7-11. G-banded karyotype of female with trisomy 18 syndrome, designated 47,XX, + 18. Note 3 chromosomes 18: total of 47 chromosomes. (From Summitt, R.L.: Pediatr. Ann. **2**:40, 1973.)

Table 7-3. Anomalies of the trisomy 18 syndrome

Area	Common (50% or more of patients)	Less common (10-50% of patients)	Unusual but mentioned
General	Females (78%)		
Amniotic fluid, placenta	Polyhydramnios, small placenta	Single umbilical artery	
Growth			
Fetal Postnatal	Birth weight under 6 lb; failure to thrive		
Central nervous system	Apparent mental deficiency; hypertonicity		Small or aplastic cerebellum; microgyria; cerebral hemiatrophy; defect of corpus callosum; meningomyelocele, hydrocephalus
Cranium	Prominent occiput	Widely patent fontanels or metopic suture	Overriding sutures
Ears and eyes	Low-set, usually malformed ears	Ptosis of eyelid, inner epicanthic folds; small palpebral fissures; corneal opacity	Coloboma of iris, downward slant
Mandible, nose, and mouth	Micrognathia, narrow palatal arch	Small oral opening, cleft in lip or palate, narrow palate, short philtrum	Choanal atresia
Arms and hands	Fingers flexed, index overlaps third or fifth overlaps fourth; digital pattern, low arches on fingertips	Simian crease, single crease fifth finger; hypoplasia of fingernails; ulnar or radial deviation of hand; flaccidity or hypoplasia of thumb; phocomelia, oligodactyly	Syndactyly third and fourth fingers; polydactyly, cleft deformities
Feet	Hallux short or dorsiflexed, rocker-bottom, clubfoot	Syndactyly second and third toes	Cleft deformities
Thorax	Short sternum	Wide chest or wide-spread nipples	Hemivertebra; rib anomaly
Pelvis, hips, anus	Small pelvis, limited hip abduction	Malposed or funnel-shaped anus	Dislocated hip
Cardiovascular	Ventricular septal defect; patent ductus arteriosus	Atrial septal defect, bicuspid aortic or pulmonic valves; nodularity of valve leaflets; pulmonic stenosis or atresia	Coarctation of aorta; anomalous coronary ostia; transposition; tetralogy; dextrocardia, right aortic arch; ventricular septal hypertrophy; aberrant right subclavian artery; arteriosclerosis with medial calcification
Lung			Bilobed right lung; supernumerary fissures, right lung; agenesis, right lung
Renal	Malformation	Horseshoe, unilateral, or double kidney, double ureter	Hydronephrosis, polycystic (small cysts)
Gastrointestinal	Meckel diverticulum; heterotopic pancreatic tissue		Tracheoesophageal fistula; pyloric stenosis; incomplete rotation of colon; omphalocele
Genitals	Male—cryptorchidism	Female—prominent clitoris, small labia	Ovarian hypoplasia; uterus bilocularis
Diaphragm, muscle	Inguinal hernia	Eventration of diaphragm, areas of muscle hypoplasia and aplasia	
Skin, etc.	Prominent cutis marmorata, hypoplastic nails	Redundancy, downy hair forehead and back	Hemangioma

Modified from Smith, D.W.: Autosomal abnormalities, Am. J. Obstet. Gynecol. **90:**1055, 1964.

Table 7-4. Anomalies of the trisomy 13 syndrome

Area	Common (50% or more of patients)	Less common
General	Apneic spells; death within 3 months (69%)	
Central nervous system	Profound mental deficiency; deafness; seizures; agenesis external olfactory apparatus	Hypertonia, hypotonia, fusion of frontal lobes, agenesis corpus callosum, cerebellar hypoplasia
Cranium	Sloping forehead	Microcephaly, wide sagittal suture
Eyes	Microphthalmos and/or colobomas, epicanthal folds, hypertelorism	Hypoplastic supraorbital ridges; slanting palpebral fissures; cataracts with cartilage formation; absent eyebrows
Ears	Abnormal helices or low set	
Mouth and mandible	Cleft lip or palate	Micrognathia, narrow palate; cleft tongue
Skin	Capillary hemangiomata	Localized scalp defect; loose skin at neck; pilonidal dimple
Hands	Distal palmar axial triradii; horizontal palmar crease; hyperconvex narrow fingernails; flexion or overlapping of fingers	Retroflexible thumb; ulnar deviation of hand; synostosis fifth finger; oligodactyly; cleft deformity
Feet	Polydactyly, hands or feet; posterior prominence of heels	Dermal-hallucal arch fibular pattern; syndactyly, hypoplastic toenails, clubfeet
Cardiac	Malformation, including rotational anomaly, ventricular septal defect, auricular septal defect, patent ductus arteriosus, anomalous pulmonary venous return, bicuspid aortic valve, overriding aorta, pulmonic stenosis	
Abdominal	Accessory spleen, large gallbladder; incomplete rotation of colon, appendiceal diverticuli	Umbilical hernia, inguinal hernia; omphalocele; heterotopic pancreatic tissue
Renal		Hydronephrosis; double pelvis; polycystic disease
Genitals		
Male	Cryptorchidism, abnormal scrotum	
Female	Partially bicornate uterus	
Other	Nuclear appendages in polymorphonuclear leukocytes; persistent fetal or embryonic (Gower II) hemoglobin	Small areolae; single umbilical artery; situs inversus lungs; cysts of thymus; calcified pulmonary arterioles; limited hip abduction; cebocephaly

Modified from Smith, D.W.: Autosomal abnormalities, Am. J. Obstet. Gynecol. **90:**1055, 1964.

Table 7-5. Major clinical features of the trisomy 8, trisomy 9, and trisomy 22 syndromes

Feature	Trisomy 8	Trisomy 9	Trisomy 22
General	Mental retardation, short stature, decreased weight, vertebral anomalies	Mental retardation	Growth retardation, mental retardation, hypotonia, deafness
Craniofacies	Dysmorphic skull, prominent forehead, dysplastic ears, strabismus, plump nose with broad base, low-set ears, everted lower lip, high palate, cleft soft palate, micrognathia	Microcephaly, abnormal cranial sutures, prominent forehead, deep-set eyes, protuberant ears, prominent nose, fishmouth, micrognathia	Microcephaly, low-set or malformed ears, preauricular appendages or sinuses, cleft palate, micrognathia, atretic ear canals, epicanthal folds, downward slanting eyes, fishmouth, hypertension, flat nasal bridge, epicanthal folds
Thorax	Congenital heart disease	Congenital heart disease	Congenital heart disease, abnormal or low-placed nipples, 13 pairs of ribs
Abdomen and pelvis	Urinary tract anomaly, narrow pelvis	Urinary tract anomaly	Renal agenesis, imperforate anus
Limbs	Patellar dysplasia, limited joint mobility, deep flexion creases on palms and soles	Congenital hip-knee dislocation, clinodactyly, digital hypoplasia, nail hypoplasia, syndactyly, simian palmar creases, absent B and C palmar digital triradii	Cubitus valgus, fingerlike or malapposed thumbs, dislocated hips, deformed lower limbs

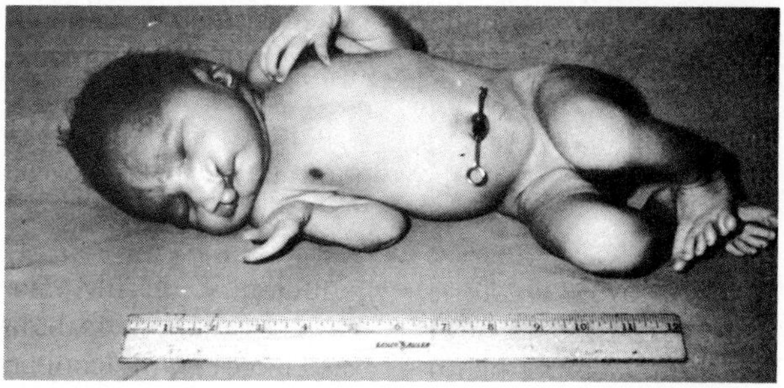

Fig. 7-12. Male infant with trisomy 13 syndrome.

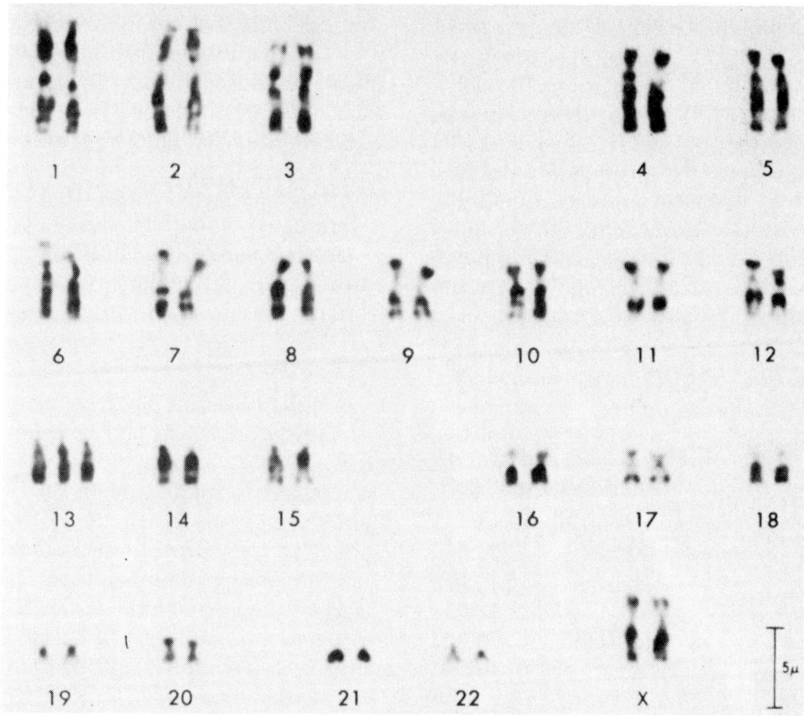

Fig. 7-13. G-banded karyotype of female with trisomy 13 syndrome, designated 47,XX, + 13. Note 3 chromosomes 13: total of 47 chromosomes. (From Summitt, R.L.: Pediatr. Ann. **2:**40, 1973.)

somy 22. Table 7-5 summarizes the findings in those three syndromes. Reported cases of each are too few to establish relationships with parental age.

Trisomy for portions of a number of other autosomes has been observed often enough to allow the delineation of several "partial trisomy" or "duplication" syndromes. These are ordinarily the result of segregation of a structurally abnormal chromosome in a parent who carries a balanced structural rearrangement.

Double aneuploidy. Rare instances of double trisomy have been reported, including XXX–Down syndrome, trisomy 18–Down syndrome, and XXY–Klinefelter syndrome–Down syndrome (double aneuploidy, with aneuploidy being defined as any number of chromosomes other than a multiple of the haploid number 23). Patients with a double aneuploidy show stigmas of both syndromes. The karyotype of a patient with double trisomy includes 48 chromosomes.

MOSAICISM

Mosaicism is the condition in which cell lines of more than one karyotype exist in a single person, all cell lines having been derived from a single fertilized ovum. It is known to occur in patients with any one of the three trisomies previously discussed, as well as in those with other chromosome anomalies (e.g., a patient in whom two cell lines, one normal and one with 47 chromosomes and trisomy 18, exist). Such an abnormality arises from an error in mitosis in the embryo. Patients may have only a few of the stigmas of the syndrome, although correlation between proportions of cell types and clinical severity is extremely poor.

AUTOSOMAL MONOSOMY

Autosomal monosomy exists when one complete autosome is absent from the diploid set. In its nonmosaic form this is an extremely rare abnormality, and it appears safe to generalize that humans tolerate monosomy much more poorly than chromosome excess. Three cases of nonmosaic monosomy for a chromosome of the G group have been reported, but none of these was critically analyzed with current banding techniques.

Mosaic monosomy G has been described, and absence of a portion of chromosome 21 is well known. The phenotypes attributable to these abnormalities are presented in the section on deletion. Nonmosaic monosomy may result from loss of a chromosome from the fertilized ovum before or at the time of the first mitotic division, or from meiotic nondisjunction leading to the exclusion of both members of a homologous chromosome pair from the germ cell.

Monosomies other than G monosomy have not been described in liveborn humans. Only a few autosomal monosomies have been described in the products of spontaneous abortion, suggesting either that monosomy is a rare occurrence or is highly lethal so early in pregnancy that it does not result in recognizable pregnancy.

DELETION (PARTIAL MONOSOMY)

Deletion, compatible with life in at least some instances, results from loss of a portion of a chromosome. If the deletion occurs after fertilization, mosaicism for the deletion will be

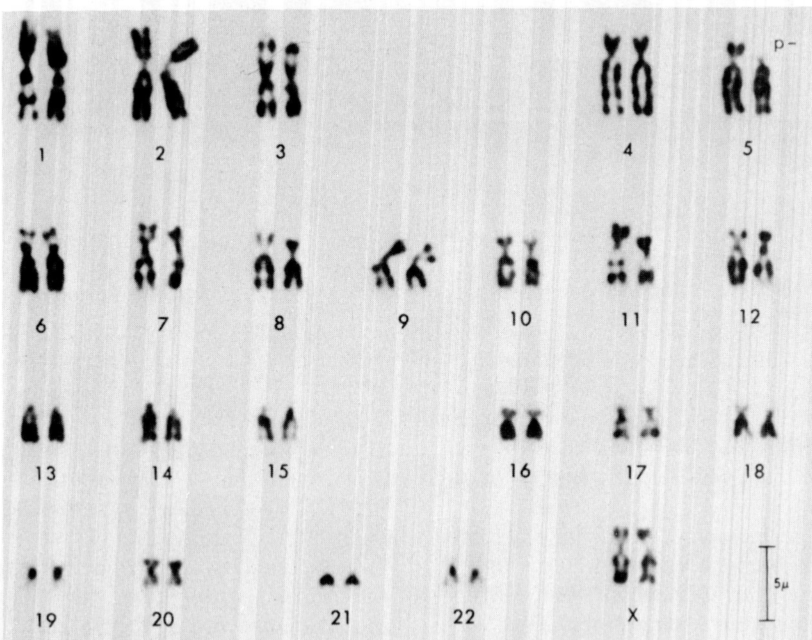

Fig. 7-14. G-banded karyotype of female with deletion of the short arm of chromosome 5, designated 46,XX,del (5) (p11). (From Summitt, R.L.: Pediatr. Ann. **2**:40, 1973.)

found. The best-known deletion is that of a portion of the short arm of chromosome 5 (Fig. 7-14), first described by Lejeune and associates as producing a syndrome of mental retardation, prenatal and postnatal growth retardation, and multiple anomalies including microcephaly, large frontal sinuses, downward slanting palpebral fissures, hypertelorism, inner epicanthal folds, low-set ears, syndactyly, short metacarpals and metatarsals, and a characteristic peculiar high-pitched cry in infancy resembling the sound made by a kitten. The unusual cry led Lejeune and associates to term the condition the *cri du chat (cat cry) syndrome*. A sizable number of cases have been reported since Lejeune's original description, and the prognosis for lon-

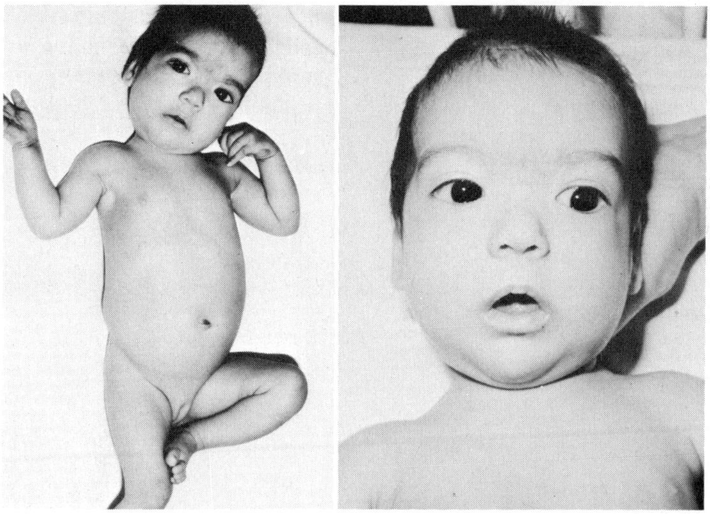

Fig. 7-15. Infant with deletion of short arm of chromosome 5 and cri du chat syndrome.

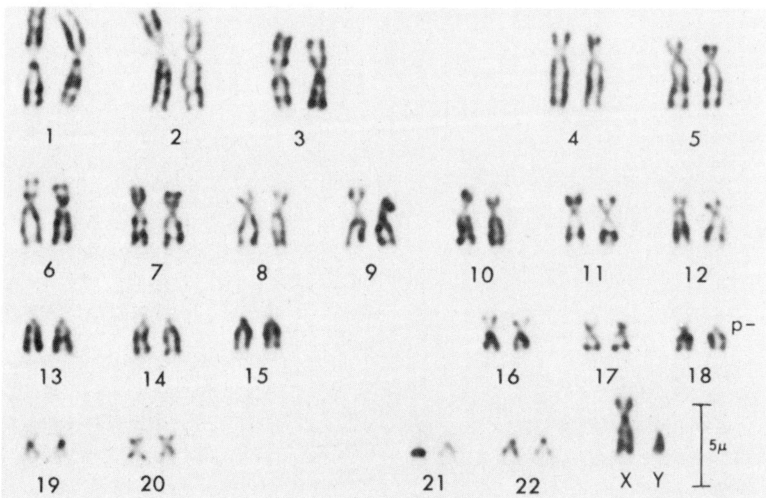

Fig. 7-16. G-banded karyotype of female with deletion of the short arm of chromosome 18, designated 46,XX,del (18) (p11).

gevity seems relatively good. The characteristic cry disappears after early infancy. An infant with this condition is shown in Fig. 7-15.

Deletions of the short or long arms of a number of autosomes have now been described, including those involving the short arm of chromosome 4 and the short arm of chromosome 18. Patients with deletion of the short arm of chromosome 4 share a number of phenotypic features with those suffering from the cri du chat syndrome; however, the former lack the characteristic cry in infancy and have a lower birth weight, more profound mental retardation, cleft palate, colobomas, hypospadias (in affected males), scalp defect, and hypoplastic dermal ridges. The phenotypes of those with deletion of the short arm of chromosome 18 (Fig. 7-16) are variable, and mental retardation may be mild. Most patients have delayed speech development and articulation defects. Deletion of portions of the long arm of chromosome 18 produces a phenotype that includes significant mental retardation, variable anomalies of the external ears, midfacial flatness with deep-set eyes, "carp" mouth, prognathism, long tapering fingers, and, according to some, a preponderance of whorl patterns on fingertips. Deletions of portions of the long arm of chromosome 13 have been reported, as have a few involving a portion of the long arm of chromosomes 21 and 22. The morphologic similarity between chromosomes 21 and 22 formerly led to problems in defining the del(21q) and del(22q) syndromes. However, banding studies have allowed delineation of the two syndromes, and the following outline gives phenotypic features of the long arm 21 deletion and long arm 22 deletion syndromes.

21 Deletion syndrome

Hypertonia
Downward-slanting eyes
Prominent nasal bridge
Micrognathia
Skeletal malformations
Growth retardation
Nail anomalies
Hypospadias
Inguinal hernia
Cryptorchidism
Pyloric stenosis

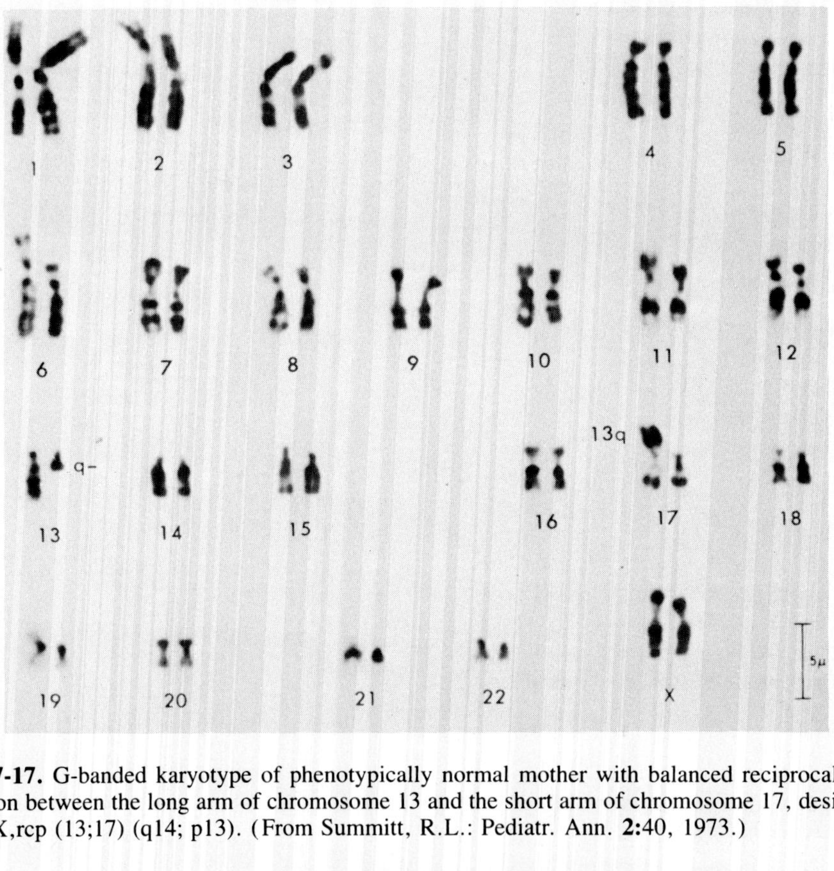

Fig. 7-17. G-banded karyotype of phenotypically normal mother with balanced reciprocal translocation between the long arm of chromosome 13 and the short arm of chromosome 17, designated 46,XX,rcp (13;17) (q14; p13). (From Summitt, R.L.: Pediatr. Ann. **2**:40, 1973.)

22 Deletion syndrome

Hypotonia	Ptosis of eyelids
Epicanthal folds	Bifid uvula
Syndactyly of toes	Clinodactyly

Features common to both syndromes

Mental retardation	Highly arched palate
Microcephaly	Large or low-set ears

Some deletions take the form of *ring chromosomes,* which are formed by a deletion from each arm of a chromosome, followed by fusion of the ends of the centric fragment.

OTHER STRUCTURAL ABNORMALITIES

Translocation. Among 48,650 infants in several newborn chromosome surveys a significant structural aberration of the autosomes was found in 99 infants. Eighty-eight of these were balanced structural rearrangements, indicating that about 1 in 550 liveborn infants harbors a balanced translocation, or structural rearrangement. These balanced translocations are the result of breaks in 2 or more chromosomes with erroneous reunion of the broken segments. Such events usually cause no phenotypic effects, since they entail no loss or gain of net chromosomal mass; however, offspring of such translocation carriers (translocation heterozygotes) may be abnormal. A portion of the germ cells produced by such a person could lead to a chromosomally unbalanced offspring. The identification of such persons is important for purposes of genetic counseling.

Available data indicate that if an inherited reciprocal translocation is ascertained through a family member with an unbalanced form of the translocation, the risk for the birth of another child with an unbalanced form of the translocation is approximately 10% to 20% if the mother carries the balanced translocation, and 5% to 10% if the father is the carrier. If the family is ascertained fortuitously through a balanced carrier of the translocation, the risk of an infant with an unbalanced form is much lower.

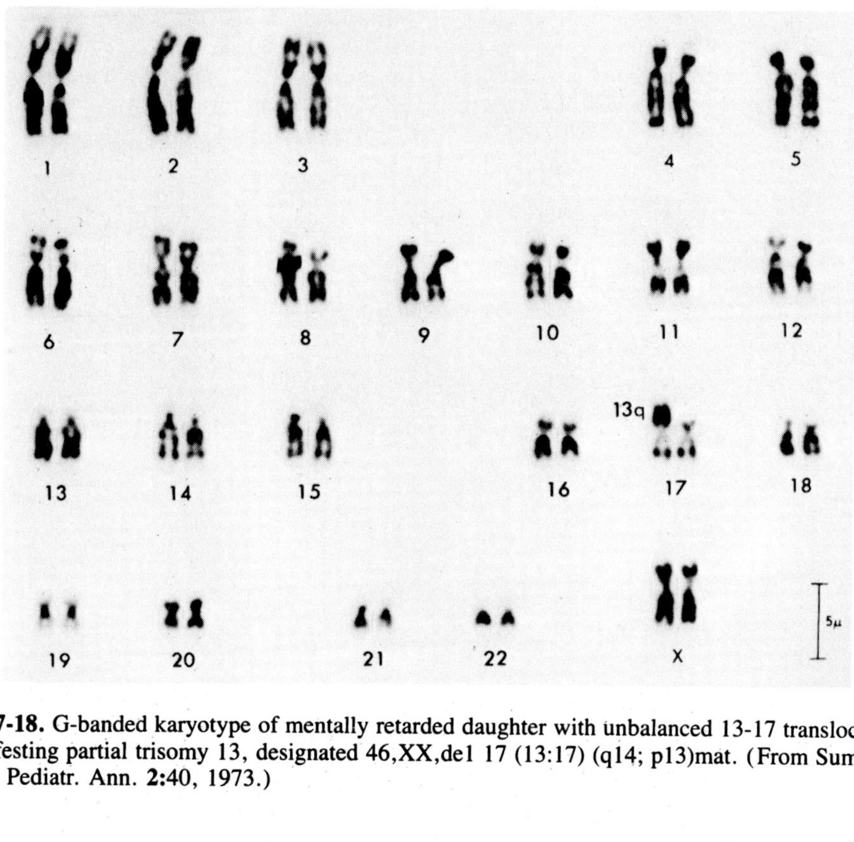

Fig. 7-18. G-banded karyotype of mentally retarded daughter with unbalanced 13-17 translocation manifesting partial trisomy 13, designated 46,XX,del 17 (13:17) (q14; p13)mat. (From Summitt, R.L.: Pediatr. Ann. **2**:40, 1973.)

Fig. 7-17 is the karyotype of a phenotypically normal mother who carries a balanced reciprocal translocation between the long arm of chromosome 13 and the short arm of chromosome 17. The mother is normal. Fig. 7-18 is the karyotype of her mentally retarded daughter with multiple anomalies. She has received her mother's normal chromosome 13 but has also received her chromosome 17 with the attached long arm of 13. Thus the daughter has a duplication of a portion of the long arm of chromosome 13 and probably deficiency of a portion of the short arm of chromosome 17. A large number of similar types of chromosome rearrangement are known in humans, involving almost every chromosome in the karyotype.

Inversion. An inversion is the result of two breaks within the same chromosome, followed by reunion of the breaks, with the segment of the chromosome between the two breaks having rotated on its own axis so that its ultimate orientation is the reverse of the original (Fig. 7-19). If the inversion is paracentric (both breaks on the same side of the centromere), it is not detectable by older techniques but should be detectable by banding techniques. A pericentric inversion (one break on each side of the centromere) is detectable if the two breaks are not equidistant from the centromere. In this case the arm ratio of the chromosome, and thus its appearance, is altered. Although several pericentric inversions have been detected, and although some of their hosts are abnormal, a cause-and-effect relationship for the abnormalities is difficult to establish in any specific instance. The vast majority of carriers of pericentric inversions are phenotypically normal. However, meiosis in a carrier of a pericentric inversion may lead to offspring with duplication-deficiency states resulting from crossing-over between the inverted segment of the abnormal chromosome and its normal homologue.

POLYPLOIDY

The term *polyploidy* describes a karyotype in which the chromosome number is an exact multiple of the haploid number of 23 but is other than 46. Polyploidy is a rare abnormality in liveborn infants. Most are mosaic, with a normal cell line and a polyploid line. A number of triploid (69 chromosomes) infants, some mosaic, and rare mosaic infants with a tetraploid (92 chromosomes) cell line have been described. At least 22 nonmosaic triploid infants have been reported, and the pattern of anomalies is constant enough to constitute a syndrome. Its features include low birth weight for gestational age, primordial shortness of stature, broad nasal bridge, low-set, malformed ears, eye defects (microphthalmia, ptosis, and colobomas), renal

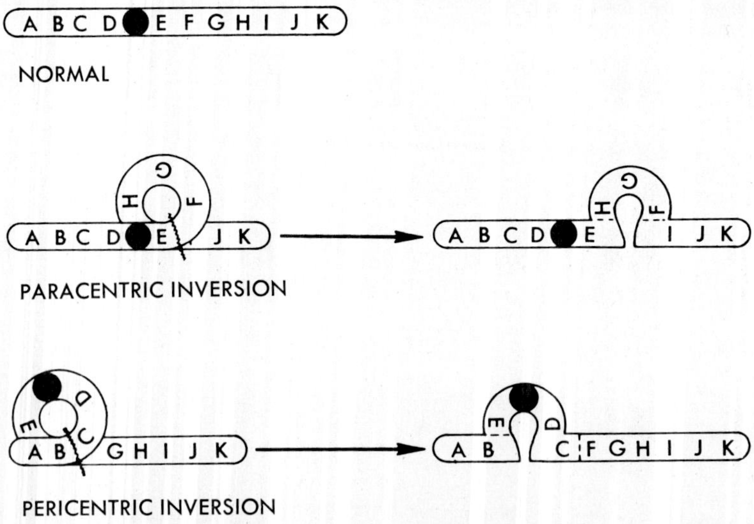

Fig. 7-19. Mechanism of chromosomal inversion. (From Summitt, R.L.: G.P. **36:**96, 1967.)

abnormalities, syndactyly, simian palmar creases, intersex genitalia with testicular interstitial cell hyperplasia in affected males, and neonatal death.

Triploidy and tetraploidy are frequent abnormalities in the products of spontaneous abortion; they accounted for 23% of 1863 chromosomally abnormal abortuses, the abnormal ones accounting for about 50% of those studied. It would appear therefore that whereas polyploidy is rare in liveborn infants, it is not uncommon at conception and may affect as many as 1.8% of all conceptions.

CHROMOSOME ABNORMALITIES AS A CAUSE OF MENTAL DEFICIENCY AND CONGENITAL ANOMALIES

Studies at the University of Wisconsin and the University of Tennessee of patients with mental deficiency and at least three congenital anomalies (patients who cannot be placed clinically in any known syndrome) showed that approximately 10% have significant discernible chromosome abnormalities. Therefore the clinician dealing with mentally deficient children with anomalies (even minor ones) should consider the possibility of a chromosome abnormality in the differential diagnosis.

CHROMOSOME ABNORMALITIES IN SPONTANEOUS ABORTION

The subject of the role of chromosome abnormalities in spontaneous abortion has been approached from two perspectives.

1. Couples have been studied after the woman has had three or more spontaneous abortions. It appears that in 2% to 5% of such couples one member has a balanced structural rearrangement of the chromosomes that would predispose to chromosomally unbalanced conceptions, some terminating in spontaneous abortion. In addition, an inordinate number of spontaneous abortions occurs among pregnancies in some families when one parent is a known carrier of a balanced structural rearrangement of the chromosomes.

2. Multiple studies of the products of spontaneous abortion have revealed that at least 50% of such products have a significant chromosome abnormality. These include trisomy for virtually every chromosome in the karyotype (especially 13, 16, 18, and 21) in 52% of the abnormal products—the most frequent single category of abnormalities. The most frequent *single* abnormality, encountered in 18% of those abortions that are chromosomally abnormal, has been 44 autosomes plus only 1 *sex* chromosome, an X. This karyotype is designated 45,X. Triploidy has been found in 17%, tetraploidy in 6%. It is reasonable to presume a cause-and-effect relationship between the chromosome abnormalities and the spontaneous abortion, and it can thus be concluded that chromosome abnormalities are a significant cause of fetal mortality.

If one considers the frequency with which spontaneous abortion occurs and the frequency of specific chromosome imbalances among those abortions, it can be calculated that as many as 80% of all 21-trisomic conceptions do not survive pregnancy, only 20% being live-born infants with Down syndrome. The in utero lethality of the other well-known trisomies is considerably higher than that for trisomy 21. Furthermore, it appears that the 45,X karyotype is highly lethal, only 1 of 500 such conceptions being born alive.

Data are also now accumulating on the chromosome complement of two consecutive spontaneous abortions by the same mother. It appears that if the first abortus had a chromosome abnormality, the probability of a chromosome abnormality in the second abortus is significant. This is particularly striking for trisomy. Jacobs has reported 22-trisomic second abortuses in 29 women whose first abortus was trisomic. The majority of these women were older, suggesting that their recurrent chromosomally abnormal abortions are age dependent.

CHROMOSOME ABNORMALITIES IN NEOPLASMS

The first well-established relationship between a specific chromosome abnormality and a neoplastic process is that between chronic myelogenous leukemia and the Philadelphia (Ph^1) chromosome. The Ph^1 chromosome was originally thought to be the result of a deletion of most of the long arm of chromosome 22. However, more recent studies have shown that the Ph^1 chromosome does not involve a simple deletion but instead a reciprocal translocation in which a major portion of the long arm of chromosome 22 is translocated to the long arm of another chromosome, most often chromosome

9, and a short segment of the long arm of chromosome 9 is translocated to chromosome 22. The manner wherein such a chromosome rearrangement is related to the neoplastic process is unclear, but recent studies have shed some light on this question. Recently a number of genes have been identified that have the property of transforming normal cells into neoplastic cells. These genes are called *oncogenes*. Several such oncogenes have been found in human tumor cell lines and some have been assigned to specific chromosomes, and even to specific bands within those chromosomes. The human oncogene, *c-abl,* has been mapped to band q34 of chromosome 9, the site of the breakpoint in chromosome 9 involved in the formation of the Ph^1 chromosome. Furthermore, this oncogene has been shown to be translocated to the short chromosome 22, providing molecular documentation that the Ph^1 chromosome is the result of a *reciprocal* translocation. In addition, the assignment of the oncogene *c-abl* to the breakpoint of chromosome 9 and its translocation to the recipient chromosome 22 (Ph^1 chromosome) provides exciting and important initial insight into the part played by chromosome abnormalities in the etiology of the neoplastic process. In chronic myelogenous leukemia the translocation that produces the Ph^1 chromosome is found only in hematopoietic tissue. The mechanism that induces the translocation is unknown, but the translocation is an *acquired* chromosome abnormality, not present at birth.

Since the discovery of the Ph^1 chromosome in chronic myelogenous leukemia, other chromosome aberrations have been found to be specific for other neoplasms. Translocations involving chromosomes 8 and 2 and chromosomes 8 and 14 have been found, limited to tumor cells, in two types of Burkitt lymphoma. In each of these two types of translocation, reciprocity has been demonstrated, with the long arm of chromosome 8 contributing a larger segment to the long arm of chromosome 2 or 14 than the reciprocal. The breakpoint in chromosome 8 in both tumor types is located at the site of the *c-myc* oncogene, which is translocated to either chromosome 2 or chromosome 14. The breakpoints in chromosomes 2 and 14 have been mapped to positions in close proximity to immunoglobulin genes.

In the above two examples, chromosome translocations, present only in the cells of the neoplasm itself, have been implicated in the etiology of the neoplasm. It may be that the translocation process results in the activation of previously inactive genes, the activation of those genes in some way producing neoplasia.

A *deletion* involving the long arm of chromosome 6 has been found in some cases of acute lymphoblastic leukemia. Here again the chromosome abnormality is limited to the leukemic cells. In such cases the breakpoint in chromosome 6 has been mapped to bands q21 to q25, the location of the *c-myb* oncogene.

Aniridia, or absence of the iris of the eye, occurs as an isolated inherited defect, with an autosomal dominant mode of inheritance. Aniridia, however, is known to occur in association with Wilms tumor or gonadoblastoma. The aniridia-Wilms tumor association is accompanied by varying degrees of mental retardation, various dysmorphic features, and ambiguous genitalia. A number of such cases have been reported, in which an interstitial deletion has been found to involve the short arm of chromosome 11. In those patients reported, the chromosome abnormality is *constitutional,* not limited to the tumor. The deletions in reported cases have been of varying extents but have in all cases included band 11p13. In one patient with Wilms tumor *without* aniridia a similar deletion was reported, but it was limited to cells from the tumor. The oncogene, *c-ras*, has been localized to the 11p11—p15 region of the short arm of chromosome 11. Although no association has been drawn between the aniridia-Wilms tumor association and the *c-ras* oncogene, a deletion of the chromosome band 11p13 in the aniridia-Wilms tumor association raises interesting possibilities. The gene for the enzyme, catalase, has also been mapped to band 11p13, and in patients with the aniridia-Wilms tumor association and the 11p13 deletion, catalase activity is only *half* that found in normal controls. It should be noted that the mutant gene in autosomal dominant aniridia has been mapped to the short arm of chromosome 2. Therefore two loci, one in the short arm of chromosome 2 and the other in the short arm of chromosome 11, are in some way related to aniridia. However, Wilms tumor occurs in only those cases of aniridia with the 11p13 deletion.

One more example of a chromosome deletion

in association with a neoplasm deserves mention. Retinoblastoma is a rare malignant tumor of the eye that occurs in young children. This tumor may be inherited in an autosomal dominant manner, in which case it is bilateral; or it may be nonhereditary, in which case it is unilateral. The hereditary bilateral form accounts for approximately 10% of cases, 90% being of the sporadic, noninherited variety. Based on recently acquired information, an estimated 2% to 10% of all cases of retinoblastoma are associated with and the result of a chromosome abnormality. The chromosome abnormality that results in retinoblastoma is a deletion of a portion of the long arm of chromosome 13. The deletion is virtually always interstitial, and variable in extent, but uniformly includes band 13q14. Most cases of retinoblastoma associated with a 13q deletion are the result of a de novo deletion and thus are sporadic; however, some are hereditary on the basis of segregation of an hereditary parental balanced chromosome rearrangement involving chromosome 13. In the cases mentioned here, the 13q deletion is *constitutional,* not limited to tumor cells. No oncogene has been mapped to the long arm of chromosome 13. However, the gene for the enzyme, esterase D, has been mapped to band 13q14 of the long arm of chromosome 13. In cells from patients with retinoblastoma and a 13q14 deletion, esterase D activity has been shown to be only 50% of that in normal cells. Whether enzyme levels have anything to do with susceptibility to retinoblastoma, or whether the gene for esterase D is closely linked to a retinoblastoma gene in 13q14, is unknown. Interesting insight has been provided by a patient reported by Benedict and associates. Their patient had retinoblastoma. Cells from three tissues of the patient exhibited 50% of normal esterase activity. However, no chromosome deletion could be discerned, even using high-resolution banding techniques. The authors hypothesized that a deletion existed but was too small to be visible. In addition, cells from the tumor itself contained multiple and various chromosome abnormalities. Common to all tumor cells, however, was monosomy for chromosome 13. Esterase D assay demonstrated *no* esterase D activity in cells from the tumor. These findings were interpreted as meaning that the normal (undeleted) chromosome had been lost from the tumor cells, leaving the chromosome 13 that contained the submicroscopic deletion. The gene governing retinoblastoma was completely absent, as was the esterase D gene. The significance of this case is that it presents suggestive evidence that the retinoblastoma gene is recessive and that both relevant alleles must be lost (in Benedict's case one from deletion and the other from monosomy) for retinoblastoma to develop.

Cytogenetic findings in cancer suggest two "classes" of genes related to cancer. One class includes the cellular oncogenes, the translocation of which results in abnormal gene activation (exemplified by chronic myelogenous leukemia and Burkitt lymphoma). The second class of "cancer genes" includes those the loss of which results in malignancy. This class may be exemplified by the aniridia-Wilms tumor association and retinoblastoma.

An interesting and important group of conditions is known, each inherited in an autosomal recessive manner, and in each of which a tendency to spontaneous chromosome aberrations has been observed. These are Bloom syndrome, Fanconi pancytopenia syndrome, ataxia-telangiectasia (Louis-Bar syndrome), and xeroderma pigmentosum. Each is also characterized by an increased incidence of malignant neoplasia.

Bloom syndrome is characterized by severe prenatal and postnatal growth retardation, variable immunodeficiency, and an increased facial sensitivity to ultraviolet irradiation, leading to a telangiectatic erythematous facial rash. The incidence of cancer or leukemia in affected patients is approximately 1 in 6. From the cytogenetic viewpoint Bloom syndrome is characterized by spontaneous chromosome breakage, exchanges between homologous chromosomes, and increased exchanges between sister chromatids. A "chromosome breakage factor" has recently been reported in the plasma of affected patients.

The Fanconi pancytopenia syndrome includes a variable pattern of failure of all elements of the bone marrow associated with short stature, abnormal skin pigmentation, and congenital limb, cardiac, and renal defects. The pancytopenia is not congenital but appears at various ages from 17 months to the early third decade of life. Death may result from the progressive pancytopenia and its complications or from leukemia or another malignant neoplasm. Increased chromosome breakage is a consistent finding in lymphocytes cultured from affected patients, and exchanges between nonhomologous chromosomes have been observed. The increase in sister chromatid exchanges found in cells from patients with Bloom syndrome is not observed in the Fanconi pancytopenia syndrome. Clones (distinct, stable subpopulations) of cells containing abnormal chromosome complements have been observed in lymphocytes, skin fibroblasts, and bone marrow cells from affected patients. In addition, cultured cells from patients are hypersensitive to chromosome-breaking agents.

The features of ataxia-telangiectasia are first discernible in early childhood. These features include progressive cerebellar ataxia and other neurologic manifestations, oculocutaneous telangiectasia, frequent and severe respiratory infections, abnormalities of the lymphoid tissue, and an immunodeficiency state. IgA is decreased or absent. The incidence of malignant neoplasms, predominantly involving the reticuloendothelial tissue, is increased in affected patients. Chromosome breaks and rearrangements occur in ataxia-telangiectasia, but are discernible to varying degrees in different stages of the disease. Rearrangements include dicentric and abnormal monocentric chromosomes, and the appearance of clones of abnormal cells. Chromosomes 7 and 14 have been involved preferentially in the rearrangements in observed clones.

Xeroderma pigmentosum is characterized by profound skin sensitivity to ultraviolet light. Homozygous affected patients appear normal at birth, but exposure to sunlight leads to progressively severe injury to the skin. Changes include freckles of various sizes and pigmentation, progressive dryness, telangiectasia, atrophy, and keratosis. Photophobia may be intense; corneal ulceration and scarring may lead to blindness, and the eyelids may become scarred and ectopic. The skin damage progresses relentlessly to the formation of large numbers of squamous and basal cell carcinomas, leading to death before age 30. Genetic heterogeneity exists in xeroderma pigmentosum. Convincing evidence of a defect in the DNA repair mechanism has been found in cells of xeroderma patients. No increase in chromosome breaks or rearrangements occurs in xeroderma pigmentosum patients, but clones of pseudodiploid cells with translocations have been observed in cultured fibroblasts and lymphocytes.

Chromosome changes have also been described in incontinentia pigmenti, Rothmund-Thomson syndrome, and basal cell nevus syndrome.

One additional condition deserves mention; Prader-Willi syndrome. Although the etiology of Prader-Willi syndrome and the question of whether it is genetically determined remain unclear, recent evidence points to a chromosome abnormality as causative in at least a proportion of cases. Surveys of patients diagnosed clinically as having Prader-Willi syndrome show that approximately 50% have an abnormality involving chromosome 15. The most common abnormality is an interstitial deletion of chromosome 15, usually with breakpoints in bands 15q11 and 15q13, although other abnormalities involving 15 have been reported. The absence of a discernible chromosome abnormality in about half of clinically diagnosed cases of Prader-Willi syndrome suggest nosologic heterogeneity in this condition.

INDUCED CHROMOSOME ABNORMALITIES

In this era of attention to environmental factors in the causation of human disease, the role of certain agents in the induction of chromosome damage (breaks and rearrangements) has become a matter of concern. The action of ionizing irradiation in the production of such damage has been well documented; Uchida presented evidence that ionizing irradiation in mothers has led to an increase in the frequency of nondisjunction, resulting in trisomy in their offspring. Mutagenic properties of various chemicals have been evaluated for some time by measuring their ability to induce chromosome aberrations in cultured cells. Recent studies of mutagens have turned to measurement of the incidence of sister chromatid exchanges in cultured cells.

INDICATIONS FOR CHROMOSOME ANALYSIS

The responsibility for deciding to do a chromosome analysis rests with the physician. A few basic indications for such investigation may be listed, although the reader is cautioned that all such rules have their exceptions and that each patient must be evaluated individually.

1. To substantiate a clinical diagnosis of Down syndrome and to delineate the cytogenetic mechanism involved. While the diagnosis of Down syndrome can be made on clinical grounds, the long-term impact of such a diagnosis on the patient and the family makes it mandatory that the clinical diagnosis be substantiated by chromosome analysis. In addition, when all factors have been considered, chromosome analysis is the only way to discover those cases that involve a translocation and thus may indicate a situation with a high recurrence risk.
2. To substantiate a clinical diagnosis of other established syndromes.
3. The presence of various combinations of the following:
   a. Low birth weight for gestational age
   b. Postnatal failure to thrive
   c. Mental retardation
   d. Multiple congenital anomalies (may be minor anomalies)
4. Extended family studies in families in which structural chromosomal rearrangements are found.
5. Couples who have experienced recurrent spontaneous abortion.
6. To substantiate a clinical diagnosis of the following:
   a. Turner syndrome
   b. Klinefelter syndrome
7. Short stature and sexual infantilism in the female.
8. Delayed adolescence and small testes in the male
9. Sterility.
10. Primary amenorrhea.
11. Any patient with abnormal sex differentiation.
12. Products of spontaneous abortion. Such studies on *every* spontaneous abortion are probably impractical.
13. To confirm the diagnosis in a patient suspected of having one of the chromosome breakage syndromes.
14. To confirm the diagnosis in a patient suspected of having Prader-Willi syndrome.
15. To aid in the diagnosis of one of the neoplasms or neoplasm-related syndromes in which a characteristic chromosome aberration has been shown to exist as a constitutional abnormality in the affected patient or limited to the neoplasm itself.
16. To confirm or refute a clinical diagnosis of fragile-X-linked mental retardation.

The conditions in nos. 6 through 11 are discussed in Chapter 22.

PRENATAL CHROMOSOME ANALYSIS

Chromosome analysis has been performed efficaciously and with low risk on the fetus in utero for over a decade. Amniotic fluid is obtained by transabdominal amniocentesis, and the cells contained in the fluid are cultured for chromosome analysis and accurate assessment of the fetal karyotype. Although chromosome analysis on cultured amniocytes has added a new dimension to the field of clinical genetics and genetic counseling, it has had the disadvantage of not being feasible until the second trimester of pregnancy, most often in the sixteenth week or later. A new technique, the efficacy and safety of which is being widely tested at this time, may allow assessment of the fetal karyotype, as well as the diagnosis of other genetic disorders, in the first trimester of pregnancy and within a few hours after obtaining the sample. This technique involves the insertion of a small plastic cannula through the cervical os into the uterus. The location of the chorion frondosum is ascertained by ultrasonography, and the cannula is guided to that location under real-time ultrasonography. The cannula contains an ultrasound-visible obturator; when the chorion frondosum is reached, the obturator is removed and tissue from the chorionic villi aspirated into a sterile syringe. Direct preparations for chromosome analysis, for analysis of cellular enzyme activity, or for restriction enzyme analysis of recovered DNA, can be made. Furthermore, cells may be cultured from the sample for further analysis. Either technique allows for results within a few hours to a few days, significantly sooner than results are obtained in amniocentesis. In all likelihood, chorionic villus biopsy for prenatal genetic diagnosis will become a routinely applicable procedure in the near future.

Prenatal diagnostic studies for the detection of chromosome abnormalities is not practical or applicable in every pregnancy, but their availability should be made known to pregnant women or women contemplating pregnancy who fall within one of the following categories:

1. Any woman who is known to carry a balanced chromosome structural rearrangement or whose mate is known to carry a balanced chromosome structural rearrangement.
2. Any woman to whom a previous trisomic infant has been liveborn, or who has had a trisomic embryonic or fetal death. In addition, prenatal chromosome analysis is commonly offered to women who have had a liveborn infant with a chromosome abnormality other than trisomy.
3. Any woman who becomes pregnant at an older age. The usual practice is that this applies to women 35 years of age or older.

In any of these situations the discovery of a normal fetal chromosome complement will relieve the anxiety of the parents involved. If the findings are abnormal, therapeutic abortion is offered to the parents.

Robert L. Summitt

SELECTED READINGS

Bonné-Tamir, B.: Human genetics: part B, medical aspects, New York, 1982, Alan R. Liss, Inc.

Boue, J.G., et al.: Retrospective and prospective epidemiological studies in 1500 karyotyped spontaneous human abortions, Teratology **12:**11, 1975.

Cervenka, J., and Koulischer, L.: Chromosomes and human cancer, Springfield, Ill., 1973, Charles C. Thomas, Publisher.

Chicago Conference on Standardization in Human Cytogenetics, Birth Defects **2:**2, 1966.

German, J.: Chromosomes and cancer, New York, 1974, John Wiley & Sons, Inc.

Hamerton, J.L.: Human cytogenetics, vols. I and II, New York, 1971, Academic Press, Inc.

Hook, E.B., and Cross, P.K.; Interpretation of recent data pertinent to genetic counseling for Down syndrome: Maternal-age-specific-rates, temporal trends, adjustments for paternal age, recurrence risks, risks after other cytogenetic abnormalities, recurrence risk after remarriage. In Willey, A.M., et al.: Clinical genetics: problems in diagnosis and counseling, New York, 1982, Academic Press, Inc.

Hook, E.B., and Porter, I.H.: Population cytogenetics: study in humans, New York, 1977, Academic Press, Inc.

Jacobs, P.A.: Human population cytogenetics, In de Grouchy, J., et al., editors: Human genetics, Proceedings of the Fourth International Congress of Human Genetics, Amsterdam, 1972, Excerpta Medica Foundation. pp. 232-242.

Jacobs, P.A.: Recurrence risk for chromosome abnormalities. In Epstein, C.J., et al., editors: Risk, communication, and decision making in genetic counseling, Birth Defects original article series, **15-5c:**71-80, 1979.

Kajii, T., et al.: Banding analyses of abnormal karyotypes in spontaneous abortion, Am. J. Hum. Genet. **25:**539, 1973.

Ledbetter, D.H., et al.: Chromosome 15 abnormalities and the Prader-Willi syndrome: a follow-up report of 40 cases, Am. J. Hum. Genet. **34:**278, 1982.

Magenis, R.E., et al.: Parental origin of extra chromosome in Down's syndrome, Hum Genet. **37:**7, 1977.

Paris Conference on Standardization in Human Cytogenetics, Birth Defects **8:**7, 1972.

Rowley, J.D.: A new consistent chromosomal abnormality in chronic myelogenous leukaemia identified by quinacrine fluorescence and Giemsa staining, Nature **243:**290, 1973.

Rowley, J.D.: Nonrandom chromosomal abnormalities in hematologic disorders in man, Proc. Natl. Acad. Sci. USA **72:**152, 1975.

Rowley, J.D.: Human oncogene locations and chromosome aberrations, Nature **301:**290, 1983.

Sandberg, A.A.: The chromosomes in human cancer and leukemia. New York, 1980, Elsevier-North Holland, Inc.

Simoni, G., et al.: Efficient direct chromosome analysis and enzyme determinations from chorionic villi samples in the first trimester of pregnancy, Am. J. Hum. Genet. **63:**349, 1983.

Summitt, R.L.: Autosomal syndromes, Pediatr. Ann. **7:**431, 1978.

Summitt, R.L.: Cytogenetic disorders. In Jackson, L.G. and Schimke, R.N., editors: Clinical genetics: a sourcebook for physicians, New York, 1979, John Wiley & Sons, Inc.

Therman, E.: Human chromosomes, New York, 1980, Springer-Verlag, New York, Inc.

Williamson, R., et al.: Direct gene analysis of chorionic villi: a possible technique for first-trimester antenatal diagnosis of haemoglobinopathies, Lancet **2:**1125, 1981.

Yunis, J.J.: New Chromosomal syndromes, New York, 1977, Academic Press, Inc.

Yunis, J.J.: The chromosomal basis of human neoplasia, Science **221:**227, 1983.

8 Genetic Counseling

Genetic counseling has been defined as a communications process that deals with human problems associated with the occurrence, or the risk of occurrence, of a genetic disorder in a family. It involves an attempt by appropriately trained professionals to help the person or family who seek counsel to (1) comprehend the medical facts, including the diagnosis, the probable course of the disorder, and the available management; (2) appreciate the way heredity contributes to the disorder and the risk of occurrence or recurrence in specified relatives; (3) understand the options for dealing with the risk of occurrence or recurrence; (4) choose the course of action that seems appropriate to them in view of their risks and their family goals and act in accordance with that decision; and (5) make the best possible adjustment to the disorder in an affected family member or to the risk of occurrence or recurrence of that disorder.

The genetic counseling information given a family obviously depends on the pattern of inheritance exhibited by the disease in question. Accurate genetic counseling depends on two factors:

1. An accurate diagnosis. For example, familial hypophosphatemic rickets and a second condition, metaphyseal dysplasia, have some clinical and radiographic similarities. The former is inherited in an X-linked dominant manner, whereas the latter is inherited as an autosomal dominant. Unless the correct diagnosis (which may depend on blood chemical determinations) is made, misinformation may be given concerning recurrence risks. Incorrect recurrence risk information can be disastrous.

2. Knowledge of the genetic mode of the mutant allele in question in the family under consideration. Similar phenotypes may be produced by two or more different gene mutations *(genetic heterogeneity)*. For example, evidence exists to indicate that osteogenesis imperfecta may be inherited in some instances in an autosomal dominant manner and in other instances as an autosomal recessive. Only knowledge of the effect of the mutant allele and of the pattern of inheritance in the specific family will allow accurate counseling. The following paragraphs will discuss the various patterns of inheritance, an understanding of which is essential in counseling.

Many conditions involving the central nervous system and the endocrine system, a number of metabolic and skeletal disorders, and several conditions presenting in the newborn period have a genetic basis. For instance, achondroplasia is inherited in an autosomal dominant manner, phenylketonuria (PKU) in an autosomal recessive manner, familial hypophosphatemic rickets in an X-linked dominant manner, and the Lesch-Nyhan syndrome in an X-linked recessive manner. A condition such as congenital hypertrophic pyloric stenosis, although it does not follow simple mendelian rules of inheritance, also exhibits a familial pattern.

Humans are diploid organisms; that is, their chromosomes and therefore their genes occur in pairs, one member of each pair having been contributed by each parent. Fortunately, most contributed genes are of the normal variety. However, a mutant allele of a gene is occasionally passed to an offspring from a parental gamete. If the mutant allele is located in an autosome and if it is *dominant,* it will ordinarily manifest its effect (its *phenotype*) when present in the *heterozygous* state, that is, in a single dose, paired with the normal *allele,* or alternate form of a gene (e.g., the normal allele and the mutant allele of a gene). On the other hand, if the mutant allele is *recessive,* it will manifest its effect only when present in a "double dose," that is, in the *homozygous* state. A recessive mutant allele generally appears in the homozygous state only when mating occurs between two heterozygotes. The same general rules hold for genes located in the X chromosome (X-linked genes), except that the male possesses only one X. If a mutant allele of a gene located in the X chromosome is contributed to a male by his mother, he will ordinarily manifest the effect of that allele, whether it is dominant or recessive. An X-linked mutant allele in the male is not paired with a modifying normal allele and is said to be *hemizygous*. Occasionally a mutant allele may be present but not manifest its effect, in which case it is said to be *nonpenetrant*. An allele that manifests its effect in 80% of those who possess it is said to be 80% penetrant. The severity of the effect of a mutant allele may vary in different persons who possess that allele; that is, the *expressivity* of an allele may vary.

AUTOSOMAL DOMINANT INHERITANCE

The inheritance of an autosomal dominant mutant allele in humans occurs most often in a mating between a heterozygous affected person and a homozygous unaffected mate (Fig. 8-1). In considering all such matings, about half the offspring are affected, regardless in most cases of the sex of the offspring. In considering one mating, the product of each individual pregnancy, regardless of sex, has a 50% probability of being affected. A general set of rules governing autosomal dominant inheritance in humans, as set forth by Roberts, includes the following:

1. Every affected person has an affected parent.
2. The two sexes are ordinarily affected with equal frequency.
3. Affected persons married to unaffected persons produce, on the average, affected and unaffected offspring in equal proportions.
4. The unaffected children of affected persons, when they marry unaffected persons, have only unaffected offspring.

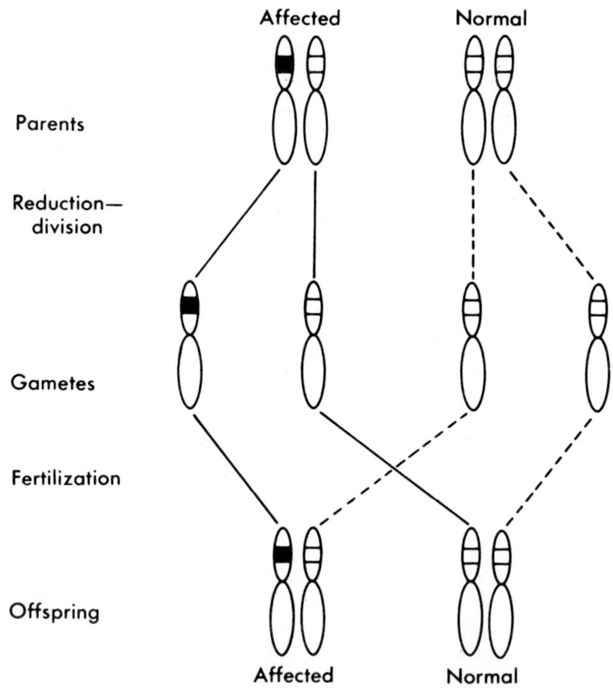

Fig. 8-1. Mating diagram representing a mating between an affected person heterozygous for an autosomal dominant mutant allele and a homozygous unaffected person. In this and subsequent mating diagrams the rodlike structure with a near-central constriction represents a chromosome and the blocked-off segment represents the gene locus in question. If the "gene-block" is shaded, it is the mutant allele; if unshaded, it is the normal allele.

The reader should keep in mind that, as is the case with most rules in biology, each of these rules has its exceptions. In general, as a consequence of these rules, a pedigree of autosomal dominant inheritance will present a vertical distribution of affected cases (Fig. 8-2), that is, affected cases in more than one generation and in more than one sibship within a given generation.

One of two types of counseling situation is ordinarily encountered in regard to autosomal dominant inheritance. In the first type a couple (or individual) seeks advice *because one of the couple (or the individual) is affected with a condition inherited in an autosomal dominant manner.* In such a situation, if the diagnosis and genetic mode can be established with certainty, the couple (or individual) should be advised that with any pregnancy the risk of an affected offspring is 50%. However, it may actually be less if the mutant gene is less than 100% penetrant. In the second type of counseling situation *a couple, both of whom are unaffected, seek advice because they have produced an offspring who has a condition inherited in an autosomal dominant manner.* The counselor must again be as sure as possible that the diagnosis is correct and must be certain that this is not a genetically heterogeneous phenotype (a condition that may be inherited in more than one manner). In addition, the counselor must be as sure as possible that both members of the couple are free of the mutant allele, that is, that neither bears a *nonpenetrant* dominant mutant allele. These problems may be difficult to overcome, particularly the latter two. If the counselor is satisfied concerning these three points, the couple may be informed that their child with the autosomal dominantly inherited condition is affected as the result of a *new spontaneous mutation* and that their risk of producing another affected offspring is, for all practical purposes, negligible. For the potential offspring of their affected child, however, the rules hold and the probability that any one will be affected is again 50%.

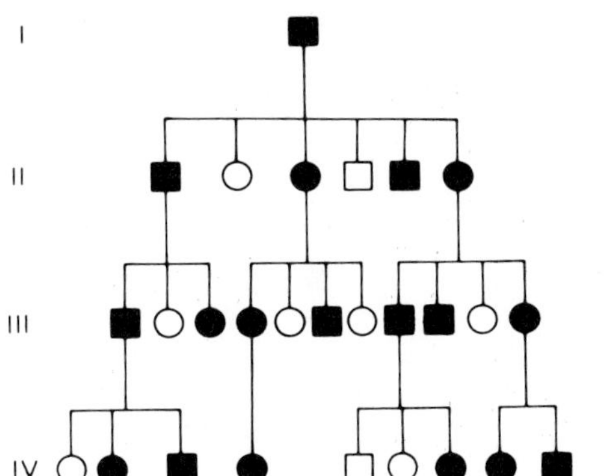

Fig. 8-2. Idealized pedigree demonstrating autosomal dominant inheritance, with vertical distribution of affected cases. A square signifies a male; a circle, a female. A shaded-in symbol indicates that the person is affected.

A few examples of conditions discussed in this book that are inherited in an autosomal dominant manner include achondroplasia (p. 969), neurofibromatosis (p. 796), and osteogenesis imperfecta (p. 966). As a rule of thumb, autosomal dominant mutations often produce phenotypic abnormalities in structure, in contrast to autosomal recessive mutations, which often produce enzyme deficiencies that lead to metabolic abnormalities and their resultant complicated phenotypes.

AUTOSOMAL RECESSIVE INHERITANCE

An autosomal recessive mutant allele may be transmitted through multiple generations of a family without detection as long as it occurs only in the heterozygous state (Fig. 8-3). Ordinarily, only in a mating of two heterozygotes does a homozygous-affected offspring occur (Fig. 8-4). As indicated in Fig. 8-4, when considering all matings between two heterozygotes, approximately one fourth (25%) of offspring are affected, regardless of sex. When considering a single mating between two heterozygotes, the risk of an affected offspring with any pregnancy is 25%, regardless of sex. A general set of rules governing autosomal recessive inheritance in humans, as set forth by Roberts, includes the following:

1. Affected persons ordinarily have parents who are unaffected.
2. On the average, 25% of the offspring of heterozygous parents are affected, 25% are homozygous unaffected, and 50% are also unaffected but heterozygous.
3. If the abnormality is rare, an unduly high proportion of marriages between blood

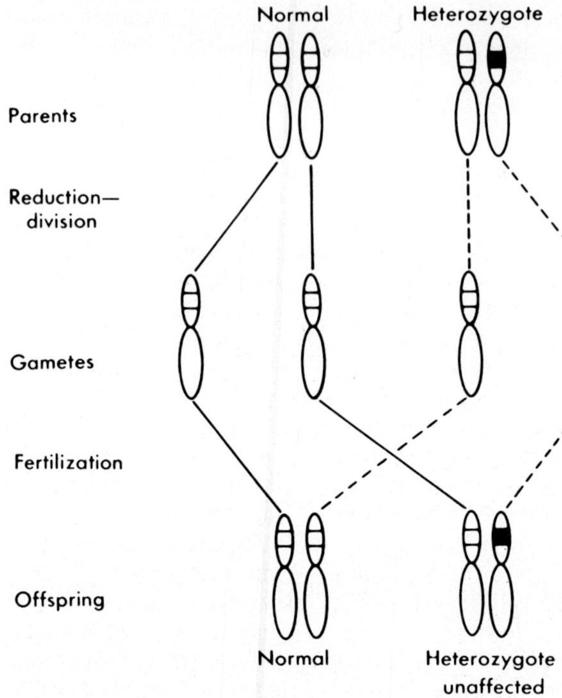

Fig. 8-3. Mating diagram representing the transmission of a mutant autosomal recessive allele in a "hidden state," which occurs in a mating between a heterozygote and a homozygous unaffected person.

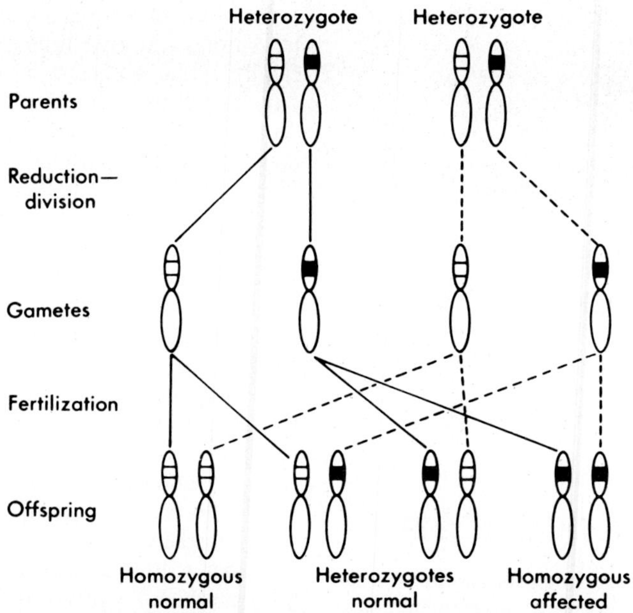

Fig. 8-4. Mating diagram representing a mating between two persons unaffected by, but heterozygous for, the same autosomal recessive mutant allele.

relatives is found among the parents of affected persons.

4. Affected persons who marry unaffected persons ordinarily have only unaffected offspring.
5. Affected persons who marry affected persons have only affected offspring.

In contrast to the vertical distribution of affected cases in pedigrees demonstrating autosomal dominant inheritance, the distribution of affected cases in autosomal recessive pedigrees is horizontal (Fig. 8-5), and affected cases are most often confined to a single sibship. When one considers the small size of many human sibships, it is logical that many instances of conditions inherited in an autosomal recessive manner are sporadic, that is, the only occurrence in the sibship (or the first occurrence). Unless the examining physician is well informed and alert, he may incorrectly conclude that the patient has a nongenetic condition or a new dominant mutation. An extensive discussion of consanguinity is not within the scope of this chapter. Suffice it to state that if a mutant allele is rare, the probability of a mating between two unrelated heterozygotes is low; on the other hand, if, for example, first cousins marry, the probability of their both having inherited the same autosomal recessive mutant allele from a common grandparent significantly increases the chance of their both being heterozygous for the same mutant allele.

The usual counseling problem encountered in conditions inherited in an autosomal recessive manner is that in which the affected infant or child is presented to the physician by unaffected parents. The family history is usually negative for similar occurrences outside the immediate sibship of the patient. If no affected siblings are known, the mode of inheritance in a specific family may be difficult to determine, unless the diagnosis can be firmly established and unless genetic heterogeneity can be excluded. Parental consanguinity supports an autosomal recessive hypothesis in a specific case. If autosomal recessive inheritance can be firmly established, the parents should be informed that the risk of an affected offspring with any subsequent pregnancy is 25%.

Examples of conditions discussed in this book that are inherited in an autosomal recessive manner include the various forms of congenital virilizing adrenal hyperplasia (adrenogenital syndrome, p. 582), cystic fibrosis of the pancreas (p. 670), Hurler syndrome (p. 658), and some of the inherited aminoacidopathies (p. 645).

In general, conditions inherited in an autosomal recessive manner are severely disabling and are often lethal in early infancy. Thus diagnosis must be established as early as possible, or the opportunity may disappear. In some instances therapy, if begun early in the life of the patient, may mitigate the effect of the mutant gene. This is true for phenylketonuria (p. 645) and for galactosemia (p. 646). Techniques for the study of cells from amniotic fluid obtained by transabdominal amniocentesis have made possible the in utero diagnosis of certain conditions that are inherited in an autosomal recessive manner. If such a diagnosis is made, genetic counseling can be accomplished "before the fact," the parents can be appropriately informed, and a therapeutic abortion can be offered.

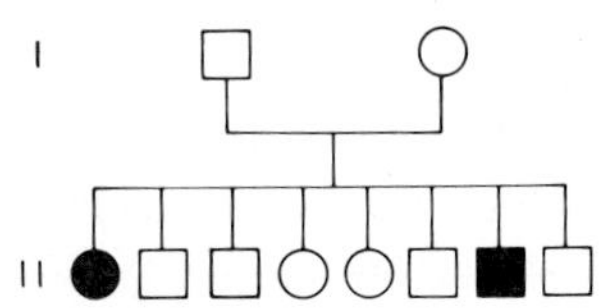

Fig. 8-5. Idealized pedigree demonstrating autosomal recessive inheritance, with horizontal distribution of affected cases.

X-LINKED DOMINANT INHERITANCE

Many conditions in humans have been known for years to be inherited in a sex-linked manner. Such a condition is the result of a mutant allele borne by the X chromosome and is thus more appropriately referred to as an *X-linked condition*. The inheritance of an X-linked dominant mutant allele in humans is observed in one of two types of mating. The first is a mating between a female heterozygous for the mutant allele (and manifesting its effect because it is dominant) and a male whose one X chromosome bears the normal allele of the gene and who is thus unaffected (Fig. 8-6). In considering all such matings, one half of the offspring are affected regardless of sex. On the average, males are more severely affected. In considering a single such mating, the product of each pregnancy,

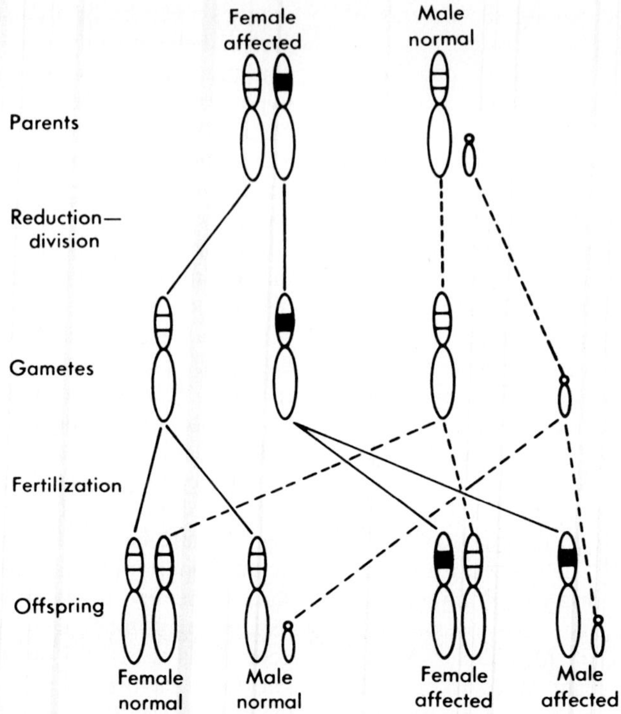

Fig. 8-6. Mating diagram representing a mating between an affected female heterozygous for an X-linked dominant mutant allele and an unaffected male. The larger chromosome here represents the X chromosome; the smaller chromosome represents the Y chromosome.

regardless of sex, has a 50% chance of being affected. The second type of mating is that between an unaffected female and a hemizygous affected male (Fig. 8-7). In considering all such matings, none of the sons can be affected because the affected father contributes his Y chromosome to all his sons, but all the daughters will be affected because each receives her affected father's only X chromosome. Male-to-male transmission of an X-linked allele does not occur. Rules governing X-linked dominant inheritance in humans, as set forth by Roberts, include the following:

1. If the affected person is a female, one half of her offspring (on the average) will be affected, regardless of sex.
2. If the affected person is a male, *none* of his male offspring will be affected, but *all* his female offspring will be affected.
3. An affected male ordinarily has an affected mother.
4. An affected female ordinarily has one affected parent, but it can be either mother or father.
5. An unaffected person cannot transmit the abnormality to his or her offspring.

The counseling for X-linked dominant inheritance depends on which member of the couple seeking advice is affected. If the wife is affected, the couple is advised that the offspring of each pregnancy, regardless of sex, has a 50% chance of being affected. If the husband is affected, they should be advised that the male offspring of any pregnancy will not be affected but that the female offspring of any pregnancy will be affected with *100% probability*. In some situations two normal parents may seek advice because a child has a condition inherited in an X-linked dominant manner. If the diagnosis and genetic mode can be established and if the counselor can be certain that neither parent (particularly the mother) carries a nonpenetrant mutant allele, then the affected child is the result of a new spontaneous mutation; the couple can be assured that the recurrence risk is, for all practical purposes, negligible.

Conditions that are inherited in an X-linked

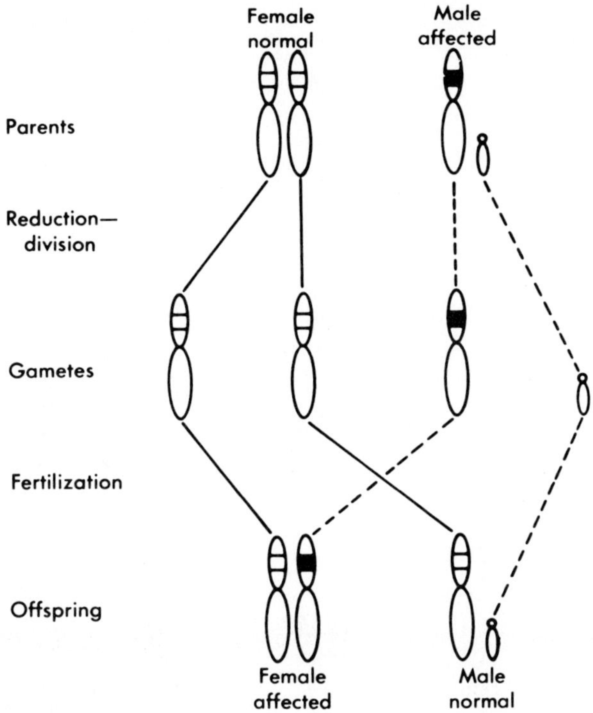

Fig. 8-7. Mating diagram representing a mating between an affected male hemizygous for an X-linked dominant mutant allele and a homozygous unaffected female.

dominant manner include familial hypophosphatemic rickets and Albright hereditary osteodystrophy (pseudohypoparathyroidism).

X-LINKED RECESSIVE INHERITANCE

By the very nature of gene effects, only the hemizygous male is ordinarily the victim of a condition inherited in an X-linked recessive manner. As in X-linked dominant inheritance, two types of mating are of importance in X-linked recessive inheritance. The first is the mating between a heterozygous (but phenotypically normal) female and an unaffected male (Fig. 8-8). In general, the female contributes her X chromosome that bears the mutant allele to half of her offspring, regardless of the sex of the offspring. The daughters who receive the mutant X-linked allele, like the mother, are phenotypically normal heterozygotes. Any son who receives the mutant allele will manifest its effect. Thus in considering a single mating, the risk of an affected daughter is zero, but the risk that any male offspring will be affected is 50%. The overall risk of an affected offspring with any pregnancy, without consideration of the sex of the offspring, is 25%. The second important mating type is that between a homozygous unaffected female and a hemizygous affected male (Fig. 8-9). No offspring is affected, but all the daughters are heterozygous for the mutant allele. The risk of an affected offspring in any given pregnancy is zero. Rules governing X-linked recessive inheritance in humans include the following:

1. Ordinarily, only males are affected.
2. Every affected male has a heterozygous carrier mother.
3. On the average, half of the male offspring of a heterozygous female are affected and half are unaffected.
4. On the average, half of the female offspring of a carrier female are also heterozygous carriers, and half are homozygous unaffected.
5. An affected male cannot transmit the abnormality to his male offspring, but all his daughters are heterozygous carriers.

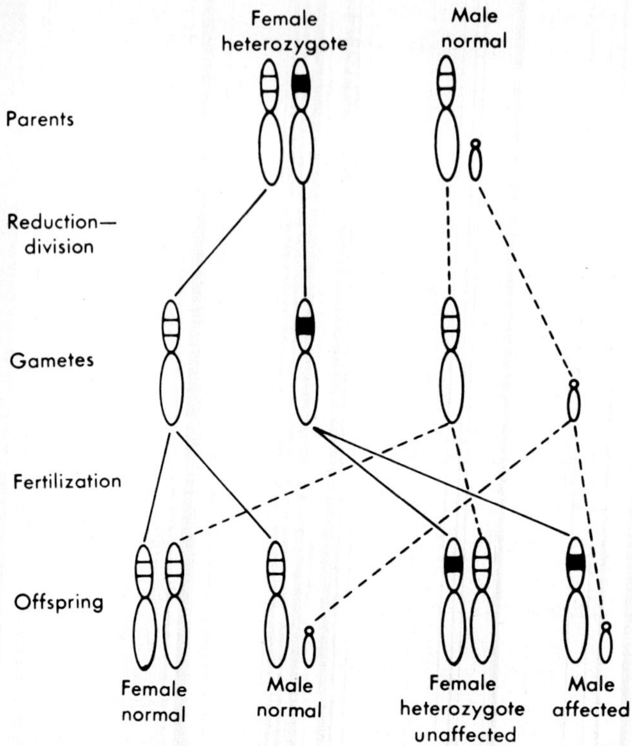

Fig. 8-8. Mating diagram representing a mating between a female unaffected by, but heterozygous for, an X-linked recessive mutant allele and an unaffected male.

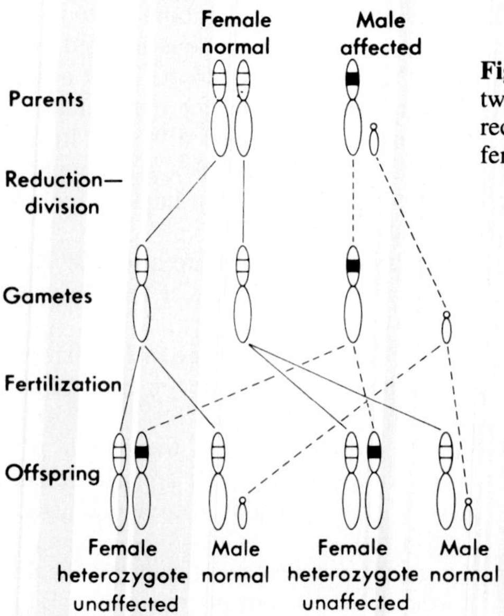

Fig. 8-9. Mating diagram representing a mating between an affected male hemizygous for an X-linked recessive mutant allele and a homozygous unaffected female.

6. Unaffected male offspring of proved heterozygous mothers cannot transmit the abnormality.
7. Affected female offspring ordinarily occur only when an affected male marries a heterozygous female.

Two types of counseling situations pertain in X-linked recessive inheritance. The first occurs when a couple, both of whom are unaffected, consult the genetic counselor because they have produced an affected son. If the mother's family history includes other affected males, the counselor may conclude that she is heterozygous for the mutant allele and has contributed it to the son. If her family history is negative, the question of whether she is heterozygous for the mutant allele or whether her son's condition is the result of a new spontaneous mutation may be difficult to answer. In a few conditions the female heterozygote may be detectable by means of special techniques. If the mother is heterozygous, the couple should be counseled that a female product of any subsequent pregnancy will be unaffected but that a male product of any subsequent pregnancy has a 50% chance of being affected. The second counseling situation arises when a couple seeks advice because the husband is the victim of an X-linked recessive condition. Such a couple should be advised that no offspring will be affected but that *every* daughter will be heterozygous for the mutant allele and that the risks just mentioned will apply to her when she reaches reproductive age.

Conditions discussed in this book that are inherited in an X-linked recessive manner include hemophilia A and B (pp. 524 to 527), Duchenne and Becker types of muscular dystrophy (pp. 820 and 822), Hunter syndrome (p. 659), the Lesch-Nyhan syndrome (p. 668), and some cases of mental retardation.

Interesting and important information has recently been acquired on the last of these examples. That the frequency of mentally retarded males exceeds that of mentally retarded females has been known for some time. This difference has been shown to be, at least in part, the result of several forms of mental retardation inherited in an X-linked manner. Among the X-linked forms of mental retardation are those patients with so-called nonspecific X-linked mental retardation. A chromosome *fragile site* has been found in the distal long arm of an X chromosome in cultured lymphocytes and fibroblasts from affected males and heterozygous females in a proportion of pedigrees demonstrating this nonspecific X-linked mental retardation. The fragile site appears as an attenuated segment in band q27-q28 of the involved chromosome, with the result that the terminal band of the long arm of the X appears as a satellite and the fragile site appears as a stalk. The *fragile X chromosome* (Fig. 8-10) is visible in varying, usually small, proportions of cells from affected males. In obligate heterozygous females the fragile X is seen usually in an even smaller proportion of cultured cells. This "fragile-X-linked mental retardation" apparently constitutes a distinct nosologic entity among the genetically heterogeneous category of nonspecific X-linked mental retardation. A characteristic phenotype has been described for this condition, although its complete definition remains uncertain. Features include long facies, prominent forehead and chin, flat midfacial region, thick lips, highly arched palate, and large, sometimes malformed ears. Mental retardation in affected males is usually of moderate to severe degree, and is associated with a major speech defect. Prominent among phenotypic features is megalotestes, resulting from increased interstitial fluid. In some pedigrees heterozygous females manifest varying degrees of mental retardation.

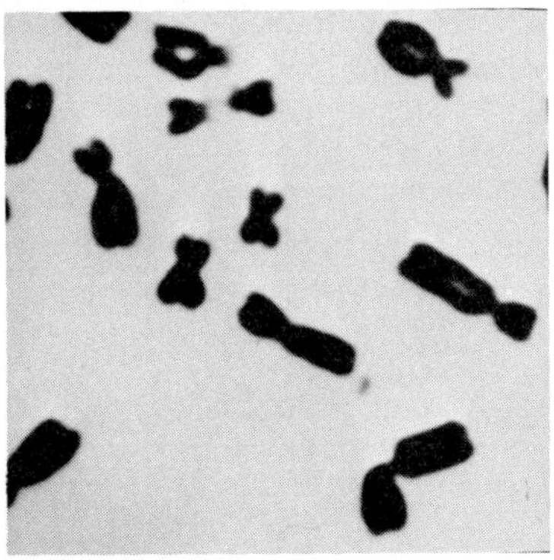

Fig. 8-10. Portion of homogeneously stained metaphase cell showing X chromosome that demonstrates q27-28 fragile site. Affected chromosome is medium-sized submetacentric near center of figure. Note small dots of chromatin separated from end of long arms. Barely visible "stalk" joining these dots to end of chromosome is *fragile site*.

Although *fragile-X-linked mental retardation with megalotestes* may well constitute an important newly recognized mendelian entity associated with a chromosome marker, much is yet to be learned about it. Intellectually normal males with the Xq27-28 fragile site have been reported. Whereas the fragile X chromosome has been demonstrated in cultured amniocytes, the applicability of this technique for prenatal diagnosis remains fraught with uncertainty. The culture conditions are known to affect the demonstrability of the fragile X. It is much more frequent in cells cultured in folic acid-deficient medium. The role played by folic acid or folic acid deficiency in the expression of the phenotype in this condition remains to be determined, as does its possible role in prevention or treatment of the mental retardation.

Fragile X-linked mental retardation should be kept in mind in the differential diagnosis of mental retardation, and appropriate chromosome analysis requested to investigate the possibility.

In utero diagnosis is possible in a few X-linked recessive diseases by means of studies conducted on cells obtained by amniocentesis. Prenatal sex diagnosis can be made by a chromosome analysis of such cells. If the fetus is a female, she will not be affected; if it is a male, he has a 50% chance of being affected. For a few conditions a firm diagnosis can be made by specialized studies on cultured cells from amniotic fluid or on a sample of fetal blood. If the fetus is found to be affected, a therapeutic abortion may be offered.

POLYGENIC INHERITANCE: EMPIRIC RISKS

Some conditions in humans are known to occur with familial distribution, but their inheritance patterns do not conform to the rules governing mendelian inheritance already discussed. That they are genetically determined (and inherited) is supported by their more frequent occurrence in both members of identical twin pairs than in nonidentical twin pairs of the same sex. Based partly on evidence gained through study of other organisms, these conditions are thought to be the result of the cooperative action of several mutant genes, not just one; that is, they are *polygenic* in origin. A few such conditions are congenital hypertrophic pyloric stenosis, cleft lip with or without cleft palate, cleft palate alone, and abnormalities of the spinal axis such as anencephaly and spina bifida. In a couple one of whom is affected, or both of whom are unaffected but have produced one affected child, recurrence risks such as 50% or 25% cannot be quoted. Empiric recurrence risk figures have been derived largely from the observation of the frequency of recurrence in the subsequent offspring of couples who have produced one affected child. Recurrence risks for each of the abnormalities mentioned fall within a range of 2% to 8%, compared with a primary risk of 0.1% to 0.2% (Table 8-1).

COUNSELING FOR CHROMOSOME ABNORMALITIES

Counseling for chromosome abnormalities is considered briefly in Chapter 7.

OTHER ASPECTS OF GENETIC COUNSELING

The responsibilities of genetic counselors are obvious. To be effective, they must be able to communicate with frightened, tense parents; they must have knowledge of the field in which they are working; and they must be familiar

Table 8-1. Risk of occurrence and recurrence of common malformations

Malformation	Primary risk (%)	Affected sibling (%)	Affected parent (%)	Affected sibling and parent (%)	Two affected siblings (%)
Cleft lip ± palate	0.1	4	4	17	9
Cleft palate	0.02	2	6	15	
Clubfoot	0.3	3-8		10	
Hip dislocation	0.1	5			
Spina bifida cystica	0.15-0.25	2-5	2-5		
Anencephaly	0.1-0.2	2-5			
Pyloric stenosis	0.2-0.3	6			

with, and have at hand, the diagnostic techniques necessary to confirm their clinical impressions.

Currently available techniques that permit mass screening for the presence of genetic disease and of heterozygotes for recessive mutant genes and that permit in utero diagnosis and selective abortion open up much wider possibilities for the genetic counselor in the prevention of genetic disease. At the same time, these new horizons introduce an entirely new series of questions as to who should be screened, how screening should be implemented, and the proper place for interruption of pregnancy.

Legislation requiring the screening of all newborn infants for phenylketonuria has been enacted in most states in the United States; in a few, screening for galactosemia and other conditions is routine. This type of genetic screening is probably the least controversial because, particularly in the cases of phenylketonuria and galactosemia, the consequence of delay in treatment is mental retardation. On the other hand, if diagnosis is made early in infancy and proper treatment instituted, mental retardation may be prevented. In addition, screening for these diseases involves no social or ethnic implications—it involves search for *disease,* not unaffected heterozygotes, and involves a potentially *treatable* condition in most cases.

Population screening for the heterozygous state of the autosomal recessive allele in such conditions as Tay-Sachs disease and sickle cell anemia is currently technically feasible and under way. Other heterozygote screening will doubtless soon be possible. Because Tay-Sachs disease is most frequent in Jews of eastern European origin and sickle cell anemia in blacks of African origin, such screening raises questions regarding ethnic discrimination. That one should desire to know whether he or she is heterozygous for a lethal recessive gene for purposes of reproductive planning is ideal. However, such knowledge should not be forced on anyone. Heterozygote screening is certainly acceptable and desirable as long as it is carried out on a voluntary basis and is accompanied by an effective program of education for the susceptible population. It allows genetic counseling at a time ideal for prevention, that is, "before the fact."

In utero diagnosis of chromosome abnormalities is discussed in Chapter 7. In addition, as mentioned previously in this chapter, in utero diagnosis is possible for an increasing number of conditions, a list of which follows:

Disorders of lipid metabolism
- Abetalipoproteinemia
- Adrenoleukodystrophy
- Cerebellar ataxia, juvenile
- Cholesterol ester storage disease
- *Fabry disease
- *Farber disease
- *Gaucher disease
- *Generalized gangliosidosis (G_{M1} gangliosidosis, type 1)
- *Ichthyosis, X-linked (placental steroid sulfatase deficiency)
- *Juvenile G_{M1} gangliosidosis (G_{M1} gangliosidosis, type 2)
- *Tay-Sachs disease (G_{M2} gangliosidosis, type 1)
- *Sandhoff disease (G_{M2} gangliosidosis, type 2)
- Juvenile G_{M2} gangliosidosis (G_{M2} gangliosidosis, type 3)
- G_{M3} sphingolipodystrophy
- *Krabbe disease (globoid cell leukodystrophy)
- Lactosyl ceramidosis
- *Mucolipidosis type I (sialidosis)
- *Mucolipidosis type II (I cell disease)
- Mucolipidosis type III
- *Mucolipidosis type IV
- *Metachromatic leukodystrophy
- *Niemann-Pick disease, type A
- Niemann-Pick disease, type B
- Niemann-Pick disease, type C
- Refsum disease
- Tangier disease
- *Wolman disease

Mucopolysaccharidoses
- *Hurler syndrome (MPS I-H)
- Scheie disease (MPS I-S)
- Hurler-Scheie disease (MPS I-HS)
- *Hunter disease (MPS II, A)
- *Hunter disease (MPS II, B)
- *Sanfilippo syndrome (MPS III, A)
- *Sanfilippo syndrome (MPS III, B)
- Morquio syndrome (MPS IV)
- *Maroteaux-Lamy syndrome (MPS VI, A)
- *Maroteaux-Lamy syndrome (MPS VI, B)
- β-Glucuronidase deficiency (MPS VII)

Amino acid and related disorders
- *Argininosuccinic aciduria
- Aspartylglucosaminuria
- *Citrullinemia
- Cystathioninuria
- *Cystinosis
- *Cystinuria
- *Glutaric aciduria, type II
- Hartnup disease
- Histidinemia
- Homocystinuria
- Hyperargininemia

---

*Prenatal diagnosis made.

Amino acid and related disorders—cont'd
- Hyperlysinemia
- Hypervalinemia
- Iminoglycinuria
- *Isovaleric acidemia
- Branched chain ketoaciduria (maple syrup urine disease)
  - *Severe infantile
  - Intermittent
- Methylmalonic aciduria
  - Vitamin B_{12} responsive
  - *Vitamin B_{12} unresponsive
- Methylenetetrahydrofolate reductase deficiency
- Ornithine-α-ketoacid transaminase deficiency
- Ornithinemia (gyrate atrophy of retina)
- *Propionyl-CoA carboxylase deficiency (ketotic hyperglycinemia)
- Succinyl-CoA: 3-ketoacid-CoA transferase deficiency

Disorders of carbohydrate metabolism
- *Fucosidosis
- *Galactokinase deficiency
- *Galactosemia
- Glucose-6-phosphate dehydrogenase deficiency
- *Glycogen storage disease, type II
- Glycogen storage disease, type III
- *Glycogen storage disease, type IV
- Glycogen storage disease with phosphorylase kinase deficiency
- Mannosidosis
- *Phosphohexose isomerase deficiency
- *Pyruvate decarboxylase deficiency
- Pyruvate dehydrogenase deficiency

Miscellaneous disorders
- Acatalasemia
- *Acute intermittent porphyria
- *Adenosine deaminase deficiency
- *Adrenal hyperplasia caused by 21-hydroxylase deficiency
- Androgen insensitivity syndrome
- Chediak-Higashi syndrome
- *Chronic granulomatous disease
- *Congenital erythropoietic porphyria
- *Congenital nephrosis
- *Duchenne muscular dystrophy
- Ehlers-Danlos syndrome, type IV
- Ehlers-Danlos syndrome, type V
- *Ellis-Van Creveld syndrome
- *Epidermolysis bullosa
- *Familial hypercholesterolemia
- *Fanconi pancytopenia syndrome
- *Fragile X-linked mental retardation
- Glutathionuria
- Hemoglobinopathies
- *Hemophilia A
- Hemolytic anemia VIII
- Hyperammonemia, type II
- Hyperthyroidism
- *Hypophosphatasia
- *Hypothyroidism
- *Ichthyosis, epidermolytic hyperkeratosis
- *Ichthyosis, lamellar

*Prenatal diagnosis made.

Miscellaneous disorders—cont'd
- Leigh encephalopathy
- *Lesch-Nyhan syndrome
- *Lysosomal acid phosphatase deficiency
- Lysyl-protocollagen hydroxylase deficiency
- *Meckel syndrome
- *Menke disease
- Methyltetrahydrofolate methyltransferase deficiency
- *Myotonic muscular dystrophy
- Nucleoside phosphorylase deficiency (with immunodeficiency)
- Orotic aciduria
- *Osteogenesis imperfecta (severe autosomal recessive form)
- Osteopetrosis
- Protoporphyria
- Saccharopurinuria
- Severe combined immunodeficiency disease
- *Sickle cell anemia
- Sulfite oxidase deficiency
- Skeletal dysplasia
- *Thalassemia
- Vitamin B_{12} metabolic defect
- *Von Willebrand disease
- Wiskott-Aldrich syndrome
- *Xeroderma pigmentosum
- Zellweger syndrome

Congenital malformations
- *Any chromosome anomaly (Chapter 7)
- *Neural tube defects
  - Anencephaly
  - Spina bifida
- *Oomphalocele

In couples who have previously produced an affected child or who have shown themselves to be at risk through family or population screening, the women are candidates for in utero diagnostic procedures, as indicated in the following outline:

- Pregnancies at risk for chromosome aberrations (Chapter 7)
- Pregnancies at risk for single gene disorder
  - Serious untreatable inborn metabolic or other disorder
  - Treatable genetic defects in which treatment must be instituted early
  - Serious X-linked conditions
- Pregnancies at risk for neural tube defects
  - Mother has previously produced affected offspring
  - Affected parent
  - Parent with roentgenographically demonstrated complex spina bifida occulta
  - Mother who has elevated serum AFP level

Many of the above conditions are detectable on the basis of enzyme analysis in cultured amniocytes obtained by transabdominal amniocentesis in the second trimester of pregnancy,

*Prenatal diagnosis made.

or cultured cells obtained from biopsy of the chorionic villi in the first trimester; some by radiographic examination of the fetus in utero; some by amniotic fluid alpha-fetoprotein determination; some by ultrasonography; and some by examination of fetal skin or blood samples obtained by fetoscopy. The newly developed techniques of restriction enzyme analysis of polymorphisms in DNA extracted from cultured or uncultured amniocytes have made possible the in utero diagnosis of a number of hemoglobinopathies without the risk incurred by fetoscopy and fetal blood sampling. These same techniques will undoubtedly further broaden the spectrum of conditions diagnosable in utero.

Neural tube defects (anencephaly and meningomyelocele) deserve special mention in a discussion of prenatal diagnosis. They are relatively common malformations and are diagnosable by a combination of amniotic fluid alpha-fetoprotein (AFP) assay and ultrasonography. Women at an increased risk over the general population, on the basis of a previously affected offspring, may seek prenatal diagnosis. However, even though the general population risk is relatively high (see Table 8-1), amniocentesis cannot be made routine in all pregnancies. Measurement of AFP in the serum of the pregnant woman has been shown to be effective as a screening procedure for neural tube defects and other malformations associated with an open skin defect. Maternal serum AFP measurement will soon become a procedure routinely offered to the pregnant woman. If the serum AFP is elevated, an ultrasonogram is done and, if indicated, the patient is offered confirmatory amniocentesis.

As in chromosome disorders, if an affected fetus is found, termination of pregnancy may be offered; on the other hand, if the fetus is found to be unaffected, the pregnancy can continue with considerably relieved parents. It should be mentioned that *no* in utero diagnostic procedure guarantees a *normal* infant because a large number of genetic and nongenetic conditions are not amenable to such procedures.

Robert L. Summitt

SELECTED READINGS

Antonarakis, S.E., et al.: Genetic diseases: diagnosis by restriction endonuclease analysis, J. Pediat. **100:**845, 1982.

Fraser, F.C.: Genetic counseling, Am. J. Hum. Genet. **26:**636, 1974.

Fuhrman, W., and Vogel, F.: Genetic counseling, ed. 3, New York, 1983, Springer-Verlag, New York, Inc.

Golbus, M., et al.: Prenatal genetic diagnosis in 3000 amniocenteses, N. Engl. J. Med. **300:**157, 1979.

Golbus, M.S.: The current scope of antenatal diagnosis, Hosp. Pract. **17:**179, 1982.

Kelly, T.E.: Clinical genetics and genetic counseling, Chicago, 1980, Year Book Medical Publishers, Inc.

Milunsky, A.: Prenatal diagnosis of genetic disorders, N. Engl. J. Med. **295:**377, 1976.

National Institute of Child Health Development Amniocentesis Registry: The safety and accuracy of mid-trimester amniocentesis, U.S. Department of Health, Education, and Welfare, pub. no. (NIH) 78-190, Washington, D.C., 1978, U.S. Government Printing Office.

Simpson, J.L., et al.: Genetics in obstetrics and gynecology, New York, 1982, Grune & Stratton, Inc.

Tariverdian, G., and Weck, B.: Nonspecific X-linked mental retardation—A review, Hum. Genet. **62:**95, 1982.

Thompson, J.S., and Thompson, M.W.: Genetics in medicine, ed. 3, Philadelphia, 1980, W.B. Saunders Co.

9 Nutrition and Nutritional Disturbances

Recently the role of nutrition in growth, development, and maintenance of health has received increased attention by health providers and a better-informed public. Significant changes have been made in infant feeding practices, such as delaying the introduction of solid foods and reducing salt intake. Despite this progress, children frequently do not receive a diet adequate in the nutrients necessary for optimal body metabolism. Supplemental vitamins given to cover dietary inadequacy may not be sufficient, since there are probably several nutrients that have not yet been discovered. Certain foods taken in excess may be harmful by promoting obesity, diabetes, atherosclerosis, or other pathologic processes.

This chapter presents a summary of the current knowledge concerning nutritional requirements of infants and children and disorders resulting from failure to meet these requirements.

NUTRITIONAL REQUIREMENTS

Water

Water is necessary for life. A severe deficiency can develop rapidly from inadequate intake or excessive loss. On the basis of body weight, the turnover of water is 2 to 3 times greater in infants than adults because of the infants' higher metabolic rate, limited capacity for renal conservation, and insensible loss from the relatively larger skin and alveolar surface areas. The usual amount of water required for maintenance calculated by body surface area is 1500 ml/m^2/day. Table 9-1 shows the water requirement based on body weight and age. A small amount of water (12 g/100 kcal) is produced by the oxidation of food. Depending on the rate of growth, 1% to 3% of the water consumed is retained by the body. Under normal circumstances 40% to 50% of ingested water is eliminated by the skin and lungs, 5% to 10% through the intestinal tract, and the remainder by the kidneys, which can concentrate urine only to about 700 mOsm/L in the infant, compared to a maximum of 1400 mOsm/L in the older child or adult.

Many factors affect the water needs of infants and children, such as the amount of fluid, protein, and minerals in the diet, the solute load to the kidneys, and the metabolic rate. During ordinary conditions the sensation of thirst helps keep a balance between water intake and output. Fever, tachypnea, exercise, perspiration, vomiting, and diarrhea increase the need for water.

Energy

The energy value of foods is expressed as the kilocalorie (kcal), the amount of heat necessary to raise the temperature of 1 kg water from 14.5° C (58.1° F) to 15.5° C (59.9° F).

A positive energy balance is required for growth, maintenance of basal organ metabolic function, and physical activity. The energy from food for the average child 6 to 12 years of age is used in the following way: 50% for basal metabolism, 25% for physical activity, 10% for fecal loss, 12% for growth, and 3% to 5% for specific dynamic action of food. Energy costs of growth have been estimated to be between 5 and 8 kcal/g of tissue gained. Foods vary in their available energy. When used by the body as energy sources, 1 g fat produces 9 kcal,

Table 9-1. Average daily requirements of water expressed in terms of weight and age

Age (years)	Water (ml/kg)
0-1	150
1-3	125
4-6	100
7-9	75
10-12	75
13 or older	50

whereas 1 g protein and 1 g carbohydrate each yields 4 kcal. Carbohydrate and fat are the major sources of energy. Recommended energy intakes for children of various ages are given in Table 9-2. Caloric requirements can also be predicted from body surface area; the average person requires approximately 1500 kcal/m^2 body surface/24 hr. Exercise can increase appreciably the caloric requirement.

The decisive criteria of the adequacy of the diet to meet energy needs is the growth of the child. If energy content of the diet is inadequate, the child will fail to gain weight at a normal rate. If energy needs are exceeded, obesity will ensue.

Protein and amino acids

Amino acids derived from protein are essential for the synthesis of structural proteins, enzymes, antibodies, and hormones. Nine amino acids are classified as essential: histidine, leucine, isoleucine, lysine, methionine, phenylalanine, threonine, tryptophan, and valine. In addition, in low birth weight infants arginine, cystine, and possibly taurine are essential. The absence of just one of these amino acids will result in a negative nitrogen balance. In contrast, an excessive protein intake during the first month of life could result in neurologic damage.

Recommended daily intakes of protein for children are shown in Table 9-2. Requirements for essential amino acids are largely regulated by the growth requirements of the infant or child. The protein in milk, fish, poultry, beef, and pork has a higher nutritive value than the protein in vegetables, in which the essential amino acid content is less complete.

Unless sufficient calories are provided in the diet in the form of fat and carbohydrate, protein will be deaminated and used for energy. Protein intakes greater than 20% of the total calories will increase the requirement for water for renal solute load and may precipitate dehydration in the infant. Excessive protein in the older child is an economically and metabolically inefficient method of providing calories.

Fat

In infancy, 40% to 50% of the energy requirement is met with calories from fat. In older children fat provides approximately 40% of the energy consumed. Polyunsaturated linoleic acid is an essential nutrient for both children and adults. It is necessary for growth, prostaglandin synthesis, reproduction, platelet function, and normal skin and hair. Essential fatty acid deficiency is manifested by dry flaky skin, thrombocytopenia, poor hair growth, failure to thrive, difficulty in healing, increased susceptibility to infection, and elevated levels of eicosatrienoic acid. Ingestion of excessive linoleic acid may cause injury to cell membranes by accelerated

Table 9-2. Mean heights and weights* and recommended protein and energy intake† at various ages

Category	Age (years)	Weight (kg)	Weight (lb)	Height (cm)	Height (inches)	Protein (g)	Energy needs (kcal)	Range of needs (kcal)	Energy (kcal/kg)
Infants	0.0-0.5	6	13	60	24	kg × 2.2	kg × 115	(95-145)	115
	0.5-1.0	9	20	71	28	kg × 2.0	kg × 105	(80-135)	105
Children	1-3	13	29	90	35	23	1300	(900-1800)	100
	4-6	20	44	112	44	30	1700	(1300-2300)	85
	7-10	28	62	132	52	34	2400	(1650-3300)	86
Men	11-14	45	99	157	62	45	2700	(2000-3700)	60
	15-18	66	145	176	69	56	2800	(2100-3900)	42
Women	11-14	46	101	157	62	46	2200	(1500-3000)	48
	15-18	55	121	163	64	46	2100	(1200-3000)	38

*The data in this table have been assembled from the observed median heights and weights of children. From Food and Nutrition Board: Recommended dietary allowances, ed. 8, Washington, D.C. 1980, National Academy of Sciences–National Research Council. Reproduced with the permission of the National Academy of Sciences, Washington, D.C.

†Energy allowances for children through age 18 are based on median energy intakes of children of these ages followed in longitudinal growth studies. The values in parentheses are 10th and 90th percentiles of energy intake to indicate the range of energy consumption among children of these ages.

peroxidation. The minimal requirement for linoleic acid is 1% of the total calories. An optimum intake of linoleic acid would constitute 3% to 5% of the calories. In addition, linolenic and arachidonic acids may be essential in infants. Dietary fat also serves as a carrier for the fat-soluble vitamins, makes the diet palatable, and provides satiety.

Carbohydrates

Carbohydrates are a major source of energy. They are a constituent of cell structure, antibodies, serum carrier glycoproteins, glycogen, and roughage. Unused carbohydrate is converted to fat.

Carbohydrate cannot be considered a dietary essential, since it can be synthesized from amino acids and the glycerol moiety of fat. Ingestion of less than 5% of the daily caloric needs may result in ketosis and loss of protein for growth and tissue repair. It is recommended that 25% to 55% of the calories in the diet be supplied by carbohydrates. Excessive use of sucrose should be avoided to prevent dental caries.

Vitamins

Vitamins are essential cofactors required for normal metabolism. Most cannot be synthesized by the body and must be supplied by the diet. On the basis of solubility, vitamins are divided into 2 groups: fat-soluble and water-soluble. The fat-soluble vitamins A, D, E, and K are absorbed and transported in a manner similar to lipids. Any condition that results in malabsorption of fat may also result in malabsorption of these vitamins. Excessive ingestion of vitamin A, D, or K may lead to toxicity. The body is much less able to store water-soluble vitamins. Therefore their removal from the diet will result more quickly in a clinically recordable deficient state.

The most desirable method of ensuring adequate vitamin intake is by providing a well-balanced diet. Vitamin supplements should be used discriminately. Recommended daily allowances of vitamins are found in Tables 9-3 and 9-4.

Vitamin A. Several biologically active compounds are collectively known as vitamin A. Carotenoids of variable biologic activity as Vitamin A precursors are found in plants. The most studied metabolic function of vitamin A is its role in visual adaptation to changes in light. Other known functions are to protect and regulate cell membranes and to promote skeletal and soft tissue growth by its influence on protein synthesis.

Preformed vitamin A occurs only in animal foods. The vitamin A precursor carotenoids are found chiefly in deep orange, yellow, and green fruits and vegetables.

Vitamin D. The most important antirachitic compounds are ergocalciferol (vitamin D_2) and cholecalciferol (vitamin D_3). Cholecalciferol is

Table 9-3. Recommended daily dietary allowances for fat-soluble vitamins

	Age (years)	Vitamin A		Vitamin D		Vitamin E (mg alpha TE)‡
		(μg RE)*	(IU)	(μg)†	(IU)	
Infants	0.0-0.5	420	1400	10	400	3
	0.5-1.0	400	2000	10	400	4
Children	1-3	400	2000	10	400	5
	4-6	500	2500	10	400	6
	7-10	700	3300	10	400	7
Men	11-14	1000	5000	10	400	8
	15-18	1000	5000	10	400	10
Women	11-14	800	4000	10	400	8
	15-18	800	4000	10	400	8

From Food and Nutrition Board: Recommended dietary allowances, ed. 8, Washington, D.C., 1980, National Academy of Sciences–National Research Council. Reproduced with the permission of the National Academy of Sciences, Washington, D.C.

*Retinol equivalents: 1 retinol equivalent = 1 μg retinol or 6 μg beta carotene.

†As cholecalciferol: 10 μg cholecalciferol = 400 IU vitamin D.

‡Alpha tocopherol equivalents: 1 mg d-alpha-tocopherol = 1 alpha TE.

formed by the conversion of the provitamin 7-dehydrocholesterol in the skin by sunlight.

Vitamin D maintains normal serum calcium levels and facilitates mineralization of the bone. The recommended intake is 400 IU vitamin D daily. This amount will cover the requirements of infants and children without exposure to sunlight.

Most of the various forms of cow's milk marketed in the United States are fortified with 400 IU of vitamin D per quart. Human milk contains both a fat-soluble and a water-soluble conjugate of vitamin D with sulfate. It now appears that most of the vitamin D in human milk is water-soluble and is present in amounts adequate to prevent the young infant from acquiring rickets.

Vitamin E. Vitamin E represents a group of fat-soluble compounds essential for the human infant, but whose role in the nutrition of the older child and adult is still uncertain. Alpha tocopherol promotes the greatest tissue retention relative to the other vitamin E compounds. The natural tocopherols are found in greatest concentration in seed oils. Tocopherols are important natural antioxidants in foods and tissue and are especially important in preventing peroxidation of lipids.

Vitamin K. The only known function of vitamin K is its role in maintaining a normal clotting mechanism.

The richest sources of vitamin K are green leafy vegetables. The bacterial flora of the intestinal tract also produce vitamin K. The safe and adequate daily dietary intake of vitamin K is shown in Table 9-6.

Vitamin C. Ascorbic acid has many functions. L-Ascorbic acid is the active form. Among its known metabolic functions is its role as a coenzyme, or cofactor, in reactions in which the rate of the reaction is important. Ascorbic acid is important for the normal development of fibroblasts, osteoblasts, and odontoblasts. It aids in the conversion of folic acid to folinic acid. Vitamin C facilitates the gastrointestinal absorption of iron and calcium. In its role as an antioxidant it protects vitamins A and E and the polyunsaturated fatty acids. It is necessary for the formation of ground substance, the synthesis of collagen, and the metabolism of tyrosine and tryptophan.

Thiamine. Thiamine (vitamin B_1) functions in metabolic reactions as the coenzyme thiamine pyrophosphate. The requirement for this vitamin is determined by the carbohydrate and caloric content of the diet because of thiamine's vital role in the metabolism of carbohydrate and its participation in the citric acid cycle. Recommendations for different age groups are based on the provision of 0.2 to 0.5 mg/1000 kcal consumed.

Table 9-4. Recommended daily dietary allowances for water-soluble vitamins

	Age (year)	Ascorbic acid (mg)	Thiamine (mg)	Riboflavin (mg)	Niacin (mg NE)*	Vitamin B_6 (mg)	Folacin† (μg)	Vitamin B_{12} (μg)
Infants	0-0.5	35	0.3	0.4	6	0.3	30	0.5‡
	0.5-1.0	35	0.5	0.6	8	0.6	45	1.5
Children	1-3	45	0.7	0.8	9	0.9	100	2.0
	4-6	45	0.9	1.0	11	1.3	200	2.5
	7-10	45	1.2	1.4	16	1.6	300	3.0
Men	11-14	50	1.4	1.6	18	1.8	400	3.0
	15-18	60	1.4	1.7	20	2.0	400	3.0
Women	11-14	50	1.1	1.3	15	1.8	400	3.0
	15-18	60	1.1	1.3	14	2.0	400	3.0

From Food and Nutrition Board: Recommended dietary allowances, ed. 8, Washington, D.C., 1980, National Academy of Sciences–National Research Council. Reproduced with the permission of the National Academy of Sciences, Washington, D.C.

*1 NE (niacin equivalent) = 1 mg niacin or 60 mg dietary tryptophan.

†Folacin allowances refer to dietary sources as determined by *Lactobacillus casei* assay after treatment with enzymes ("conjugases") to make polyglutamyl forms of the vitamin available to the test organism.

‡The RDA for vitamin B_{12} in infants is based on average concentration of the vitamin in human milk. The allowances after weaning are based on energy intake (as recommended by the American Academy of Pediatrics) and consideration of other factors such as intestinal absorption.

Riboflavin. Riboflavin (vitamin B_2) is a precursor of two enzymes, flavin mononucleotide (FMN) and flavin adenine dinucleotide (FAD), essential to a number of oxidative enzyme systems. Therefore riboflavin is involved in many reactions of intermediary metabolism involving protein, fat, and carbohydrate.

Because of its involvement in energy metabolism, requirements for riboflavin are based on caloric intake. The recommendation at all ages is 0.6 mg riboflavin/1000 kcal.

Rich sources of riboflavin are meats, eggs, green leafy vegetables, legumes, and whole grains.

Niacin. Niacin (nicotinic acid) is an essential component of coenzyme I (nicotinamide adenine dinucleotide) and coenzyme II (nicotinamide adenine dinucleotide phosphate). These coenzymes are essential for the transfer of hydrogen in the intercellular respiratory mechanism of all cells. They are essential in metabolic reactions involving carbohydrate, fat, and protein. The requirement of niacin is related to energy metabolism and is 6.6 mg/1000 kcal for children and adolescents.

The amino acid tryptophan (in the presence of adequate amounts of pyridoxine) can be converted to niacin and fulfill a portion of the body's requirement.

Pyridoxine. Three chemically related compounds—pyridoxine, pyridoxal, and pyridoxamine—serve the metabolic function of vitamin B_6. The physiologically active form, pyridoxal-5′-phosphate, is important in protein, carbohydrate, and lipid metabolism. This coenzyme is used in nearly all enzymatic reactions involving nonoxidative degradation and interconversion of amino acids.

The requirement for pyridoxine is probably related more to protein content than to caloric content of the diet. An intake of 0.09 to 0.015 mg/g of protein may be used as an approximation of the requirement.

Folacin. The most important clinical function of folacin (folic acid) is its role in the synthesis of the purine and pyrimidine compounds, which are used for the formation of nucleoproteins. The absence of an adequate supply of nucleoproteins explains the megaloblastic anemia that results from a deficiency of this vitamin (see Chapter 20).

Major sources of folacin are meats and leafy green vegetables. Goat's milk contains very little folacin, and deficiency may develop in children using it as a major foodstuff.

Vitamin B_{12}. Vitamin B_{12} (cyanocobalamin) coenzyme forms are involved in many metabolic processes in protein, fat, and carbohydrate metabolism. It facilitates the synthesis of folic acid enzymes. Cyanocobalamin is essential for the synthesis of DNA because of its participation in the synthesis of purines and pyrimidines.

Cyanocobalamin occurs only in animal foods. Strict vegetarian diets will lead to a deficiency of vitamin B_{12}. Nursing infants of strict vegetarians are susceptible to this deficiency and will manifest megaloblastic anemia and neurologic dysfunction (see Chapter 20).

Biotin. Biotin plays an important regulatory role in carbohydrate and fat metabolism as a component of carboxylating enzymes including pyruvate/carboxylase and acetyl coenzyme A carboxylase. The recommended daily dietary allowance for biotin has not been established; however, Table 9-6 provides an estimate believed to be safe and adequate.

Panothenic acid. Panothenic acid is a component of coenzyme A and as such is important in gluconeogenesis and in the metabolism of carbohydrates and fatty acids. In Table 9-6 the estimated safe and adequate dietary allowance of this vitamin is shown.

Minerals

Minerals are inorganic nutrients that play important roles in the regulation of body fluids, acid-base balance, and metabolic processes. Minerals may function as catalysts and are found as constituents of enzymes and hormones. The major minerals, because of their relative abundance in the human body, are sodium, chloride, potassium, calcium, phosphorus, magnesium, and sulfur. Other minerals found in smaller quantities in the body are iron, zinc, iodine, copper, manganese, fluoride, chromium, selenium, and molybdenum. The minerals most likely to be deficient in the diet are calcium, iron, iodine, and possibly zinc in early infancy.

Zinc deficiency. Zinc plays an important role in nucleic acid metabolism and cell growth and repair. It is a component of insulin and of several enzymes important in metabolism, including alkaline phosphatase, carbonic anhydrase, thymidine kinase, carboxypeptidase, lactic dehydrogenase, DNA polymerase, and RNA polymerase.

Severe zinc deficiency in infants who possess an autosomal recessive inherited defect in their ability to metabolize zinc (acrodermatitis enteropathica), will result in failure to thrive in infancy. These infants have diarrhea, steatorrhea, alopecia, and pustulous skin lesions involving body orifices, the head, and the extremities. If the diet is not supplemented with zinc the failure to thrive may become profound and may cause death.

Zinc deficiency may result from a diet high in phytate and fiber, which reduces zinc absorption, causes intestinal malabsorption, and increases the urinary loss of zinc. In patients with Crohn disease and cystic fibrosis, intestinal malabsorption may lead to zinc deficiency. Hyperzincuria may cause zinc deficiency in patients with chronic renal disease, diabetes mellitus, sickle cell disease, acute viral hepatitis, chronic alcohol ingestion, and cirrhosis. Zinc deficiency is characterized by failure to thrive in infants and impaired growth velocity and delayed sexual maturation in children and adolescents. Other clinical features include lethargy, anorexia, irritability, hypogeusesthesia, depression, alopecia, delayed wound healing, dwarfism, hypogonadism, increased susceptibility of infection, corneal opacities, and hypertriglyceridemia.

There is some evidence that suggests that maternal zinc deficiency may cause malformations in the fetus. Zinc deficiency has been described in children with achondroplasia and in the fetal-alcohol syndrome. Recent studies indicate that some children with constitutional growth delay have decreased concentrations of zinc in their serum and hair. The efficacy of treating these children with zinc remains to be established. We are treating a 6-year-old child with hypoparathyroidism and mucocutaneous moniliasis (autoimmune polyglandular syndrome, type I) who had low serum levels of calcium, magnesium, and zinc. The cause of the zinc deficiency in this patient is thought to be intestinal malabsorption of zinc from steatorrhea and reduced serum 1,25-dihydroxyvitamin D_3, a hormone that increases intestinal absorption of zinc.

Administration of elemental zinc at a dosage of 100 mg daily for 2 to 3 months will correct most cases of zinc deficiency.

• • •

Recommended daily allowances of calcium, phosphorus, magnesium, iron, zinc, and iodine are provided in Table 9-5. Estimated safe and adequate daily dietary intake of selected trace elements are given in Table 9-6.

INFANT FEEDING

Growth during early infancy is very rapid, requiring ideal nutritional status. Too often society and industry have dictated feeding practices that have not always been in the child's best interest. Nutritional counseling should be given to the parents to influence long-term health of the family.

Human milk

Human milk provides the full-term infant with all necessary nutrients, including taurine and polyamines, that may be essential for the growing infant. It is important that the mother

Table 9-5. Recommended daily dietary allowances for minerals

	Age (year)	Calcium (mg)	Phosphorus (mg)	Magnesium (mg)	Iron (mg)	Zinc (mg)	Iodine (μg)
Infants	0.0-0.5	360	240	50	10	3	40
	0.5-1.0	540	360	70	15	5	50
Children	1-3	800	800	150	15	10	70
	4-6	800	800	200	10	10	90
	7-10	800	800	250	10	10	120
Men	11-14	1200	1200	350	18	15	150
	15-18	1200	1200	400	18	15	150
Women	11-14	1200	1200	300	18	15	150
	15-18	1200	1200	300	18	15	150

From Food and Nutrition Board: Recommended dietary allowances, ed. 8, Washington, D.C., 1980, National Academy of Sciences-National Research Council. Reproduced with the permission of the National Academy of Sciences, Washington, D.C.

Table 9-6. Estimated safe and adequate daily dietary intakes of additional selected vitamins and minerals*

		Vitamins			Trace elements†					
	Age (years)	**Vitamin K (μg)**	**Biotin (pg)**	**Pantothenic acid (mg)**	**Copper (mg)**	**Manganese (mg)**	**Fluoride (mg)**	**Chromium (mg)**	**Selenium (mg)**	**Molybdenum (mg)**
Infants	0-0.5	12	35	2	0.5-0.7	0.5-0.7	0.1-0.5	0.01-0.04	0.01-0.04	0.03-0.06
	0.5-1	10-20	50	3	0.7-1.0	0.7-1.0	0.2-1.0	0.02-0.06	0.02-0.06	0.04-0.08
Children and adolescents	1-3	15-30	65	3	1.0-1.5	1.0-1.5	0.5-1.5	0.02-0.08	0.02-0.03	0.05-0.1
	4-6	20-40	85	3-4	1.5-2.0	1.5-2.0	1.0-2.5	0.03-0.12	0.03-0.12	0.06-0.15
	7-10	30-60	120	4-5	2.0-2.5	2.0-3.0	1.5-2.5	0.05-0.2	0.05-0.2	0.1-0.3
	11+	50-100	100-200	4-7	2.0-3.0	2.5-5.0	1.5-2.5	0.05-0.2	0.05-0.2	0.15-0.5
Adults		70-140	100-200	4-7	2.0-3.0	2.5-5.0	1.5-4.0	0.05-0.2	0.05-0.2	0.15-0.5

From Recommended Dietary Allowances, Washington, D.C., 1980, Food and Nutrition Board National Academy of Sciences–National Research Council.
*Because there is less information on which to base allowances, these figures are not given in the main table of the RDA and are provided here in the form of ranges of recommended intakes.
†Since the toxic levels for many trace elements may be only several times usual intakes, the upper levels for the trace elements given in this table should not be habitually exceeded.

be well nourished during pregnancy and lactation. Studies on the bioavailability of iron in breast milk indicate that the amounts present in milk of well-nourished mothers will provide all the infant's needs for at least the first 4 to 6 months of life. Vitamin D is also adequate, and recent information on the water-soluble form of vitamin D in breast milk supports this observation. However, if the mother is not well nourished, vitamin supplements and iron should be given to the nursing infant. Evidence exists to support the immunologic protective factors of breast milk. Breast-fed infants have a lower incidence of common infections. Allergic manifestations such as atopic dermatitis and gastrointestinal symptomatology are less frequent in the infant who is fed human milk.

The suitability of human milk as the sole nutrient source for the premature infant is still controversial. For nutritional requirements of the premature infant see *Textbook of Pediatric Nutrition* listed under "Selected readings" at end of chapter.

There are few contraindications to breastfeeding. The infant who is unable to suck, such as one with cleft lip or palate, and the very premature or ill infant may still receive human milk as nourishment through manual or breast pump extraction of mother's milk. Drugs taken by the mother may prove to be a contraindication. A mother who does not desire to feed her infant by breast should have her feelings respected, and care should be taken not to make her feel guilty.

The main determinant for successful breast feeding is an adequate milk supply. Factors largely responsible for this are adequate diet, rest, and emotional well-being of the mother, as well as complete emptying of the breast after each feeding. Frequent nursing will aid in the establishment of an adequate milk supply, and most infants will be capable of setting their own schedules.

Infant formulas

When human milk is not available for the infant, the best alternative is one of the commercial infant formulas based on a modified cow's milk protein base. The formulas mimic human milk in caloric distributions among fat, carbohydrate, and protein. All are vitamin fortified and are available with iron added. Major difficulties with their use arise from errors associated with dilution of the concentrate commonly employed and from intolerance to cow protein. Many problems associated with formulas probably relate to the technique of their administration to the infant. Because the mother is often the one in control of volume of feedings, the infant may be overfed or underfed.

Infant formulas for special use. Soy protein–based formulas have had increasing use as an infant food over the past few years. The indications for use of these products are intolerance to cow protein formula and intolerance to lactose, the sugar present in both human milk and the cow protein–based formula. Infants appear to grow at normal rates when fed soy-based formulas.

Nutramigen and Pregestimil, which contain casein hydrolysate as the protein source, should be reserved for infants who are unable to tolerate the cow protein–based or soy-based formula.

Cow's milk and infant feeding. Cow's milk is marketed in various forms: Whole (4% butterfat), evaporated (4% butterfat), 2% (2% butterfat), skim (0.1% butterfat), and dry skim milk powder. None of these products is a desirable infant beverage during the first year of life. Unless the milks are fortified with vitamins D and C, deficiencies of these vitamins may occur. Iron, fluoride, and zinc are not present in recommended amounts. Use of the low-fat forms may well result in poor growth because of deficient calories, and essential fatty acid deficiency can occur with skim milk. Evaporated milk is the more suitable form for infant consumption if economic factors preclude the use of an infant formula. The heat process renders the protein less antigenic and the butterfat more digestible. Most evaporated milk products are vitamin D fortified. Dilution of evaporated milk with water (1½ parts water to 1 part evaporated milk) and the addition of carbohydrate to about 5% will result in a formula with a protein and mineral content more similar to that of human milk, thereby providing a lower renal solute load.

The introduction of foods other than human milk or formula into the infant's diet in the first year continues to be an area of pediatric nutrition in which marked differences in practice are observed.

From a nutritional standpoint, there is little to be gained by the introduction of foods other than milk before 6 months of age. The nutrients of human milk or infant formula adequately meet the needs of infants. The introduction of additional foods may result in either excesses or deficiencies of fat, protein, and carbohydrate. Excess of carbohydrate-derived calories is common because of the popularity of fruits and cereals as infant foods.

Foods other than milk may be provided by the use of commercially prepared foods for infants. Except for dry cereal, all varieties of commercially prepared foods are more expensive than human milk or infant formula when compared on a basis of cost per 100 kcal. Home-prepared foods, while economically more reasonable, can lead to excessive caloric and salt intake.

A suggested infant feeding schedule for the first year of life is presented in Table 9-7. Nutritional advice should be given on an individual basis. Probably one of the most reasonable evaluation tools to determine readiness of the infant for foods other than milk is developmental staging.

After the child has reached his first birthday, the goals of optimal nutrition should be (1) providing a diet that has optimal nutrients for the growth and energy needs of the child; (2) continuing to introduce new foods, with decreasing emphasis on milk or formula as the major nutrient; and (3) fostering behaviors that will lead to a lifelong appreciation of nutritious foods in reasonable amounts.

Table 9-7. Suggested schedule for the introduction of solid foods

Age (months)	Infant food*
0-6	Human milk or infant formula—no solid food
6-7	Rice cereal
7-8	Fruits†—applesauce, pears, peaches, bananas
8-9	Vegetables†—carrots, squash, beans, peas, beets, spinach, sweet potatoes
9-10	Meats†—beef, lamb, chicken
10-12	Finger foods*—cottage cheese, toast, crackers

*Avoid citrus fruits, wheat, and other foods containing gluten.
†Introduce one new food at a time at intervals of 1 week.

NUTRITIONAL DISTURBANCES

Periodic nutritional assessment should be provided for all children by health care professionals. It should include questions designed to determine the child's nutritional needs and how they are being met by the diet, a physical examination emphasizing growth assessment with anthropometry, and selected laboratory tests such as for hemoglobin, serum albumin, and cholesterol levels. Abnormal findings such as monotonous or bizarre diet, physical signs suggesting nutritional disorders, obesity, failure to grow at a normal rate, or abnormal laboratory studies should lead to more detailed nutritional assessment. The assistance of a dietitian is available through many hospitals and public health departments.

Overnutrition

Obesity (see also pp. 106 and 107). Overabundance of dietary calories in relation to the needs of the child for growth, maintenance, and activity will lead to the obese state and is the cause of most obesity in children. This so-called exogenous obesity is the major malnutrition problem in the American population. The diagnosis of obesity should be based on a combination of observations. Probably the best indicators are measurements of subcutaneous fat by caliper technique and weight-height ratios.

Prevention of the obese state is at present the most effective means of approaching the problems of weight control. Various dietary manipulations, drugs, and behavior modification have been used as treatment modalities. At present, the best results in weight reduction appear to come from an approach that combines dietary modifications to decrease caloric intake, exercise, and behavior modifications. Care must be taken not to restrict caloric intake to levels that will compromise the growth of the child. The reference for a weight management workbook for adolescents and a leader's guide called Shapedown is provided at the end of the chapter.

Undernutrition

Protein-energy malnutrition is caused by inadequate food intake or diseases that interfere with digestion, absorption, or use of food. It can be thought of as a spectrum with marasmus, caused by a predominant energy deficiency, on one end and kwashiorkor (sugar baby), a predominant protein deficiency, on the other end. Chronic protein and calorie malnutrition or acute protein deficiency in an infant or child with marasmus results in a condition termed *marasmic-kwashiorkor*.

Marasmus. Severe inadequate caloric intake in infants result in a condition termed *marasmus*. There is a marked discrepancy in weight for height. At first the infant fails to gain weight, then there is a progressive weight loss. The loss of subcutaneous fat results in loose wrinkled skin with poor turgor. The abdomen is distended or flat, the muscles are atrophic, the pulse is low, and the temperature is frequently subnormal. The infant is listless with poor physical activity. Constipation or diarrhea is frequently present. Intercurrent infections are common.

Parenteral fluid therapy may be necessary initially to restore renal function and correct dehydration. At first oral feedings should be small and low in calories. The usual milk formulas are satisfactory and are preferable to solid foods for initiating treatment. The diet should be increased slowly until caloric requirements are met. Supplements of vitamins or amino acids may be necessary. Any remediable coexistent systemic disease should receive appropriate therapy. If the malnutrition occurs early in life short stature and decreased head circumference may be present even after nutritional rehabilitation has occurred.

Kwashiorkor. In kwashiorkor the fundamental deficiency is a lack of dietary protein containing adequate amounts of all the essential amino acids, but caloric undernutrition and vitamin and mineral deficiencies often coexist. This disease is seen most commonly between the ages of 1 and 5 years following weaning from the breast. The underlying cause is failure to provide an adequate dietary source of protein to substitute for milk protein, the major protein source before weaning. Although rare in the United States, kwashiorkor is prevalent in many underdeveloped countries.

Initial clinical signs and symptoms are obscure. Retardation of growth is usually the first explicit manifestation. Loss of weight occurs despite edema from hypoalbuminemia. The hair becomes sparse, depigmented, or reddish yellow, and eventually course. A variety of skin manifestations has been observed with inflammatory changes and desquamation. Dyspigmentation of the skin is common. The abdomen is distended, and the liver is enlarged usually with fatty infiltration. Progressive irritability, apathy, and misery ensue. Infections are frequent and poorly tolerated. Serum glucose, essential amino acids, potassium, magnesium, and cholesterol are frequently decreased, whereas growth hormone may be elevated.

Initial therapy should consist of reestablishing renal function, correcting dehydration and electrolyte imbalance, and giving appropriate antibiotics for bacterial infections. Lactose should be avoided early because of disaccharidase deficiency. Gradually, a diet rich in proteins of high biologic quality should be introduced. Multiple vitamins and minerals including chromium, magnesium, and iron are needed. Treatment of parasitic infestations, if not severe, can wait until management of the malnutrition is underway. Residual stunted growth and perceptual defects are common.

Failure to thrive. *Failure to thrive* is a term used to describe infants who lack adequate growth in weight and height for no apparent reason. Dietary deprivation is often found to be responsible. However, in many instances an inadequate home environment is present, resulting in emotional deprivation or physical abuse. Such infants have growth failure and psychomotor and phychosocial retardation. A thorough medical history and physical examination should be done. Unless organic disease is suspected, few laboratory tests should be obtained early in the diagnostic workup. Screening tests include urinalysis, urine culture, serum electrolytes, complete blood count, thyroid profile, tuberculin test, and stool examination. Further evaluation may be required if weight gain does not begin within 2 to 3 weeks. In the absence of organic disease most of these children gain weight rapidly in the hospital. When the family situation is favorable, improvement continues after discharge. However, when family dysfunction is present, temporary or permanent placement in a foster home may be necessary.

Deficiency of fat-soluble vitamins

Vitamin A deficiency. Deficiency of vitamin A from inadequate dietary intake is rare in the United States. However, deficiency can occur in patients with impaired digestion and absorption of fat and the fat-soluble vitamins. This can occur in chronic intestinal, pancreatic, or hepatic diseases or from prolonged use of mineral oil.

Vitamin A deficiency may cause anemia, growth failure, and mental retardation. Metaplastic keratinizing changes in the mucosa of the respiratory passages increase vulnerability to respiratory infections, and similar changes in the urinary tract may lead to pyuria and hematuria. Epithelial metaplasia causes follicular hyperkeratosis of the skin. Cornification of the conjunctiva and lacrimal glands produces dryness of the conjunctiva (xerophthalmia). The dry conjunctival surfaces are injected and have a dull, hazy appearance. Gray plaques termed *Bitot's spots* may be seen on the bulbar conjunctiva. Photophobia is prominent and infection often ensues, producing a purulent discharge from and even ulceration of the cornea. This may progress to destruction of the eye or may heal with scarring. Keratomalacia may develop. An increase in intracranial pressure may occur, leading infrequently to hydrocephalus. Older children often complain of night blindness.

For mild primary vitamin A deficiency the diet should be corrected and the recommended daily allowances of vitamin A should be given as a supplement. When significant evidence of deficiency is present, 20,000 to 50,000 IU vitamin A should be given daily for a short period of time. When fat absorption is poor, water-miscible preparations must be used.

Vitamin D deficiency rickets. Vitamin D deficiency rickets results from inadequate exposure to sunlight or faulty intake or absorption of the vitamin. This leads to impaired intestinal absorption of dietary calcium and phosphate from the intestinal tract and decreased reabsorption of phosphate by renal tubule cells. Thus these minerals are lost in increased amounts in the feces and urine. The serum phosphorus level is decreased, the serum calcium level is usually normal but may be reduced, and the serum alkaline phosphatase level is elevated. Failure of normal maturation and degeneration of cartilage cells and failure of normal mineralization of cartilaginous and osseous matrix result in softened, rarefied bone, which is responsible for many of the skeletal deformities.

Rickets is found primarily in rapidly growing infants, particularly premature infants. Most patients are between 6 and 18 months of age. However, there have been recent reports of premature infants weighing less than 1300 g in whom nutritional rickets developed during their stay in a neonatal unit. Because of their small size, these infants received an inadequate volume of formula to provide an adequate vitamin D intake. Early rickets may produce only craniotabes, slight enlargement of costochondral junctions, and slight thickening of wrists and elbows. Serum calcium, phosphorus, and phosphatase determinations and radiographs of the long bones may be required to detect early rickets. Advanced rickets produces weakness of bones, relaxation of ligaments, and decrease in muscle tone. Craniotabes, delay in closure of the fontanels, bossing of the skull, rachitic rosary, pigeon breast and Harrison's groove, kyphosis, scoliosis, lordosis, disturbed growth of the pelvis, epiphyseal enlargements at the wrists and ankles, and bowing of the extremities may all become more noticeable. Development of the dentition may be delayed, and combined deformities of the spine, pelvis, and legs may result in rachitic dwarfism. Relaxation of ligaments produces knock-knees, hyperextension of the knees, weak ankles, and scoliosis. Relaxation of muscles of the abdominal wall causes the characteristic potbelly.

Histologic changes in the bones and chemical changes in the serum develop several weeks before the appearance of radiographic changes. The distal ends of the ulna and radius are the optimal sites for the demonstration of the earliest lesions. The principal diagnostic features are rarefaction and irregular fraying of the epiphyseal plate and rarefaction of the shaft (Fig. 9-1); these lead to widening, cupping, and fraying of the distal ends of the long bones, with a double periosteal contour along the shaft. The epiphyseal plate appears much wider, since the large rachitic metaphysis does not mineralize and therefore does not appear on the radiograph.

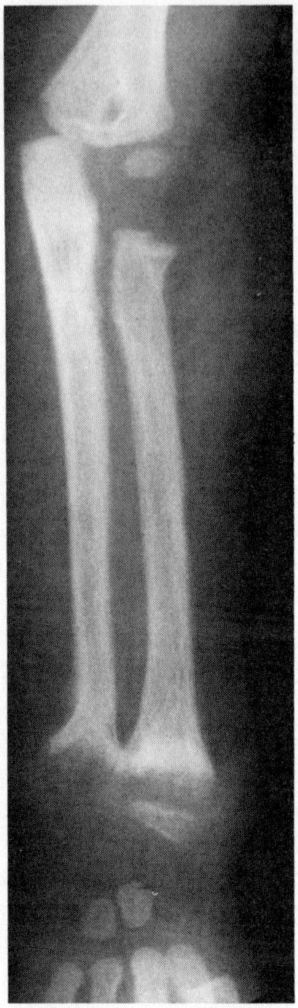

Fig. 9-1. Rickets in a 17-month-old child. Note coarsening of trabecular structures in demineralized bone. Metaphyses are splayed, and there is widening of epiphyseal line. (Courtesy Dr. W. Webster Riggs, Le Bonheur Children's Medical Center, Memphis.)

Doses of vitamin D should be given orally. There is no standardized dosage, but administration of approximately 1500 to 5000 IU daily will produce radiographic evidence of healing within 2 to 4 weeks. Permanent skeletal deformities persist if the disease exists into the advanced stages.

Tetany associated with vitamin D deficiency is rarely seen. However, treatment with vitamin D can cause deposition of calcium in rachitic bones so rapidly that it may temporarily reduce the serum calcium level and cause hypocalcemic tetany. Calcium should be administered intravenously if convulsions have occurred; if there have been no convulsions, it may be given orally.

Vitamin D–resistant rickets and other metabolic disturbances with osseous lesions resembling rickets must be differentiated from vitamin D deficiency rickets.

Vitamin E deficiency. Deficiencies have occurred in human infants with low intakes of vitamin E and in children with steatorrhea who fail to absorb vitamin E. Children with cystic fibrosis of the pancreas, biliary atresia, and infants of low birth weight are especially prone to the development of vitamin E deficiency. This deficiency has been clinically recognized by demonstration of low concentrations of tocopherol in plasma, excessive creatinuria, and increased hemolysis of erythrocytes in dilute solutions of hydrogen peroxide.

Hemolytic anemia has been reported in premature infants with low serum concentrations of vitamin E and in vitro hemolysis.

The requirement of vitamin E is related to the amount of polyunsaturated fatty acids in the diet. Plasma concentrations of alpha tocopherol of 1 mg/dl can be maintained by a diet containing 0.4 mg vitamin E per gram of polyunsaturated fatty acid. Both human milk and commercial infant formulas meet this requirement of vitamin E. Vitamin E intake of 5 IU (3.3 mg) daily is recommended for a 9 kg infant whose diet contains 4% to 7% of the calories as linoleic acid.

Low birth weight infants should receive a formula that provides 0.7 IU of vitamin E/100 kcal and a minimum of 1.0 IU/g linoleic acid. In addition, supplementation of the diet with 5 IU of a water-miscible preparation of vitamin E is recommended. Infants and children with chronic steatorrhea should also be given vitamin E supplementation using a water-miscible preparation.

Vitamin K deficiency. At 2 to 3 days of age, mild deficiency of vitamin K results in hypoprothrombinemia in many infants, particularly those who are breast-fed. In approximately 1 in 400 infants the deficiency is severe enough to produce clinical manifestations of bleeding. The coagulation abnormality can be corrected with the administration of vitamin K.

Vitamin K deficiency may result from decreased intestinal bacterial synthesis of the vitamin during the course of broad-spectrum antibiotic therapy or in conditions interfering with fat absorption, such as obstructive lesions of the biliary tract and the malabsorption syndromes. Even in the presence of adequate amounts of vitamin K, severe liver malfunction or competitive inhibition of vitamin K by coumarin-type drugs may prevent use of the vitamin to produce prothrombin and other coagulation factors.

Deficiency of vitamin K produces a defect of blood coagulation that may be associated with hemorrhagic manifestations. The lesions are usually purpuric, but internal bleeding may occur. Mild deficiency is corrected by the oral administration of 1 to 2 mg daily of vitamin K; the water-soluble preparations should be used for patients who absorb fat poorly. In patients with active bleeding vitamin K should be given parenterally in a dosage of 5 mg daily. In liver disease fresh frozen plasma or fresh blood should be given. Hemorrhagic disease of the newborn is discussed on p. 306.

Deficiency of water-soluble vitamins

Scurvy: vitamin C deficiency. Scurvy results from prolonged deficiency of vitamin C. It is seen almost exclusively in infants fed a cow's milk formula without adequate supplement of vitamin C, fruit juices, or vegetables, and only rarely in breast-fed infants or those on a highly restricted diet.

The major manifestations are bone changes and a hemorrhagic tendency. Most patients with this condition are between 6 and 15 months of age. General symptoms of pallor, irritability, poor appetite, and failure to gain weight precede local symptoms. In most instances the legs exhibit tenderness first, particularly about the knees. There is aversion to movement of the extremities, resulting in pseudoparalysis. The hips and knees are held in semiflexion, and the feet are externally rotated, producing the typical "frog position." Similar tenderness and swelling in other bones near joints may be noted. Costochondral beading and sternal depression occur. These symptoms result from subperiosteal hemorrhage and other bony changes. The gingiva becomes spongy and hemorrhagic, and bleeding may occur into the skin, bowel, and urine. Retro-orbital hemorrhage may produce unilateral exophthalmos. Moderate anemia and low-grade fever are usually present.

Radiographic changes (Fig. 9-2) include osteoporosis of the epiphyseal center, which leaves a white ring at its periphery (Wimberger circle); calcified spurs on the metaphyseal side of the epiphyseal center; a wide calcified zone of provisional calcification (Fraenkel line); a translucent zone of metaphyseal rarefaction on the diaphyseal side of the metaphysis; ground-glass appearance of shaft with thinning of cortex; and subperiosteal hemorrhage and subsequent calcification.

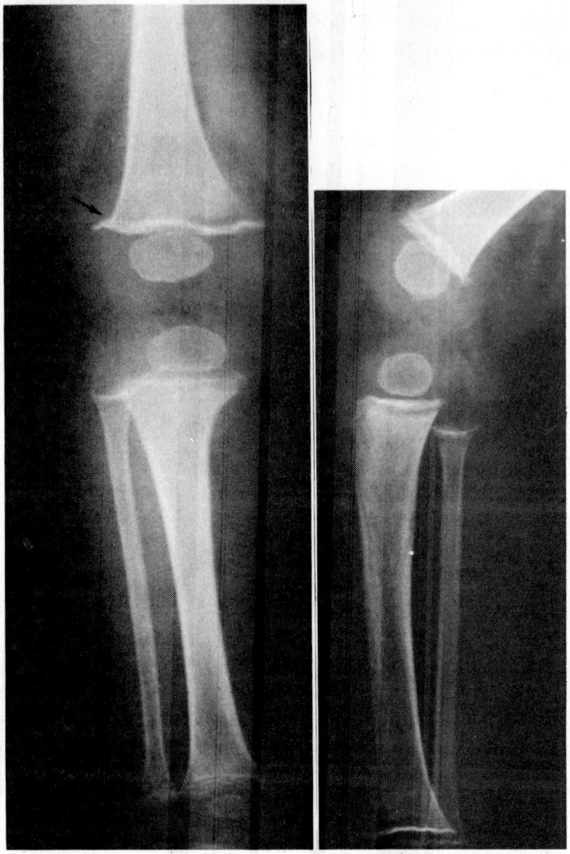

Fig. 9-2. Scurvy in an 8-month-old infant. Note diffuse demineralization and irregular, dense provisional zones of calcification, which end in spurs *(arrow)*. Shaftward are transverse radiolucent bands ("scurvy lines"). (Courtesy Dr. W. Webster Riggs, Le Bonheur Children's Medical Center, Memphis.)

Rapid healing occurs with daily administration of 100 mg or more of ascorbic acid.

Beriberi. In beriberi, thiamine deficiency leads to degenerative changes manifested by polyneuritis and cardiopathy. Thiamine requirements increase during pregnancy and lactation, and beriberi may occur in breast-fed infants of mothers whose diet is deficient in thiamine. The most common cause of thiamine deficiency in the United States is chronic alcoholism.

Prodromal symptoms of apathy, irritability, anorexia, vomiting, and constipation are nonspecific and difficult to detect. Severe manifestations result when cardiac involvement produces a failing heart manifested by cardiomegaly, tachycardia, dyspnea, and hepatomegaly. Serous effusions and dependent edema may occur in the absence of cardiac or renal complications or hypoproteinemia. Early manifestations of beriberi include neuritis, both motor and sensory hyperesthesia, and areflexia. Ptosis and laryngeal nerve paralysis may occur. Paralytic symptoms are rare.

Parenteral administration of 10 mg thiamine twice daily often produces dramatic improvement in patients with severe beriberi, although complete cure may require several weeks. Oral administration of 5 mg thiamine daily is also effective in less severe instances. The use of whole vitamin B complex is recommended to ensure correction of possible coexisting deficiencies. Thiamine-deficient mothers should also receive 50 mg daily.

There are some rare disorders that may respond to high doses of thiamine, including a rare form of maple syrup urine disease, Leigh encephalopathy, chronic lactic acidosis, and a type of megaloblastic anemia that does not improve with vitamin B_{12} or folate administration.

Pyridoxine deficiency. Primary dietary deficiency of pyridoxine is rare. It has occurred, however, in infants fed formulas lacking vitamin B_6 or in which vitamin B_6 was destroyed by faulty heat sterilization. Isoniazid is also known to increase the requirement for pyridoxine. Rare instances of pyridoxine dependency in which the person requires large amounts of this vitamin have been reported as occurring in early infancy and in adolescence.

Pyridoxine deficiency chiefly affects the nervous system, causing irritability, aggravated startle responses, staring spells, opisthotonus, repeated seizures, and abnormal electroencephalogram tracings. Poor weight gain and hypochromic anemia also occur. Infantile pyridoxine dependency is apparently a hereditary disorder; familial occurrences have been reported. In some instances intrauterine convulsions were noted by the mother, indicating difficulty even before birth. The course in the infant is usually progressive, and without treatment mental retardation or death may occur.

Pyridoxine-dependent convulsions are not responsive to ordinary anticonvulsant therapy. Early recognition and treatment with 10 to 100 mg pyridoxine intravenously or intramuscularly result in prompt relief and subsequent normal development. Daily maintenance with 4 to 10 mg pyridoxine orally is often needed. Treatment may be required indefinitely for the dependent variety. Prognosis is related directly to the interval between onset of symptoms and treatment.

Riboflavin deficiency. Riboflavin deficiency is rare in the United States. Manifestations commonly involve the eye, with corneal vascularization, seborrheic dermatitis (especially of the nasolabial folds), and cheilosis and angular stomatitis of the lips and corners of the mouth. Glossitis may also occur. Riboflavin deficiency usually occurs in combination with other vitamin deficiencies.

Pellagra. The deficiency disease of niacin is pellagra, characterized early by anorexia, apathy, weakness, and paresthesias progressing to the classic triad of dermatitis, diarrhea, and dementia. The dermatitis occurs chiefly on exposed or traumatized areas of the body, and photosensitivity is common. Pellagra is most likely to occur in patients on diets based chiefly on corn (a deficient foodstuff for both niacin and tryptophan) and in those with cirrhosis of the liver or chronic diarrheal disease.

A dose of 50 to 300 mg/24 hr of niacin should be administered. The diet should be corrected, and multivitamin supplementation should be given to correct possible associated vitamin deficiencies.

Hypervitaminoses

Hypervitaminosis A. Acute poisoning usually follows a single massive dose of vitamin A of several hundred thousand units. Nausea and vomiting are the principal symptoms, but lethargy and bulging of the anterior fontanel also occur. These symptoms subside rapidly, and there are no residual effects.

Chronic poisoning follows prolonged excessive intake of vitamin A. Affected infants are usually over 1 year of age. The blood vitamin A level becomes elevated. Anorexia, nausea, headache, and hepatosplenomegaly occur early. Pruritus is frequent, the skin becomes dry and scaly, and alopecia may result. Hyperostosis and a painful periostitis are characteristic and lead to increasing irritability, decreased movement, and tender swellings over the involved bones. These symptoms are usually reversible with decrease in vitamin A intake, but permanent crippling skeletal changes have been reported. In the differential diagnosis one must consider infantile cortical hyperostosis (Caffey disease).

Hypervitaminosis D. Vitamin D poisoning may be acute or chronic. Vomiting, dehydration, and fever are common in the acute form; coma, convulsions, abdominal cramps, and bone pain occur in the more severe acute form. Common early symptoms of the chronic form are lassitude, anorexia, thirst, and urinary urgency with or without polyuria. Vomiting, diarrhea, and abdominal discomfort occur later. The serum calcium and phosphorus levels are increased. Hypercalcuria occurs and, in the absence of polyuria, the urine Sulkowitch test is often strongly positive. Nephrocalcinosis leads to progressive renal insufficiency. Metastatic calcifications are found in blood vessels, kidneys, heart, gastric wall, lungs, adrenal glands, and other soft tissues. An increase in the width and density of the zones of provisional calcification, cortical thickening, and osteoporosis may be seen in radiographs of the long bones. Treatment includes reduction in vitamin D intake and a temporary low-calcium diet during the early phase. It is possible that chronic idiopathic hypercalcemia of infancy is caused by idiosyncrasy to this vitamin in certain infants.

Hypervitaminosis K. Excessive dosage of vitamin K may be harmful to low birth weight infants and those with glucose-6-phosphate dehydrogenase deficiency. Water-soluble vitamin K analogues in large dosages have resulted in hemolytic anemia, jaundice, and kernicterus.

NUTRITIONAL SUPPORT FOR THE CHILD WITH CHRONIC ILLNESS

Nutritional support for the child with chronic illness who is often unable or unwilling to take adequate nutrition orally is a matter of much importance and a field of pediatric nutrition in which many advances are now being made. Enteral nutrition provided by nasogastric or nasoduodenal tube can be used to furnish nutrients for maintenance needs and for the excessive needs generated by the disease process if the intestine is functional. In those cases in which the intestine is not available for use or cannot be expected to handle very large amounts of nutrients, intravenous nutrition may prove of vast importance in the final outcome of the patient.

Intravenous nutrition. Total parenteral nutrition (TPN) is a lifesaving procedure that is still in its infancy. It uses a central venous catheter and fusion pump to deliver the hypertonic infusate. Short-term intravenous feedings can also be given using scalp veins or other peripheral veins.

Several groups of patients should be considered as candidates for parenteral nutrition:

1. Patients with surgical gastrointestinal problems that preclude oral feeding. Most notable among this group are infants with gastroschisis, intestinal atresia, complicated omphalocele, bowel fistulas, and peritonitis.
2. Patients with chronic diarrhea or malabsorption syndrome. In these patients, TPN allows the bowel to rest so that, after a period of time, nutrients given by mouth can be absorbed and used.
3. Patients with acute renal failure. When only essential amino acids and glucose are provided, the need for dialysis is reduced.
4. Patients with inflammatory bowel disease. The use of TPN may allow patients to have a complete or partial remission or be prepared for surgery.
5. Low birth weight infants. Although parenteral nutrition has several potential advantages, this procedure should be considered investigational and used for patients unable to tolerate enteral feedings.

The complications associated with the use of TPN are numerous and should be completely understood by any physician undertaking it. Sepsis is common and markedly increases with duration of therapy. Metabolic complications include acidosis, elevated blood levels of glucose, ammonia, amino acids, calcium, cholesterol, and triglycerides and decreased blood levels of glucose, magnesium, copper, calcium, and linoleic acid. Dehydration may result from osmotic diuresis. Intensive monitoring of the nutritional therapy and proper technique are necessary for the success of parenteral nutrition.

Intravenous nutritional solutions can be designed to provide a patient's total fluid and nutritional needs as closely as possible. At the present time, these needs may be met by various form of amino acid solutions and by intravenous fat emulsions.

Parenteral alimentation by a peripheral vein can be a valuable adjunct to supplement oral feedings or for short-term nutrition in patients with gastrointestinal pathology. The principal difficulty with this route of administration is the extreme hypertonicity of the parenteral nutritional solution, which quickly causes thrombophlebitis and necessitates frequent change of intravenous sites. Intravenous fat emulsions are of great value in peripheral hyperalimentation because of their high caloric content and low osmolarity. The soybean oil product Intralipid (Cutter Laboratories) contains 1.1 calories/ml. The essential fatty acids provided by the fat emulsion are known to be important for the structure of cell membranes and in the synthesis of prostaglandins, thromboxanes, and prostacyclins. The maximal dose of fat emulsions is thought to be 4 g/kg/24 hr (or 30% to 40% of total calories) in adolescents and adults. Only 10% of the total daily calories need to be given to ensure that the essential fatty acids are given.

The seemingly simple technique of TPN is deceptive. Its proper execution is facilitated by a team approach to patient management. TPN with a central venous catheter should be administered only in a setting in which the patient can be intensively monitored.

George A. Burghen

REFERENCES

Mellin, L.: Shapedown—weight management program for adolescents, San Francisco 1983, Balboa Publishing Co.

Mellin, L.: Shapedown—leader's guide—weight management program for adolescents, San Francisco, 1983, Balboa Publishing Co.

National Academy of Sciences: Recommended dietary allowances, rev. 9, Washington, D.C., 1980, U.S. Government Printing Office.

O'Brien, D., editor: Pediatric nutrition handbook, Evanston, Illinois, 1979, American Academy of Pediatrics.

Suskin, R.M., editor: Textbook of pediatric nutrition, New York, 1981, Raven Press.

SELECTED READINGS

Applebaum, R.M.: The modern management of successful breast feeding, Pediatr. Clin. North Am. **17:**203, 1970.

Committee on Nutrition, American Academy of Pediatrics: Commentary on breast-feeding and infant formulas, including proposed standards for formulas, Pediatrics **57:**278, 1976.

Committee on Nutrition, American Academy of Pediatrics: Iron supplementation for infants, Pediatrics **58:**765, 1976.

Fisher, J.E., editor: Total parenteral nutrition, Boston, 1976, Little, Brown & Co.

Fomon, S.J.: Infant nutrition, ed. 2, Philadelphia, 1974, W.B. Saunders Co.

Fomon, S.J.: Nutritional disorders of children, U.S. Department of Health, Education, and Welfare, pub. no. (HSA) 76-5612.

Gerrard, J.W.: Breast-feeding: second thoughts, Pediatrics **54:**757, 1974.

Heird, W.C., and Winters, R.W.: Total parenteral nutrition, J. Pediatr. **86:**2, 1975.

Jelliffee, D.B., and Jelliffee, E.F.P.: Breast is best; Modern meanings, N. Engl. J. Med. **297:**912, 1977.

McMillan, J.A., et al.: Iron sufficiency in breast-fed infants and the availability of iron from human milk, Pediatrics **58:**686, 1976.

Neumann, C., and Jelliffee, D.B., editors: Nutrition in pediatrics, Pediatr. Clin. North Am. **24:**1, 1977.

Pipes, P.L., editor: Nutrition in infancy and childhood, ed. 2, St. Louis, 1981, The C.V. Mosby Co.

Schneider, et al., editors: Nutrition support of medical practice, New York, 1977, Harper & Row, Publishers, Inc.

10 Fluid and Electrolyte Homeostasis

Clinical alterations in fluid and electrolyte homeostasis are encountered frequently in the practice of pediatrics. In no other area of clinical medicine is there a closer relationship between an understanding of altered *physiology* and *clinical* therapy. It is no surprise that much of today's knowledge of clinical disorders in fluid and electrolyte disturbances has been the product of pediatric scientists; nor is it surprising that mastery of clinical management of electrolyte disturbances is one of the benchmarks of an accomplished practicing pediatrician.

A physician's goal in managing any child with altered fluid and electrolyte balance is to restore physiologic homeostasis. In this chapter, general approaches to problems of altered extracellular and intracellular composition are provided. When one understands the pathophysiology of fluid and electrolyte disturbances, a rational therapy may be instituted even if the precise clinical etiology of the disturbance is unknown. As the clinician develops experience in fluid management and studies disorders of body physiology and chemistry, these general approaches may serve as the foundation on which rational analysis and management can be based.

COMPOSITION OF BODY FLUID COMPARTMENTS

Water is the principal constituent of body fluids and is distributed intracellularly and extracellularly. Total body water content and the relative distribution of the major physiologic fluid compartments during childhood are shown in Fig. 10-1. Children, particularly during infancy, have a relatively greater water content than do adults. At birth, nearly 80% of body weight is water. Adipose tissue contains little water; for this reason the relative body water weight declines with the significant accumulation of fat during the first year of life. Extracellular water is distributed between the interstitial fluid and plasma water and quantitatively exceeds intracellular water until 3 months of age. The ratio of intracellular to extracellular fluid becomes more stable after 3 months of age.

Important chemical differences exist between intracellular and extracellular fluids (Fig. 10-2). The extracellular fluid primarily contains sodium, chloride, and bicarbonate, whereas intracellular ions are potassium, magnesium, phosphates, sulfates, and proteins. The concentration of extracellular solutes is controlled within narrow limits by the kidney. The concentration of solutes varies slightly between plasma and interstitial water, reflecting the Gibbs-Donnan effect created by impermeable plasma proteins. Intracellular volume and ionic composition are maintained by active membrane transport processes. Because vascular and cellular membranes are freely permeable to water, osmotic equilibrium is maintained throughout the body fluid compartments.

Access to the intracellular fluid space requires initial fluid entry into the extracellular compartment. The distribution space of any administered fluid will depend on its osmolar content. Isotonic (solute concentration equal to extracellular fluid) fluids will remain in the extracellular fluid compartment. Within the extracellular fluid compartment, intravenous fluids containing colloid (impermeant molecules, usually protein) will remain in the vascular space, whereas noncolloidal isotonic solutions will distribute to both the interstitial and vascular spaces. Hypotonic fluids, on the other hand, will distribute throughout body fluid compartments.

BASAL FLUID AND ELECTROLYTE REQUIREMENTS

Intake of water with an electrolyte content equal to daily losses is required to maintain body fluid homeostasis. The amount of water required

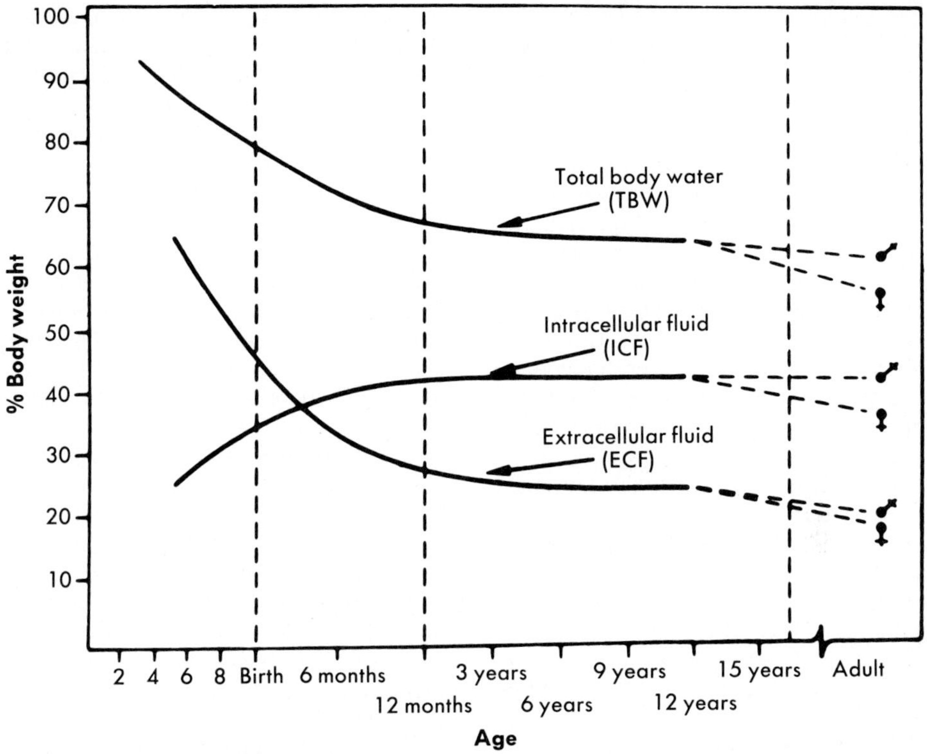

Fig. 10-1. Body water compartments during childhood. (From Winters, R.W.: The body fluids in pediatrics, Boston, 1973, Little, Brown & Co.)

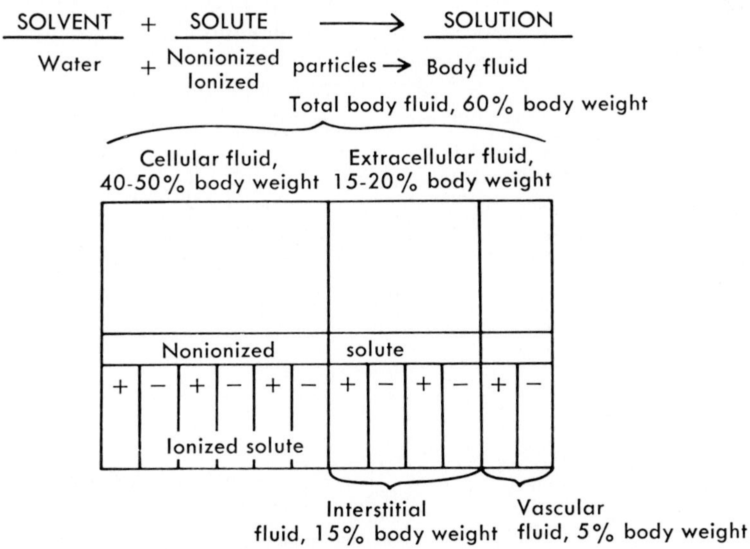

Fig. 10-2. Diagrammatic representation of body fluids. (From Etteldorf, J.N., and Sweeney, M.J.: Pediatr. Clin. North Am. **9:**133, 1962.)

for this "maintenance" fluid is determined by water losses expended in the dissipation of metabolic heat. Obligatory water losses occur as insensible water losses, urine production, and stool water. Insensible water losses represent approximately 45% of the daily maintenance requirements and occur through the evaporation of water through the interstices of the skin and through the exhalation of pulmonary water vapor. These insensible water losses are electrolyte free. Heat (and therefore water) balance is a product of both the metabolic rate (heat production) and the surface area per body mass (heat loss). Younger children have a higher metabolic rate in part because of the large relative surface area available for heat loss.

Maintenance fluid volumes may be computed on the basis of body weight, body surface area, or caloric expenditure. Use of caloric expenditure as a frame of reference is a simple and physiologically sound method of estimating fluid requirements. Based on data reported by Holliday and Segar (1957), daily caloric expenditure may be estimated from body weight as follows:

1. 100 kcal/kg for the first 10 kg body weight
2. 50 kcal/kg for the next 10 kg body weight
3. 20 kcal/kg for each additional kilogram greater than 20 kg

Thus a 7 kg hospitalized infant would expend 700 calories (7 × 100 kcal/kg) per day. The estimated daily caloric expenditure for a 22 kg child would be 1540 calories (100 kcal/kg × 10) + (50 kcal/kg × 10) + (20 kcal/kg × 20). The components of maintenance water requirements are shown in Table 10-1. Insensible water losses account for approximately 45 ml/100 kcal and urine losses average 55 ml/100 kcal; therefore water replacement is 100 ml for each 100 kcal. Under usual conditions with normal renal function, maintenance fluid calculations do not consider stool water losses, sweat losses, and gain of water of oxidation. Therefore an 8 kg child's maintenance water volume per day is 800 ml (8 × 100 kcal/kg = 800 kcal = 800 ml).

Basal water requirements will be modified by alterations in the metabolic rate or by altered water losses. The most common alteration in caloric expenditure is fever. With each degree (centigrade) increase in body temperature, daily caloric expenditure and daily total fluid requirements will increase by 12%. Hypothermia will decrease caloric expenditure in a similar fashion. Any hypermetabolic state, such as salicylism, hyperthyroidism, or burns, will greatly increase daily caloric expenditure and maintenance water needs. Water losses will increase with hyperventilation and decrease with use of a mist tent or inhalation of humidified air through a mask or endotracheal tube.

Maintenance solute requirements are generally limited to sodium, chloride, and potassium. Bicarbonate may be indicated if acidosis is present. Sodium is replaced at 3 mEq/100 kcal and potassium requirements are approximately 2 mEq/100 kcal. Both of these cations are usually administered as chloride salts; however, 1 mEq of bicarbonate may be given with each 4 mEq chloride. In anuric states, no electrolyte replacement should be given because insensible water losses are free of electrolytes. Most commercial intravenous fluids are provided as 5% dextrose solutions.

Example: Maintenance requirements for a 10-kg child. (Basal condition without fever, tachypnea or sweating)
Volume = 10 kg × 100 kcal/kg = 1000 kcal = 1000 ml

Table 10-1. Usual maintenance water requirements

	Source of water	ml/100 kcal/24 hr
Losses	Insensible	
	Skin	30
	Pulmonary	15
	Urine	55
	Stool	0-10
Gain	Water of oxidation	12
Average total maintenance water requirement		100 ml/100 kcal/24 hr

Electrolyte = Sodium 3 mEq/100 kcal for 1000 kcal = 30 mEq
Potassium 2 mEq/100 kcal for 1000 kcal = 20 mEq
Order: Give 1000 ml of 5% dextrose with 30 mmole sodium chloride and 20 mmole potassium chloride over 24 hours

A second, frequently used reference for calculating maintenance fluid replacement is body surface area. Computation of body surface area requires both height and weight measurements plus a reference nomogram. The daily fluid replacement using this reference is 1500 ml/m^2 body surface area per day. The electrolyte composition is similar to the previous recommendations (Na^+ = 30 mEq/L; K^+ = 20 mEq/L).

Example: A 30-kg child whose height is 130 cm, is hospitalized and has a temperature of 38° C (100.4° F). Body surface area is 1.0 m^2. The increase in body temperature of 1 ° C will increase total requirements by 12%.
Maintenance fluids:
1500 ml/m^2 × 1.0 m^2 = 1500 ml as 5% dextrose with 30 mmole/L NaCl and 20 mmole/L KCl. However, the increase in body temperature will increase basal fluid losses by 12%. The additional requirements will be 12% × 1500 ml or 180 ml. The final maintenance fluid replacement will be 1500 + 180 or 1680 ml of 5% dextrose with 30 mmole/L NaCl and 20 mmole/L KCl per 24 hours.

DEFICIT IN BODY FLUIDS AND ELECTROLYTES

Deficits in body water and electrolytes usually occur from excessive gastrointestinal losses, although rarely renal or sweat losses may lead to dehydration. A hallmark of a body fluid deficit is the reduction in body weight within a 48-hour period; consequently, dehydration is frequently graded as the percentage of body weight loss. In young children "mild" dehydration represents a 5% reduction, "moderate" is a 10% reduction, and "severe" dehydration is a 15% loss of body weight. In disturbances of body fluids, water and electrolytes may be lost in proportional quantities with no disturbance in extracellular fluid osmolality (isotonic dehydration), sodium may be lost to a greater degree than water with reduction of serum sodium concentration below 130 mEq/L (hypotonic dehydration), or water losses may exceed solute loss, resulting in hypertonicity of the extracellular fluid (hypertonic dehydration, serum sodium greater than 150 mEq/L). In both isotonic and hypotonic dehydration, clinical manifestations of dehydration will reflect decreased extracellular and vascular volume. In "mild" or 5% dehydration, the skin and mucous membranes will be dry, the heart rate will increase by 10% above basal, the urine will be concentrated, and the child will be unable to generate tears while crying. The blood pressure and refilling of distal capillary beds will be normal.

In "moderate" or 10% dehydration, the elasticity of the skin (skin turgor) will be reduced, the pulse rate will increase further, the eyeballs will be sunken and the anterior fontanel will be depressed. Oliguria and an orthostatic drop in blood pressure will be present. A slight delay in refilling of distal capillary beds will occur and the extremities may become cool. In "severe" or 15% dehydration the skin is mottled and cool and usually the child is very lethargic. Skin turgor is extremely poor, mucous membranes parched, and pulse rapid and weak. Blood pressure is reduced and urine output is scant, with elevation of the blood urea nitrogen. Compression of the digital capillary beds demonstrates marked delay in capillary refilling. Severe dehydration is a medical emergency. Although reduction in body fluids may be estimated by clinical signs, there is no better measure of water deficits than an accurate determination of acute weight reduction.

In recent years, oral glucose-electrolyte solutions have emerged as a successful mode of treatment for children with diarrhea and have supplanted intravenous therapy in many instances. The World Health Organization (WHO) has developed an oral hydrating solution that contains (in millimoles per liter): sodium (Na), 90; potassium (K), 20; bicarbonate, 30; chloride (Cl), 80; and glucose, 111. This hydrating solution may be effective despite mild degrees of vomiting or altered extracellular sodium concentration. A large volume of oral fluid is required; the intake during the first day of therapy should equal the estimated fluid deficit volume plus the daily maintenance fluid volume and continuing losses. Oral hydration with this solution is not indicated as the initial therapy when the degree of dehydration exceeds 10% or if the patient is in shock. Oral hydration is often unsuccessful when diarrheal losses exceed 10 ml/kg/hour, with glucose intolerance, or if vom-

Table 10-2. Composition of frequently used replacement or hydrating solutions

	mEq/L			
	Na	K	Cl	mOsm/L
Oral solutions				
Pedialyte	30	20	30	400
Gatorade	21	2.5	17	410
WHO	90	20	80	333
Breast milk	7	13	11	133
Intravenous solutions				
Ringer's lactate	130	4	109	274
0.9% NaCl (normal saline)	154		154	292
$D_5$0.45% NaCl (half normal saline)	77		77	432
$D_5$0.25% NaCl	39		39	350
D_5W (5% dextrose)				278
3% NaCl	513		513	969

iting persists. The safety of this therapy in the first 3 months of life has not yet been determined. As physicians in the United States become familiar with the WHO solution, fewer children will receive parenteral fluid therapy for uncomplicated diarrheal dehydration.

A number of solutions are available for oral and intravenous infusion (Table 10-2).

A general approach to intravenous therapy for fluid and electrolyte deficits follows four steps:

1. Restoration of circulation—emergency, within 1 hour
2. Repair of water and sodium deficits—first 8 hours
3. Provision of basal or maintenance requirements and ongoing loss—next 16 hours.
4. Repair of potassium deficits—several days

The speed with which these steps are accomplished may depend on the type and severity of electrolyte disturbance.

Restoration of circulation (step 1) is an emergency consideration and should be accomplished within a 10 to 15-minute period for severe circulatory compromise. Infusion of an extracellular fluid is required. Either Ringer's lactate or 0.9% NaCl should be infused at a rate of 20 ml/kg. This volume may be repeated if required for severe circulatory collapse. Blood or plasmanate may also be infused at a rate of 10 ml/kg.

Repair of isotonic dehydration

Isotonic dehydration accounts for approximately 65-70% of children admitted to hospitals for dehydration. The signs of dehydration have been discussed previously. The usual schedule for repair of deficits and provision of maintenance (Steps 2 and 3) is shown in the following example. For convenience, maintenance fluid requirements are provided on the basis of admission weight.

EXAMPLE

A child is admitted to the hospital for dehydration. The admission weight is 10 kg. The clinical signs suggest a moderate degree of dehydration, and the child is known to have lost 1 kg in the previous 36 hours. The serum sodium concentration is 140 mEq/L and potassium is 4.0 mEq/L.

The deficit is calculated as 1000 ml because the child has lost 1000 gm body weight. The sodium deficit is 135 to 140 mEq because 1 liter of extracellular fluid is lost. Maintenance fluid requirements are considered to be 100 kcal/kg or 1000 kcal = 1000 ml. The total sodium deficit will be replaced throughout the first 24 hours as 0.45% NaCl. This solution will allow repair of both the small intracellular and large extracellular deficit. This sodium provision in the first day fails to totally replace the deficit plus the maintenance requirements; however, this deficiency in sodium replacement is insignificant. Potassium replacement begins after urine flow is established and is generally given as either 20 or 40 mmol/L depending on the serum potassium concentration.

FLUID ORDERS

Deficit volume—Repair in first 8 hours as 1000 ml $D_5$0.45% NaCl with 20 millimole/L KCl

Maintenance volume—Provide during the next 16 hours as 1000 ml $D_5$0.45% NaCl with 20 millimole/L KCl

HYPONATREMIA

Hyponatremia is defined as a serum sodium concentration less than 130 mEq/L. Several physiologic alterations may cause hyponatremia. In hyponatremic dehydration there is a reduction in total body water with a relatively greater reduction in extracellular sodium. Decreased serum sodium may also be the result of increased total body water with normal total body sodium. This is the situation in the syndrome of inappropriate antidiuretic hormone secretion. A low serum level may occur with an excess of total body sodium with a greater excess in total body water. Patients with congestive heart failure and peripheral edema frequently have this abnormality. Finally, a low sodium level may be found with normal total body water and normal total body sodium levels. Such "factitious" hyponatremia accompanies hyperlipidemia or hyperglycemia. Obviously the appropriate management of hyponatremia depends entirely on the specific physiologic abnormality. A diagnostic approach to patients with hyponatremia is outlined below.

Approach to a patient with hyponatremia (serum sodium less than 130 mEq/L)

Step 1. Determine serum osmolality
- A. Isotonic "pseudo" hyponatremia
  - 1. Hyperlipidemia or hyperproteinemia
- B. Hypertonic hyponatremia
  - 1. Hyperglycemia or mannitol excess
- C. Hypotonic hyponatremia—proceed to Step 2

Step 2. Assess extracellular fluid volume
- A. Hypovolemia (sodium losses exceed water loss)
  - 1. Urine sodium <20 mEq/L
    - a. Extra renal (usually gastrointestinal) losses
  - 2. Urine sodium >20 mEq/L
    - a. Renal salt losing
- B. Isovolemia (Water Gain)
  - 1. Urine sodium <20 mEq/L
    - a. Psychogenic or iatrogenic water loads
  - 2. Urine sodium >20 mEq/L
    - a. Syndrome of inappropriate ADH secretion
- C. Hypervolemia (water gain in excess of sodium gain)
  - 1. Urine sodium <20 mEq/L)
    - a. Heart failure, liver disease, nephrosis
  - 2. Urine sodium >20 mEq/L
    - a. Acute renal failure with fluid overload

Repair of hyponatremic dehydration

Children with hyponatremic dehydration (serum sodium less than 130 mEq/L) will demonstrate the classic manifestations of extracellular volume depletion. The clinical assessment of the severity of dehydration is therefore similar to that in children with isotonic dehydration. Neurologic dysfunction is an additional, and many times predominant, clinical manifestation of hyponatremia. A rapid reduction in extracellular osmolality will cause entry of water into the intracellular compartment and produce cerebral edema. Symptoms include seizures, agitation, altered consciousness, and weakness. When hyponatremia occurs slowly or is a chronic phenomenon, the degree of brain swelling is less and patients may be asymptomatic.

Therapy for children with hyponatremic dehydration requires the estimation of both the body water deficit and the total sodium deficit. Water deficits are estimated by either acute weight loss or clinical signs. The estimation of the sodium must consider the current body sodium deficit plus the sodium deficit in the fluid losses. Current total body sodium deficit is calculated with the following formula:

Desired $[Na^+]$ − actual $[Na^+]$ ×
Body weight (kg) × volume of distribution =
(135 − actual $[Na^+]$ × weight × 0.6

EXAMPLE:
Serum Na 120 mEq/L in a 10 kg child
(135 mEq/L − 120 mEq/L) × 10 kg ×
0.6 ml/g = 15 × 6 = 90 mEq

The amount of sodium required to increase the serum sodium in the current extracellular fluid to 135 mEq/L is 90 mEq. Sixty percent of body weight or approximately the entire body space is used as the volume of sodium distribution because the osmotic pressure of infused solute will be distributed throughout the total exchangeable body water. In addition to the above calculations, one must remember that the fluid deficit also represents an additional isotonic sodium deficit that must be replaced.

Correction of hyponatremia in a dehydrated patient requires the intravenous infusion of fluids that have an osmolality greater than the serum osmolality. Normally, the serum osmolality is tightly controlled by the action of antidiuretic hormone (ADH) on renal water excretion. In order for the kidney to begin to correct a decreased serum osmolality, water must be excreted in excess of solute excretion. This can only occur in the absence of ADH. In the dehydrated state, ADH secretion will always be high. Therefore the kidney is unable to excrete solute-free water until the dehydration is repaired. For this reason, correction of hyponatremia in a dehydrated child is not accomplished by solutions such as 0.45% NaCl (half-normal saline).

On the other hand, rapid infusion of hypertonic solutions (such as 3% or 5% NaCl) will produce acute shrinkage of brain cells. For this reason, if the patient is asymptomatic, rapid "bolus" infusions of hypertonic salt should be avoided. Rather, the sodium deficit may be repaired during the first 24 hours.

If the patient is having seizures sufficient concentrated saline should be infused to raise the serum sodium by 10 mEq/L over 30 to 60 minutes. For reference, 1 ml of 3% NaCl equals 0.5 mEq Na^+.

EXAMPLE

A child is admitted to the hospital weighing 10 kg. He has lost 1 kg of body weight in the previous 36 hours. The serum sodium level is 120 mEq/L and the serum potassium level is 4.0 mEq/L.

Calculations

Deficits:

a. Fluid loss is 1 kg = 1000 gm = 1000 ml
b. Sodium deficit: (Desired sodium concentration is 135 mEq/L)
Current deficit = (135 mEq/L − 120 mEq/L) × 10 × 0.6 = 90 mEq
Isotonic deficit = 135 mEq (in isotonic losses) total sodium deficit is 90 mEq + 135 mEq = 225 mEq

Maintenance

Fluid = 10 kg × 100 kcal/kg = 1000 kcal × 100 ml/100 kcal = 1000 ml

Electrolyte requirements = 3 mEq Na^+/100 kcal, 2 mEq K^+/100 kcal

Management plan

The isotonic fluid deficit will be replaced during the first 8 hours of therapy. The current body sodium deficit (90 mEq) will be replaced during the entire 24-hour period. Therefore (90 mEq/24 hr) or approximately 3.5 mEq/hour will be added to the intravenous fluids throughout the first 24-hour period.

Deficit repair in first 8 hours

1000 ml of 5% dextrose with 135 mEq Na^+ (isotonic loss) plus (8 hr × 3.5 mEq/hr, current body Na^+ deficit = 28 mEq). Therefore the total solution concentration = 163 millimole NaCl plus 20 millimole KCl.

Maintenance plus sodium replacement in next 16 hours

1000 ml of 5% dextrose with 30 mM NaCl (maintenance) plus (16 hr × 3.5 mEq/hr sodium deficit) = 56 mEq Na^+. Therefore total sodium concentration = 86 millimole NaCl plus 20 millimole KCl.

HYPERNATREMIC DEHYDRATION

In the practice of pediatrics, dehydration with a serum sodium of greater than 150 mEq/L is not uncommon. This type of dehydration poses unique challenges in recognition and management because of the nature of body water compartment deficits. When dehydration occurs with an increased serum sodium, intracellular water shifts to the extracellular compartment thereby preventing the signs of circulatory and subcutaneous tissue fluid depletion. For this reason, the clinician must carry a high index of suspicion in patients who are at increased risk for developing hypernatremic dehydration.

Hypernatremic dehydration occurs most frequently in the first 2 years of life. Infants in the first 3 months of life are predisposed to developing relative body water deficits because of an inability to maximally concentrate urine. Later in infancy, hypernatremia may be more common because fluid intake ceases earlier in the course of the disease and at this age the child depends on caretakers to provide water to sate his thirst. Hypernatremic dehydration develops more commonly in the winter months when children have a greater number of rotavirus infections and the environment may predispose to a greater insensible water loss in dry heated apartments.

Because hypernatremic dehydration is primarily an intracellular deficit, central nervous system manifestations predominate. Clinical symptoms include marked irritability, lethargy, tremulousness, increased deep tendon reflexes, shrill cry, and seizures. As in hyponatremia the more rapidly the serum sodium changes, the more dramatic the intracellular dessication and neurologic manifestations. When the brain shrinks, pathologic changes occur, including subarachnoid and intracerebral hemorrhages and venous thromboses. Other manifestations of hypertonic dehydration include fever and a doughy texture to the skin. Whenever the clinical history in an infant suggests that the degree of dehydration should be greater than indicated by the physical examination, the diagnosis of hypernatremic dehydration should be suspected. In estimating the degree of dehydration in a hypernatremic child, it should be assumed that at least a 10% reduction in body weight has occurred. If signs of circulatory impairment are present, then the degree of dehydration is assumed to be 15% or greater.

Several metabolic abnormalities are associated with hypernatremic dehydration. Hyperglycemia is a frequent complication of hypernatremia, and acidemia tends to be more severe in hypernatremic dehydration. Calcium levels in serum are also depressed and may lead to seizures. The most profound abnormality, however, is the generation of new intracellular osmols in both brain and muscle. These so-called idiogenic osmols appear to be the result of the breakdown of intracellular peptides and proteins to amino acids. These idiogenic osmols have important implications in clinical management. Rapid reduction in extracellular sodium will thus result therefore in cerebral swelling and additional central nervous system insult.

The goal of management in hypertonic dehydration is to lower the serum sodium slowly (15 mEq/L/24 hours), repair water deficits over 48 hours, and prevent further central nervous system insult. To accomplish these ends, a sodium concentration of 20 to 35 mEq/L is recommended in the replacement fluids. An example of a therapeutic management plan is offered.

EXAMPLE:

A 5 kg infant has lost 500 gm as a result of diarrheal losses over 24 hours. The serum sodium concentration is 170 mEq/L and the serum potassium is 3.0 mEq/L.

Calculations

Deficit volume = 500 ml. The goal of therapy is to replete water deficits over 48 hours; therefore the daily deficit replacement during the first 48 hours is 250 ml/24 hours.

Maintenance

100 kcal/kg × 5 = 500 kcal = 500 ml/day

Repair of hypernatremic dehydration requires special considerations in addition to a slower rate of deficit repletion. First, the recommended sodium concentration is 20 to 35 mEq/L, and the potassium concentration is usually 40 mEq/L. The anion content may contain chloride and either acetate or lactate, depending on the degree of acidosis. The dextrose concentration is reduced to 2.5% because of the problem of hyperglycemia. Finally, 10 ml of 10% calcium gluconate should be added to each 500 ml of intravenous fluid. (This prevents the use of bicarbonate as a base in the rehydration fluids.)

Management plan for the first 24 hours

750 ml of 2.5% dextrose with 30 mEq/L Na^+, 40 mEq/L K^+, 50 mEq/L Cl^-, 20 mEq/L acetate, 10 ml of 10% calcium gluconate is administered evenly over 24 hours (i.e., 31 ml/hr). A similar plan is appropriate for the second 24 hours of therapy.

NOTE: If emergency repletion of the circulation is required, a 5% albumin solution should be infused at 20 ml/kg.

ACID-BASE ABNORMALITIES

Clinical acid-base abnormalities are the result of both the pathophysiologic mechanisms that raise or lower the hydrogen ion activity of body fluids and the body's defense mechanisms, which protect the pH and return pH toward normal. The two primary pathophysiologic forces that act to alter pH are metabolism and respiration. Processes that bring about a change in HCO_3^- concentration, the numerator of the Henderson-Hasselbalch equation, result in either metabolic acidosis or alkalosis. Changes in the respiratory or denominator component of the equation, measured as the $PaCO_2$, result in respiratory acidosis or alkalosis. The body's defense mechanisms against pH change consist of chemical buffers (primarily $H_2CO_3 - HCO_3^-$) and renal and respiratory compensation and correction. The latter occurs when the primary disease process causing the acid-base disorder is cured or modified so that the lungs can correct the respiratory component or the kidneys can correct the metabolic component of the Henderson-Hasselbalch equation.

The Henderson-Hasselbalch equation is as follows: pH = pK + log (H_2CO_3). H_2CO_3 is present in blood in minute quantities and is not regularly measured in clinical laboratories. Because H_2CO_3 is in equilibrium with CO_2 in solution, which is in turn dependent on the PCO_2, the term $S + PCO_2$ is substituted. S is the solubility coefficient for CO_2 and H_2CO_3. Rewriting the equation pH = pK + log ($HCO_3^- \div S \cdot PCO_2$) allows one to recognize that the (HCO_3^-) is primarily affected by the kidneys and the $S \cdot PCO_2$ is primarily affected by the lungs. Through physiologic mechanisms that alter (HCO_3^-) (renal) and $S \cdot PCO_2$ (respiratory), the body's pH is maintained at a constant 7.40 ± 0.05.

Because the body defense mechanisms can never "overcompensate," a respiratory acidosis cannot be converted to an alkaline pH by metabolic compensation or a metabolic alkalosis cannot be converted to an acid pH by respiratory compensation. Use of the Henderson-Hasselbalch equation will allow determination of the primary nature of an acid-base abnormality. When it is determined that a child has a primarily metabolic etiology of the perturbation in body pH (seen as a change in the numerator of the Henderson-Hasselbalch equation), then a systematic clinical approach can be directed toward assigning a specific diagnosis and planning therapy. In metabolic alkalosis there is a net gain of bicarbonate or a loss of acid; metabolic acidosis, on the other hand, is caused by a gain of acid or loss of bicarbonate.

Metabolic acidosis

Metabolic acidosis is a pathophysiologic state characterized by a gain of strong acid or loss of HCO_3^- from the extracellular fluid (ECF) through renal or extrarenal mechanisms. The net result is a decrease in HCO_3^- (the numerator of the Henderson-Hasselbalch equation). HCO_3^- can be decreased by the addition of a strong acid to body fluids, which is buffered by HCO_3^-, by the loss of HCO_3^- from body fluids through the gastrointestinal tract or kidneys, or by rapid dilution of the extracellular fluid space.

Anion gap. A concept that is helpful in categorizing the cause of metabolic acidosis is that of the "anion gap." Unmeasured anions, or the anion gap, can be calculated as follows: (plasma Na concentration) − (plasma Cl^- + HCO_3^- concentrations) = anion gap. The normal range is 10 to 14 mmole per liter. The anion gap is slightly greater in early infancy because the serum HCO_3^- concentration is normally 20 to 22 mEq/L.

An increase in the anion gap (unmeasured anions) is always present when metabolic acidosis is caused by the addition of acid from either external or internal sources. When HCO_3^- is lost from the gastrointestinal tract or kidney in excess of simultaneous chloride losses, the plasma HCO_3^- falls and plasma chloride concentration rises to that the anion gap remains unchanged. When plasma HCO_3^- is decreased by expanding ECF volume with a nonbicarbonate solution, plasma chloride concentration also rises as plasma HCO_3^- falls and the anion gap remains unchanged.

The differential diagnosis of metabolic acidosis is best approached by using the above anion-gap concept to divide the causes into two groups; normal anion gap metabolic acidosis and increased anion gap metabolic acidosis. External losses of HCO_3^- from the gastrointestinal tract or kidneys produce a normal anion gap, whereas an increased anion gap acidosis is caused by the addition of acid to the body stores at a rate that exceeds the kidney's ability to excrete it. Table 10-3 lists common causes of metabolic acidosis according to the anion-gap concept.

Correction of mild degrees of acidosis associated with dehydration is usually readily achieved by repair of deficits with saline solutions. When acidosis is severe, arterial pH $<$ 7.25, or acidemia occurs in small infants (in whom a low glomerular filtration rate slows the absolute excretion of acid by the kidneys), administration of base as bicarbonate, acetate, or lactate is warranted. In general the goal of base therapy is to restore the serum bicarbonate concentration to a concentration of 18 to 20 mEq/L. Bicarbonate replacement requirements can be

Table 10-3. Gap-nongap metabolic acidosis

Anion gap: Normal	Anion gap: Increased
Gastrointestinal loss of HCO_3	Increased acid production
Diarrhea	Diabetic ketoacidosis
Loss of small bowel or pancreatic fluids	Lactic acidosis; starvation
Ureterosigmoidostomy	Inborn errors of metabolism
Anion-exchange resins	Alcoholic ketoacidosis
	Nonketotic hyperosmolar coma
Renal loss of HCO_3	Ingestion of toxic substances
Carbonic anhydrase inhibitors	Salicylate overdose
Renal tubular acidosis	Paraldehyde poisoning
	Methyl alcohol ingestion
	Ethylene glycol ingestion
Miscellaneous	Failure of acid excretion
Dilutional acidosis	Acute renal failure
Addition of HCl	Chronic renal failure
Hyperalimentation acidosis	

calculated by determining the mEq/L increment desired and considering the volume of distribution to be 50% of body weight, which includes extracellular fluid volume and some intracellular buffer requirements.

Metabolic alkalosis

Metabolic alkalosis is a pathophysiologic state characterized by a net gain of HCO_3^- a loss of nonvolatile acid (H^+) from the extracellular fluid, or a loss of extracellular fluid containing a chloride concentration disproportionately greater than that of HCO_3^-.

HCO_3^- can be added to the extracellular fluid by the oral or intravenous administration of HCO_3^- or by the administration of a precursor of HCO_3^- such as lactate, citrate, or acetate at a rate greater than the body's daily acid production. It has recently been shown that HCO_3^- is absorbed from the skin in quantities sufficient to produce metabolic alkalosis.

Hydrogen ion can be lost from the extracellular fluid by way of the gastrointestinal tract or the kidneys or by shifting into cells in response to significant deficits of potassium.

When fluid containing chloride in greater concentration and HCO_3^- in lesser concentration than the extracellular fluid is lost from the body, extracellular fluid volume becomes concentrated and HCO_3^- concentration rises. Clinical situations such as chloride-diarrhea, diuretic use or abuse, and chloride loss through sweating in cystic fibrosis or through the kidneys in Bartter syndrome can lead to metabolic alkalosis through chloride loss. It has also been shown that a chloride-deficient diet in infancy may lead to metabolic alkalosis.

In defense of a rise in pH, the body attempts to restore pH to normal by buffering with H^+ derived from phosphates and proteins, by alveolar hypoventilation causing CO_2 retention and a rise in Pa_{CO_2}, and by rapid excretion of excess HCO_3^- through the kidneys.

The factors that tend to increase HCO_3^- reabsorption and in turn interfere with renal correction of the plasma HCO_3^- in metabolic alkalosis are the unavailability of adequate amounts of chloride ion, contraction of the extracellular fluid volume, an excess of mineralocorticoid activity, potassium depletion, and hypercapnia.

Metabolic alkalosis can be classified in two categories, depending on the status of the extracellular fluid volume and the availability of sodium chloride. Sodium chloride-responsive causes of metabolic alkalosis occur in association with a contracted extracellular fluid volume, whereas the sodium chloride–resistant causes include diseases that produce mineralocorticoid excess or, as in the case of licorice ingestion, simulate hyperaldosteronism. Table 10-4 classifies sodium chloride–responsive and sodium chloride–resistant forms of metabolic alkalosis.

POTASSIUM DEFICITS

All dehydrated children have some degree of potassium deficit. Because 98% of the body's potassium stores are located intracellularly, relatively little information about body potassium balance is gleaned from the concentration of potassium in the serum. Furthermore, an inverse relationship exists between blood pH and extracellular fluid potassium because extracellular potassium exchanges with intracellular hydro-

Table 10-4. Metabolic alkalosis

NaCl-responsive (urine Cl <10 mmol/L)	NaCl-resistant (urine Cl >20 mmol/L)
Gastrointestinal disorders	Excess mineralocorticoid activity
Vomiting	Hyperaldosteronism
Gastric drainage	Cushing syndrome
Chloride diarrhea	Bartter syndrome
Villous adenoma of colon	Excess licorice intake
Diuretic therapy	Profound potassium depletion
Cystic fibrosis	Unclassified
Chloride-deficient diet	Alkali administration
$NaHCO_3$ application to skin	Milk-alkali syndrome
	Nonparathyroid hypercalcemia

gen ions. A decrease or increase in blood pH by 0.1 pH units is associated with an increase or decrease in potassium of 1.0 mEq/L. In general, total daily potassium replacement should not exceed 4 mEq/kg/day and should be administered as continuous infusion rather than rapid boluses. Repair of potassium deficits should be accomplished over a 3- to 4-day period. When renal function is impaired, potassium should be administered with extreme caution and normally is not added to intravenous fluids.

APPROACH TO SERUM ELECTROLYTE ABNORMALITIES

Determination of electrolyte and mineral concentration in the serum (extracellular fluid) is an integral part of the evaluation of children seen in a pediatric practice. Not uncommonly, either an elevated or depressed value is encountered. In most instances, the pathogenesis of the disorder can be determined by a logical assessment, even if the physician is unaware of the specific disease entity. In our previous discussion of hyponatremia, for instance, a systematic assessment determined if the decreased sodium concentration was factitious, dilutional, or the result of sodium depletion. A rational therapy could then be instituted as the specific diagnosis was being confirmed.

In general, when an abnormal concentration of a serum mineral or electrolyte (other than sodium) is discovered, one of three primary pathologic processes is responsible. First, there may be an abnormal intake of the electrolyte into the body. Secondly, there may be a shift of the electrolyte within body water compartments. Finally, there may be altered losses or excretion. A surprising number of clinical electrolyte problems are readily solved with this approach. An example of the relatively frequent problem of hypokalemia (serum potassium less than 3.5 mEq/L) demonstrates the usefulness of this type of clinical analysis.

EXAMPLE

A 7-year-old child with cystic fibrosis is admitted to the hospital with pneumonia. Intravenous antibiotics are administered. On the third hospital day the serum potassium concentration is noted to be 2.5 mEq/L.

Question 1 Is intake deficient? If the child has been chronically ill with a poor appetite, perhaps potassium intake was deficient. A careful history revealed that the child had a good appetite until immediately before admission. Furthermore, the serum potassium concentration was normal at the time of admission and potassium provisions were adequate in the hospital.

Question 2 Was there a shift of extracellular potassium into the intracellular compartment? Alkalosis will cause a shift of potassium intracellularly. The blood pH and serum bicarbonate were normal both at the time of admission and on the third day of hospitalization; therefore another cause of hypokalemia was sought.

Question 3 Was there an increased loss of potassium? Potassium may be lost in either stool or urine. In this child with the aid of pancreatic extract therapy, there was no diarrhea or other intestinal losses. Urine potassium concentration is easily measured and is exceedingly helpful in assessing hypokalemia. If there is inadequate intake or increased extrarenal potassium losses, the concentration of potassium in the urine will be low (<10 mEq/L). In this patient the urinary potassium concentration was high. A number of renal and extrarenal disorders may lead to excessive potassium loss; however, a review of the hospital chart revealed that the child was receiving carbenicillin sodium as therapy for the pulmonary infection. Carbenicillin increases urinary potassium excretion by acting as a poorly reabsorbed anion in the distal nephron. This patient's hypokalemia was a complication of carbenicillin therapy.

A detailed discussion of diseases, drugs, and hormones that increase renal potassium excretion is beyond the scope of this chapter; however, the etiology of hypokalemia based on this clinical assessment is described below. The above example illustrates how quickly the mechanism of hypokalemia can be determined, thereby directing attention in this patient to the potential explanations of renal potassium wasting.

Etiology of hypokalemia

- I. Inadequate intake
  - A. Protein-calorie malnutrition
  - B. Anorexia nervosa
  - C. Parenteral fluids devoid of potassium
- II. Extracellular to intracellular shifts
  - A. Metabolic or respiratory alkalosis
  - B. Insulin
  - C. Hypokalemic periodic paralysis
- III. Excessive losses
  - A. Renal
    1. Renal tubular acidosis
    2. Bartter syndrome
    3. Fanconi syndrome
    4. Diuretics

5. Hyperaldosteronism
6. Anionic drugs (Carbenicillin)
7. Cushing syndrome

B. Gastrointestinal
1. Diarrhea
2. Vomiting
3. Intestinal fistulae
4. Chronic laxative use
5. Potassium exchange resins

F. Bruder Stapleton
Shane Roy III

The authors respectfully recognize the pioneering investigations and invaluable teaching in the area of fluid and electrolyte metabolism by James N. Etteldorf, M.D., the previous author of this chapter.

SELECTED READINGS

Etteldorf, J.N., and Sweeney, M.J.: Dehydration and metabolic acid-base disturbances: diagnosis and treatment, Pediatr. Clin. North Am. **9:**133, 1962.

Feig, P., and McCurdy, D.K.: The hypertonic state, N. Engl. J. Med. **297:**1444, 1977.

Finberg, L., et al.: Water and electrolytes in pediatrics: physiology, pathophysiology and treatment, Philadelphia, 1982, W.B. Saunders Co.

Gruskin, A.B.: Fluid therapy in children, Urol. Clin. North Am. **3:**277, 1976.

Holliday, M.A., and Segar, W.E.: The maintenance need for water in parenteral fluid therapy, Pediatrics **19:**823, 1957.

Humes, H.D., et al.: Disorders of water balance, Hosp. Pract. **14:**133, 1979.

Winters, R.W.: The body fluids in pediatrics, Boston, 1973, Little, Brown & Co.

11 Immunization Procedures

Immunization against infectious organisms is an important public health measure. It has become so much a part of routine pediatric health care that it is frequently taken for granted; yet a leading health authority considers immunization against infectious organisms an example of the highest form of modern medical technology in the sense that it has the capacity to almost completely prevent certain illnesses (Thomas, 1971). Other aspects of medicine that are generally considered by the public to be areas of high technology, such as organ transplant and specialized care units, actually represent expensive makeshift efforts to compensate for the incapacitating effects of certain diseases.

Because immunization against infectious organisms has been so successful, the public has lost some of its dread of the diseases caused by these organisms. As a result, it has become increasingly apparent that large segments of the pediatric population have failed to complete the recommended course of immunizations. Because of this, a number of states are requiring that a completed course of immunizations be a requisite for admission into the school systems.

The best source of information about recommended immunization practices in the pediatric age group is the *Report of the Committee on Infectious Diseases* (The Red Book).* Rather than discussing the specific details readily found in this source, this chapter will cover some of the more general aspects of immunization.

BACKGROUND

Vaccination against smallpox was practiced by the Chinese centuries ago. In Western Europe, modern immunology originated in the studies of Edward Jenner in the late eighteenth century when he introduced vaccination against cowpox as a means of protection against smallpox. The attempt to immunize animals against infectious organisms was the stimulus for much of the work of Pasteur and Koch. The use of routine immunization against bacterial organisms such as pertussis, diphtheria, and tetanus became commonplace during the 1920s, 1930s, and 1940s.

Vaccines against common pediatric viral illnesses were developed during the 1950s and 1960s. In recent years there has been a resurgence of interest in bacterial vaccines because organisms resistant to antimicrobials have become an increasingly common problem.

TYPES OF IMMUNIZATION

Passive immunization

Passive immunization refers to the administration of antibody from an exogenous source to another subject. It provides temporary immunity and is only effective if the disorder is preventable by adequate levels of serum antibody and if this antibody is given before or early in the incubation period of the organism.

Antibody for passive immunization may be obtained from humans or animals. No serum of animal origin should be given until a history of allergies to the animal species is obtained, scratch testing is done, and intradermal testing is accomplished to determine if the patient is sensitive to that serum. The scratch test should be performed with a 1:100 saline dilution of the serum. If it is negative after 30 minutes, then 0.1 ml of the 1:100 saline dilution can be administered intradermally.

From the time of the skin test through the actual injection of the serum, a syringe containing 1 ml of 1:1000 epinephrine should be on hand.

In addition to acute anaphylactic reactions to serum administration, more chronic reactions

*American Academy of Pediatrics, P.O. Box 927, 141 Northwest Point Road, Elk Grove Village, Ill. 60007.

Table 11-1. Indications for human immune serum globulin for passive immunization

Indication	Purpose	Intramuscular dose	Comment
Standard human immune globulin (HIG)			
Hepatitis A	Prevention	0.02-0.04 ml/kg	
Measles	Prevention	0.25 ml/kg	
Human special immune globulin			
Hepatitis B	Prevention	0.06 ml/kg	Standard HIG may also be effective.
Rabies	Prevention	20 IU/kg	Give one half at site of wound, other half intramuscularly. Should be used in combination with vaccine.
Tetanus	Prevention and therapy	3000-5000 U/IM	
Varicella-Zoster	Prevention	2.0-5.0 ml	Should be used only in persons at high risk who have been exposed. 1.2-2.4 ml/kg of standard immunoglobulin may be used if V-ZIG is not available.

such as serum sickness may develop after administration of an animal serum. Whenever possible, serum of human origin is preferred to serum of animal origin. Table 11-1 lists conditions for which antisera for passive immunization are available. Equine antisera and antitoxins are available for human use against infectious agents (botulism, diphtheria, rabies, tetanus) and noninfectious agents (black widow spider and snake bite).

Two of the most important uses of passive immunization are (1) for children with hypogammaglobulinemia and (2) to prevent the development of anti-Rh antibodies in Rh-negative mothers. In the former situation human immune serum globulin is given intramuscularly or intravenously. In the prevention of Rh isoimmunization, Rho (D) immune globulin (RhoGAM) is given intramuscularly within 72 hours of a birth or abortion of an Rh-positive infant. RhoGAM consists of specific antibodies against the D antigen on the Rh-positive erythrocyte. Administration of these specific antibodies prevents the sensitization of the mother.

Active immunization

Active immunization refers to the process whereby material is administered to a subject before exposure to the infectious agent. The subject produces his own antibody against the administered material. He thus has preexisting an-

Table 11-2. Recommended schedule for active immunization of normal infants and children*

2 mo	DTP†	TOPV‡
4 mo	DTP	TOPV
6 mo	DTP	§
1 yr		Tuberculin test‖
15 mo	Measles,¶ rubella¶	Mumps¶
1½ yr	DTP	TOPV
4 to 6 yr	DTP	TOPV
14 to 16 yr	Td#—repeat every 10 years	

*From Report of the Committee on Infectious Diseases, ed. 19, American Academy of Pediatrics. Copyright American Academy of Pediatrics, 1982.

†DTP—diphtheria and tetanus toxoids combined with pertussis vaccine.

‡TOPV—trivalent oral poliovirus vaccine. This recommendation is suitable for breast-fed as well as bottle-fed infants.

§A third dose of TOPV is optional but may be given in areas of high endemicity of poliomyelitis.

‖Frequency of repeated tuberculin tests depends on risk of exposure of the child and on the prevalence of tuberculosis in the population group. For the pediatrician's office or outpatient clinic, an annual or biennial tuberculin test, unless local circumstances clearly indicate otherwise, is appropriate. The initial test should be done at the time of, or preceding, the measles immunization.

¶May be given at 15 months as measles-rubella or measles-mumps-rubella combined vaccines.

#Td—combined tetanus and diphtheria toxoids (adult type) for those more than 6 years of age, in contrast to diphtheria and tetanus (DT) toxoids which contain a larger amount of diphtheria antigen.

tibody levels to the material in question and is capable of rapidly increasing this level on subsequent vaccination against the same material.

In much of the Western world diphtheria, tetanus, pertussis, poliomyelitis, rubeola, rubella, and mumps vaccines are routinely given. Table 11-2 gives a schedule for routine active immunization of healthy infants. Table 11-3 shows the recommendations for immunization of a child not immunized in early infancy.

There is an increased effort today to inform parents and, when of appropriate age, the patient about the agents being administered and what the associated reactions to these agents might be. In general, when inactivated antigens (such as DPT) are administered, unfavorable reactions are most likely to consist of soreness at injection sites, fever, and malaise. These generally occur within 48 hours of administration of the vaccine.

Adverse reactions following live attenuated virus vaccines may occur within days to 2 to 4 weeks following vaccination.

Age of active immunization

The natural history of a disease determines when immunization is best performed. For diseases that have their greatest impact on infants, immunization is begun within weeks to months after birth. For example, pertussis rarely causes serious problems after early childhood. Therefore immunization against pertussis is recommended for infants and is not usually recommended after 6 years of age.

Another consideration is whether the recipient is capable of responding to specific antigens. For instance, infants respond poorly to polysaccaride antigens. Thus immunization with pneumococcal polysaccaride, capsular antigens from *Haemophilus influenzae,* or meningococcal vaccines frequently fail to provoke a sufficient antibody response in infants.

Infants also may fail to respond to certain vaccines because of interfering antibodies of maternal origin. Recognition of this has resulted in deferring the recommended age for immunization against measles to 15 months.

Route of immunization

The route of immunization is now recognized as an important element in the type and duration of induced immunity. Jenner's original method of inoculation was by scarification. As it turned out, this was the appropriate route to immunize against smallpox. Attempts at developing an intramuscular vaccine against respiratory syncytial virus resulted in a number of patients developing a more severe infection than nonimmunized control patients. This occurred despite the presence of adequate levels of serum antibody. Experimental studies now show that if this virus vaccine is administered intranasally, significant local IgA antibody and resistance to challenge develop.

Contraindications to vaccine administration

Serious reactions to immunizations do occur, although the frequency is very low. Most of the

Table 11-3. Primary immunization for children not immunized in early infancy*

	Under 6 years of age	6 years of age and over
First visit	DTP, TOPV, tuberculin test	Td, TOPV, tuberculin test
Interval after first visit		
1 mo	Measles,† mumps, rubella	Measles, mumps, rubella
2 mo	DTP, TOPV	Td, TOPV
4 mo	DTP, TOPV‡	
8 to 14 mo		Td, TOPV
10 to 16 mo or preschool	DTP, TOPV	
Age 14 to 16 yr	Td—repeat every 10 yr	Td—repeat every 10 yr

From Report of the Committee on Infectious Diseases, ed. 19, 1982, American Academy of Pediatrics. Copyright American Academy of Pediatrics, 1982.

*Physicians may choose to alter the sequence of these schedules if specific infections are prevalent at the time. For example, measles vaccine might be given on the first visit if an epidemic is underway in the community.

†Measles vaccine is not routinely given before 15 months of age.

‡Optional.

reported complications of vaccination can also occur independently of any vaccination.

An acute febrile illness is reason to defer immunization. Minor, nonfebrile infections such as mild upper respiratory tract infections are not contraindications. The occurrence of a severe reaction to DPT is cause for caution in administering subsequent injections. If a severe reaction to DPT should occur, future vaccination should either be deferred or the dose divided into smaller aliquots.

Children with immunodeficiency disorders should not be vaccinated with live virus vaccines. Patients who are pregnant, who have recently received gamma globulin (within 8 weeks), or those receiving immunosuppressive therapy should also avoid vaccination, particularly with live virus vaccines.

Vaccines prepared on chick or duck embryos include influenza, yellow fever, and certain rabies vaccines. Children allergic to eggs, chickens, or ducks should not receive these vaccines. These same children may also be allergic to vaccines for diseases such as measles, rubella, and mumps, which are grown on chick or duck fibroblasts. Before administering these vaccines, children with a history of possible sensitivity should be skin tested.

COMMON VACCINES

Diphtheria

Diphtheria continues to be rare in the United States. However, there have been significant outbreaks of cutaneous disease in several areas in this country. The standard vaccine is a formalin-treated toxin produced by *Corynebacterium diphtheriae*.

In primary immunization for children less than age 6 years diphtheria toxoid is given along with tetanus toxoid and pertussis vaccine (DPT). After this age diphtheria toxoid is given along with tetanus toxoid (Td). The dose of diphtheria toxoid is reduced in this preparation, thus decreasing the chance for severe reactions.

Pertussis (whooping cough)

Pertussis vaccine is made from an extract of killed whole bacteria. Pertussis is particularly severe in young infants; therefore recommendations are for immunization to begin by 2 months of age.

In addition to the adverse reactions common to both diphtheria and tetanus toxoids, pertussis vaccine has been implicated in causing convulsions. It has proved very difficult to evaluate the role of pertussis vaccine in these cases. The current recommendation is that static neurologic diseases in infants do not constitute a contraindication to pertussis vaccine. An evolving neurologic disease does represent a contraindication.

Tetanus

Immunization against the toxin produced by *Clostridium tetani* is perhaps the most effective vaccine available. Following a complete course of immunization, antitoxin titers have been found to persist for at least 20 years. It is recommended that after the initial series of immunizations boosters be given only at intervals of 10 years.

Tetanus is unusual in that the infection itself produces too little toxin to serve as an immunizing dose or a booster dose. Thus a person who develops tetanus still requires full immunization to prevent future infection.

Poliomyelitis

In the era before the introduction of poliovirus vaccine up to 20,000 cases of paralytic poliomyelitis were seen in the United States each year. Two effective vaccines were developed in the United States. The Salk vaccine consists of a formalin-inactivated vaccine administered intramuscularly. It is the standard vaccine used to protect against poliomyelitis in Sweden.

The Sabin vaccine is an attenuated vaccine consisting of three antigenic types—polio 1, 2, and 3. It is administered orally and induces an antibody response in the gastrointestinal tract as well as systemically. Trivalent oral polio vaccine (TOPV) is the recommended preparation to be used in the United States. There is a slight risk of approximately 1:9 million doses of vaccine for paralytic disease to develop secondary to the virus in the vaccine.

Rubeola (measles)

Measles vaccine consists of a live attenuated virus preparation. Because of this, measles vaccine should not be administered to an immunosuppressed patient. If exposed to measles, such a child should receive measles immune serum globulin. Tuberculin skin testing should precede or accompany the administration of measles vaccine. Measles virus temporarily diminishes cutaneous manifestations of cell-mediated immunity, and a tuberculin test performed 4 days to 4 weeks after vaccination may give false negative results.

Mumps

Mumps is usually a benign disease in children but may be accompanied by aseptic meningitis, pancreatitis, orchitis, or oophoritis. Of all the diseases for which routine immunization is given, mumps is responsible for the least morbidity. Perhaps the most distressing illness due to mumps virus is mumps orchitis. Consequently, adolescent males without a history of either mumps or immunization against mumps should be given mumps vaccine.

Rubella (German measles)

Rubella in children and adults is basically a benign disease. The sole purpose of immunization is to prevent rubella infections in pregnant females and subsequent intrauterine infection.

Current recommendations call for administration of the vaccine to both boys and girls between 15 months and puberty. There is a slightly greater chance of side effects, chiefly self-limited arthritis or arthralgia, in older children, but the vaccine is generally well tolerated. As with the other live attenuated virus vaccines, administration of the vaccine to pregnant females is contraindicated.

Other vaccines

Among the diseases for which vaccines are available but not routinely used are influenza, salmonellosis (typhoid), rabies, cholera, and tuberculosis (BCG vaccine).

Polyvalent pneumococcal polysaccaride is of limited usefulness in children. It is specifically recommended for children highly susceptible to pneumococcal infections such as children with sickle cell anemia, children who have undergone splenectomy, and children with nephrotic syndrome.

Specific recommendations for use of the hepatitis B vaccine in children have yet to be developed. It is likely that populations at risk for developing hepatitis B infection such as children requiring hemodialysis, those who receive repeated transfusions of blood products, and drug users would benefit from vaccine therapy.

Henry G. Herrod

REFERENCES

Anderson, D.C., and Stiehm, E.R.: Immunization. In Feign, R.D., and Cherry, J.D., editors: Pediatric infectious diseases, Philadelphia, 1981, W.B. Saunders Co.

Cody, C.L., et al: Nature and rates of adverse reactions associated with DTP and DT immunizations in infants and children, Pediatrics **68:**650, 1981.

Fulginiti, V.A.: Controversies in current immunization policy and practices: one physician's viewpoint, Curr. Probl. Pediatr. **6:**3, 1976.

Fulginitti, V.: Immunizations: current controversies, J. Pediatr. **101:**487, 1982.

Herman, J.J., et al.: Allergic reaction to measles (rubeola) vaccine in patients hypersensitive to eggs protein, J. Pediatr. **102:**196, 1983.

Katz, S.L.: Childhood immunizations, Hosp. Pract. **11:**49, 1976.

Report of the Committee on Infectious Diseases, American Academy of Pediatrics, ed. 19, Evanston, Ill., 1982, The Academy.

Sever, J.L.: Infectious diseases and immunizations, Rev. Infect. Dis. **4:**136, 1982.

Thomas, L.: The technology of medicine, N. Engl. J. Med. **285:**1367, 1971.

12 Injuries and Poisonings during Childhood

In the United States at the present time, injuries and poisonings are the greatest cause of morbidity and mortality from 1 year of age until age 45. During childhood, injuries account for more deaths than the next nine leading causes combined. With the advent of immunizations, antibiotics, and effective chemotherapeutic agents for childhood cancers, injuries remain as the most important cause of childhood disease, disability, and death. The purpose of this chapter is to introduce students of the medical profession to the approach of the modern field of injury control and outline some specific instances of prevention and treatment.

SCOPE OF PROBLEM

About 75 million Americans are injured every year. Table 12-1 presents the leading causes of death in 1977, according to the National Center for Health Statistics. Beyond the age of 1 year, motor vehicle injuries were the leading cause of death, accounting for over ½ of the childhood deaths from nonintentional injuries. Drownings, fire deaths, and poisonings together cause more deaths than cancer, congenital anomalies, or cardiovascular disease in children beyond 1 year of age. In most categories, deaths increase substantially after age 14; the 15- to 19-year-old age group includes nearly 50% of the nonintentional injuries, 70% of the homicides, and 90% of the suicides during childhood. Males have three times the death rate from injuries than do females, even in the youngest age group. Although injuries rank fifth in terms of overall number of deaths in the United States, motor vehicle–related deaths alone account for more potential years of life lost than from any other single cause.

Among other causes of violent deaths in children and adolescents, homicides account for nearly 3000 deaths per year; suicides add another 2000 to the total. Homicides are second only to motor vehicle crashes as a leading cause of death among all teenagers, and are the leading

Table 12-1. Violent deaths in children and adolescents in United States (1977)

	Age in years					
Cause of death	**<1**	**1-4**	**5-9**	**10-14**	**15-19**	**Total**
Nonintentional injuries	1173	3297	2967	3398	12,680	23,515
Motor vehicle injuries	253	1219	1485	1657	9085	13,699
Drowning	66	631	485	549	1075	2806
Fire	159	608	344	206	272	1589
Poisoning	18	111	30	69	446	674
Falls	54	121	50	72	234	531
Firearms (nonintentional)	1	47	104	240	390	782
Suffocation	275	168	42	37	87	609
Other	347	392	427	568	1091	2825
Homicide	108	399	188	248	1897	2840
Suicide			2	188	1871	2061
Congenital abnormalities	8420	1066	372	304	350	10,512
Malignant neoplasms	121	631	869	864	1250	3735
Influenza and pneumonia	1682	374	161	183	250	2650
Cardiovascular diseases	983	357	224	305	684	2553

From National Center for Health Statistics: Vital statistics of the United States, 1977, DHHS Pub. No. (PHS) 81-1101, Vol. II, Part A, Hyattsville, Md., 1981, U.S. Government Printing Office.

cause of death among nonwhite teenagers. At present, almost 85% of these homicides involve firearms, 75% of which are handguns.

Suicide is the third most common cause of death among teenage males and the fourth among females. As with homicides, firearms have played an important role in the increase in suicide deaths and are now the most common means of suicide in males of all ages.

Survivors of these traumatic events do not escape unscathed. In 1980, an estimated 68 million persons were injured—21 million of these were under 17 years of age. This resulted in 86,879,000 days of restricted activity, more days than for any other single cause. Injuries overall accounted for an incredible 357 days of restricted activity per 100 persons per year—over 3.5 days for every man, woman, and child in the United States. Nearly ⅓ of all impairments in function are caused by injuries, resulting in over 12,000,000 people suffering traumatic impairments in 1977. Injuries cost society over $75 billion per year in medical expenses, lost wages, and property damage.

INJURIES AND ACCIDENTS

Before examining patterns of injury in the population, just what is it that we are talking about? Throughout this chapter, injuries will refer to "damage resulting from acute exposure to physical or chemical agents." Poisonings are properly included as injuries. The term "accident" will not be used; it is an inaccurate anachronism reflecting unscientific attitudes towards injuries. "Accident" connotes randomicity, that is, events occurring at random, without pattern or predictability. The term *accident* should also be abandoned because of its moral connotations. Accidents have been viewed as rightful punishment for negligent and careless behavior.

The term *injury,* on the other hand, refocuses scientific attention on the problem—the damage to the person.

CAUSES OF INJURY AND PREVENTIVE OPTIONS

The necessary and specific agent of injury is energy transfer in the form of electrical, ionizing, mechanical, chemical, or thermal energy. Whether or not the energy transfer takes place and therefore an injury occurs depends on the combination of the host, the agent of the energy transfer (e.g., a motor vehicle, hot tap water, or an electrical cord), and the environment. Much work in the past has focused on trying to change the host—the child or his parent. Modern injury control efforts have met with much greater success by concentrating on the agent or the environment.

For many years, study of the host factors involved with childhood injuries have centered around attempts to pinpoint the "accident prone" child, that is, innate characteristics of the child that result in a greater frequence of injury. Children with impaired locomotor skills do have a greater frequency of injury. This may represent a mismatch between the developmental abilities of the child and the skills demanded by the task at hand; however, this is not "accident proneness." Other studies of the child's personality characteristics, behavior, activity, and social adjustment have been inconsistent in their ability to identify such children and predict the risk of injury.

Most serious scientists involved with injury research have now discounted the theory of "accident proneness." Although some persons in a group have higher injury rates than others, the available evidence at present indicates that over a long period of observation, this is essentially a shifting group of persons, with new persons constantly entering and leaving the group. Moreover, statistical correlations between past and future injuries are low, and a multitude of possible confounding factors inadequately controlled in previous studies may account for the high rate of injury in some groups.

The question does arise, however, of why children become members (albeit temporary) of this group of persons with repeated injuries. A number of sociocultural factors can be identified that clearly do play a role in increasing the risk of injury to a child. Maternal age has been identified as the most important predictor of injury to children in the first year of life. Infants born to teenage mothers have an approximately 50% increase in the risk of injury as compared to infants of older mothers.

Injuries and ingestions can be viewed as pediatric "social diseases" along with child abuse and neglect. Newberger studied the stress factors in the environment that led to these problems in children under 4 years of age. Injuries were found to correlate highly with current stresses in the household, such as recent moves and changes in household composition. Ingestions were more common among families encountering other childrearing problems, or where there had been mother-child separation. Other researchers have found similar results when analyzing risk-taking behavior. There is a significant correlation between injury and degree of life change as measured by such scales as the Holmes and Rahe Social Readjustment Rating Questionnaire. Other studies have shown that high rates of injury correlate with single-parent families, relatively loose parental supervision, and family stress. Children living in poverty also have higher injury rates, probably as a result of the social disruption of their lives.

Although these factors associated with higher risk of injury in children can be identified, they are not highly discriminatory. The problem lies with the fact that high-risk children represent only a small proportion, probably less than 20%, of children injured annually. The predictors cited above can identify most of these high-risk children but will have a false positive rate on the order of 75%. Programs aimed at reducing injuries in these high-risk children can be expected to have only a small impact on the total number of injuries occurring in the United States each year.

Ten basic logical strategies for reducing injuries have been developed and are listed below.*

1. Prevent the creation of the hazard in the first place
   Do not manufacture lead-containing paint
   Do not manufacture and sell handguns
2. Reduce the amount of the hazard
   Reduce the top speed capability of motor vehicles
   Reduce water-heater temperatures to below scalding levels
3. Prevent the inappropriate release of the hazard
   Use child-proof containers for drugs and potential poisons
   Lock up guns in the house
4. Modify release of the agent
   Use child seat restraints and seat belts in motor vehicles
   Manufacture flame-retardant sleepwear
5. Separate the hazard from the host in time or space
   Build bicycle paths away from streets and highways
   Have children play in playgrounds rather than the street
6. Separate the hazard with a barrier
   Install fences around swimming pools
   Use air bags in motor vehicles
7. Modify the hazard
   Incorporate an antidote into drugs
   Make crib slats closer together
8. Increase resistance to injury
   Improve training and conditioning for sports
   Use factor VIII prophylactically in children with hemophilia
9. Counter damage already done
   Improve emergency medical services
   Provide Poison Control Centers
10. Rehabilitate the injured person
    Provide rehabilitative surgery for paraplegics
    Provide support to families

In thinking about prevention of any injury, the options provide a logical framework for identifying appropriate strategies. The great value of these options is that they specify the various stages in the disease and injury process at which intervention should be considered and can be successful.

HEALTH EDUCATION

Health education efforts must be combined with attempts to modify the agent and the environment. By itself, health education has not proven a very effective method of injury control. However, when focused on specific changes parents can make to provide a safer environment for their children, education can provide the physician with the means to prevent significant harm to his patients.

Child safety counseling should be oriented to the child's developmental stage. Injuries during childhood are developmentally determined. The infant is most susceptible to falls and burns. The toddler is the victim of most of the cases of nonintentional poisoning. Preschool children are particularly susceptible to pedestrian injuries. Most injuries to school-aged children occur on the playing field. Injuries in adolescents often involve the use of drugs or alcohol. Table 12-2 shows an appropriate protocol for safety counseling at different well-child visits.

Certain principles underlie health education efforts: First, a positive approach is probably more effective than the traditional "scare tactics." Second, repeated reinforcement of injury

*Adapted from Haddon, W., Jr., and Baker, S.P.: Injury control. In Clark, D., and MacMahon, B., editors: Preventive medicine, ed. 2, Boston, 1981, Little, Brown & Co.

Table 12-2. Early childhood safety counseling schedule

Age	Introduce	Reinforce
Prenatal/Newborn	Infant car seat Smoke detector Crib safety	
2 to 4 weeks	Falls	Infant car seat
2 months	Burns—hot liquids	Infant car seat Falls
4 months	Choking	Infant car seat Falls Burns—hot liquids
6 months	Poison Burns—hot surface	Falls Burns—hot liquids
9 months	Water safety Toddler car seat	Poison Falls Burns
1 year		Poison Falls Burns
15 months	Specific to need—optional	
18 months		Poison Falls Burns
2 years	Falls—play equipment, tricycles Auto—pedestrian	Auto—restraints Poison Burns
3 years		Auto—restraints, pedestrian Falls Burns
4 years		Auto—restraints, pedestrian Falls—play equipment Burns

prevention measures is more effective than a one time contact. Third, written literature helps to increase compliance. Fourth, modeling by the physician and nurses in the hospital and office is an important education device. Finally, the ease of a safety measure is probably the most important determinant of parent (and child) compliance.

MOTOR VEHICLES

Motor vehicle fatalities are the leading cause of potential years of life lost and in 1980 accounted for 54,200 deaths. The National Transportation Safety Board estimates that 145 persons, including 12 children, die each day in vehicular collisions. The total cost of motor vehicle injuries, in 1980 dollars, is over $20 billion annually.

Among children age 1 to 14 years, motor vehicle collisions are a major cause of injury and disability and are responsible for 20% of all deaths in that age group. In 1980, approximately 90,000 children under 6 years of age and 800,000 children 6 to 16 years of age were injured by motor vehicles.

The injuries incurred in motor vehicle collisions are severe. Motor vehicle crashes result in more than 5300 spinal cord injuries every year in the United States. They are responsible for 114,000 severe facial lacerations and 25,000 severe facial fractures annually.

Among children under 13 years of age, children under 6 months of age have the highest motor vehicle fatality rate, approximately three times the rate of 6 to 12 year olds. This high death rate is most likely caused by a greater likelihood of being in the front seat or held in someone's arms.

On the positive side, a solid base of research and experience supports the conclusion that large and sustained reductions in motor vehicle crash injuries can be accomplished by approaches already at hand. The following discussion outlines some approaches of particular importance to the physician caring for children.

Seat belt and child restraint use

In recent years the greatest activity in childhood injury control, and the area of most active involvement by physicians, has been in the area of child passenger protection.

Most motor vehicle injuries to children occur within 25 miles of home, at speeds of 30 miles per hour or less, and during daylight hours. Child restraint use and the position in the car are two factors related to the risk of injury. Children are safest riding restrained in the back seat. Unrestrained children in the front seat have the highest injury rate. It is also safer to be riding restrained in the front seat than unrestrained in the back seat. Among children under the age of 5, proper use of child restraints can decrease deaths by 90% and injuries by 80%.

Traveling in the lap of an adult is one of the most dangerous positions for a small child. In a 30 mph crash, a 20-pound child is thrown forward with a force of 600 pounds. Even when subjects in test crashes know when the moment of impact would occur, they are unable to hold a dummy in their arms weighing half as much.

The best protection for children under age 4 traveling in motor vehicles is a child seat restraint. As of January 1, 1981, all child seat restraints on the market have been dynamically crash tested to provide sufficient protection in a frontal crash into a solid wall at 30 miles per hour. When used properly, child restraints meeting crash-test requirements have provided excellent protection in actual serious frontal crashes.

Optimally, these devices should be used from the time the child first rides home in the family auto. Yet studies have shown that baseline use of child seat restraints is only on the order of 7% to 10%.

A number of approaches have been used successfully by pediatricians, obstetricians, family physicians, and communities to increase child seat restraint use. Handouts given to parents by physicians emphasizing the positive benefits of child seat restraint use have been successful in improving parent acceptance. Careful studies have shown that toddlers who normally ride in a restraint seat behave much better during car trips than children who normally ride unrestrained.

Excellent films are available that can be shown to parents in waiting rooms or mothers on hospital postpartum floors discussing the advantages of child seat restraint use. Combining this with appropriate modeling behavior by the nurse at the time of hospital discharge can greatly increase use.

Many hospitals and communities have adopted loaner programs, renting restraints to parents at low cost. This is especially important for low-income families, who have the lowest rate of restraint use.

A list of acceptable devices is available from the American Academy of Pediatrics and Physicians for Automotive Safety. Children under 20 pounds may use an infant carrier or a "convertible" infant-toddler carrier. The infant is placed in the device with a safety harness; the vehicle's lap belt secures the carrier in a rear-facing position. Children 20 to 40 pounds should be transported in a toddler seat in the forward-facing position. Many of these seats have top tether straps which, when present, *must* be used for optimal protection. Children over 40 pounds can graduate to use of a lap belt fitted low across the pelvis. When the child is 55 inches tall, the shoulder harness should be added to the lap belt.

Despite the availability and safety protection afforded by these devices, the majority of children presently ride unprotected. This has led to legislative efforts to increase child seat restraint use. As of January 1, 1984, 40 states and the District of Columbia have enacted laws requiring the use of, or have instituted public education programs on, safety seats or belts for children. Tennessee was the first state to pass such a law, which became effective January, 1978. The Tennessee law now states that all children under the age of 4 traveling in their parent's car must be protected by a federally approved child seat restraint. A vigorous educational campaign, institution of loaner programs, and active law enforcement have contributed to the success of the law. Rigorous evaluation of the law has shown that use of child seat restraint increased from 8% in 1977 to 29% 2½ years later. Injury rates have decreased by 30% and death rates by 55%.

In other countries, including Australia, Canada, and many European nations, mandatory seat belt laws for all passengers have been implemented. In Victoria, Australia, seat belt use increased from approximately 15% to between 80% and 90% after enactment of legislation requiring their use. Statistics indicate that sustained enforcement and education are necessary for continued use of restraints. In the United States, only 10% of adults use seat belts while riding in a car, yet seat belt use can reduce fatalities by 50% and injuries by 65%.

Because of the difficulty of getting persons to use seat belts and restraint systems, many researchers have advocated a passive restraint system, that is, one requiring no cooperation by the occupant of the car. There are two major forms of passive restraint devices. The automatic seat belt wraps around the occupant when the door is closed. Airbags, on the other hand, inflate automatically at the instant of frontal impact and disburse crash forces effectively. In more than 800 million miles of road testing, air bags have shown to be highly effective in reducing injuries. For a system costing approximately $200 per motor vehicle, the savings are great; air bags can reduce fatalities by 70% and save 9000 lives and $5 billion annually.

Driver education and driver age

Drivers age 15 to 17 years have 2½ times the rate of collisions per 1000 registered drivers as motorists 18 years of age and older. One past strategy to decrease the rate of crashes, and presumably injuries, was driver education. The federal government has been contributing some 10% of the more than $300 million in estimated national spending for high school driver education courses. The premise underlying such expenditures has been that high school "driver ed" courses promote higher levels of safety on the highway. However, carefully done studies in Connecticut have failed to find differences in the crash experience of drivers who had driver education and otherwise similar drivers who have not. In fact, it has been found that the more driver education is provided in schools in the United States and England, the higher the percentage of 16- and 17-year-old licensed drivers on the road. Because driver education is not associated with lower fatal crash rates among those who take it, and because it permits 16- and 17-year-old persons to drive, the net result is that the more driver education is provided, the higher are the fatality rates in the 16- and 17-year-old population. In Connecticut, state funding for driver education in high schools was eliminated in 1976. In those communities dropping driver education, the licensing of 16- and 17-year-old persons decreased by 57% and the reported crashes in the overall 16- and 17-year-old population decreased by 63%.

Research has also indicated possible injury reduction payoff from restricting 16- and 17-year-old persons to daytime-only driving. Almost half of the fatal crashes involving drivers under the age of 18 occur in the 4 hours before or the 4 hours after midnight. In states imposing night-time driving curfews on teenagers under 18 years, there has been a significant decrease in crash involvement and fatalities.

Alcohol abuse and driving

More than half of all deaths from motor vehicle crashes and one third of serious injuries involve drivers with blood-alcohol concentrations of 0.10% or higher. Other drugs, either independently or in combination with alcohol, also contribute to vehicular crashes. Studies in England have found significant associations between use of minor tranquilizers and serious crashes.

The legislative approach to drunk driving has so far *not* proved highly successful. Programs to meaningfully reduce motor vehicle crash injuries by "cracking down" on drunk drivers so as to remove them from the roads at best have achieved short-term reductions in crash-related injuries. One of the most successful approaches is to raise the legal drinking age. In the middle 1970's, when Michigan lowered its legal drinking age to 18, both the number of establishments serving drinks and their hours of operation increased, as did the number of fatal and nonfatal motor vehicle crashes among 18- to 20-year-olds. In response to these findings, the legal drinking age was raised to 21. The effects of the recent national campaign against drunk driving is undetermined. To be effective, drunk-driving laws must be accompanied by increased efforts to apprehend drunken drivers and give them swift and certain penalties, instead of making penalties more severe.

FIRE AND BURN-RELATED INJURIES

Fire and burn-related injuries and deaths are an exceedingly important problem in the United States. About 6000 burn injury deaths occur each year in the United States. For both injuries and deaths, the first decade of life is the period of highest risk. Burns are second only to motor vehicle crashes in the number of years of life lost *per death,* reflecting the relatively young population involved in serious burn injuries. The likelihood of burn injury is strongly related to socioeconomic status: the lower the family income, the higher the risk of fire and burn-related injury and death. As with other types of injuries, burns are much more frequent among males than females. For instance, among children 10 to 14 years of age, males have eight times the rate of burns involving flammable substances than do females. A number of interventions for specific types of fire and burn-related deaths have proved to be effective, whereas others have been shown to be relatively ineffective.

One of the first effective interventions involved flammable fabrics. Flame burns resulting from ignition of clothing by a single source were a common, serious burn injury in small children. At least one third of those injuries involved infant sleepwear. The extent of these burns was on the average 30% of the body surface, requiring hospitalization for an average of 70 days. In 1967 the Federal Flammable Fabrics Act was passed, requiring children's sleepwear to be flame retardant. As a result of this and similar state legislation, clothing ignition burns in small children now account for only a small fraction of burns in children. Despite the withdrawal of Tris-containing clothing because of potential mutagenicity studies, federal flammability standards still apply to children's sleepwear.

Another example of vector modification resulting in substantial reduction of injury losses is tap water scalds. Scald burns account for 40% of the burn injuries in children requiring hospitalization. Unlike flame burns, children with scalds generally do not die; however, many children face long hospitalizations, multiple surgical procedures, and severe disfigurement. At least 25% of these scald burns involve tap water. A study in Seattle showed that 80% of residences surveyed had hot tap water temperatures greater than 130° F. The risk of full-thickness burns increases geometrically at temperatures above 130° F. At 150° F, a full-thickness burn will be produced in adult skin in 2 seconds. A simple and effective preventive maneuver is simply to turn down the water heater temperature to 120° F. At this setting, dishwashers and washing machines will still operate effectively, but the risk of a serious scald injury is greatly reduced. In many cities the local power company will turn down the temperature without charge. In 1980, Florida became the first state requiring new water heaters to be preset at a temperature of 125° F. Such a move can also result in substantial energy savings as well—8% to 9% savings per year with a 30° F reduction in water heater temperatures.

Nearly 70% of all fire deaths in the United States occur in private dwellings. Of these deaths, 60% are caused by smoke asphyxiation and *not* flame burns. Smoke detectors provide an inexpensive but effective method of preventing the majority of these deaths. Their effect has been well-substantiated in studies done in Canada and elsewhere. Between 1974 and 1977, the Ontario Housing Corporation installed smoke detectors in 79,000 houses and apartments in their jurisdiction. During the first 2 years of operation the detectors provided the initial warning in 85% of the fires that occurred.

At present the most common type of smoke detector is an ionization alarm. These are based on the ability of smoke to interfere with the movement of ionized particles in a chamber. They are small, inexpensive, work on a battery source, and are easily installed by the homeowner. Studies have shown that by offering information on smoke detectors in their offices, physicians can alter parental behavior with regard to smoke detector purchase and installation.

Other approaches, particularly purely educational ones, have not proved effective. The Consumer Product Safety Commission supported a large study, Project Burn Prevention, in two communities in Massachusetts. There was a widespread mass media effort to educate the public about burn risks, numerous small community presentations, and educational programs in elementary and high schools. None of the programs showed a statistically significant reduction in burn incidence or severity. The school program did result in increased knowledge about burn hazards; however, this did not result in decreased frequency of burn injury. This and similar studies indicate that product modification, rather than education, is the most effective method of decreasing the incidence and severity of fire and burn-related injuries.

DROWNINGS

In 1980, 7000 drownings, previously associated with recreational activities, occurred in the United States. For children over the age of 5, drowning ranks second only to motor vehicle injury as a cause of traumatic death.

It is often assumed that most aquatic deaths occur in swimming pools, but pools account for only 10% of all reported drownings. Lakes, rivers, and oceans are more often the site of drownings, although among children drownings have been reported in ornamental pools, bathtubs, and even pails.

Although no precise data exist on the number of water-related injuries, it is estimated that 140,000 injuries occur annually from swimming activities alone. Diving and head-first sliding into the water account for the most serious aquatic injuries because of spinal cord damage. Of the estimated 700 spinal cord injuries resulting from aquatic activities each year, the majority are sufficiently severe to result in permanent paralysis.

Prevention of drowning injuries and deaths must be approached on a number of levels. For the protection of small children, probably the most effective method is erection of barriers around pools and small bodies of water. The use of barriers 1.4 m high would prevent 75% of these injuries and deaths. Many people have advocated "water-babies" and other swimming instruction for young children. The efficacy of such techniques is untested. The potential exists for both child and parent to become less vigilant around water, possibly with tragic consequences.

Among adolescents and young adults, alcohol and drug use have been found to be involved in nearly one half of all drowning deaths. The restriction of the sale and consumption of alcoholic beverages in boating, pool, harbor, marina, and beach areas may combat this dangerous combination of activities.

More restrictive licensing of boat owners should also be considered. Coast Guard data show that although only 7% of boats involved with mishaps lacked available personal flotation devices, they accounted for 29% of the boating fatalities.

FIREARM INJURIES

Injuries to children and adolescents involving firearms occur in three different situations: nonintentional injury, suicide attempt, or assault. In each case the injury induced may be fatal or may result in permanent sequelae.

Among children under the age of 18 years, firearms are the fifth-ranking cause of death from nonintentional trauma in the United States. Twelve hundred children die each year from nonintentional gunshot wounds. An additional 8000 children and adolescents are injured annually by firearms; 25% are left with permanent sequelae, not including emotional and psychologic problems.

Nonintentional firearm injuries generally occur in a family dwelling; 85% of firearm deaths occur in the home. In gunshot fatalities in children less than 16 years of age, poverty is more closely related to shooting deaths than race or population density. Urban whites have the lowest death rate, rural whites are intermediate, and urban black children have the highest fatality rate.

Suicide is now the third most common cause of death in teenage males and the fourth for females. During the period from 1961 to 1975, the rates for children and adolescents more than doubled, accounting for over 1700 deaths per year by the end of the period. As with homicides, firearms have played an important role in this increase and are now the most common means of suicide in males of all ages. The difference in the rate of suicide between males and females is related less to number of attempts than to method. Women die less often in suicide attempts because they use less lethal means, mainly drugs. The use of firearms in a suicidal act usually converts an attempt into a fatality.

Homicides are second only to motor vehicle crashes among causes of death in teenagers over the age of 15 years. In 1976 more than 2600 children and adolescents were homicide victims; nonwhite teenagers accounted for 47% of the total, making homicides the most common cause of death among nonwhite teenagers. At present almost 85% of homicides among males involve firearms, 75% of which are handguns.

From the initiation of vital statistic records in the United States until about 1960, mortality among young adults had consistently declined. However, beginning in 1960, death rates for teenagers began to level off, and for males actually began to rise. This increase in mortality is solely due to increased rates of violent death; nonviolent causes among young adults have continued to decrease. Firearms have played an important role in all areas of this increase: nonintentional injuries, homicides, and suicides.

In the United States today there are an estimated 210 to 220 million firearms. During the 1970s over 6 million firearms were sold in the United States each year. Handguns account for only approximately 20% of the firearms in use today, yet they are involved in 90% of criminal and nonintentional firearms misuse.

There is a strong geographic correlation between ownership of firearms and the risk of firearm injury and death. Areas of the country characterized by high rates of firearm ownership have the highest rates of homicides, aggravated assaults, and nonintentional deaths involving firearms.

The data seem to indicate that, of all firearms, handguns pose the most risk to the health of children and adolescents. Regulation and elimination of handguns, rather than all firearms, would appear to be the most appropriate focus for efforts to reduce shooting injuries to children.

One approach that has been tried in the past is information and education campaigns on firearms safety. No data exist to support the effectiveness of such programs in decreasing the number of gunshot wounds in children. Regardless of the merits of safety education, firearms around the home pose a risk to children and adolescents, who have not yet developed adequate judgement for the safe handling of these weapons. Elimination of these weapons from the environment of children and adolescents is the necessary key to reduction in firearm fatalities and injuries. Furthermore, safety education will have no effect on the use of firearms in homicides and suicides. Most homicides are between relations or acquaintances and are acts of rage. Elimination of handguns would certainly not eliminate the arguments, but it would decrease the likelihood of a fatal conclusion; in an assault, the chance of death is five times greater with a firearm than with a knife.

The rate of suicide could also be decreased by eliminating handguns from the environment of adolescents. In England, until recently, domestic gas in home ovens was a common means of suicide. Reduction of the carbon monoxide content was successful in eliminating these deaths; there was not a proportionate increase in suicide deaths by other means.

POISONING

Poisoning in children and adolescents remains a huge problem in the United States. In 1977 it was the fourth most common cause of "traumatic" death, resulting in the loss of over 600 lives (Table 12-1). Among school-age children the rate has not changed appreciably over the last 15 years, but the rate among children under 5 years of age has dropped by about 60%. The majority of nonintentional ingestions occur in this 0 to 5 age group. Unlike other types of injuries, there is little sex difference in the rates for infants and small children.

Among children, drugs are the most commonly reported poisoning agent. These are responsible for over one fifth of the poisonings in the preschool age group and over two fifths in the older age group. These are followed by plants, household products, soaps, cosmetics, and pesticides in decreasing order of frequency. In the youngest age group of children, 0 to 5 years of age, the most common drugs involved are aspirin, followed by vitamins, acetaminophen, isopropyl alcohol, Dimetapp, and Desitin. Plants account for nearly one fifth of reported poisonings in infants and young children. The vast majority of these plant ingestions are harmless, but certain plants can produce serious symptoms and even death. These include red sage, the deadly nightshade, monkshood, narcissus bulbs, mountain laurel, rhododendron, jimson weed, water hemlock, and wild mushrooms. A useful list of these plants has been published and is available from the National Clearinghouse for Poison Control Centers.

Poisoning fatalities among children have dropped in recent years for a number of reasons. One of these is the contribution made by the nationwide network of regional poison control centers. Each of the more than 60 centers manages 30,000 to 40,000 poisoning episodes annually, 85% of which are handled over the phone. In addition, these centers provide quality consultation in toxicology to medical professionals dealing with the poisoned child.

Probably the largest factor responsible for reducing serious and fatal poisonings in children is the Poison Prevention Packaging Act (PPPA) of 1970, administered by the Consumer Product Safety Commission (CPSC). This act requires that products that are toxic, corrosive, an irritant, or a strong sensitizer be packaged in "special packaging," constructed to be significantly difficult for children less than 5 years of age to open. The substances covered by the act are shown in Table 12-3. Studies conducted by the Consumer Product Safety Commission have shown that the act has resulted in a 45% to 55% reduction in nonintentional ingestion of children's aspirin and a 40% to 45% reduction in ingestions of regular aspirin. For all regulated products the number of ingestions has declined by 45%, representing nearly 200,000 ingestions prevented.

Other approaches to poisoning prevention have focused on educational efforts and the use of "Mr. Yuk" stickers on household poisons. Unfortunately, recent studies have failed to show any reduction in poisoning rates and levels of household hazards in the children of families provided with "Mr. Yuk" stickers. Again, reliance for prevention of poisonings, as in other types of injuries, must be more on "passive" approaches such as the PPPA rather than educational approaches or "Mr. Yuk" stickers.

General principles of treatment of ingested poisons

Perhaps the most important principle in the management of the poisoned patient is the need for general supportive care. Few specific antidotes exist, and recovery will generally occur even without their use. However, all patients will require general supportive care, which plays the largest role in decreasing morbidity and preventing mortality.

The systematic approach to emergency care of the poisoned patient consists of: (1) assessing the nature and severity of the ingestion, (2) minimizing absorption of the toxin, (3) increasing the rate of excretion, (4) providing supportive or symptomatic care, and (5) using antidotes.

Assessing nature and severity of ingestion

The first task of the physician is to determine that a poisoning has occurred. Some patients come to the physician or emergency department

Table 12-3. Special packaging regulations

PPPA* regulation	Effective date	Characteristics of products regulated
Aspirin	8/14/72	Products containing aspirin for oral human use
Furniture polish	9/13/72	Nonemulsion liquid form, low viscosity, containing at least 10% mineral seal oil or petroleum distillates
Methyl salicylate	9/21/72	Liquid products containing more than 5% by weight
Controlled drugs	10/24/72	For oral human use
Sodium and/or potassium hydroxide	4/11/73	Dry forms at least 10% by weight; other forms at least 2% by weight
Turpentine	7/01/73	Liquid form at least 10% by weight
Kindling and/or illumination preparations	10/29/73	Prepackaged liquid, low viscosity containing at least 10% petroleum distillates
Methyl alcohol	7/01/73	Liquids containing at least 4% by weight
Sulfuric acid	8/14/73	Substances containing at least 10% by weight
Prescription drugs	4/16/74	For oral human use
Ethylene glycol	6/01/74	Liquids containing at least 10% by weight
Paint solvents	4/23/77	Solvents for paints that contain 10% or more by weight of benzene, toluene, xylene
Iron-containing drugs	10/17/78	Noninjectable animal and human drugs containing 250 mg or more elemental iron (total package)
Dietary supplements	10/17/78	Dietary supplements containing 250 mg or more elemental iron (total package)
Acetaminophen	2/27/80	Preparations for oral human use with 1 gm or more acetaminophen (total package)

From Walton, W.W.: An evaluation of the Poison Prevention Packaging Act, Pediatrics **69:**363, 1982.
*Poison Prevention Packaging Act.

with a clear history that an ingestion has occurred. However, in many other cases the child may appear with only an unexplained illness, no immediate history of ingestion, and nonspecific signs and symptoms. Poisoning should be suspected in any child with a sudden, unexplained illness or with a puzzling combination of signs and symptoms in the high-risk age group (6 months to 5 years old). Nearly any symptom can be seen with poisoning; however, some signs and symptoms are suggestive of particular toxin exposure.

Depression of the central nervous system should suggest ingestion of narcotics, sedatives, hypnotics, alcohol, salicylates, or organophosphate compounds; central nervous system stimulation is seen with antidepressants, phenothiazines, street drugs (phencyclidine, marijuana), or sympathomimetics. Miosis is seen with narcotic and organophosphate ingestion; mydriasis with amphetamines, barbituates, atropine, and cocaine. Convulsions are found with ingestion of alcohol, amphetamines, antidepressants, lead, salicylates, and organophosphates.

Instability of the vital signs can be seen in nearly any serious intoxication. Depressant drugs such as ethanol, barbituates, narcotics, and sedatives commonly produce hypothermia; hyperthermia is seen with salicylates, atropine, and tricyclics. Slowed, depressed respirations are seen with alcohol, barbiturates, narcotics, and sedative drugs, whereas salicylates, carbon monoxide, and amphetamines stimulate respiration.

Certain compounds have characteristic odors: ethanol, cyanide (bitter almond), oil of wintergreen (methyl salicylates), camphor, and hydrocarbons.

As discussed below, some compounds produce characteristic clinical pictures, such as organophosphate poisoning with pinpoint pupils, bradycardia, central nervous system depression, sweating, excessive salivation, and diarrhea. These clinical pictures are relatively easy to recognize by the experienced clinician; however, such clear clinical pictures are relatively uncommon.

Once a poisoning is suspected or confirmed, appropriate material should be sent to the laboratory for analysis. Gastric contents may contain the greatest concentration of drug but are difficult to analyze. Blood or urine should be sent for testing. The clinician should communicate to the laboratory his clinical impression of the most likely toxin to hasten identification. Usually, quantification of the poison is not necessary; identification alone is sufficient. However, serum levels are important for salicylates, acetaminophen, alcohol, carbon monoxide, organophosphates, iron, dilantin, theophylline, digoxin, and barbiturates.

Minimizing absorption of toxin

This may be the most important step in preventing a minor ingestion from leading to a serious intoxication. Early, efficient measures to prevent or limit the absorption of the toxin are essential.

Gastric emptying. If a poison has been ingested, evacuation of the stomach should be achieved unless there are specific contraindications for doing so, such as ingestion of caustics (acids or alkalis) or ingestion of a petroleum distillate having a low surface tension. Gastric evacuation should be attempted up to 24 hours after ingestion, although it will be most effective if performed within 4 hours.

Numerous studies have shown that induction of emesis is more effective than lavage in evacuation of the stomach. The method of choice is syrup of Ipecac in a dose of 10 ml for the child under 1 year, 15 ml for the 1 to 5-year-old, and 15 to 30 ml for the child over 5 or the adolescent. It should be administered with 240 ml of fluid, followed by motion of the child. It can be repeated in 30 minutes if no emesis occurs and is over 90% effective in inducing vomiting. Apomorphine is a potent parenteral drug used to induce vomiting, but probably should not be used because of the risk of respiratory depression and protracted vomiting after its use.

If the child is comatose, lacks a gag reflex, or is having seizures, gastric lavage should be performed after endotracheal intubation with a cuffed tube. The largest nasogastric tube that can be passed should be used to ensure adequate evacuation, especially of undissolved pills. The lavage should be performed using 0.45 normal saline until clear, usually requiring 10 to 12 passes or approximately 2 liters of fluid.

Activated charcoal. Further retardation of toxin absorption can be produced in most cases through the use of activated charcoal. It is an odorless, tasteless, fine, black residue from distillation of wood pulp that prevents absorption of drugs from the gastrointestinal tract by binding to its surface. There are no contraindications to its use, but it is ineffective for iron, lead, alcohol, hydrocarbons, and corrosives. It should not be given *before* Ipecac because it will inactivate the emetic. It is most effective if given within the first few hours after ingestion. Burnt toast as a substitute is ineffective, as is "universal antidote." The recommended dose of activated charcoal is 5 to 10 times the dose of the poison. For a child, a minimum of 20 g should be given; for an adolescent or adult, 50 to 100 g. The activated charcoal should be mixed with water to make a slurry and then taken orally or by means of a nasogastric tube. Recent studies have shown that multiple oral doses of activated charcoal enhanced the nonrenal excretion of phenobarbital given intravenously by adsorption through the gastrointestinal tract.

Catharsis. Laxatives may decrease the rate of absorption by increasing gastrointestinal excretion of the poison and the poison-activated charcoal complex. The cathartics generally recommended are sodium sulfate, 250 mg/kg orally up to 30 g/dose; magnesium sulfate at the same dose, or magnesium citrate, 4 ml/kg up to 300 ml/dose. The cathartic may be repeated every 1 to 2 hours as long as bowel sounds are present until there is passage per rectum of the activated charcoal. Patients with renal failure should not be given saline cathartics.

Hastening rate of excretion

Numerous methods have been used to increase the rate of excretion of poisons from the body. Of these, only diuresis, dialysis, and hemoperfusion are useful, and then only if the risks of the procedure are significantly outweighed by the expected benefits or if the recovery of the patient is seriously in doubt.

Diuresis is the most common method used for poisons that are excreted, at least in part, by the renal route. Forced diuresis by fluid administration alone may result in increased excretion but can be greatly enhanced through the use of diuretics such as furosemide (1 mg/kg/dose). Osmotic diuresis through the use of mannitol or urea will be most effective, because it blocks tubular reabsorption of the drug. Urine flow should be 3 to 5 times normal for children and 12 L/24 hours for adolescents and adults. Decreased renal function, pulmonary edema, cerebral edema, and hypotension are obvious contraindications to osmotic diuresis.

Ionized diuresis is another method used to increase excretion of certain chemicals. It relies on the fact that the drug in the ionized form will be trapped in the tubule and not be reabsorbed. Alkalinization of the urine for poisoning by weak acids such as salicylates or barbiturates can be achieved by the use of $NaHCO_3$, 1 to 2 mg/kg given intravenously over a 1 to 2 hour period to achieve a urine pH of 8.0 or greater. Acid diuresis may enhance the excretion of weak bases such as amphetamines. This can be achieved through the use of ammonium chloride, 2.75 mg/kg/dose orally every 6 hours until the urine pH is 5.0 or less.

Dialysis may be necessary for certain severe cases of poisoning. The expected duration of coma should be prolonged, other pathways of excretion unavailable, and clinical deterioration present. The toxicity of the drug should correlate with the plasma level, and the drug should be membrane permeable. Hemodialysis is the most effective method of dialysis but poses serious risks of its own to the patient. Peritoneal dialysis is more readily available and much safer, especially in the small child. Exchange transfusion may be used, particularly in the small infant, to rapidly reduce the level of a toxin.

Providing supportive care

Supportive and symptomatic care are the mainstays of treatment of the poisoned patient. In the search for specific antidotes and methods to increase excretion of the drug, attention to vital functions must not be neglected to the detriment of the patient.

Establishment of adequate respiratory exchange and maintenance of circulation are, as in the management of any patient, of first importance. Many poisons are respiratory depressants. Inadequate ventilation should be treated by endotracheal intubation, oxygen, and assisted ventilation. Hypotension or shock should be treated in the usual fashion with intravenous volume expansion. Vasopressors may be necessary for hypotension unresponsive to volume load.

Other components of supportive care include the management of seizures with valium or barbiturates, prevention of aspiration through evacuation of the stomach and use of a cuffed endotracheal tube, and prevention of cerebral edema through the use of steroids and hypertonic solutions.

Acid-base, fluid, electrolytes, and blood glucose should be monitored for derangements in these parameters. Hypoglycemia in poisonings such as ethanol or salicylate ingestion is uncommon but must be treated if damage to the patient is to be prevented.

Using antidotes

Few poisons have specific antidotes. The search for and use of an antidote should never replace good supportive care.

Antidotes are either local or systemic. As mentioned above, activated charcoal is an effective local antidote for most poisonings. Water or milk can be used as local antidotes for acids and caustics. Calcium as a gluconate, lactate, or in milk is an effective local antidote for fluoride poisoning. Sodium bicarbonate and deferoxamine are used for iron ingestion. Specific systemic antidotes will be described below for the poisonings discussed. Others are physostigmine (2 mg for adults, 0.5 mg for children intravenously) for anticholinergics, 100% O_2 for carbon monoxide, dimercaprol or calcium disodium EDTA for heavy metals (except iron), ethanol for methanol, Naloxone (0.005 to 0.01 mg/kg intravenously every 2 to 3 minutes) for narcotics, and diphenhydramine (0.5-1.0 mg/kg intramuscularly or intravenously) for phenothiazines.

Recently, successful treatment of life-threatening digitalis intoxication with digoxin-specific Fab antibody fragments has been reported. The antibody fragments appear to act at the cellular level to reverse the toxicity. With the advent of monoclonal antibodies, this general approach may prove very useful in the treatment of serious intoxications in the future.

Salicylate poisoning

Salicylates are the most frequently involved drug poisoning in children in the United States. Safety packaging has decreased ingestions by 40% to 45%; nevertheless, 300 to 400 children die each year of salicylate intoxication. At present, more than 80% of the fatal cases have occurred as the result of therapeutic overdoses, primarily in small children. Intoxication may follow the nonintentional ingestion of a single large dose of aspirin, sodium salicylate, or methyl salicylate (oil of wintergreen), or it may follow repeated small therapeutic doses of aspirin, particularly in febrile and dehydrated children. In the latter instance, the symptoms of salicylism are superimposed on the syndrome of the underlying disease and may be deceptive. Methyl salicylate usually causes severe poisoning because of its concentrated salicylate concentration (1 teaspoon equals twelve 5-grain aspirin tablets).

Pathophysiology and clinical manifestations. The signs and symptoms of salicylate intoxication are related to direct central nervous system respiratory center stimulation, uncoupling of oxidative phosphorylation and inhibition of glucose metabolism by the Krebs cycle, increased tissue glycolysis, interference with hemostasis, and later, central nervous system depression, coma, respiratory failure, and circulatory collapse.

Stimulation of the central nervous system respiratory center is universally present early in the course of salicylate intoxication and results in hyperpnea, decreased P_{CO_2}, and respiratory alkalosis. In this early phase, renal compensation occurs with excretion of bicarbonate and concomitant loss of sodium and potassium.

Salicylates also uncouple oxidative phosphorylation. The result is inefficient use of energy substrates such as glucose, increased tissue glycolysis, increased oxygen consumption and CO_2 production, and increased heat generation. Salicylates increase the formation of ketone bodies, β-hydroxybutarate, acetoacetate and acetone and increase the plasma levels of free amino acids. As a result there is a generalized aminoaciduria and predisposition to hypoglycemia.

In infants and children under the age of 4 the resulting accumulation of organic acids leads to a metabolic acidosis and is often already developed when the patient is first seen by a physician. Metabolic acidosis is especially likely to be seen in instances of chronic overdosage of salicylates, or when more than 12 hours has elapsed since acute ingestion of a single large overdose. The acid-base disturbance is thus a mixed respiratory alkalosis and metabolic acidosis, with varying degrees of compensation. An individual patient's status can only be determined by measurement of blood pH and bicarbonate concentration.

Salicylate intoxication commonly results in depletion of fluid and electrolytes. Water loss is increased through insensible pulmonary loss, sweating and hyperthermia, and an osmotic diuresis from the organic acidemia. The water loss may amount to 4 to 6 liters per square meter in severe intoxication. Renal loss of sodium and potassium accompanies the organic acidemia; loss of bicarbonate occurs during the initial respiratory alkalosis.

The altered glucose metabolism may result in hypoglycemia, normoglycemia, or hyperglycemia. Hyperglycemia is frequently seen early but may progress on to hypoglycemia with depletion of glucose stores.

Salicylates have important effects on hemostasis. These include decreased prothrombin formation, increased capillary fragility, decreased platelet adhesiveness, and decreased platelet levels.

Principal causes of morbidity in salicylate intoxication are central nervous system dysfunction, cardiac dysfunction, and pulmonary edema. Central nervous system manifestations vary from lethargy to seizures and coma, and are related to the central nervous system salicylate concentration. Congestive failure is related to acidosis, potassium depletion, and impaired myocardial metabolism. Pulmonary edema related to fluid retention or fluid overload is a late finding.

Laboratory data. As mentioned, determination of blood pH as well as serum electrolytes is mandatory. Serum calcium and glucose should also be measured. The quantitative measurement of serum salicylate levels provides the definitive diagnostic test and is indicated in all cases of suspected salicylate intoxication. The level per se correlates poorly with the severity of intoxication; symptoms are determined instead by the magnitude of the peak level and the rapidity of decline. For acute intoxication a nomogram developed by Done correlates severity of symptoms with serum salicylate concentration (Fig. 12-1). The serum level plotted on the nomogram should be obtained no earlier than

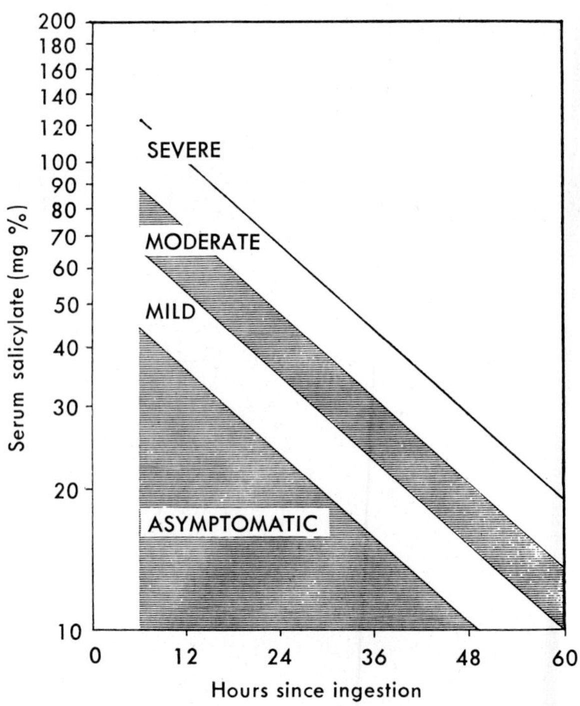

Fig. 12-1. Nomogram relating serum salicylate concentration and expected severity of intoxication at varying intervals after the ingestion of a single dose of salicylate. (From Done, A.K.: Pediatrics **26:**800, 1960.)

6 hours after the ingestion; earlier levels may not reflect the peak salicylate concentration. Alternatively, two levels can be plotted, obtained at different times to ascertain if the concentration is falling and to confirm the location on the graph. In the absence of salicylate levels the following formula provides a rough approximation of serum level: Serum level =

$$\frac{\text{Amount ingested in milligrams}}{60\% \text{ of body weight in kilograms}} \times 100.$$

An acute ingestion of 150 to 200 mg/kg usually causes symptoms.

In persons who have chronic salicylate intoxication, the serum level bears little relationship to the severity of symptoms and the nomogram *should not be used*. One should rely on the clinical picture.

Treatment. Initial treatment should be as described above, including gastric removal, catharsis, and administration of activated charcoal.

Initial intravenous fluids should be given to correct shock and establish adequate urine flow. After urine flow is established, one half to one third normal saline with 3 to 4 mEq of potassium/kg/day should be given at a rate of 3 to 5 liters/M^2/24 hours. Adequate replacement of potassium losses is necessary to correct the acidosis.

Some authors suggest alkalinizing the urine to enhance excretion of salicylate. However, a urine pH above 7.5 would be required to sufficiently increase renal clearance of salicylate. The large amount of sodium bicarbonate necessary to alkalinize urine to this point poses a serious threat of significant systemic alkalosis and therefore is not indicated in the poisoned patient. Potassium replenishment is more effective in correcting the acidosis and alkalinizing the urine than is administration of alkali. However, if the blood pH is less than 7.20, acute use of buffer may be necessary.

In patients with severe salicylate poisoning (coma, seizures, pulmonary edema), or in whom the removal of salicylate by the kidney is impaired, other procedures to remove salicylates may be indicated. Peritoneal dialysis offers the most readily available alternative. Because salicylate is protein-bound, dialysis is most effective employing a solution with 5% albumin (Albuminisol). Concentrations of glucose and electrolytes can be altered as indicated by the clinical condition of the patient.

Hemodialysis is highly effective but rarely indicated. Exchange transfusions should not be used; peritoneal dialysis is more effective and safer.

Acetaminophen poisoning

Acetaminophen is a safe and effective antipyretic/analgesic for children. Unlike aspirin, chronic poisoning with acetaminophen appears not to occur as a result of noncumulative kinetics. Nevertheless, acetaminophen is now one of the five most common drugs ingested by small children, and one of the ten most common drugs used in suicide attempts by adolescents and young adults. Differences in metabolism, however, in the two groups appear to be responsible for major differences in the incidence of toxicity.

Pathophysiology and clinical signs. Acetaminophen is rapidly absorbed from the gastrointestinal tract, with peak plasma levels occurring within 60 to 120 minutes after ingestion of tablet form and as rapidly as 30 minutes after liquid form of the drug. Acetaminophen is metabolized in the liver primarily by conjugation with glucuronide or sulfate and excreted into the urine. Approximately 4% of a dose is metabolized by means of the cytochrome P-450–mixed oxygenase system to a reactive metabolite, acetamidoquinone. This metabolite is normally conjugated with glutathione and excreted as a mercapturate conjugate.

In infants and children under 9 to 12 years of age, acetaminophen is mostly sulfate-conjugated; after this time it is predominantly glucuronide conjugated. This may explain why children under this age who take large overdoses rarely have serious toxicity. However, in adolescents and adults, when a very large overdose occurs and more than 70% of the available glutathione is used to detoxify the metabolite acetamidoquinone, this metabolite bonds to the hepatocyte macromolecules and causes hepatic necrosis. This hepatic damage is the major source of morbidity and mortality in acetaminophen overdose.

During the first 12 to 24 hours after ingestion there are nonspecific signs of nausea, vomiting, anorexia, and diaphoresis. Central nervous system depression does not occur. For many patients, symptoms of acetaminophen toxicity never progress beyond this point. However, if toxicity does ensue, during the next 1 to 4 days there is a latent phase accompanied by asymptomatic rises in liver enzymes and bilirubin, and prolongation of the prothrombin time as hepatic necrosis ensues. By 3 to 5 days after ingestion the 2% to 4% of patients with hepatic damage will manifest signs related to liver failure. Recovery, even from severe hepatoxicity, is usually complete with no residual liver functional or histologic abnormalities.

Laboratory data. Treatment of acetaminophen toxicity has been predicated on obtaining accurate plasma levels of the drug and plotting it on the nomogram developed by Rumack and colleagues at the Rocky Mountain Poison Center (Fig. 12-2). It is generally recommended that the lower line of the nomogram, plotted 25%

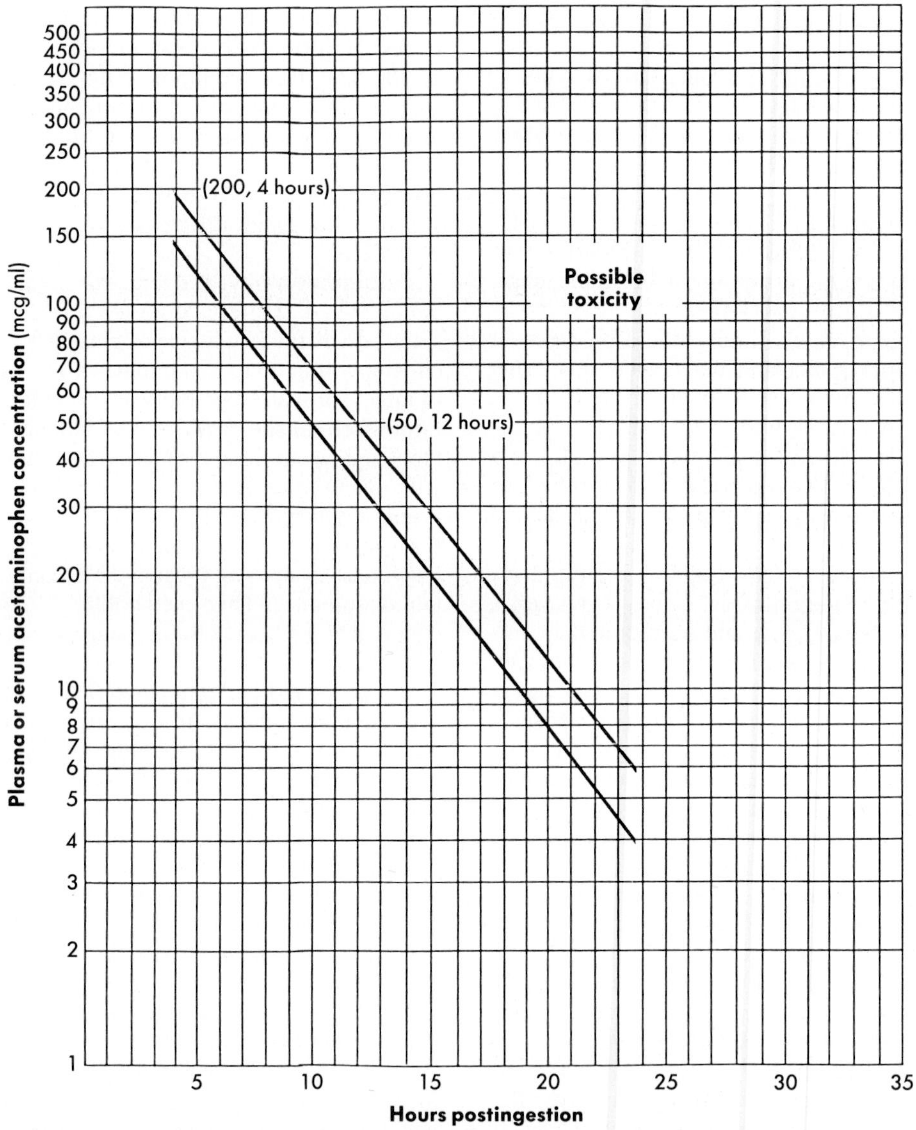

Fig. 12-2. Nomogram developed by Rumack and colleagues for use in plotting plasma levels of acetaminophen. (From Rumack, B., and Matthew, H.: Acetaminophen poisoning and toxicity, Pediatrics **55:**871-876, 1975. Copyright American Academy of Pediatrics 1975.)

below the toxicity line, be used to make treatment decisions, allowing for a margin of error. The acetaminophen assay should be delayed until at least 4 hours have elapsed since the ingestion to assure that peak acetaminophen levels have been reached. If the time from ingestion is less than 4 hours, then a second assay should be done *at least* 4 hours after ingestion.

Baseline liver function tests should be obtained on admission and repeated at 24-hour intervals until at least 96 hours have elapsed.

Treatment. Gastric emptying by Ipecac or lavage should be performed. However, activated charcoal and cathartics should *not* be used if use of the antidote, N-acetylcysteine, is anticipated because these may interfere with its effectiveness.

If the plasma levels plotted on the nomogram fall above the toxic line, indicating that hepatic damage is likely, treatment should be initiated with N-acetylcysteine (Mucomyst) orally. Mucomyst acts by replenishing the hepatic stores of glutathione or by serving as a glutathione surrogate that combines directly with the reactive metabolites and thus prevents hepatic damage. It must be started within 16 hours to be most effective. Therapy is initiated with a loading dose of 140 mg/kg orally followed by 70 mg/kg every 4 hours over a period of 68 hours (i.e., 17 maintenance doses). If the patient vomits a dose within 1 hour of dosing, repeat the dose. The 20% solution of Mucomyst is diluted with cola, juice, or water to a 5% solution and taken orally or through nasogastric tube. The oral route achieves higher hepatic levels than the intravenous route. Treatment of acetaminophen ingestion with Mucomyst should be nearly completely effective if begun within 24 hours of ingestion.

Petroleum distillate ingestions

Ingestion of petroleum products accounts for approximately 5% of nonintentional ingestions in children under 5 years of age and are responsible for significant morbidity and mortality. With the increase in sale of kerosene space heaters, the frequency of these poisonings may actually increase in the years ahead.

Pathophysiology and clinical manifestations. Toxicity from hydrocarbons is related to any or all of the following reactions: (1) pneumonia, (2) central nervous system toxicity, and (3) visceral involvement with gastrointestinal symptoms, myocardiopathy, and renal and liver toxicity.

Toxicity of these compounds is related to their viscosity. Generally, products with high viscosity and low volatility, such as mineral oil, motor oil, household oil, grease, or liquid petrolatum, are not toxic when ingested. However, products with a low surface tension, low viscosity, and high volatility have a high risk of causing pulmonary symptoms. These include gasoline, kerosene, mineral seal oil (the major ingredient of furniture polishes), mineral spirits, and naptha. Halogenated hydrocarbons (trichlorethylene, carbon tetrachloride) and aromatic hydrocarbons (toluene, xylene, benzene) are likely to cause systemic toxicity apart from pulmonary involvement.

The pulmonary involvement after hydrocarbon ingestion is not a result of gastrointestinal absorption of the chemical, but rather of aspiration, inhalation during deglutition and spread from the hypopharynx into the contiguous airway. Little or no pulmonary damage occurs when these compounds are directly instilled into the stomachs of animals in which aspiration is prevented by ligation of the esophagus. Hydrocarbons in the lungs appear to cause a diffuse, acute alveolitis, necrotizing bronchopneumonia, and interstitial inflammation. This lasts from 3 to 10 days and may be followed by a more chronic inflammation that gradually resolves over a period of several weeks. The ventilation perfusion abnormalities seen may also be caused by surfactant damage, leading to alveolar collapse and early distal airway closure.

Up to 40% of patients with hydrocarbon ingestion will have pulmonary involvement. Children who have ingested furniture polish or lighter fluid are especially likely to have symptoms and x-ray findings. Most children initially have a burning sensation in the mouth and throat, followed by gagging, choking, and coughing. If there is significant drug involvement, the child will usually become tachypneic and febrile. Respiratory symptoms usually progress during the first 24 hours of hospitalization, plateau, and subside between the second and fifth days.

Symptoms of central nervous system depression vary in severity and include generalized weakness, hypotonia, dizziness or confusion, coma, and convulsions.

Laboratory data. With pulmonary involvement, the chest x-ray initially shows perihilar densities extending into the midlung fields. These may coalesce to produce an x-ray picture of consolidation; pleural effusion may also develop. Pneumatoceles and cysts have been observed after hydrocarbon ingestion. The x-ray abnormalities reach their maximum by 72 hours and usually clear within a few days, but occasionally persist for weeks.

Arterial blood gases usually demonstrate hypoxemia with a normal or low P_{CO_2}.

Treatment. The management of the patient with hydrocarbon pneumonia must be tempered by the fact that such ingestion is generally not serious. In a study by Anas et al. of 950 children with a history of hydrocarbon ingestion, almost 90% required no treatment at all. In their series, 12% required hospitalization, 8% were symptomatic, 2% showed progression during hospitalization, and 0.2% died. Further, the duration of hospitalization is usually short, with a mean of 3 days.

The patient's clinical course over the first 6 to 8 hours after ingestion is the best predictor of subsequent severity and the need for hospitalization. The vast majority of patients who remain asymptomatic during this period will not need hospitalization, regardless of the x-ray findings. Conversely, symptoms appearing during the first 6 to 8 hours indicate the group who are likely to remain symptomatic and need hospitalization.

The child ingesting petroleum distillates should not be made to vomit, nor given any medications such as activated charcoal which might induce vomiting. Nevertheless, up to 40% of symptomatic children will spontaneously vomit.

On the other hand, many authorities recommend that in the case of ingestion of aromatic hydrocarbons or hydrocarbons with toxic additives, gastric evacuation should be performed. The best method of evacuation in these circumstances has not been determined, but may be lavage.

Treatment of hydrocarbon pneumonia is basically supportive care. Adrenal corticosteroids in hydrocarbon pneumonia have been associated with increased morbidity and should not be used. Antibiotics in controlled trials have not been shown to decrease the duration or severity of symptoms.

Iron poisoning

Iron poisoning is an extremely important cause of serious intoxications in children. The widespread use of iron and vitamin preparations and nutrient supplements presents a frequent threat to small children. Ferrous sulfate is the product most widely prescribed and the one most commonly involved in serious iron poisoning in children. Serious hazards also exist from the iron contained in prenatal vitamins and children's chewable vitamins. As little as 30 mg/kg of elemental iron can cause toxicity. Since 1978, the Consumer Product Safety Commission has required all medications containing more than 250 mg of elemental iron to be packaged in child-resistant containers.

Pathophysiology and clinical manifestations. The toxicity of iron is related to *local* effects on the gastrointestinal mucosa and *systemic* effects related to toxic levels of free iron in the circulation. Large quantities of iron are locally highly corrosive, ulcerating the gastric and intestinal mucosa from duodenum to rectum and occasionally resulting in perforations.

Iron ingestions saturate the iron-binding mechanisms of plasma and release large quantities of free iron into the circulation. This iron overloads the Kupffer cells of the liver, acts as a mitochondrial poison, and causes hepatic necrosis. Shock ensues by mechanisms not yet well established, but that may include hypovolemia, release of endogenous vasodilators, and direct vasodepressant effect on the circulation.

Classically, the toxicity of iron overdose is divided into four clinical phases. In the first 30 to 60 minutes after ingestion the signs and symptoms are related to the direct effect on the gastrointestinal mucosa, with vomiting and diarrhea (bloody in about 10% of cases). With severe intoxication this can progress on to acidemia, hypovolemia, and shock.

The second phase begins 6 to 8 hours after ingestion and lasts for 8 to 24 hours. During this phase, symptoms seem to abate.

In untreated patients with large ingestions, a third phase ensues that can have high mortality. There is severe liver injury and failure, central nervous system involvement with coma, and possibly convulsions and circulatory collapse with unresponsive shock. Survival of this third phase can result in gastric scarring and contracture, with pyloric obstruction during the 4 weeks or longer of the fourth phase of iron toxicity.

Laboratory data. Prompt and appropriate laboratory tests are key to the successful management of patients with a history of iron ingestion. The amount of drug ingested is difficult to determine by history. Fortunately, serum iron levels have been shown to correlate quite well with the probability of developing serious toxicity. A serum iron level greater than 350 μg/dl within 4 to 6 hours of ingestion or a serum iron level exceeding the total iron-binding capacity by 50 μg/dl indicates severe poisoning and the need for chelation therapy.

Other tests may also be done to determine the risk of ingestion and the presence of free iron in the circulation. A qualitative deferoxamine color test can be performed on the gastric aspirate to confirm iron ingestion. Two milliliters of gastric aspirate are mixed with two drops of 30% H_2O_2, to which is added 60 mg of deferoxamine. Iron present in the gastric aspirate will turn the solution a color from light orange to dark red.

The need for chelation therapy can be assessed by performing a chelation challenge test. Deferoxamine 15 mg/kg in 50 to 100 ml of 5% dextrose in water is given intravenously over 1 hour. A red color in the urine indicates free iron in the serum and a need for further chelation.

Other studies have been shown to correlate well with a serum iron greater than 300 μg/dl. A white blood cell count greater than 15,000/mm^3 or a blood glucose level greater than 150 mg/dl have a very high predictive value for serum iron over 300 μg/dl.

The abdominal radiograph has also been advocated as useful in identifying intact iron-containing pills. However, metals other than iron will be radioopaque, and dissolved iron tablets will usually not be visible on radiographs.

Treatment. Most patients with iron ingestion will be asymptomatic on arrival. Lovejoy and colleagues have found that the presence of vomiting has a 94% sensitivity for the presence of serious iron ingestion. Diarrhea is also quite sensitive for serious ingestion. Conversely, patients who remain asymptomatic for 6 hours after iron ingestion may be discharged with minimal risk of having a serum iron level over 300 μg/dl.

Patients with iron ingestion require gastric emptying. In those with signs of serious toxicity it is recommended that gastric lavage be performed with 1.5% bicarbonate solution, in the hopes of precipitating free iron and minimizing gastric damage. Previous recommendations of using a diluted Fleet's enema solution for lavage have led to serious hypertonic phosphate poisoning and should be discouraged. More recent recommendations are to add deferoxamine to a concentration of 2 g/l to the lavage fluid and leave a postlavage bolus of 10 grams of deferrioxamine in the stomach.

Chelation therapy with deferoxamine is indicated in any patient with a known ingestion of 25 mg/kg of elemental iron, or a serum iron greater than 350 μg/dl at 4 to 6 hours after ingestion, or a serum iron more than 50 μg/dl greater than the total iron-binding capacity of the serum. For children in shock and for those with severe poisoning the intravenous route is preferred at a dose of 15 mg/kg/hr (maximum daily dose—360 mg/kg). For those with less severe toxicity, the intramuscular route should be used because it is associated with less risk of hypotension (20 mg/kg every 4 to 8 hours). Treatment is continued until the urine color is clear and the serum iron level has returned to normal. Adequate fluid must be administered to maintain renal function. In the face of inadequate renal function, peritoneal dialysis or hemodialysis is feasible because the iron-deferoxamine complex is dialyzable.

If radiographs of the abdomen reveal iron tablets that have not been removed by lavage or emesis, operative removal by endoscopy or gastrostomy is indicated.

Organophosphates

Organophosphates are currently in widespread use throughout the world for eradication of soft-bodied insects. They are among the most poisonous substances commonly used for pest control and are a frequent source of serious poisoning in children in both rural and urban settings. The organophosphates are absorbed through the skin, lungs, conjunctivae, and gastrointestinal tract. Severe symptoms can occur from absorption by any route.

A large number of organophosphate preparations are used as pesticides. Those of moderate toxicity, requiring relatively large doses, are malathion, DDVP, EPN, dilbrom, and diazinon. Others are highly toxic: parathion, ethion, methyl parathion, demeton, and octamethyl pyrophosphoramide. Although the *mean* lethal dose for parathion is approximately 4 mg/kg, as little as 10 to 20 mg can be lethal to an adult, and 2 mg (.1 mg/kg) to a child. Toxicity is affected by the route of absorption. In decreasing order of toxicity, these are the eye, where one drop may produce severe symptoms, the lung (inhalation), the gastrointestinal tract, and the skin.

Pathophysiology and clinical manifestations. The toxicity of the organophosphates is related to their ability to inhibit the enzyme cholinesterase in all parts of the body by phosphorylation of the active site of the enzyme. This leads to local accumulations of acetylcholine, which in low concentrations acts as an excitatory substance and in high concentrations is paralytic.

Acetylcholine is the neurohormone responsible for physiologic transmission of nerve impulses from: (1) preganglionic to postganglionic neurons of both the parasympathetic and sympathetic nervous system, (2) postganglionic parasympathetic fibers to effector organs, (3) postganglionic sympathetic fibers to sweat glands, (4) motor nerves to skeletal muscle, and (5) some nerve endings in the central nervous system. Therefore the clinical manifestations of organophosphate poisoning might include any or all of the following major symptoms and signs: pinpoint pupils, excessive lacrimation, excessive salivation, bronchorrhea, bronchospasm and expiratory wheezing, hyperperistalsis producing abdominal cramps and diarrhea, bradycardia, excessive sweating, fasiculations and weakness of the skeletal muscles, convulsions, and coma.

The time of onset and severity of symptoms depend on the route of entry and total dose received. Toxic signs and symptoms develop most rapidly after inhalation and slowest after skin absorption. In severe cases the onset of symptoms is extremely rapid; without treatment death occurs within 24 hours. Death is typically caused by respiratory failure based on some combination of excessive bronchial secretions, bronchospasm, and paralysis of the muscles of respiration or paralysis of the central respiratory center. In mild cases of exposure, failure to develop signs within 6 hours indicates a low likelihood of subsequent problems.

With a history of exposure the diagnosis should be made without difficulty. However, in the absence of such a history the diagnosis may not be at all apparent. The triad of miosis, bradycardia, and muscle fasiculations should suggest the possibility of organophosphate poisoning and warrants a therapeutic trial of the antidotes discussed below.

Laboratory data. Confirmation of the diagnosis can be achieved by measurement of the red blood cell cholinesterase activity or the enzyme pseudocholinesterase produced by the liver and found in the plasma. Clinical toxicity is usually seen only after a 50% reduction in enzyme activity. The blood sugar concentration should also be monitored because hyperglycemia and glucosuria may occur.

Treatment. In the management of a patient with organophosphate poisoning, care must be taken not to contaminate medical personnel. Staff should wear gloves, masks, and aprons to protect themselves against contaminated clothing, skin, or gastric fluid of the patient.

If the poison has been ingested, gastric lavage or emesis should be performed, followed by activated charcoal and cathartics. In the case of skin contamination the patient should be washed with copious amounts of water and alcohol.

Supportive therapy should include maintenance of an airway and adequate ventilation, and establishment of an intravenous line.

The pharmacologic management of organophosphate intoxication relies on the administration of atropine and pralidoxime. Atropine is a physiologic antidote. It has no effect on inhibited cholinesterase but it does block the actions of acetylcholine on parasympathetic receptors. It thus alleviates bronchospasm and reduces bronchial secretions and miosis. However, atropine has no effect on the flaccid muscle paralysis or the central respiratory failure of severe poisoning. Atropine is indicated in *all* symptomatic patients and can be used as a diagnostic aid. It should be given intravenously and in large doses: 0.05 to 0.1 mg/kg to children and 2 to 5 mg for adolescents and young adults. It should be repeated at 5 to 10 minute intervals until signs of atropinization appear, as indicated by clearing of bronchial secretions and pulmonary rales. Therapy may require large doses over a period of several days until all absorbed organophosphate is metabolized.

For severe poisonings, characterized by reduction of cholinesterase activity to less than 20% of normal and profound weakness, restoration of enzyme activity is necessary. PAM (2-pyridine aldoxamine methiodide, pralidoxime iodide) or the pralidoxime chloride salt Protopam break the covalent bond between the cholinesterase and the organophosphate. The phosphate-colinesterase binding is initially reversible but gradually becomes irreversible; therapy with PAM or Protopam thus must be prompt. The drug should be given at a dose of 25 to 50 mg/kg intravenously over 5 to 20 minutes. If muscle weakness persists or recurs, the dose may be repeated after 1 hour, and again, if needed. Both atropine and PAM or Protopam should be given together; PAM or Protopam should not be given alone. In symptomatic organophosphate poisoning, use of barbituates, phenothiazones, theophylline, or opiates is *contraindicated.*

NONTOXIC INGESTIONS

The majority of ingestions by children are of nontoxic substances. Some are handled by parents at home; many come to the attention of the local poison control center. The list below can serve as a reference for the physician when confronted by a patient or parent with such an ingestion.

Abrasives
Adhesives (most)
Ballpoint pen inks
Bathtub floating toys
Bath oil
Battery (dry cell)
Bubble bath soaps
Candles (beeswax or paraffin)
Chalk
Cosmetics
Clay (modeling)
Crayons with AP, CP or CS 130-46 designation
Cigarettes or cigars
Caps (toy pistol)
Contraceptive pills
Dehumidifying packets
Detergents (not electric dishwasher)
Deodorants
Elmer's glue
Fish bowl additives
Fabric softeners
Hand products
Hand lotion and cream
Ink (black, blue)
Indelible markers
Incense
Lipstick
Lead pencils
Matches (book)
Mineral oil
Newspaper
Paint (indoor, latex)
Putty and silly putty
Petroleum jelly
Shampoo
Shaving cream
Sweetening agents (saccharin)
Soaps
Thermometer mercury
Toothpaste
Vitamins *(only without iron)*

Furthermore, most products swallowed by children are ingested in small amounts. The volume of a swallow has been calculated to be 0.2 ml/kg; for the child 1½ to 3 years old, the amount of one swallow is about 1 teaspoon.

Nevertheless, nontoxic ingestions should serve as warnings to the physician of the possibility of inadequate supervision or of an improper or unsafe environment. Ingestions often occur around times of family stress such as recent moves, birth of a sibling, death of a family member, or other family crisis. Intervention for these problems is as important as treatment of an ingestion.

LEAD POISONING

Lead is an extremely useful but toxic metal. The Romans and Greeks knew that lead was harmful but did little to limit their exposure through food and drink. Lead has been mined for centuries, but its dispersion in the human environment rose sharply only after the industrial revolution, and particularly since the early 1940s. Today, world lead production is 2.5 million tons per year, approximately 40% produced and nearly 50% consumed in the United States.

Concern over the possible health effects of environmental lead pollution intensified in the late 1960s after childhood lead-poisoning screening programs uncovered thousands of children with elevated blood lead levels. In the late 1960s and the early 1970s, 25% to 40% of children in inner-city slums had elevated blood lead levels. More recent data from the Centers for Disease Control seemed to indicate that this had dropped to only 5% of children screened in 1981. However, the problem appears to be still with us. Data from the National Health and Nutrition Examination Survey (NHANES), conducted between 1976 and 1980, showed that many groups continued to have a significant prevalence of elevated blood lead. Overall, 12%

of black children 6 months through 5 years old and 2% of white children had elevated blood lead values. There is a significant association with income as well: among black children in the lowest income group, nearly one fifth had elevated blood lead values.

The source of lead in these children appears to be multiple. Classically, lead-based paint has been and still is the most important "high-dose" source of lead and the most common cause of serious lead poisoning in children. One single paint flake containing 1% lead delivers an external dose of 10,000 μg. Point sources of lead emission have resulted in elevated lead exposure, principally among children living near primary or secondary lead smelters and storage battery manufacturing plants. In homes near such plants and smelters the lead content of house dust is enormously elevated (up to 100,000 parts per million). This occurs through both air pollution and exposure to clothing and shoes brought home by workers at the smelter or factory. Other sources of lead that have been postulated, although not proved, are from the burning of leaded gasoline in cars and the diet. The available evidence, however, indicates that hand-to-mouth transfer of house dust may be the major source of the more moderate degree of excessive lead exposure commonly encountered today.

Children appear to absorb higher proportions of ingested lead than do adults. Adults in a nonfasting state usually absorb 5% to 10% of ingested lead; children under 9 years of age may absorb up to 50%. Children with low-calcium diets have increased rates of lead absorption and release more lead from their bones into the blood. Experimentally, iron deficiency has been shown to increase susceptibility to lead toxicity. Similar effects have been shown as a result of diets low in protein, vitamin D, or vitamin C.

Adverse effects of lead

The major route of absorption of lead in children is the gastrointestinal tract. A single dose of lead is distributed between the blood, the bone, and the soft tissues. Owing to the inherent affinity of lead for osseous tissues, lead accumulates in bone to a much greater extent than in other tissues.

The most significant implications of the kinetic behavior of lead are its high degree of accumulation on continued exposure and its slow rate of removal when exposure ceases. In cases of long-term exposure, reduction in blood lead (PbB) is largely limited to excretion in the urine and feces. PbB is a marker of recent exposure to lead; elevations of blood lead levels in the past do not correlate well with lead levels in the present. The best measure of past exposure in lead appears to be dentine level. Lead exists in dentine in a closed storage system. Dentine lead is elevated in children with unequivocal lead poisoning, urban children living in the "lead belt," and those living in decaying homes or homes near major lead processors.

One of the most sensitive parameters of the biologic effects of lead is in the hematopoietic system. Lead affects heme synthesis in at least three ways. Aminolevulinic acid dehydratase (ALA-D) is directly inhibited, resulting in a block in utilization of ALA and in subsequent decline in heme synthesis. ALA-synthetase is derepressed, resulting in increased activity of the enzyme and increased synthesis of ALA. Finally, lead blocks the incorporation of ferrous iron into the prophyrin ring structure by inhibition of the enzyme ferrochelatase. The porphyrin chelates zinc nonenzymatically to form zinc protoporphyrin, which in turn becomes incorporated into hemoglobin. This elevation in erythrocyte protoporphyrin (EP) can be measured and provides a sensitive indicator of lead exposure.

Lead has widespread effects on other organ systems. In the kidney, lead poisoning causes an acquired Fanconi syndrome: proximal tubular dysfunction with aminoaciduria, glycosuria, and hyperphosphaturia. Early in the course of the disease these changes are reversible with treatment; continued chronic lead exposure results in progressive interstitial fibrosis.

Peripheral neuropathy is a classical manifestation of lead toxicity, particularly in adults with chronic occupational exposure. Children may also develop peripheral neuropathy, most commonly foot drop and generalized weakness.

The effects of lead poisoning on the central nervous system may occur over a wide range of blood lead levels. Historically, the only recognized central nervous system symptoms of lead poisoning were acute lead encephalopathy, but carefully done studies have documented more subtle effects at low blood lead levels as well. Acute encephalopathy occurs generally at blood levels over 80 μg/dl, manifested as reduced consciousness, seizures, coma, and death. Autopsy studies have shown this to be caused by a combination of severe cerebral edema, secondary to capillary leak, and a direct toxic effect on neurons. There is loss of neurons in the gray matter, hypothalamus, thalamus, and basal ganglia, with secondary gliosis.

Numerous studies have now pointed to the effects of lead on brain dysfunction at much lower levels than previously thought to be harmful. Psychologic impairment occurs in some otherwise asymptomatic children with repeated blood lead levels at the 40 to 80 μg/dl level. Other studies using dentine lead as an index of chronic exposure show that children with high dentine lead levels scored significantly less well on the Wechsler Intelligence Scale for Children and had more nonadaptive classroom behavior than children with lower levels of dentine lead. None of these children had overt lead poisoning. These effects on the brain may be caused by the ability of lead to inhibit neuron transmission.

Clinical features

Acute lead poisoning is rare and usually follows the ingestion of large quantities of soluble lead salts such as lead acetate or lead carbonate in a single dose. The symptoms result mainly from local irritation of the alimentary tract and include nausea, vomiting, and abdominal pain. In severe cases, leg cramps, muscle weakness, paresthesias, hemolytic anemia, coma, and death may follow. Acute poisoning resulting from the inhalation of lead oxide dust given off by the burning of battery casings produces an acute encephalopathy. This type of intoxication appears to have a better prognosis than the closely related encephalopathy of chronic plumbism described below.

Symptoms and signs of chronic lead poisoning vary. The degree of exposure, age of the child, rate of intestinal absorption of ingested lead, and rate and degree of transport of lead from bone to blood and soft tissues affect the symptomatology. The onset is insidious. Early manifestations include irritability, lethargy, weight loss, anemia, pallor, headache, sporadic vomiting, constipation, and colicky abdominal pain. Progression of lead poisoning results in severe lead encephalopathy manifested by rapidly increasing papilledema, personality and mood changes, cranial nerve palsies, cerebellar ataxia, persistent vomiting, convulsions, and stupor or coma. In such severe cases a mortality of 20% or more has been reported, and in those patients who recover from this stage, severe residual injury to the central nervous system is common. Peripheral neuropathy is rarely seen in children.

Hematologic abnormalities include hypochromic microcytic anemia, basophilic stippling, increased numbers of target cells, and red fluorescence of erythrocytes examined under ultraviolet light. Urinalysis may reveal mild glycosuria and aminoaciduria. Plain films of the abdomen may reveal radiopaque material, indicating the ingestion of foreign substances that may contain lead. Increased radiologic density at metaphyses of long bones can usually be demonstrated, chiefly at the knees and wrists. When encephalopathy is present, skull radiographs often show suture separation; the cerebrospinal fluid is under increased pressure and has a normal glucose content, an increased concentration of protein, and, less uniformly, increased numbers of cells, generally less than 100 lymphocytes/mm^3.

Diagnostic evaluation

Most children with elevated blood lead levels are now identified through screening of high-risk groups. Currently the most useful screening tests are erythrocyte protoporphyrin (EP) and blood lead (PbB) determinations. These are most commonly collected by capillary blood samples; confirmation requires venous blood determinations. These two tests represent different parameters of undue lead absorption. PbB determination is a measure of the internal dose of lead and EP determination is an indicator of adverse metabolic effect. EP determination is less subject to laboratory error and provides a better indicator of risk of lead poisoning. EP is also elevated in iron deficiency and the rare case of erythropoietic protoporphyria.

Children may be arbitrarily divided into four classes based on their EP and PbB determination results (Table 12-4). Class IV children are at urgent risk of lead poisoning and should have immediate medical evaluation within 24 hours. Class III children are at high risk. They are asymptomatic and require quick confirmation

Table 12-4. Risk classification for asymptomatic children

Test results		Erythrocyte proptoporphyrin (μg/dl whole blood)			
		≤49	50-109	110-249	≥250
Blood lead (μg/dl)	≤29	1	1a	Ia	EPP*
	30-49	1b	II	III	III
	50-69	†	III	III	IV
	≥70	†	†	IV	IV

From Centers for Disease Control: Preventing lead poisoning in young children, U.S. DHEW (PHS), Atlanta, 1978.
*EPP = Erythropoietic protoporphyria.
†Combination of results not generally observed; retest with venous blood immediately.

and more complete diagnostic evaluation. Class II children are considered at moderate risk for lead poisoning; they are usually asymptomatic and should be retested at 3-month intervals. Children in class I are considered normal, although two subgroups exist in Class I. Class Ia children have iron deficiency, and class Ib children appear to have transient, stable, or declining blood lead levels.

Confirmatory tests for children in classes III and IV and any child with symptoms include repeated venous PbB and EP determinations, and complete blood count with smear. Radiography of the abdomen may reveal radiopaque foreign material within the intestine in one third of patients, but only if such material has been ingested in the last 24 to 36 hours. Examination of the long bones for deposition of lead in the metaphyses correlates with the degree and duration of exposure.

Children in class IV or who are symptomatic should be treated and should not receive a provocative chelation test. The chelation test is useful when other tests indicate undue lead absorption but without definite poisoning. In this test, 1000 mg of CaEDTA/M^2 is injected intramuscularly in divided doses at 12-hour intervals, and urine collected for 24 hours. A ratio of lead excreted to EDTA given (μg Pb/mg CaEDTA) greater than 1 is indicative of a fivefold increase in the mobile fraction of the total body lead burden and an indication for treatment.

The test can also be modified for outpatient use. A single, intramuscular dose of 50 mg/kg of CaEDTA (maximum dose = 1000 mg) followed by a quantitative 6 to 8–hour collection of urine can be done. Under these conditions an excretion ratio (μg Pb/mg CaEDTA) greater than .5 is considered "positive."

Treatment

The major aim of therapy is the reduction of the concentration of lead in the blood and tissues. Excessive lead intake must be stopped immediately and environmental sources of lead identified. Cooperation with the social services department and public health officials is often necessary to remove the hazard from the house.

Chelation therapy is used to remove excessive body burdens of lead. Patients are usually hospitalized, at least for the initial course of chelation. For children with other signs of severe poisoning, treatment should begin with D^{10}/w (10 to 20 ml/kg) over 1 to 2 hours. If this fails to initiate urine flow, mannitol at a dose of 1 to 2 g/kg should be infused at the rate of 1 ml/minute. After urine flow has been established, fluids should be restricted to basal requirements to avoid cerebral edema. Chelation therapy is then started with 2,3-dimercapto-propanol (BAL) and CaEDTA at a dose of BAL 500 mg/M^2/24 hours and CaEDTA 1500 mg/M^2/24 hours, intramuscularly at separate sites every 4 hours for 5 days. In patients with only mild symptoms BAL may be stopped in 2 to 3 days. Monitor urinalysis daily and serum BUN, calcium, and creatinine on days 1 and 5.

After 4 to 5 days of therapy, toxicity of CaEDTA increases and the output of mobilizable lead decreases. Therapy should be discontinued on all patients for a minimum of 48 to 72 hours. The chelation is then repeated with CaEDTA alone and the urinary lead is measured. If the excretion ratio exceeds 1, the entire 5-day course is completed. As many chelations as are necessary to reduce the body burden of lead are performed, providing adequate waiting periods occur between each chelation. When the value falls to less than 1 further chelation can be deferred.

An alternative is substituting d-pencillamine in children who are old enough to comply. Although not approved by the FDA for this purpose, it has been shown to be an effective agent in reducing chronic blood lead. The drug is started at a low dose and doubled weekly until a dose of 20 to 40 mg/kg/24 hours is achieved. The child is then maintained for 3 to 6 months on this dose.

Frederick P. Rivara

REFERENCES

Anas, N., et al.: Criteria for hospitalizing children who have ingested products containing hydrocarbons, J.A.M.A. **246:**840-843, 1981.

Arena, J.M.: Poisoning, ed. 3, Springfield, Ill., 1974, Charles C Thomas, Publisher.

Berg, M.J., et al.: Acceleration of the body clearance of phenobarbital by oral activated charcoal, N. Engl. J. Med. **307:**642-644, 1982.

Berger, L.R.: Childhood injuries: recognition and prevention, Curr. Probl. Pediatr. **12:**1-59, 1981.

Bergman, A.B., editor: Preventing childhood injuries: report of the Twelfth Ross Roundtable on Critical Approaches to Common Pediatric Problems, Columbus, Ohio, 1982, Ross Laboratories.

Centers for Disease Control: Preventing lead poisoning in young children, U.S. DHEW (PHS), Atlanta, 1978.

Chisholm, J.J., and O'Hara, D.M., editors: Lead absorption in children: management, clinical and environmental aspects, Baltimore, 1982, Urban Schwarzenberg, Inc.

Clarke, A., and Walton, W.W.: Effect of safety packaging on aspirin ingestion by children, Pediatrics **63:**687, 1979.

Dietz, P.E., and Baker, S.P.: Drowning: epidemiology and prevention, Am. J. Public Health 64:303, 1974.

Done, A.K.: Aspirin overdosage: incidence, diagnosis and management, Pediatrics **62**(suppl.):890-897, 1978.

Eade, N.R., et al.: Hydrocarbon pneumonitis, Pediatrics **54:**351-357, 1974.

Feck G, et al.: An epidemiologic study of burn injuries and strategies for prevention, Atlanta, 1978, U.S. Centers for Disease Control.

Feldman, K.W., et al.: Tap water scalds in children, Pediatrics **62:**1, 1978.

Fergusson, D.M., et al.: A controlled field trial of a poisoning prevention method, Pediatrics **69:**515-520, 1982.

Gaudreault, P., et al.: The relative severity of acute versus chronic salicylate poisoning in children. A clinical comparison, Pediatrics **70:**566-569, 1982.

Gleason, M.N., et al.: Clinical toxicology of commercial products, ed. 3, Baltimore, 1969, Williams & Wilkins.

Haddon, W., and Baker, S.P.: Injury control. In Preventive and community medicine, Clark, D., and MacMahon, B., editors: Boston, 1981, Little, Brown & Co.

Insurance Institute for Highway Safety: Children in crashes, Washington, D.C., 1980, The Institute.

Insurance Institute for Highway Safety: Policy options for reducing the motor vehicle crash injury cost burden, Washington, D.C., 1981, The Institute.

Lacouture, P.G., et al.: Emergency assessment of severity in iron overdose by clinical and laboratory methods, J. Pediatr. **99:**89-91, 1981.

McLoughlin, E., et al.: Project burn prevention: outcome and implications, Am. J. Pub. Health **72:**241, 1982.

McLoughlin, E., et al.: One pediatric burn unit's experience with sleepwear-related injuries, Pediatrics **60:**405, 1977.

Mahaffey, K.R., et al.: National estimates of blood lead levels: United States, 1976, N. Engl. J. Med. **307:**573, 1982.

Mofenson, H.C., and Greensher, J.: The nontoxic ingestion, Ped. Clin. North Am. **17**(3):583-590, 1970.

National Safety Council: Accident Facts, Chicago, 1982, National Safety Council.

Needleman, H.L., et al.: Deficits in psychologic and classroom performance of children with elevated dentine lead levels, N. Engl. J. Med. **300:**689, 1979.

Newberger, E.H., et al.: Pediatric social illness: toward an etiologic classification, Pediatrics **60:**178, 1977.

Pearn, J.D., et al.: Drowning and near drowning involving children: a five year total population study from the city and county of Honolulu, Am. J. Pub. Health **69:**450, 1979.

Peterson, R.G., and Rumack, B.H.: Pharmacokinetics of acetaminophen in children, Pediatrics **62**(suppl.):877-879, 1978.

Reisinger, K.S., and Williams, A.F.: Evaluation of programs designed to increase the protection of infants in cars, Pediatrics **62:**280, 1978.

Reisinger, K.S.: Smoke detectors: reducing deaths and injuries due to fire, Pediatrics **65:**718, 1980.

Rivara, F.P.: Epidemiology of childhood injuries. I. Review of current research and presentation of conceptual framework, Am. J. Dis. Child **136:**399, 1982.

Rivara, F.P., and Stapleton, F.B.: Handguns and children: a dangerous mix, J. Dev. Behav. Pediatr. **3:**35, 1982.

Robertson, L.S.: Crash involvement of teenaged drivers when driver education is eliminated from high school, Am. J. Pub. Health **70:**599, 1980.

Robotham, J.L., and Letman, P.S.: Acute iron poisoning—a review, Am. J. Dis. Child **134:**875, 1980.

Rumack, B.H., and Peterson, R.G.: Acetaminophen overdose: incidence, diagnosis, and management in 416 patients, Pediatrics **62:**(suppl.):898-903, 1978.

Rutter, M.: Raised lead levels and impaired cognitive/behavioral functioning: a review of the evidence, Develop. Med. Child. Neurol. **22**(suppl. 42):1, 1980.

Saracino, M, et al.: The epidemiology of poisoning from drug products, Am. J. Dis. Child **134:**763-765, 1980.

Scherz, R.G.: Restraint systems for the prevention of injury to children in automobile accidents, Am. J. Pub. Health **66:**451, 1976.

Smith, T.W., et al.: Treatment of life-threatening digitalis intoxication with digoxin-specific Fab antibody fragments, Experience in 26 cases, N. Engl. J. Med. **307:**1357-62, 1982.

Temple, A.R.: Pathophysiology of aspirin overdosage toxicity, with implications for management, Pediatrics **62**(suppl.):873-876, 1978.

Venturelli, J., et al.: Gastrotomy in the management of acute iron poisoning, J. Pediatr. **100:**768-769, 1982.

Walton, W.W.: An evaluation of the Poison Prevention Packaging Act, Pediatrics **69:**363-370, 1982.

Zarvon, M.R.: Poisoning from pesticides: diagnosis and treatment, Pediatrics **54:**332-336, 1974.

13 Child Abuse and Neglect

The unfortunate human tendency toward violence, starting when Cain killed Abel, constitutes a somber page in the archives of history. The record of mankind is replete with accounts of child abuse and neglect. None is more vivid than those of Charles Dickens, epitomized in his novels *Oliver Twist* and *David Copperfield*. The severely adverse conditions under which children often lived and worked during the industrial revolution as well as the dark fate of many of Europe's children during World War II are modern examples of massive child abuse and neglect.

As is generally true of the progress of the human race, growing awareness of the worth of children, their rights, and their need for proper nurture and protection has come by fits and starts; by no means have these concepts been advanced steadily and consistently. Nevertheless, in most of the world, society's conscience in regard to children has been awakened. Like other countries the United States has become aware of the need for children to be properly nurtured, protected, and permitted to achieve their maximum potentials physically, intellectually, emotionally, and socially. However, the current incidence of child abuse and neglect constitutes a startling example of how far we have yet to go to achieve these ideals.

The immense problem of child abuse and neglect in the United States has received particular attention since 1962, when Kempe coined the phrase "the battered child syndrome." Kempe et al. (1962) reported on this problem, surveying more than 300 cases in 71 hospitals. Previously, Caffey (1946), Silverman (1953), and Woolley and Evans (1955) had called attention to various components of the syndrome. However, international recognition of the syndrome stems from Kempe's report.

There are four major facets of child abuse and neglect: (1) physical abuse, (2) mental abuse, (3) sexual abuse, and (4) neglect (physical, emotional, educational, medical, or social). Various combinations of these four aspects often exist in the individual case. A national definition of child abuse and neglect was stated in Public Law 92-247, S. 1191, of January 31, 1974:

> The term "child abuse and neglect" means the physical or mental injury, sexual abuse, negligent treatment, or maltreatment of a child under the age of eighteen by a person who is responsible for the child's welfare, under circumstances which indicate the child's health or welfare is harmed or threatened thereby.

The magnitude of the problem is difficult to assess because for every case detected and reported there are undoubtedly many others that escape recognition. It has been estimated that there are probably a million or more American children who annually suffer abuse and/or neglect. It is further estimated that, of this huge number, 60,000 children each year are seriously injured, perhaps as many as 3000 are killed, and that 20% to 30% of those repeatedly physically traumatized suffer permanent injuries, particularly of the central nervous system. Such lasting neurologic impairment may cause mental retardation, brain damage, abnormal behavior, acquired cerebral palsy, epilepsy, blindness, and other defects. In addition, it has been reported that as many as 10% to 15% of all children less than 5 years of age who are brought to emergency rooms because of trauma are actually suffering from child abuse (nonaccidental trauma).

Although physical abuse has received the greatest attention and publicity, further exploration of the total syndrome continues to reveal the high incidence of neglect, mental abuse, and sexual abuse. Cases of neglect outnumber those of physical abuse in a ratio of about 3:1. Sexual abuse occurs far more commonly than was generally suspected, is often hidden, and may elude diagnosis. Mental abuse is extremely common and may exist as an isolated component of the abuse and neglect syndrome or in association with one of the other elements, such as physical abuse.

ETIOLOGY

Child abuse and neglect occur in all strata of society. They are not limited to any particular race, cultural or educational background, or socioeconomic status. However, they are detected and reported far more often in families who are economically and socially underprivileged. The probable reasons for this are that such families more frequently take their children for medical care to public or university hospitals, emergency rooms, or clinics, where greater knowledge of child abuse and neglect and a higher index of suspicion prevail than is commonly found in the offices of private physicians or private community hospitals; and poorer families generally suffer from a greater degree of chronic stress and an increased frequency of intercurrent crises. Furthermore, under the close relationships that often exist in the private practice setting, the physician may find it difficult to believe that the parents—often well-educated, personable, and apparently "good" parents—could be guilty of abuse and neglect. Even if this is believed to be true, there is a reluctance to report the milder cases and a tendency to take necessary protective action only when abuse and neglect are flagrant.

Certain well-known high-risk factors set the stage for child abuse and neglect. Chief among them is the psychologic makeup of the parents, described in more detail later. The great majority of abusive or neglectful parents have themselves been abused and neglected as children. They learn patterns of abuse and neglect early in life and subsequently have a striking tendency to marry individuals who grew up in similar circumstances. Such spouses more readily accept abuse and neglect in the family and to a high degree do not give psychologic support to the abusive marital partner when crises and tensions arise. Childhood experiences of abuse and neglect have instilled in such parents feeling of unworthiness and rejection, often combined with underlying hostility. Very importantly, early in life they have lost basic trust in people and are unable to establish warm, friendly relationships within the family or in their neighborhood, school, church, business, and social contacts. They become isolated and withdrawn and develop social clumsiness to the degree that they are incapable of reaching out to others when under stress. As crises and tensions arise and frustration and irritation increase, they find no help from others and may finally erupt in violence toward the child. Thus the self-perpetuating vicious circle of child abuse is observed: abused and neglected children growing up to become abusive and neglectful parents who in turn produce a new generation of children who subsequently abuse and neglect their children.

There are numerous other high-risk factors, including unwanted pregnancies, premarital pregnancies, forced marriages, pregnancies in the early teen years, pregnancies characterized by illness or other abnormalities, difficult deliveries, and the birth of a premature or physically or mentally handicapped baby. Another factor of high interest is the rigid separation of premature or ill newborn infants from their parents, especially the mother. A particular example is an infant placed in the intensive care nursery whose parents are not permitted to visit the baby or touch and hold him to establish the paternal- and maternal-infant bonding so important to warm, loving acceptance of the child. Even if such a separation is for only a short time, proper bonding may not take place. Recognition of the need for bonding is the chief basis for the recent more liberalized visiting privileges of parents of newborn babies.

Situational high-risk factors also include poverty with its associated chronic tensions and crises, ethnic and social isolation, single-parent homes, broken marriages, and disintegration of the family so that mutually supportive relationships between family members and close relatives are lacking. Indeed, in the child abuse and neglect field one is continually impressed with the tenuous and often nonexistent relationships between members of the extended family.

Thus it is clear that three major factors interrelate to cause child abuse and neglect: (1) the nature of the parents, (2) the child, and (3) chronic tensions and intermittent crises that trigger violence or neglect.

Characteristics of abusive parents

Parents who abuse and neglect their children have been studied by psychologists and psychiatrists to discover what unique psychologic characteristics they possess that predispose them to abusive and neglectful behavior. Although much of the investigation that has been conducted has been largely observational and interpretational rather than experimentally controlled, a considerable amount of useful descriptive information has been accumulated. The collection of these data has led to the development of stimulating and insightful psychologic theory about the dynamics of child abuse and neglect.

It is estimated that no more than 10% of abusive and neglectful parents suffer from some form of mental disorder that can be classified under the diagnostic category of psychosis. Thus the great majority of these parents are not so disturbed as to be thought of as having lost substantial contact with reality. Various forms of mental disorders are present in the approximately 10% who are judged to be psychotic.

Among the most potentially dangerous of psychotic parents are those who suffer from paranoid schizophrenia. These parents experience some form of delusional thinking that may be either persecutory and/or grandiose in nature. Paranoid schizophrenic parents very often are found to represent a significant threat to their children because of their impairment in reality testing ability and reasoning and their concomitant exaggerated fear and underlying hostility. These parents may easily involve their children in their delusional thinking and may project onto the children their hostility and anger in such a way as to justify, in their minds, punitive behavior toward them.

Other forms of schizophrenia can also severely impair a parent's ability to satisfactorily care for his children. Furthermore, parents suffering from other forms of psychosis (e.g., affective disorders and organic brain syndrome) generally represent potential threats to their children in the form of abuse or neglect. Some important characteristics of patients who are suffering from a serious mental or emotional problem include loss of orientation as to time, person, and place; bizarre speech, including inconsistent or illogical thought progression; delusional thinking; auditory and visual hallucinatory experiences; feelings of unrealness; extreme mood states (elation or depression) and rapid mood swings; and inappropriate affectual expression.

The physician who encounters parents who exhibit one or more of these symptoms (or other psychotic symptoms) should always refer them for psychiatric evaluation and should examine the children carefully for signs of abuse and neglect. Such parents almost always need immediate psychiatric care, including placement on psychotropic medication and possibly hospitalization. The physician should inform the local child protection agency of his concern about the welfare of the children of these parents when the children show physical or emotional signs of abuse or neglect. Even in cases in which the children show no overt signs of abuse or neglect the physician should ensure that another responsible adult in the family is willing to assume responsibility for their well-being. When such an adult is not available, the children should generally be at least temporarily removed from the home and placed with responsible relatives or in a foster home until the disturbed parent is treated and evaluated as to his ability to provide adequate child care. Matters of this nature can best be handled by contacting the local child protection agency.

One other notable form of psychopathology that deserves particular mention is the antisocial (formerly often labeled psychopathic) personality. These individuals lack sufficient internal systems of behavior control (i.e., moral and social conscience) to adequately monitor and inhibit their antisocial impulses. Such persons generally make very poor parents and fail to provide their children with proper parental modeling and care. Most of these individuals are unable to form close, lasting emotional attachments to other people and are self-centered and superficial in their social and familial relationships. They frequently abuse and/or neglect their children (including sexual abuse) and have a very poor prognosis for change through treatment. Characteristics also often include drug and alcohol abuse, prostitution, and antisocial and criminal behavior.

When the physician comes into contact with such persons, he should be particularly alert to the possibility of child abuse and neglect. The most likely place for encountering such parents would be in the emergency room of a hospital. When the children of such parents are brought in for medical treatment, it is usually only after the child has suffered a serious physical injury that requires immediate medical attention. The emergency room behavior of these parents may include general apathy toward the child and his injuries and hostility toward and lack of cooperation with hospital personnel.

The great majority of abusive and neglectful parents do not suffer from a diagnosable psychiatric disorder; however, by no means are they psychologically healthy or well-adjusted individuals. Instead they are individuals with significant deficits in their ability to cope with stress and handle the problems that normally arise in the course of family living. As stated previously, one of the most prevalent characteristics of abusive and neglectful parents is that they were abused and/or neglected as children. We estimate that approximately 80% or more of abusive and neglectful parents were significantly abused or neglected as children. These parents grew up with ineffective parental models and were deprived of the love, attention, and concern necessary for healthy psychologic growth and development.

Parents who were physically abused as children experienced life under unstable and often chaotic family conditions. Their parents demonstrated poor methods of dealing with stress and often exhibited frequent outbursts of anger and aggression toward them. When they misbehaved as children, they were taught (via modeling) that physical punishment often took on extreme forms and was accompanied by verbal abuse as well. Parents who were treated in such a fashion as children frequently exhibit deficits in their ability to handle stress and difficulty in giving and receiving love. Those who were neglected as children developed without proper parental attention to their physical and emotional needs.

Besides the physical trauma suffered as children, these parents accrued psychologic scars as the result of the inflicted abuse and neglect. One such psychologic maladjustment is that they develop strong, unfulfilled dependency needs that remain with them into adult life. It has been noted by researchers that abusive parents often expect and demand too much too soon from their children in both a physical and emotional sense. They may possess unrealistic expectations of the developmental capabilities of their children, and may demand that very young children be capable of feats considerably beyond their behavioral repertoire. As an example, an abusive mother may expect her 6-month-old child to be toilet trained before he can walk and may become quite angry and upset with the child when he soils his diaper.

Emotionally these parents often demand from their children the love, attention, concern, and understanding that they lacked as children. This has been described by investigators as a role-reversal phenomenon, in that the abusive parent may psychologically take on the role of the child and expect the child to behave as the parent in the family. Failure of these children to live up to their physical and emotional expectations may lead to severe frustration and result in aggression toward the child. Significantly lacking in such parents is true empathy for the emotional and physical needs of the child and a realistic and practical understanding of his emotional and physical capabilities. Furthermore, there appears to be a lack of awareness that the child is a separate entity with his own unique needs, thoughts, and feelings.

Another characteristic of abusive and neglectful parents is their relative psychologic immaturity as adults. This may well be associated with stunted personality development as children and adolescents because of the physical and emotional abuse they suffered from their parents. These individuals may not have developed the capacity for mature, independent adult functioning and may well remain egocentric in their mode of interaction with the world about them. Because of their easily hurt feelings, strong needs for love and attention from others, inability to delay gratification, and failure to put their children's needs before theirs, they are unable to deal with the stresses of being a parent.

Many abusive and neglectful parents suffer from a poor self-image and low self-esteem. Often they grew up with a sense of personal incompetence and are easily threatened and upset when they encounter problems with their children. In many cases they may lack confidence in their ability to handle problems, and they see themselves as inadequate individuals. Poor self-esteem may have its beginning in a childhood where the parents belittle the children and constantly remind them of their failures and shortcomings. In times of stress they may accept these personality inadequacies and behave accordingly.

It is likewise thought that abusive and neglectful parents experience difficulty in deriving pleasure and enjoyment from their relationships with other people, including most prominently their relationships with their children (DHEW, 1975). These deficits in experiencing pleasure are also frequently evident in the relationship with the spouse. A high percentage of abusive parents experience marital disharmony and do not derive much emotional support and encouragement from their mates. Their marriages may be held together more by financial need or mutual strong emotional dependency rather than by love and concern. It is not unusual for such individuals to experience conflict in their sexual relationships. Marital conflict and dissatisfaction add to the stresses of living and significantly increase the potential for abusive and neglectful parental behavior.

Abusive and neglectful parents seldom have strong support systems in their lives. Their friendships are typically few and rather shallow, and they usually do not have extended family support. Often they are quite emotionally and socially isolated and have no one to turn to for help in times of need. A lack of extended family support is particularly notable. A family with access to relatives who take an interest in the children and who are willing to occasionally care for them has less of a potential for child abuse and neglect.

Drug and alcohol abuse are estimated to be factors in a significant percentage of child abuse and neglect cases. Estimates vary according to the population studied but are generally thought to range between 10% and 40% of all cases reported. Parents who are dependent on alcohol or drugs are less able to meet the physical and emotional needs of their children. They demonstrate less control over their impulses (e.g., sexual, aggressive) and exercise poorer judgment than when they are in a nondrug state. Alcohol abuse has been specifically identified as a frequent factor in the sexual abuse of children and in maternal child neglect.

Mental retardation, ranging from severe to borderline, is estimated to be a contributing factor in a significant percentage of neglect cases. Exact figures are not available, but it has been our finding that many neglectful mothers have a low level of general intelligence and have specific deficits in knowledge of child care practices and the general physical and emotional needs of children at various ages. Frequently compounding this lack of intelligence in neglectful parents are general apathy, chronic emotional immaturity, lack of family support, poor judgment and reasoning, and a history of neglect and abuse as children. The result is parents who are not emotionally and intellectually capable of providing adequate care for their children and who do not appreciate the problems the children manifest (e.g., failure to thrive). Mental retardation in itself, unless it is severe or profound in degree, does not necessarily lead to the probability of abusive or neglectful behavior. Of particular importance in cases of mild and moderate parental mental retardation is the previously discussed extended family support. A mildly retarded young woman with competent sibling and parental support may make a good mother for her children.

A significant portion of physically abusive parents maintain a strong belief in the value of physical punishment as the most effective means of discipline. Many of these parents rationalize their punitive behavior and explain that the child's actions merited such severe punishment. Many, in fact, go so far as to maintain that they are doing their child a favor by punishing him so severely. In defense of their behavior these parents may state that if children are not treated so severely they will not grow up to be "good citizens" but in contrast will be "spoiled" and "unruly."

Sexual abuse is an area of particular complexity in the child abuse and neglect syndrome. Sexual abuse can take many forms, ranging from violent acts of sexual attack from strangers to incestuous sexual contact between a parent or stepparent and child. Likewise, the age of the child can vary from infancy to adolescence. The following remarks indicate some of the psychologic characteristics of parents who engage in sexual relations with their children, including both their biologic children and their stepchildren.

Sexual abuse continues to represent an area in need of much more research and clinical study. Growing awareness in recent years of the enormity of the problem has led to much more professional attention than was previously afforded. Despite this, there continues to be controversy as to the degree and kind of psychologic disturbance in the offenders and the severity of the psychologic impact on the victims. Although the area of sexual abuse is in need of much more study regarding the contributing social and psychologic characteristics of sexually abusive parents, a moderate degree of descriptive information is available.

It is now generally accepted that in the vast majority of cases, the victim, whether it be a very young child or an adolescent, is not responsible for seductively attracting the molester. Quite to the contrary, these children are in many cases either seduced into performing sexual acts by the adult or physically coerced into such involvement. It is likewise increasingly apparent that sexual molestation can take on many forms with children of a variety of ages. Therefore, to accurately study the problem, one must examine subgroups of molesters according to the sex and age of the child, the offender's relationship to the child, and the frequency, chronicity, and type of abuse.

It has been estimated that 75% of all sexual molestation occurs between the child and someone he knows well (Caylor, 1978). Contrary to common belief, the greater threat to children is the psychologically maladjusted parent, close relative, or friend of the family rather than the disturbed stranger. It serves as testimony of our denial and selective consciousness regarding the fallibility of parents fulfilling their caretaking responsibilities that we have been so oriented toward informing children of the dangers that exist for them out of the home and away from the family. Commensurate with increased societal awareness that good parenting skills are not innate and that parents are often ill-prepared for the process of parenting has been our increased cognizance that children are all too frequently victimized by the very societal unit that is designed to protect them from harm and promote their healthy psychologic development.

The exact incidence of sexual abuse is still unknown, but its prevalence is undoubtedly staggering in proportion. As recently as 1975 there were only 6372 reported cases of incest in the United States (American Humane Society, 1975). The 1980 figures show 33,600 cases reported nationally, but workers in the field are all too aware that we still are only seeing the "tip of the iceberg." It has been estimated that there are three to six hundred thousand cases of sexual abuse annually (American Humane Society, 1980). The vast majority of cases are no doubt not reported by the victims, the family, or professionals who learn of the problem. Possibly more alarming than the number of victims who choose not to report are the number of professionals who rationalize not dealing with the problem. It is as though sexual abuse is a problem that nearly everyone abhors but few are willing to directly acknowledge and address.

Likewise, many myths still exist about the forms that sexual abuse takes. Past estimates were that the ratio of girls who were sexually abused to boys was approximately between 10 and 12 to 1 (De Francis, 1969). Furthermore, it was assumed that the vast majority of boys who were molested were molested by nonrelated homosexual adult men. These figures are reflective of our difficulty in viewing the parent-child relationship, in particular the mother-child relationship, as seriously pathologic. It is now apparent that a large percentage of sexual abuse cases involve male victims. Fritz et al. (1981) state that the girl to boy ratio is more in the realm of 2 to 1 and that approximately 60% of male molestation involves female offenders. Furthermore, it has been documented that sexual abuse does occur between same-sex parents and children as well.

It is also most unfortunate that so many parents, relatives, and professionals still question the validity of reports from child victims. Traditionally, it has been unthinkable to entertain the belief that parents could sexually abuse their own child. Even Freud was reluctant to believe his adult patients when they reported sexual abuse occurring when they were children and instead interpreted this as fantasy material (Freud, 1953). The extensive experience of workers in the field indicates that it is rare for an adolescent to fabricate such a report and even rarer for a young child to create such a story when there is no basis for it in reality. When reports are made by the child they should be taken seriously, and a complete investigation should be conducted.

As with physical abuse and neglect, workers are finding that a significant percentage of adults who sexually abuse their children were sexually abused themselves as children. Additionally, many of these adults select victims of approximately the same age as they were when they were abused. This recapitulation of abuse is evidence of the fixation in the parent's own psychosexual development as a result of having been abused as a child. It has furthermore been found that a significant number of adolescents who are sexually abusive to younger children were sexually abused at a younger age. The generational repetition of learned maladaptive patterns of sexually aggressive behavior is of obvious importance in treatment and prevention programs.

Although subtypes are still being identified by researchers, there is a growing suggestion that sexually molesting adults can be categorized in at least two ways: those in whom there is developmental fixation and those in whom there is developmental regression (Sgroi et al., 1982). Those who are developmentally fixated include pedophilic adults who have an established preference for younger children, often of a particular age. These adults tend to molest not only their own children but also other children with whom they have established some regularity of contact. Sgroi et al. hypothesize that alcohol abuse is not as significant a problem in these individuals as it is in the other type. Developmentally regressive offenders can be viewed as engaging in sexual relations with children as a regression from their more typical pattern of adult heterosexual relationships. In these individuals, there frequently are significant stresses within the family and marital dyad that lead to a turning to younger individuals for sexual contact. In these cases, alcohol and drug usage may play a prominent role. Quinsey et al. (1979) comment that many cases of incest may fall into this latter category in which "situational" circumstances and "opportunism" may play a greater role than inappropriate sexual preferences.

The degree of personality disturbance in sexually abusive parents varies from particular dysfunction in the psychosexual realm to more pervasive personality and ego impairment. Generally speaking, the younger the object of gratification and the more physically aggressive the attack, the greater the extent of psychopathology in the offender. This is not to suggest that parents who engage in only nonintercourse sexual molestation of older children are without serious psychologic problems, only that their degree of impairment tends to be relatively less severe and possibly more receptive to intervention. Perpetrators of violent sexual attacks on very young children often have severe psychologic disturbance and may be either psychotic or borderline psychotic in their psychologic makeup. Although much less is known about mothers who sexually abuse their sons or daughters, those seen by us often suffer from a borderline personality disorder and had engaged the child in a symbiotic relationship with them. In general, many sexually abusive parents have a limited capacity for mature objective relations and are immature, narcissistic individuals with poor impulse control and judgment.

Danton (1979) has compared incestuous and nonincestuous molesters of male children and found that both groups appear to be motivated in part by fears of heterosexual inadequacy. He also found both groups to consist of despondent, emotionally rigid, and inhibited individuals who experience feelings of emotional and social alienation. In contrast, the incestuous group appeared to be more socially introverted, whereas the nonincestuous molesters appeared to be functioning at a more psychosexually immature level.

It is important when examining the problem of sexual abuse not to focus exclusively on the psychopathology of the offender. It has been repeatedly learned that incestuous sexual abuse is not simply the result of a disturbed individual but is a product of a disturbed family unit as well. Despite the common initial report by spouses of the abusers that they had no knowledge of such activity, it is highly unlikely that this is indeed the case. In most families the sexual abuse has become a family secret that is not talked about in or out of the family, but is common knowledge of both spouses and siblings of the victim.

One rather commonly found form of sexual abuse occurs in an unstable family unit in which the mother whose children are of latency or adolescent age marries or lives with a man who sexually molests her children. In many such families the mother may be quite emotionally dependent on her husband or boyfriend and is passively supportive of his behavior. These mothers' own psychologic needs for love and attention appear to outweigh their concern for their children, and they are reluctant to challenge the husband or boyfriend over the impropriety of his behavior. In some cases, the mother may actually use her daughter(s) as a means of keeping her husband or boyfriend in the home, particularly when she experiences sexual maladjustment with her mate and feels unable or unwilling to meet his sexual needs. The finding of sexual disturbance between the wife and husband in these families is high. In this kind of family sexual abuse usually is detected when the child confides in a relative or other person outside the family unit (e.g., a school counselor).

Very often when parents learn through social agency contact that the child has informed outsiders of the advances of the father or stepfather, they become very upset with the child and blame the child for the disruption of the family. The blame of breaking up the family can be emotionally traumatizing to the child. Emotional problems of these children are discussed later in more detail.

The stepfathers or live-in boyfriends in such families are usually quite emotionally and socially unstable, immature individuals who lack sufficient cognitive, moral, and social restraints over their behavior. In incestuous family relationships many of these men seem to be shy, introverted, passive males who have few social contacts and who are quite family oriented. However, in other cases, these males may be antisocial personalities who act out in a variety of ways and who view their children as objects for their own gratification.

It must be reiterated that sexual abuse can occur in a variety of forms and that sexually abusive parents may not show any obvious psychologic disturbance. In fact, many overtly appear to be relatively normal and well-adjusted individuals who are respected and well-liked by their relatives and family. As previously stated, this is an area where more research and study are needed.

Characteristics of abused children

The way the parents regard the child and the way the child acts may contribute to abuse and neglect. There may be underlying hostility to the child and lack of paternal- and maternal-infant bonding because of such conditions as unwanted pregnancy, premarital conception, forced marriage, or pregnancy, labor, or delivery characterized by physical and psychologic difficulties. Other factors include a child of the "wrong" sex (not the sex the parents desired), a child who resembles a hated relative (psychologic transference), a malformed or chronically handicapped child whose care places great psychologic and financial stress on the parents, and a child who for one reason or another (e.g., colic) cries with unusual frequency. Premature infants are especially vulnerable to abuse and neglect, either through failure to establish maternal-infant bonding or through parental apprehension concerning their ability to take care of the fragile baby. The hyperactive child, with his ceaseless driven behavior, short attention span, and destructiveness, may so irritate the parents that temper control is lost and violence occurs. The child who is not truly hyperactive but only normally active and exuberant may also irritate parents who have a low frustration threshold and lack the knowledge of child development to recognize that the child's behavior is normal.

As the abused child grows older, he may react to abuse with passive acceptance and fear or compensate with aggressive behavior and talking back to his parents. Such actions pour fuel on the fire and aggravate the abuse. Saddest of all is the child who is somewhat slower than normal in his development and has even more difficulty than the normally developing child in meeting the ill-founded, excessive expectations of his parents developmentally or in learning to play his part in the abnormal parental requirements of role-reversal.

Chronic stress and crises

The psychologic characteristics of abusive and neglectful parents have been commented on previously, indicating their particular vulnerabilities to stress and crises. Situational high-risk factors have also been discussed. Although economically secure parents may abuse their children, a very large percentage of abuse and neglect cases occurs in families who have difficulty making ends meet and live in poverty or on the ragged edge of public dependence. Unemployment, frequent loss or change of jobs, repeated change of residence, marital discord, and a generally unstable and sometimes chaotic style of living form a pattern in many instances.

Against the stressful background of this chronically precarious existence, intermittent crises occur that increase parental frustration, tension, and despair. The abusive parent may then take out his or her frustration on the child. Sometimes the abuse is triggered by the child's incessant crying, as from an earache, or the whimpering and irritability sometimes accompanying severe gastroenteritis or other illnesses.

PSYCHOLOGIC SYMPTOMS OF ABUSED CHILDREN

The psychologic impact of abuse and neglect on children can produce a variety of symptoms according to a number of factors, including the type and severity of the abuse, the age of the child, and the chronicity of the abuse. In general, children who are physically and emotionally neglected do not develop the feeling of being loved and valued as an individual. They may be plagued by feelings of insecurity, have a poor self-concept, and feel depressed and anxious. Emotionally abused children in particular often suffer low self-esteem and a poor self-image as a result of the verbal abuse inflicted by their parents. Children who are told they are stupid or who are chronically scapegoated for family problems do not develop the self-confidence and feeling of intrinsic self-worth and value that normal children do. They may feel quite despondent, as well as angry and resentful, as a result of the mistreatment they receive at home.

Physically abused children show many of the above symptoms of emotional maladjustment as well as a tendency to act out in an angry and aggressive manner in their interaction with peers. Severely physically abused children may demonstrate fear or great anxiety when around the abusive parent and not seek out the parent for comfort or protection when emotionally stressed or physically hurt. These children are also generally passive, socially isolated and withdrawn, and chronically emotionally anxious when around others. Often, abused and neglected children perform poorly in school because of the problems they experience at home. They may have difficulty concentrating on their schoolwork and lack the achievement motivation of normal children.

It is particularly important for pediatricians to note that sexually abused children often have unexplained psychosomatic and behavioral complaints and that sexual abuse often is not identified as a problem at the time of referral. Young children who have been chronically sexually abused often demonstrate various symptoms of emotional and social maladjustment. These children are frequently anxious, emotionally immature, and tend to regress when distressed. They may also demonstrate aloofness and a reluctance to become involved with peers. In particular, they often show signs of a masked underlying depression in the form of sleeping and eating disturbances, irritability and nervousness, difficulty concentrating in school, and consequent poor academic performance. These children may also run away from home and be truant from school. It was noted by Kempe (1978) that boys who have been seduced into incestuous relationships with their mothers, fathers, or grandparents are particularly prone to the development of serious emotional problems. The normal psychologic growth and development of these children is severely disrupted, and an unusually high number of them become psychotic when confronted with stress.

Adams-Tucker (1982) states that emotional disturbances in sexually abused children tend to be more severe under the following circumstances: "(1) the abuse began at an early age and was long-standing; and (2) when the abused child was a teenager, even though the abuse may have been limited to one time and may have been recent."

Groth (1976) has commented that the potential danger the sexual abuse has for the victim can be examined on the basis of four factors: (1) the nature of the relationship between the victim and offender, (2) the chronicity or duration of the sexual relationship, (3) the type of sexual abuse, and (4) the degree of physical coercion involved in the commission of the offense. The negative impact is viewed as greater the closer the relationship between offender and victim (parent as opposed to stranger), the longer the period of abuse, the more intimate the sexual contact (intercourse as opposed to exhibitionism), and the more violent the sexual act.

Adolescent children who are physically abused may act out in a variety of ways and may engage in various forms of rebellious behavior. These include socially delinquent behavior, poor school performance, fighting, sexual acting out, and possibly drug and alcohol abuse. In addition, a large number of these adolescents run away from home in an attempt to escape from their problems. Sexually abused adolescent females often appear to be more severely emotionally traumatized by incestuous relations with the father or stepfather than occurs when younger girls are so exploited. They may be particularly prone toward engagement in various forms of acting out, including promiscuous sexual and delinquent behavior.

These adolescents may feel quite justifiably resentful and hostile toward the abuser, and these feelings can generalize to their relationships with other males. Sexually abused girls often have underlying masked depression associated with their acting-out behavior. The symptoms of these depressions are similar to those previously described and include vague somatic complaints, tension, irritability, difficulty concentrating in school, and sleeping and eating disturbances. Although many are sexually promiscuous, most of them experience deep sexual conflicts and are not orgasmic through sexual intercourse. These problems may well accompany them into adulthood and only later manifest themselves in multiple psychiatric disturbances and marital and heterosexual difficulties. It is noted that females who have been sexually abused as adolescents may not only develop strong feelings of sensitivity to exploitation by males but also a distrust of females as a result of the lack of protection by their mothers.

The self-esteem of sexually abused girls is often quite low, and they are particularly susceptible to the development of feelings of guilt and shame about their experiences, especially when they realize through peer relations that what has happened to them is considered to be culturally abnormal and very unacceptable. A large percentage of such girls attempt to escape from their intolerable home environment, either through running away or perhaps marrying at an early age. These girls can be particularly psychologically traumatized if they are impregnated by the father, stepfather, or other male relative. The realization or fear of being pregnant with their father's child can cause serious depression and even lead to suicidal behavior.

CLINICAL MANIFESTATIONS

Physical abuse or neglect can be minimal, moderate, or severe at the time the physician or other individual observes the child, Injuries may be single or multiple.

Physical abuse

Bruises are the most common evidence of physical abuse and must be distinguished from those accidentally acquired. They most often result from unduly severe spankings or whippings and are most frequently located on the buttocks and on the posterior surfaces of the thorax, lumbar area, thighs, and calves. The severity and the locations of these lesions are the chief indicators of abuse. As regards severity, they go far beyond the bounds of ordinary redness inflicted by the usual spanking. There are often extensive ecchymotic areas. The fact that they are not limited to the buttocks indicates that the spanking was really a beating or that the child struggled wildly to avoid the blows and the perpetrator missed the mark.

The shape and size of the bruises can indicate the instrument used. The favorite whipping weapon is the folded electrical extension cord. It leaves telltale U-shaped ecchymoses. Whipping with a strap or belt leaves bandlike marks the size of the object employed. At times the buckle end of the belt is used, leaving a clear buckle-shaped mark on the child. Severe spanking with the hand may result in a handprint lesion. Grabbing the struggling child to hold him while he is being whipped or beaten often leaves thumb- and finger-shaped ecchymotic marks on the arms.

Bruises in unusual locations should immediately arouse suspicion of abuse. Most accidentally acquired bruises are on the anterior or lateral surfaces of the legs or on the knees, elbows, outer surfaces of the arms, or the forehead. Bruises on the neck may be caused by throttling or choking the child. Ecchymoses of the ears may result from cuffing, pulling, or twisting the ears. Bruises about the orbit may be caused by direct blows. Bruising and lacerations of the gums and inner surfaces of the lips also result from blows. Bruising of the external genitalia is rarely accidental and is often caused by abuse.

When a child has been repeatedly struck or beaten over a short period of time the various sets of bruises have a different color pattern that is helpful in dating their time of occurrence. This is important not only in the diagnosis of abuse but may also assist in determining who abused the child. For example, the presence of fresh bruises would exonerate anyone who had not been in contact with the child within the past few days, but fading bruises would not. A helpful color scheme (Table 13-1) for dating bruises was developed by Wilson and modified by Schmitt.

In addition to bruises, one may also observe *welts, abrasions,* and, much less frequently, *lacerations.*

Burns constitute another common lesion of child abuse. The parents usually give a most implausible or changing account of how the "accident" occurred. Two types of burns are notoriously indicative of child abuse: the cigarette burn and the dunking burn. When abusive parents burn the child with a lighted cigarette, they usually choose a site that will not be easily viewed by others who might report the abuse. Thus cigarette burns can be found on the soles of the feet or on areas not seen when the child is dressed. In the fresh state cigarette burns are easily diagnosed by their rounded shape and their appearance. When such burns become infected, they resemble lesions of pyoderma, but the distinction is usually easily made. When healed, they leave rounded scars that closely resemble healed, deep-seated, impetiginous lesions.

Dunking burns occur when an extremity or the small child's buttocks and neighboring parts are deliberately forced into and held down in hot water. The evidence of abuse consists of the precise line of demarcation of the burn, instead of the irregular edge and neighboring splash burns that consistently occur when such a hot water burn is accidentally acquired.

Burns of the palm caused by a hotplate or

Table 13-1. Dating of bruises

Age	Color
0-2 days	Swollen, tender
0-5 days	Red, blue
5-7 days	Green
7-10 days	Yellow
10-14 days	Brown
2-4 weeks	Clear

From Schmitt, B.D., Child abuse/neglect, Evanston, Ill., 1979, American Academy of Pediatrics, modified from Wilson, E.F., Pediatrics **60:**750, 1977. Copyright American Academy of Pediatrics, 1977.

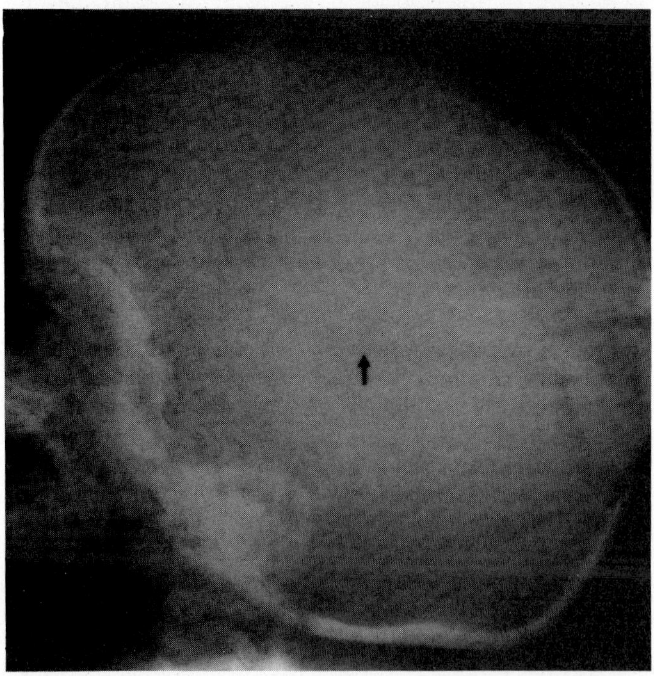

Fig. 13-1. Gaping parietal skull fracture is characteristic of severe trauma. Child abuse should be suspected when the type of fracture does not agree with the clinical information. The parents related vague, mild trauma in this case. (Courtesy Dr. W. Webster Riggs, Le Bonheur Children's Medical Center, Memphis.)

griddle, those of the feet caused by a floor furnace grating, or those of the buttocks caused by an electric heater present more of a diagnostic problem. When really accidental, such burns occur chiefly in toddlers and young children. When seen in infants too young to be up and about or in preschool children who have reached the age of reasonable discretion, such burns immediately arouse the suspicion of child abuse and neglect.

Fractures, chiefly of the extremities, skull, or ribs, constitute another important component of the child abuse syndrome. Fractures occur in about 15% to 20% of such children. Child abuse and neglect should always be included in the differential diagnosis when the story of how the fracture occurred seems highly implausible, the parents differ in their accounts, or the story changes with subsequent retelling. Most important is consideration of the developmental capacities of the child. Fractures in children less than age 2 years should especially arouse concern regarding physical abuse, since such youngsters rarely break bones accidentally. Especially suspect are the accounts of parents that the child only a few weeks or months of age broke his leg by kicking the crib or getting his leg caught in the side rails or broke his arm by rolling off a couch onto a rug.

Fractures may be single or multiple, minimal or severe. Most strongly suggestive of physical abuse is the presence of several fractures in various stages: perhaps one well healed, another healing, and a third constituting the fresh fracture for which the child is being seen. Another strongly suggestive indication of abuse is that

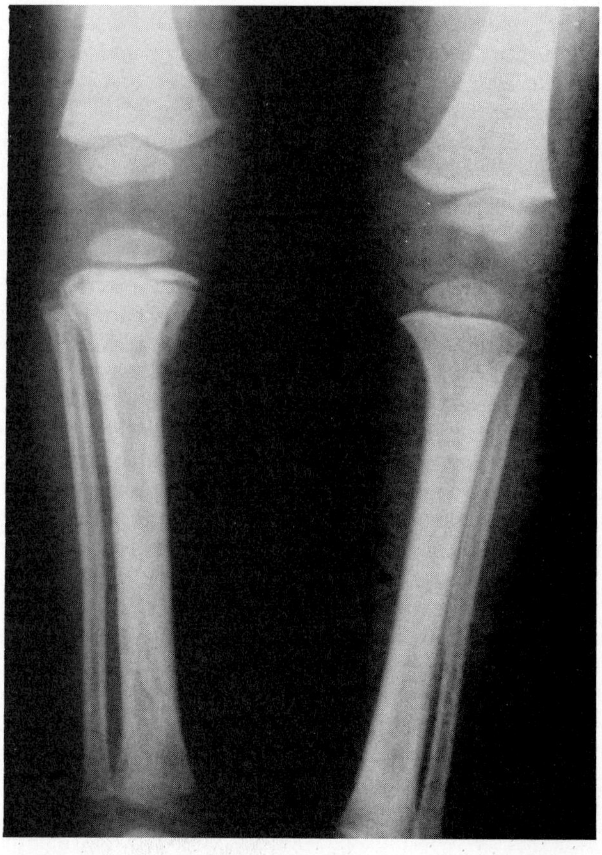

Fig. 13-2. Fragmentation of the right proximal tibial metaphysis represents healing injury by twisting or jerking of the leg, unlike natural trauma at this age. The sclerosis about both midtibial shafts suggests healing from trauma sustained at a date earlier than the injury of the right proximal tibia. Demonstrating evidence of two separate episodes of trauma is characteristic of child abuse. (Courtesy Dr. W. Webster Riggs, Le Bonheur Children's Medical Center, Memphis.)

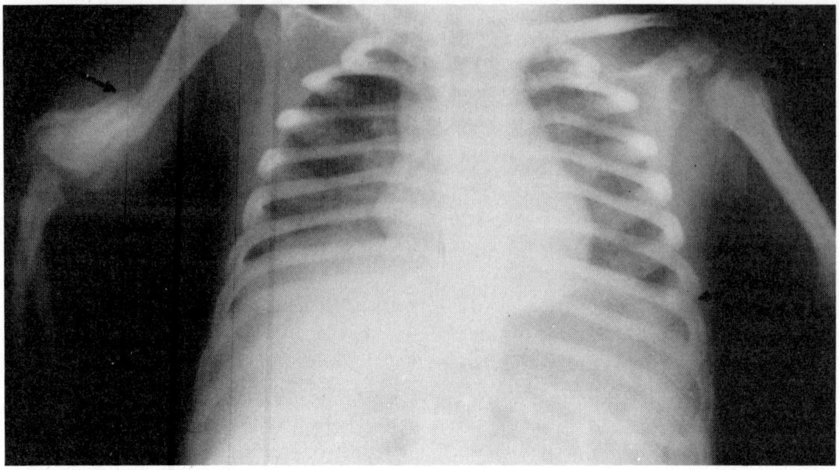

Fig. 13-3. Healing fracture of the left sixth rib would suggest child abuse in a small child who has no abnormal metabolic state. The fragmentation of bones about the left shoulder and about the right distal humerus would corroborate the suspicion. (Courtesy Dr. W. Webster Riggs, Le Bonheur Children's Medical Center, Memphis.)

the fresh fracture already shows radiographic evidence of healing when the child is first brought for medical attention, meaning there were approximately 10 or more days between the injury and the attempt to seek medical attention. Such an unwarranted delay is characteristic of child abuse. Skull fractures are caused by direct blows by the hand or fist of the perpetrator or by hitting the child's head against a hard object. Rib fractures are fairly common in young infants who are abused. Fractures of the extremities are usually caused by twisting, jerking, or striking the extremity. Although a transverse fracture may occur, it is more common to see a greenstick or spiral fracture. Figs. 13-1 to 13-4 indicate some of the common radiographic findings in children who have suffered child abuse.

Injuries of the central nervous system occur when the child is struck on the head by the abuser, the head is slammed against a hard object, or, in the case of small infants, the baby is shaken vigorously. These injuries can result in edema of the brain, hemorrhage from torn blood vessels, accumulation of blood, permanent neurologic syndrome, mental retardation, or death. Subdural hematoma is a particularly common result of severe head trauma.

Trauma to the eye may result in traumatic cataract, retinal hemorrhage, retinal detachment, or blindness.

Blows inflicted in anger may knock teeth out or break them and may cause damage to the lips and gums.

Injuries to the thorax may cause fractured ribs, pneumothorax, bleeding into the pleural cavity or elsewhere, and damage to the lungs.

Abdominal injuries from severe blows to the abdominal wall may result in laceration of the liver or spleen, rupture of the stomach or duodenum, intramural hematoma of the bowel wall, or traumatic pancreatitis sometimes followed by a pseudocyst of the pancreas. Severe blows over the kidney may cause rupture of the kidney and intrarenal hemorrhage.

Traumatic *injuries to the genitalia* may also be present.

Mental abuse

Mental abuse consists of continually scapegoating, picking on, criticizing, and denigrating a child, thereby instilling attitudes of worthlessness, inferiority, resentment, hostility, and hopelessness. The spirits of such children may become crushed, and they may become withdrawn, detached, lonely, and forever lacking the ability to form warm attachments and friendships. Under the repeated tongue-lashing and criticism by the parent the hostility and resentment of the child may flare up in self-defense, further aggravating the mental abuse by the parent. In other instances the child simply becomes

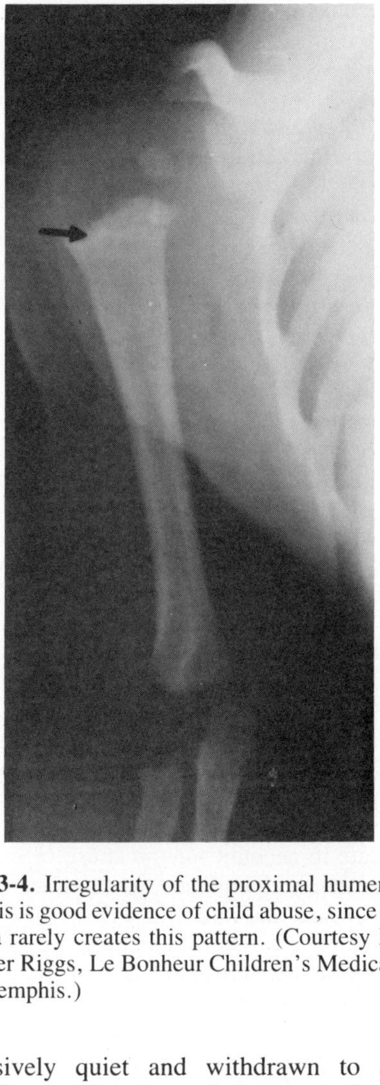

Fig. 13-4. Irregularity of the proximal humeral metaphysis is good evidence of child abuse, since natural trauma rarely creates this pattern. (Courtesy Dr. W. Webster Riggs, Le Bonheur Children's Medical Center, Memphis.)

excessively quiet and withdrawn to avoid, through passivity, the verbal storms of the parent. One way or another the child's personality becomes seriously affected, perhaps for life. Mental abuse also includes abandonment of children in public places, locking them in cellars, closets, attics, or small rooms, and in other ways terrorizing them. It also includes ignoring the child, as if he did not exist, and failing to afford the warm, affectionate support and protection the child needs.

Sexual abuse

Sexual exploitation of children occurs far more commonly than is generally suspected, is greatly underreported, and is difficult to prove. The victim is usually a girl, and the perpetrator is usually the father, stepfather, or boyfriend of the mother. Such abnormal sexual relationships take many forms, including exposure of genitalia, fondling the child's genitalia, masturbation, oral-genital sex practices, sodomy, and true intercourse. The child may show evidence of vulvitis, vaginitis, or venereal disease (gonorrhea particularly). Venereal disease in a prepubertal child is always highly suggestive of sexual abuse.

Neglect

Deliberate child neglect must be distinguished from failure, because of ignorance or poverty, to provide the child the necessities of life such as proper food, clothing, housing, and medical attention. This distinction can usually be made readily by careful study of the parents and the family situation.

Neglect may be manifested by excessively poor skin hygiene, persistent severe diaper rash, prolonged cradle cap, malnutrition, or failure to thrive. The child may be inappropriately dressed for the weather, and the clothing may be excessively dirty and in disrepair. The neglected infant or young child may be passive, withdrawn, apathetic, almost expressionless, and rarely smiling. He may seem listless and tired and remain quiet for long periods of time. On the other hand, he may be apprehensive, anxious, and fearful of strangers. He may be indifferent to affection, or he may desperately crave affection from strangers.

Neglectful parents often feed infants irregularly and inadequately, which leads to malnutrition and failure to thrive. It has been estimated that 20% to 50% of all infants who have the syndrome of failure to thrive are the victims of neglect caused by environmental deprivation. It is remarkable how rapidly they gain weight when admitted to the hospital, are fed well, and are given tender loving care. In view of the frequency of child neglect as a cause of the failure to thrive syndrome, psychosocial evaluation of the family should be initiated immediately.

Other aspects of neglect include leaving children by themselves for long periods of time, possibly in locked rooms, failure to afford a stimulating home environment and contacts with other children, necessary for adequate development of the child's personality and social responsiveness, failure to obtain necessary medical attention (immunizations, serial health screening, etc.), and lack of interest in the child's school attendance.

DIAGNOSIS

In view of the danger to the child, the diagnosis must be established as soon as possible to protect the child and his siblings from continued exposure to abuse or neglect and to seek to rehabilitate parental attitudes and feelings so that the home becomes safe. Severe cases of abuse and neglect may be so flagrant that the diagnosis is readily established, and there may even be a confession by the parents or witnesses to verify abuse or neglect. The majority of cases are not so clear-cut, although most of them are readily diagnosable once the possibility is entertained and adequate evaluation of the child and family is performed. In some cases the local child protective service (an arm of the state Department of Family Services or Human Services or similar name) has already investigated the family and has determined that abuse or neglect has occurred.

Many parents who repeatedly abuse or neglect their children take them for medical attention to a different hospital emergency room or clinic for each episode so that no one hospital will have a record of recurrent abuse. Therefore, when abuse is finally suspected, it may prove helpful to probe for such visits to other hospitals. Some cities have a confidential registry of children suspected of or known to be victims of abuse. When such a registry exists, a telephone call may verify that the child has already been identified or is suspected to be a case of child abuse or neglect.

On the other hand, parents who are abusing their children may repeatedly bring them to clinics or emergency rooms during times when they show no sign of injury, have only a mild cold, or have some other exceptionally slight complaint. It has been shown that for some parents these repeated visits for superficially insignificant reasons are actually a cry for help—a sign that they hope someone will talk with them and help them solve the family's child abuse problem.

When evaluating a child to determine whether injuries are truly accidental or the result of abuse or neglect, it is important to avoid an aggressive, accusatory, punitive approach. Such tactics constitute a real affront to parents who did not really abuse their child. Furthermore, a harsh approach is unjustified even in the abuse case. When questions are too aggressively put in an underlying attitude of accusation, abusive parents are even less likely than usual to give information and often become defensive and hostile.

The real purpose of the diagnosis is to facilitate protection and treatment of the abused child and at the same time create a receptive attitude in the psychologically distorted parents toward subsequent management of the family and the situation. Turning the parents off with the wrong approach denies them the opportunity for help they so often desperately crave. Moreover, if the abuse is severe, the juvenile court and in some cases the police will enter the picture. If there is to be punishment for abuse, this is within the province of the law, not health professionals.

Despite their innate disapproval of abuse and neglect and sometimes righteous indignation, health professionals, social service workers, and others involved should cultivate a calm helpful approach in the diagnosis and management of child abuse and neglect.

Perhaps the most important lead to a diagnosis of abuse is what is termed the *implausible story* given by the parent(s) as to how the injuries or neglect occurred. The history may be totally inadequate to account for the abuse or neglect; the history may change on repetition; one parent may contradict the other. In cases where there may have been a neutral caretaker or observer of the abuse, such a person's account may differ sharply from that of the parents, who may be combining to hide the facts.

Abusive parents often explain bruises by saying that the child just bruises easily, falls repeatedly, or fell from a couch, table, or bed. Fractures in infants only a few weeks or months old are often ascribed to the child kicking the side of the crib, an arm of leg being caught between the side rails of the baby bed, or the rough play of a slightly older sibling. In one of our recent cases a 2-month-old child was said to have broken his humerus by rolling over on the couch, and the "snap could be heard across the room." In another instance a family dog (a small one) was said to have fractured the arm of a child only a few weeks old by jumping on the couch and romping and playing with the infant; a few weeks later this child was admitted to the hospital with a fractured skull, subdural hematoma, convulsions, and severe brain damage. Cigarette burns are usually ascribed to the child touching or walking into a lighted cigarette or playing with one.

The implausibility of the story may also relate to the child's developmental state. When injuries are said to have occurred through actions the child could not possibly have performed, one immediately suspects child abuse. Examples are alleged rolling off couches or beds when the infant is not old enough to roll over, falling while running when the child is not old enough to run, and so on.

Helfer et al. (1976) suggested four particular questions that should be asked when attempting to separate accidental from nonaccidental (abuse) injuries.

1. *When did the accident take place and where?* One needs to know the day and time the injury occurred. Vague answers or the inability to answer this question indicates that the parents or caretakers were not present at the time of injury or do not want it known they were absent. Delay in bringing the child for medical attention is highly suggestive of abuse. A common statement is that the child seemed perfectly normal when put to bed but could not move an arm or leg the next morning. Abused children who have sustained fractures may be brought to emergency rooms days after the injury occurred, with the parents' vague excuse that they did not realize the injury had happened or was serious.

2. *Who was caring for the child at the time of the accident, and who saw the accident occur?* The parent or other informant might give vague answers to this question, seeking to camouflage his own responsibility or to protect the real abuser, who may be the other parent, a so-called boyfriend or girlfriend, or an older sibling.

3. *How did the accident take place?* Detailed information is sought as to how the accident occurred. Examples of the implausible story have already been given; the injuries are not adequately explained by the account given and in terms of the child's developmental state.

4. *What did the child do after the accident, and how did you manage the child?* Abusive parents often minimize the effect of the injury on the child, often stating that they did not realize the seriousness of it. They say that this in turn caused them to delay seeking medical attention. Such a story is quite at variance with what nonabusive parents do: they immediately rush the child to the physician or the emergency room when suspicious of serious injury.

The way abusive parents act in the emergency room, clinic, or physician's office may be highly suggestive of abuse or neglect. Such parents may have a shallow affect, as if not really interested in the child and the severity of his injuries or neglect. They may appear passive and unconcerned. In contrast to normal parents, who hover over their child, are anxious, answer questions readily, and want to be near the child when he is examined, abusive parents may reluctantly give information, show little interest in the examination, and may even leave the room to have a soft drink or smoke a cigarette. On the other hand, abusive parents may show bristling defensiveness and hostility when asked about the injuries or neglect, openly resenting the implication that they have abused or neglected their child.

Physical examination of the abused or neglected child may reveal lesions of the type previously discussed.

Radiographic studies should be performed in cases of physical abuse and should not be limited to the site of a fresh fracture. Full skeletal radiographic surveys should be performed, particularly in children less than 3 years of age, who more often have multiple skeletal lesions of varying stages of healing. The finding of such lesions makes the diagnosis of child abuse certain. Radiographic findings in child abuse are indicated in Figs. 13-1 to 13-4.

In view of the frequent association of subdural hematoma and child abuse, full skeletal surveys should be obtained in all infants diagnosed as having subdural hematoma, and evidence of subdural hematoma should be sought in all infants who are victims of physical abuse (careful neurologic examination, head circumference, special diagnostic procedures).

The importance of full skeletal surveys was exemplified in one of our recent cases in which a 2-month-old infant was brought to the emergency room with a fracture of the arm. He was seen by a new orthopedic resident not alert to the possibility of child abuse. The fracture was set, and the child was seen by a second resident 2 weeks later and found to be doing well. One month later he was brought back to the hospital badly battered, and he subsequently died. The radiologist had suspected child abuse at the first visit, had taken additional radiographs, and had dictated the findings, but the resident did not notify the hospital child abuse team. We now require the radiologist to telephone the senior supervising pediatric resident in the emergency room and the resident or other physician who ordered the radiographs as soon as evidence of child abuse is noted. The senior supervising resident promptly telephones the medical social worker on call for the emergency room, who in turn immediately becomes involved in the case.

Although there are other entities, some quite rare, that cause skeletal lesions superficially suggesting child abuse, a skilled radiologist—especially a pediatric radiologist—can usually make the differential diagnosis easily. Some of the conditions to be considered are congenital syphilis, scurvy, osteogenesis imperfecta, infantile cortical hyperostosis, congenital indifference to pain, and Menkes kinky hair syndrome.

In the hospital or clinic setting the social service department should be informed immediately when child abuse is strongly suggested or evident. The medical social worker is of inestimable value in dealing with the family, in obtaining family background information that is of great help, especially in borderline cases, and is the individual who may be given the responsibility of fulfilling the state law by promptly notifying the child protective service (of the state Department of Family Services, or Human Services, or similar name). The child protective service promptly assigns one of its own social workers to collaborate with the hospital social worker. The information obtained by both these social workers is greater than either one could obtain alone. When the child leaves the hospital, the chief responsibility for following the family rests with the child protective social worker and the state department.

TREATMENT

Physically abused children, especially those less than 3 years of age, should be admitted to the hospital for treatment of their injuries and to permit a thorough evaluation of the family situation by the hospital medical social worker and the child protective service agency. For older children with minimal trauma, hospitalization is perhaps not always necessary if the child can be placed immediately in a safe environment—foster care in the home of a reliable relative or in a licensed foster home. The extent of the injuries in these older children is a factor to be considered, and, if they are moderate to severe, hospitalization is indicated. Likewise, serious cases of neglect and those of moderate degree in infancy indicate hospitalization. Milder cases of neglect in infants and older children may often be managed safely in the home under protective supervision of the child protective agency. There is less indication for hospitalization in cases of mental or sexual abuse, but this depends on their severity.

In the first-contact diagnostic phase at the emergency room, clinic, or office level, the decision is made whether to hospitalize the child, based on the preceding criteria. Parents often accept without question the need for hospitalization, and some welcome it as a relief from their intolerable burden of abuse or neglect and as an opportunity to be helped. Others resent the idea of hospitalization or even refuse to permit admission. In such a circumstance the physician and perhaps the social worker explain as kindly as possible why admission is indicated, emphasizing the need for a complete evaluation of the child and treatment of his condition. The simple statement that the injuries are difficult to explain in view of the history given and that further studies are needed for the child's welfare may suffice to obtain agreement on hospitalization. If the parents continue to refuse, the medical social worker or other designated person telephones a representative of the child protective service, who then quickly obtains from the local juvenile court or other authority an order making the child a ward of the court and mandating that the child be admitted.

Once the child is admitted, agreeably or otherwise, treatment of the injuries or the effects of neglect is begun. The medical management of the case is of course under the direction of the child's physician or an assigned physician, if the family does not have a private doctor or he is not on the particular hospital's medical staff. Treatment of the injuries and neglect follows standard high quality procedures. If the private physician is not closely associated with the in-hospital management of the child, he should be kept fully informed, not only of the child's condition but also of plans for disposition.

Since there are often medicolegal aspects of child abuse and neglect, it is essential for possible subsequent court hearings that the hospital record be very thorough and precise, especially as pertains to description of the injuries or the degree of neglect. Color photographs should be made of the child and the externally visible lesions as documentation of the nature and severity of the injuries. To refute the allegation that the child has an unusual tendency to bruise and bleed, blood coagulation tests should be performed. Generally, these include bleeding time, platelet count, prothrombin time, and partial thromboplastin time. The radiographs previously mentioned also constitute important court evidence of skeletal trauma.

Detailed progress notes should be made in the chart, concerning not only the medical aspects of the case but also the behavior and attitudes of the parents when visiting the child. Their regularity in visiting is a factor in determining their degree of concern for and interest in the child.

The discharge summary should be particularly thorough. If there is definite agreement by the staff that physical abuse or neglect exists, it is very important that these diagnoses be stated positively in the discharge summary. Nothing weakens a case in court more than a vaguely written summary and a questionable or weak diagnosis of abuse or neglect. The words "probable" or "possible" abuse or neglect should be strictly reserved for truly questionable cases.

During the hospitalization the medical social worker and the child protective service social worker collaborate in their work-up, the latter evaluating the home situation, affording the family helpful social services as needed, and specifically arranging for temporary foster care after discharge, when indicated.

If the hospital has a child abuse and neglect team, as it should if it admits children suffering from abuse or neglect, the team can be used to help make recommendations concerning disposition of the child and subsequent treatment of the family, seeking to help them become psychologically rehabilitated and to make the home safe for subsequent return of the child.

Various arrangements for long-term therapy of the abuse and neglect family exist in different communities. Our Center for Children in Crisis, sponsored by the Le Bonheur Children's Medical Center and the University of Tennessee Center for the Health Sciences, affords multidisciplinary, comprehensive evaluations of abused and neglected children and their families referred to the Center by the county office of the Tennessee Department of Human Services (DHS). Families and their children are evaluated in depth from the pediatric, social service, psychologic, and psychiatric viewpoints. Staffing conferences are then held, resulting in final group recommendations concerning long-term treatment of the family and whether the child should remain at home or be placed with safe relatives or in a licensed foster home. Immediately following the staff conference the parents are informed of the recommendation. Copies of the Center's complete work-up are then sent to the Department of Human Services and to the geographically appropriate community mental health center where long-term treatment will take place. Copies may also be required by the local juvenile court. Confidentiality of reports is essential.

Representatives of the Center for Children in Crisis, the seven mental health centers, the Department of Human Services, and the juvenile court meet periodically to monitor the progress of the community's child abuse and neglect program and to perfect the degree of collaboration between the various agencies mentioned. In addition, the child abuse and neglect committee of the Le Bonheur Children's Medical Center meets monthly in association with representatives from the Department of Human Services to monitor the progress of abused and neglected children discharged from the hospital.

Some of the major aspects of long-term therapy with abuse and neglect families follow.

Therapy with parents

Abusive and neglectful parents and their children can be helped by psychologic treatment as well as through the provision of comprehensive social services. Physically abusive parents need strong support systems built into their environment to aid them in modifying their injurious behaviors. Each family unit must be evaluated individually as to the nature of their problems and what kind of help is needed. This not only includes the assessment of the individual characteristics of each person in the family but also assessment of how family members interact with each other. Without comprehensive analysis of the family unit, treatment will not be effective in changing maladaptive patterns of living.

Physically abusive parents very often have severe marital problems that contribute to their personal discontent as well as their tendency to abuse. The husband and wife may show little support to one another in their attempts to deal with the children. In this regard *marital therapy* can be useful in helping parents face these problems and improve their ability to communicate and interact in a more rewarding and healthy manner. Likewise, problems such as sexual maladjustment can be addressed and treated appropriately. In cases where a lack of communication between family members is one of the primary problems, *family therapy* may be helpful.

Both abusive and neglectful parents often greatly benefit from *special classes* designed to strengthen their parenting skills. Such classes include explanation of the child's emotional and physical development as well as the teaching of proper child management approaches. In many cases abusive parents can be taught to use alternative methods (behavior modification) of controlling their children's behavior so that resort to physical punishment is not necessary. Neglectful parents, in particular, often benefit from therapy aimed at teaching them how to enjoy themselves in their relationships with their children.

Lay therapists—nonprofessionals trained to be companions for abusive and neglectful parents—have been found to represent effective means of aiding families in distress. These lay people are usually well-adjusted women of similar socioeconomic background to the parent who have successfully raised children of their own (i.e., school age or older). They provide concrete services for these parents (e.g., taking the mother to the store) in addition to serving as models of appropriate parental behavior. Lay therapists working in conjunction with professionals may well represent the most effective combination of treatments for abusive and neglectful parents.

Parents who exhibit serious emotional problems, aside from their abusive or neglectful behavior, may require *individual psychotherapy* directed at helping them work through and better understand their conflicts. Parents who exhibit extreme anxiety, tension, or evidence of a thought disorder may need treatment by psychotropic medication as well. Therefore therapists should be provided in conjunction with the other needed family services.

Parents Anonymous and Parents United are support groups that are operated by parents who have respectively either physically abused or sexually abused their children. These groups often constitute an integral part of a treatment program for such families. They are growing in numbers throughout the country and can be found in most areas.

Sexual abuse can be a difficult problem to treat successfully. In incestuous sexual abuse cases it is often wise to separate the offending parent from the child until the parent and child are treated and the home environment can be made safe for the child. This is best done by having the parent removed from the home as opposed to removal of the child. However, this is dependent on the nature of the approach of the legal system in handling these cases. In areas of the country where the legal system is not designed for early and rapid confession of the offender, it may be necessary to remove the child from the home and place him with a relative or in a shelter home. Treatment needs to include intensive work with the mother in a relationship in which she has passively supported the father's or stepfather's behavior. Although a moderate degree of success has been found in rehabilitation of these families, it is unfortunate that a significant percentage of these children may never be able to return to the home. However, as techniques for modifying maladaptive individual and family behavior improve, and professionals become more adept at working with these families, the percentage of successfully treated cases will rise.

Therapy with children

Children who have been severely physically abused need a variety of services. In some cases in which the parents do not show potential for rehabilitation, the children may be placed in the care of a responsible relative or in foster care. This, however, is usually not done unless their current home environment is potentially quite threatening to their emotional and physical well-being and their parents do not show motivation for treatment. These children are usually helped by the change in environment if the environment in which they are placed provides them with consistent love, attention, and protection. In many cases in which temporary placement outside the home is necessary, the child can later be successfully reintegrated into the home if the parents have demonstrated improvement through therapy. With infants and very young children a simple change in environmental conditions may be all that is needed.

Children who exhibit emotional and social maladjustment as a consequence of being abused may be helped by *individual psychotherapy* experiences. *Play therapy* in the form of working through unresolved conflicts with the parent(s) and other authority figures has been found to be successful. Also, *behavior therapy* instituted with the aid of teachers and parents (or foster parents) can be helpful in modifying maladaptive behavior tendencies (e.g., aggressive acting out).

Group therapy experiences with an emphasis on socialization and experiencing appropriate emotional relationships with adults and peers also is effective in overcoming the effects of physical abuse and neglect as well as sexual abuse. One particular form of group therapy that has been successfully used in the treatment of sexually abused latency-age females emphasizes a "guided regression" wherein the therapists help the child gain emotional catharsis by verbally describing feelings associated with the experienced trauma (McQuiston and Schrant, 1977).

Group therapy also is effective in helping both adolescent male and female victims of sexual abuse openly discuss their problems. Often such adolescents feel inhibited in individual therapy from making disclosures about their traumatic experiences, but gain enough support and encouragement in group therapy to do so. The support of peers who have had similar experiences can be a strong factor in helping these adolescents begin to relate experiences that they have found to be frightening, confusing, and guilt provoking.

Adolescents who have been physically abused may also benefit from individual and group therapy experiences, as well as a change in home environment when necessary. Adolescent girls who have been sexually abused need to be provided with a safe protective environment in which they are not forced to interact with the abusive father or stepfather. As with all abused and neglected children, the individual wishes and desires of the child should be taken into careful consideration when planning any treatment program. A child who voices strong objection to remaining in or leaving the home should be carefully listened to. Adolescent girls who have been sexually abused may greatly benefit from supportive psychotherapy with a warm and empathetic female therapist.

Therapy with victims of physical and sexual abuse often needs to center on their mistrust of adults, their damaged self-esteem, and their feelings of anxiety and guilt. It is particularly important with victims of sexual abuse to help them explore their conflicting feelings about their own sexuality and their often disturbed view of the nature of sexual relationships. Therapy with these children must always be conducted with reference to the developmental tasks they are facing at their particular age, and at a level that they are developmentally capable of understanding. Therapy with these children is often a long and time-consuming undertaking that may not show benefits for some time.

It must be understood that treatment of abused children and their parents should be coordinated whenever the family unit is still intact or whenever there is hope of reuniting the family. *Family therapy* is often an important component of treatment of abused and neglected children. The timing of such intervention, however, can be critical, particularly in the case of sexually abused children. Our experiences have been that bringing the entire family together to discuss the incidents in the early phases of treatment can often be too anxiety provoking for the family to handle, and may only lead to an early termination of therapeutic efforts. Family therapy, however, can be a powerful and effective treatment intervention after individual family members have gained sufficient strength and stability to address the subject matter. Furthermore, it is our conviction that family therapy should always be a prerequisite to returning children to a family from which they have been removed because of concern for their safety and physical or emotional well-being.

If treatment is to be successful, the needs of

the family as a whole must be taken into consideration, and all persons or agencies involved in providing services to any family member must be cognizant of this. Furthermore, it is imperative that all agencies providing services to the family communicate openly with each other and work toward mutually agreed on goals.

PREVENTION

The ultimate objective and society's moral obligation is to seek to prevent child abuse and neglect before it begins. Perhaps this utopian ideal can never be achieved, considering man's inhumanity to man, the tremendous socioeconomic, cultural, and educational disadvantages of large segments of the population, and the human and financial resources that would be necessary. Nevertheless, effective preventive methods must be developed and carried out comprehensively if there is to be a significant reduction in abuse and neglect.

It is not sufficient merely to educate the public and the health professionals in the causes, recognition, and reporting of cases of child abuse and neglect, and the problem cannot be solved by the best of diagnosis and treatment after abuse and neglect have occurred. Secondary prevention of subsequent abuse and neglect can, of course, be achieved by proper programs, but there will always be a large number of parents who, for reasons already explained, are psychologically destined to abuse their children.

The key to the problem, as Gray et al. (1977) have shown, is to determine the significant indicators that can be used to predict that a specific parent is likely to be abusive or neglectful, and having so identified the individual(s), to establish a preventive program. They evaluated a group of pregnant women as to their upbringing, feelings about their pregnancy, expectations for the unborn child, attitudes toward discipline, availability of support systems, and present living conditions. A questionnaire was also administered to each mother before or soon after the birth of her baby.

During delivery, and especially immediately after the birth of the baby, observations were made concerning the mother's reactions to the baby (and the father's reactions, if present at time of delivery). Chief observations concerned how they looked at the baby (warmly accepting or rejecting, etc.) and what they said and did. Observations and/or interviews were also conducted in the early postpartum period.

From these studies the mothers were divided into two groups: (1) mothers considered to have a high risk for abnormal parenting practices and (2) mothers considered to have a low risk in this regard. Twenty-five high-risk mothers were placed in a "nonintervention" group and twenty-five high-risk mothers in an "intervention" group. Twenty-five low-risk mothers were placed in the nonintervention group as controls; this meant that the investigators did nothing unusual for the family after discharge, and the families received the usual pediatric care available in the community.

Intervention included assigning the mother and child to a single pediatrician for postdischarge infant care for the next 2 years. The pediatrician thus had continuous contact with the family for well-child supervision and telephoned the mother between serial health visits. A public health nurse visited the homes weekly. Lay health visitors (also called lay therapists) visited the homes frequently, gave emotional and other support and companionship to the mothers, and afforded liaison with the professional health system. When necessary, referrals were made to special medical facilities or mental health clinics.

At the end of approximately 2 years of follow-up there were five children in the high-risk nonintervention group who suffered abuse and neglect of sufficient severity to require hospitalization (fractured skull, fractured femur, subdural hematoma, third degree burns, and barbiturate ingestion). No child in the high-risk intervention or low-risk nonintervention group suffered an injury caused by abnormal parenting practices sufficient to merit hospitalization. The incidence of other aspects of abuse and neglect was also higher in the high-risk nonintervention group than in the others.

The above research findings have been cited at length to indicate that a practical model already exists for primary prevention of child abuse and neglect. It obviously needs to be more widely applied.

James G. Hughes
John A. Hunter

REFERENCES

Adams-Tucker, C.: Proximate effects of sexual abuse in childhood: report on 28 children, Am. J. Psychiatry **139:**10, 1982.

Caffey, J.: Multiple fractures in the long bones of infants suffering from chronic subdural hematoma, Am. J. Roentgenol. **56:**163, 1946.

Caylor, S.P.: The sexual abuse of children: the crime nobody wants to talk about, The Record **41**(6):7, 1978.

Danton, J.H.: MMPI profile configurations associated with incestuous and non-incestuous child molesting, Psychol. Rep. **45,** 1979.

DeFrancis, V.: Protecting the child victim of sex crimes by adults, Denver, 1969, The American Humane Assoc.

Freud, Sigmund: Psycho-analysis: collected papers, vol. V, London, 1953, Hogarth Press, Ltd.

Fritz, G.S., et al.: A comparison of males and females who were sexually molested as children, J. Sex Marital Ther. **7**(1):54, 1981.

Gray, J.D., et al.: Prediction and prevention of child abuse and neglect, Int. J. Child Abuse Neglect, vol. **1,** 1977.

Groth, N.A.: Guidelines for the assessment and management of the offender in sexual assault: The victim and the rapist, In Walker, M.T., et al., editors: Lexington Books, Lexington, Mass., 1976.

Helfer, R.E., et al.: Child abuse and neglect: the family and the community, Cambridge, Mass., 1976, Ballinger Publishing Co.

Kempe, C.H.: Sexual abuse, another hidden pediatric problem, Pediatrics **62:**382, 1978.

Kempe, C.H., and Helfer, R.E.: Helping the battered child and his family, Philadelphia, 1972, J.B. Lippincott Co., Inc.

Kempe, C.H., et al.: The battered child syndrome, JAMA **181:**17, 1962.

McQuiston, M., and Schrandt, R.: Improving parent-child relationships through parent didactic/play group, Paper presented at symposium on Treatment of the Abused and Neglected Child, Part II, Oct., 1977, Denver, Colo.

Quinsey, V.L., et al.: Sexual preferences among incestuous and nonincestuous child molesters, Behav. Ther. **10,** 1979.

Rodriguez, A.: Handbook of child abuse and neglect, Flushing, N.Y., 1977, Medical Examination Publishing Co., Inc.

Sgroi, S.M., et al.: Child sexual abuse: the offense, the offender, and the victim, Workshop presented at Georgetown University, Washington, D.C., March 26, 1982.

Silverman, F.M.: The roentgen manifestations of unrecognized skeletal trauma in infants, Am. J. Roentgenol. **69:**413, 1953.

U.S. Department of Health, Education, and Welfare: Child Abuse and neglect: the problem and its management, I. An overview of the problem, pub. no. (OHD) 73-30073, Washington, D.C., 1975, U.S. Government Printing Office.

Woolley, P.V., Jr., and Evans, W.A., Jr.: Significance of skeletal lesions in infants resembling those of traumatic origin, JAMA **158:**539, 1955.

14 The Pediatric History and Physical Examination

GENERAL CONSIDERATIONS

The fundamentals of diagnosis are (1) skillful history taking, (2) careful physical examination, (3) keen powers of observation, (4) wise selection of laboratory and other technical procedures, and (5) good analytic judgment. None of these is more important than obtaining an excellent history. On this alone a diagnosis can be made in a large percentage of cases.

The ability to obtain a good pediatric history and to conduct an adequate physical examination is not only basic to the diagnosis of disease but is also essential in the evaluation of the normal child, especially the child who has slight deviations from the usual that still fall within the normal range. Yet more errors are made because of inadequate history taking and superficial physical examinations than any other cause.

This chapter discusses the diagnostic approach to the child, emphasizing attitudes and actions of the physician that have bearing on securing cooperation of the parents and the child, how to proceed with the taking of the history, and ways of conducting the physical examination that will make it a more pleasant and less traumatic experience.

OBTAINING THE PEDIATRIC HISTORY

The details of a good pediatric history include information concerning (1) present illness, (2) mother's health during the pregnancy, (3) events of labor and delivery, (4) condition of the child in the neonatal period, (5) growth and development, (6) immunizations, (7) diet and feeding history, (8) previous diseases and whether residual defects occurred, (9) previous operations or hospitalization, (10) child's mental level, (11) child's emotional adjustments, and (12) family history.

Those unfamiliar with pediatrics often consider it a disadvantage that small children cannot describe their symptoms accurately. Actually, the experienced physician frequently finds this helpful. At least the true illness does not have a superimposed veneer of subjective reactions. The pediatrician is accustomed to deal with the relatively pure manifestations of disease in the young and learns to rely on factual findings. As the child grows older, obtaining a history and securing cooperation in the physical examination usually become progressively easier. Toward the end of childhood these procedures do not differ greatly from those employed with adult patients.

There is a tendency to hurry through history taking, to get on with the physical examination, and often to depend unduly on tests and laboratory procedures. A good history is the launching pad to the diagnosis.

Actually, there are few things as interesting in medicine as a properly taken history. There is a certain sameness about "red throats," inflamed eardrums, stiff necks, and other objective evidences of illness, but no two children are just alike, and, especially, no two informants are alike. One is educated, articulate, and accurate. Another with less background can hardly tell a clear story. One is calm; another is frantic. One is sensibly cooperative, another emits information as if under duress, and the next goes on and on in a torrent of talk. From the standpoint of sheer human interest this panorama of people makes any history taking interesting.

The perceptive physician will also find in history taking excellent opportunities for evaluating parent-child relationships, attitudes toward disease and toward possible hospitalization, the degree to which cooperation in management of the child is likely to be obtained, and many other things that clarify the total picture of the sick child in the family group.

Not uncommonly, the physician detects by the way the history is presented, by the way the parent acts, and by the way the child behaves in the examining room that the real disturbance is not organic but emotional. This may serve to avoid pursuit of a diagnosis that does not exist, such as investigating vague, recurrent abdominal pain or functional headache through endless tests until one finally realizes that the problem was emotional all along.

History taking has a special connotation in regard to the new patient. It marks the point of the first contact with the child and the parents. From the moment the first words are spoken, possibly over the telephone, impressions are being formed regarding the competence of the physician. In the office the ease and intelligence with which he diplomatically obtains the history are noted by observant parents. It makes a considerable difference whether he permits the parents to tell their story and listens attentively or interrupts and interrogates incessantly, thus destroying the historical continuity of events on which the diagnosis may hinge; whether he seems rushed and too busy, actually giving medical *inattention* rather than the medical attention for which physicians are noted; whether he respects the sensibilities of the parents in not forcing sensitive questions about family life that they may not wish to discuss at the moment; whether he takes notes quietly and efficiently or scribbles hurriedly, frequently asking the parents to slow down; whether he seems sympathetic and understanding or critical; whether by the way he speaks and looks at the child he shows warmth and friendliness toward children; and, by far the most important of all, whether he exhibits assurance and self-confidence.

Although the atmosphere of the private office and the educational level and attitudes of the usual private patient are conducive to the rapid establishment of good rapport between physician and patient, this is often not true in the crowded public clinic. The parent and sick child may have come a long way by bus, often across half the city. The long delay under crowded circumstances often follows. Social service interviews—certainly necessary—may prolong the interval between arrival and seeing the physician. There are the elevators, the reporting at the clinic desk, the period of time in the waiting room, and finally, at long last, the call to the examining room to see the physician. Seeing large numbers of patients daily, clinic personnel may have had their natural sympathies for the sick beaten down somewhat. Small wonder that when the physician enters the room, he often finds a tired parent and a tired child—a parent who may have developed resentment for what seems an impersonal system of seeing the sick.

The physician should appreciate these things when entering the examining room in such a clinic, realizing that as the first physician seeing the child the impression given will be of special importance to parent and child. The history should be obtained and the physical examination conducted with the same courtesy and consideration as in the private office, and every skillful technique at the physician's command should be used. Not only does one wish because of personal standards to handle the situation gracefully and well, but basically and importantly one seeks to influence the parents to cooperate in treatment of the child, to bring him back for subsequent evaluations, and to appreciate the services of the clinic. Many children who do not return fail to come back because something occurred that alienated the parents. In permitting this to happen the physician has penalized the child.

The attitude and manner of the physician should be friendly, yet dignified, courteous, and noncritical. Students and house staff in medical training should particularly beware of developing hostile attitudes toward patients seen en masse, attitudes that will carry over into practice. One hears too often of "ignorant, uneducated" parents. Physicians should remember that their cultural, educational, and social backgrounds are often far different from those of the patients they treat and that their very training and responsible position obligate them to make all allowances. It is part of being a physician to understand people and why they act as they do. We cannot have two sets of manners—one for the country club and one for the clinic. When confronted with parents who seem hostile, resentful, or uncooperative, the physician should remember that they are often concealing their insecurity, tensions, apprehensions, and possible guilt feelings regarding the sick child. If the physician shows sincerity and skill, most parents will cooperate. The quickest way to alienate parents is to show irritation. Doctors who show resentment toward patients need counseling themselves.

While the history is being taken, the physician seeks to establish a friendly relationship with the child. The physician who is a parent has a certain advantage, but all who like children can learn the simple informal things that tend to please and calm them.

It is legitimate to offer the tense young child a Band-aid, a balloon, two tongue depressors to make an airplane, or some other bribe. Praising a pretty dress, a hairdo, or anything else pleasing to the child also helps. Somewhat older children would be insulted by such techniques. The skilled physician will know how to pitch comments to the child's level of interest.

Let us assume that the physician is entering the examining room where a frightened young child is waiting with his mother. Although it may appear rudimentary and decidedly informal, the experience of seasoned pediatricians has shown that the following approach, taking advantage of many "tricks of the trade," yields dividends.

On entering the room the physician greets the parent courteously, introduces himself if necessary, makes some pleasant remark to or about the child, and sits down as promptly as possible. By sitting down he becomes less threatening in the eyes of the child. He keeps his voice reasonably low, remembering that small children are sometimes frightened by a stranger's loud voice. Although the physician glances from time to time at the child and, if skilled, may learn much about the illness in this way, he avoids looking steadily into the eyes of the child. Small children often become frightened if stared at fixedly.

Since the mother represents to the child security in a threatening situation, the physician permits the child to sit in the mother's lap or, if a bit older, to stand close to her side. If the child becomes upset and continues to be so despite this approach, it is best to proceed quickly to the examination. Few mothers can give an intelligent history while their children are crying and clinging to them. During the examination there will be opportunities to ask questions, and often the child quiets down as soon as it is over and he is back in his mother's arms. If the child is accompanied by two people, it may be preferable to obtain the history from the mother in one room while the second person is with the child in another room.

Although it is customary to teach students to take a very complete history and then to examine the patient, there are circumstances in which the time devoted to history taking should be shortened and the additional information obtained during the physical examination or at its conclusion. If the child is acutely ill with a clearly apparent condition, it is generally advisable to direct the history taking to the pertinent points, obtaining the additional information immediately afterward. The parents are concerned about the child and want the diagnosis settled as quickly as reasonably possible. They may be so upset that they do not want at this time to take up all the small points of the past history, which often bear no relationship to the present complaint. A disconcerting aspect of pediatrics to persons beginning its study is this necessity to modify the approach to the history in view of circumstances of the moment. Nevertheless, a good pediatrician obtains a good history, although possibly going about obtaining it in a way that seems unorthodox to persons who deal with adults.

CONDUCT OF THE PHYSICAL EXAMINATION

General comments

Newborn infants and those up to about 6 months of age often do not exhibit apprehension on being examined. The main group of children who show tension and lack of cooperation in the examining room are those from 1 to 4 years of age. Depending on the emotional maturity of the child, this age range may be extended in the case of overly dependent children or reduced for those who are more independent and sociable.

Before the examination begins, the physician invariably washes and warms hands and instruments. All parents appreciate this but especially those who worry about the germs a physician may carry from the last patient examined. At the end of the examination the hands and instruments are washed again.

In the examination of the young apprehensive child it is a great mistake to remove him immediately from his mother's arms. Much of the examination can be done, and done well, with the child sitting in the mother's lap or standing close by. Beginners in pediatrics tend to sweep the child out of the mother's arms and place him on the table, generally leading to crying and struggling that could have been avoided.

When it is necessary to place the small child on the table, the mother should be permitted to stand nearby where he can see her. At first he should be permitted to assume whatever position he prefers rather than to be forced automatically into the traditional supine position. Many children prefer to sit to be examined, and some even like it better if they are standing. The physician goes along with these preferences up to a point, but not to the extent of preventing a thorough examination. He examines the child in whatever position is needed for a particular purpose.

Some children feel reassured if they cannot see the physician (ostrich technique). The small child may be held in the mother's arms with his head on her shoulder, and the physician can conduct part of the examination by remaining behind the child.

Regardless of how patient the physician is, some children will not be pacified by such measures and will continue to be upset. In such a situation it is better to proceed quickly, to restrain the child adequately, and to conduct the examination rapidly, although accurately.

If it becomes necessary to force the issue in the case of the uncooperative, frightened, or rebellious child, sufficient help should be mobilized for restraint. When the child sees that further struggle is useless, acquiescence may follow. At any rate the period of being upset will be shortened. It is not a kindness to wheedle with a terrified child. Whenever restraint is used, the mother should be told that it is necessary. One may evaluate whether it is wise to send the mother out of the room. Sometimes this results in rapid improvement of the child's behavior; sometimes it only adds to the fright.

Children exhibit a variable degree of modesty, ranging from those who have no compunctions about disrobing to boys who will not even unbutton their shirts if their sisters are in the room. The child's modesty should be respected as much as possible, since it may be based on family custom. However, when undue modesty is shown, the physician may tactfully inquire concerning this, because it may relate to other aspects of the child's behavior that may present problems. Regardless of the child's reluctance, a complete physical examination must be made, and this will require inspecting and examining the various parts. If the child objects, this can still be done tactfully, exposing one part after another. Obviously the best examination is one in which all the clothing is removed except shorts.

Beginning the examination

The physical examination begins as soon as the physician enters the room. He notes whether the child seems well or sick, malnourished, pale, breathing abnormally, cyanotic or jaundiced, or shows any other visible abnormality. A glance tells the practiced physician much about the patient. Furthermore, attitudes the child exhibits toward the parent and the examiner and attitudes the parent exhibits toward the child and the physician give evidence of the emotional balance of the child and parent-child relationships. The inexperienced physician often makes the mistake of starting palpation, percussion, or auscultation before thorough inspection and may miss the obvious in searching for the obscure.

Inspection also gives excellent evidence of the neuromuscular status and mental level of the small child, since developmental diagnostic techniques are based largely on observation. Thus one evaluates the child's abilities in the four fields of developmental diagnosis: motor, language, personal-social, and adaptive.

Examining instruments should be kept out of sight as much as possible, because they add to the child's fear. When brought out for use one by one, the small child is frequently reassured by being permitted to play with them, as if with toys. The usual trick with the otoscope is to shine the light and permit the child to "blow out the light," turning it off as he blows. The percussion hammer is played with as a toy hammer. The blood pressure cuff is "only a little balloon in a bag." The stethoscope is like a telephone. Unfortunately, there is no way to make the tongue depressor attractive; it is the most feared of the nefarious devices.

The small child usually becomes more apprehensive as the physician moves closer to make physical contact. If the child is in the mother's lap, there is generally less fright. The physician should move toward the child slowly, with reassuring remarks.

If the child is not upset when the examination begins, it may prove profitable to examine first the site of suspected pathologic condition, provided this cannot be examined just as well if the child is crying. For example, if the history indicates the presence of a heart murmur, perhaps a gentle approach and auscultation of the heart may permit evaluation of the murmur before the child begins to struggle and cry. The same would be true for a suspected abdominal mass. In this case it may be convenient to have the small child put his arms around the mother's neck, and then from behind the child the physician passes his warmed hands lightly around the child's abdomen, palpating gently and then more deeply. Information gained in this way may be better than that obtained after the child tenses his abdominal muscles with crying.

Naturally, if the presenting complaint indicates a painful lesion, such as an inflamed joint, examining it first would be an error. The same would be true for oral or pharyngeal lesions that involve the most dreaded part of the examination. Furthermore, if a child has a deformity, it is not the kindest thing to focus on it first. Approaching the primary abnormality first carries the risk that the physician will become so preoccupied in evaluating it that the remainder of the examination suffers.

Sometimes just letting the mother put the child through his paces is the best way to start the examination. For instance, much can be learned by remaining quietly seated and observing the mentally retarded child in action or watching the cerebral palsied child move about the room. With hyperkinetic children it is important to permit them to roam the examining room in their often ceaseless, uncontrolled, driven behavior so that the physician may make the diagnosis by simply observing their actions.

Let us assume that none of these peculiar obstacles to a straightforward pediatric examination applies to the child under consideration. If so, one may begin by examining the lower leg of the child as he sits on the mother's lap. The purpose at the moment is not really the examination of the leg but simply to make the first physical contact at a rather remote spot—a peninsula of the body, as it were—and to make it as gently as possible to allay apprehension. It helps to avoid looking directly in the child's eyes. If the child does not become frightened, one then goes on to examine other areas in whatever sequence seems least upsetting.

Although the front of the chest may be auscultated easily by passing the chest piece of the stethoscope between the mother and the clutching child, the mother may have to turn the child around sideways in her lap. Closing the eyes at this point often makes one seem less dangerous to the tense young child. Percussion usually worries small children more than auscultation and should follow it.

After examination of the extremities, abdomen, genitalia, and chest, in whatever order seems easiest, examination of the neck and head follows. Last of all come the examinations of the ears, nose, and throat.

Examination of the ears, nose, and throat

In examination of the ears, nose, and throat (see also p. 988) it is essential that the light be as bright as possible; otherwise, many errors are made in the interpretation of eardrums, nasal mucosa, and mouth and throat. The flashlight and the electric otoscope are the equipment of the pediatrician, but the headband and mirror are as sacred to the otolaryngologist as is the turban to the Hindu. Examination of the throat is often best achieved by placing the child in such a position that daylight affords the illumination. This decreases the chance of overinterpretation of pharyngeal hyperemia.

The ears. Letting the small child play with the otoscope a few moments may save time and make the examination easier. The physician lets the child "blow the light out." Looking briefly at the mother's ears or examining the ears of an older sibling also present is often reassuring.

In the actual examination of the child's ears the tip of the speculum is touched lightly to one ear and then to the other, is then inserted slightly into the external meatus, and then the inspection of the canal and drum takes place. One should use the largest speculum that will fit the external meatus so that better vision will be obtained and to avoid the necessity of inserting the speculum deeply into the canal. Proper examination does not involve inserting the tip of the speculum more than a slight distance into the canal. Pulling lightly on the external ear in the proper direction straightens the canal. Determining mobility of the eardrum by pneumatoscopy is an essential part of the examination.

If the child is sick, especially with an upper respiratory tract infection with fever, the physician must visualize fully both eardrums because of the well-known fact that otitis media may exist without pain. Often cerumen obstructs the view and must be removed. Usually it does not fill the canal, and it can be removed with an ear spoon or small ring curet. If this is necessary, the procedure should be deferred until the rest of the examination has been completed, since it is often painful. After the child is restrained suitably and the speculum of the otoscope is inserted, the cerumen is lifted out until the drum can be seen fully. The physician should invariable tell the parent without the child hearing the remark that sometimes it is impossible to avoid scratching the lining of the canal and that this may result in blood appearing on the tip of the curet as it is withdrawn. Parents not prepared may be upset to observe a drop of blood on the instrument or welling from the auditory canal. There are two parts of the physical examination in which the physician should invariably mention the possibility of blood: removing cerumen from ear canals and doing a digital rectal examination on a small infant.

As is true when any painful procedure is necessary, the child who is old enough to understand should be told in simple terms what has to be done, why it has to be done, and that it will hurt some, but not much. He is also told that the doctor will tell him when the painful part of the procedure is about to begin. The interval between predicting pain and inflicting pain should be short. Children find it hard to forgive a physician who does not tell them when they are going to be hurt. They may be difficult patients to examine for a long time to come.

The handle of the ring curet or ear spoon is held so lightly between the thumb and forefinger that if the child should make a sudden movement toward the physician, the tip would not perforate the drum. If the canal is filled with dry impacted cerumen, it will be necessary to use an ear syringe or some other irrigating device.

If the child with impacted cerumen is being examined only for routine purposes, or if there are causes for the child's illness that are obviously not related to the upper respiratory tract, it may be preferable to defer painful cleaning of the canal until a later date, possibly after the cerumen has been softened by appropriate ear drops or by a cerumenolytic agent.

The nose. Examination of the nose often frightens children more than examination of the ears because the examiner's face is so close to theirs. Again, demonstration on the mother or an older sibling may allay apprehension. The physician remarks and demonstrates that the speculum will not be thrust into the nose, but that only the upper rim of the nostril will be lifted to obtain a good view. As in examination of the ear, the largest speculum that will fit the nostril is employed.

The throat. The throat examination includes the lips, gums, teeth, tongue, buccal mucosa, palate, tonsillar pillars, tonsils, and pharynx. In the child too small to cooperate the tongue depressor is a necessity. However, older cooperative children can often be persuaded to open their mouths widely and say the traditional "ah." Having the mother or older sibling give a quick demonstration may help. The physician must become accustomed to evaluating everything very quickly. Frequently, having the child thus voluntarily display the pharynx gives a better view than is obtained by use of the tongue depressor. Some children are so adept that they seem to be turning the back of the throat inside out.

The best approach to the cooperative child is to try to examine the pharynx in the manner described before the tongue depressor is even exhibited. Once children see this feared instrument, they tend to rebel. However, the depressor will invariably be needed to visualize properly the teeth, gums, and portions of the buccal mucosa.

If the child refuses to cooperate or is unable to reveal the pharynx fully (this ability varies from child to child even when they are fully cooperative), the physician will, of course, have to employ the tongue depressor. Children frequently thrust their tongues out to make the examination easier. Actually, this makes it more difficult. The tongue should be in the usual position. The depressor is passed over the base of the tongue, which is then drawn slightly forward and depressed, a maneuver that tends to minimize the gag reflex. The depressor may also be passed a little to one side of the tongue, the tongue is pushed to the opposite side to permit visualization of that side of the pharynx, and the procedure is then repeated on the opposite side. This technique also minimizes gagging.

Children who clench their teeth and resist

throat inspection will require forceful examination with adequate restraint. They can be made to open their mouths if the tongue depressor is passed between the inner surface of the cheek and the teeth and if strong pressure with a horizontal swinging motion is employed. Eventually the teeth fly apart, and the physician quickly inserts the tongue depressor far enough back to cause a gag reflex, revealing the pharynx.

Although examination of the throat has been listed as the last item in the physical examination of frightened children, there are times when it should be the first, as in children who dread the procedure so much that they are tense and fearful until this part of the examination is over.

The small child's throat is best examined with him sitting in the mother's lap. She holds him upright with his back firmly against her, holds his right hand in her left hand, his left hand in her right hand, and presses down so firmly on the child's thighs that he cannot slide downward or forward. The child's head is controlled by the physician's left hand on the head and forehead. With infants about 1 to 2 years of age the mother may hold the child on her lap, sitting upright and with his back firmly against her, take both of the child's small hands in one of her hands, and with her other hand on the forehead press the child's head back firmly against her chest.

Examination of the chest

Other than the standard inspection, palpation, percussion, and auscultation, there are no special methods of examining the chests of infants and children. However, it is helpful to remember that the chest wall of the infant and young child is so thin and mobile that it rather accurately reflects by its respiratory excursions underlying disease. Sometimes slight differences in excursions between the two sides of the chest can be noted more easily if, with the child lying on his back, one observes from the foot of the child with the eyes slightly above the level of the child's chest.

Examination of the abdomen

How to examine the abdomen of the small child seated on his mother's lap or embracing her has already been discussed. With the older more cooperative child the examination is best conducted with the patient lying on his back, knees drawn up, arms to his side, and head slightly elevated on a pillow. If he will then open his mouth and "pant like a puppy," the abdominal wall will become even more relaxed. The important ingredients of the abdominal examination are a warm hand and a reassuring manner. The physician who has had experience with small children will develop a patter of conversation during the abdominal examination that will also tend to relax the child.

Because it is embarrassing to press on the abdomen of an infant who has just been fed and to have the milk gush up, it is wise to ask whether the child has just been fed and to take precautions if he has been.

Examination of the rectum

If a rectal examination is necessary, the parent should be told why it is needed and so should the child who is capable of understanding. If the patient is a small infant, one should tell the mother that the procedure will hurt only a little and that, at times, a drop of blood may be on the examining finger as it is withdrawn. This is because of the frequency with which rectal examinations in small infants reveal an anorectal shelf, and passing the finger through the tightened area often makes slight tears that bleed. Also, if the finger is inserted too rapidly, a slight anal fissure may be created.

If children are old enough to understand, they should be told that they are going to have an examination, "Like having your temperature taken. It won't really hurt or only a little. You may feel like you're going to have a bowel movement. But it won't take long." Obviously, if the child is an infant, modesty is of no concern; but it is often a great concern to somewhat older children, especially girls. Yet, one sometimes sees on ward rounds an older child's hospital gown drawn up above the hips and the rectal examination done without any draping at all. The proper procedure is to drape the legs. Absorbent paper, a diaper, or a towel is placed underneath the buttocks. The perineal area and the anal margin are inspected before the finger is inserted, and the physician should look especially for a fissure.

The child is not permitted to see the finger cot or rubber glove and the tube of lubricant. The cot is placed on the finger and ample lubricant is applied. Now the physician holds a diaper or small towel over the patient's genitalia so that if the examining finger presses against a full bladder, sudden voiding of urine will not be so obvious, making the doctor look like a novice. The diaper or towel is also there for another purpose—so that when the finger is slowly withdrawn any blood or feces will not be visible to the parent, and in case a moderate amount of feces comes out it can be caught in the diaper or towel. One may as well make a smooth production out of what is not really a pleasant task.

The usual mistake is to insert the finger too rapidly or in the wrong direction or to fail to use sufficient lubricant. The physician begins by simply pressing the tip of the finger directly into the anus pointed toward the navel and holds it there with gentle pressure. The anal sphincter, recognizing the presence of an intruder, goes into a defensive spasm. The spasm cannot be maintained, and the sphincter soon relaxes. The finger then slides in easily, as if drawn upward. The digital examination is then conducted as gently and as rapidly as possible.

The physician should withdraw the finger slowly, allowing the straining bowel to release its pressure gradually so that when the finger is finally removed, there will not be a sudden expulsion of feces. When the tip of the finger is just within the anus, the physician stops, waits a few moments, then withdraws the finger entirely, observes whether blood, mucus, or feces is on it, and tidies up the patient.

CONCLUSION

In concluding these general remarks on examining children, some of the commonest errors should be mentioned. They include failure to examine the genitalia because of modesty on the part of the patient and undue willingness of the physician to gloss over this part of the examination, failure to examine the feet properly, failure to observe the gait, failure to plot height and weight on growth charts and head circumference in infants and younger children, failure to determine blood pressure, skimpy neurologic examinations, and accepting defeat too readily in examining eyegrounds.

Although many things that have been said in this presentation may appear exceptionally trivial to the uninitiated, the experienced pediatrician who values rapport with children and parents uses all or most of the maneuvers and approaches discussed.

James G. Hughes

SELECTED READING

Barness, L.A.: Manual of pediatric physical diagnosis, ed. 5, Chicago, 1980, Year Book Medical Publishers, Inc.

15 The Newborn: Perinatal Pediatrics

Perinatal pediatrics embraces events that begin at the moment of conception and continue throughout the neonatal period. In the past, interest in this continuum was fragmented among embryologists, physiologists, obstetricians, anesthesiologists, and pediatricians. The latter's traditional preoccupation with postnatal phenomena has led logically to an equivalent concern for their prenatal origins, particularly those of the fetal period. Material based on this concept will be summarized at the outset in a general description of perinatal phenomena, which are discussed in more detail subsequently.

The patient is invisible for approximately 9 months, yet may be affected by an array of disorders involving genetic, nutritional, metabolic, pharmacologic, immunologic, or infectious factors. In most of these categories some kind of maternal involvement must precede the fetal effect, whether or not the former is discernible. Transmission to the fetus also implicates the placenta; indeed, the origins of some fetal and neonatal illnesses are restricted to abnormalities of that organ. Although analysis of amniotic fluid components has become available for the diagnosis of certain fetal disorders, familiarity with the history is still fundamental to these diagnoses, all of which require consideration of the present pregnancy, the course and outcome of previous pregnancies, maternal illness prior to the current gestation, and family histories of the mother and father. Historical facts and maternal physical findings sometimes indicate a high-risk pregnancy, which requires intensive observation of mother and fetus during gestation and throughout labor and of the infant after birth.

Parturition is a tumultuous experience for the fetus, even when it progresses normally. The stress it produces is associated with profound alterations of placental gas exchange patterns, of acid-base balance in blood, and of cardiovascular activity in the fetus. During abnormal labor fetal stress is exaggerated, and if the changes are sufficiently intensified and protracted, adjustment to extrauterine life is impaired and intact survival is jeopardized. These catastrophes can often be avoided if procedures are available to monitor fetal cardiac function and acid-base status of blood. Many of them can be anticipated by contemporary obstetric practices. The risk of trauma, although usually averted by obstetric skill, is nevertheless enhanced by some mechanical difficulties of labor, specific types of physical injury being related to certain types of abnormal labor and fetal presentation. Quite apart from the tumult of separation from the mother, the fetus may also be adversely affected by anesthetic and analgesic agents administered to her; this must also be taken into account during postnatal evaluation of a sick neonate.

The first breath normally occurs at the moment the head is exteriorized, often before the entire body is delivered. The fetal lungs are aerated within a fraction of a second thereafter, and evacuation of alveolar fluid occurs rapidly. At the same time slower changes are initiated that, if uninterrupted, will ultimately convert the fetal circulation to an adult pattern. Most infants compensate for the asphyctic effects of normal delivery. They also activate thermoregulatory mechanisms as countermeasures to an inordinate loss of body heat.

These changes are usually effected with little if any difficulty, but many infants need help. Failure to breathe properly requires swift and adept resuscitation in the broadest sense of the term, that is, artificial ventilation, external cardiac massage, expansion of intravascular volume, and provision of ambient heat to decelerate loss of body heat.

Nursery management of newborn infants varies from intensive care of sick babies to routine care of those who are healthy and at term. Accurate interpretation of physical signs and laboratory data largely depends on appreciation of the features that distinguish neonates from older infants. Thus the diagnostic alternatives suggested by many neonatal physical signs (dyspnea, cyanosis, jaundice, convulsions, hepatomegaly, abdominal distention) are dissimilar to those encountered later in infancy, and the significance of laboratory data also differs remarkably. The simple matter of hemoglobin concentration is a dramatic example; levels considered normal for infants several months of age are indicative during the early postnatal hours of disastrous fetal blood loss. Also, blood glucose levels that are normal during the first days of life are dangerously low for older infants.

Age-dependent differences exist between neonates themselves, and here the concern is with gestational age. The disabilities of premature infants have long been appropriately emphasized, whereas the plight of inordinately small but mature infants was not widely recognized until the early 1960s. Realization that at birth coevals may vary considerably in weight has led to abandonment of birth weight as a reliable index of gestational age. Thus, depending on fetal growth rate and length of gestation, newborn infants may be mature or premature, small, large, or normal for gestational age. Because several postnatal disorders depend on birth weight–gestational age relationships, they can be anticipated or more easily recognized if the significance of abnormal fetal growth is appreciated.

Three points may thus be gleaned from these general considerations. First, birth of a healthy newborn infant is the culmination of many antecedent events that must transpire without disruption. Second, an understanding of these events is prerequisite to the diagnosis of prenatal and postnatal illness. Third, it is as inappropriate to consider the neonate a small child as it is to consider the child a small adult.

PRENATAL ASPECTS: THE FETUS

Fetal growth. Normal intrauterine growth proceeds through three phases: predominant hyperplasia, a declining rate of hyperplasia associated with increasing hypertrophy, and predominant hypertrophy. Embryonic growth, which ceases after the twelfth week, is largely the result of hyperplasia (cellular proliferation). As cellular cytoplasm and intercellular material accumulate later, growth is largely a function of hypertrophy (cellular enlargement).

Growth rate is at first linear and rapid. It slows at about the thirty-eighth week, accelerates immediately after birth, and slows again during late infancy. In early life, growth is therefore a heterogeneous process that involves varying rates of cellular proliferation and enlargement. Deleterious influences may be exerted during phases of hyperplasia, hypertrophy, or both. Congenital rubella is acquired by the embryo early in pregnancy. It therefore exerts its effects primarily on hyperplasia; cell counts in various organs are subnormal. The effects of toxemia are exerted late in gestation, thereby impairing hypertrophic growth; cell counts are somewhat diminished, but the major effect is diminution of cell size (cytoplasmic mass). These latter findings, which are characteristic of severe malnutrition during the first year of postnatal life, are generally believed to indicate intrauterine malnutrition when they occur in neonates. In the infant with congenital rubella, proper postnatal nutrition is unlikely to restore a normal cell number; limitation of growth potential is permanent. However, intrauterine malnutrition may be reversible if proper postnatal nutrition is available. Permanent limitation in growth of the brain follows severe intrauterine malnutrition in animals.

The normal decrement in growth rate that occurs at about the thirty-eighth week of gestation is not caused by loss of fetal growth potential. Rather, postnatal resumption of the rapid rate that existed in the first 38 weeks suggests that normally the intrauterine milieu becomes less capable of supporting fetal growth and is therefore more vulnerable to factors that interfere with maternofetal transfer of nutrient. The fetal effects of mild or moderate malnutrition may thus be more profound late in gestation, when normally the capacity to sustain growth is marginal. Thus, in maternal preeclampsia, placental volume and weight diminish toward term as villous surface area and exchanging tissue progressively decrease. In the extreme, normal gas exchange may be affected; more often the resultant principal deficiency is in the transfer of nutrient to the fetus.

Placental circulation. Although the placenta

functions as a single organ, it comprises embryonic tissue (chorion) and maternal tissue (decidua basalis). Primitive chorionic villi from the embryo are embedded in endometrium within a week after implantation, and villous capillaries are formed from angioblastic mesoderm that invades these structures. Meanwhile the villi increase in number and penetrate more deeply into the endometrium; uterine vessels are eroded in the process, and an intervillous space is formed, which is filled with maternal blood surrounding the villi. Fetomaternal exchange transpires at this site. The intervillous space receives spurts of blood from the tips of uterine arteries. Venous blood returns through vessels that drain the intervillous space and course laterally through the decidua basalis. Direction of blood flow is maintained by an arteriovenous pressure gradient. On the fetal side two umbilical arteries enter the placenta near the center of its surface, branch successively, and then terminate at the villous capillary loops. Blood returns through veins that coalesce repeatedly to form a single umbilical vein (pp. 252 to 253).

Metabolic exchange between the fetus and mother depends on an intact circulatory apparatus. Structural disruption may occur gradually or abruptly in relation to several fetal and maternal disorders before or during labor or as a result of anomalous vascularization.

Fetal gas exchange. Assuming structural integrity of placental vessels, fetomaternal exchange of oxygen and carbon dioxide is governed by factors that influence the partial pressures of these gases in the maternal and fetal circulations at the intervillous space. Gaseous transfer occurs by simple diffusion and therefore in the direction of existing pressure gradients. At the intervillous space, diffusion of oxygen from mother to fetus is the result of higher maternal arterial Po_2, whereas the gradient of carbon dioxide pressure from fetal to maternal blood drives diffusion of that gas in the opposite direction. Fetal asphyxia may result from impairment of maternal blood flow associated with hypotension or, as in another example, from obstruction of fetal blood flow caused by compression of the umbilical cord. Reduction of effective surface area over which both circulations come into apposition may occur from abruptio placentae; the immediate life-threatening effects on the fetus are the result of inadequate gas exchange. A variety of clinical conditions involving obstetric misadventure ultimately lead to aberrations of gas exchange. These conditions are described in subsequent sections.

Amniotic fluid. At term the fetus is enveloped in 700 to 1200 ml amniotic fluid, which has accumulated at a rate of 25 to 50 ml weekly. Early in pregnancy the fluid is essentially a dialysate of maternal extracellular fluid; later its primary source is the fetal urinary tract and, to a minor degree, the respiratory and gastrointestinal tracts. The constant turnover of amniotic fluid involves complex water and solute exchanges, precise details of which have yet to be elucidated. Egress of fluid is largely through the gastrointestinal tract, into which it gains entry by fetal swallowing. From this site, absorption into the fetal bloodstream ensues. Normal volume of amniotic fluid is thus primarily regulated by absorptive activity of the fetal gastrointestinal tract and excretory function of the urinary tract. Accumulation of 2000 ml or more (hydramnios) is associated with esophageal atresia, presumably because flow of fluid during swallowing is obstructed in the fetus. Hydramnios is also associated with anencephaly, apparently because effective swallowing is absent. In contrast, an inordinately small amount of amniotic fluid, or absence of it (oligohydramnios), is characteristic of renal agenesis, since addition of fetal urine to amniotic fluid is precluded.

Most descriptions of the components of amniotic fluid are based on analyses performed at term. Information on changes related to fetal maturation is scant. Approximately 2% solids are present, half of which is protein. Cellular content is of fetal origin and increases as pregnancy progresses. Several diagnostic techniques have used chemical analysis of fluid and morphologic or histochemical attributes of cells for identification of fetal abnormalities.

Fetal circulation. The fetal circulatory structure differs from neonatal and adult patterns in three major aspects: high pulmonary vascular resistance, which causes minimal lung perfusion (approximately 5% of total cardiac output); low vascular resistance in the placental circulation, which receives approximately 50% of total cardiac output; and presence of right to left shunts within the heart (foramen ovale) and between the pulmonary artery and aorta (ductus arteriosus).

Oxygenated blood returns from chorionic villi

and enters the fetal abdomen through the umbilical vein. Most of the blood passes to the inferior vena cava after traversing the ductus venosus, whereas a smaller portion perfuses liver substance (left lobe). At a point just before the inferior vena cava enters the heart, blood has converged from the ductus venosus (highest oxygen saturation), from liver substance (reduced oxygen saturation), from the distal portion of the inferior vena cava (which drains the lower body), and from the portal vein (lowest oxygen saturation). At the cardiac orifice the main current of blood from the inferior vena cava is directed into the left atrium by the upper edge of the foramen ovale (crista dividens), where it mixes with the small quantity of blood from the pulmonary veins, further lowering oxygen saturation. Blood then flows to the left ventricle, from where its major distribution is to the coronary arteries and the head by way of arteries from the aortic arch; little of it passes to the descending aorta. The smaller portion of blood in the right atrium is mixed with venous blood from the head (superior vena cava) and the myocardium (coronary sinus). This mixture flows to the right ventricle and thence through the main pulmonary artery, where the current divides so that most blood enters the ductus arteriosus into the distal aortic arch and through the descending aorta to the lower part of the body. Hypogastric arteries branch from the iliac arteries and course on each side of the bladder into the umbilical cord, where they appear as two umbilical arteries. These terminate in capillary loops in the placental villi. A smaller portion of blood from the right ventricle continues through branches of the pulmonary artery to the lungs and is returned to the left atrium through pulmonary veins.

Mixing of well-oxygenated and desaturated blood thus occurs at the juncture of the ductus venosus with the inferior vena cava, within the right atrium, and at the junction of the ductus arteriosus with the aorta.

Fetal evaluation. Clinical examination of the fetus was limited a number of years ago to palpation through the maternal abdominal wall and auscultation of fetal heart tones, both of which yield little useful information. The increasing use of ultrasound has largely eliminated the need for radiologic examination. As better understanding of the prenatal origins of neonatal disease emerges, the need for penetration of natural barriers to fetal evaluation becomes more urgent. Several ingenious methods are sufficiently safe and informative to justify extensive application; others require further development. Many fetal deaths can be prevented, and a considerable number of intrapartum hazards can be avoided (or at least attentuated) if data on fetal status can be obtained.

Ultrasound is virtually indispensable for the estimation of fetal growth and age. Ultrasonography is also useful for the identification of multiple fetuses and certain congenital anomalies (such as anencephaly), demonstration of fetal presentation, and localization of the placenta. It produces no maternal discomfort, it is not harmful to the fetus, and it eliminates the hazards of radiation that are inherent in x-ray diagnosis.

Above frequencies of human hearing (approximately 18,000 cps), sound waves can be focused like light beams. The frequency of ultrasound for intrauterine visualization is 2,000,000 to 5,000,000 cps (2 to 5 MHz). Low frequencies penetrate to greater depths but they produce suboptimal resolution of images; high frequencies produce sharper images but penetrate less deeply. Because resolution is significantly improved at higher frequencies and images of deeper tissues are required during pregnancy, the choice of frequencies is a compromise between the need for deeper penetration and desirability of the highest possible resolution. Tissues of differing density impose varying degrees of impedance to the directional passage of ultrasonic waves. When two adjacent tissue masses differ in their impedance, ultrasonic waves rebound (echo) at the interface of the two tissue masses. The greater the difference in impedance, the greater the quantity of rebounded ultrasound. Energy in reflected waves, sensed by a transducer, is converted to voltage that is amplified and displayed as white images on a screen or is photographed as a permanent record. If there is no difference in the *acoustic density* of adjacent tissue masses, echoes are not produced and the resultant image is black. For obstetric use the real-time scanner is preferred. Fetal movements are visualized at 15 to 30 frames per second, and continuous scan of the entire fetus is feasible.

A gestational sac is identifiable by ultrasound at 5 weeks after the last menstrual period, thus providing the earliest evidence of an existing pregnancy. The embryo is first visible at 6 to 7 weeks. During the first trimester (embryonic period) fetal maturity is estimated by measurement of crown-rump length. Before the fourteenth gestational week, close prediction of delivery date is possible in approximately 95% of patients. Beyond the first trimester, fetal maturity is estimated by measurement of the fetal head in its biparietal diameter. After 28 weeks, interpretation of biparietal diameters is considerably less reliable because of increased variation in head growth from one fetus to another. Identification of fetal undergrowth (intrauterine growth retardation) requires comparison of head measurements with those of the abdomen at the level of umbilical vein.

Visualization of the fetus by ultrasound has established a diagnostic capability that was virtually nonexistent. Ultrasonography provides direct visualization of the placenta, thus enabling accurate identification of placenta previa. Ultrasonography is indispensable for the diagnosis of numerous congenital anomalies; the major ones are often discernible at 15 to 16 weeks gestation.

Amniotic fluid analysis (amniocentesis) is a standard procedure for evaluation of the fetal state in certain high-risk pregnancies. The procedure was first used widely for study of amniotic fluid in rhesus (Rh)-incompatible pregnancies. Properly executed, amniocentesis is virtually devoid of serious complications.

Amniotic fluid analyses are largely concerned with determination of pulmonary maturity, the assessment of the severity of Rh disease, and identification of genetic disorders. Earlier, a number of determinations were attempted for the assessment of fetal maturity, but the clinical usefulness of these procedures has proven to be at best equivocal. Creatinine concentrations, viscosity and osmolarity, and staining of cells for fat content are examples of attempts to evaluate maturity of the fetus. Because of their inconsistent results, coupled with the advent of ultrasonography, these procedures are not frequently used at present. A number of hereditary and metabolic disorders are identifiable by tissue culture of cells from amniotic fluid or by biochemical analysis. The diagnosis of *erythroblastosis fetalis* and assessment of its severity are accomplished by spectrophotometric analysis of amniotic fluid for bilirubin content.

The *lecithin-sphingomyelin* (L/S) *ratio* in amniotic fluid is a valuable indicator of pulmonary maturity. Lecithin is the major phospholipid constituent of pulmonary surfactant, and elaboration of the latter substance reaches mature proportions at 35 or 36 weeks of gestation. The level of lecithin in amniotic fluid rises as a consequence of increased surfactant production, and because the level of sphingomyelin does not rise at the same rate, an enlarging ratio of lecithin to sphingomyelin progresses to exceed 2.0 at 35 or 36 gestational weeks. This ratio reflects mature surfactant activity in alveoli, and there is thus little likelihood that hyaline membrane disease (respiratory distress syndrome) will occur after birth. Medium or low ratios indicate a strong possibility of impending hyaline membrane disease, although some infants are unaffected in spite of a low L/S ratio.

Surfactant is produced by type II alveolar cells, beginning at about 20 gestational weeks. The most important phospholipid in mature surfactant is phosphatidylcholine (lecithin), which is usually present in functional quantities at approximately 35 weeks. Thus at 35 weeks the quantity of lecithin in amniotic fluid increases abruptly. The production of sphingomyelin, which is not a surfactant phospholipid, changes little during pregnancy; it is therefore a reliable baseline to which the quantity of lecithin can be related. Both lecithin and sphingomyelin are present in approximately equal concentrations until about 30 to 32 gestational weeks. The L/S ratio is generally 1.0 during this period. Between 30 and 34 weeks, lecithin production increases more than that of sphingomyelin, and the resultant L/S ratio may be at approximately 1.2 to 1.5.

The L/S ratio is currently the most reliable predictor of hyaline membrane disease, but immature ratios are sometimes confusing because 20% to 25% of such fetuses do not have the disease postnatally. Mature ratios, however, are considerably more reliable predictors; very few such fetuses will develop hyaline membrane disease after birth.

Development of pulmonary maturity, and thus a mature L/S ratio, may be accelerated or retarded in association with a number of maternal or fetal conditions. Mature ratios before 35 weeks have been reported in the presence of maternal toxemia, hypertensive renal or cardiovascular disease, sickle cell anemia, narcotic addiction, and advanced maternal vascular diabetes (classes D, E, and F). All these conditions are associated with intrauterine growth retardation and presumably an increased elaboration of fetal corticosteroids in response to the stress they produce. Increased corticosteroid levels are thought to stimulate production of mature surfactant in type II alveolar cells. The same phenomenon is believed by some investigators to be operative in the presence of prematurely ruptured membranes, which is often associated with accelerated lung maturity. In contrast, pulmonary maturity is impeded in association with the less advanced stages of maternal diabetes, Rh incompatibility (particularly in the presence of hydrops), and in the smaller of identical twins.

Phosphatidylglycerol determination substantially increases the accuracy of L/S ratio interpretations. Phosphatidylglycerol is a component of surfactant; it appears at approximately 36 weeks and increases steadily thereafter. The presence of phosphatidylglycerol is probably the most reliable indicator of lung maturity that is now available.

The *foam stability test* (shake test) is an admirably simple procedure that is based on the capacity of surfactant to stabilize bubbles that are created by the vigorous shaking of amniotic fluid mixed with 95% ethanol in a test tube. A complete ring of bubbles that persists for 15 minutes correlates well with a mature L/S ratio. However, the absence of bubble stability is not as reliable an indicator of immature L/S ratios. In such circumstances pulmonary immaturity should be verified by performance of an L/S ratio. The shake test has been applied postnatally to neonatal gastric aspirate, as well as tracheal and hypopharyngeal secretions. The results are similar to those from amniotic fluid testing.

Monitoring of fetal status during labor has been greatly facilitated by availability of a technique for obtaining *blood from the fetal scalp.* The procedure is usually restricted to pregnancies in which there is high risk of fetal asphyxia (diabetes mellitus, toxemia, elderly gravida, postmaturity, and erythroblastosis) or clinical evidence of fetal distress (abnormal heart rates and meconium-stained amniotic fluid). A diminished blood pH and presence of base deficit are the most reliable biochemical indicators of fetal distress. Determinations of Po_2 and Pco_2 are not such reliable indications of distress because they are so frequently evanescent, whereas changes in hydrogen ion concentration are more persistent. Fetal acidosis is a result of carbon dioxide retention and accumulation of lactic acid. The latter is a reflection of oxygen deprivation and the ensuing degradation of glucose to lactic acid (anaerobic glycolysis). If oxygen deprivation and carbon dioxide retention are mild and transient, decline in pH is insignificant, if it occurs at all. Assessment of acid-base status must be performed repeatedly to ascertain its significance. The impression of life-threatening asphyxia based on the single set of data obtained during temporary stress could erroneously lead to surgical interference. A pH below 7.2 in two consecutive samples is believed to indicate necessity for immediate delivery, assuming absence of maternal acidosis has been demonstrated.

Maternal excretion of estriol is sometimes an indicator of fetal well being. The adrenals of the fetus are the principal source of estriol precursors, and ultimate conversion to estriol is accomplished in the placenta. Estriol levels thus reflect the functional status of the fetoplacental unit. Daily urinary content increases from 0.1 mg in the first trimester to at least 12 mg during the last trimester. Fetal distress is present if serial determinations demonstrate a gradual or abrupt fall from previous levels. During the third trimester, values below 12 mg/24 hr suggest fetal difficulty; levels below 3 to 4 mg indicate fetal death or anencephaly. The literature concerning estriol determinations for fetal well-being is at best unsettled. There is agreement that interpretation of results is confounded by day-to-day variations. There is some disagreement on which determination is a more reliable predictor, plasma or urinary estriol. The value of estriol determinations as an index of fetoplacental function has been well established in cases of diabetic pregnancies.

Fetal heart rate (FHR) *monitoring* is yet another useful procedure for early detection of fetal distress. Bradycardia is a well-known response to asphyxia, but tachycardia usually occurs first. Beside these changes, the pattern of slowed rate in relation to uterine contractions is an important aid in the early detection of asphyctic changes. A drop in rate normally appears with the onset of contractions and disappears with their termination (early deceleration). This pattern is reproducible by manual application of pressure to the fetal head and was experimentally eliminated by administration of small doses of atropine into the fetal buttock. It is thus apparently caused by circulatory changes in the brain stem attendant to pressure exerted on the head by uterine contractions and transmitted to the heart by way of the vagus nerve. An abnormal pattern of bradycardia, which is indicative of fetal jeopardy (asphyxia), consists of delayed onset of return to normal rate beyond the end of contractions (late deceleration). This pattern is not reproducible by application of pressure to the head, and it is only partially eliminated by atropine. Late deceleration is abnormal in any circumstance. Its lowest point appears after the peak of a uterine contraction; the return to baseline occurs well after the end of the contraction. The onset of the contraction compromises perfusion of a placenta that may already be marginally functional. Mild hypoxemia appears early during this process and the response is an adrenergic fetal hypertension. A baroreceptor vagal response then gradually slows the heart. The delayed appearance of this type of deceleration in relation to the onset of contraction is attributed to the interval of time required for the development of mild hypoxemia. In the presence of a dysfunctional placenta, oxygen exchange becomes significantly impaired and fetal hypoxemia eventually produces lactic acidosis. Now, the pattern of late deceleration becomes a consequence of depressed myocardial activity during the recurrent episodes of hypoxemia associated with uterine contractions.

A third decelerative pattern is called variable deceleration. This interval of bradycardia bears no relationship to uterine contractions and thus appears irregularly and for variable lengths of time. Variable deceleration is caused by cord compression. If sufficient external pressure is applied to the cord, occlusion of the arteries increases resistance to blood flow from fetus to low-resistance placental circuit. Fetal hypertension follows; a baroreceptor response is mediated by the vagus nerve, and bradycardia ensues. The duration of bradycardia is related to duration of cord compression. In instances of protracted compression, hypoxemia and metabolic acidosis are produced to cause myocardial depression. Cord compression is usually evanescent however, and in these circumstances the vagal baroreceptor response ceases abruptly and the heart rate returns to baseline quite rapidly.

Beat-to-beat variability of heart rate is an intrinsic characteristic of normal heart rate tracings. Variability is produced by opposition of sympathetic and parasympathetic influences on the sinoatrial node. On a routine tracing beat-to-beat variability is seen as recurrent differences in R-R intervals. The presence of variability on the fetal heart rate tracing is a reassuring indication of fetal well-being. In the presence of abnormal decelerations, preservation of variability suggests that the fetus is not in significant jeopardy. The disappearance of variability however, is a sinister sign of hypoxemia regardless of the presence or pattern of deceleration unless another known cause for the change is identifiable. These nonhypoxemic causes are narcotics, sedatives, local analgesics, parasympathetic drugs or beta-adrenergic blockers, fetal sleep, or heart block.

The nonstress test (NST) for fetal well-being entails assessment of fetal cardiac reactivity to fetal movement. Normally, the cardiac rate increases by 15 or more beats during periods of fetal movement on at least two occasions during a 20-minute observational period. This is called a *reactive* NST. The test is nonreactive if the heart rate does not increase with movement. If there are no fetal movements, and the baseline fetal heart rate is normal, the test is deemed suspicious. The NST is widely used for high-risk pregnancies. Nonreactive or suspicious results may indicate a need for the oxytocin challenge test. The NST records externally the fetal cardiac activity, fetal movements, and uterine contractions by using transabdominal electronic instrumentation.

The *oxytocin challenge test* (OCT) is performed for the prediction of fetal jeopardy during labor in the presence of chronic uteroplacental insufficiency. The test is usually first performed for maternal hypertension, advanced diabetes, or intrauterine growth retardation from any cause. Oxytocin is administered intravenously in dilute solution until three uterine contractions per minute are produced. The fetal heart rate is monitored externally. If late deceleration appears and persists, the test is positive.

Delivery is performed soon thereafter if fetal lung maturity is demonstrated. The incidence of false positive results is 25%. If the test is negative (no late decelerations), the absence of fetal jeopardy can be inferred reliably.

Effects of drugs on the fetus. Metabolic mechanisms that transform the chemical structure of drugs are minimally operative in the fetus. The placenta generally accommodates maternofetal transfer of most drugs. The degree to which a drug may cross the placenta is largely dependent on its molecular weight, lipid solubility, extent of ionization, and protein binding. Beyond its diffusibility, the accumulation of a drug in the fetus is determined by maternal dosage, duration of administration, and rate of maternal elimination and therefore maternal blood levels.

In addition to the degree of fetal drug accumulation, the time of administration during gestation is pivotal. During the embryonic period, when organogenesis is most active, extensive damage may occur. It is at this time that the most disastrous malformations are produced. Severe growth retardation without specific malformation may also occur during the embryonic period. Drugs administered late in pregnancy are dependent on fetal and neonatal capacity for chemical transformation. Effects of short-acting barbiturates and meperidine (Demerol) given to the mother before delivery may be enhanced and protracted in the neonate because of inadequate oxidative activity (barbiturates) and glucuronidation (meperidine) in the liver. Since gaseous anesthetic agents are excreted through the lungs, respiratory distress at birth may increase the effects of these retained agents. Another type of pharmacologic hazard is exemplified in the inadvertent injection of mepivacaine into the fetus during caudal analgesia, a rare event. In such infants, bradycardia, cyanosis, convulsions, and death occur. Mepivacaine also traverses the placenta with ease. High fetal blood levels may seriously depress the infant at birth. Chlorpropamide, a sulfonylurea, crosses the placenta and persists in the neonate to cause prolonged and intractable hypoglycemia and convulsions, thus presenting a serious hazard to the infant as a result of inappropriate therapy for maternal diabetes.

Narcotic withdrawal syndrome has long been known in infants of mothers addicted to morphine or heroin and in mothers under treatment with methadone for narcotic addiction. The widespread use of narcotics among young people (of whom one third are female) has steadily yielded a large number of affected neonates since the mid-1960s. The narcotic withdrawal syndrome occurs in at least 50% of the offspring of addicted mothers. The incidence of affected infants is as high as 75% if the duration of maternal addiction is over a year. The onset of symptoms is generally within the first few days of life; the closer the last maternal dose to birth of the infant, the later the onset of symptoms. The higher the dose, the more likely are signs of neonatal withdrawal. The likelihood of withdrawal disorders decreases as the interval between the last dose and birth increases beyond 24 hours.

The signs in affected babies include vomiting, diarrhea (often severe, dehydrating, and life threatening), sweating, hypothermia or hyperthermia, and agitative central nervous system signs such as irritability, hyperactivity, hypertonia, hyperreflexia, myoclonus, and seizures. Infants are often of low birth weight—either small for gestational age and mature, or premature. Induction of glucuronyl transferase activity in utero by morphine or heroin is apparently the basis for a low incidence of hyperbilirubinemia. Induction in the fetus of surfactant synthesis in type II alveolar cells apparently diminishes the incidence of hyaline membrane disease in prematurely born babies. The signs of methadone withdrawal are similar to, but more severe and protracted than those described for heroin. Treatment with phenobarbital, paregoric, chlorpromazine, or diazepam is relatively effective; overall mortality is approximately 4%.

The *fetal alcohol syndrome* and *acute neonatal alcohol withdrawal syndrome* are, respectively, the result of chronic and acute maternal alcoholism. The fetal alcohol syndrome affects almost half the infants born of alcoholic mothers. It comprises a constellation of anomalies that include fetal undergrowth, small palpebral fissures, epicanthal folds, microcephaly, dislocated hips, cardiac malformations, and restricted joint mobility that is particularly notable at the elbows and the hands.

Infants born of inebriated mothers have about the same blood alcohol levels as does maternal blood. Their breath reeks of alcohol. After several hours they become irritable and hyperactive, and these signs may progress to tremors and seizures. After approximately 72 hours, rather profound lethargy occurs over the next 2 days. This is followed by a normal neonatal demeanor. Treatment of alcohol withdrawal utilizes the same drugs listed for therapy of narcotic withdrawal.

Table 15-1 includes a list of maternal medications that may be harmful to the fetus and the newborn.

Effects of maternal illness on the fetus and the newborn. Table 15-1 lists maternal illnesses that may adversely affect fetal outcome. In some instances available data are limited to a few case reports, but the evidence at least suggests maternofetal association.

High-risk pregnancy. If the delivery of currently known techniques for obstetric and neonatal care were utopian, most perinatal deaths would be averted. Over 70% of infant deaths in the United States (death under 1 year of age) occur during the neonatal period (first 28 days of life). More than 90% of neonatal deaths occur during the first 7 days. The earliest deaths are usually associated with misadventure during pregnancy, labor, and delivery. Since 1950, progress in reduction of infant perinatal mortality in this country has lagged behind that in most other well-developed nations. This comparison may be of great concern, but the discrepancy in perinatal deaths between white and nonwhite populations in the United States should be an even greater cause of professional disquietude. Prematurity and perinatal death are approximately twice as frequent for the nonwhite as for the white population. The background of this end result is complex and multifactorial, and although there are no quick solutions, means by which pregnancy wastage can be reduced are at hand. The delivery of this care to those who need it most is still a major problem.

Because a major portion of the infant perinatal mortality is related to maternal antecedents, and because reduction of deaths has been accomplished in some localities when these are identified early, an awareness of the factors that cause high-risk pregnancy is of fundamental importance. Once identified, application of presently known techniques to the management of high-risk women and their infants will avert or attentuate fetal and neonatal catastrophe. A pregnancy is considered high risk when certain conditions or events impose hazards to the mother herself and to the intact survival of her fetus or infant. Factors in high-risk pregnancy are presented in Table 15-1 and in the following outline:

- General factors
  - Age of mother less than 16 years, over 40 years
  - Primigravida over 35 years
  - Weight less than 45 kg (100 pounds), over 90 kg (200 pounds)
  - Height less than 158 cm (63 inches)
  - Malnutrition, acute or chronic
- Previous pregnancy experience
  - Grand multiparity (more than 6 pregnancies lasting more than 20 weeks)
  - Cesarean section or midforceps delivery
  - Prolonged labor (over 24 hours)
  - Premature labor, delivery
  - Postmature labor, delivery
  - Abnormal product of pregnancy
    - Spontaneous abortion
    - Stillbirth
    - Neonatal death
    - CNS disorder (any type)
    - Major anomaly (any type)
- Medical or obstetric factors
  - Toxemia
  - Hypertensive cardiovascular disease
  - Diabetes (gestational, overt)
  - Rheumatic heart disease
  - Congenital heart disease
  - Peripheral vascular disease
  - Pulmonary insufficiency (acute or chronic)
  - Rh sensitization
  - Idiopathic thrombocytopenic purpura
  - Sickle cell disease
  - Other blood dyscrasia
  - Neoplasm
- Convulsive disorder
- Collagen disease
- Thyroid, parathyroid disorders, other endocrinopathies
- Rubella, cytomegalovirus, toxoplasma, herpes, and syphilitic infection
- Kidney infection
- Amnionitis
- Bleeding during second, third trimesters
- Multiple pregnancy
- Incompetent cervix
- Hydramnios, oligohydramnios
- Drug addiction
- Habitual cigarette smoking

INTRAPARTUM ASPECTS: EFFECTS OF LABOR

The fetus who has thrived normally throughout pregnancy is well equipped to withstand the stresses of normal labor and can compensate for them within a short time after birth. Often, however, the normal course of pregnancy is marred

Text continued on p. 265.

Table 15-1. Maternal abnormalities and associated fetal and neonatal disorders

Maternal factors	Fetal, neonatal disorders
ANTEPARTUM	
Metabolic	
Diabetes mellitus	Prematurity*
	Hyaline membrane disease
	Hyperbilirubinemia
	Hypoglycemia
	Macrosomatia
	Hypocalcemia
	Renal vein thrombosis
	Polyhydramnios
	Congenital anomalies
	Intrauterine growth retardation
Gout	Hyperuricemia (transient, asymptomatic)
Malnutrition	Intrauterine growth retardation
Porphyria	Porphyrinuria (transient, asymptomatic)
Endocrine	
Addison disease	Prematurity
	Intrauterine growth retardation
Chronic hypoparathyroidism	Hyperparathyroidism (intrauterine and postnatal)
Primary hyperparathyroidism	Neonatal tetany (hypocalcemia)
	Hypomagnesemia
Thyroid	
Goiter (nontoxic)	Goiter
Hyperthyroidism (untreated)	Hyperthyroidism (goitrous or nongoitrous)
Hyperthyroidism (treated)	Goiter (nontoxic)
	Hyperthyroidism (goitrous or nongoitrous)
	Hypothyroidism (goitrous or nongoitrous)
Hypothyroidism	CNS defects
	Hypothyroidism
Cardiac	
Congestive failure	Prematurity
	Asphyxia†
Hypertensive cardiovascular disease	Asphyxia
	Intrauterine growth retardation
Pulmonary	
Asthma (intractable) or any disorder associated with hypoxemia and hypercapnia	Asphyxia
	Prematurity
	Intrauterine growth retardation
Gastrointestinal	
Regional ileitis	Prematurity
Renal	
Polycystic kidney disease	Polycystic kidney disease
Chronic glomerulonephritis	Prematurity
	Intrauterine growth retardation
	Asphyxia
Neurologic	
Myasthenia gravis	Myasthenia gravis
Status epilepticus	Asphyxia

From Korones, S.B., and Lancaster, J.: High-risk newborn infants: the basis for intensive nursing care, ed. 3, St. Louis, 1981, The C.V. Mosby Co.
*Prematurity = gestational age less than 37 completed weeks.
†Asphyxia = hypoxemia, hypercapnia, low pH.

Table 15-1. Maternal abnormalities and associated fetal and neonatal disorders—cont'd

Maternal factors	Fetal, neonatal disorders
ANTEPARTUM—cont'd	
Hematologic	
Blood incompatibility (Rh, ABO, other)	Erythroblastosis fetalis
Idiopathic thrombocytopenic purpura	Idiopathic thrombocytopenic purpura (transient)
Leukemia (acute)	Prematurity
Megaloblastic anemia	Hazards of abruptio placentae
Sickle cell anemia	Low birth weight Intrauterine growth retardation
Anemia (iron deficiency)	Low birth weight, prematurity
Skin	
Pemphigus	Bullae (transient)
Neoplastic	
Hodgkin disease	Hodgkin disease
Ovarian tumors (complicated)	Prematurity
Collagen disease	
Lupus erythematosus (acute)	Systemic lupus erythematosus
Lupus erythematosus (subacute)	Syndrome of congenital heart block, fibroelastosis, fibrosis of liver, spleen, kidney, adrenals
Infection (antepartum or intrapartum)	
Viral	
Coxsackie	Coxsackie infection (encephalomyocarditis)
Cytomegalic inclusion disease	Cytomegalic inclusion disease
Hepatitis (SH)	Neonatal hepatitis
Herpesvirus infection	Herpesvirus infection
Measles	Measles
Mumps	?Congenital anomalies
Poliomyelitis	Poliomyelitis
Rubella	Congenital rubella syndrome
Smallpox	Smallpox
TRIC agent (cervicitis)	Inclusion blenorrhea
Vaccinia (primary vaccination)	Generalized vaccinia
Varicella	Varicella
Western equine encephalomyelitis	Western equine encephalomyelitis
Protozoan	
Candidiasis (vaginal)	Thrush
Malaria	Malaria
Toxoplasmosis	Toxoplasmosis
Trypanosomiasis	Trypanosomiasis
Bacterial	
Acute pyelonephritis	Prematurity Bacterial infections
Enteropathogenic *E. coli* (carrier)	Diarrhea (enteropathogenic *E. coli*)
Gonorrhea	Gonorrheal infection (usually ophthalmia)
Listeriosis	Listeriosis
Pneumococcal meningitis	Pneumococcal meningitis
Salmonellosis	Salmonellosis
Septicemia (any organism)	Septicemia (any organism)
Shigellosis	Shigellosis
Syphilis	Congenital syphilis
Tuberculosis	Tuberculosis
Typhoid fever	Typhoid fever

Table 15-1. Maternal abnormalities and associated fetal and neonatal disorders—cont'd

Maternal factors	Fetal, neonatal disorders
ANTEPARTUM—cont'd	
Obstetric and gynecologic	
Amputated cervix	Prematurity
Incompetent cervix	Prematurity
Toxemia	Prematurity
	Intrauterine growth retardation
	Hypoglycemia
	Hypocalcemia
	Aspiration syndrome
	Polycythemia
	Asphyxia
Pharmacologic	
Alcohol	Low birth weight
	Developmental delay
	Microcephaly
	Small palpebral fissures
	Maxillary hypoplasia
	Cardiac anomaly (ventricular septal defect, patent ductus arteriosus)
	Abnormal palm creases
Aminopterin and amethopterin	Multiple anomalies
	Abortion
	Intrauterine growth retardation
Ammonium chloride	Acidosis
Androgen (methyl testosterone)	Masculinization of females
	Advanced bone age
Barbiturates	Withdrawal syndrome
	Diminished sucking
	Diminished serum bilirubin
Cephalothin	Direct Coombs positive test
Chlorambucil	?Renal agenesis
Chlorothiazide	Thrombocytopenia
	Salt and water depletion
Chloroquine	?Retinal damage
	Death
	Mental retardation
Chlorpromazine	Depression
	Lethargy
Chlorpropamide	Hypoglycemia (protracted)
	Increased fetal wastage
Cigarette smoking	Intrauterine growth retardation
	Increased neonatal hematocrit
	Increased mortality caused by abruptio previa
	Mental retardation
Diazepam (Valium)	Hypothermia
Dicumarol	Fetal hemorrhage and death
Diphenylhydantoin (Dilantin)	Hypoplastic phalanges
	Diaphragmatic hernia
	Cleft lip
	Coloboma
	Pulmonary atresia
	Patent ductus arteriosus
Estrogen	Masculinization of females
	Carcinoma of vagina and cervix (years later)
	Advanced bone age
Ethchlorvynol (Placidyl)	Irritability, jitteriness (withdrawal symptoms)

Table 15-1. Maternal abnormalities and associated fetal and neonatal disorders—cont'd

Maternal factors	Fetal, neonatal disorders
ANTEPARTUM—cont'd	
Pharmacologic—cont'd	
Hexamethonium bromide	Paralytic ileus
Insulin shock	Death
Intravenous fluid (copious, hypotonic)	Hyponatremia Convulsions Edema
Lithium	Lithium toxicity (cyanosis, hypotonia), congenital heart disease
Lysergic acid diethylamide	Chromosome damage
Magnesium sulfate	Hypermagnesemia CNS depression Peripheral neuromuscular blockage
Meperidine (Demerol)	Placental vasoconstriction CNS and respiratory depression
Mepivacaine	Bradycardia Convulsions Apnea Death Depression Tachycardia Flaccidity Metabolic acidosis Hypoxemia
Methimazole	Goiter
Morphine, heroin, methadone	Withdrawal symptoms (tremors, dyspnea, cyanosis, convulsions, death) Intrauterine growth retardation Lower serum bilirubin
Naphthalene (mothballs)	Hemolytic anemia (in G-6-PD deficiency)
Nitrofurantoin	Hemolytic anemia (in G-6-PD deficiency)
Nortriptyline	Urinary retention (bladder)
Potassium iodide	Goiter
Primaquine	Hemolytic anemia (in G-6-PD deficiency)
Progestins	Masculinization of female infants Advanced bone age
Propanolol	Low Apgar scores, hypoglycemia, bradycardia
Propoxyphene (Darvon)	Hyperactivity Sweating Convulsions Withdrawal symptoms
Propylthiouracil	Goiter
Quinine	Thrombocytopenia Abortion
Radioactive iodine	Hypothyroidism Thyroid destruction
Reserpine	Obstructed respiration caused by nasal congestion Lethargy Bradycardia Hypothermia
Salicylates	Neonatal hemorrhage caused by platelet dysfunction
Sedatives (excessive during labor)	CNS depression and respiratory distress
Steroids (adrenocortical)	Increased incidence of fetal death Adrenal suppression Accelerated fetal lung maturation (betamethasone) ?Cleft palate

Table 15-1. Maternal abnormalities and associated fetal and neonatal disorders—cont'd

Maternal factors	Fetal, neonatal disorders
ANTEPARTUM—cont'd	
Pharmacologic—cont'd	
Streptomycin	Deafness, eighth nerve damage
Stilbestrol	Adenocarcinoma of vagina in adolescents
Sulfonamides (long-acting)	Kernicterus at low bilirubin levels
Tetracyclines (after first trimester)	Tooth stain, enamel hypoplasia (primary teeth) Temporarily inhibited linear growth (premature infants)
Thalidomide	Phocomelia and other anomalies Death
Tolbutamide (Orinase)	Thrombocytopenia, bilirubin displacement from albumin
Vitamin D (excessive)	?Hypercalcemia (supravalvular aortic stenosis, mental retardation, osteosclerosis)
Vitamin K (excessive)	Hyperbilirubinemia
INTRAPARTUM	
Cord pathology	
Inflammation	Bacterial infection Umbilical vein thrombosis (asphyxia)
Meconium staining	Asphyxia
Prolapsed cord	Asphyxia
Single umbilical artery	Congenital anomalies Intrauterine growth retardation
True knot	Asphyxia
Velamentous insertion, vasa previa	Intrauterine blood loss
Rupture of normal cord (precipitous delivery), varices, aneurysm	Intrauterine blood loss
Fetal membrane, amniotic fluid	
Amnion nodosum	Renal agenesis Severe obstructive uropathy (bilateral) Intrauterine parabiotic syndrome (small twin)
Amnionitis	Infection, usually bacterial
Early membrane rupture	Bacterial infection Prematurity Prolapsed cord
Meconium stain (fluid or membranes)	Asphyxia Aspiration syndrome Pneumonia
Oligohydramnios	Postmaturity Renal agenesis and dysplasia Polycystic kidney Urethral obstruction Intrauterine parabiotic syndrome (small twin) Fetal death
Polyhydramnios	High gastrointestinal obstruction Spina bifida Hydrocephalus Anencephaly Achondroplasia Hydrops fetalis Intrauterine parabiotic syndrome (large twin)
Placenta	
Placenta previa	Prematurity Asphyxia Prolapsed cord Intrauterine blood loss

Table 15-1. Maternal abnormalities and associated fetal and neonatal disorders—cont'd

Maternal factors	Fetal, neonatal disorders
INTRAPARTUM—cont'd	
Placenta—cont'd	
Abruptio placentae	Prematurity Asphyxia Intrauterine blood loss
Fetomaternal transfusion	Intrauterine blood loss (chronic or acute) Asphyxia
Incision during cesarean section	Intrauterine blood loss (acute)
Placental insufficiency	Asphyxia Intrauterine malnutrition
Multilobed placenta (rupture of communicating vessels)	Intrauterine blood loss (acute)
Complications of labor	
Breech delivery	Asphyxia Intracranial hemorrhage Visceral hemorrhage (adrenal, kidney, spleen) Spinal cord trauma Brachial plexus injury Bone fracture (clavicle, humerus, femur) Epiphyseal injury (proximal femur or humerus) Characteristic posture Edema, ecchymosis of buttocks, genitalia, and lower extremities
Face and brow presentation	Edema, ecchymosis of face Asphyxia Characteristic posture (head retraction)
Transverse presentation	Asphyxia, trauma
Precipitate delivery	Asphyxia, trauma Intracranial hemorrhage
Prolonged labor	Asphyxia, trauma Bacterial infection
Uterine inertia	Hazard of prolonged labor
Uterine rupture	Asphyxia
Uterine tetany	Asphyxia
Shoulder dystocia	Asphyxia Brachial plexus injury Fractured clavicle Fractured humerus
Manual version, extraction	Asphyxia Bone fractures Brachial plexus injury, spinal cord trauma
Forceps (high or mid)	Asphyxia Cephalhematoma Intracranial hemorrhage
Multiple gestation	Asphyxia (usually second twin) Prematurity Intrauterine growth retardation Intrauterine parabiotic syndrome (fetofetal transfusion) Hypoglycemia (smaller twin) Congenital anomalies Bacterial infection (first or both twins)

by misadventure during labor, with adverse consequences to the neonate that include asphyxia, trauma, or hemorrhage (blood loss). If the fetus has developed and grown suboptimally for any reason, he is ill-prepared for the trials of normal parturition, much less labor gone awry.

Asphyxia during labor. The asphyctic state comprises hypoxemia (low PaO_2), hypercapnia (increased $PaCO_2$), and acidemia (low pH). The end stage of normal labor inevitably involves varying degrees of asphyxia as a function of increasingly impaired placental gas exchange, which is inherent in the process of maternofetal separation. Low blood pH is a consequence of carbon dioxide retention (respiratory acidosis) and organic acid accumulation, primarily lactic and pyruvic acids, (metabolic acidosis). At birth the lungs of healthy infants expand promptly, carbon dioxide elimination and increased oxygen saturation are accomplished rapidly, and within several hours pH is near normal. Compensatory activity is largely limited to pulmonary excretion of carbon dioxide. These changes may be exaggerated beyond normal limits by impairment of maternal or fetal circulation and by acid-base imbalance and hypoxemia in the mother. In these circumstances, recovery from asphyxia is delayed or impossible without assistance. The abnormal asphyctic state is common to several specific obstetric conditions, which are discussed subsequently.

Trauma of labor and delivery. Occasionally, trauma is inevitable in certain abnormalities of labor or presentation at delivery; the most adept obstetric management can at best minimize the unfortunate consequences. Several traumatic lesions are recognizable in the neonate; their effects may range from transient insignificance to permanent disability or death. Neonatal trauma of labor and delivery is listed in the following outline:

- Skin, subcutaneous tissue, muscle
  - Edema of presenting part; caput succedaneum (vertex); edema and cyanosis of buttocks and perineum (frank breech), of feet (footling), and of upper extremity
  - Cephalhematoma
  - Subgaleal hemorrhage (diffuse scalp hemorrhage)
  - Sternocleidomastoid hemorrhage (hematoma)
  - Subcutaneous fat necrosis (pressure necrosis)
  - Skin abrasion
  - Ecchymosis or petechiae in skin
- Bone
  - Molding of skull
  - Fracture (linear or depressed) of skull
  - Fracture of clavicle, humerus, femur
  - Epiphyseal separation (humerus most common)
- Central nervous system
  - Subdural hematoma
  - Hemorrhage into brain substance
  - Spinal cord injury
- Ocular
  - Subconjunctival hemorrhage
  - Retinal hemorrhage
  - Corneal injury
- Peripheral nerves
  - Brachial plexus: Erb palsy (upper, C5, C6), Klumpke palsy (lower, C8, T1), or both
  - Diaphragmatic paralysis (associated with Erb palsy if roots of C3, C4, C5 are injured)
  - Horner syndrome (associated with Klumpke palsy)
  - Facial palsy
  - Radial palsy (associated with subcutaneous fat necrosis over lateral aspect of arm just above elbow)
- Visceral injury
  - Liver (subcapsular, parenchymal hemorrhage)
  - Kidney (perirenal, parenchymal hemorrhage)
  - Adrenals (hemorrhage may extend to perirenal area)
  - Rupture of stomach

Blood loss during labor and delivery. Tears in fetal vessels of the placenta or cord may cause life-threatening loss of blood. Fetal blood loss also occurs in placenta previa and abruptio placentae. Recognition and treatment are discussed on pp. 265 and 266.

Obstetric abnormalities associated with asphyxia. Dystocia, abnormal presentations, premature separation of placenta, uterine tetany, and compression of the cord are the commonest obstetric disorders associated with fetal asphyxia.

Prolongation of labor because of mechanical factors is known as *dystocia*. Total length of labor should not exceed approximately 20 hours. The second stage for a multipara is considered prolonged if it exceeds an hour and for a primipara if it exceeds 2 hours. Progress of labor may be impeded by disproportion between the maternal pelvis and the size of the fetus (contracted maternal pelvis, fetal hydrocephalus, fetal macrosomia), uterine inertia, and abnormal presentation. One or more of these factors may coexist; perinatal mortality rises sharply in their presence.

Premature separation of the placenta (abruptio placentae) occurs when the placenta, implanted at a normal site, is detached from the uterine wall early in labor—after the twentieth gestational week. Separation before the twentieth week is an abortion. The extent of separation varies, ranging from a few millimeters in diameter to detachment of the entire surface. Multiparity and toxemia of pregnancy are common predisposing conditions. There is no apparent relationship to age of the mother. Bleeding may be obvious if it occurs from the vagina (external hemorrhage), or it may be inapparent (concealed hemorrhage). In the former, blood escapes between the fetal membranes and uterine wall and thence through the cervix and vagina, whereas in the latter, blood is confined behind the placenta by intact attachment of its margins. Concealed hemorrhage is more sinister for both mother and fetus; it is common in toxemia of pregnancy. As a result of abruptio, interference with maternal placental circulation causes serious fetal asphyxia or death. Premature birth is a frequent outcome of abruptio placentae.

Uterine tetany (prolonged contractions) interferes with blood flow through the intervillous space and increases ischemia of the fetal brain by virtue of sustained pressure on the head. During such episodes fetomaternal gas exchange is seriously diminished and fetal asphyxia ensues.

Placental implantation in the lower uterine segment is *placenta previa*. Malposition in relation to the internal os is the basis for a descriptive classification. Total placenta previa exists when the internal os is completely occluded, partial placenta previa involves partial obstruction of the internal os, and low implantation refers to a placental margin that is palpable in the region of the internal os but does not encroach on it. In the Collaborative Perinatal Study the incidence of placenta previa among approximately 60,000 pregnancies was 0.5%. Increasing age of gravida is a prominent predisposing factor, and the incidence in multiparas is thus twice that of primiparas. Vaginal hemorrhage, the most frequent maternal sign, does not often appear before the seventh gestational month. Placental attachment is easily disrupted when the thinner wall of the lower uterine segment becomes increasingly attentuated as pregnancy progresses. Onset of labor accelerates the previously slow process of placental detachment. The principal cause of perinatal mortality from placenta previa is premature birth, but other serious effects include asphyxia from early placental detachment, fetal blood loss, and prolonged labor resulting from obstructed passage of the fetal head.

Fetal blood flow is partially or completely obstructed when *cord compression* occurs. This is a common event when compression is spontaneously relieved and the fetal effects are insignificant and imperceptible. Sustained occlusion results in serious fetal asphyxia. It is most often caused by prolapse of the cord (occult or apparent) and by the cord wrapping tightly around the fetal neck or body, which stretches umbilical vessels thereby diminishing their caliber. Complete occlusion of the cord totally depletes fetal oxygen supply within 2½ minutes. Milder compression affects the umbilical vein more extensively; the wall is thinner and pressure is lower than in the arteries; fetal oxygenation is reduced because fetal blood return from the placenta is reduced.

Obstetric abnormalities associated with trauma. Labor shorter than 3 hours in duration is termed *precipitate labor*. The principal threat to the fetus is subdural hematoma, which usually results from a torn tentorium cerebelli. Sudden anteroposterior compression of the skull causes commensurate expansion in the bitemporal direction, which stretches and tears the tentorium. Less frequently, bitemporal compression elongates the anteroposterior diameter, thereby causing rupture of the bridging veins.

Breech extraction predisposes to several traumatic lesions, particularly in large babies. *Fracture of the femur* occurs in footling deliveries when vigorous traction is applied to the legs. Difficulty in delivery of the shoulders may lead to *fracture of the clavicle;* if the arm is manipulated roughly during attempts to deliver a shoulder, *fracture of the humerus occurs*. Excessive traction along the longitudinal axis of the lower or upper extremities may result in *epiphyseal separations* at the upper end of the femur or humerus. Excessive lateral displacement of the neck during delivery results in traumatic *tear of the sternocleidomastoid muscle* and hematoma formation in the muscle belly, which is apparent a few weeks after birth as a fibrous mass. The various types of *brachial plexus injury* (Table 15-1) follow similar displacement of the neck, which is incurred while the body is deflected by manipulation from below, before delivery of the head. Excessive traction on the feet stretches the vertebral column and may lead to *spinal cord injury* at any level.

POSTNATAL ASPECTS: THE NEONATE

The first breath

On his emergence from an aquatic thermoneutral intrauterine environment, several changes befall the infant, the most crucial of which is adaptation to respiration in a gaseous milieu. Before the respiratory apparatus can normally assume and sustain this function, several prerequisites must be satisfied: stimulation of initial respiratory movements; entry of air against several impedent forces; establishment of alveolar stability to preserve a constant gas-liquid interface (functional residual capacity); increase of pulmonary blood flow; and redistribution of cardiac output. Although these events transpire simultaneously, they lend themselves well to sequential description.

Stimulation of initial respiratory movement. The stimuli to the first respiratory movement are primarily chemical and thermal. The most active chemical stimuli are provided by asphyctic changes in blood (low oxygen and high carbon dioxide tensions, low pH) that excite the medullary respiratory center directly or by neural transmission from peripheral chemoreceptors in the carotids and aorta. Asphyxia of normal birth stimulates respiration, but profound and prolonged asphyctic changes are severely depressive. Thermal factors are probably also important in triggering the first respiratory movement; sudden chilling of the infant probably excites peripheral neural receptors, which transmit impulses to the respiratory center. Emergence from an intrauterine environment of slightly over 37° C (98.6° F) to an ambient temperature in the delivery room of 21° to 23° C (70° to 75° F) is undoubtedly a powerful stimulus. Tactile sensation is of little significance in the initiation of respiration; and although no harm is inflicted by the traditional slaps on heels or buttocks if the infant is depressed, the time expended is better used for more effective resuscitative measures.

Entry of air and expansion of lungs. Initial entry of air into the lungs is opposed by surface tension forces, viscous forces of fetal lung fluid, and inherent elasticity of pulmonary tissue.

Surface tension forces are a significant impedent to initial expansion of alveoli and to maintenance of the expanded state. In the normal infant, surface-active forces are counteracted by surfactant, a lipoprotein film that coats the alveolar surface and is produced by alveolar lining cells. It is probably present in functional quantities at approximately 20 weeks of gestation. In the absence of surfactant, inward pressure produced by surface tension forces would tend to collapse the alveolus. Since this pressure increases as the radius of the alveolus diminishes, smaller alveoli would collapse, emptying air into the larger ones less likely to collapse. The fixed relationship between inward alveolar pressure and the size of alveoli is altered by surfactant. As the film of surfactant is condensed during alveolar deflation, surface tension forces are more effectively counteracted; complete collapse is avoided. When surfactant lining is stretched during alveolar expansion, surface-active forces in the wall are less effectively neutralized. Without surfactant, not only is initial alveolar expansion impaired but also alveoli that do expand tend to collapse at end expiration. The lungs of premature infants who die of hyaline membrane disease are surfactant deficient.

Another opposing factor to the first entry of air is viscosity of fluid in the fetal tracheobronchial tree and alveoli. This fetal lung fluid is elaborated by alveolar lining cells. The fluid lends itself to absorption across alveolar walls by virtue of its low protein content compared to that of amniotic fluid, and its lesser viscosity. Absorption occurs principally into alveolar capillaries, although about one third of the fluid is taken up by lymphatic channels in the interalveolar space. Egress of fetal fluid is dependent on expansion of alveoli and dilation of capillaries and lymphatics. The fall in pulmonary vascular pressure and the increased blood flow that ensues facilitate absorption and ultimate evacuation of fluid from alveoli. The rate of absorption is unknown, but it is undoubtedly slowed in asphyxic states (which entail diminished alveolar blood flow), thereby compounding ventilatory difficulties. Part of the lung fluid is lost through the mouth at delivery as a result of the well known thoracic squeeze exerted on the infant during passage through the cervix and vagina. This is undoubtedly of secondary importance, since establishment of normal respiration after delivery by elective cesarean section is so common.

Inherent elasticity of pulmonary tissue is probably a minor source of impedance to the first breath, as indicated by small intrathoracic pressure changes that govern normal respiration once it is established.

Maintenance of alveolar stability. Alveolar stability requires retention of a volume of air at end expiration (functional residual capacity) and thus maintenance of alveolar expansion. In the normal neonatal lung the volume of functional residual air 10 minutes after birth is equal to that at 5 days of age. Surfactant is indispensable to formation and preservation of functional residual capacity because it prevents alveolar collapse. In the mature lung a stable alveolar volume at end expiration is established after the first few breaths; subsequent respiration can proceed easily with relatively small pressure changes. In contrast, the surfactant-deficient lung begins each inspiration from a state of collapse just as the first one did, thereby requiring inordinately large energy expenditure for each breath (about the amount required for a vigorous cry). A stable alveolar volume facilitates continuous gas exchange during the expiratory phase, which would be impossible with alveolar collapse.

Increased pulmonary blood flow. The fetal lungs are perfused by only 5% to 10% of cardiac output, mainly because of higher intravascular pressure in the pulmonary circuit than in systemic vessels. After the onset of respiration, blood flow through the lungs increases as a result of vasodilation and thus lowered pulmonary vascular resistance; pressure in the left atrium rises as it receives a greater volume of blood, and the foramen ovale closes abruptly when pressure in the left atrium exceeds that of the right atrium. The ductus arteriosus closes by constriction in response to heightened arterial $Pa{O_2}$, but this is a more gradual process. The fetal pattern, in which the right and left circulations had passed through their respective sides of the heart in parallel, is thus converted to a mature pattern, in which continuity of right and left is in series. The transformation of flow through the heart and great vessels depends on dilation of pulmonary capillaries and arterioles. Dilation occurs in response to increased alveolar and arterial $P{O_2}$ and decreased $Pa{CO_2}$, which were at asphyctic levels before the first breath. Impaired ventilation causes oxygen deprivation, hypercapnia, and acidemia, all of which result in sustained constriction of pulmonary arterioles (increased intravascular pressure) and a tendency to revert to fetal shunts.

• • •

In summary, establishment of normal ventilation requires an intact central and peripheral neural apparatus to stimulate first respiratory movements, the presence of functional quantities of surfactant to facilitate initial and sustained expansion of the lungs, and prompt correction of the asphyxia of normal birth for pulmonary vasodilation and redistribution of cardiac output.

Thermoregulation

Theoretical and practical considerations. The association of increased mortality with severe hypothermia in premature infants was well described as early as 1900, but the practical implications of thermal homeostasis have become increasingly clear only in the last few decades. In humans, deep body temperature (core temperature) normally does not vary more than 0.3%. This rigid homeostatic requirement is in contrast to variations tolerated in hydrogen ion concentration (10% to 20%) and to fluctuations of blood glucose content (up to 50%).

Thermal stability is maintained by regulating rates of heat loss and production. The four modalities by which the body loses heat are convection, radiation, evaporation, and conduction; each is significant in the care of newborn infants. Loss of heat by *convection* is governed by temperature gradients between body surface and ambient (surrounding) air. The extent of this loss is generally determined by temperature and velocity of air in the incubator or in the nursery. Thermal dissipation by *radiation* is largely independent of the temperature of ambient air. It occurs from the body surface to relatively distant objects that are cooler than skin temperature. Thus, even if the temperature of ambient air is high, significant heat loss may occur if incubator walls are inordinately cool. *Evaporative heat loss* results from expenditure of thermal energy to convert liquid on an exposed surface to a gaseous state (amniotic fluid, sweat, water of expired air). These losses are augmented in low relative humidity and are minimized in high humidity. *Conductive heat loss* is the result of direct contact between the body surface and a cooler solid object. In the usual nursery environment, heat loss by radiation accounts for approximately 60% of the total and evaporation in expired air for approximately 10% to 15%; the remainder is lost by convection. Conductive losses are ordinarily of little significance.

The newborn, particularly the low birth weight baby, has difficulty maintaining body temperature because of predisposition to heat loss rather than inability to produce it. Heat loss is four times greater per unit of body weight than in adults, primarily because of the greater ratio of surface area to body weight. At birth, weight of full-term infants is 5% that of adults, whereas body surface is 15%; the smaller the infant is, the more discrepant will be the difference. In addition to these dimensional factors, a greater propensity to heat loss is created by a paucity of subcutaneous tissue, particularly in low birth weight infants. Conduction of heat from viscera to skin is enhanced. Thus heat is rapidly dissipated from the neonate because it is readily transferred from the body core to the skin (internal thermal gradient) and thence from a disproportionately extensive surface area to the environment.

In normal circumstances the thermogenic capacity of the newborn approximates that of the adult. Heat production depends primarily on increased metabolic rate (nonshivering thermogenesis), which entails increased rates of oxygen consumption. Shivering occurs with a rapid fall in rectal temperature, but this is exceptional. Except for brown fat, the sites of thermogenesis have not yet been clearly delineated; heart, liver, brain, and skeletal muscle are probably important. The fascinating role of brown adipose tissue has been convincingly demonstrated in rabbits, whereas in humans the evidence is all but direct. Brown fat, a specialized thermogenic tissue that is more cellular than white fat, appears in the fetus at about 26 to 30 weeks' gestation and usually continues to increase in quantity for several weeks after birth. In humans, superficial deposits are situated in the anterior mediastinum, posterior cervical triangles, the interscapular region, the axillae, and at deeper levels along the vertebral column around the kidneys and adrenals. Several lines of evidence indicate a thermogenic role in human infants. At necropsy, brown fat is depleted in infants known to experience cold stress, whereas it remains unchanged in others. Skin temperatures over subcutaneous depots are higher than in other areas during cold stress, approximating deep body temperature.

Heat loss is diminished by vasoconstriction in the skin, which decreases conduction from the body core to superficial layers. The more mature infant can also assume flexion postures that shield a significant amount of surface from environmental exposure, and this too is a rather effective impediment to thermal dissipation. During prolonged cold stress, the overriding need is for replenishment of thermal stores, and this is attempted with heat production by linear increase in metabolic rate as ambient temperature falls. At environmental temperature of about 23° C (73.4° F) oxygen consumption increases considerably, but body temperature falls nevertheless because heat loss exceeds production. At a warmer ambient temperature such as about 29° C (84.2° F) heat loss is less, and the augmented metabolic rate successfully maintains rectal temperature at a normal level. Increased oxygen consumption is inherent in the hypermetabolism that creates heat as its byproduct. Increased metabolic rate is inhibited by hypoxia. Under experimental conditions, infants who breathe 15% oxygen fail to respond. Hypercapnea, acidosis, and symptomatic hypoglycemia also exert an inhibitory influence. The effects of hypoglycemia are probably a consequence of disrupted central nervous system function. Anencephalic infants, for example, do not increase oxygen consumption when exposed to cold. Prematurity lessens the response somewhat but mostly as a function of small body size rather than gestational age. Thermoreceptors in the skin provide an immediate stimulus to hypermetabolism on exposure to cold; the receptors of the face are particularly sensitive. The role of the sympathetic nervous system is not yet known in detail but is apparently significant. Norepinephrine is a powerful thermogenic agent in humans and animals. Infusion of norepinephrine into animals causes heightened metabolic activity in brown fat. Catecholamine excretion increases in human infants during periods of cold stress.

The principal metabolic penalties of cold exposure are metabolic acidosis, depletion of energy stores, decreased blood glucose concentration at 4 to 6 hours, increased oxygen deprivation in distressed infants, and pulmonary vasoconstriction. The well-nourished, vigorous full-term infant withstands cold stress for a reasonable period. The small-for-dates baby whose hepatic glycogen stores are already depleted at birth and whose rate of heat loss is high can ill afford the metabolic expenditure imposed by cold stress. Compensation for metabolic acidosis is accomplished by pulmonary excretion of carbon dioxide; if ventilatory function is compromised, acidosis caused by hypothermia compounds that of asphyxia. Furthermore, respiratory distress implies hypoxia, which itself impairs heat production; body temperature continues to fall unless environmental countermeasures are instituted. Even if, as is usual, the infant successfully maintains normal body temperature, the oxygen cost will eventually be intolerable.

Planning for optimal care requires cognizance of the unique thermoregulatory problems encountered by newborn infants. Simple measures will provide a suitable microenvironment in which heat loss by radiation and convection can be minimized in the delivery room and nursery. Evaporative losses are greatest at birth, when the infant is covered with amniotic fluid; thorough drying of body and scalp will obviously minimize this effect. A radiant heat lamp, placed at an appropriate distance above the resuscitation table, is effective in conserving body heat while permitting maximum accessibility to the infant. The baby should be wrapped in a warm blanket for transfer to the nursery in a previously heated incubator. Bathing of vigorous infants in the nursery should be delayed at least 4 hours; for depressed infants a longer delay is indicated, depending on restoration of normal skin temperature. These practices make for a very real difference in promptness of recovery from asphyxial birth stress. Infants who are allowed to dissipate body heat in the delivery room and who are then bathed on arrival in the nursery do not recover normal body temperature, even at the end of 8 hours. Their core temperature drops about 2.5° C (4.5° F) at the end of 1 hour. In contrast, optimally managed infants achieve normal temperature by the end of 3 hours, and the fall in core temperature is less than 1° F by the end of the first hour.

In the nursery, failure to provide a thermal environment for small babies (1750 g or less), particularly those who are ill, results in lowered rates of survival. A neutral thermal environment controls loss of body heat at a level commensurate with minimal oxygen consumption at rest. Convective heat loss is minimized by traditional measures that control the temperature of incubator air. However, loss by radiation is insidious; a considerable amount of heat is lost even when temperature of ambient air is appropriate. This can be minimized by ascertaining that the temperature of incubator walls is not inordinately low, perhaps because of placement in the path of air from an air conditioner or because of proximity to cold windows or walls. Skin temperature of approximately 36° C (97° F) correlates fairly well with minimal oxygen consumption. There is also evidence that when temperature of the inner surface of the incubator wall is more than 1.5° C (2.8° F) below that of the skin, oxygen consumption increases. This may be the most reliable method by which to monitor the neutrality of thermal environment. Equipment currently in common use provides servo-controlled temperature of incubator air, set at skin temperature of 36° C (97° F), in response to a thermistor attached to skin of the epigastrium. If the infant is prone, the system will obviously be inaccurate.

Considerations of thermoregulatory problems appropriately emphasize hypothermia, but increased body heat, although less frequent, is also troublesome. Oxygen consumption rises sharply with slight elevation of body temperature. Overheating may result from improper operation of equipment, from placing an incubator in direct sunlight, or from infection.

In summary, thermal lability is a handicap to the normal full-term infant and is a hazard to the small infant, mature or premature. The homeothermic response to cold increases heat production by increasing the metabolic rate and oxygen consumption. This response is impaired by depressed central nervous system function, asphyxia, and hypoglycemia. Sustained hypermetabolism with reduced availability of oxygen results in metabolic acidosis. Survival rates of small infants can be increased by minimizing heat loss in the delivery room and in the nursery.

The cold-stressed infant presents several characteristic clinical signs. Although the metabolic penalties of cold are activated when the temperature falls only slightly, the clinical signs appear only after a more severe decline occurs in body temperature. When rectal temperature is approximately 32° C (90° F) the body is cold to the touch; the skin is bright red because hemoglobin gives up oxygen less readily at low temperatures (the oxyhemoglobin dissociation curve shifts to the left), and the baby appears deceptively healthy; respiration is slow and shallow; bradycardia is profound. Spontaneous activity is almost absent, and the response to painful stimuli is feeble or absent. Edema of the face and extremities is sometimes apparent, and sclerema of the cheeks and buttocks is common. These are the signs of severe cold stress, and they are rarely encountered in most nurseries. Less severe thermal deprivation produces clinical manifestations that are associated with metabolic insults. Increased need for oxygen causes tachypnea and perhaps cyanosis. Hypoglycemia can precipitate coma or lethargy, or less often, jitteriness and convulsions. Metabolic acidosis may cause pallor and also may contribute to tachypnea.

The temptation to warm a cold infant rapidly is difficult to resist. Too often hot-water bags and overheated incubators are brought into action with great vigor. The resultant rapid rise in body temperatures now causes repeated apneic episodes that may require resuscitative measures. The proper treatment of cold-stressed infants requires a gradual rise in body temperature. The temperature of the incubator is best maintained no more than 1.5° C (2.7° F) higher than the infant's skin temperature, in spite of a subnormal rectal temperature. Oxygen is given in concentrations necessary to raise the arterial Po_2 to normal levels. Bicarbonate is administered intravenously for correction of metabolic acidosis (p. 291), and intravenous dextrose is used for hypoglycemia (p. 326).

Evaluation and treatment in the delivery room

Apgar score. In 1953 Virginia Apgar introduced a simple, semiquantitative method for clinical evaluation of newborn infants immediately after birth. The score is based on observations of heart rate, respiration, muscle tone, reflex irritability, and color. Scores of 0, 1, or 2 are assigned to each item; the lower the score, the more depressed the infant (Table 15-2). Low scores generally correlate well with severe acidosis. Evaluations are made at 1 and 5 minutes after birth, disregarding delivery of the placenta. The vast majority of infants achieve scores of 7 or more at 1 minute and 8 or more at 5 minutes. Several prognostic correlations have been based on the Apgar score; 5-minute evaluation is the better predictor. Neonatal mortality and morbidity and neurologic abnormality at 1 year of age are highest among infants whose scores range from 0 to 3. Frequency distribution of low scores is inversely related to birth weight, which itself is some indication of outcome. The combination of scores and birth weight increases prognostic value. In the Collaborative Perinatal Study, among infants under 2000 g in weight who scored 0 to 3, the incidence of neurologic abnormality at 1 year was approximately 20%, whereas among infants over 2500 g with identical scores the incidence was 2.7%. The influence of Apgar scores on infants of equal birth weight can be appreciated by comparing those under 2000 g with scores of 0 to 3 to infants of equal weight who scored 7 to 10. In the former group, incidence of neurologic disorder at 1 year of age was 20%; in the latter group it was approximately 6%.

Resuscitation at birth. Resuscitative efforts must include administration of oxygen, stimulation of cardiac activity (if absent), rapid correction of low pH, and prevention of excessive loss of body heat. The Apgar score is a de-

Table 15-2. Apgar scoring chart

Sign	Score 0	Score 1	Score 2
Heart rate	Absent	Slow (below 100)	Over 100
Respiratory effort	Absent	Slow, irregular; hypoventilation	Good; crying lustily
Muscle tone	Flaccid	Some flexion of extremities	Active motion, well flexed
Reflex irritability	No response	Cry; some motion	Vigorous cry
Color	Blue, pale	Body pink, hands and feet blue	Completely pink

pendable indicator of the type of resuscitation required. One-minute scores of 3 or less (no respiratory effort, heart rate of less than 100) require immediate intubation and positive pressure ventilation, external cardiac massage if heartbeat is absent, and sometimes the intravenous administration of alkali. Scores of 4 to 6 at 1 minute (poor respiratory effort, heart rate over 100) require administration of oxygen by mask with intermittent positive pressure.

There is little if any indication for use of stimulant drugs in an asphyxiated infant. The margin of safety is small and the salutory effects doubtful. The most effective stimulant to respiration is oxygen.

The procedures that should be used for effective resuscitation are outlined here. The oropharynx of all infants, whether depressed or not, should be suctioned with a bulb syringe or rubber catheter. This is best performed with the infant supine, head down slightly and turned to one side.

Intubation. The chin is slightly forward. The head should be held squarely in the midline position. With battery case upward, a laryngoscope is held in the left hand; the blade is inserted toward the hypopharynx along the right side of the oral cavity and is moved toward the midline to displace the tongue to the left.

As the blade is advanced, the epiglottic rim becomes visible. The tip of the blade should come to rest in the cul-de-sac (vallecula) between the base of the tongue and epiglottis.

Slight upward movement of the battery handle away from the operator will protrude the mandible and raise the tip of the blade, thus exposing the glottis, which becomes visible as a dark longitudinal slit limited posteriorly by pink arytenoid cartilage.

If suction is necessary, a catheter should be inserted attached to a DeLee trap at the operator's end; the operator should suck on the trap during insertion. The catheter is advanced into the trachea to aspirate fluid. In the presence of meconium, removal of particulate matter is effective only with the use of an endotracheal tube. The operator must apply gentle suction through his masked mouth. The suction is maintained as the endotracheal tube is withdrawn and repeated reinsertion and suction is usually necessary.

A resuscitation bag is attached to the endotracheal tube, and the lungs are insufflated manually. As a rule, 100% oxygen should be flowing into the bag. We have found the Penlon bag to be a satisfactory instrument.

Effective delivery of air is ascertained by adequate excursion of the chest wall and auscultation of the anterolateral thorax on each side. The rate of insufflation should be maintained at approximately 40 per minute.

External cardiac massage. Manual depression of the sternum forces blood into the aorta; release of sternal depression fills the heart with venous blood. External cardiac massage should be instituted if a heartbeat is not present after three or four insufflations. It should always be performed at end expiration. If administered during inspiratory intervals, the risk of pneumothorax and pneumomediastinum is notably enhanced. Excessively vigorous external massage may cause rupture of the liver and fatal hemorrhage. The effectiveness of cardiac massage should be verified by palpating femoral pulses.

Correction of acidosis. Profound asphyxia involves metabolic acidosis, which requires rapid administration of alkali and glucose while respiratory and cardiac resuscitation are in progress. Infusion of alkali is of little use unless effective cardiac activity has been restored. The umbilical vein should be cannulated.

Dilute 3 ml/kg body weight of a 0.9 m solution of sodium bicarbonate with an equal amount of 10% glucose or water, and infuse into the umbilical vein over a period of 3 minutes. The need for subsequent alkali therapy is determined by repeated blood gas and pH determinations.

The use of sodium bicarbonate for resuscitation imposes some degree of significant risk. The establishment of alveolar ventilation is a primary prerequisite. This can be judged clinically, if immediate blood gas data are not available, by ascertaining adequate chest wall excursion and listening for normal breath sounds. In the presence of inadequate ventilation with already elevated CO_2 levels, the administration of bicarbonate generates additional CO_2 that cannot be eliminated through the lungs. The infant is in essence a closed system, and blood pH falls as CO_2 accumulates. Thus alkali should be withheld from infants whose ventilatory adequacy is in doubt. Another significant risk of bicarbonate administration is the abrupt rise in serum osmolality that results. Undiluted, commercially available sodium bicarbonate contains 1400 mOsm/L; an abrupt rise in serum osmolality is inevitable. It can be minimized by slow administration of a diluted preparation. Experimental evidence in animals indicates that intraventricular hemorrhage results from abrupt hyperosmolality. Clinical evidence strongly suggests a higher incidence of intraventricular hemorrhage among premature infants who receive alkali during resuscitation. Sodium bicarbonate therapy is undoubtedly risky, yet when blood pH is below 7.15 the potential short-term benefits may well overshadow the risks. However, the fact is that most infants who require resuscitation in the delivery room can be managed effectively without the use of alkali therapy.

Prevention of body heat loss. Exposure of asphyxiated infants to usual delivery room temperatures causes tremendous heat loss in a short period of time. Metabolic acidosis is accentuated, and respiratory compensation is less effective. The infant should be wiped dry immediately after birth. A source of radiant heat is indispensable. It should deliver heat to the surface of the table on which resuscitation is administered, thus minimizing thermal losses even though the infant is completely exposed and accessible for treatment. Placing the infant in an incubator or wrapping with warm blankets limits accessibility for resuscitative efforts.

The procedures just outlined for management of asphyxiated infants in the delivery room are applicable in the nursery if apneic episodes occur.

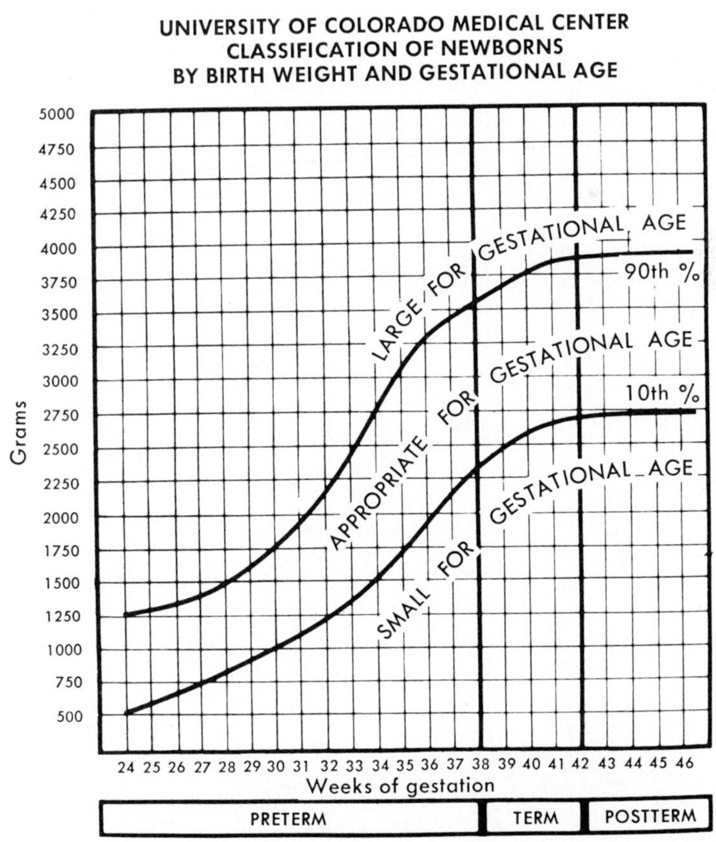

Fig. 15-1. A practical classification of newborn infants by weight and gestational age. (From Battaglia, F.C., and Lubchenco, L.O.: J. Pediatr. **71:**159, 1967.)

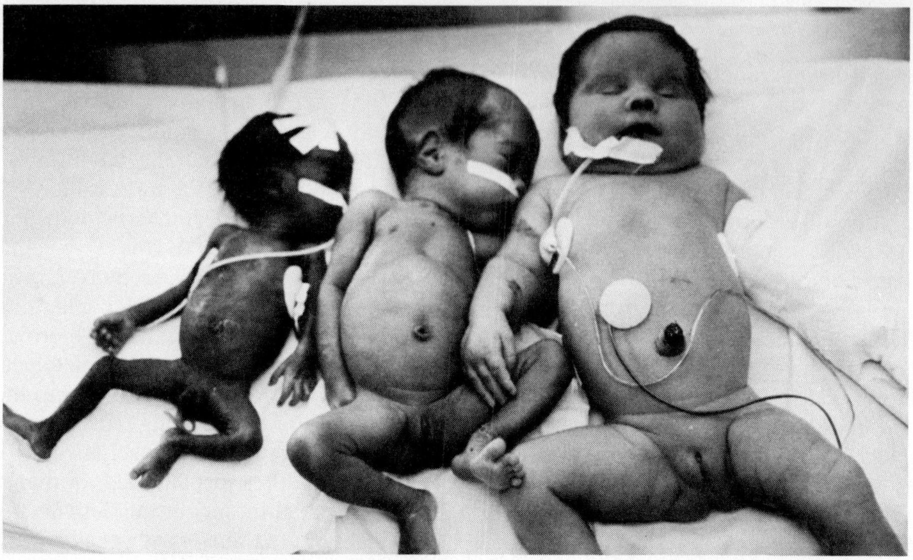

Fig. 15-2. Three babies, same gestational age, weigh 600, 1400, and 2750 g, respectively, from left to right. (From Korones, S.B.: High-risk newborn infants, ed. 3, St. Louis, 1981, The C.V. Mosby Co.)

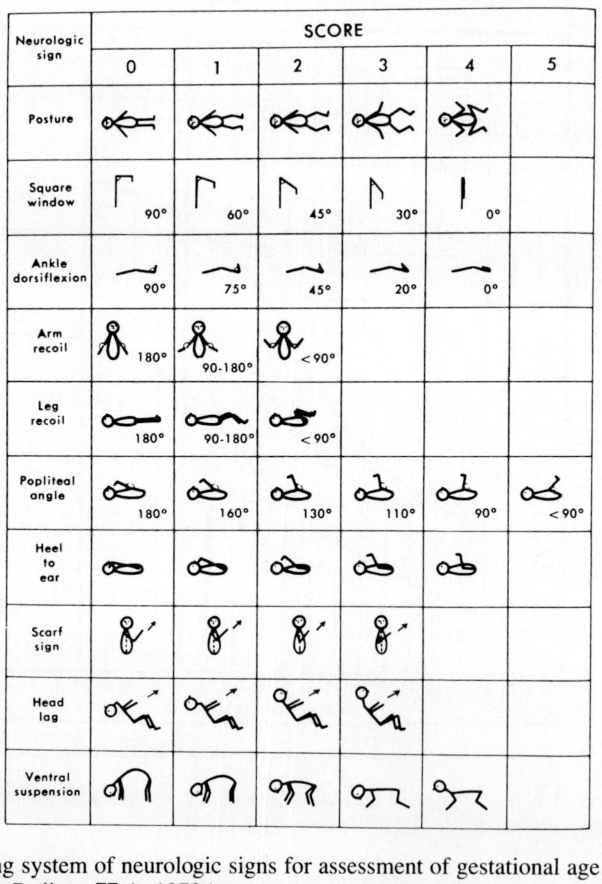

Fig. 15-3. Scoring system of neurologic signs for assessment of gestational age. (From Dubowitz, L.M.S., et al.: J. Pediatr. **77:**1, 1970.)

Birth weight and gestational age

Variations in size and weight for gestational age are the result of numerous factors that influence fetal growth. These relationships are associated with a predisposition to certain disorders in the neonatal period and to outcomes later in life. Several important diagnostic and therapeutic considerations are predicated on assessment of growth status at birth.

A low birth weight (LBW) infant is 2500 g or less at birth, regardless of gestational age. A premature infant is one who is born before completion of the thirty-seventh gestational week, regardless of birth weight. Low birth weight may be the result of delivery before term when intrauterine growth had been normal, or delivery at any time (usually close to term) when prenatal growth was impaired. Accelerated growth rate in utero often occurs in fetuses of diabetic mothers, and, as a result, birth weight over 2500 g is noted in a premature infant. Delivered near term, such infants are frequently oversized for their gestational age.

Variations in size of coeval infants are expressed as percentiles of distribution in a population or as standard deviations from the mean.

SOME NOTES ON TECHNIQUES OF ASSESSMENT OF NEUROLOGIC CRITERIA

Posture: Observed with infant quiet and in supine position. Score 0: Arms and legs extended; 1: beginning of flexion of hips and knees, arms extended; 2: stronger flexion of legs, arms extended; 3: arms slightly flexed, legs flexed and abducted; 4: full flexion of arms and legs.

Square window: The hand is flexed on the forearm between the thumb and index finger of the examiner. Enough pressure is applied to get as full a flexion as possible, and the angle between the hypothenar eminence and the ventral aspect of the forearm is measured and graded according to diagram (Fig. 15-3). (Care is taken not to rotate the infant's wrist while doing this maneuver.)

Ankle dorsiflexion: The foot is dorsiflexed onto the anterior aspect of the leg, with the examiner's thumb on the sole of the foot and other fingers behind the leg. Enough pressure is applied to get as full flexion as possible, and the angle between the dorsum of the foot and the anterior aspect of the leg is measured.

Arm recoil: With the infant in the supine position the forearms are first flexed for 5 seconds, then fully extended by pulling on the hands, and then released. The sign is fully positive if the arms return briskly to full flexion (Score 2). If the arms return to incomplete flexion or the response is sluggish it is graded as Score 1. If they remain extended or are only followed by random movements the score is 0.

Leg recoil: With the infant supine, the hips and knees are fully flexed for 5 seconds, then extended by traction on the feet, and released. A maximal response is one of full flexion of the hips and knees (Score 2). A partial flexion scores 1, and minimal or no movement scores 0.

Popliteal angle: With the infant supine and his pelvis flat on the examining couch, the thigh is held in the knee-chest position by the examiner's left index finger and thumb supporting the knee. The leg is then extended by gentle pressure from the examiner's right index finger behind the ankle and the popliteal angle is measured.

Heel to ear maneuver: With the baby supine, draw the baby's foot as near to the head as it will go without forcing it. Observe the distance between the foot and the head as well as the degree of extension at the knee. Grade according to diagram (Fig. 15-3). Note that the knee is left free and may draw down alongside the abdomen.

Scarf sign: With the baby supine, take the infant's hand and try to put it around the neck and as far posteriorly as possible around the opposite shoulder. Assist this maneuver by lifting the elbow across the body. See how far the elbow will go across and grade according to illustrations (Fig. 15-3). Score 0: Elbow reaches opposite axillary line; 1: Elbow between midline and opposite axillary line; 2: Elbow reaches midline; 3: Elbow will not reach midline.

Head lag: With the baby lying supine, grasp the hands (or the arms if a very small infant) and pull him slowly towards the sitting position. Observe the position of the head in relation to the trunk and grade accordingly. In a small infant the head may initially be supported by one hand. Score 0: Complete lag; 1: Partial head control; 2: Able to maintain head in line with body; 3: Brings head anterior to body.

Ventral suspension: The infant is suspended in the prone position, with examiner's hand under the infant's chest (one hand in a small infant, two in a large infant). Observe the degree of extension of the back and the amount of flexion of the arms and legs. Also note the relation of the head to the trunk. Grade according to diagram (Fig. 15-3). If score differs on the two sides, take the mean.

From Dubowitz, L.M., Dubowitz, V., and Goldberg, C.: Clinical assessment of gestational age in the newborn infant, J.Pediatr. **77:**1, 1970.

Gestational age is plotted against birth weight to derive percentile curves from the Colorado Intrauterine Growth Chart (Fig. 15-1), which is presently the most widely used reference standard. Infants below the tenth percentile are considered small for gestational age (intrauterine growth retardation, small-for-dates), and those above the ninetieth percentile are large for age at birth. Fig. 15-2 shows three infants, each of 32 weeks gestational age, whose weight is widely discrepant. From left to right their birth weights were respectively 600 g (SGA), 1400 g (AGA), and 2750 g (LGA).

Estimation of gestational age by history. There is as yet no generally accepted laboratory parameter to indicate the precise age at birth. Clinical parameters currently in use can provide an estimate that is within 2 weeks of dates obtained reliably from the last menstrual period.

The keystone for assessment of the length of pregnancy is still the maternal menstrual history. Gestational ages are in reality ''menstrual age,'' since they are calculated from the first day of the last menstrual period (LMP), rather than from the time of implantation, which may not occur until 2 weeks later. Menstrual histories are generally reliable, and prevailing tendencies to be distrustful of their accuracy are unjustified. Three sources of inaccuracy should be recognized, however: (1) irregularity of menses does not provide a basis for a predictable repetitive pattern; (2) short intergestational intervals preclude reestablishment of regular menstruation; and (3) postconceptional bleeding early in pregnancy is erroneously reported as the last menstrual period.

Estimation of gestational age by physical examination. Postnatal assessment of gestational age is possible by examination for certain external characteristics and neuromuscular signs. The procedure that is universally employed was described by Dubowitz et al. in 1970 (pp. 274 and 275). The examination is easily performed in 5 to 7 minutes. The resultant estimate of gestational age is apparently accurate within 2 weeks, and measurements are valid up to 5 days of age. Fig. 15-3 illustrates the neurologic responses elicited and the scores assigned to each. Table 15-3 describes the external features and their appropriate scores. The combined scores add up to a maximum total of 70. Fig. 15-4 is a graph that correlates the total score to gestational age. A score of 50 thus indicates a gestational age of 38 weeks; 20 corresponds to 30 weeks.

Intrauterine growth retardation (small-for-dates infants, dysmaturity, intrauterine malnutrition). Impairment of fetal growth is associated with a variety of disorders in the mother, fetus, and placenta. Most of the identifiable factors are as follows:

- Maternal factors
  - Low socioeconomic status
  - Toxemia
  - Hypertensive cardiovascular disease
  - Chronic renal disease
  - Diabetes (advanced)
  - Malnutrition
  - Cigarette smoking
  - Heroin addiction
  - Alcohol
  - High-altitude residence
- Fetal factors
  - Multiple gestation
  - Congenital malformation
  - Chromosomal abnormality
  - Chronic intrauterine infection
    - Rubella
    - Cytomegalovirus
- Placental factors
  - ''Placental insufficiency''
  - Vascular anastomoses (twin to twin)
  - Single umbilical artery
  - Abnormal cord insertion
  - Separation
  - Massive infarction
  - ? Vascular anomalies and tumors
  - ? Site of implantation
  - Avascular chorionic villi

Maternal factors

Low socioeconomic status. Poverty or near-poverty profoundly influences the incidence of babies who are small for gestational age. Maternal social class, parity, age, and in particular maternal height are interrelated and additive when statistical analysis is undertaken. The association of small stature and poor fetal outcome is undoubtedly indirect. Aside from genetically determined short stature in any social class, there is a repeatedly observed association between height and social class, suggesting that short stature is at least in part the result of poor nutrition during the growth period in childhood. Short stature may thus merely signify the many unfavorable circumstances that characterize poverty.

Toxemia of pregnancy. Toxemia of pregnancy is a maternal disorder characterized by gener-

Table 15-3. Scoring system for external criteria

External sign	Score* 0	1	2	3	4
Edema	Obvious edema of hands and feet; pitting over tibia	No obvious edema of hands and feet; pitting over tibia	No edema		
Skin texture	Very thin, gelatinous	Thin and smooth	Smooth; medium thickness. Rash or superficial peeling	Slight thickening. Superficial cracking and peeling especially of hands and feet	Thick and parchmentlike; superficial or deep cracking
Skin color	Dark red	Uniformly pink	Pale pink; variable over body	Pale; only pink over ears, lips, palms, or soles	
Skin opacity (trunk)	Numerous veins and venules clearly seen, especially over abdomen	Veins and tributaries seen	A few large vessels clearly seen over abdomen	A few large vessels seen indistinctly over abdomen	No blood vessels seen
Lanugo (over back)	No lanugo	Abundant; long and thick over whole back	Hair thinning especially over lower back	Small amount of lanugo and bald areas	At least ½ of back devoid of lanugo
Plantar creases	No skin creases	Faint red marks over anterior half of sole	Definite red marks over > anterior ½; indentations over < anterior ⅓	Indentations over > anterior ⅓	Definite deep indentations over > anterior ⅓
Nipple formation	Nipple barely visible; no areola	Nipple well defined; areola smooth and flat, diameter <0.75 cm	Areola stippled, edge not raised, diameter <0.75 cm	Areola stippled, edge raised, diameter >0.75 cm	
Breast size	No breast tissue palpable	Breast tissue on one or both sides, <0.5 cm diameter	Breast tissue both sides; one or both 0.5-1 cm	Breast tissue both sides; one or both >1 cm	
Ear form	Pinna flat and shapeless, little or no incurving of edge	Incurving of part of edge of pinna	Partial incurving whole of upper pinna	Well-defined incurving whole of upper pinna	
Ear firmness	Pinna soft, easily folded, no recoil	Pinna soft, easily folded, slow recoil	Cartilage to edge of pinna, but soft in places, ready recoil	Pinna firm, cartilage to edge; instant recoil	
Genitals					
Male	Neither testis in scrotum	At least one testis high in scrotum	At least one testis right down		
Female (with hips ½ abducted)	Labia majora widely separated, labia minora protruding	Labia majora almost cover labia minora	Labia majora completely cover labia minora		

From Dubowitz, L.M.S., et al.: Clinical assessment of gestational age in the newborn infant, J. Pediatr. **77:**1, 1970; adapted from Farr, V., et al.: Dev. Med. Child Neurol. **8:**507, 1966.
*If score differs on two sides, take the mean.

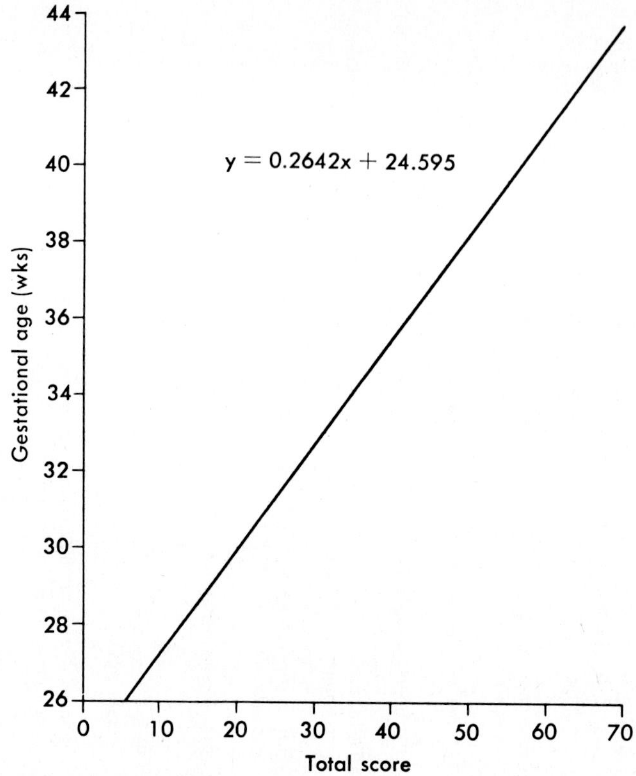

Fig. 15-4. Graph for reading gestational age according to total score derived from evaluation of neurologic signs and external characteristics. (From Dubowitz, L.M.S., et al.: J. Pediatr. **77:**1, 1970.)

alized vascular involvement in which diminution of uterine and placental blood flow impair the function of the placenta. Undergrowth for gestational age is a common outcome of toxemic pregnancies. Cellular abnormalities are characterized by diminished cytoplasmic mass in most organs, particularly the liver and adrenals. The brain is usually less affected than other organs. Gross and microscopic appearance of tissues in affected infants closely resembles that of infants who died during the first year of life from postnatally acquired malnutrition. The number of cells in most organs is diminished little, if at all. The diminutive size of these organs is attributable to the diminished cytoplasmic mass.

Advanced diabetes. In advanced form, diabetes involves generalized vascular damage that impairs normal placental blood flow. Women with early-onset diabetes are more likely to give birth to a small-for-dates infant in contrast to the macrosomic infants born of mothers whose diabetes is not as severe.

Malnutrition of the mother. Maternal malnutrition is probably a significant contributory factor to fetal undergrowth, particularly in severely deprived populations. It is quite likely that long-standing maternal malnutrition is an important cause of fetal undergrowth in low socioeconomic populations. The results of animal experiments strongly suggest a significant role of maternal malnutrition in faulty fetal growth. It has been shown to impair cellular growth in the human placenta and as a result these placentas are smaller than those of normally nourished women. The growth-limiting effect on the placenta is most profound in the villi. It is thus conceivable that these anatomic shortcomings exert a functional effect by reducing the total capacity of the placenta to transfer nutrition to the growing fetus. Epidemiologic data in humans strongly suggest that maternal malnutrition results in fetal undergrowth. There is widespread belief that growth is influenced not only by maternal nutritional status before pregnancy but also during the pregnancy. The rate of maternal weight gain during pregnancy seems to be related to infant birth weight and length. Furthermore, in nutritionally deprived populations, enhanced intake during pregnancy is associated with a significant increase in mean birth weight.

The incidence of small-for-dates babies among moderate *smokers* is twice that of nonsmokers; among heavy smokers it is three times as great. The outcome seems to be related to the number of cigarettes smoked and the duration of the insult. Birth weight and body length are both reduced. At 7 years of age children of smoking women are shorter than controls and have a higher incidence of educational difficulties, regardless of social class, maternal age, or parity. The statistical association of maternal smoking and the incidence of intrauterine growth retardation is among the most direct and unequivocal of all the maternal factors thus far scrutinized for this purpose. Fetal undergrowth probably does not occur if the mother ceases smoking at the onset of pregnancy, but consumption of as few as five cigarettes a day may affect fetal growth.

Narcotic addiction. Approximately half the babies born of maternal addicts are low birth weight infants; 40% of these infants are small-for-dates. Affected infants are small by virtue of a reduced number of cells, indicating early growth impairment of the hypoplastic variety. Diminutive size is therefore largely a function of fewer than normal cells rather than diminished cytoplasmic mass. The effect of heroin and morphine is probably independent of malnutrition.

Alcohol. Consumption of alcohol during pregnancy produces the *fetal alcohol syndrome*. In addition to severe growth deficiency a constellation of structural defects has been noted that includes microcephaly, short palpebral fissures and microphthalmia, epicanthal folds, micrognathia, malformed and immobile joints, dislocation of the hips, cardiac malformations, and malformations of the central nervous system. Mental retardation occurs in almost half of affected infants.

Fetal factors

Multiple gestation. The rate of intrauterine growth in normal singletons diminishes at 36 to 38 weeks. This effect is more pronounced in twins and begins earlier, at approximately 35 weeks. This slowed growth rate has been attributed to progressive diminution in the effective transfer of nutrients across the placenta, perhaps as a function of placental aging. Tissue abnormalities in twins support the notion that nutritional deficiency late in pregnancy is responsible for their small size. Thus subnormal organ weights are primarily a function of diminished cytoplasmic mass. Ordinarily, growth retardation is seen in twins who are delivered after 35 weeks. Before that age, growth parallels that of singletons.

Major congenital malformations and chromosomal abnormalities. A high incidence of fetal undergrowth is associated with congenital and chromosomal abnormalities. This is the hypoplastic variety of growth retardation in which mitotic activity is impaired and the number of cells is therefore reduced. Among small-for-dates infants, major congenital anomalies are severalfold increased compared to those who are appropriately grown for age.

Chronic intrauterine infections. Impaired fetal growth is virtually a hallmark of infections that begin early in pregnancy, particularly during the first trimester. Rubella is the archetypal example of this phenomenon; infections caused by cytomegalovirus are similarly implicated. Hypoplastic growth retardation is identical to that described for congenital malformations.

Placental factors

Placental insufficiency. Insufficiency of the placenta is a concept that is frequently invoked to explain the occurrence of fetal malnutrition. It implies impaired exchange from mother to fetus, particularly suboptimal delivery of nutrients and hormones to the fetus. There are several well-defined pathologic lesions in the placenta that seem to be associated with placental insufficiency, but they occur in only a few instances. These lesions include extensive fibrosis, occlusion of fetal vessels in the villi, large hemangiomas, and early separation. Maternal diabetes and toxemia are apparently associated with placental insufficiency.

Intrauterine parabiotic syndrome (fetofetal

transfusion). The syndrome of fetofetal transfusion is relatively infrequent, occurring in but a small percentage of identical twins. It is a direct result of placental arteriovenous anastomoses between the two fetuses. Blood is transferred from artery to vein (twin to twin) and the extent of blood transfer from one sibling to the other depends on the number of anastomoses that are present. The discrepancy in blood volume between the two infants at birth may or may not be associated with differences in weights. At birth the donor twin is pale as a consequence of diminished red cell mass. The recipient twin is plethoric and polycythemic. The anemic twin may be in shock at birth if blood loss to his sibling was acute; more often the infant is hypoxic as a result of chronic intrauterine anemia. Blood volume in the recipient twin is increased and the polycythemia may cause congestive heart failure as a result of cardiac overload, hyperbilirubinemia because of excessive red cell sequestration, and convulsions as a result of diminished perfusion of the brain.

Single umbilical artery. The presence of only one umbilical artery is sometimes associated with a variety of major congenital anomalies, most commonly in the urinary tract. Numerous investigations have reported the incidence of single umbilical artery to vary from 0.2% to 2% of all births. Among such infants 20% to 65% have congenital anomalies. In some series the incidence of congenital malformation is not higher in infants with single umbilical artery than in normal controls.

Small-for-dates infants. Small-for-dates infants may appear asthenic; subcutaneous fat is diminished in almost all, although on gross inspection this is apparent in only half of them. Those who are not depressed are considerably more vigorous than premature infants of equal birth weight. They are sometimes polycythemic (hematocrit over 60 vol%), presumably because of chronic hypoxia in utero, but the skin is pale nevertheless. Asphyxia at birth may be severe; acidosis is both metabolic (lactic acid accumulation) and respiratory. Massive aspiration of meconium causes pulmonary difficulty, thus prolonging the duration or accentuating asphyctic changes. Hypoglycemia (glucose less than 20 mg/dl) may appear within 48 hours because of depletion of glycogen stores. The respiratory distress syndrome (hyaline membrane disease) rarely if ever occurs in the undergrown infant delivered at term. Massive aspiration of meconium is the usual cause of respiratory distress. Ball valve mechanisms throughout the lung are established by aspirated material, and emphysema ensues. In the extreme the trapping of air leads to pneumothorax, pneumomediastinum, or both.

Responsible management begins with identification of the discordance between weight and age at birth. This can be demonstrated by plotting length of gestation against birth weight on an intrauterine growth chart. Anticipatory observation and therapy of the entire gamut of complications is then possible. Feedings initiated early in infants who can accept them will probably prevent or attenuate hypoglycemia. Feedings should be offered as soon after birth as is feasible. Blood glucose levels should be monitored at frequent intervals for the first 48 hours, even in the absence of symptoms. Administration of alkali and the treatment of hypoglycemia are discussed on pp. 291 and 326. Chest films should be obtained repeatedly if respiratory distress persists; if it worsens, pneumothorax and pneumomediastinum are suspect. Antibiotics are given if radiodensities suggest pneumonia. Small-for-dates infants are likely to lose inordinate amounts of body heat; an adequate thermal environment is indispensable (pp. 268 to 271).

Intrauterine growth acceleration (large for gestational age; macrosomia). High birth weight is defined as 4000 g or more. At any birth weight and gestational age, infants who plot at or above the 90th percentile on intrauterine growth charts are considered large for gestational age. Except for mothers with advanced, vascular diabetes, excessive size is the rule among offspring of diabetic mothers. However, these infants comprise a small fraction of all macrosomic babies. Excessive weight may be a result of genetic predisposition. It is also apparently associated with maternal prepregnancy weight and is probably proportional to weight gain during pregnancy. Multiparous mothers give birth to large infants three times as often as do primiparous mothers. Babies who have transposition of great vessels are usually large for gestational age for reasons that are not currently understood. A number of infants plot above the 90th percentile on growth curves because of miscalculation of the last menstrual period. The source of error is most often the occurrence of postconceptional bleeding, which is thought to be the last menstrual period. The estimated date of confinement (EDC) is thus approximately 1 month beyond the actual date. Born at term, the infant is considered premature, and his term birth weight places him above the 90th percentile.

The mortality rate for macrosomic babies born at term is higher than for those of normal weight. Furthermore, their large size imposes mechanical difficulties during labor and delivery. The need for midforceps and cesarean section is increased, the latter because of the common occurrence of fetopelvic disproportion. Injuries include fractured clavicle, brachial plexus palsy, facial paralysis, and depressed skull fracture, together occurring in 15% of oversized babies. Shoulder dystocia is frequent.

Physical examination of the neonate

Several dramatic physical findings, which may arouse unnecessary parental apprehension, are often observed in normal neonates. The physician should be prepared to state that a given finding does not imply disease and that it will or will not disappear. Erythema toxicum must therefore be distinguished from staphylococcal pyoderma. A prominent interparietal fontanel or a wide metopic suture must not be erroneously labeled as a skull defect. The red stain on a diaper caused by uric acid crystals in urine should not be confused with gross hematuria. A mucosanguinous vaginal discharge or edema of the scrotum must be explained to anxiously inquiring parents, as must the spontaneous disappearance of cephalhematoma.

Proportions, contour, and posture. The trunk of the normal newborn infant is cylindric. The head circumference is slightly larger than that of the chest and averages 33 to 35.5 cm (13 to 14 inches). The circumference of the chest is usually 30.5 to 33 cm (12 to 13 inches). The sitting height (crown-rump measurement) is roughly equal to the head circumference. These values may vary, but their relationship to each other is fairly constant. The head circumference should not be significantly smaller than the chest or crown-rump measurements. When the head circumference is inordinately greater than the chest or crown-rump measurements, hydrocephalus must be suspected. The relationship of the head measurement to the crown-rump measurement is probably more reliable than that of the head to the chest measurement. The *posture* of the newborn child is the result of in utero position. In cephalic deliveries the head is flexed, and the chin rests on the upper part of the sternum. The vertebral column is flexed. The arms are adducted to the thorax, the elbows are flexed, and the forearms are pronated. The hips and knees are flexed, and the feet are characteristically dorsiflexed. Several variations of this in utero posture have been linked to abnormal contours of long bones and the cranium. Variations in posture associated with more unusual presentations are striking. After a brow presentation the infant's head is extended and his neck is long. In frank breech deliveries the legs are extended at the knees, the head is somewhat flattened on top, and the neck is elongated compared to the neck of an infant born from the usual cephalic presentations.

Skin. At birth the skin is covered with patches of gray-white caseous material called *vernix,* which, if not removed, will dry and disappear after several hours. The subsequently exposed skin is blush red. At the end of the first day the soft red skin becomes dry and flaky. *Jaundice* may be evident on the second or third day in approximately one half of normal newborn infants and disappears by the fifth to seventh day. *Edema* of the subcutaneous tissue is commonly present and is most clearly evident about the eyes, the face, the dorsa of the hands and feet, and the legs. It disappears after several days. *Peripheral cyanosis* of the hands, feet, and circumoral region is frequently present at birth and for a variable number of days thereafter. It is probably caused by venous stasis. In contradistinction to generalized cyanosis it is not the result of a hypoxic state. Localized cyanosis may be seen over presenting parts, such as a prolapsed upper extremity. *Cutis marmorata* is a purple reticulated pattern frequently noted in the skin when the infant is exposed to a cool atmosphere. *Mongolian spots* are irregular areas of deep blue pigmentation, usually distributed over the sacral and gluteal regions, which fade after several weeks. They may be so extensive as to involve much of the infant's back. They are extremely common in black neonates and in infants of southern European stock. *Telangiectatic nevi,* also known as stork bites, are almost universal in newborn infants and are evident over the lower occiput and the back of the neck, the upper eyelids, the nasion, alae nasi, and upper lip. They are deep pink and flat and are easily blanched. They disappear between the first and second years. *Subcutaneous fat necrosis* is caused by trauma from forceps or manipulation. It is a sharply demarcated firm mass of variable size. It is attached to the overlying skin, which is occasionally reddish purple, but is free of attachment to underlying tissues. *Harlequin color change* is a peculiar discrepancy in color between the two longitudinal halves of the infant in which one side is paler than the other. This phenomenon may be elicited by placing the infant on his side for several minutes. The colors will be reversed when the infant is placed on the other side. In the supine position, color distribution is normal. *Lanugo* is fine hair, characteristic of the neonatal period, which is best seen on the shoulders, back, forehead, and cheeks. *Milia* are distended sebaceous glands seen as minute white papules on the cheeks, chin, and nose. They disappear spontaneously. *Sudamina* are distended sweat glands usually seen on the face, which cause tiny vesicles on the skin surface. *Erythema toxicum* is a pink papular rash found on the thorax, back, diaper area, and abdomen. Frequently the papules appear purulent and are confused with pyoderma. A smear of the fluid in the lesion will reveal many eosinophils when Wright stain is used. Toxic erythema appears on about the second day and may persist for several days thereafter. The etiology is unknown.

Head. The contour of the head is characteristic because of a relatively small face, large calvarium, and prominent frontal and parietal eminences. The bones of the calvarium are separated by bands of connective tissue, the sutures, along which several widened areas, the *fontanels,* are easily palpable. Six of these fontanels are located at each of the corners of the two parietal bones. Two of these, the *anterior* and *posterior fontanels,* are in the midline. The former is at the junction of the coronal and sagittal sutures, whereas the latter is at the junction of the lambdoidal and sagittal sutures. The two *anterolateral fontanels* are at the junctions of the squamosal and coronal sutures, and the two *posterolateral fontanels* are at the junction of the squamosal and lambdoidal sutures. Occasionally a *parietal (sagittal) fontanel* is palpated midway between the anterior and posterior fontanels along the sagittal suture. The *metopic fontanel* is a widening of the metopic suture at the midline of the upper forehead. It is sometimes continuous with the anterior fontanel. The metopic fontanel may be continuous with the *glabellar fontanel* immediately anterior to it. In the vast majority of infants the anterior fontanel has closed by 18 months of age. Occasionally it persists to 2 years of age. The posterior fontanel is closed by 6 weeks of age. *Physiologic craniotabes* is caused by pliability of the skull, most frequently demonstrated at the margins of the parietal and occipital bones along the lambdoidal suture. When pressure is applied to this area, the resultant snapping sensation is classically likened to the forceful indentation of a ping-pong ball. *Molding* of the head is almost always present to some degree, ranging from barely perceptible to grotesque. This results from several forces exerted during the birth process and is influenced also by the mode of presentation of the head. The usual cephalic presentation causes flattening of the forehead, with a gradual rise to an apex in the midparietal region and an abrupt drop at the posterior skull. In a brow presentation the forehead is unusually prominent, and in a breech delivery the vertex is often flattened. For several hours after birth the bones of the calvarium may overlap each other at their margins as a result of the compression that causes molding. By the end of the first or second day the normal contour of the skull is more nearly in evidence. *Caput succedaneum* is an edematous swelling of that portion of the scalp that first presents itself. *Cephalhematomas* are unilateral or bilateral accumulations of extravasated blood between the periosteum and the underlying bone first noted at the end of the first or second day. The parietal bones are most frequently involved.

Eyes. *Chemical conjunctivitis* with purulent exudate occurs on the first day as a result of silver nitrate instillation in the eyes at birth. The purulent discharge disappears 1 or 2 days later. *Subconjunctival hemorrhage* occurs at the limbus. It may be crescent shaped or may form a red halo about the entire iris. *Retinal hemorrhages* have been reported in 20% of full-term infants. They are flame shaped, irregular, or round. No residual defects have been reported from subconjunctival or retinal hemorrhages. Most neonates begin to lacrimate at 2 to 3 weeks of age.

Mouth. *Inclusion cysts,* gray round lesions seen at the gum margins, are frequently thought to be teeth. They disappear in a few weeks. *True teeth* are occasionally seen at birth in the lower central incisor position. These are normal teeth that have erupted prematurely. They are rarely supernumerary. When they appear to be in danger of spontaneous detachment, as is usual, they should be removed to prevent aspiration. *Epstein pearls,* also known as *Bohn pearls,* are small white papules on the hard palate on each side of the midline; they disappear in several weeks. Parents sometimes think these lesions represent early thrush. *Bednar aphthae* are found at the posterior margin of the hard palate close to and on either side of the midline. They are round or oval-shaped gray ulcers probably caused by vigorous use of coarse gauze in cleansing the mouth at birth. Because this practice has been generally discontinued, these lesions are now rarely seen. They may be evident on the second day of life. The *frenulum of the tongue* arises from the lingual base in the midline and attaches to the ventral lingual surface for varying distances toward the tip. When the frenulum is attached far forward, protrusion of the tongue causes a concavity at the tip. This does not interfere with nursing nor does it produce a speech defect later in childhood. "Clipping the tongue" by incising the frenulum is rarely indicated; severance of the profunda linguae vein may result in considerable hemorrhage and, furthermore, creates a portal of entry for infection. The *frenum of the upper lip* is a band of pink tissue that courses from the inner surface of the upper lip to the maxillary alveolar ridge in the midline. It is often thick, and at its point of attachment on the alveolar ridge a deep notch will be found that disappears as the maxilla grows.

Throat. The throat is incompletely visualized when the tongue is merely depressed, since such attempts are met with strong reflex protrusion. An excellent view of the posterior pharynx is obtained by stimulating the baby to cry and gently depressing the chin without the use of the tongue depressor. Depression of the tongue while the infant is crying is also effective. The uvula may not be visible when retracted upward and posteriorly as the infant cries.

Chest. The anteroposterior and lateral diameters of the thorax are equal. The ribs are so flexible that slight sternal retraction may be evident during inspiration. The xiphoid cartilage frequently points ventrad and is thus seen as a small protrusion at the lower end of the sternum. *Breast enlargement* appears in many infants on the third day. By the end of the first week the engorged breasts may secrete a milklike substance, "witches' milk." Massaging the breasts with various preparations is a common lay practice that may cause breast abscess. *Supernumerary nipples* without glandular tissue are common. These are usually inferior and slightly medial to the normal nipples. The normal infant's *lungs* may emit fine crepitant rales at the end of inspiration. Respirations are predominantly abdominal, with little activity of the rib cage. Shallow respirations or momentary apnea followed by deep inspirations may be seen in normal infants.

Heart. The heart rate of the normal neonate is usually between 100 and 180. Ninety percent of murmurs heard during the first week of life are not associated with cardiac anomalies. Occasionally the typical murmur of a patent ductus arteriosus may be heard during the first day, only to disappear hours later. Major cardiac malformations have been demonstrated at autopsy in infants in whom murmurs were not detectable during life.

Abdomen. The normal cylindric contour of the abdomen should be carefully noted. *Abdominal distention* may be generalized, as in intestinal obstruction. *Localized bulging* in one or both flanks is often apparent in hydronephrosis. A grotesque deviation from the normal contour is seen in congenital absence of the abdominal musculature. In this condition the anterior aspect of the abdomen is depressed, whereas the intestines, covered only by skin and subcutaneous tissue, bulge pendulously from the flanks. *Diastasis recti* is a separation of the rectus muscles, 1 to 2 cm in width. With rare exception the edge of the *liver* is palpable as far as 2 cm below the right costal margin. In some infants the *spleen* tip is palpable. The *kidneys* can be felt under ideal conditions of complete relaxation. This is more easily accomplished on the left. On the right only the lower pole can be felt. Palpation of the lower abdomen should not be neglected. A distended *bladder* that remains palpable following feeble micturition is suggestive of an obstructive lesion at the bladder outlet. The *umbilical cord* is lustrous blue-white at birth. Within 24 hours it becomes dull and yellow-brown and then black-brown and dry. In this gangrenous state it sloughs from the point of attachment at the end of 1 week. *Umbilical hernia* is a skin-covered protuberance at the umbilicus. The herniation occurs through a round defect in the abdominal wall 0.5 to 1 cm or greater in diameter and comprises greater omentum and small intestine. The protuberance may not be visible at birth, but the muscle defect is easily demonstrated. Umbilical hernias are common. They are particularly frequent in black infants and have been reported in approximately one half of a large series of Italian infants. The vast majority of umbilical hernias disappear spontaneously at the end of the first year. Some observers report correlation between size of defect and necessity for surgical repair.

Male genitalia. The prepuce covers the entire glans and is not retractable in many infants. Frequently the *external meatus* cannot be visualized. Even at 6 months of age the prepuce is not fully retractable. This is not caused by adhesions but rather by the slow development of free space between the prepuce and the glans. The temptation to break up adhesions should be resisted. When the ventral surface of the glans is not covered by preputial tissue, some degree of *hypospadias* is invariably present. *Epithelial pearls,* 1 or 2 mm in diameter, are occasionally seen at the tip of the prepuce. The scrotum may be small or large and pendulous. Edema of the scrotal wall is common. It disappears in several days. Noncommunicating *hydrocele* occurs frequently. In the scrotum it is usually unilateral, and it resolves within several months. *Inguinal hernia* is rarely manifested before 2 weeks of age in a full-term infant. In premature infants it is more likely to become apparent early. The *testes* are usually palpable in the scrotum or in the inguinal canal.

Female genitalia. In the full-term infant the labia minora and the clitoris are often more prominent than the labia majora. In premature babies this is invariable. The *hymenal tag* comprising labia minora and hymenal tissue is occasionally large as it protrudes from the floor of the vagina. It disappears in several weeks. A milk-white glistening vaginal discharge may be seen during the first week. Sometimes it is blood tinged or composed of whole blood. This is a physiologic manifestation of maternal hormonal influences that disappears within 2 weeks.

Central nervous system. It is important to make as many observations as possible without disturbing the infant. Reflexes requiring greater degrees of disturbance should be elicited toward the end of the examination. Increased or decreased *spontaneous movements* must be noted. *Motor activity* should also be observed for symmetry, gross tremulousness, myoclonic jerks, and convulsive movements. A bright light is directed to each eye for the *blink reflex* that is present even with the eyes closed. The *grasp reflexes* are elicited in the palms and soles by placing a finger at the bases of the fingers and toes that respond by flexion. The *rooting reflex* is elicited by stroking the angles of the lips with the finger. The infant turns the head to the side of the stimulus. Recently fed or lethargic infants may merely purse their lips. The normal *suck* reflex is elicited by placing a sterile nipple in the mouth. Recently fed infants respond more feebly than hungry infants. *Head control* in the newborn infant is more effective than is generally realized. With the infant in the supine position the examiner lifts the infant slowly by the forearms to a sitting position. As traction is exerted, the shoulder and arm muscles contract, followed by flexion of the neck muscles. In the sitting position the head may fall forward, but attempts to elevate it will usually be noted a few seconds later. The *Moro reflex* as generally practiced is elicited by slapping the examining table or jerking the underlying blanket. As described originally by Moro, however, the stimulus is a sudden movement of the head in relation to the position of the spine. Responses are more consistently elicited when the infant is held in the supine position with one of the examiner's palms beneath the sacrum and the other placed beneath the occiput and upper back. The head is allowed to drop backward through an angle of 30 degrees when support of the occiput is withdrawn. The normal response comprises abduction of the arms and extension of the elbows, wrists, and fingers, followed by adduction of the arms and flexion of the elbows and fingers.

Simultaneous reflex movement of the legs is of variable extent. The Moro response should be evaluated for symmetry and overall vigor. The *eyes* are observed for their normal central position at rest and for contraction of the pupils to light. Paralysis of *extraocular movements* is demonstrated by holding the child upright and moving him horizontally from left to right in relation to the examiner. Normally, conjugate deviation is noted in the direction of the movement. The fundi are examined after mydriasis is accomplished with 1% or 2% homatropine. *Transillumination of the skull* is performed in a dark room. An ordinary flashlight with a rubber cuff attached to the lighted end is pressed against the infant's head. A normal circular flare of red light approximately 1 to 2 cm is usually noted. This is best seen in the frontal area and in the region of the anterior fontanel. Little or no light is seen at the occipital and temporal regions. Excessive light conduction may be indicative of hydranencephaly, porencephaly, subdural hematoma, or severe hydrocephalus.

Respiratory disorders

Periodic breathing. Short apneic episodes of 10 to 20 seconds duration, which alternate with rapid deep respiration for intervals of similar duration, are observable in most premature infants who are otherwise well. This pattern is of such frequent occurrence that it is interpreted as a normal phenomenon, an assumption that has not been documented. Periodic breathing generally appears during active (REM) sleep and disappears during quiet sleep. It rarely occurs during the first 24 hours of life and usually disappears when 36 postconceptional weeks or 2 kg (about 4.4 pounds) body weight are attained. In contrast to prolonged apnea, heart rate and body temperature are unchanged and cyanosis never occurs. The causes and significance of this respiratory pattern have not been determined.

Apnea of prematurity. Prolonged apneic episodes (duration of 20 seconds or more) result from a wide variety of underlying causes and are a source of great concern in any premature nursery. They may occur on any day of life, and in many instances a contributory factor cannot be demonstrated. Overall mortality of premature infants who are apneic from any cause is approximately 70%; in full-term infants the mortality is 15%. Bradycardia, cyanosis, and respiratory acidosis are common during prolonged episodes, in contrast to periodic breathing. Administration of oxygen is frequently of little benefit, although tactile stimulation often triggers resumption of respiration. Apneic episodes may occur in hyaline membrane disease and respiratory insufficiency of prematurity, in infections such as septicemia, pneumonia, and meningitis, in intraventricular hemorrhage, from a large left to right shunt across the ductus arteriosus in premature infants, in hypoglycemia and hypocalcemia, during seizures or infrequently as a sole manifestation of them, during cold stress, and in association with numerous other and less frequent disorders. These disease processes must be ruled out before the diagnosis of *apnea of prematurity* can be made. The smallest premature babies are most often affected. The cause and pathogenesis are incompletely understood. Severe episodes are associated with bradycardia or cardiac arrest and cyanosis.

The simplest therapy is tactile stimulation, to which most infants respond readily. Pulsating water beds are also effective but no one knows why they are. Constant positive airway pressure (CPAP) is almost universally successful in eliminating or drastically reducing apneic episodes; yet the mechanism of its action is also not understood. Theophylline and caffeine are the only recommended pharmacologic agents and both are usually effective. A priming dose of theophylline (5.5 mg/kg) is followed by a maintenance dose of 1.1 mg/kg every 8 hours. Blood levels should be obtained frequently and the dose adjusted accordingly. Therapeutic levels of theophylline vary from 6.5 μg/ml to 12.0 μg/ml. Caffeine levels should also be obtained because part of the theophylline is metabolized to caffeine, which accumulates and is itself effective. Toxicity to theophylline is indicated most often by a heart rate in excess of 180 beats/min. Irritability, seizures, naturesis, diuresis, and rarely hematemesis also occur. Caffeine is thought to be more effective by some investigators. Toxicity is infrequent and it is easier to administer. A loading dose of 10 mg/kg is followed by maintenance with a single daily dose of 2.5 mg/kg given either intravenously or orally. Therapeutic blood levels vary from 5 to 20 μg/ml.

Respiratory distress syndrome type II (transient tachypnea of the newborn). Infants affected with respiratory distress syndrome type II (RDSII) are usually mature or nearly so. Their respiratory distress begins at birth or shortly thereafter, and it is characterized by retractions, tachypnea, and grunting. If cyanosis in room air is discernible, it usually disappears when the infant is placed in relatively small increments of ambient oxygen concentration. Respiratory distress may resolve in 1 to 2 days or less, or it may persist for 4 or 5 days.

The chest film is characterized by generalized overexpansion of the lungs that is clearly identifiable by noting flattened diaphragms. Dense streaks radiate from the hilar areas, and occasionally one or several patches of density are apparent. The streaks represent interstitial fetal lung fluid and distended lymphatic vessels. Although the literature frequently alludes to a clinical resemblance of RDS II to hyaline membrane disease, there is actually little basis for confusion. The roentgenographic appearances of both disorders are quite dissimilar; the fundamental discerning feature is the state of lung expansion. The lungs of an infant with RDS II are well-expanded, and more often they are overexpanded. The hallmark of hyaline membrane disease is underexpansion. These changes are generally discernible on most chest films with little equivocation. There is general agreement that failure to completely evacuate fetal lung fluid is the cause of this syndrome.

Blood pH may be moderately depressed, P_{CO_2} may be somewhat, if at all, elevated, and the base deficit is usually 10 mEq/L or less. It is characteristic of the clinical course that initial correction of metabolic acidosis with bicarbonate rarely requires repetition. Although the clinical appearance of respiratory distress simulates hyaline membrane disease, transient tachypnea of the newborn is a different entity with a far more favorable outlook. Mortality attributable to this disorder has not been seen. However, several instances of spontaneous pneumothorax in infants with this syndrome have been encountered.

Respiratory distress syndrome (RDS; hyaline membrane disease). Hyaline membrane disease is an acute disorder that is symptomatic at birth or soon thereafter. Primarily characterized by respiratory distress, it occurs virtually exclusively in premature infants, affecting approximately 20% to 25% of them. The shorter the gestational age and the lower the birth weight, the higher the incidence. Thus between birth weight of 1000 g and 1500 g, approximately 57% of infants have been observed to be affected. Case fatality is quite variable from one institution to another. Advances in therapy, particularly in the application of end expiratory positive pressure, have diminished the percent mortality. Overall, 15% to 20% of affected infants do not survive. Most of them expire as a result of complications such as intracranial hemorrhage, infection, air leak syndromes, bronchopulmonary dysplasia, and decompensated patent ductus arteriosus.

Fig. 15-5 depicts in general terms the pathogenesis of the disease as it is currently understood. Partial persistence of the fetal cardiopulmonary state is indicated in *1* as the neonate is born with surfactant deficiency and increased pulmonary vascular resistance. The latter would normally lessen considerably if lung expansion

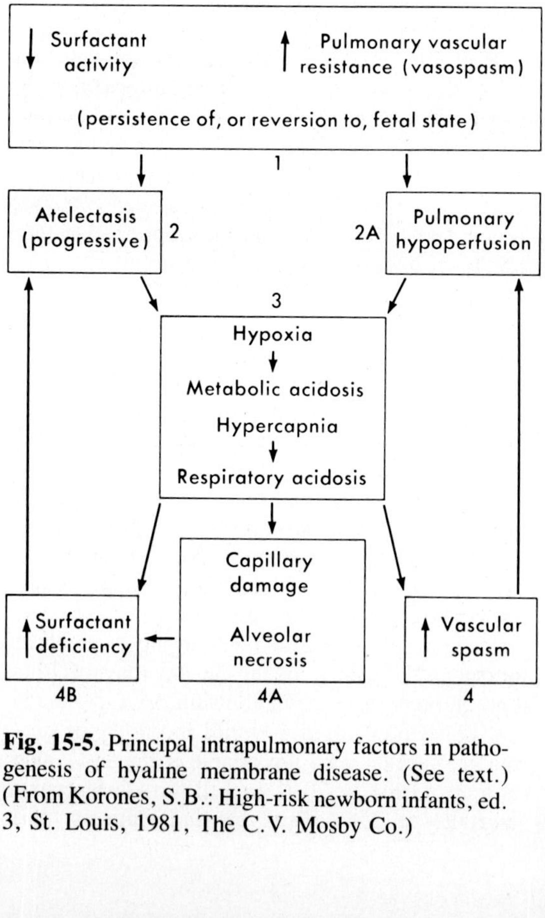

Fig. 15-5. Principal intrapulmonary factors in pathogenesis of hyaline membrane disease. (See text.) (From Korones, S.B.: High-risk newborn infants, ed. 3, St. Louis, 1981, The C.V. Mosby Co.)

and oxygen intake were feasible with relative ease. Atelectasis, indicated in *2*, progresses in response to the predominance of surface-active forces that are not counterbalanced by normally requisite surfactant activity, and commensurately, pulmonary hypoperfusion increases as a consequence of progressive vasoconstriction because of inadequate tissue oxygen supply. The biochemical aberrations that are produced as a result of failure to breathe normally *(3)* accentuate surfactant deficiency *(4B)* by producing capillary damage and alveolar cell necrosis *(4A)*. Atelectasis becomes more extensive *(2)*. These same biochemical changes intensify vasospasm *(4)*, which accentuates the existing hypoperfusion *(2A)*. The most effective available method for intervention is the use of end-expiratory positive pressure, which eliminates atelectasis to a degree that permits adequate alveolar ventilation and the establishment of functional residual capacity.

The importance of surfactant deficiency and its association with prematurity and perinatal distress are universally acknowledged, but the specific factors leading to its diminution have not been demonstrated. The end result of surfactant deficiency is failure of proper lung expansion and absence of alveolar stability (collapse at end-expiration, atelectasis). Cardiovascular effects of poor expansion with the first breath and with those that follow have been well described. Essentially, and in varying degrees, the fetal pattern of cardiopulmonary circulation persists after birth in that pulmonary vascular resistance is elevated (because of vasoconstriction and failure of capillaries to dilate), thus diverting blood from the lungs. Compliance of the lung is significantly diminished. Collapse of alveoli and poor lung perfusion cause diminished gas exchange. Some expanded alveoli, which receive air extremely well, are not supplied with sufficient blood, whereas other alveoli in a collapsed state are poorly ventilated and are of little use even if blood supply is optimal. The predominant effect is from poor alveolar ventilation caused by widespread atelectasis. Overall, the balance of ventilation and perfusion is thus abnormal. Oxygen intake is decreased, and retention of carbon dioxide is increased. Continued hypoxia is associated with metabolic acidosis, whereas accumulation of carbon dioxide causes respiratory acidosis. Blood gas and pH values are similar to those of asphyxiated fetuses before birth, that is, low PO_2, high PCO_2, and low pH.

The hallmarks of morphologic pathology are atelectasis and eosinophilic hyaline membranes in aerated alveoli and alveolar ducts. Atelectasis is diffuse, but emphysematous areas are often interspersed throughout the lung. Hyaline membranes are absent in the lungs of infants who die in the first few hours of life, whereas atelectasis is extensive. In infants who die of unrelated causes, hyaline membrane fragments are visible up to 10 days after recovery from the disease. The hyaline membrane is undoubtedly of endogenous origin, probably derived from blood and necrotic alveolar epithelial cells.

RDS occurs almost exclusively in premature infants. Infants of diabetic mothers are apparently more frequently affected. Fetal asphyxia during labor plays an important role in predisposition to the disease among premature infants. RDS appears to be more frequent in antepartum hemorrhage (placenta previa, abruptio placentae), in association with compression of the cord, and among infants of toxemic mothers.

Some degree of respiratory distress is usually identifiable immediately after birth. Eighty percent of RDS infants are dyspneic by the end of 1 hour, and Apgar scores are low in a majority of them. Signs of respiratory distress are not specific for RDS, but the diagnosis may be assumed if other causes are shown to be absent in a premature infant whose chest film displays typical abnormalities. Laboratory evidence in support of the diagnosis includes an L/S ratio less than 2.0 or a negative shake test performed on amniotic fluid, gastric aspirate, or tracheal or pharyngeal secretion. Tachypnea is the rule, but occasionally slow respirations are observed. Retraction of the chest wall is usually most prominent at the lower sternum; occasionally the upper chest appears overexpanded. The alae nasi dilate with each inspiration. Expiratory grunting is common, often appearing as a sigh. The expiratory grunt is a fascinating phenomenon, which raises arterial PO_2 by maintaining some degree of alveolar expansion at end expiration. With closure of the glottis by the epiglottis during deflation, the egress of air is momentarily blocked, thus raising intrapulmonary pressure at end expiration. Sudden release of the epiglottis results in a rush of air that produces the characteristic grunt by vibration of the vocal cords. Auscultation of the lungs reveals diminished air exchange, harsh breath sounds, and crepitant rales (occasionally). Cyanosis while breathing room air may be relieved by increasing ambient oxygen unless the disease is severe. Increasing cyanosis despite oxygen administration is a sign of severe disease. Bradycardia (less than 100 beats/min) is often a terminal event. Murmurs are seldom detectable during the period of respiratory distress. Cardiomegaly is sometimes evident on radiography. Hypotension in the systemic circulation is common, particularly in the early hours of the disease. The skin is often gray or dusky; this seems to be related to peripheral vasoconstriction. Edema, although common among unaffected premature infants, is even more frequent in RDS. Pitting edema of the dorsa of the hands and feet seems to be peculiar to these infants. It is seldom present at birth, appears within 24 hours, and disappears by the end of the fifth day.

Hypothermia is correctable in infants who are mildly or moderately affected, but it is often irremediable in severely involved babies. Incubator temperatures up to 35° C (95° F) may be necessary to maintain body temperature.

Central nervous system signs are few. Affected infants are usually flaccid and hypoactive. In the presence of severe disease they lie in frog-leg position, head to one side and mouth open.

The radiograph is characteristic, but variations of the classic pattern occur frequently. Diffuse and patchy atelectasis conveys a radiograph of underexpanded lungs in which a reticulogranular pattern (caused by focal atelectasis) is discernible. The hilar regions are more uniformly opaque for varying short distances toward the periphery; air bronchograms are evident within these dense areas. Air bronchograms are often visible behind the cardiac shadow in normal infants. In RDS they are also discernible in other pulmonary areas, particularly in the upper lobes. This radiologic pattern may occasionally precede the onset of severe symptoms, but often it does not appear until 12 to 24 hours after birth. Severity of disease cannot be estimated consistently from the radiologic appearance of the lungs.

Recovery begins at 5 to 10 days of life. During this phase peripheral edema disappears, meconium is passed more frequently, and urine output increases. The continuous murmur of a patent ductus arteriosus is often detected for the first time.

Pneumonia due to group B streptococcus (GBS) may closely resemble RDS. The chest film may be identical in both disorders. The onset and the manifestations of respiratory distress are often indistinguishable. Apnea in the first few hours is more likely in GBS pneumonia; lung compliance is often less reduced; and leukopenia with neutropenia strongly suggests the presence of GBS infection.

Complications of RDS include infections, intracranial hemorrhage, hyperbilirubinemia, and cardiac failure caused by a left to right shunt through a patent ductus arteriosus. A massive left to right shunt may occur during the recovery period, when gradual dilation of pulmonary arterioles reduces pulmonary vascular pressure below systemic blood pressure. The resultant gradient leads to hyperperfusion of the lungs and subsequent pulmonary edema. The superiority of medical management versus surgical ligation of the ductus is still controversial.

Preventive measures. Thus far, the most promising direct approach to the prevention of RDS is the administration of certain pharmacologic agents to the mother before the birth of her premature infant. Corticosteroids are among the most prominent of these agents. There is good (but as yet inconclusive) evidence that the administration of corticosteroids to mothers who are in premature labor diminishes the incidence of RDS. Betamethasone and dexamethasone appear to be the most active preparations. Their effect seems to be limited to infants whose gestational age is 32 weeks or less. Steroids have been shown in animals to accelerate lung maturation by attachment to receptor sites on type II alveolar cells to subsequently enhance production and/or release of surfactant. Thyroxin, aminophylline, and heroin produce similar effects. In humans the incidence of RDS is diminished when appropriate doses of steroids are given between 1 and 7 days before delivery.

Therapeutic measures

General comments. Therapy of hyaline membrane disease is complex. Management of severely affected infants, who inevitably develop complications of the disease and of the therapy itself, is the most demanding of all the commitments of a neonatal intensive care unit. The physician must be experienced, knowledgeable, and circumspect in making decisions, yet quick to change the plan when the situation requires it. Major responsibility befalls the nurse. Of all caregiving personnel, the nurse's attention to the infant must be most intense and unflagging. Nurses must be capable of inserting an endotracheal tube rapidly when the tube already in place becomes dislodged or occluded. They should be able to start intravenous infusions and collect arterial blood samples. They must anticipate deterioration and certainly recognize it when it occurs. Their effectiveness is directly proportional to their knowledge of the disease and their alertness to the many details involved in its adequate therapy. A laboratory capable of determining blood gases and pH within minutes of sample collection is indispensable, and it must be manned by personnel around the clock every day. Furthermore, laboratory personnel must be trained to understand the clinical significance of data they generate. In short, management of respiratory distress syndrome in particular and neonatal intensive care in general cannot be effective (much less justified) without the expertise of several disciplines—the so-called team approach. The involvement of people in such a program of therapy is most important. The availability of equipment ranks next in importance. Superior personnel can often improvise to overcome the absence of some forms of equipment. Superb equipment is obviously useless without the type of personnel just described.

Specific procedures. Management is concerned with provision of optimal ventilation, maintenance of acid-base balance, hydration, normal body temperature, blood volume, and nutrition.

Respiratory support. Exceptionally, respiratory support may simply require an increment in fraction of inspired oxygen (FiO_2) in a plastic hood, or more often it may be complex in that some form of mechanical ventilatory support is essential. In either event assiduous monitoring of arterial blood gases and pH is the only reliable method for evaluation of the effectiveness of therapy. These determinations are essential after any change in respiratory therapy, no matter how frequent or, in the absence of change in therapy, at least every 4 hours. In general, we attempt to maintain PaO_2 between 50 and 70 torr, pH above 7.25, and $PaCO_2$ between 45 and 50 torr. Unless the infant is obviously in severe distress, cyanotic in oxygen and apneic, we first try the simplest of measures—an increased FiO_2 in a hood for an infant who breathes spontaneously. If the PaO_2 falls below 50 to 60 torr in an FiO_2 of 0.60 (60% oxygen concentration), and provided $PaCO_2$ has not risen above 60 torr, we initiate constant positive airway pressure (CPAP). In 1971 Gregory introduced CPAP for the treatment of hyaline membrane disease. Gas exchange is significantly improved by this method, which in essence maintains varying degrees of lung expansion at end expiration, depending on the amount of applied positive pressure. The distention of collapsed but perfused alveoli provides a greater surface for effective gas exchange; the maintenance of positive pressure at end expiration increases functional residual capacity. The benefits of this procedure are reflected in an increased PaO_2 where hypoxic levels had existed previously. CPAP has reduced the mortality of RDS significantly. Its effectiveness depends on the infant's ability to ventilate spontaneously. If the infant cannot maintain an adequate tidal volume, $PaCO_2$ will rise even if PaO_2 remains within satisfactory limits. When carbon dioxide retention elevates the $PaCO_2$ above 60 torr, a mechanical ventilator must be used. The respiratory acidosis produced by severe hypercapnia is often eliminated within minutes after an appropriately set ventilator is applied.

Oxygen therapy. Retrolental fibroplasia (RLF) and bronchopulmonary dysplasia are the two known significant complications of oxygen overdosage. RLF is caused primarily by hyperoxemia in premature babies. It rarely occurs in infants whose gestational age is over 37 weeks. The precise PaO_2 that is toxic has not been documented nor has the critical duration of toxic levels been established. Most neonatologists attempt to keep PaO_2 below 90 to 100 torr. *The development of RLF is directly related to the PaO_2, not to the percent concentration of inspired oxygen.* Infants with hyaline membrane disease are actually less likely to have RLF, in spite of the frequency with which a high FiO_2 must be provided, because their disorder militates against the achievement of high arterial oxygen tensions. It is rather the nonhyaline membrane disease premature in need of increased environmental oxygen concentrations because of recurrent apnea who is most likely to become involved. *Measurement only of the FiO_2, and maintenance of this concentration below 40%, is no assurance against the appearance of RLF. Arterial oxygen tensions must be determined for adequate surveillance. Without them oxygen therapy for premature infants is dangerous.*

Oxygen monitoring. FiO_2 is monitored continuously with an oxygen analyzer whether the infant is in a hood or on a respirator. PaO_2 is traditionally determined on arterial blood samples that are drawn from the aorta through an umbilical artery catheter or from puncture of a peripheral artery, most commonly the right radial artery. Capillary blood is less desirable for this purpose.

Transcutaneous oxygen measurements ($TcPO_2$) are now widely used for continuous monitoring of PaO_2. The core of this device is its electrode, which is in essence a Clark electrode similar to the standard devices used in laboratory blood gas analyzers. The skin electrode is heated to a servocontrolled temperature that ranges from 42° to 44° C, depending on the age of the infant and the manufacturer of the apparatus. The heated electrode warms subepidermal tissue to dilate loop capillaries. This assures, in usual circumstances, adequate perfusion. The warmed capillary blood releases oxygen more readily because the oxygen-hemoglobin dissociation curve is shifted to the right in response to local hyperthermia. Furthermore, the warmed skin becomes increasingly porous and hyperperfused. The net effect of these factors is diffusion of oxygen through skin at PaO_2 levels that closely approximate aortic values. The skin electrode senses diffused oxygen and registers accordingly. A large number of studies have compared $TcPO_2$ to aortic PO_2 and with few exceptions, correlation coefficients have ranged from 0.90 to 0.96.

$TcPO_2$ is spuriously low when the skin is underperfused, as in impending or blatant shock or severe cold stress. The monitor indicates a need for more voltage to maintain servocontrolled skin temperature and this in itself may be a valuable sign of potential catastrophe.

Skin monitoring obviously reduces the number of blood samples required for adequate PaO_2 assessment, but blood samples are nonetheless essential for assessing $PaCO_2$ and pH. We have found that the value of transcutaneous monitoring is greatest in acutely ill infants for whom a more rapid optimal adjustment of respirator settings is feasible, and also in babies with chronic lung disease (bronchopulmonary disease) whose reaction to the pain of skin puncture completely negates the validity of arterial PO_2 determinations. Another advantage of the $TcPO_2$ is its instant display of hypoxemia during the performance of procedures or at the inception of a catastrophic event. Thus a danger point is more easily recognized during endotracheal suction or exchange transfusion or with the onset of pneumothorax or septic shock. One can also expect fewer intervals of hyperoxemia with the continuous monitoring afforded by the $TcPO_2$.

Bronchopulmonary dysplasia (BPD) is directly related to FiO_2 breathed for protracted periods, rather than to arterial oxygen tension. BPD is a progressive, chronic lung disease that follows mechanical ventilation with high concentrations of oxygen and with the use of an endotracheal tube. All tissues of the lung are involved. Barotrauma caused by mechanical ventilation is generally accepted as a principal causative factor. In the vast majority of instances, hyaline membrane disease precedes the onset of BPD, but other acute pulmonary disorders may also be antecedent. Wilson-Mikity syndrome, pneumonia, apnea of prematurity, cardiac arrest following ligation of a ductus arteriosus, and meconium aspiration have all been observed as precursors to BPD. Whether preceded by hyaline membrane disease or some other pulmonary disorder, BPD is virtually always associated with mechanical ventilation through an endotracheal tube that also involves high concentrations of administered oxygen. The relative significance of these three factors (mechanical ventilation, endotracheal tube, and high FiO_2) has yet to be satisfactorily delineated. There are no magic figures for the concentration of administered oxygen that can be considered toxic or for the duration of its administration. If mechanical ventilation is required, prevention of BPD entails use of the lowest FiO_2 and airway pressure that will also provide adequate alveolar gas exchange.

BPD is characterized in the early phase by necrosis of alveolar lining cells and adjacent capillary endothelium, accompanied by edema of interstitial connective tissue. Continued thickening of interstitial tissue ensues, and emphysematous areas alternate with atelectatic ones. The chest film in the early phase is characterized by diffuse haziness of both lungs, which in the extreme appear opaque ("white-out"). Later, rounded areas of radiolucency are intermingled with dense opaque strands. The lungs are eventually overdistended, often to an astounding extent. The outcome is in some question if there is progressive right ventricular hypertrophy on ECG. This finding often portends cor pulmonale. At its onset bronchopulmonary dysplasia causes increased FiO_2 requirements at a time in the progress of hyaline membrane disease therapy that one would expect diminished oxygen requirement. The need for higher environmental oxygen concentrations increases progressively and usually must be maintained for 6 to 8 weeks. Gradual reduction of FiO_2 is eventually possible.

Acid-base balance. Mixed respiratory and metabolic acidosis is the rule. Respiratory acidosis results from retention of carbon dioxide. Metabolic acidosis is a result of increased production of the organic acid end products of anaerobic glycolysis (principally lactic acid). This is usually the most important contributory factor to the low pH values in RDS. Intravenous infusion of sodium bicarbonate ($NaHCO_3$) is used to elevate the pH when it falls below 7.25. This affects metabolic acidosis and has no direct neutralizing influence on the respiratory component. The only effective therapy for the hypercapnea of respiratory acidosis is mechanical ventilation. Sodium bicarbonate actually raises PCO_2, which (except in the most severely affected infants) is usually excreted through the lungs, at least partially. The dose of intravenous $NaHCO_3$ depends on assessment of the infant's acid-base status. This is generally stated in terms of *base excess,* which is calculable on the Siggaard-Andersen nomogram if two of the following three parameters are known: PCO_2, pH, and plasma bicarbonate. Hemoglobin concentration must be determined, regardless of the parameters used (pp. 1024-1025).

Base excess expresses the hydrogen ion concentration (acidity) of whole blood in milliequivalents per liter. Negative (−) base excess (base deficit) indicates increased hydrogen ion concentration, whereas a positive (+) base excess indicates increased alkalinity (as in overdosage of intravenous bicarbonate). Normal values range from +8 to −8 mEq/L. Base excess is a negative value in infants with metabolic acidosis. The quantity of $NaHCO_3$ (in milliequivalents) necessary to elevate the pH toward normal is derived from the following formula:

$$\text{mEq NaHCO}_3 = \text{Negative base excess} \times 0.3 \times \text{Body weight (kg)}$$

Sodium bicarbonate is available in ampules as a 7.5% solution that contains 0.88 mEq $NaHCO_3$/ml. For ease of calculation one may consider that 1 ml of this solution contains 1 mEq $NaHCO_3$. Initially one third to one half of the calculated dose may be administered by intravenous push over a period of several minutes, but only after the 7.5% solution has been diluted with 10% dextrose water or water for injection to one half of its original concentration. The remainder is given by intravenous drip. An infusion pump delivers the calculated dose with acceptable accuracy. Use of sodium bicarbonate should be minimal. Metabolic acidosis, unless unusually severe, is remediable by provision of adequate oxygenation. This is a matter of proper ventilatory support. Use of sodium bicarbonate is thought to acutely elevate serum osmolality, which appears to be associated with an increased occurrence of intraventricular hemorrhage.

Sodium bicarbonate should not be used in the presence of hypercapnea (PCO_2 over 60). Inability to exhale carbon dioxide on hand causes the enhanced retention of additional carbon dioxide that is generated by the administered bicarbonate. In this circumstance, bicarbonate therapy paradoxically results in diminution of blood pH as a function of an accentuated respiratory acidosis.

Blood gas and pH determinations must be repeated frequently in moderately or severely ill infants, and subsequent doses of $NaHCO_3$ should be given accordingly.

Body temperature. Maintenance of a neutral thermal environment is of crucial importance. The increased oxygen requirement incurred by suboptimal environmental temperature control is of sufficient magnitude to affect outcome adversely. Because skin temperature close to 36° C (97° F) correlates fairly well with minimal oxygen consumption, maintenance of this level is essential. Ambient incubator temperatures between 33° to 35° C (91.4° and 95° F) are often required to accomplish this end.

Blood volume. Circulating blood volume is often decreased in infants who are severely affected by hyaline membrane disease. In such instances, blood pressure is low, hematocrit is subnormal (less than 45 to 50 vol%), and tachycardia is present (rate over 160 beats/min). More often, soon after birth the blood pressure and hematocrit are normal, but tachycardia is evident. If blood is not infused, most of such infants will soon become hypotensive, while the hematocrit drops to levels below 40 vol% within 2 to 3 hours. We administer whole blood (20 ml/kg of body weight) to infants who have only tachycardia during the first day of life. In most instances the heart rate drops to normal (120 to 160 beats/min). We also attempt to maintain the hematocrit at 45 to 50 vol% throughout the course of the disease.

Nutrition. During the first 24 to 48 hours, caloric needs are partially met by continuous intravenous infusion of 10% dextrose water; thereafter, parenteral alimentation with an amino acid and dextrose solution and a lipid solution are given intravenously, but feeding of formula through a nasogastric tube should be instituted as soon as possible, that is, after diminution of dyspnea, passage of meconium, and voiding of urine. Gastric emptying time is prolonged in infants with RDS. Therefore the interim between feedings should initially be no less than 3 hours. The baby is fed by nasojejunal tube when the weight is below 1500 g.

Persistent fetal circulation (PFC syndrome); persistent pulmonary hypertension; persistent pulmonary vasospasm. Persistent fetal circulation (PFC syndrome) in the immediate postnatal period is caused by pulmonary arteriolar constriction. It is seen as a component of a number of clinical entities; it is also a clinical entity in its own right. Pulmonary vasoconstriction raises pulmonary artery pressure above that of the aorta; a right-to-left shunt across the ductus results. Right atrial pressure is usually higher than that of the left atrium; right-to-left shunting also occurs at this level. Furthermore, the arteriolar constriction results in pulmonary hypoperfusion, and the total quantity of oxygenated blood leaving the lungs is thereby reduced. In essence the fetal pattern of cardiopulmonary circulation either persists after birth or reappears with hypoxia in the postnatal period. These pulmonary vascular phenomena are components of a number of clinical entities such as hyaline membrane disease, RDS II, pneumonia (especially group B streptococcal), diaphragmatic hernia, and cold stress. It may also follow injudicious decrements in FiO_2 for babies receiving oxygen therapy.

Depending on the severity of vasoconstriction, treatment may vary from simple hood oxygen to mechanical ventilation and the production of a respiratory alkalosis, as well as the administration of tolazoline.

The diagnosis of persistent pulmonary vasospasm or, more commonly, persistent fetal circulation (PFC) is justifiable when pulmonary vasospasm and its associated right-to-left shunts are demonstrated in the absence of other associated disorders. Persistent pulmonary vasospasm occurs in infants who are at or near term. In the vast majority there is a history of perinatal asphyxia, and Apgar scores are usually 5 or below at 1 or 5 minutes. The onset of clearly abnormal respiration may be delayed for as long as 12 hours, but in most instances tachypnea is evident within an hour after birth. Retractions are usually minimal, if at all present, thus indicating good lung compliance. Cyanosis in room air occurs soon after delivery. Auscultation of the lungs indicates normal air exchange and there are no overt signs of cardiac abnormalities. Systemic blood pressure is normal. The response to oxygen may be satisfactory initially, but in severe cases hypoxemia ultimately develops within a few hours.

The chest film is usually normal, save for slight cardiomegaly in an occasional instance. Dense streaks may emanate from the hilar regions to the peripheral lung fields and occasionally the lungs are marginally overexpanded.

As a rule, arterial oxygen tensions are subnormal but $PaCO_2$ levels are normal or reduced. Simultaneous blood gas specimens from the right radial artery and from the aorta will indicate the likelihood of a right-to-left shunt across the ductus arteriosus. If the PaO_2 from the right radial artery (preductal sample) is below 50, the aortic PaO_2 will be at least 15% lower if a clinically significant right-to-left ductal shunt is present.

A substantial number of babies with persistent pulmonary vasospasm can be satisfactorily oxygenated in an oxygen hood. This failing, mechanical ventilatory support is indicated. In the primary form of this disorder, that is, pulmonary vasospasm in the virtual absence of parenchy-

mal involvement, the use of end-expiratory positive pressure is contraindicated. Failure to oxygenate an affected infant indicates severe pulmonary hypoperfusion caused by vasospasm. Hyperventilation is frequently successful. Pa_{CO_2} levels between 25 and 30 with an associated pH of approximately 7.50 usually dilates pulmonary vasculature sufficiently for adequate oxygenation. In the secondary form of pulmonary vasospasm, that is, in the presence of parenchymal involvement (hyaline membrane disease, group B streptococcal pneumonia) low levels of P_{CO_2} are frequently impossible to achieve by hyperventilation. In either primary or secondary vasospasm, the failure of hyperventilation indicates the use of tolazoline. Tolazoline is an alpha-adrenergic blocker that apparently also acts directly on smooth muscle to dilate blood vessels in the pulmonary and systemic circuits. Its administration is often associated with hypotension. A drop in systolic blood pressure of approximately 10 torr is to be expected. We administer the drug in an intravascular bolus of 2 mg/kg, mixed with 10 ml/kg of plasmanate. The response is virtually always satisfactory if the primary form of pulmonary vasospasm is present or in most instances of vasospasm associated with meconium aspiration. A second bolus is frequently necessary and, this failing, we give a third bolus followed by a continuous intravenous infusion of 2 mg/kg/hr. Tolazoline causes a wide variety of undesirable side effects that include hypotension, extreme tachycardia, gastric hemorrhage, and renal failure.

Meconium aspiration syndrome. Acute intrauterine asphyxia causes fetal gasping movements and passage of meconium. Fetal aspiration of amniotic sac contents may thus cause obstruction of the respiratory tract at any level. If this material is lodged in the upper tract, it can be removed by suction. More often, aspirated material fills alveoli and bronchioles, causing widespread atelectasis; if obstruction is partial (ball valve), regional emphysema is the result of air trapping. Respiratory distress, which is noted at birth, is presumably a continuation of preexisting intrauterine asphyxia, as indicated by the presence of meconium in the amniotic fluid. Sudden fetal gasping occurs in utero in response to asphyxia. Although some meconium aspiration occurs at the time, *most of it occurs with the first few breaths and thereafter* during delivery. Aspiration of meconium-stained fluid is thought to occur at this time. Chest film reveals a flattened diaphragm and increased anteroposterior diameter of the thorax, both of which are the result of regional air trapping. Linear densities, which emanate from the hilar areas, are separated by lobular hyperaeration, giving an overall honeycomb appearance. Densities of varied and irregular contour represent atelectasis and retention of fetal lung fluid. The course of the disease often simulates that of respiratory distress syndrome (RDS). Rapid respiration and retraction of the chest wall are characteristic. Blood gas and pH values indicate combined respiratory and metabolic acidosis.

Meconium aspiration syndrome is considered an aftermath of fetal asphyxia. Although considerable difficulty is caused by obstruction of airways by particulate matter, there is a prominent vasospastic component to this disorder in most infants affected by it. Presumably, the pulmonary vasospasm (or PFC) is the result of fetal asphyxia, which also triggers the passage and aspiration of meconium in utero. In most instances of associated pulmonary vasospasm a significant difference between preductal and postductal Pa_{O_2} is demonstrable. Failure to oxygenate an infant by the usual modalities requires consideration of tolazoline therapy.

In the delivery room, resuscitative efforts may be lifesaving; the procedure is presented in detail elsewhere in this chapter (pp. 271 to 273). A critical difference in the resuscitative procedure for meconium aspiration, as opposed to that for other types of respiratory depression, is the removal of meconium from the respiratory tract. This must be accomplished rapidly before insufflation is begun. An endotracheal tube must be used. The small caliber of a suction catheter of DeLee trap precludes effective aspiration of the larger (and the most dangerous) particles of meconium. With his mask in place, the operator exerts gentle suction with his mouth through the inserted endotracheal tube. This must be maintained as the tube is withdrawn. The procedure should be repeated using a new tube each time, until meconium is no longer seen in the aspirated material. Adequately performed, this procedure will almost eliminate the probability of severe respiratory distress from meconium aspiration.

We do not perform endotracheal suction on every meconium-stained infant. Rather, we be-

lieve it is indicated only in those babies who also have some degree of respiratory distress. Other aspects of therapy are similar to those described for the respiratory distress syndrome.

Choanal atresia. Complete or partial (unilateral and bilateral) obstructions are caused by a membranous covering or a thick bony plate over the choanae (posterior nares). Because the neonate does not usually breathe through his mouth, severe respiratory distress is the result. The first breath may be normal, since it is ordinarily taken through the mouth, but cyanosis and retractions ensue when the infant attempts normal respiration. Thick mucoid secretion may fill the nares and pharynx. The lesion is demonstrable by failure to pass a catheter or probe past the choanal level. Lipiodol drops instilled in the nose demonstrate the obstruction radiographically. Complete obstruction is more easily demonstrated by failure to visualize intranasally instilled methylene blue in the pharynx. An oral airway, which induces mouth breathing, must be maintained pending ultimate removal of the obstruction by surgical means.

Micrognathia with glossoptosis. Micrognathia with glossoptosis is most often seen in Pierre-Robin syndrome (mandibular hypoplasia, cleft palate, and glossoptosis) and in Treacher-Collins syndrome (mandibulofacial dysostosis). Posterior displacement of the tongue impedes passage of air, and an oral airway is often necessary for relief. Obstruction is more severe when the infant is supine. Anterior fixation of the tongue by surgical means is required when these measures are ineffective.

Oropharyngeal masses (usually ranulas) are blue cysts beneath the anterior part of the tongue, commonly arising from the minor salivary glands. The cysts, which are single or multiple, may displace the tongue posteriorly to interfere with normal respiration. Because they are unilocular, aspiration effectively relieves the obstructive element.

Tumors in the neck exert extrinsic pressure on the hypopharynx, larynx, or trachea. Cystic hygroma, congenital goiter, hemangioma, and branchial cleft cysts are the most frequently encountered lesions.

Laryngeal web. A membranous obstruction above, below, or at the level of the vocal cords may be complete or partial. If obstruction is complete, the infant fails to take the first breath in spite of initially vigorous attempts. If it is partial, there is respiratory stridor. Laryngoscopy reveals the obstructive membrane, which may be perforated as an emergency procedure pending tracheostomy and complete surgical removal. The cause of stridor must be determined by laryngoscopy immediately after birth. Simple epiglottic or laryngeal flaccidity must be differentiated from serious laryngeal lesions such as a *web, vocal cord paralysis, subglottic hemangioma, cysts,* and *tumors.*

Extrinsic pressure on the trachea by anomalous great vessels (see also pp. 440 and 910). Vascular rings that constrict the trachea, major bronchi, and esophagus comprise varying arrangements of anomalous blood vessels: aberrant subclavian artery, anomalous innominate artery, double aortic arch, or right aortic arch. Resultant impingement causes feeding difficulties and respiratory obstructive phenomena, which may not appear until the postneonatal period. A severely affected infant who is dyspneic because of inspiratory obstruction prefers to retract the head for relief, and movement to a neutral or flexed position increases respiratory distress. Respirations marked by inspiratory crow and expiratory wheeze are characteristic of airway obstruction caused by a vascular ring. Esophageal encroachment causes regurgitation of feedings, often with aspiration. The lesion must be demonstrated radiographically. Plain films occasionally demonstrate tracheal narrowing above the carina. Barium swallow is probably the most valuable procedure for depicting esophageal impingement. Contrast tracheogram and angiography may be necessary to delineate the anomaly in more detail.

Agenesis of the lung. Pulmonary agenesis is usually unilateral; the left lung is more frequently involved. Complete absence of one lung is often compatible with normal life unless it is associated with other major anomalies, which is the case in nearly 50% of the patients. Symptoms appear during the newborn period in only 20% of affected infants. Breath sounds are absent or diminished in the involved hemithorax, although they may be prominent when the contralateral lung extends across the mediastinum. The cardiac impulse and the trachea are then displaced toward the involved side. The functional lung is hypertrophied rather than emphysematous. Occasionally a considerable amount

of fluid replaces the atretic lung, and complete opacification of the hemithorax is evident on chest film. Malformations of thoracic vertebrae (hemivertebrae and other anomalies) are often radiographically visualized. Bronchograms and angiocardiograms reveal absence of the bronchial tree and the corresponding pulmonary vasculature.

Hypoplasia of the lungs. In several teratogenic syndromes, hypoplasia of the lungs is a prominent component. The commonest syndrome is *diaphragmatic hernia* (pp. 888 and 889), in which the total number of bronchi are reduced although each gives rise to the usual quantity of alveoli. Hypoplasia of the lungs is also seen in *renal agenesis* (Potter syndrome), in which development of the lung is considerably retarded for gestational age. Bronchi are prominent, and alveolar air spaces are diminished in number. The renal and pulmonary malformations are incompatible with life. These infants (three fourths are male) have a characteristic senile facies. A prominent infraorbital skin fold originates at the inner canthus and curves downward and laterally. The eyes are widely spaced; the nose is prominent; the ears are anomalous and large and are set in a low position. In half the infants other anomalies of various organ systems are present, particularly in the heart. Death usually occurs within 12 hours after birth. Oligohydramnios is common because the urinary source of amniotic fluid is absent. The placenta is studded on its fetal surface with small yellow-gray plaques (amnion nodosum).

Wilson-Mikity syndrome. The etiology of the diffuse pulmonary disorder called Wilson-Mikity syndrome is unknown. Death occurs in half the affected infants, although others recover slowly over a period of several months. All reported infants have weighed less than 2500 g at birth; most weight less than 1500 g. Symptoms may appear at birth or as late as 35 days of age. Cyanosis usually disappears when oxygen is administered. Retractions are seen occasionally, but in most instances only slight tachypnea accompanies the cyanosis.

Radiographic features are distinctively characterized by a lacework pattern of linear densities (thickened pulmonary interstitial tissue) that course between radiolucent areas of hyperaerated cysts 2 to 10 mm in diameter. Overall lung volume is increased; cardiovascular structures are normal. Specific therapy is unknown, and steroids are ineffective. Increased concentration of ambient oxygen is indicated for cyanosis.

Congenital pulmonary lymphangiectasia. Congenital pulmonary lymphangiectasia is characterized by severe, generalized dilation of pulmonary lymphatics, which causes respiratory distress at birth or soon after. Most affected infants are born at term, and most die by 8 days of age. A mixture of other congenital anomalies occurs in half these infants, but lymph anomalies in other organs have not been noted except in one case. Chest film reveals hyperaeration of both lungs and diffuse mottled densities that simulate focal atelectasis.

Lung cysts. Pulmonary cysts may be congenital or acquired; the latter are apparently far more common. They cause respiratory distress by expansion and impingement on adjacent alveoli or bronchial structures; if they are intraluminal, the distal airway is obstructed. Solitary or multiple cysts may be peripheral or close to major bronchi. Partial obstruction of a bronchus may cause lobar emphysema. As a rule, only one lobe or one entire lung is involved. There is no predilection for any particular portion of the lung. Symptoms are sometimes absent, but more often tachypnea and respiratory distress are present in varying degrees of severity. When larger bronchi are compressed, wheezing and stridor are audible. Infection occasionally develops in one or more cysts. In most cases the congenital or acquired nature of the lesion is indeterminate. Cuboidal cells, cartilage, and smooth muscle are present in both types. Acquired cysts are most often associated with pneumonia, which in most cases is caused by staphylococci, although other bacteria may be involved occasionally. A single large, tense, air-filled cyst can be confused with lobar emphysema or pneumothorax. Multiple cysts simulate emphysematous blebs, but the latter are usually present bilaterally. In most cases the cysts disappear spontaneously over a period of months or years. If respiratory distress is severe or progressive, surgical intervention is indicated.

Congenital cystic adenomatoid malformation. This unusual cystic malformation of the lung has been reported in over 50 infants. A minority have survived. Many of those who died were stillborn or died shortly after birth. Hydramnios and anasarca are prominent features in the stillborn group.

One or two lobes are affected, but bilateral disease has not been reported. Gross pathologic appearance is characterized by impressive enlargement of the affected lobe, which contains clusters of cysts separated by solid areas. The lining of the cyst is cuboidal or pseudostratified columnar epithelium.

Acute respiratory distress is the rule. Shift in mediastinal contents is common. Diminished breath sounds are perceptible in the involved lung. The radiographic appearance varies from lucent air-filled cysts within areas of water density to an opaque hemithorax if two lobes are involved. The overall impression in most films is that of a pulmonary mass that contains cystic areas. Treatment requires surgical excision of the affected lobe. Ten infants have been operated on; eight have survived. Surgery is indicated if respiratory distress is present.

Tracheoesophageal fistula (pp. 886 to 888). Tracheoesophageal fistula exists in several variations. In 85% of affected infants there is segmental atresia of the esophagus associated with an upper blind pouch; the lower esophagus empties into the stomach normally while communicating with the trachea or a bronchus through a fistula. In another form, segmental esophageal atresia is present without a fistulous communication. The H-type fistula, which is well known but rare, is a connection between a normal esophagus and trachea. Other variants of combined tracheoesophageal malformations have been reported sporadically.

A characteristic triad of symptoms suggests the presence of the commonest variant of tracheoesophageal fistula: accumulation of secretions in the mouth and hypopharynx, repeated regurgitation of feedings, and continuous or sporadic respiratory distress. Other indications of the diagnosis are distended abdomen resulting from entry of an inordinate quantity of air into the stomach through the fistula between the trachea and lower esophageal segment, atelectasis of the right upper lobe, and a history of hydramnios. Surgical correction should be performed as early as possible.

Diaphragmatic hernia (pp. 888 and 889). Herniation of abdominal organs through a congenital defect in the diaphragm causes severe respiratory distress, which is usually present at birth. The left side is involved four times more often than the right. Most herniations occur through the posterolateral portion of the diaphragm (foramen of Bochdalek). The esophageal hiatus and the retrosternal area (foramen of Morgagni) are considerably less frequent sites of herniation.

Abdominal viscera including intestine, stomach, and spleen displace the lung when left-sided involvement occurs; the gastrointestinal tract occupies most of the space preempted from the lung. On the right side the liver is the primary herniated abdominal organ. In either case the mediastinum often deviates to the contralateral side. Pulmonary hypoplasia commonly accompanies diaphragmatic hernia.

Symptoms of ventilatory compromise are present at birth or shortly thereafter. Onset has also been noted later in infancy and childhood. In the most severe involvement, the infant gasps at birth and fails to establish respiration. More commonly, dyspnea is persistent and is often associated with cyanosis, which may progress as the intestine in the chest expands because of normal entry of gas. Severity of symptoms depends on the magnitude of herniation. The pattern of respiratory distress is identical to that caused by any other neonatal disorder.

Invariably, attention is directed to the infant's illness because of respiratory difficulty. Displacement of the cardiac impulse to either side of normal is the most helpful of all physical signs for immediate realization that the usual resuscitatory efforts will not suffice to restore normal respiration. Although the scaphoid abdomen is classically described as a major indication of diaphragmatic hernia, in fact it is often barely perceptible. A truly scaphoid abdomen results from massive herniation of abdominal viscera. Diminished breath sounds in the involved hemithorax are the rule. Dullness to percussion is frequently present. Tympany is perceptible if significant gaseous distention of the intestine has occurred. In right-sided involvement only dullness can be expected.

The chest film confirms the diagnosis. Occasionally the intestines impart a multicystic appearance to the left hemithorax. Absence of the diaphragmatic margin is often discernible. Mediastinal displacement and the presence of inappropriate structures in the thorax are readily visible.

Surgical correction of the defect must be performed with dispatch. Delay in the diagnosis may be fatal, yet even after surgery a substantial number of infants die, apparently because of severe pulmonary hypoplasia. Some infants do not survive to the time surgery is initiated.

Pulmonary vasospasm has been reported as a major cause of distress and poor oxygenation in affected infants. Apparently morbidity and mortality, formerly attributed to hypoplasia of the lung on the affected side, is more a function of pulmonary vasospasm and hypoperfusion than anything else. These infants have responded to tolazoline therapy.

Congenital lobar emphysema. Emphysema of one lobe causes respiratory distress, which may be sufficiently severe soon after its inception to require emergency lobectomy. Only one lobe is usually affected, but multilobar involvement occurs occasionally. The right upper and middle lobes are most frequently involved.

Any emphysematous change in the lungs is a result of their failure to deflate normally; egress of air is impeded to some extent. In congenital lobar emphysema the causes of this impedance are variable, although an overdistended lobe is always the end result. Absent or deficient cartilage localized to one bronchus is a frequent cause of lobar emphysema. Aspiration of particulate matter of any type, or inflammatory exudate, may set up a check value mechanism that results in retention of air. Intraluminal cysts and extrinsic pressure on a bronchus by tumors and anomalous blood vessels have also been identified as the underlying lesions of lobar emphysema.

Symptoms usually appear after the first week of life, but tachypnea and some wheezing may be noted earlier. Severe symptoms are uncommon during the first days after birth. Respiratory distress is at least moderately severe at its onset, and rapid progression may threaten life within a few hours. Retractions and cyanosis are common. Breath sounds are diminished on the affected side, and tympany is elicited on percussion over the same area. Displacement of the cardiac impulse suggests mediastinal shift.

Chest films demonstrate severe emphysema of one or more lobes with varying degrees of compression atelectasis in the adjacent ones. The mediastinum is often deviated to the contralateral hemithorax.

Once the diagnosis is established, immediate bronchoscopy is indicated. If overdistention is caused by aspirated particulate matter, relief of symptoms will follow its removal, but this is infrequent. Excision of the affected lobe should be accomplished without delay if bronchoscopy is ineffective. Rarely, lobar emphysema is identified in an asymptomatic infant in whom bronchoscopy should be performed but lobectomy deferred until symptoms appear. On rare occasions the overdistention slowly disappears spontaneously.

Extraneous air syndromes (air leak). Extraneous air syndromes are a group of clinically recognizable disorders produced by alveolar rupture and the subsequent escape of air to tissues in which air is not normally present. Following are the sites in which extraneous air has been reported.

Site of extraneous air	Syndrome
Pulmonary interstitium (perivascular sheaths)	Interstitial emphysema
Alveoli-trabeculae-pleura	Pseudocysts
Pleural space	Pneumothorax
Mediastinum	Pneumomediastinum
Pericardial space	Pneumopericardium
Perivascular sheaths (peripheral vessels)	Perivascular emphysema
Vascular lumens (blood)	Air embolus
Subcutaneous tissue	Subcutaneous emphysema
Retroperitoneal connective tissue	Retroperitoneal emphysema
Peritoneal space	Pneumoperitoneum
Intestinal wall	Pneumatosis intestinalis
Scrotum	Pneumoscrotum

Although most of these syndromes have long been known to occur spontaneously, their incidence increased as the use of ventilatory support became widespread, particularly since the advent of end-expiratory positive pressure. Air leak syndrome now constitutes the most frequent life-threatening complication of ventilatory assistance. The capacity for instant recognition, evaluation, and relief of these disorders is a primary requisite for personnel who assume responsibility for sustained neonatal ventilatory support.

All these air leak syndromes have a common pathogenesis in that they are initiated by rupture of overdistended alveoli. Air escapes to interstitial tissue *(interstitial emphysema)* and migrates within perivascular sheaths to the hilum. From there air may extend into the mediastinum *(pneumomediastinum)*. It may also enter the pleural space *(pneumothorax)* or, rarely, the pericardial space *(pneumopericardium)*. Pneu-

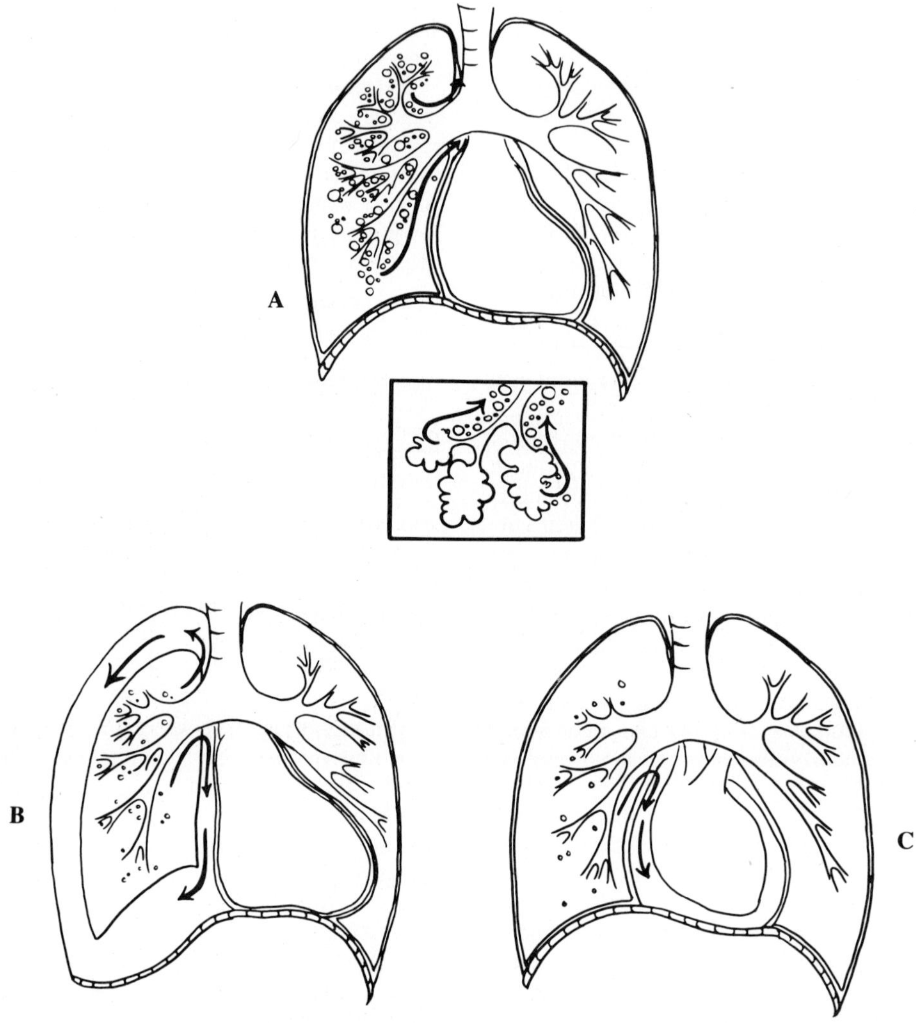

Fig. 15-6. A, Air in interstitial lung tissue. Ruptured alveoli are indicated in framed alveoli at bottom. Air dissects from alveoli along vascular sheaths to hilus and thence to pleural space. (See x-ray film in Fig. 15-7, *A*.) **B,** Pneumothorax, indicating origin of air in lung tissue and its pathway to inflate pleural space. Heart shifts to left because of high pressure created in right chest. (See x-ray film in Fig. 15-7, *B*.) **C,** Course of air from lung to pericardial space. Distended pericardial space causes cardiac tamponade, small heart. (See x-ray film in Fig. 15-7, *C*.) (From Korones, S.B.: High-risk newborn infants, ed. 3, St. Louis, 1981, The C.V. Mosby Co.)

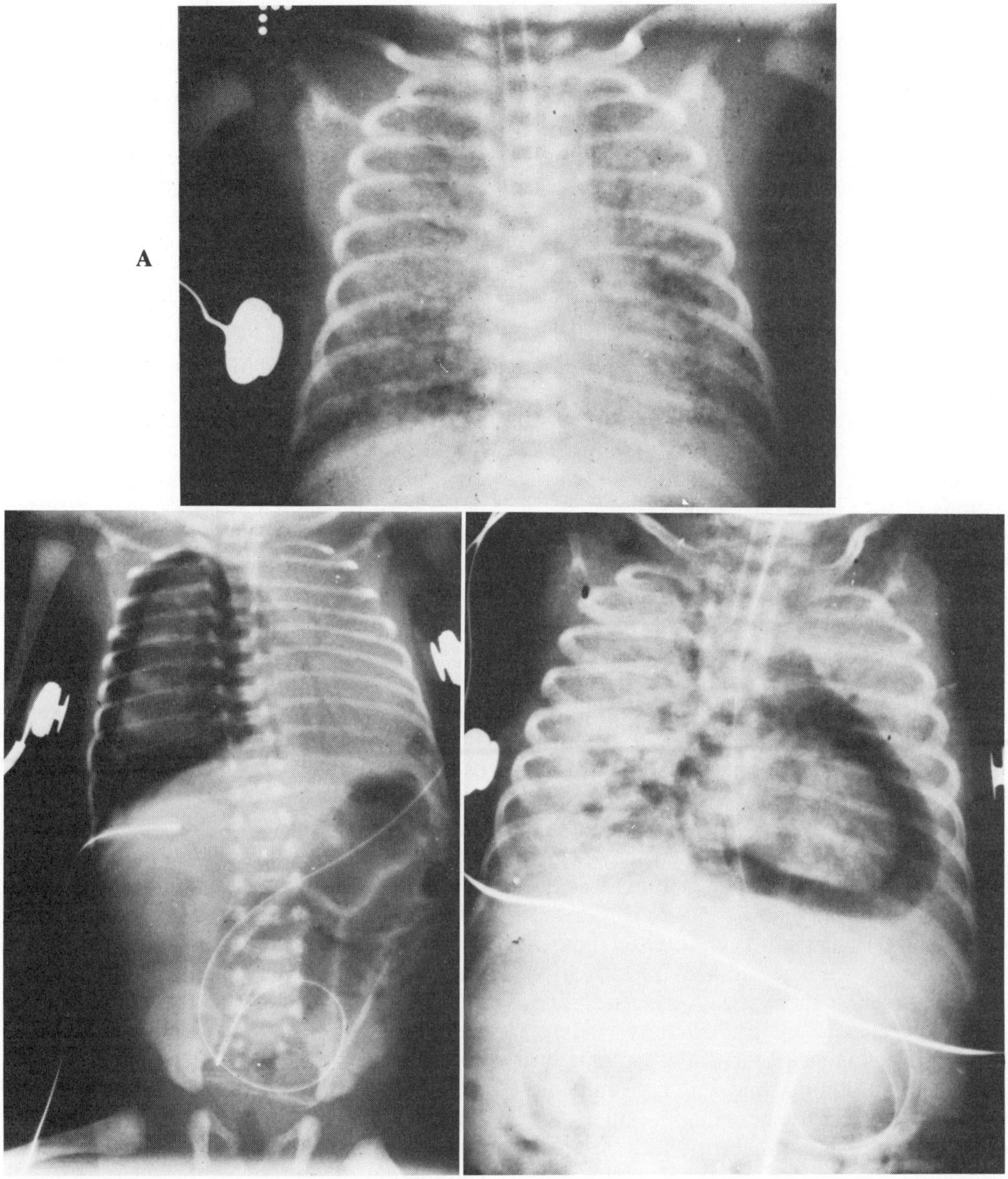

A

B

C

Fig. 15-7. A, Interstitial emphysema. Multiple lakes of radiolucency (air), varying in size, impart a spongy appearance to lungs. (See Fig. 15-6, *A*.) **B,** Tension pneumothorax, right pleural cavity. The dense right lung is collapsed by pressure in pleural space created by air accumulation. Air-filled pleural cavity is darkest area that envelops right lung. (See Fig. 15-6, *B*.) **C,** Pneumopericardium. Dark halo of air fills pericardial space, outlining the heart itself. Note interstitial emphysema in right lung, indicated by large lakes of air. (See Fig. 15-6, *C*.) (From Korones, S.B.: High-risk newborn infants, ed. 3, St. Louis, 1981, The C.V. Mosby Co.)

moperitoneum is the result of migration of mediastinal air through the diaphragm by way of periesophageal or perivascular tissue into the peritoneal cavity. *Air embolus* occurs when extremely high pressures are used for ventilatory assistance. Air is apparently injected directly into blood vessels at the time of alveolar rupture.

Fig. 15-6 depicts the pathways of air, and Fig. 15-7 presents the corresponding chest films.

Interstitial emphysema regularly precedes the other extraneous air disorders. It is often not perceivable, however, if air does not accumulate in the pulmonary interstitial tissue. When it does, ongoing respiratory support becomes inadequate. The infant may suddenly become cyanotic; the $Pa{O_2}$ falls and the $Pa{CO_2}$ rises because transfer of gases between alveolar membranes and capillaries is impeded by intervening aggregations of air. The x-ray film is diagnostic. Rarely, only one lung is involved; as a rule, both are involved. The lungs contain numerous small radiolucent areas (interstitial air) that create an overall spongy appearance (Fig. 15-7, *A*). The diagnosis can be made only by x-ray examination. A substantial number of affected infants will soon develop pneumothorax or pneumomediastinum as interstitial air follows the pathogenetic course already described.

Some pneumothoraces are not symptomatic, or if symptoms appear, the course is often quite mild. They are usually severe when they occur as complications of ventilatory therapy. Tachypnea may be the only abnormal sign. On the other hand, the abrupt intrusion into the pleural space of a large volume of air is a dramatic life-threatening event. Tachypnea, grunting, and generalized cyanosis are immediately evident; sometimes the cyanosis appears more gradually. The affected hemithorax may bulge prominently. Tension displaces the hemidiaphragm downward, and severe abdominal distention appears immediately. The heart and mediastinum are displaced to the unaffected side of the chest, and as a result, the cardiac sounds and impulses cannot be identified in their usual location. They may be perceived in the right chest if there is a left-sided pneumothorax or far laterally against the left wall if the pneumothorax is on the right. The shift in apical impulse is the most valuable diagnostic sign. Confirmation is possible only by x-ray examination because an identical clinical appearance may be produced by diaphragmatic hernia. On the radiograph of a pneumothorax, the lung on the affected side appears collapsed by air in the pleural space, and varying degrees of mediastinal displacement are apparent (Fig. 15-7, *B*).

Early recognition of pneumothorax is sometimes facilitated by changes in voltage on an electrocardiographic oscilloscope. The RS voltage decreases substantially (by 40%), often before clinical signs can be detected.

Another effective method for rapid diagnosis involves transillumination of the chest. If a significant amount of air has accumulated, the involved area clearly transilluminates when a high-intensity fiberoptic light source is applied to the chest. We have identified pneumothorax within 1 or 2 minutes with this method.

In the evaluation of an infant with respiratory distress, locating the position of the cardiac impulse is of fundamental importance. If it is abnormal, a thoracentesis tray should be readied immediately. The release of pleural air is lifesaving. During the time preceding thoracentesis, the nurse should administer 100% oxygen through a hood or a tight-fitting mask. Positive-pressure ventilatory assistance through an endotracheal tube may increase the pneumothorax and should thus be avoided, if possible, pending establishment of continuous pleural suction through a chest tube. Breathing 100% oxygen may hasten the resolution of pleural air or at least retard further accumulation. This response occurs over a 6- to 12-hour period, and although this therapy is extremely valuable, it should not be considered appropriate treatment for tension pneumothorax. After the emergency release of pleural air by needle aspiration, a chest tube must be inserted and connected to continuous suction under water.

Pneumomediastinum usually produces mild, sometimes moderately disturbing, symptoms. Severe distress may result from a massive accumulation of air around the heart, which impairs venous return from the inferior and superior venae cavae by compression of these vessels. Tachypnea is the most frequent sign; occasionally cyanosis is apparent. Nurses often call attention to the possibility of pneumomediastinum by finding it difficult to locate the heartbeat. Cardiac sounds are distant and barely audible as a result of accumulation of air around the heart. There is no mediastinal shift; the breath sounds are normal. Sometimes air may spread to the subcutaneous tissue of the neck, where it causes visible swelling and a "crunchy" sensation when palpated (crepitus). The chest film is diagnostic. Lateral views reveal a collection of air directly beneath the sternum, displacing the cardiac shadow posteriorly. Sometimes a black halo, which is cast by mediastinal air, may be seen around the cardiac border in the frontal view. Since the thymus overlays the mediastinum, the thymus is frequently elevated by the air that is interposed between the thymic and cardiac shadows (Fig. 15-8). This is called the "batwing" sign on x-ray film.

Needle aspiration for removal of mediastinal air is ineffective, nor has any form of constant suction been shown to be valuable. Administration of 100% oxygen is the treatment of choice.

Acid-base imbalance and blood gas abnormalities may occur in pneumomediastinum or pneumothorax, particularly in the most profoundly affected babies. These biochemical deviations are similar to those of hyaline membrane disease. They are treated in the same fashion as described previously.

Pneumothorax, and probably pneumomediastinum as well, occurs with the first few breaths as a consequence of spontaneous alveolar rupture in normally expanded portions of a lung that fails to expand in other segments. In such circumstances excessive distending pressure is applied to the normal alveoli during the forceful initial breaths. X-ray surveys have shown pneumothorax in 1% or 2% of all normal newborns who had no other difficulties and who were generally asymptomatic. They required no treatment. Spontaneous pneumothorax has long been reported also as a complication of meconium aspiration, hyaline membrane disease, pneumonia, and pulmonary hypoplasia associated with renal anomalies and with diaphragmatic hernia. Pneumothorax as a consequence of overzealous positive-pressure resuscitation is less frequent than is generally supposed.

Pneumopericardium was a rare clinical entity until recently. Only 13 cases had been reported in English medical literature from 1942 to 1974. Now it probably occurs far more often than it is reported. It rarely appears alone, generally being associated with pneumomediastinum or pneumothorax. Of 17 cases in the English literature, 11 expired. Most of them also had hyaline membrane disease, and all but 1 had previously been resuscitated by bag. The infant with pneumopericardium becomes cyanotic abruptly. Because air in the pericardial space produces cardiac tamponade, the heart sounds are severely muffled or cannot be heard at all. In our four babies, all were receiving mechanical ventilation. There was thus no perceptible change in respiratory pattern. Cyanosis was profound, but the most impressive manifestation was total inaudibility of heart sounds in the presence of continued cardiac activity, as seen on the oscilloscope. Cardiac tamponade causes pulse pressure to decrease; the pulses may not be palpable, and blood pressure is therefore low or unobtainable. The x-ray film (Fig. 15-7, *C*) is dramatic. A dark halo, varying in thickness with the amount of accumulated air, surrounds the heart completely, separating it inferiorly from the diaphragm. External to and encasing the halo, the parietal layer of the pericardium is often visible because the pericardial space is distended.

Treatment must be applied immediately, since untreated affected infants die in minutes. A pericardial tap must be done to evacuate the air. A repeat tap may be necessary, or a catheter may be required to provide for egress of air that continues to accumulate.

Pulmonary hemorrhage. Lung hemorrhage is a component of several syndromes, and in most instances the etiology is unknown. Pulmonary infection, usually bacterial, has been cited most frequently as an underlying cause. An association with kernicterus has been observed by some investigators but not by others. Pulmonary hemorrhage occurs in infants with congenital heart disease if increased perfusion of the lung is present (wide patency of the ductus arteriosus). Cold injury of sufficient severity to lower the body temperature several degrees Fahrenheit has been noted in association with pulmonary hemorrhage, but there is no experimental evidence for a relationship between these events. The bleeding caused by hemorrhagic disease of the newborn may involve the lungs.

Pulmonary hemorrhage occurs most frequently in premature infants. It is marked by sudden onset of respiratory distress, cyanosis, and issuance of blood from the nose and mouth in about half the affected infants. The radiographic findings include nodular densities, homoge-

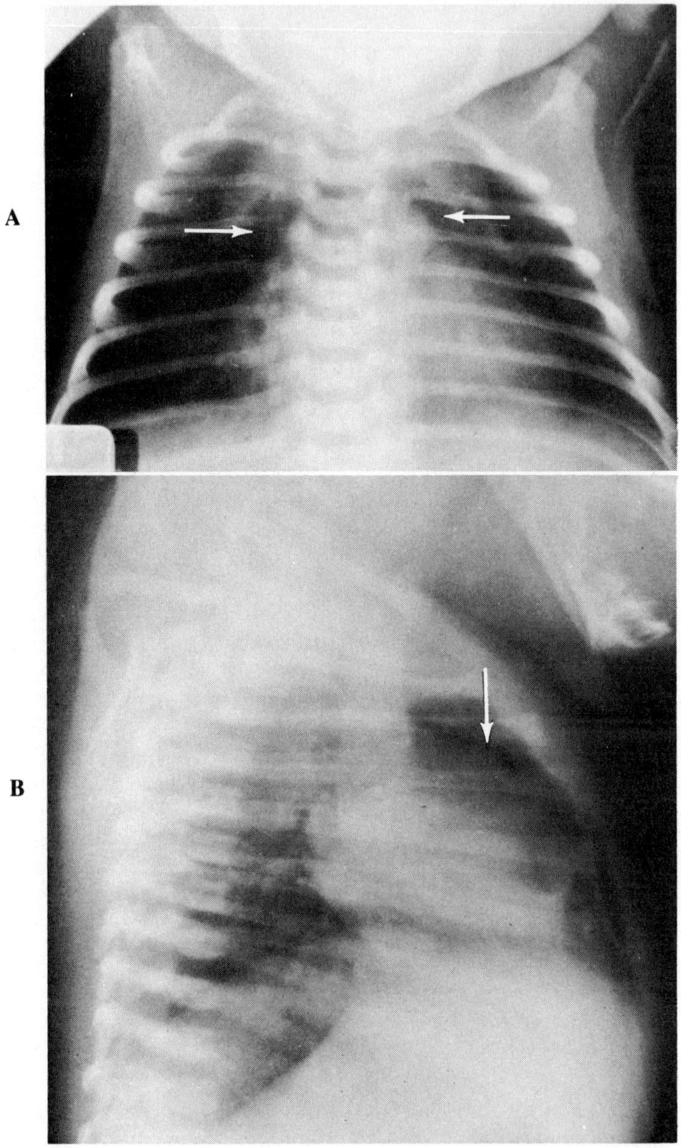

Fig. 15-8. Pneumomediastinum. **A,** Anteroposterior view. The "batwing" shadow of the thymus is above mediastinal air. The air *(arrows)* separates the thymic shadow and the cardiac shadow beneath it. **B,** Lateral view. Mediastinal air *(arrow)* is visible in the darkest area immediately beneath the sternum. Since air is situated between the heart and the anterior chest wall, the intensity of heart sounds is substantially diminished. (From Korones, S.B.: High-risk newborn infants, ed. 3, St. Louis, 1981, The C.V. Mosby Co.)

neous opacification, and a reticulogranular pattern, none of which is a specific indication of pulmonary hemorrhage.

Although pulmonary hemorrhage is obviously a serious and sometimes catastrophic event, in our experience most infants survive it. One may be mislead by the appearance of an impressive quantity of gross blood during endotracheal suction. In most instances this is the result of trauma from the passage of the catheter.

We have rarely encountered a significant drop in hematocrit associated with an episode of pulmonary hemorrhage; certainly not to the extent that is regularly seen with massive intraventricular hemorrhage. We surmise that this is caused by the nature of the "hemorrhage" into the lung. In most instances it has shown to be hemorrhagic pulmonary edema with hematocrit that may be as low as 10%.

Sheldon B. Korones

Hematologic disorders in the newborn period

Some hematologic disorders during the newborn period deserve special mention. They may have special features with regard to pathogenetic mechanisms, clinical presentation, and treatment. The most frequent of these disorders is anemia, but bleeding problems and diseases of the leukocytes may also occur.

Anemia

The usual cause for anemia during the newborn period is hemolytic disease. Most frequently the hemolysis is caused by factors extrinsic to the red cell, but some congenital red cell defects may be associated with hemolytic disease immediately after birth.

Isoimmune hemolytic disease. If the fetal erythrocytes have an antigen not shared by the mother, there is the possibility that maternal antibodies of the immunoglobulin G (IgG) type, directed against that antigen, can cross the placenta and cause an isoimmune hemolytic disease in the infant. The severity of this hemolytic disease may vary considerably. In some instance the disease may be so mild that only jaundice results from increased bilirubin formation. In other infants the destruction of red cells may be so great that life-threatening anemia results. In all cases the diagnosis must be confirmed by demonstration of the presence of maternal antibody on the infant's erythrocytes.

Rh incompatibility was formerly the most frequent cause of severe isoimmune hemolytic disease in this country. It is a disease in which the full cycle from recognition to understanding of its pathogenesis, development of therapy, and finally institution of an effective program of prevention encompassed the period of one generation. Today it should be a rare cause of hemolysis in a newborn. There are several antigens in the Rh system, but the one most frequently involved in this disease is designated D. Less frequently involved are the antigens C and E. Because of the importance of the D antigen, persons possessing it on their red cells are designated Rh positive, and those without the D antigen are termed Rh negative. The frequency of Rh-negative persons varies with race, being 15% in whites, 7% in blacks, and 1% in Chinese. The risk of Rh incompatibility is therefore greatest among whites.

Sensitization of an Rh-negative mother carrying an Rh-positive infant may occur if fetal red cells enter the maternal bloodstream. This event usually happens at the time of delivery, when small amounts of fetal blood can cross the placenta. Thus a firstborn infant is rarely affected by this disease, but subsequent fetuses may be at risk if maternal antibodies have been formed against the Rh antigen.

The clinical features may range from severe anemia to mild neonatal icterus. If the fetus has been severely affected by anemia in utero, congestive heart failure may result, and at birth the infant may have hydrops fetalis with severe edema or may even be stillborn. In less severe degrees of anemia, the infant may be pale at birth and demonstrate such evidences of extramedullary hematopoiesis as hepatosplenomegaly. In milder forms of the disease the infant may have no difficulties at birth, but within the first 24 to 48 hours may manifest evidence of hemolysis be becoming icteric. Some infants with this disease have no difficulties during the first week of life, only to become progressively anemic during the second to fourth weeks of life to the point of requiring transfusions.

In the infant who is pale at birth or who becomes icteric during the first 24 hours, laboratory studies should be done to determine the cause. Rh incompatibility will be associated with varying degrees of anemia, reticulocytosis, and presence of nucleated red cells on the blood smear. There will be increasing values of bilirubin, almost all of which are the indirect fraction. The maternal antibody coating the infant's red cells can be demonstrated by the Coombs test, and the mother can be found to be Rh negative and the infant Rh positive.

Treatment for this disease, when necessary, is exchange transfusion for correction of severe anemia, as well as for reduction of bilirubin levels to prevent the development of kernicterus. Indications for exchange transfusion in Rh-incompatible isoimmune hemolytic disease are presented in Table 15-4. If the infant has no difficulty during the immediate neonatal period but becomes severely anemic subsequently, then simple transfusions with packed erythrocytes are sufficient. If the infant is at high risk of being stillborn or having hydrops fetalis because of severe intrauterine anemia, an intrauterine transfusion may be given. Infants at high risk for this complication can be detected by the presence of increasing levels of bilirubin in the amniotic fluid. These determinations can be made by amniocentesis, beginning about the twenty-eighth week of pregnancy. Intrauterine transfusions are done by introducing a polyethylene catheter through the maternal abdominal wall and uterus and into the fetal peritoneal cavity. The red cells are effectively absorbed from the peritoneal cavity into the fetal circulation.

Therapy for this disease is rarely needed today because of the availability of an effective method for prevention of maternal sensitization by fetal erythrocytes. For unsensitized Rh-negative mothers giving birth to Rh-positive infants, a high titer human anti-D gamma globulin is given within 48 to 72 hours of delivery. This antibody rapidly removes the fetal Rh-positive erythrocytes from the maternal circulation before recognition and antibody production can begin.

ABO incompatibility between mother and infant rarely produces severe hemolytic disease. Even where the maternal fetal incompatibility in the ABO system has the potential for ABO hemolytic disease, in only 5% of the infants will any evidence for erythrocyte sensitization be found. Because preformed anti-A and anti-B antibodies are present in persons lacking these erythrocyte antigens, it is possible for the firstborn infant to be affected. Antibodies must be IgG in nature, however, to cross the placenta, and the usual naturally occurring anti-A and anti-B antibodies are IgM in nature, accounting in part for the low frequency of disease in newborns.

The major clinical feature of ABO hemolytic disease is the onset of jaundice within the first 24 hours of birth. Pallor is uncommon at any stage of the disease, and the signs or symptoms related to anemia do not occur. Splenomegaly of any degree is uncommon.

The laboratory findings include a normal hemoglobin value or minimal degrees of anemia. Reticulocytosis will be slight, if at all present, and a characteristic feature of the blood smear is the presence of spherocytes. A direct Coombs test can be demonstrated in about half the affected infants, but a greater frequency of antibody presence can be demonstrated by eluting the antibody from the infant's red cells and demonstrating their presence by an indirect Coombs test with adult red cells. The incompatibility between fetus and mother in the ABO system can be demonstrated, and is usually found to be an infant with A cells and a mother with 0 cells.

Table 15-4. Indications for therapy of isoimmune hemolytic disease of the newborn

Clinical condition	Therapy	Timing
Early anemia, congestive failure	Exchange transfusion	Immediately after birth
Early anemia, no congestive failure, cord blood Hb <10 g/dl	Exchange transfusion	As soon as possible after birth
Early anemia, no congestive failure, cord blood Hb 10 to 12 g/dl	Exchange transfusion	Early exchange on clinical indication only
Cord blood Hb > 12 g/dl	None	Early exchange not desirable or necessary
Serum bilirubin concentration 20 mg/dl or greater	Exchange transfusion	Whenever this serum bilirubin concentration is reached
Hemoglobin concentrations <7 g/dl during second to fourth wk	Simple transfusion	As this degree of anemia develops

Treatment is directed to the icterus, with the only concern being the prevention of kernicterus in the infant. Less than 10% of infants with ABO incompatibility disease develop significant increases in bilirubin values. For most infants, prevention of bilirubin increase by phototherapy is adequate, and only rarely is an exchange transfusion to reduce bilirubin levels necessary.

Minor group incompatibilities between mother and fetus can occasionally produce isoimmune hemolytic disease in the newborn period. These incompatibilities may occur in any of the minor group antigens, such as M, Kidd, and Kell. The sensitization may result from fetal erythrocytes entering maternal circulation at delivery, as is the case for Rh sensitization. In some instances, sensitization of the mother has occurred from transfusion of blood containing the antigen. With this in mind, caution should be used in transfusing women before and during the childbearing period. Treatment of isoimmune hemolytic disease caused by these minor group incompatibilities is outlined in Table 15-4 according to the principles for Rh incompatibilities.

Infections. Severe hemolytic anemia caused by infections during the newborn period is usually related to such intrauterine infections as cytomegalic inclusion disease, rubella, toxoplasmosis, and syphilis. Of these, the most frequent cause is cytomegalic inclusion disease, which can present during the newborn period with anemia, icterus, hepatosplenomegaly, and frequently petechiae and purpura. Bacterial sepsis can also be associated with hemolysis, but the degree is rarely severe. In infants having hemolysis as a consequence of infection, there will be anemia, reticulocytosis of moderate degree, and icterus. Usually the bilirubin will be increased in both the direct and indirect fractions. The Coombs test is negative. On physical examination the characteristic features of the specific infection will be found. If the anemia is severe, blood transfusions may be necessary. If the indirect bilirubin level increases to ranges associated with kernicterus, an exchange transfusion may be needed.

Intrinsic erythrocyte abnormalities. Infants with congenital spherocytosis and elliptocytosis may have sufficient hemolysis in the newborn period to produce anemia and jaundice. In hereditary spherocytosis the characteristic spherocytes will be seen on blood smear. In infants with elliptocytosis, however, striking deformity of the red cells and fragmentation is characteristic, and the elliptocytosis of later life may not be found. Pyruvate kinase deficiency may be associated with neonatal hemolysis, but it is unusual for a deficiency of glucose-6-phosphate dehydrogenase (G-6-PD) to cause difficulties at this age. In infants in whom intrinsic erythrocyte abnormalities produce hemolysis in the newborn period, blood transfusions and even exchange transfusion may be necessary if indicated by severe anemia or icterus. Hemoglobinopathies do not cause hemolysis during the newborn period because of the predominance of fetal hemoglobin in the infant's red cells.

Blood loss. Anemia in the newborn can result from bleeding through the placenta into the maternal circulation or loss of blood from the placenta or cord at delivery. These infants will appear pale, and if sufficient blood has been lost, they may also have the clinical features of hypovolemic shock. If chronic transplacental blood loss has occurred in utero, the infant may have the microcytic hypochromic anemia of iron deficiency. Treatment with blood transfusions may be necessary if the clinical condition warrants. For further discussion of blood loss see pp. 265 to 266 and pp. 307 to 308.

Bleeding disorders

Thrombocytopenia. An incompatibility of platelet antigens may result in isoimmune neonatal thrombocytopenic purpura because of the presence of maternal antiplatelet antibodies directed against the infant's platelets. The infant will demonstrate petechiae and purpura shortly after birth, and there may be bleeding from mucous membranes or the gastrointestinal tract. For the severely affected infant, an exchange transfusion with fresh whole blood may be needed to reduce the antibody titer, followed by transfusions of compatible platelets. The disease is self-limited; within a few weeks the maternal antibody disappears, and the platelets subsequently return to normal levels.

Thrombocytopenia may be a feature of intrauterine infections such as cytomegalic inclusion disease, rubella, and syphilis. Bacterial sepsis, if associated with disseminated intravascular coagulation, may also cause thrombocytopenia. Congenital amegakaryocytic thrombocytopenia may sometimes be associated with bleeding in the newborn period, as can the Wiscott-Aldrich syndrome.

Plasma factor deficiencies. Vitamin K is necessary for the synthesis of prothrombin and factors VII, IX, and X by the liver. It is obtained from dietary sources and is also produced by bacterial flora of the gut. In the immediate newborn period, before an adequate dietary source is offered and before bacterial flora are established, there may be a period of a few days in which the infant has an inadequate source of vitamin K. It is the usual practice now to give each newborn an injection of vitamin K (0.5 mg intramuscularly) at birth, which prevents deficiency of the vitamin K–dependent clotting factors from developing. If this vitamin is not given, especially in breast-fed infants, the deficiency may lead to bleeding manifestations such as ecchymosis and gastrointestinal bleeding, usually occurring from the second to seventh day of life. The condition can be diagnosed by the lack of vitamin K administration and the presence of prolonged plasma prothrombin time and partial thromboplastin time. The condition is rapidly corrected within 4 to 6 hours by the intravenous administration of 0.5 to 1 mg vitamin K. For treatment of a severe acute bleeding problem, fresh plasma and blood transfusions may be necessary if indicated clinically.

Infection during the newborn period may be associated with disseminated intravascular coagulation. In addition to the characteristic features of the specific infection, the infant may develop petechiae, purpura, and frank hemorrhage from mucous membranes or the gastrointestinal tract. There may also be deep tissue hemorrhage or bleeding into the lungs or brain. On blood smear decreased numbers of platelets and fragmentation of erythrocytes will be found. Hemolytic anemia may be associated. The prothrombin time, partial thromboplastin time, and thrombin time will be prolonged, and fibrin split products can usually be demonstrated. Treatment is for the underlying cause, but blood transfusions may be necessary to correct blood loss. If effective treatment can be directed to the disease causing the disseminated intravascular coagulation, the clotting problem will stop spontaneously and no further therapy is needed. Attempts to stop the bleeding with heparin, cryoprecipitate, and platelets are frequently unsuccessful if the primary disease cannot be alleviated.

In infants with severe neonatal hepatitis, a deficiency of clotting factors produced in the liver may occur. In addition to the vitamin K–dependent factors (prothrombin, VII, IX, and X), factor V will also be depleted. There will be prolongation of the prothrombin time and partial thromboplastin time, with minimal if any correction from the administration of vitamin K. For these infants the resulting bleeding problem is usually not of primary clinical concern. If necessary, blood transfusions and fresh plasma may be administered.

Congenital plasma factor deficiencies rarely cause difficulty in the newborn period unless surgical trauma such as circumcision has taken place. If there should be prolonged and unexplained bleeding from the umbilicus, or following circumcision or needle puncture, further studies should be done to determine whether a congenital plasma factor deficiency is present.

Leukocyte disorders

At birth there can be considerable variation in the total white blood count, with values ranging from 4000 to 40,000. In the first few days of life the neutrophilic granulocytes predominate, but by the end of the first week in the normal infant lymphocytes predominate.

Neutropenia. Isoimmune neutropenia may occur if there has been maternal sensitization to a neutrophil antigen present on infant cells but absent on the maternal neutrophilic granulocyte. The neutrophil concentration may be less than $500/mm^3$, and these infants may develop severe bacterial infections. The process is self-limited because the maternal antibody disappears from the infant's circulation during the first weeks of life. Severe lifelong congenital neutropenia may also present during the neonatal period with bacterial infections. In all septic infants complete blood counts with leukocyte differentials should be obtained to exclude those rare infants with neonatal neutropenia.

Congenital leukemia. Rarely, leukemia may be present at birth or become evident shortly thereafter. Such infants are generally pale and have petechiae. Hepatosplenomegaly may be present. White blood counts are generally markedly increased, and on blood smear the cells are predominantly blast forms. The prognosis for congenital leukemia is poor. Congenital leukemia may occur in infants with Down syndrome, but the development of a myeloid leukemoid reaction is more likely. The infant with Down syndrome may have a markedly increased white blood count, with many myeloblasts present on blood smear. Usually there is minimal, if any, anemia and no associated thrombocytopenic purpura. Although the blood leukocytes are predominantly blast cells, the bone marrow, although showing a myeloid hypoplasia, has strikingly good differentiation of all cell forms. The discrepancy between the appearance of the blood and bone marrow is a useful diagnostic clue. No therapy is indicated for this myeloid leukemoid reaction in infants with Down syndrome.

Alvin M. Mauer

Fetal and neonatal blood loss

Hemorrhage may occur in utero before labor, during parturition, or soon after birth. It may be associated with fetal bleeding into the maternal circulation or into a twin, with obstetric misadventure or rupture of anomalous vessels of the cord and placenta, or with enclosed hemorrhage. The resultant blood loss may be exsanguinating. Loss of 30 to 50 ml causes acute shock, which can be fatal if simple transfusion is not administered immediately. Causes of perinatal blood loss are listed as follows:

- Cord
  - Rupture of varices or aneurysms
  - Traumatic rupture of normal cord
  - Torn vessels with velamentous insertion
- Placenta
  - Incision into fetal side during cesarean section
  - Placenta previa
  - Abruptio placentae
  - Multilobed placenta with interlobar vessels
- Fetal blood loss
  - Fetomaternal (acute or chronic blood loss)
  - Fetofetal (into twin, acute or chronic blood loss)
- Enclosed hemorrhage
  - Intracranial hemorrhage
  - Ruptured liver
  - Ruptured spleen
  - Adrenal hemorrhage
  - Retroperitoneal hemorrhage
  - Subaponeurotic (scalp) hemorrhage
  - Cephalhematoma
  - Pulmonary (massive) hemorrhage

Acute hemorrhage may result from any of the conditions listed in the outline, although fetomaternal and fetofetal transfusions are more likely to cause chronic blood loss. Signs of distress are recognizable at birth, or they may be delayed for as long as 6 hours. Repeated hematocrit or hemoglobin determinations are thus necessary if antecedent events suggest occurrence of significant hemorrhage, since a normal result at birth is not a certain indication that all is well. Clinical signs include pallor, cyanosis (unrelieved by oxygen), tachycardia (rate above 160 beats/min), feeble or absent pulses, gasping, and tachypnea (occasionally with retractions). The cry is weak, and spontaneous activity is absent or diminished. Superficial examination is suggestive of severe asphyxia. The true hemorrhagic nature of the distress is discernible by cyanosis and pallor that persist in spite of oxygen administration, by presence of tachycardia rather than the bradycardia characteristic of asphyxia, and by increased respiratory rate in contrast to slow breathing in an asphyxiated infant. The diagnosis of blood loss is established by demonstrating low hemoglobin or hematocrit values. Anemia may not be apparent for several hours after birth, when hemodilution first occurs as a result of fluid shift from extravascular to intravascular spaces. Spuriously normal hemoglobin levels may be obtained from capillary heel prick specimens if peripheral circulatory stasis is severe; venous blood samples are therefore preferred under such circumstances. Hemoglobin concentration of 12 g/dl or less indicates blood loss. Reticulocytes are normal or slightly elevated. Red cells appear macrocytic or normal on a smear of peripheral blood.

Transfusion of whole blood is urgent if acute blood loss has occurred. Rapid infusion of approximately 20 ml should be accomplished. Usually the infant's condition improves dramatically, but if the degree of improvement is unsatisfactory, slower infusion of half the original quantity of blood is essential. Assiduous attention to optimal oxygenation and prevention of heat loss are important.

The commonest cause of neonatal anemia is probably passage of fetal erythrocytes into the maternal circulation. *Fetomaternal hemorrhage* of some degree is said to occur in half of all pregnancies, but only in relatively few infants is the process sufficiently severe to cause anemia and shock. In the extreme, stillbirth may result. Protracted fetomaternal hemorrhage (chronic blood loss) may be associated with slowly developing anemia and compensatory adjustment of circulating blood volume. At birth affected infants are thus pale and anemic but misleadingly vigorous. Several reports describe infants who are pale but apparently well, with hemoglobin concentrations as low as 5 g/dl. Fetomaternal hemorrhage may also cause acute blood loss, with clinical signs and laboratory findings as previously described.

The peripheral blood smear from an infant whose blood loss was chronic reveals hypochromic and microcytic erythrocytes, in contrast to the essentially normal appearance of red cells in acute hemorrhage. Nucleated red blood cells are increased in both types of blood loss. Reticulocytes are more likely to be increased in chronic blood loss. Treatment of chronic fetal hemorrhage may require transfusion of packed red cells, but often iron therapy alone is sufficient.

Fetofetal (twin-to-twin) transfusion occurs in a monochorionic placenta, which is present in approximately 70% of monozygotic twin pregnancies. Vascular anastomoses between twins occur from artery to artery, vein to vein, or artery to vein; the last arrangement gives rise to fetofetal transfusion. Blood loss from a donor twin is usually chronic in nature and should be suspected if the discrepancy in hemoglobin values between infants is 5 g/dl or more. The donor twin is generally smaller than the recipient, but discordant size is not regularly present. Oligohydramnios and anemia occur in the donor, polyhydramnios and polycythemia in the recipient. Donor hemoglobin may be as low as 4 g/dl, and reticulocytes and nucleated red cells are elevated. The recipient's hemoglobin ranges from 20 to 30 g/dl, and the resultant polycythemia may cause respiratory distress, cardiac failure, convulsions, hyperbilirubinemia, and on occasion, kernicterus. Treatment of polycythemia is discussed on p. 309.

Enclosed hemorrhage is a common cause of anemia during the first 3 days of life. Subarachnoid, subdural, and intraventricular hemorrhages may be sufficiently severe to cause low hemoglobin concentrations, although the other effects of these lesions are predominantly conspicuous. *Hemorrhage into the scalp* is particularly pernicious, sometimes resulting in profound blood loss with hemoglobin concentration as low as 3 g/dl. The scalp is boggy and edematous, obscuring sutures and fontanelles and extending over the forehead to impart a blue suffusion to the skin. Deficiency in vitamin K–dependent clotting factors or factor VIII (antihemophilic) are identifiable in many affected infants, and in addition there is a high incidence of difficult traumatic labor. The condition becomes apparent from 30 minutes to 4 days after birth. Pallor increases, and in severe hemorrhage, shock ensues. Demonstration of a defective clotting mechanism must be sought. Treatment includes transfusion and administration of deficient clotting factors.

Bleeding into the liver, spleen, adrenals, kidneys, and retroperitoneal region is associated with traumatic labor, particularly breech deliveries. Hemorrhage into the liver also results from needlessly vigorous external cardiac massage. It may be contained by Glisson's capsule, or it may rupture through it into the peritoneum. Blood accumulates within the liver for a day or two, at which time the infant may appear well, although perhaps somewhat pale. Shock occurs abruptly when the capsule ruptures, thereby removing the tamponade of external pressure, which had been inhibiting free hemorrhage. The liver is often palpably enlarged, either locally or diffusely, and the upper abdomen appears distended, particularly after rupture of the capsule.

Identification of adrenal hemorrhage is facilitated by presence of a palpable flank mass, which often gives the impression of an enlarged kidney because blood tends to accumulate in the perinephric area. Rupture of the spleen may occur during traumatic delivery, from severe enlargement in erythroblastosis fetalis, or during exchange transfusion.

Enclosed hemorrhage causes the signs of shock that have been described, and degradation of extraneous blood subsequently causes hyperbilirubinemia. Treatment is at first primarily concerned with replacement of blood volume by administration of whole blood. Phototherapy should be used when serum bilirubin is 10 mg/dl or more. Occasionally exchange transfusion is necessary.

Polycythemia

Polycythemia and hypervolemia may arise from four possible sources: excessive transfusion of placental blood into the infant at birth; continuous transfer of maternal blood to the fetus in utero; transfusion from a donor twin in utero; and increased fetal erythropoiesis. Cardiac failure and respiratory distress occur in affected infants; these events seem to be related to hypervolemia, pulmonary hypertension, and increased viscosity of blood. Convulsions have also been attributed to polycythemia.

The placental source of excess blood is provided at the time of birth. In the full-term infant, during the first 5 minutes of life an average of 165 ml blood is transferred from the placenta if the baby is held below the introitus after delivery, thereby increasing blood volume by 60%. Approximately 40 ml is transfused during the first 15 seconds. Two thirds of the volume is lost from the vascular space by transudation of plasma during the ensuing 4 hours.

Maternal transfer of blood to the fetus occurs frequently, usually in minute quantities. Exaggeration of this process may cause neonatal polycythemia. The mechanism of fetofetal transfusion was described in relation to hypovolemia and anemia in the donor twin. The recipient fetus, on the other hand, is in jeopardy from the effects of hypervolemia. Polycythemia has also been observed in association with chronic intrauterine hypoxia and congenital adrenal hyperplasia, as well as among infants of diabetic mothers.

Upper limits of normal hemoglobin concentration and hematocrit are difficult to define precisely because infants with high values are often asymptomatic, whereas some with lower values become ill. Trouble should be anticipated if the hematocrit exceeds 65 vol%.

Treatment is by partial exchange transfusion calculated to lower the hematocrit to 50%.

Disorders of bilirubin metabolism (see also pp. 351 to 355)

Hyperbilirubinemia. According to adult norms, hyperbilirubinemia occurs in most neonates, although jaundice is apparent in only half of them. The precarious balance between bilirubin formation and excretion is another example of the handicaps to survival imposed by functional limitations of immaturity. At any given moment an abnormally increased total quantity of bilirubin in the intravascular and extravascular compartments represents imbalance between pigment formation and capacity of the liver to excrete it. Approximately 85% of total bilirubin is formed from degradation of red cells, 1 g hemoglobin yielding 35 mg bilirubin. Breakdown of hemoglobin occurs in reticuloendothelial cells (particularly of the spleen) after sequestration of phagocytized aged erythrocytes.

In plasma, bilirubin is bound to albumin, 16 mg pigment to 1 g protein. This implies that serum bilirubin concentration of approximately 80 mg/dl can be bound to circulating albumin, when such is not actually the case. Bilirubin levels are rarely as high as 80 mg/dl, and albumin-binding capacity is always surpassed at much lower levels. Competition for binding sites by other metabolites such as free fatty acids is a constant occurrence; the truly available binding activity for bilirubin is thus considerably less than calculated. Bound bilirubin remains in the vascular compartment, whereas unbound pigment leaves the blood to permeate extravascular tissue. The migration to tissues is reversible by infusion of albumin, which by lowering tissue content augments serum concentration. Serum bilirubin levels are therefore not simply governed by rates of formation and excretion but also by binding with albumin, which undoubtedly is the principal determinant of distribution between serum and tissue.

Existence of *direct reacting* and *indirect reacting* bilirubin has been known for over 50 years, but the chemical differences between them were first demonstrated only a few decades ago. The direct component is bilirubin glucuronide (conjugated bilirubin); because it is water soluble, it is excreted through liver and kidneys and is incapable of tissue permeation. The indirect form is free bilirubin (unconjugated), which is lipid soluble and thus not excretable in bile or urine. It has high affinity for extravascular tissue, particularly subcutaneous and other fatty deposits.

Conjugation of bilirubin with glucuronide radicals transpires in hepatic cells by a series of enzymatic reactions. In the last of these reactions, uridine diphosphate glucuronic acid (UDPGA) and free bilirubin are converted to bilirubin glucuronide and uridine diphosphate (UDP) by the enzymatic activity of glucuronyl transferase. Antecedent formation of UDPGA depends on availability of adequate quantities of glucose, and since the reaction is strictly aerobic, adequate oxygenation is also essential. Oxygen deprivation during asphyctic states is therefore deleterious to these reactions. Some degree of glucuronyl transferase hypoactivity is common to all neonates. Neonatal bilirubin excretion is only 1% or 2% of the adult capacity as a result of this diminished enzyme activity, and this is the principal cause of most cases of neonatal hyperbilirubinemia. In a smaller number of infants, excretion is impaired by direct damage to liver cells.

Glucuronyl transferase activity, deficient at birth, tends to increase gradually, probably approaching adult levels between the second and fourth weeks of extrauterine life. Because at birth red cell breakdown presents a larger load of pigment to the liver than it is able to conjugate and excrete, serum unconjugated bilirubin accumulates. In addition, a significant amount of bilirubin is absorbed from the upper intestine into the enterohepatic circulation and is transported back to the liver. The neonate apparently has a greater capacity to absorb bilirubin from the upper intestine than the adult. Bilirubin glucuronide, deposited in the upper intestine as a component of bile, is converted to unconjugated bilirubin by the activity of bilirubin glucuronidase, an enzyme in the gut mucosa. The alkaline pH in this segment of the gut also contributes to conversion of conjugated bilirubin to the unconjugated form.

In the full-term infant peak levels occur between the second and fourth days and in premature infants on the fifth or sixth days. This is the mechanism of physiologic jaundice. The same events can produce high serum levels, which thus require exchange transfusion, particularly in premature babies. Physiologic jaundice is therefore a clinical concept of great utility in that it implies no need for therapy, but it is nevertheless difficult to define precisely because it occasionally assumes dangerous proportions and is then obviously not physiologic. The attributes of physiologic jaundice concern the time it appears and subsides and the peak concentrations of serum bilirubin. Jaundice is clinically apparent at bilirubin levels of approximately 5 mg/dl. The characteristics of physiologic jaundice in infants who are otherwise well include (1) appearance in term infants after 24 hours and disappearance by the end of the seventh day, (2) appearance in premature infants after 48 hours and disappearance by the end of the tenth day, (3) serum unconjugated bilirubin concentration of 12 mg/dl or less in mature or premature infants, higher levels suggesting either an exaggeration of physiologic handicaps or disease, (4) daily increments of serum bilirubin no greater than 5 mg/dl, and (5) direct bilirubin concentration less than 1 mg/dl. Fulfillment of these criteria does not always indicate that purely physiologic processes are operative; bilirubin conjugation and excretion may be unusually efficient, for instance, even in the presence of hemolytic disease.

Disorders that cause neonatal jaundice are many and diverse. In all instances listed in the outline (pp. 311 to 312) hemolysis exceeds capacity to conjugate the pigment, parenchymal liver damage impairs excretory function, or a combination of both factors exists.

The classic examples of *intravascular hemolysis* are Rh and ABO maternal-fetal incompatibilities. Although hemolysis proceeds in utero, unconjugated bilirubin is cleared across the placenta from fetus to mother by an unknown mechanism that probably involves selective activity. Jaundice at birth is thus exceptional, but in severe disease it may appear as soon as 30 minutes later. *Chemical hemolysins* cause severe jaundice. The administration of large doses of vitamin K_3 to mother or infant is a well-documented example. Maternal ingestion of mothballs (naphthalene) and even infant inhalation of the vapors cause hemolysis in G-6-PD–deficient persons. *Extravascular hemolysis* occurs most often from extensive ecchymosis associated with birth trauma. Hemolysis of large collections of blood in cephalhematomas, particularly when bilateral, results in formation of bilirubin quantities that are not totally excretable. The *Crigler-Najjar* syndrome is a rare, heritable, permanent deficiency of glucuronyl transferase. Hemolytic factors have been excluded as pathogenetic. Unconjugated hyperbilirubinemia persists throughout life and is a consequence of an inability to form bilirubin glucuronide. Death from kernicterus is the rule during the first week, unless exchange transfusions are performed. Most infants who survive suffer severe brain damage, and occasionally kernicterus develops later in childhood. Bilirubin concentrations remain in excess of 20 mg/

dl throughout life. *Transient familial neonatal hyperbilirubinemia* (Lucey-Driscoll syndrome) occurs in all the infants from a single mother. Severe unconjugated hyperbilirubinemia develops during the first few days and subsides between the second and third weeks. Sera from mothers and infants contain abnormally large amounts of an unidentified factor that inhibits glucuronyl transferase activity in vitro. Jaundice is often a result of *bacterial and nonbacterial infections,* particularly those in which hepatic damage occurs. Morphologic abnormalities may not be demonstrated at necropsy or in liver biopsy material, but changes have been noted in most of the infections listed in the outline (p. 320). Infection is the commonest cause of conjugated hyperbilirubinemia during the neonatal period; when the latter is demonstrated, extensive efforts to identify an infectious process are essential. *Neonatal hepatitis* is probably of viral etiology, although this has not yet been established. Diffuse giant cell transformation, which is regularly noted, is a nonspecific response to other types of hepatic injury. Clinical and laboratory characteristics are similar to those of biliary atresia and congenital nonbacterial infections. The latter are discussed on pp. 319 to 322. *Biliary atresia* (pp. 354-355) is difficult to identify in the neonatal period and later in infancy because differentiation from hepatitis is often confounding. Jaundice may appear during the first week or later; half the affected infants are not icteric until the second week. Hyperbilirubinemia is conjugated, but in the first days of life, glucuronyl transferase deficiency also causes notable accumulation of unconjugated bilirubin. Later, indirect bilirubin remains elevated as a result of hepatocellular damage. Associated with these cellular changes are elevations of serum glutamic oxaloacetic and glutamic pyruvic transaminase levels. Biliary atresia has been traditionally regarded as a developmental anomaly. Demonstration of the lesion in congenital rubella suggests that intrauterine virus infection may be a significant etiologic factor. *Infants of diabetic mothers* are predisposed to hyperbilirubinemia. The factors that favor its occurrence are prematurity, perinatal asphyxia, and hypoglycemia. *Galactosemia* causes conjugated hyperbilirubinemia. Hepatomegaly and severely impaired liver function are confusing unless appropriate diagnostic tests are performed. *"Breast milk jaundice"* is an interesting condition in which unconjugated hyperbilirubinemia appears during the second or third week. Bilirubin concentrations range from 15 to 25 mg/dl. Jaundice disappears at 3 weeks or may persist to the tenth week, even if breastfeeding is not interrupted. When feeding is discontinued, bilirubin levels fall rapidly over the ensuing few days. Kernicterus has not been reported in association with this syndrome; affected infants are well in all other respects. Breast milk from mothers of affected infants contains a pregnanediol that inhibits activity of glucuronyl transferase in vitro, but the mother's serum does not contain inhibitory factors.

Causes of neonatal jaundice are as follows:

- Increased bilirubin production
  - Intravascular hemolysis (unconjugated hyperbilirubinemia)
    - Hemolytic disease of the newborn (Rh, ABO, others)
    - Polycythemia (large placental transfusion, fetofetal transfusion, maternal-fetal transfusion)
    - Abnormalities of red cells
      - Hereditary spherocytosis
      - Enzyme deficiencies (G-6-PD deficiency and others)
      - Pyknocytosis
      - Hemoglobinopathy (Barts, Zurich)
    - Chemical hemolysis (vitamin K analogues, maternal naphthalene ingestion in G-6-PD deficiency)
  - Extravascular hemolysis; enclosed hemorrhage (unconjugated hyperbilirubinemia)
    - Petechiae, ecchymoses
    - Hematoma
    - Hemorrhage
    - Intraventricular hemorrhage
- Impaired hepatic function
  - Deficient glucuronyl transferase (unconjugated hyperbilirubinemia)
    - Physiologic
    - Crigler-Najjar syndrome
    - Transient familial neonatal hyperbilirubinemia
  - Infection (conjugated, unconjugated hyperbilirubinemia)
    - Bacterial (septicemia, syphilis, pyelonephritis)
    - Nonbacterial
      - Toxoplasmosis
      - Cytomegalovirus (CMV)
      - Rubella
      - Herpes simplex
      - Coxsackie
      - Neonatal hepatitis
  - Metabolic factors (unconjugated hyperbilirubinemia)
    - Hypoxia
    - Hypoglycemia
      - Infants of diabetic mothers
    - Galactosemia (conjugated)
    - Hormonal influence

"Breast milk jaundice"
Hypothyroidism
Biliary obstruction (conjugated, unconjugated hyperbilirubinemia)
Biliary atresia
Choledochal cyst
Miscellaneous (unconjugated hyperbilirubinemia)
Pyloric stenosis
Intestinal obstruction

Kernicterus (bilirubin encephalopathy). Kernicterus, the gravest complication of hyperbilirubinemia, results from damage to the central nervous system caused by deposition of unconjugated bilirubin in brain cells. The neurologic symptoms, which appear from the second to the tenth day, are those of severe depression (lethargy, diminished deep tendon reflexes and Moro response, hypotonia, absent suck) or excitation (opisthotonos, twitching, convulsions, high-pitched cry). Occasionally the anterior fontanel bulges. Many infants die; those who survive are likely to manifest severe neurologic damage after a 3-month period of apparent recovery. The neurologic deficits in later childhood are varied; they may be severely crippling or rather subtle. The pathology of kernicterus indicates that injury may affect learning, memory, and adaptive behavior. Perceptual function may be impaired, even though subnormal IQ or cerebral palsy is absent.

The principal determinant of bilirubin traversal of the blood-brain barrier is the extent to which it is bound to albumin in plasma. Conjugated bilirubin is not implicated in kernicterus. Normally the albumin-binding capacity for bilirubin is such that only minute amounts are unbound. The unbound pigment increases when serum bilirubin levels surpass the capacity of albumin to bind it, when the pigment is displaced by competitive substances of metabolic origin (free fatty acids) or by drugs (sulfonamides, salicylates), and if hypoproteinemia is present. Although there is a relationship between the height of bilirubin levels and incidence of kernicterus, it is nevertheless an indirect one. In the presence of high binding capacity, kernicterus will occur at higher levels of pigment in serum; conversely, with low binding capacity from whatever cause the danger point of serum bilirubin concentration is lowered considerably. Diminished tolerance to pigment levels is well demonstrated in competitive displacement of bilirubin by sulfisoxazole, which causes kernicterus at relatively low pigment concentrations.

In spite of the variables that affect the development of kernicterus, serum bilirubin determination generally continues to serve best as a basis for deciding whether to perform an exchange transfusion. Until a quantitative determination of albumin-binding capacity becomes feasible in hospital laboratories everywhere, traditional reliance on bilirubin levels must continue, but necessarily in combination with assessment of all factors pertinent to a particular infant's hyperbilirubinemic state.

The aim of therapy for hyperbilirubinemia is to prevent kernicterus; it includes measures directed primarily at underlying disorders and procedures concerned with actual removal of excess pigment (exchange transfusion [pp. 304, 312 to 313, and 352], phototherapy, and administration of barbiturates).

Phototherapy effectively diminishes serum content of unconjugated bilirubin. It is the blue segment of the light spectrum (420 to 500 nm) that effectively dissipates bilirubin. The commonly used fluorescent bulbs (Daylight or Cool White) deliver relatively little energy in the blue segment. Fluorescent bulbs especially designed to provide a significant quantity of blue light have been found to be more effective. Regardless of the light source used, the minimum therapeutic dosage of blue light is considered to be $4 m\mu W/cm^2/nm$. Relatively inexpensive photometers are available to measure specifically the blue light delivered to the skin surface. The effectiveness of phototherapy apparatus should be monitored periodically with the use of these instruments. Phototherapy is used in some units for routine prophylaxis against hyperbilirubinemia, particularly in infants below 1500 g birth weight. It is obviously useful for ABO incompatibility, in which exchange transfusions are frequently avoided or forestalled if phototherapy is begun at an appropriately early time. Phototherapy is used similarly in many facilities for Rh disease, and the data indicate that fewer early (first 12 hours of life) and late transfusions are necessary with its use. However, it should be considered that in removing bilirubin with phototherapy, the vulnerable red cells remain in circulation for ultimate hemolysis. The result is a progressive anemia in spite of the safe levels of serum bilirubin that are maintained by phototherapy. In our experience there has been frequent prolongation of hospital stay because of continuous or precipitous decline in hemoglobin. A need has arisen for one or more multiple simple transfusions because of the progressive anemia. Thus we believe it best to withhold phototherapy in Rh disease until the first exchange transfusion has been performed and the "target" red cells have been removed. Phototherapy is applied subsequently and the need for additional exchange transfusions is diminished. With an infant under light, diminution of jaundice is no cause for complacency; etiologic diagnosis must be sought before and after initiating therapy. Generally, serum indirect bilirubin concentration should be at least 10 mg/dl before initiating therapy in term infants; between 6 and 8 mg/dl in small babies. The lights are not a substitute for exchange transfusion once the need for the latter has been established. Phototherapy may possibly avert repeated transfusions if applied immediately after the first one. Serum bilirubin levels should be followed assiduously throughout the period of therapy. The average fall in pigment concentration after 8 to 12 hours of therapy is 3 to 4 mg/dl. Rebound elevations may occur after therapy is discontinued.

The most important immediate untoward effects of phototherapy include increased metabolic rate, hyperthermia, and significantly increased loss of water through the skin. Metabolic rate increases, and the caloric requirement rises. There may be difficulty in meeting caloric needs if intestinal transit time is increased sufficiently to cause loose stools. Hyperthermia (and the loose stools) increases water losses, and the daily fluid requirement therefore increases. In premature infants insensible water losses may increase by as much as 50%. Urine may darken because photodegradation products are water soluble and are thus excreted by the kidneys.

Some minor side effects include loose dark stools, dark urine, green skin color (which soon fades), rash, and priapism. Jaundice diminishes noticeably over skin surfaces exposed to light; a striking contrast is provided by persistent jaundice in unexposed areas. That natural light conditions affect serum bilirubin levels has been documented in a study in Finland some years ago where, through the year, seasonal daily duration of daylight varies from 3 to 22 hours. Premature babies born during the "light" half of the year had significantly lower bilirubin levels than those born during the "dark" half of the year. None of them received phototherapy. Environmental light undoubtedly also influences the effect of phototherapy. Factors such as the number of windows in a nursery, the light they admit, the position of the baby in relation to windows, and the geographic location of the hospital must all be considered in evaluating the results of phototherapy.

A warning issued by the Food and Drug Administration has called attention to the protective effect of a plastic barrier between phototherapy lights and babies. Without a plastic shield, ultraviolet light from fluorescent bulbs has caused skin erythema. Commercial lights have plastic shields built into the apparatus. The plastic walls of an incubator are also protective. Phototherapy should thus be used only with plastic interposed between light and baby. The erythema caused by ultraviolet light suggests that the retina would also be jeopardized in the absence of a surface that filters out the ultraviolet light.

The infant's eyes are shielded from the intense light he receives during phototherapy. No evidence from human eyes has indicated that light is injurious, but microsopic injury to retinal cells has been observed in monkeys exposed to phototherapy (without shielding eyes) for 3 to 7 days. The extent of the damage was well correlated with the duration of exposure. Pharmacologic stimulation of hepatic bilirubin clearance may be an additional useful form of therapy. Phenobarbital has been used most often for this purpose. The mechanism by which it lowers serum unconjugated bilirubin is unknown. It has been administered to mothers several days before delivery, to infants several days later, and perinatally to both. In animals, phenobarbital is known to stimulate hepatic detoxifying activity for several substances, including steroids in the neonate and in the fetoplacental unit. The data so far available do not justify use of barbiturates or any other substance for the purpose of enhancing hepatic bilirubin excretion.

Infectious disease

General considerations

Infections are a major cause of perinatal mortality and morbidity. Because of several unique attributes, perinatal infection should be discussed in a separate context from infectious disease in later life. Thus some agents (e.g., rubella and herpes virus) produce devastating changes in the fetus and newborn, but in older children they cause benign disease or none at all. The converse also applies; some organisms that threaten life in later infancy and childhood (e.g., *Haemophilus influenzae* and meningococcus) rarely constitute a problem during the perinatal period. Interpretation of diagnostic serology in older children is not applicable to neonates. Immunologic response is immature, and the presence of maternal antibodies obviously does not reflect the infant's experience with infection. Identification of infectious disease also requires a specialized clinical orientation because the signs are subtle and nonspecific. A septicemic premature infant may merely be lethargic and hypoactive. Fever, a hallmark of disease in older infants and children, is ordinarily imperceptible in the newborn infant, whereas cough is unusual even if extensive pneumonitis is rampant. Epidemiologic considerations must include maternal influences inherent to prenatal life and the relatively defenseless state of the infant in respect to nursery environment and the demeanor of nursery personnel.

Host defenses: immunity

Resistance to infection is multifactorial. Most studies of perinatal responses to infection have attempted to characterize the developmental aspects of humoral antibody production (immunoglobulins).

Of the three major immunoglobulins (IgG, IgA, IgM), only IgG normally traverses the placenta from maternal to fetal circulation. Traversal is not dependent on molecular size (which is smallest for IgG) but rather is the result of a selective process. Other proteins of even lower molecular weight, such as albumin or growth hormone, are not transferred across the placenta. Maternally derived IgG initially appears in the fetus during the third gestational month, and it accumulates progressively throughout pregnancy. Because length of gestation is a significant determinant, IgG levels in premature infants are generally lower than in those born at term. At birth, IgG concentration in serum of a normal full-term infant is equivalent to, or slightly higher than, that of the mother. Most antitoxins and most antibodies against gram-positive bacteria and viruses are of the IgG type; maternal and neonatal titers are thus similar. Maternally bestowed IgG is steadily depleted after birth at a time when the infant's capacity to synthesize it increases. The total concentration falls from a mean of 1000 mg/dl at birth to approximately 400 mg/dl about 3 months later, when the decline in total IgG is arrested by the increased capacity to synthesize it. Thereafter, concentrations increase gradually, and at 1 or 2 years of age they are close to adult values.

IgM is first produced by the fetus during the third gestational month. Normally only small quantities are elaborated; in the presence of infection, synthesis increases. The normal IgM content of cord serum is below 20 mg/dl, but intrauterine infection often results in much higher levels. Because IgM is not maternally derived, abnormally high levels reflect an immunologic response to infection intrinsic to the fetus. Augmented levels may result from any antigenic stimulus and are thus no more indicative of a specific infectious agent than an increased erythrocyte sedimentation rate would be in older children. Specific etiologic diagnosis is provided by fluorescent antibody (FA) techniques, which are employed to demonstrate antibodies in the IgM fraction.

Immaturity of the complement system and defective phagocytic activity of granulocytes are also characteristic limitations of perinatal defense against infection. The latter finding is a result of deficient opsonic activity in plasma rather than limitations to the phagocytic cells. Adult leukocytes in serum from premature infants exhibit similar deficiencies; phagocytic activity is normal when leukocytes from premature infants are placed in adult serum.

Bacterial infections

Infections are acquired before, during, or after birth. Prenatal infection is acquired by the transplacental or ascending routes; the latter is more frequent. Bacteria comprising normal flora of the vaginal and intestinal tracts gain access to amniotic fluid and membranes through the cervix. The fetus is thus exposed to infection, but disease may not ensue. Organisms gain entry by way of the mouth and nose to the lungs and intestinal tract or by way of placental vessels directly into the bloodstream. The ascent of organisms is facilitated by rupture of membranes, and the possibility of fetal disease is enhanced as the interval between membrane rupture and delivery is lengthened.

Several procedures have been contrived in an effort to identify at birth those infants exposed to infection in utero; these procedures are predicated on the presence of acute inflammatory cells in amniotic membranes, in the umbilical cord, or in the aspirate of gastric contents. Sole reliance on these tests is not justified as an indication for antibiotic therapy of infants.

Postnatally acquired infections occur in sporadic or epidemic form. Nursery epidemics are initiated or extended by hospital personnel, infant cohorts, or the physical environment. Serious infection resulting from staphylococci, enteropathogenic *Escherichia coli, Pseudomonas aeruginosa,* and *Salmonella* have occurred repeatedly in widespread epidemics.

Pneumonia. Pneumonia is the commonest of the serious neonatal infections. It has been cited as the primary cause of death in 10% to 20% of neonatal autopsies. Peak incidence is during the second and third days; half of all cases occur during the first week of life. Although infection takes place in many infants with normal obstetric histories, most seem to be associated with some obstetric abnormality, the most frequent of which are early rupture of membranes, prolonged duration of labor, maternal infection, and uncomplicated premature delivery. The interrelations of these abnormal events and the relative importance of each have not been determined. Estimates of the time at which early rupture of membranes is hazardous to the fetus have varied widely from 6 to 48 hours before delivery. Early rupture of membranes, combined with prolonged labor, is apparently more hazardous than either of these factors separately.

Bacteria that most often cause intrauterine pneumonia are derived from normal flora of the maternal intestinal and genital tracts. *E. coli* and other enteric organisms, staphylococci, and Group B streptococci are the commonest offenders. Pneumonia acquired postnatally is caused by hospital strains of penicillin-resistant staphylococci, *P. aeruginosa,* enteric bacilli, and several other bacterial agents of less frequent occurrence.

Symptoms of intrauterine pneumonia are evident at birth or within the first 48 hours of life. When in distress at birth, these infants are flaccid, inactive, pale, or cyanotic. Respirations, if spontaneous, are shallow and ineffective and may be delayed for several minutes, requiring vigorous resuscitative measures. Once established, respirations are then rapid and shallow, with slight or moderate retractions that are seldom as striking as those of hyaline membrane disease. Repeated apneic episodes are characteristic, particularly if the infection is severe. Breath sounds may be diffusely or regionally diminished. Crepitant rales are diffuse or localized, and when respirations are shallow, they may be perceptible only when full inspiration is forced by stimulating a cry. Percussion notes are unreliable. Temperature elevation, often absent, is more likely to occur in full-sized rather than in small infants. Subnormal temperatures are not unusual in premature infants.

Clinical signs of postnatally acquired pneumonia usually appear after 48 hours of life, although the onset is somewhat earlier in premature infants. Some of these infants may have been hypoxic at birth for reasons unrelated to infection. Tachypnea, poor feeding, or aspiration during feeding are the commonest presenting signs. Retractions, if present, are not severe; flaring of alae nasi indicates air hunger. Recovery is more frequent in postnatal than in congenital pneumonia.

The chest film may reveal extensive homogeneous opacification in a major portion of both lungs, which probably represents infection acquired many days before birth. Another pattern consists of patchy opacities of varying size about the hilar areas; from these, smaller patches and linear densities extend radially to the periphery of the lung. In advanced disease, patches are large and coalescent. The chest film in postnatal pneumonia is most often characterized by one or more irregular areas of consolidation. Pneumatoceles (regional obstructive emphysema) and pleural exudation suggest staphylococcal infection but are sometimes caused by other infections as well.

Peripheral blood studies and cultures of the throat and nasopharynx seldom provide useful data. Except for Group B streptococcus, blood cultures are positive in only a minority of affected infants. IgM levels are almost always high, but the increase may not occur until several days after onset.

Choice of antibiotics is somewhat influenced

by whether the infection was acquired prenatally or postnatally. Gentamicin and penicillin or ampicillin are used for antenatal infections. Nafcillin or methicillin and polymixin (an aminoglycoside) are preferred for postnatal infection. Dosage and schedules are listed in Table 15-5.

Septicemia. The incidence of septicemia has not diminished since the introduction of antibiotics, but the frequency of distribution of several etiologic agents has changed remarkably. Before 1944, Group A beta hemolytic streptococcus was predominant. Since then, coliform organisms have caused a preponderance of these infections. Among the gram-positive cocci, Group B beta hemolytic streptococci and staphylococci are most frequent. Among the coliform organisms, *E. coli, Klebsiella-Aerobacter, Pseudomonas,* and *Proteus* predominate. Isolated reports of infection from uncommon etiologic agents appear continuously. Staphylococcal septicemia is considerably less common than it was 25 to 30 years ago. Case fatality was 90% before antibiotics were available but has since fallen to a range of 13% to 45%. Premature infants are most often affected. The ratio of male to female involvement is approximately 2:1.

Symptoms are characteristically vague. One expects chills, abrupt onset of fever, and prostration in older infants, but the newborn infant may merely lose vigor, refuse feedings, and cease to gain weight or is simply reported by nurses to be "doing poorly." Lethargy, diminished spontaneous activity, and pallor are additional nebulous signs of disease. These responses, however subtle, are usually recognizable, although their relation to septicemia is inconstant. Other abnormal manifestations are less subtle and are as wide-ranging as the blood stream itself. Fever is an infrequent sign. Abdominal distention, probably caused by paralytic ileus, may be prominent. Abnormal patterns of respiration, which mimic those of intracranial and pulmonary disorders, occur in 20% to 30% of septicemic infants. Apnea, tachypnea, and cyanosis are the usual signs. Jaundice at some time during the course of illness has been reported in 20% to 60% of cases. Enteric gram-negative organisms are particularly likely to cause jaundice. Attempts to correlate skin lesions with specific etiologic agents are seldom successful. Pustules, furuncles, and subcutaneous abscesses may represent metastatic

Table 15-5. Antibiotics of choice

	First week of life or premature			Full-term infant over 1 week of age		
Agent	**Dosage**	**Route**	**Schedule**	**Dosage**	**Route**	**Schedule**
Penicillin	50,000-100,000 units/kg/day	IM, IV	q8h or q12h	50,000-300,000 units/kg/day	IM, IV	q6h or q8h
Ampicillin	50-100 mg/kg/day	IM, IV	q12h	150-200 mg/kg/day	IM, IV	q8h
Methicillin	100 mg/kg/day	IM, IV	q8h	200 mg/kg/day	IM, IV	q6h
Nafcillin	100 mg/kg/day	IM, IV	q12h	200 mg/kg/day	IM, IV	q6h
Carbenicillin	225 mg/kg/day	IM, IV	q8h	300 mg/kg/day	IM, IV	q6h
Kanamycin	15 mg/kg/day	IM, IV	q12h	25 mg/kg/day	IM, IV	q8h or q12h
Gentamicin	5 mg/kg/day	IM, IV	q12h	7.5 mg/kg/day	IM, IV	q8h
Tobramycin	4 mg/kg/day	IM, IV	q12h	5 mg/kg/day	IM, IV	q6h or q8h
Polymyxin B	3 mg/kg/day	IM, IV	q12h	4 mg/kg/day	IM, IV	q8h
Neomycin	50-100 mg/kg/day	PO	q6h	50-100 mg/kg/day	PO	q6h
Colistimethate	5 mg/kg/day	IM	q12h	8 mg/kg/day	IM	q8h
Chloramphenicol	25 mg/kg/day	IV	q8h	50 mg/kg/day	IV	q6h
Nystatin	200,000-400,000 units	PO	q6h	200,000-400,000 units	PO	q6h
Amikacin	15 mg/kg/day	IM, IV	q12h	22.5 mg/kg/day	IM, IV	q8h
Moxalactam	100 mg/kg/day	IV	q12h	150 mg/kg/day	IV	q8h

Adapted from Feigin, R.D., and Callanan, D.L.: Postnally acquired infections. In Fanaroff, A.A., and Martin, R.J., editors: Behrman's Neonatal-Perinatal Medicine, ed. 3, St. Louis, 1983, The C.V. Mosby Co.

phenomena most often associated with streptococcal and staphylococcal infection, or less often with *E. coli* and *P. aeruginosa*. Staphyolococci may cause scattered black areas of gangrenous dermatitis. Erythema multiforme has been seen in septicemia resulting from streptococci, staphylococci and other organisms as well. *P. aeruginosa* often causes a lesion, characterized by purple cellulitis, that evolves into a gangrenous ulcer. *P. aeruginosa* may also cause impetiginous lesions of green or purple hue. A peculiar diffuse, indurated, erythematous rash occurs in septicemia resulting from *Achromobacter, Alcaligenes faecalis, P. aeruginosa, E. coli,* and *Proteus*. Petechiae and ecchymoses are uncommon and are in fact more suggestive of disease caused by cytomegalovirus, Coxsackie, rubella viruses, or toxoplasmosis. Enlargement of the liver is common.

Signs of meningitis occur in approximately 15% of cases (convulsions, altered state of consciousness, irritability, paralysis, spasticity, and fullness of fontanel).

Infection of the umbilical cord indicated by erythema and induration of surrounding skin and occasionally by purulent exudation is an early sign in about 10% of septicemic infants.

Clinical impressions of septicemia must ultimately be confirmed by recovery of organisms from the blood. Etiologic agents are recovered from spinal fluid in one third of affected infants, although only half of these exhibit neurologic abnormalities. Rapid morphologic identification is feasible when Gram stain is applied to the centrifuged sediment. Other laboratory procedures are of limited value but are nevertheless informative. Examination of urine is often neglected. Culture and Gram stain are often rewarding. Cultures of the throat, nasopharynx, and umbilicus are of little diagnostic value, except when purulent exudation is present in the latter. High direct bilirubin concentration is suggestive of infection. IgM levels are elevated.

The clinician (and the patient) can ill afford to await identification of the offending organism, but cultures of blood, spinal fluid, and urine must be made before treatment is begun. Penicillin or ampicillin plus gentamicin together are active against approximately 90% of organisms that infect the neonate. *P. aeruginosa* may be resistant to these antibiotics. In hospitals in which this organism is known to be a relatively frequent cause of infection, polymixin, colistin or, carbenicillin should be added to this regimen, particularly if the onset of disease occurred after 72 hours. It should also be added if, after 24 hours of therapy, the infant is notably worse. Dosage and route of administration of antibiotics are listed in Table 15-5.

Meningitis. Almost half the cases of meningitis in children occur in the first year of life; during this period the incidence is highest in the first month. It has been observed seventeen times more frequently in premature than in full-term infants. The preponderant involvement of males, as noted for septicemia, has not been regularly observed for meningitis. The etiologic agents are similar to those cited for septicemia. *Diplococcus pneumoniae, Haemophilus influenzae,* and meningococcus are rare in the neonate. Abnormal obstetric histories, most commonly involving premature birth, occur in over half the patients. Other frequently mentioned obstetric complications include early rupture of membranes, birth trauma, and maternal infection.

Symptoms of meningitis are similar to those of septicemia. Fullness of the anterior fontanel is the commonest specific sign of central nervous system disease; stiffness of the neck is rare. Convulsions and coma may occur in over half the patients, opisthotonos in more than a fourth of them.

Abnormalities of spinal fluid do not differ from those of older age groups. Cell content, predominantly polymorphonuclear leukocytes, may vary from under twenty to several thousand per cubic millimeter. A predominantly mononuclear response is produced by *Listeria monocytogenes*. Sugar content is usually low; protein is increased. Organisms are evident on gram-stained sediment in most instances. The results of blood cultures are positive in 75% of affected infants.

In all large series, fatality rates of 30% to 50% are the rule. Severe neurologic handicaps are noted in the majority of survivors.

Gentamicin and penicillin or ampicillin are drugs of choice. If polymixin is indicated (as in *Pseudomonas* meningitis), it must be administered intrathecally, because it does not appear in spinal fluid when given by any other route.

Diarrhea. Epidemic diarrhea of the newborn is a syndrome comprising several acute and highly communicable primary diarrheal disorders of varying etiology but with similar clinical and epidemiologic expression. Several bacterial agents are known to cause the syndrome, most important of which is enteropathogenic *E. coli*. *Salmonella* and *Shigella* occur much less frequently.

Serologic techniques have identified 140 serogroups of *E. coli* based on the antigenic structure of the cell wall. These groups are further divided into serotypes. Diarrheal syndromes are caused by approximately 14 strains, which are identified by agglutination techniques. The most common strains are 026:B6, 055:B5, 0111:B4, and 0127:B8. Several strains of *Salmonella* and *Shigella* have been identified in nursery epidemics. Typhoid and paratyphoid have not been isolated from stools in any of the reported outbreaks. Staphylococcal enteritis has been reported in epidemic form.

Early signs of disease are the same regardless of the etiologic organism (diarrhea, refusal to feed, weight loss, diminished spontaneous activity, and lethargy). Blood, pus, and mucus in stools are rare, except in shigellosis, which is itself uncommon. As these signs progress in severity the infant becomes toxic, dehydrated, and acidotic. Fluid is lost even more rapidly when vomiting ensues and when stools become more liquid and more frequent. An ashen gray color or pallor is indicative of vasomotor collapse. Mild forms of the disease are not unusual and are characterized by protracted diarrhea and simple reluctance to feed.

Institutional outbreaks of diarrhea are usually propagated by hospitalized infants. Disease spreads from one bassinet to an adjacent one. Feces of infected infants contain enormous quantities of organisms and contamination may thus occur by way of hands and gowns of attending personnel. Enteropathogenic *E. coli* has been recovered from the nasopharynx of infected infants, suggesting transfer or organisms through the air. Maternal carriers may impart these organisms to their offspring during the birth process. A constant reservoir of carriers in the community has been postulated, since despite stringent precautions during and after an epidemic, organisms may still be cultured with unchanged frequency from inpatients. Once an infected infant is admitted to the nursery or pediatric ward, intramural spread of infection is virtually inevitable.

Diarrheal stools should be cultured as soon as they appear. The diagnosis is clinically self-evident, but bacteriologic data from stool culture must establish cause. If staphylococcal infection is considered, Gram stain of a fecal smear is indispensable to the diagnosis, whereupon a preponderance of gram-positive cocci, to the exclusion of enteric bacilli, will be evident.

An affected infant must be transferred to an isolation facility promptly; diarrhea in a newborn infant is infectious until proved otherwise. Dehydration may occur in a few hours; replacement of fluids and correction of severe acidosis are thus urgent considerations. Antibiotic therapy for *E. coli* enteritis is relatively simple and effective. Neomycin is probably most effective. Polymixin B has been used with neomycin and without it. Some strains have become resistant to neomycin.

Conjunctivitis. Infection of the conjunctivae may be acquired during the birth process or from the nursery environment. Epidemics of conjunctivitis caused by *Staphylococcus aureus* or *P. aeruginosa* are not unusual. The most serious form of conjunctivitis is caused by *Neisseria gonorrhoeae*. *E. coli* and other enteric organisms may also be etiologic.

Purulent conjunctival exudate resulting from gonococcus may appear from the second to the fifth day of life and sometimes later. Conjunctivitis caused by other bacterial agents appears at any time after the second or third day of life. In its mildest form the infection causes "sticky eyes," with little or no conjunctival edema or scleral injection. In severe cases, exudate is copious and thick, conjunctivae are swollen and red, and periorbital edema with purplish suffusion is often present.

One percent silver nitrate is generaly instilled into eyes at birth for prevention of gonococcal conjunctivitis. Bacterial conjunctivitis is treated by local instillation of an ointment containing neomycin, bacitracin, and polymixin. The gonococcal variety must be treated with intramuscular penicillin, plus local application of penicillin ophthalmic ointment.

Omphalitis. The umbilical stump is a portal of entry for all types of bacteria. Inflammation may herald disseminated infection. In severe infection purulent or serosanguinous exudate is present. In milder infections there is no visible discharge, but redness and induration of the periumbilical skin are obvious. Slight periumbilical erythema without induration is usually benign. Redness of the skin and edema of subcutaneous tissue over the umbilical vein indicates cellulitis and subjacent infection. Rarely, omphalitis is externally invisible. If the umbilicus is infected, systemic administration of antibiotics should be instituted after the blood and a cut surface of the cord are cultured.

Pyelonephritis. Neonatal renal infection occurs as a complication of septicemia, as a consequence of anomalies of the central nervous system that produce bladder paralysis, in association with a congenital anomaly of the urinary tract, and as the sole manifestation of disease. Contrary to prevailing impressions, most neonatal renal infection is not associated with congenital malformations.

Pyelonephritis is seldom considered in the differential diagnosis of the infected neonate. In one study the diagnosis was overlooked in approximately 85% of cases identified at autopsy among infants up to several months of age. Its prevalence in the neonatal period is not insignificant. The clinical appearance, usually far from striking is characterized by little more than failure to gain, anorexia, and apathy. When pyelonephritis is associated with septicemia, the symptomatology of the latter predominates. Jaundice with direct hyperbilirubinemia is particularly frequent in this combination of infections. Sex incidence apparently favors males impressively. Metabolic acidosis and elevated blood urea nitrogen (BUN) level are common. Diagnosis depends on demonstration of pyuria and bacteriuria. Until organisms are identified and their sensitivities defined, therapy should be initiated with gentamicin and ampicillin. A urine sample should be obtained by suprapubic puncture.

Treatment of overt disease. Ampicillin and gentamicin are generally the antibiotics of choice. Pending results of bacterial cultures, these preparations should be administered when onset of systemic infection occurs prior to 48 or 72 hours. Onset at later ages implies greater likelihood that hospital-acquired organisms are etiologic (penicillin-resistant staphylococcus, *Pseudomonas*). For these later infections nafcillin is indicated, and polymixin, colistimethate or carbenicillin with gentamicin deserves serious consideration. All systemic infections should be treated for at least 10 days.

Prophylactic treatment. Regardless of other findings, ampicillin and gentamicin should be administered soon after birth to all babies in whom amniotic membranes have ruptured more than 48 hours before delivery. Individual evaluation is required before similar treatment is given when membranes have ruptured between 12 and 48 hours before birth. Cultures of blood, pharynx, and groin are taken before onset of treatment, which is then maintained for 5 days in asymptomatic infants and longer if there is evidence of disease.

Congenital syphilis. See pp. 736 to 740.

Viral infection

The thirteen viruses that have been implicated in the causation of perinatal infection are listed in Table 15-6. Fetal damage, with a few exceptions, is a result of disease produced by transmission of virus across the placenta from mother to fetus. This may occur early in gestation to cause chronic intrauterine disease, as in the case of rubella or cytomegalovirus, or it may occur close to delivery to cause disease that is first apparent a few days after birth, as in the case of varicella-zoster, Coxsackie group B, or small pox viruses. Another pathogenetic mechanism involves ascent of virus into amniotic fluid from an infected cervix and vagina, or exposure of the fetus to these same infected structures during the descent of birth. Herpesvirus hominis infection is most commonly acquired in this fashion.

Maternal virus infections may exert the following variety of effects on the fetus: abortion or premature birth solely caused by maternal toxicity, death (and thus abortion or stillbirth) due to intrinsic disease, congenital malformations, establishment of chronic intrauterine infection that continues into postnatal life, tissue destruction and inflammatory processes, intrauterine growth retardation, postnatal persistence of virus in an asymptomatic neonate, and unaffected fetus or neonate. Rubella, cytomegalovirus, and herpesvirus hominis infections are of primary interest.

Rubella. Estimates of the fetal risk imposed by maternal rubella vary from one epidemic to another. A summary of fifteen prospective studies reported between 1946 and 1961 provides the following mean percentages of fetal risk: maternal infection during the first gestational month results in 33% incidence of affected infants; during the second month 25% are affected; and during the third and fourth months, 9% and 4%, respectively, are abnormal. Overall risk

Table 15-6. Maternal infections affecting the fetus or newborn

Infection	Effect
Rubella	Congenital cardiovascular anomalies, cataracts, micropthalmia, glaucoma, deafness, hepatitis, jaundice, hepatosplenomegaly, pneumonitis, meningoencephalitis (chronic), microcephaly, myocardial necrosis, thrombocytopenia, inguinal hernia
Cytomegalovirus	Microcephaly, hydrocephalus, encephalitis, chorioretinitis, hepatitis, jaundice, hepatosplenomegaly, thrombocytopenia, pneumonitis, intracranial calcification, congenital heart disease, inguinal hernia
Herpesvirus hominis	Herpetic rash, hepatitis, jaundice, meningoencephalitis, pneumonitis, thrombocytopenia, coagulopathy, keratoconjunctivitis, chorioretinitis, cerebral calcification
Coxsackie group B	Meningoencephalitis, myocarditis, hepatitis, jaundice, thrombocytopenia
Varicella-zoster	Varicella rash, pneumonitis, hepatitis
Smallpox	Variola rash, pneumonitis, hepatitis, meningoencephalitis
Vaccinia	Vaccinia rash, pneumonitis, hepatitis, stillbirth
Poliomyelitis	Spinal or bulbar polio similar to adult, myocarditis, pneumonitis, stillbirth, abortion
Rubeola	Measles as in later life (usually benign), stillbirth, abortion
Western equine encephalitis	Meningoencephalitis
Mumps	Congenital parotitis, congenital malformations (?)
Hepatitis B	Asymptomatic hepatitis (HB Ag positive); acute hepatitis
Influenza	No proved effect; congenital malformation (?), anencephaly (?)

during the first trimester is approximately 20%.

Rubella virus was first identified in the laboratory in 1961. In 1964 a severe nationwide rubella epidemic was followed by the birth of thousands of affected infants. Newly described virologic and serologic techniques were applied to clinical observations, and, as a result, new concepts of the congenital rubella syndrome evolved.

Maternal rubella is asymptomatic in approximately half the affected women; clinical signs of acquired infection are difficult to interpret in sporadic cases. History of infection, whether positive or negative, is therefore inaccurate because of the high incidence of asymptomatic infections and the difficulty in diagnosis of sporadic ones. The severity of fetal disease is not related to presence or absence of maternal signs.

The congenital rubella syndrome is a chronic viral infection that begins in utero and persists in many infants for several months after birth. Rubella virus has been recovered from abortuses, placentas, and amniotic fluid, and from throat, urine, meconium, conjunctival fluids, and spinal fluid of live newborn infants. At necropsy the virus has been grown from almost every organ of the body as well as from surgically extirpated ductus arteriosus, cataractous lens, and liver. Although the majority of infants do not harbor virus beyond the third month of life, it may persist in some for several months or years longer. Persistently infected infants were first reported to be a source of contagion in 1965 when small epidemics among hospital personnel were traced to them. Pregnant women are thus at risk when exposed to such infants.

The clinical signs are varied. Intrauterine growth retardation is prominent in a majority of infants. Cardiac anomalies are present in most; their commonest lesions are persistent patent ductus arteriosus and peripheral pulmonic stenoses. Septal defects occur alone or in combination with other cardiac malformations. Severe myodardial damage, which is intractable to vigorous medical therapy, has also been observed. Electrocardiograms resemble those of adults with myocardial infarction, and in some instances they suggest that myocardial disease originated in utero. In the eyes unilateral or bilateral cataracts are the commonest lesions. Other eye involvement includes microphthalmia, glaucoma, and transient corneal clouding, which clears in several weeks. Purpura and thrombocytopenia may occur in 40% to 80% of infants. Hepatosplenomegaly is common, and in some infants obstructive jaundice also occurs. Rubella virus causes hepatitis in the neonatal period, which may later progress to cirrhosis. Indirect hyperbilirubinemia results from hemolysis; enlargement of the liver and spleen is primarily related to extramedullary hematopoiesis. Interstitial pneumonitis is another component of the syndrome. Spinal fluid contains abnormally high protein levels and increased numbers of leukocytes, predominantly lymphocytes, even though abnormal neurologic signs are uncommon in the neonatal period. Long bone radiographs reveal longitudinal and ovoid radiolucent areas in the metaphyses, particularly in the distal femurs and proximal tibias.

The postneonatal course of congenital rubella is troublesome. Approximately 20% of patients die within the first year. Neurologic abnormality, identifiable in approximately 80% during the first year, is persistent in 66% at 18 months of age. Coordination of rehabilitative efforts is indispensable because the defects affect so many organ systems.

Diagnosis in the neonatal period is possible solely on clinical grounds and serologic confirmation by demonstration of rubella IgM antibodies. Beyond this age, demonstration of HI or neutralizing antibodies is reliable for establishing the diagnosis.

Cytomegalovirus. Congenital cytomegalic inclusion disease is caused by transmission of virus from the maternal bloodstream to the fetus. During pregnancy maternal seroconversion to cytomegalovirus apparently occurs in about 6% of women, yet the incidence of congenital disease is considerably less frequent. Maternal viruria at term has been demonstrated in 2% to 4% of pregnant women, but only a minority of their infants were affected. Virus has been recovered from asymptomatic neonates, although follow-up studies did not reveal neurologic abnormalities in all instances. The significance of virus shedding in an apparently healthy infant is not yet known with certainty. Despite these gaps in knowledge, fetal cytomegalovirus disease is considered a major cause of perinatal morbidity and mortality resulting from infection.

Maternal infection is usually imperceptible. Signs of disease in the infant are present at birth or soon after. As in rubella, herpes, and toxoplasmosis, infection from cytomegalovirus is widespread. Intranuclear inclusions appear in cells of almost every organ in the body. Intrauterine growth retardation is often prominent. Other clinical effects are most apparent in blood, liver, and central nervous system. Hemolysis causes anemia, reticulocytosis, increased nucleated red cell counts, and jaundice. Hepatosplenomegaly is largely a function of extensive extramedullary hematopoiesis. Thrombocytopenia, skin petechiae, and ecchymoses are frequent. Hepatic necrosis superimposes direct hyperbilirubinemia on the icteric effects of hemolysis and causes elevation of serum transaminase as well. Involvement of the brain, ultimately leading to microcephaly, is often most severe in ependymal and subependymal cells of the lateral ventricles; calcifications evident on skull films are thus characteristically periventricular. Calcification in the brain may also assume a more diffuse pattern; neither of these arrangements is distinguishable from toxoplasmic infection. Chorioretinitis has been described repeatedly; most retinal lesions are at the periphery of the fundus. Pneumonitis may occur but is infrequent. Congenital heart disease is not uncommon. Survivors are usually neurologically abnormal.

The best laboratory methods for establishing the diagnosis are isolation of virus from urine and demonstration of specific IgM antibodies by indirect fluorescence. Viruria persists for months or years after birth. Inclusion-bearing cells ("owl-eye cells") in urine are also diagnostic of the disease, but unfortunately they are present in fewer than 20% of infants with documented infection. There is no effective treatment currently available.

Herpesvirus hominis. Like most other agents that infect the newborn, herpesvirus hominis produces a wide spectrum of clinical signs. The disseminated form is fatal in 96% of affected infants. Several nondisseminated forms comprise varying combinations of central nervous system, skin, and eye involvement. In the aggregate the case fatality rate in nondisseminated herpes is 25%, but in over half the survivors there is residual damage to the eye or central nervous system.

The virus has been classified into type 1 and type 2. The former is responsible for the vast majority of herpetic lesions on the lips, in the oral cavity, and in the skin "above the belt." Type 2 virus seems to cause almost all herpetic genital disease and skin lesions in the lower part of the body. Approximately 95% of neonatal infections are caused by the type 2 virus. Exposure to virus occurs during the descent of parturition or before onset of labor as a result of ascending infection from the cervix or external genitalia. If transmission across the placenta occurs, it is apparently rare, having been reported in only a few cases in which such a pathogenesis was suggested.

Disseminated infection primarily involves the liver, adrenals, brain, blood, and lung, although microscopic lesions occur in almost every organ of the body. Initial symptoms appear at birth or as late as 21 days later. Generalized infection is suggested by fever in approximately one third of the cases. Other common signs include hepatosplenomegaly, hepatitis with jaundice (which may be associated with direct hyperbilirubinemia), bleeding diathesis, and neurologic abnormalities. Vesicular skin lesions are the most obvious diagnostic portents, occurring in about one third of patients. They are sparsely distributed over the body, although they occasionally appear in clusters. Bleeding from the gastrointestinal tract, needle punctures, and circumcisions usually heralds death within 24 to 48 hours.

Nondisseminated disease implies absence of clinical or pathologic evidence of visceral involvement. Abnormal neurologic findings, with or without involvement of skin or eyes, are the most common clinical expression of this form of the disease. Convulsive phenomena (generalized or focal) are the most frequently observed. Bulging fontanel, abnormal muscle tone, opisthotonos, and coma are less common. Spinal fluid abnormalities include elevated protein content and pleocytosis (predominantly lymphocytes). Eye lesions usually occur in association with other manifestations, but on occasion they may be the only affected sites. Keratitis, conjunctivitis, and chorioretinitis may occur alone or in varying combinations. Skin lesions are not infrequently the sole manifestations of infection. Every infant so involved has survived, although psychomotor retardation was residual in some. Herpetic skin lesions may recur repeatedly for as long as 2 years after birth.

The most serious disabling sequelae are neurologic, consisting of microcephaly, hydrocephalus, porencephalic cysts, and varying degrees of psychomotor retardation. Ocular sequelae, occasionally associated with total blindness, include corneal scars and residual scars of chorioretinitis.

Diagnosis is elusive in the absence of skin lesions. Microscopic examination of scrapings from the margins of lesions in the skin reveals multinucleated giant cells and intranuclear inclusions. The latter can only be confused with varicella-zoster or smallpox infection. The virus is identifiable in vesicle fluid by electron microscopy within 1 hour after specimen collection or by tissue culture methods within 2 days after inoculation. Specific IgM antibodies have been demonstrated by indirect fluorescence. Arabinosyladenine (ARA-A) reduces mortality significantly, particularly for the localized forms of the disease. It is given intravenously in a dose of 15 mg/k/day over a period of 12 hours, for 10 days.

Protozoan infection: toxoplasmosis

Although usually asymptomatic in the mother, infection caused by *Toxoplasma gondii* is transmitted through the placenta to produce devastating effects in the fetus. Symptoms appear in the infant at birth or soon after. The organism may enter every type of cell in the body except the erythrocyte. The resultant clinical signs may thus vary widely. Central nervous system involvement produces an array of neurologic abnormalities, ranging from convulsions to severe hypotonia and coma, microcephaly, or hydrocephalus. Skull films reveal diffuse, comma-shaped intracranial calcifications. Chorioretinitis is evident in most infants; lesions usually cluster about the posterior pole of the fundus. Microphthalmia is also common. Other signs include hepatosplenomegaly, jaundice (direct or indirect hyperbilirubinemia), petechiae and ecchymoses in the skin (thrombocytopenia), and pallor (anemia). The fatality rate in the neonatal period is approximately 12%. Neurologic abnormalities are extremely common among survivors.

Serologic diagnosis is feasible immediately after birth if specific IgM antibodies can be demonstrated by fluorescent techniques.

Infected neonates should be treated, whether or not they are symptomatic. Seroconversion or toxoplasma IgM should indicate infection in the asymptomatic infant if treatment is initiated. Therapy is with pyrimethamine 1 mg/k/d orally for the first day and 0.5 mg/k/d for 30 days thereafter. Sulfadiazine is also given for 30 days in a dose of 25 mg/k/d.

Metabolic disorders

Carbohydrate metabolism. The fetus derives glucose directly from maternal blood by facilitated diffusion across the placenta. Glycogen is stored in the placenta during early gestation and then primarily in the liver later on. Early in pregnancy placental hoards of glycogen are high, and enzymes required for glucose release are present. At 20 to 24 weeks of gestation the liver assumes most of the glycogenolytic function, its stores having steadily accumulated while those of the placenta gradually decreased. Continuous augmentation of glycogen stores occurs in the heart and skeletal muscle as pregnancy proceeds to term. At birth hepatic glycogen is twice the adult concentration; in skeletal muscle it is three to five times greater, and in the heart it is approximately ten times the adult concentration. Cardiac glycogen is rapidly depleted during asphyctic episodes; a direct relationship exists between stores at birth and ability to survive such encounters.

Nutriment flows steadily to the fetus in utero, but after birth caloric needs must ultimately be supplied from external sources. It may be hours or days before expenditure of energy is even partially replenished by nutrition from external sources. In the meantime the energy cost of respiration, thermoregulation, and muscle activity is reflected in an abrupt decrement of glycogen stores. Obviously, intrauterine malnutrition on which asphyxia is superimposed is a serious threat to survival in terms of depleted carbohydrate stores. By the end of the third postnatal hour, liver glycogen concentration, for example, is normally only 10% of values at birth. It rises gradually thereafter to attain adult levels by the end of the second or third week. In infants with respiratory distress the work of survival causes exhaustion of glycogen reserve, almost complete depletion having been demonstrated in postmortem analysis of the heart, liver, and diaphragm.

The normal neonate can tolerate some fasting without resultant biochemical derangement. Carbohydrate stores are used for the first 2 or 3 days; later fat is probably a principal source of energy. The blood sugar at any given moment is a reflection of hepatic release of glucose (glycogen breakdown, gluconeogenesis) and its utilization by peripheral tissue. Normal output of glucose from the liver depends on adequate glycogen stores, effective activity of enzymes concerned with glucose production from glycogen and other sources, and the activity of glucagon, epinephrine, and adrenocorticoids. Utilization by peripheral tissues is abnormally increased by the metabolic response to cold stress, by acidosis, and by hypoxemia.

Hypoglycemia. Low blood sugar is a symptom, never a disorder in itself. Hypoglycemia must be defined in terms of gestational age (term or premature) and postnatal age. In premature infants, plasma sugar is abnormally low at 25 mg/dl or less; in term infants 35 mg/dl or less is hypoglycemic during the first 3 postnatal days, and 45 mg/dl is the lower limit of normal thereafter. Wide fluctuations normally occur in response to numerous influences, one of the most obvious of which is feeding. The method of specimen handling is important and is probably a common cause of spuriously low blood sugar values. Glycolysis in blood stored at room temperature is twice as rapid in the neonate as in the adult. Thus in samples from premature infants that are stored at room temperature for 3 hours, glucose concentration falls approximately 15 mg/dl/hr.

Hypoglycemia may be a symptom of several underlying disorders of diverse origin, which are listed in Table 15-7.

Hypoglycemia occurs when levels of glycogen stores are low, gluconeogenesis in the liver is diminished, available insulin is excessive, or carbohydrate regulating hormones such as cortisol, epinephrine, and glucagon are insufficient. In rare circumstances, enzyme deficiencies in the liver impair the release of glucose, thus causing hypoglycemia.

Transient symptomatic hypoglycemia of the neonate. Toxemia of pregnancy and twin pregnancy are the only prenatal conditions that portend neonatal transient symptomatic hypoglycemia. Among these toxemic mothers the incidence of fetal compromise from complications of labor and delivery is high. Male infants are affected twice as frequently as females. A majority of infants (approximately 65%) are below the tenth percentile on the Colorado Intrauterine Growth Curves and are thus small-for-dates. Hypoglycemia is a major threat to the intact survival of undergrown infants and to the smaller of twins, particularly when the discrepancy in birth weight is 25% or more. Among twins, hypoglycemia is unrelated to fetofetal transfusion, birth order, or maternal toxemia. Affected infants, beside their underweight, are short for gestational age, although length is less frequently influenced than weight. Head size is least

Table 15-7. Causes of neonatal hypoglycemia

Clinical entity	Effect	Duration
Intrauterine malnutrition	Low liver glycogen store	Transient
Transient symptomatic hypoglycemia	Low liver glycogen store	Transient
Fetal asphyxia	Low liver glycogen store	Transient
Cold stress	Low liver glycogen store	Transient
CNS hemorrhage	Unknown	Transient
CNS malformation	Unknown	Transient
Adrenal hemorrhage	Ineffective catecholamine response	Transient
Infants of diabetic mothers	Increased plasma insulin activity	Transient
Erythroblastosis	Increased plasma insulin activity	Transient
Glycogen-storage disease (types I and II)	Defective glycogen breakdown	Protracted
Glycogen synthetase deficiency	Low liver glycogen store	Protracted
Hereditary fructose intolerance	Defective fructose metabolism	Protracted
Galactose intolerance (galactosemia)	Defective conversion of galactose to glucose	Protracted
Leucine intolerance	Hyperinsulinism	Protracted
Islet cell tumor	Hyperinsulinism	Protracted
Beckwith-Wiedemann syndrome	Hyperinsulinism	Protracted

often affected. The brain of an infant who was malnourished in utero weighs five to seven times more than the liver, whereas in normally nourished infants the ratio is 3:1. The liver is among the most profoundly affected organs in the malnourished fetus; the brain is least implicated.

Most infants are well in the hours after birth. Symptoms usually appear between 24 and 72 hours of age, but occasionally onset may occur as early as 3 to 6 hours or as late as 7 days postnatally. The symptoms are not specific for hypoglycemia, but their presence in a small-for-dates infant is an unequivocal indication for blood sugar determination. Clinical signs may be characterized by hyperactivity of the central nervous system (tremors, jitteriness, twitches, generalized convulsions) or by depressed activity (apathy, lethargy, hypotonia, refusal to feed, feeble cry). Other signs include cyanosis, apnea or irregular respirations, and eye rolling. Some infants are polycythemic, and in a few hypocalcemia may coexist. Urine and spinal fluid are usually normal, except for low sugar content in the latter.

Management of infants at risk requires frequent blood sugar determinations during the hours when difficulties are most likely to occur. Any infant whose placement on intrauterine growth curves is indicative of growth retardation should be monitored assiduously for low blood sugar. Treatment comprises intravenous glucose administration and adrenocorticoids, if necessary, according to details described in the next section devoted to infants of diabetic mothers. Reliance should not be placed on orally administered glucose solutions.

Follow-up of infants reveals that neurologic deficit is identifiable in 30% to 50% of untreated symptomatic hypoglycemics.

Infants of diabetic mothers. Before the introduction of insulin over 50 years ago, few diabetic women conceived, and among those who did, the outcome of pregnancy was often catastrophic for mother and fetus. Pregnancy in diabetic women is now commonplace, and in the past 20 years screening during pregnancy has identified affected women whose diabetic diathesis was unsuspected in the nonpregnant state. As a result of more effective management (particularly during gestation) and an increased number of diabetic pregnancies, offspring of diabetic mothers are numerically significant, and the serious problems they pose are a major challenge to the care of high-risk infants. Approximately 1 in 500 to 1 in 1000 pregnancies concerns frankly diabetic women, and approximately 1 in 120 pregnancies involves maternal gestational diabetes. Perinatal infant mortality and morbidity are inordinately high. Stillbirth rates are high early in the third trimester, and they diminish to lowest levels at 36 and 37 weeks, after which there is an abrupt rise of considerable magnitude. For this reason diabetic pregnancies are interrupted at 36 and 37 weeks.

The following classification of maternal diabetes introduced by White is a universal reference based on duration of diabetes before pregnancy, age of onset, and extent of vascular disease:

Class A	Highest probability of fetal survival; no insulin, little dietary regulation; includes gestational diabetes
Class B	Onset at 20 years of age or more; duration less than 10 years before pregnancy; no vascular disease
Class C	Onset between 10 and 19 years of age; duration between 10 and 19 years; minimal vascular disease (retinal arteriosclerosis, calcification of vessels in the legs only)
Class D	Onset before 10 years of age; duration 20 years or more; moderately advanced vascular disease (diabetic retinopathy, transient albuminuria, and hypertension)
Class E	Characteristics of Class D, plus calcification of pelvic vessels
Class F	Characteristics of Class D, plus nephritis

Class A is the commonest form; it includes gestational diabetes. This type of diabetes is an abnormality of glucose tolerance in an asymptomatic mother, which reverts to normal within 6 weeks postpartum. Fetal survival is most likely in Class A diabetes, least likely in Class F. Women in the latter category often give birth to small-for-dates babies.

At necropsy, hypertrophy and hyperplasia of the beta cells in pancreatic islet tissue are hallmarks of infants of diabetic mothers. This is accompanied by infiltration of eosinophils in over half the autopsies. Content of extractable insulin is increased in proportion to the degree of islet hyperplasia. Visceral enlargement is primarily noted in the heart and liver, less striking in adrenals and kidney. Extramedullary hematopoiesis is more intense than expected for gestational age. Macrosomia is largely the result of increased deposition of fat and not, as previously believed, of edema. In fact, total body water is significantly diminished. In contrast to visceral enlargement, weight and volume of the brain are less than expected for infants of similar body weight and gestational age.

Neonatal problems include hypoglycemia, hypocalcemia, hyperbilirubinemia, respiratory distress syndrome, congenital anomalies, and renal vein thrombosis.

At birth, blood glucose in cord blood is 80% or more of the maternal level. Within an hour after birth, glucose concentration normally drops to a mean of 40 to 50 mg/dl. The rate of decline is greater in infants of mothers with gestational diabetes (Class A), and even more rapid if maternal diabetes is insulin dependent (Classes B through F). Between 4 and 6 hours of age, blood sugar frequently rises to normal neonatal values. Levels below 30 mg/dl occur in approximately half the infants of diabetic mothers; the period of greatest jeopardy is the first 6 hours of life. One in 5 of these hypoglycemic infants is symptomatic. In a few infants symptomatic hypoglycemia occurs at 12 to 24 hours after a previously uneventful course. The symptoms are not specific; they are also observed in infants with normal glucose concentrations (lethargy, hypotonia, poor suck, apnea, rapid respiration, pallor, cyanosis, convulsions, or coma).

Hypocalcemia (less than 7 mg/dl) is a relatively common occurrence, and, as in hypoglycemia, there is poor correlation with clinical signs (irritability, coarse tremors, twitches, convulsions). Furthermore, low serum calcium is often observed in premature infants of nondiabetic mothers, particularly those subjected to perinatal stress.

Hyperbilirubinemia and respiratory distress syndrome, although more frequent than in control infants of like gestational age, are similar in characteristics and modes of therapy. Renal vein thrombosis may be unilateral or bilateral and is sometimes associated with calcification. Palpation of a renal mass and presence of hematuria and proteinuria strongly suggest the diagnosis. An array of congenital anomalies has been reported in offspring of diabetic mothers. The incidence of malformations is higher than in controls, perhaps threefold or more. In the Collaborative Perinatal Study the incidence of congenital heart disease was almost three times greater among offspring of diabetic mothers than among those of nondiabetic mothers.

There is no well-defined explanation for the spectrum of abnormalities in offspring of diabetic mothers. Maternal hyperglycemia (and resultant fetal hyperglycemia) are postulated to cause macrosomia and later neonatal hypoglycemia. Fetal hyperplasia of islet cells and hyperinsulinism occur in response to elevated blood sugar. Excessive insulin causes increased tissue uptake of glucose and increased deposition of fat (macrosomia). Continued hyperactivity of islets after birth, when the generous supply of maternal glucose is eliminated, leads to accelerated rate of glucose depletion in the neonate and thus to hypoglycemia. This hypothesis does not satisfactorily explain obesity of infants whose mothers are prediabetic, or the increased incidence of congenital anomalies, immature function for gestational age, diminished size of the brain, hypocalcemia, or renal vein thrombosis.

Intensive care is essential for management of these infants. The precise nature of the maternal diabetic state should be known well before onset of labor. Resuscitative procedures in the delivery room and management of hyperbilirubinemia and of hyaline membrane disease are no different from those for other infants. Since, as a rule, lowest blood glucose levels occur between 1 and 4 hours after birth, determinations on cord blood and on capillary blood from heel prick at 1, 2, 4, and 6 hours are essential. The frequency of subsequent determinations depends on results obtained. Distressed infants and any baby of a severely affected mother should immediately be given 10% glucose by way of the umbilical vein by continuous drip at a rate that delivers 65 to 70 ml/kg body weight daily. Treatment is indicated for other infants when blood sugar falls below 20 mg/dl at any time.

The intravenous treatment for hypoglycemia is initiated with the infusion of a 10% glucose solution at a rate of 8 mg/k/min. If a more concentrated solution is to be used, the same rate of administration of glucose should be calculated. If the infant is symptomatic, rapid infusion of 250 to 300 mg/k of glucose as a 10% solution can be given over 1 to 3 minutes. This is followed by continuous infusion at the rate of glucose administration mentioned previously. An unsatisfactory response indicates an increase in the amount of glucose to be administered, generally in 2 mg/k/min increments until 12 to 14 mg/k/min has been reached. If euglycemia has not been achieved, at 12 to 14 mg/k/min, hydrocortisone is given in a dose of 10 mg/k/d divided in two administrations intravenously, intramuscularly, or orally. Alternatively, prednisone is given in a dose of 2 mg/k/d. Steroids are given for 3 to 5 days and subsequently tapered over a period of 48 hours. The infusion of glucose should be maintained while the steroid dose is reduced.

Hypocalcemic tetany is treated initially with intravenous injection of 10% calcium gluconate (1 to 1.5 ml/kg body weight). Injection must be given slowly while heart rate is monitored electronically or by auscultation. If heart rate decelerates below 100 beats/min, administration of calcium gluconate should be discontinued; treatment may subsequently be resumed, if symptoms require, after normal heart rate is present for 30 minutes. Because infiltration of tissues causes necrosis and calcification, scalp infusion should be avoided. The patient is given calcium orally as soon as feasible.

Hypoglycemia complicating erythroblastosis fetalis (Rh incompatibility). For several years a preoccupation with the dramatic cardiopulmonary and central nervous system complications of erythroblastosis fetalis obscured the significance of hypoglycemia as a hazard of the disease. Low blood glucose levels have been observed in approximately 30% of severely to moderately affected erythroblastotic infants and in 5% of all erythroblastotic infants regardless of severity. Hypoglycemia is more frequent if cord hemoglobin is below 10 g/dl. It occurs before or after exchange transfusion, usually during the first day of life. Clinical signs, when present, are identical to those previously described for hypoglycemia from other causes.

The postmortem finding of islet cell hyperplasia in erythroblastotic infants has been known for 35 years, but only recently has it become evident that insulin content of pancreatic tissue and plasma is elevated. The cause of hyperinsulinism is unknown.

Blood glucose levels should be monitored every 4 to 6 hours during the first day and regularly thereafter for 3 days. Procedures involved in diagnostic surveillance and in therapy are similar to those previously described for infants of diabetic mothers.

Hypocalcemia. The causes of neonatal hypocalcemia are multiple and often enigmatic. Low serum calcium levels during the first 2 days of life are frequently asymptomatic. When clinical signs appear, they are predominantly those of neuromuscular irritability (twitching, tremors, and focal or generalized convulsions). Convulsive episodes frequently begin when the infant is taken up for a feeding; they vary in duration from several seconds to 10 minutes. Minor stimuli may provoke convulsions or twitches, while in the interim the infant is often uncomfortably restless.

Two peaks of incidence are identifiable—the first 24 or 48 hours and the fifth to tenth days of life. The causes of these temporal groups are apparently different. Typically, the infant with early hypocalcemia has experienced perinatal asphyctic stress and is premature or small-for-dates, and pregnancy was complicated by abruptio placentae, placenta previa, toxemia, or diabetes. Low serum calcium levels are rather frequent in infants of diabetic mothers. Early hypocalcemia is seldom associated with tetany, but other signs are occasionally discernible in the form of vomiting, abdominal distention, edema, high-pitched (squeaky) cry, intermittent cyanosis, and apnea. The true relationship of these signs to hypocalcemia itself is still debatable.

Classic neonatal tetany usually appears between the fifth and tenth days in well-nourished term infants who are fed artificial formula. A dietary cause for this form of hypocalcemia is widely accepted, but etiologic details have not yet been completely elucidated. The high phosphate load in cow's milk formula is thought to be the most significant precipitating factor, the calcium-phosphate ratio rather than the absolute quantity of phosphate being of greatest importance. The ratio in human milk is 2.25:1, whereas in cow's milk it is 1.35:1. Feeding cow's milk causes high serum phosphate levels. The neonatal response to increased serum phosphate is characterized by suboptimal parathyroid activity and diminished renal excretion of phosphate. Hypocalcemia is apparently a direct result of hyperphosphatemia, whereas parathyroid inadequacy fails to raise the serum calcium level. Calcium-phosphate ratios have been altered in commercial formulas; this form of neonatal tetany is now rare.

Clinical signs are those of neuromuscular excitability, as previously described. Laryngospasm and carpopedal spasm, common in older age groups, are rare in the neonate. Chvostek's sign is of no interpretive value because it is so common in normal babies.

Maternal hyperparathyroidism is an infrequent cause of neonatal hypocalcemia, but the association has been described regularly in numerous study series. Serum calcium determination should be obtained from mothers of all hypocalcemic infants, particularly those of late onset.

Laboratory data establish the diagnosis. Serum calcium level below 7 to 8 mg/dl (3.5 to 4 mEq) is abnormal. The early-onset type may not be characterized by elevated serum phosphate concentration, but in the late tetanic form of hypocalcemia, serum phosphate is regularly elevated above 7 mg/dl.

The treatment of hypocalcemia is described on p. 326. Intravenous calcium is not necessary for the asymptomatic disorder; addition of calcium salt to formula is adequate.

Hypomagnesemia. The clinical manifestations of hypomagnesemia are indistinguishable from those of hypocalcemic neuromuscular excitability. Reports of neonatal tetany caused by low serum magnesium concentrations have increased in frequency. Normal serum magnesium in the neonate varies from 1.2 to 1.8 mEq. Hypomagnesemia may occur in association with low serum calcium levels or without it. It may occur during or after exchange transfusion in which magnesium is bound to citrate in the donor blood, in infants of diabetic mothers and in infants whose mothers are affected by malabsorption syndrome. Serum magnesium determinations are essential for evaluation of any infant with neuromuscular hyperexcitability, but particularly in those with known hypocalcemia who fail to respond to treatment or whose serum phosphate concentration is normal. Treatment results in prompt disappearance of tetany or convulsions. An intramuscular dose of 50% magnesium sulfate (0.2 ml/kg body weight) is given every 4 hours for the first day. Repeated assessment of serum magnesium levels is essential, and subsequent therapy is continued accordingly. Oral supplementation (30 mEq/24 hr) may be required for several days to 2 weeks. Often the associated hypocalcemia is corrected solely by magnesium therapy.

Miscellaneous disorders

Neonatal convulsions. Neonatal convulsive phenomena vary considerably in extent and intensity from minor localized muscle twitching to vigorous generalized seizures; there is little relationship between type of seizure and nature or severity of the abnormality that causes it. Underlying pathologic states of diverse origin may be categorized as asphyctic, traumatic, metabolic, pharmacologic, infectious, and teratologic.

Asphyctic and traumatic causes are related to intrauterine hypoxia and to injuries associated with the birth process, such as intracranial hemorrhage. Postasphyxial cerebral edema is also associated with neonatal convulsions. Metabolic factors include hypoglycemia (associated with maternal diabetes and intrauterine growth retardation), hypocalcemia, and hypomagnesemia. Blood chemistry determinations should establish the presence of these deficiencies. Hypothermia and cold injury are also ictogenic. Pyridoxine dependency is rare.

Among pharmacologic causes, narcotic withdrawal symptoms are well known in babies of addicted mothers. Protracted hypoglycemic seizures may occur in neonates whose diabetic mothers received sulfonylureas during pregnancy. Inadvertent injection of mepivacaine into the fetal scalp during caudal analgesia causes convulsions. Maternal administration of copious amounts of hypotonic fluid during labor may result in hyponatremia and seizures.

Teratogenic considerations include numerous malformations of the central nervous system. Perhaps most prominent are hydranencephaly (demonstrated by skull transillumination), porencephaly (similarly demonstrated if the lesion is large and close to the cortical surface), agenesis of corpus callosum (demonstrated by pneumoencephalography), and vascular anomalies (demonstrated by angiography).

Central nervous system disease caused by nonbacterial agents (cytomegalovirus, toxoplasmosis, herpes simplex, and Coxsackie virus group B) and bacterial infections (meningitis and septicemia) also cause seizures during the neonatal period.

Retrolental fibroplasia (p. 977). An increased incidence of retrolental fibroplasia has been noted in recent years, commensurate with increasingly vigorous oxygen therapy for the respiratory distress syndrome. The disease occurs in premature infants whose retinal vessels have not yet grown outward to reach the ora serrata. Completion of this vascularization process occurs by the end of the eighth gestational month. Retrolental fibroplasia is characterized by retinal neovascularization and edema, followed by retinal detachment and fibrosis. In the extreme the end result is blindness. The vascular changes are caused by hyperoxemia. An absolutely safe upper limit of arterial oxygen tensions has not been documented, but there is general agreement that arterial PO_2 beyond 90 to 100 mm is dangerous.

The acute phase begins with constriction, then dilatation and tortuosity of retinal vessels at the periphery of the fundus. Neovascularization soon occurs; cloudy vitreous and some hemorrhage ensue. The acute phase culminates in retinal detachment, which may be either complete or restricted to the periphery. Spontaneous regression is unlikely once retinal detachment occurs. The acute phase transpires over a period of several weeks, but more rapid progression is not unusual.

The cicatricial phase is irreversible. Fibrosis occurs after retinal detachment, and the extent of residual scars may vary from small areas in the retina to complete pupillary occlusion. Corneal opacities, cataracts, and secondary glaucoma may complicate severe cases.

Sheldon B. Korones

SELECTED READINGS

Black, P.J., and Barkhan, P.: The blood and bone marrow during growth and development. In Davis, J.A., and Dobbing, J., editors: Scientific foundations of paediatrics, ed. 2, Baltimore, 1981, University Park Press.

Fox, W.W., et al.: The respiratory system. In Fanaroff, A.A., and Martin, R.J., editors: Behrman's neonatal-perinatal medicine, ed. 3, St. Louis, 1983, The C.V. Mosby Co.

Harris, T.R.: Physiologic principles. In Goldsmith, J.P., and Karotkin, E.H.: Assisted ventilation of the neonate, Philadelphia, 1981, W.B. Saunders Co.

Heim, T.: Homeothermy and its metabolic cost. In Davis, J.A., and Dobbing, J., editors: Scientific foundations of paediatrics, ed. 2, Baltimore, 1981, University Park Press.

Hislop, A., and Reid, L.: Growth and development of the respiratory system: anatomical development. In Davis, J.A., and Dobbing, J., editors: Scientific foundations of paediatrics, ed. 2, Baltimore, 1981, University Park Press.

Korones, S.B.: Complications. In Goldsmith, J.P., and Karotkin, E.H.: Assisted ventilation of the neonate, Philadelphia, 1981, W.B. Saunders Co.

Korones, S.B.: High risk newborn infants: the basis for intensive nursing care, ed. 3, St. Louis, 1981, The C.V. Mosby Co.

Oski, F.A.: The hematologic aspects of the maternal-fetal relationship. In Oski, F.A., and Naiman, J.L.: Hematologic problems in the newborn, ed. 3, Philadelphia, 1982, W.B. Saunders Co.

Oski, F.A.: Anemia in the neonatal period. In Oski, F.A., and Naiman, J.L.: Hematologic problems in the newborn, ed. 3, Philadelphia, 1982, W.B. Saunders Co.

Hematologic disorders in the newborn period

Clarke, C.A., and Cantab, S.D.: Prevention of rhesus isoimmunization, Lancet **2:**1, 1968.

Hall, J.G., et al.: Thrombocytopenia with absent radius (TAR), Medicine (Baltimore) **48:**411, 1969.

Jensen, A.H.-B., et al.: Evolution of blood clotting factor levels in premature infants during the first 10 days of life: a study of 96 cases with comparison between clinical status and blood clotting factor levels, Pediatr. Res. **7:**638, 1973.

Kanto, W.P., Jr., et al.: ABO hemolytic disease: a comparative study of clinical severity and delayed anemia, Pediatrics **62:**365, 1978.

McIntosh, S., et al.: Neonatal isoimmune purpura: response to platelet infusions, J. Pediatr. **82:**1020, 1973.

Mull, M.M., and Hathaway, W.E.: Altered platelet function in newborns, Pediatr. Res. **4:**229, 1970.

Naiman, L.J.: Current management of hemolytic disease of the newborn infant, J. Pediatr. **80:**1049, 1972.

Nammacher, M.A., et al.: Vitamin K deficiency in infants beyond the neonatal period, J. Pediatr. **76:**549, 1970.

Sutherland, J.M., et al.: Hemorrhagic disease of the newborn, Am. J. Dis. Child. **113:**524, 1967.

16 Digestive System

This chapter is divided into sections discussing the upper gastrointestinal tract, small intestine and colon, liver, and pancreas. Each section reviews common symptoms and disorders that affect children.

UPPER GASTROINTESTINAL TRACT

Vomiting

Vomiting is initiated by stimulation of the central vomiting center in the dorsal lateral reticular formation in the medulla. Afferents to this center may come from the chemoreceptor trigger zone in the floor of the fourth ventricle initiated by drugs, toxins, or metabolic derangements, from peripheral sites (gastrointestinal tract from antrum to colon, biliary tract, mesenteric vasculature, peritoneum, heart, and pharynx), or from supramedullary receptors that cause psychic vomiting and vomiting in response to tastes and odors, from vestibular disease, and from "motion sickness." In contrast to true vomiting, which involves forceful contraction of abdominal musculature with closed pylorus and open lower esophageal sphincter, regurgitation and gastroesophageal reflux are effortless phenomena. They are included here as vomiting because initially the three are difficult to differentiate.

Vomiting is a symptom of a variety of disorders that range from quite benign to lethal.

- I. Central vomiting center
  - A. Drugs, toxins
  - B. Metabolic causes
    1. Diabetic ketoacidosis, diabetes insipidus, lactic acidosis
    2. Phenylketonuria, maple syrup urine disease, methylmalonic acidemia
    3. Hereditary fructose intolerance, glactosemia
    4. Urea cycle defects
    5. Uremia, renal tubular acidosis
    6. Pregnancy, congenital adrenal hyperplasia
- II. Supramedullary receptors
  - A. Psychogenic vomiting, tastes and odors
  - B. Vestibular disease, "motion sickness"
  - C. Increased intracerebral pressure
    1. Subdural effusion or hematoma
    2. Meningoencephalitis
    3. Cerebral edema or tumor, Reye syndrome
    4. Hydrocephalus
- III. Peripheral receptors
  - A. Pharyngeal
    1. Gag reflex
  - B. Gastric
    1. Peptic ulcer disease
    2. Motility disorder
  - C. Intestinal
    1. Infectious gastroenteritis
    2. Enterotoxin
    3. Appendicitis
    4. Carbohydrate and protein intolerance
  - D. Intestinal obstruction
    1. Bezoar
    2. Pyloric stenosis
    3. Web
    4. Superior mesenteric artery syndrome
    5. Atresia
    6. Meconium ileus
    7. Intusseception, volvulus, adhesions
    8. Meconium plug, Hirschsprung disease
  - E. Biliary
    1. Cholecystitis
  - F. Pancreatic
    1. Pancreatitis
  - G. Peritoneal
    1. Peritonitis
- IV. Regurgitation: esophageal disease
  - A. Neuromuscular
    1. Pharynogoesophageal dysphagia
    2. Esophageal body motility disorders
    3. Achalasia
    4. Gastroesophageal reflux
  - B. Structural
    1. Congenital malformation
    2. Stricture

Normal infant "spitting" is a physiologic gastroesophageal reflux that disappears as infants mature. It may be recognized by history and observation of feeding and is not associated with weight loss, respiratory problems, esophagitis, or apnea. This normal reflux may be exacerbated by poor feeding technique, including allowing air to be sucked through the nipple, inadequate burping, or shaking of the infant.

Observing feeding and vomiting is helpful in determining its cause. The choking caused by upper esophageal motility disorders can be differentiated from the "tipping over and pouring out" of achalasia, the effortless regurgitation caused by gastroesophageal reflux, and the projectile vomiting of pyloric stenosis. The child with an acute surgical abdomen or a metabolic cause for vomiting usually will be sick, as opposed to the child with reflux. Acute onset points to problems such as toxic ingestions, infections, or acute abdomen. Vomiting of bilious material should suggest intestinal obstruction, whereas the vomiting of partially digested food hours after eating suggests a gastric motility disorder or outlet obstruction. Early identification of signs of increased intracranial pressure may be lifesaving. Vomiting of particular foods may suggest specific metabolic disorders, as in galactosemia or hereditary fructose intolerance. Diarrhea suggests an infectious gastroenteritis or a partial obstruction. The menstrual and sexual history may suggest pregnancy, and a history of stress may suggest psychogenic vomiting.

The most common early complication of vomiting is dehydration with abnormalities in electrolyte and acid base balance, especially hypokalemic metabolic alkalosis. Chronic vomiting may produce malnutrition. Aspiration and Mallory-Weiss tears are potentially dangerous complications of vomiting.

In general, treatment of the cause of vomiting is more important than treatment of the vomiting itself. However, vomiting may have enough independent morbidity that the symptom itself requires treatment. Currently, metoclopramide is one of the most useful drugs for control of vomiting. Other drugs used for symptomatic treatment of vomiting are diphenhydramine, phenothiazine, and tetrahydrocannabinol.

Hematemesis. Vomiting of blood, either red (unaltered by gastric acid) or brown, coffee-ground appearing (denatured by acid), may occur from any lesion proximal to the ligament of Treitz. The most common causes of gastrointestinal bleeding are listed below.

I. Hematemesis
    A. Esophagitis
    B. Mallory-Weiss syndrome
    C. Gastritis
    D. Gastric ulcer
    E. Duodenal ulcer
    F. Esophageal varices
II. Melena
    A. Esophagitis
    B. Gastritis
    C. Gastric ulcer
    D. Duodenal ulcer
    E. Crohn disease
    F. Ulcerative colitis
    G. Angiodysplasia
    H. Polyps
    I. Henoch-Schönlein purpura
    J. Meckle diverticulum
    K. Blood dyscrasias
    L. Infectious colitis
III. Hematochezia
    A. Hemorrhoids
    B. Anal fissure
    C. Ulcerative colitis
    D. Polyps
    E. Crohn disease
    F. Angiodysplasia
    G. Infectious colitis

Gastrointestinal bleeding must be carefully differentiated from ingested blood that often comes from the lungs or upper respiratory tract.

Anorexia and dysphagia

Anorexia, or the absence of desire to eat, may be caused by any systemic illness, although the pathophysiology of this phenomenon is unclear. It may also be psychogenic such as anorexia nervosa or a child's response to forced feeding. Various drugs may cause anorexia, including aminophylline, sulfasalazine, and various antineoplastic agents. Dysphagia or other gastrointestinal symptoms may initially appear as anorexia. Because the act of eating has produced discomfort, the patient may appear disinterested in eating.

Dysphagia, or inability to suck, eat, or swallow, may be caused by structural lesions that result in mechanical narrowing or discomfort or by neuromuscular disorders. These are enumerated below.

I. Structural or mechanical narrowing
    A. Gross structural lesions, including congenital deformities
        1. Palate: cleft
        2. Tongue: macroglossia, cyst, lymphangioma, other tumor
        3. Nasopharynx: choanal atresia
        4. Mandible: micrognathia
        5. Temporomandibular joint: ankylosis
        6. Pharynx: cyst, diverticula
        7. Esophagus: atresia, web, stenosis, vascular ring

- B. Inflammatory (infectious, allergic, corrosive) acquired conditions
  1. Stomatitis
  2. Pharyngitis
  3. Esophagitis or stricture
- II. Neuromuscular deficits
  - A. Prematurity
  - B. Mental retardation
  - C. Cerebral palsy
  - D. Werdnig-Hoffmann disease
  - E. Muscular dystrophy
  - F. Myasthenia
  - G. Pharyngeal (cricopharyngeal, oropharyngeal, pharyngoesophageal) discoordination
  - H. Achalasia
  - I. Guillain-Barré syndrome
  - J. Diphtheria
  - K. Tetanus
  - L. Polio
  - M. Riley-Day syndrome
  - N. Prader-Willi syndrome
  - O. de Lange syndrome

Symptomatology may define the etiology of dysphagia. Structural lesions are characterized by the earlier onset of dysphagia for solids than for liquids, whereas the opposite is true for neuromuscular lesions. Whether the symptoms are static or progressive may narrow the differential diagnosis. The association of other neuromuscular symptoms will point to a neuromuscular etiology and may also suggest the specific diagnosis.

Diagnosis of gross structural lesions causing dysphagia is aided by endoscopy. Visualization and biopsy of inflammatory lesions are useful. A barium esophagram will demonstrate those lesions visible in profile. A cine-esophagram and manometry are helpful in neuromuscular disorders.

Specific therapy, often surgical, is available for some causes of dysphagia. If therapy is not available, nutrition must be delivered either by nasogastric tube, by gastrostomy, or parenterally.

Ingestion of a foreign body

Small children frequently ingest foreign bodies. A surprising variety of objects such as nails, tacks, pins, pennies, and dimes will safely pass out of the stomach and transit the bowel without difficulty if enough time is given. Larger coins such as nickels and quarters occasionally get caught in the esophagus and, if they get to the stomach, frequently will not pass through the pylorus. One can often remove coins from the esophagus by passing a Foley catheter beyond the coin, blowing up the Foley balloon, and withdrawing the catheter and coin. Coins and foreign bodies that remain in the stomach more than 1 month should be removed by flexible endoscopy. Nickels, which are corrosive, and some sharp objects should be removed more quickly. Only rarely will a foreign body pass out of the stomach and get caught in the terminal ileum, which requires surgical removal.

Abdominal pain

Pain is the sensation resulting from noxious stimulation of peripheral receptors. The type and intensity of the perceived pain will depend on the stimulus, the affected tissue, and several psychophysiologic factors. Abdominal pain may derive from the injury of any of the abdominopelvic organs or from referred sensory input. Also, injury to abdominal organs may cause pain to be referred to other locations.

Abdominal pain may be separated into visceral and parietal pain. Visceral pain is felt when an abdominal viscus is stimulated. The principal stimuli that result in visceral pain are stretching or tension in the wall of the gut or other hollow viscus or stretching of the capsule of a solid viscus. Inflammation can also result in visceral pain. The pain is usually dull, aching or crampy, nausea producing, and poorly localized. It is not accompanied by tenderness and is not exacerbated by movement. Localization is very poor, and pain is almost always felt in the midline at, above, or below the umbilicus. Since tenderness is absent, the physical examination will often fail to localize the site of disease unless a mass or enlarged viscus is evident. Its onset is acute because rapidly developing physical distortion of the viscus is required for its production. Parietal pain is produced by noxious stimulation of the parietal peritoneum. Inflammation, chemical agents, and physical stimuli all can produce parietal pain. The pain is usually intense, sharply localized, and accompanied by direct or rebound tenderness. The patient often lies perfectly still in an attempt to relieve the discomfort. Localization is precise, and finding an associated area of tenderness pinpoints the area of disease.

Referred pain is felt in areas supplied by the same neurosensory segment as the diseased tissue. Central mixing of peripheral input results in pain sensation in remote areas. The pain is often intense, sharply localized, and involving the skin. Generally, referred pain appears as the stimulus worsens. Pain may be referred from the abdomen, as with pancreatic, duodenal, and gallbladder pain to the back, or to the abdomen, as with pneumonia.

Acute abdominal pain, the "acute abdomen," occurring in a child who has been unaffected by chronic or recurrent pain, suggests the recent onset of a disease process that produces a noxious stimulus to visceral or parietal receptors. A partial listing of diseases that can produce acute abdominal pain follows.

- I. Visceral causes
  - A. Intestinal obstruction, partial or complete
    1. Intussusception
    2. Incarcerated hernia
    3. Intestinal volvulus
    4. Fecal impaction
    5. Adhesions
    6. Congenital anomalies
  - B. Urinary tract distention
    1. Ureteral obstruction
    2. Renal distention (pyelonephritis)
  - C. Hepatic-biliary distention
    1. Hepatitis
    2. Acute steatosis
    3. Gallstone
    4. Choledochal cyst
- II. Peritoneal causes
  - A. Generalized peritonitis
  - B. Localized peritonitis
    1. Appendicitis
    2. Abdominal abscess
    3. Pancreatitis
    4. Peptic ulcer
    5. Pelvic inflammatory disease, Fitz-Hugh-Curtis syndrome
    6. Inflammatory bowel disease
    7. Meckel diverticulitis
    8. Cholecystitis
- III. Extraabdominal causes
  - A. Thoracic
    1. Pneumonia
    2. Esophagitis
    3. Asthma
  - B. Metabolic
    1. Diabetes mellitus
    2. Acute intermittent porphyria
  - C. Miscellaneous
    1. Abdominal epilepsy
    2. Muscle contusion

Care must be taken to exclude the possibility of one of the surgical disorders, as delay in diagnosis may compromise chances of successful surgery. Acute appendicitis commonly causes difficulty in this regard, but an occasional unneccesary exploration to exclude the disease is preferable to missing one that causes a rupture that could have been prevented.

Recurrent abdominal pain is a symptom complex that affects 10% to 15% of school-aged children. Pain is usually periumbilical or epigastric in location and bears no constant temporal relationship to any intestinal function. It occurs any time, but rarely awakens the patient. Pallor, tiredness, anorexia, headache, and vomiting are frequently associated, and affected children miss an average of 1 in 10 days of school. The physical examination is usually normal, but occasionally mild epigastric tenderness is found. Despite its importance, its causes remain enigmatic. Fewer than 10% of cases are specifically diagnosed.

In the 90% of cases of recurrent pain in which no specific diagnosis can be made, the pain is termed *functional* and is thought to reflect difficulties in coping with stressful situations. It is the child's signal of distress. Many times there are family problems, such as marital discord, psychiatric illness, or hypochondriasis, or problems in school. Many affected children are perfectionists. Also, there may be a relationship to the irritable colon syndrome: family histories are often illustrative, and the patients commonly have a typical stooling pattern.

Organic causes of recurrent pain are numerous but constitute only a small fraction of the total cases. Among the recognized causes are primary acquired lactase deficiency, urinary tract disease, inflammatory bowel disease, chronic hepatitis, pancreatitis, and migraine. Heretofore, peptic disease has been given minor consideration in the genesis of recurrent pain in children, but recently it has been found to be more important. Gastroduodenoscopy has demonstrated a spectrum of disease, including gastritis or duodenitis and peptic ulcer, much of which would have remained undiagnosed by conventional radiographic techniques. It is impossible at this time to determine the fraction of children with recurrent pain who suffer with peptic disease, but it is of major importance.

Gastroesophageal reflux and reflux esophagitis

Reflux of gastric material into the esophagus occurs occasionally in most people, especially postprandially. The lower esophageal sphincter and gravity provide the main antireflux forces, which must combat the tendency of intragastric pressure to cause gastroesophageal reflux. Pathologic gastroesophageal reflux occurs when abnormalities in the lower esophageal sphincter function and increases in intragastric pressure allow episodes of gastroesophageal reflux that are more frequent or longer than normal.

Gastroesophageal reflux may have almost any of the varied symptoms outlined below.

I. Regurgitation
   A. Vomiting
   B. Rumination
   C. Wet pillow
   D. Waterbrash
   E. Halitosis
   F. Failure to thrive, malnutrition, weight loss
II. Esophagitis
   A. Heartburn
   B. Dysphagia
   C. Anemia, hematemesis, hemoccult-positive stool
   D. Irritability
III. Pulmonary symptoms
   A. Pneumonia
   B. Bronchitis
   C. Asthma
   D. Cough
   E. Abcess
   F. Atelectasis
   G. Apnea, sudden infant death syndrome, laryngospasm, stridor
IV. Neuropsychologic symptoms
   A. "Seizures," "spells," mouthing, staring
   B. Dystonia, Sandifer syndrome
   C. Irritability

Diagnostic evaluation begins with a careful history and observation of feeding and emesis or other symptom. The most useful diagnostic tests depend on the question to be answered. If the question is "Is there pathologic gastroesophageal reflux?", the most helpful test is the esophageal pH probe evaluation, scintiscan and barium swallow being much less sensitive and specific. If the question is "Are the child's symptoms caused by esophagitis?", the Bernstein test (if "heartburn" is the symptom), or the pH probe is most helpful. If the question is "Is the gastroesophageal reflux causing esophagitis?", esophageal biopsy is far more sensitive than endoscopy or barium swallow. If the question is "Is a low pressure present in the lower esophageal sphincter and does it respond to bethanecol?", then manometry is indicated.

Gastroesophageal reflux therapy falls into three categories outlined below.

I. Conservative
   A. Positioning
      1. Upright
      2. Elevation of head of bed
      3. Prone
   B. Meals
      1. Small (but frequent may be detrimental)
      2. Thickened (but unproved)
      3. Not before reclining
   C. Weight loss
      1. Loose clothing
   D. Avoid (because of detrimental effect on lower esophageal sphincter pressure)
      1. Fat
      2. Chocolate
      3. Alcohol
      4. Nicotine
      5. Peppermint
      6. Spearmint
      7. Theophylline
      8. Isoproterenol
      9. Sedatives
      10. Irritants and acid food (citrus, tomato, coffee)
   E. Ingest (because of beneficial effect on lower esophageal sphincter pressure)
      1. Antacids
      2. Proteins
II. Medical
   A. Antacid therapy
      1. Antacids
      2. Cimetidine
   B. Barrier
      1. Alaginic acid or antacid
   C. Lower esophageal sphincter pressure
      1. Bethanechol
      2. Metoclopramide
      3. Domperidone
III. Surgical
   A. Fundoplication (Nissen operation)
   B. Treatment of complications
      1. Stricture dilation
      2. Bowel interposition

Conservative therapy, in addition to being the background on which other therapy is added, is useful temporizing treatment for infants whose "developmental" gastroesophageal reflux is without pathologic effect on weight, esophageal mucosa, or pulmonary function. Reassurance is a large portion of the therapy in such patients. A combination of bethanecol or metaclopramide with the conservative therapy will help patients with pathologic gastroesophageal reflux caused by decreased lower esophageal sphincter pressure. Antacid therapy will help many patients because of the tendency of gastric acidity to cause esophagitis and decrease the lower esophageal sphincter pressure. Patients whose pathologic gastroesophageal reflux continues in spite of maximal medical management and who continue to lose weight or to have esophagitis or pulmonary symptoms will usually benefit from surgical therapy such as the Nissen procedure.

Corrosive esophagitis

Esophagitis may be caused by ingestion of caustic substances that are commonly alkali (sodium hydoxide—lye; sodium carbonate—nonphosphate detergents; etc.), but may be acid as well. Symptoms include acute onset of oral and chest pain, drooling, and vomiting. If perforation and mediastinitis do not occur, initial symptoms will usually resolve over several days, but may be followed later by increasing dysphagia as stricture forms (see below). Because oral burns can occur in the absence of esophageal burns and vice versa, endoscopy within the first 24 hours is imperative for determining management. Patients with esophageal burns require observation in the hospital and may benefit from antacid therapy, steroids, antibiotics, or early dilation. Patients who do not respond adequately to medical management of their esophageal burns may require chronic esophageal dilation or surgical replacement of the esophagus.

A relatively minor type of caustic esophageal burn may be caused by various ingested medications such as several antibiotics, nonsteroidal anti-inflammatory agents, potassium (including liquid forms), and chemotherapeutic agents (fluorouracil). They occur when prolonged contact with the mucosa is allowed by structural or motility disturbances of the esophagus, or by the patient's failure to take medication with adequate liquid while in an upright position. Since these burns are usually neither deep nor circumferential, they most often resolve without sequelae if the predisposing condition is corrected.

Stricture

Chronic esophagitis or severe acute caustic esophagitis may produce circumferential scarring, or stricture, of the esophagus. Symptoms of esophageal stricture are dysphagia and regurgitation, and diagnosis is by barium esophogram or endoscopy. Treatment of esophageal strictures with intermittent dilation, although not pleasant, usually obviates the need for surgery. Surgical treatments include stricture resection and intestinal interposition.

Peptic ulcer disease

The term *peptic ulcer disease* has in the past been used to describe chronic idiopathic ulcer disease of the duodenum and stomach. More accurately, the term should refer to a spectrum of idiopathic diseases of the stomach and duodenum that includes functional dyspepsia, gastritis, duodenitis, gastric ulcer, and duodenal ulcer. Until recently, this group of diseases was rarely diagnosed in children, but the use of upper gastrointestinal endoscopy has led to more frequent recognition. Now peptic ulcer disease is recognized to affect all age groups, including infants and children.

The etiology of peptic ulcer disease is unknown but includes hypersecretion of gastric acid, an abnormal mucus barrier in the stomach and duodenum, reduced mucosal resistance to back diffusion of hydrogen ions, bile reflux, and abnormal gastric and duodenal motility. Increased incidence of peptic ulcer disease in some families suggests that hereditary factors may be important. Psychosomatic factors may be important, but the exact psychodynamics involved are not defined. Caffeine, cigarette smoking, aspirin, and alcohol also predispose a person to have peptic ulcer disease. Steroid therapy has been implicated by some observers as causing ulcer, but careful analysis of large groups of patients with rheumatoid arthritis receiving steroid treatment has failed to support this association.

The most common symptom in peptic ulcer disease is pain that is chronic, rhythmic, periodic, and usually in the epigastric area. It may last for days or weeks only to disappear for weeks or months before returning. The pain may be relieved by eating or by using antacids. The patient with peptic ulcer disease is often awakened at night by pain. Location and severity of pain does not correlate well with severity of pathology in peptic ulcer disease. Vomiting is a prominent complaint and intermittent diarrhea is occasionally observed. The only physical finding of importance in peptic ulcer disease is tenderness in the epigastrium.

Diagnosis of peptic ulcer disease depends on upper gastrointestinal endoscopy or upper gastrointestinal barium x-ray studies. Endoscopy allows inspection and biopsy of the mucosa, making it useful in diagnosing gastritis, duodenitis, and ulcer. Barium upper gastrointestinal x-ray studies may demonstrate ulcer craters and spasm but lack sensitivity. The use of air-contrast technique increases the efficiency of x-ray studies.

The cornerstones of therapy in peptic ulcer disease are antacids, histamine-2 receptor blockers, and anticholinergics. The histamine-2 receptor blocker cimetidine is very effective, making it the most prescribed drug in the world. Cimetidine reduces acid production by gastric parietal cells, allowing healing of injured mucosa. The drug is given in doses of 200 to 300 mg before meals and at bedtime. Antacids are time-honored and effective therapy for peptic ulcer disease if used properly. They are given every 2 to 4 hours in acute disease and, when symptoms are decreased, four times a day, 1½ hours after meals and at bedtime. The anticholingergic drug propantheline may be used to reduce gastric acid secretion. A new drug, which works by coating the injured mucosa, is sucralfate. Diet therapy plays little role in ulcer therapy. Patients with peptic ulcer should be allowed a regular diet and encouraged to eat at regular hours.

Recurrence of peptic ulcer disease is characteristic and represents one of the major problems in therapy. Long-term, low-dose medication may be required to prevent recurrence of disease and to reduce symptoms. Complications of peptic ulcer disease include melena, hematemesis, gastric outlet obstruction, and rarely, perforation.

SMALL INTESTINE AND COLON

Diarrhea

Diarrhea was defined by Hippocrates as an abnormal frequency and liquidity of fecal discharge: both frequency and liquidity must be abnormal before the definition is satisfied. A more explicit definition would be fecal water excretion in excess of 100 g/m^2/day. Disorders that cause diarrhea may be classified in several ways, but they act to produce diarrhea in a limited number of ways: by causing intestinal secretion, through osmotic forces, or by interfering with normal fluid absorption.

Normal fluid balance in the small bowel is preserved by a balance of absorptive and secretory forces. Fluid absorption is a principal function of villus epithelium, whereas secretion takes place in the crypts. Secretion normally proceeds at a rate equal to 4 to 5 times the ingested fluid volume, but absorption compensates and there is no net fluid movement into the small intestine. Most of the remaining fluid is absorbed in the colon so that fecal fluid output is one tenth to one fifteenth of intake. Anything causing secretion to increase to the point that absorption by the small intestine and colon cannot compensate will result in diarrhea. Some of the diseases in which this occurs are listed below.

- I. Osmotic diarrhea
  - A. Non-absorbable solute
    - 1. $MgSO_4$, mannitol, lactulose
  - B. Malabsorbed solute
    - 2. Carbohydrate malabsorption
- II. Secretory diarrhea
  - A. Bacterial enterotoxin (exotoxin)
    - 1. Cholera (experimental model)
    - 2. *Escherichia coli* (traveler's diarrhea)
  - B. Viral enteritis
    - 1. Piglet diarrhea (experimental model)
    - 2. Human rotavirus
    - 3. Norwalk agent
  - C. Tumor-hormone associated
    - 1. Zollinger-Ellison syndrome
    - 2. Vasoactive intestinal polypeptide producing tumor (pancreatic cholera)
    - 3. Neural crest tumors
    - 4. Medullary thyroid carcinoma
  - D. Polyposis coli
  - E. Malabsorbed secretagogue
    - 1. Dihydroxy-bile acids
    - 2. Hydroxy-fatty acids
- III. Salt H_2O malabsorption
  - A. Congenital chloride diarrhea
  - B. Colitis
    - 1. Ulcerative colitis
    - 2. Hirschsprung disease
  - C. Malabsorbed inhibitors of absorption
    - 3. Dihydroxy-bile acids
    - 4. Hydroxy-fatty acids
- IV. Disorders with multiple causality
  - A. Maldigestion syndromes
  - B. Generalized malabsorption syndromes
    - 1. Gluten-sensitive enteropathy
  - C. Inflammatory bowel disease
  - D. Acute nonbacterial enteritis
  - E. Bacterial enterocolitis
    - 1. Shigellosis
    - 2. Salmonellosis

Some diseases, such as cholera, cause massive fluid losses that continue even during periods when nothing is taken by mouth, and absorption is unaffected. Treatment can be effected by oral rehydration using fluids such as those endorsed by the World Health Organization. Others are associated with absorptive defects and are not as easily treated.

Osmotically active substances that are ingested and not absorbed cause diarrhea by pulling water into the gut. Some, such as $MgSO_4$ and sorbitol, are not normally absorbed and will result in diarrhea whenever ingested in quantity. Carbohydrates are the most important nutrient that may be malabsorbed and cause osmotic diarrhea. Patients with primary or secondary lactase deficiency or other carbohydrate malabsorption syndromes experience cramps and diarrhea on ingesting the malabsorbed sugar; normally absorbed sugars have no effect. Carbohydrates that enter the colon undergo fermentation, producing smaller, more osmotically active carbon fragments and enhancing the inward movement of water. Organic acids are formed, and the fecal pH drops to below 5.0. Measuring stool pH and reducing substances may help to diagnose carbohydrate malabsorption as the cause of diarrhea. Hydrogen produced during fermentation can be detected in the breath and is a sensitive indicator of carbohydrate malabsorption. Also, such diarrhea ceases when oral intake is stopped.

Failure of normal fluid absorption is an infrequent cause of diarrhea. Congenital chloride diarrhea is a rare condition in which the normal anion exchange mechanism in the ileum and colon is nonfunctional, resulting in the fecal excretion of enormous volumes of isotonic fluid with chloride concentrations of 100 to 120 mEq/L. This results in hypochloremic metabolic acidosis, which requires lifelong treatment with large oral loads of sodium chloride and potassium chloride. Other diseases that may occasionally demonstrate similar physiology are diffuse colitis (the degree of alkalosis correlates with the severity of the disease), bile salt malabsorption (these detergents interfere with colonic fluid absorption), and cystic fibrosis (the mechanism is not known).

Many diseases produce diarrhea by more than one mechanism, making it difficult to understand the pathophysiology. However, simple diagnostic tests are often very helpful. Allowing the patient nothing by mouth and observing the response will indicate the dependency of the diarrhea on oral intake. Measuring stool electrolytes, osmolality, and pH and reducing substances yields much information. If the osmolality is greater than twice the level of sodium and potassium, the diarrhea has an osmotic component. A high chloride level suggests a failure of fluid absorption. Low pH and positive reducing substances indicate carbohydrate malabsorption. Specific diagnosis depends on finding a pathogen in the stool, the histopathology, and the results of radiographic examinations or other investigations, but knowing the pathophysiology will help direct treatment.

Because diarrhea is a symptom of many disorders, effective treatment depends on accurate diagnosis of etiology. In general, correction of fluid and electrolyte abnormalities should be the primary concern (see Chapter 10). It is important in this regard to remember ongoing fecal fluid loss when calculating maintenance fluid requirements, especially when dealing with a patient with secretory diarrhea. Special attention should be given to potassium depletion because of fecal potassium loss and enhanced aldosterone production with potassium excretion in the urine. Once fluid and electrolyte balance is corrected, one should investigate the cause of diarrhea before initiating specific therapy.

Malassimilation and failure to thrive

Failure to thrive is a term applied to infants and children who exhibit subnormal growth, which can be symmetric (height, weight, and occipitofrontal circumference are equally diminished) or asymmetric. Failure to thrive secondary to gastrointestinal disease is usually asymmetric and produces thin children who appear undernourished. In such a patient, several pathophysiologic conditions must be considered. The first possibility is that inadequate nutrients are being delivered to the tissues. This can result from exogenous malnutrition, as is common in the Third World, or in child neglect; anorexia, as can be seen in psychosocial deprivation and in infants with systemic disease; excess regurgitation, as with pyloric stenosis; or malassimilation. The second possibility is that, once absorbed, nutrients are being wasted. This occurs with loss from the body, as with extensive dermatoses, burns, and renal tubular disorders. Conditions that prevent nutrient use, such as chronic systemic acidosis and micronutrient deficiency, also result in waste. The final possibility is excess nutrient requirement. Hypermetabolism, as with hyperthyroidism and severe skeletal muscle hypertonia, produces excessive nutrient use. Although not the only cause of failure to thrive, gastrointestinal disease should be considered first in the apparently undernourished infant.

Gastrointestinal disease produces undernutrition by causing anorexia, vomiting, or malassimilation of nutrients. The first two are discussed elsewhere in this chapter. Malassimilation of nutrients results from maldigestion or malabsorption, which are discussed here. Specific disorders causing malassimilation are listed below.

- I. Isolated defects
  - A. Fat malabsorption
    - 1. Hepatobiliary
      - a. Various cholestatic disorders
    - 2. Pancreatic
      - a. Congenital lipase deficiency
      - b. Congenital colipase deficiency
    - 3. Proximal mucosal
      - a. Abetalipoproteinemia
      - b. Lymphangiectasia
    - 4. Distal mucosal
      - a. Bile salt malabsorption (Crohn disease, resection)
  - B. Carbohydrate malabsorption
    - 1. Pancreatic
      - a. Congenital amylase deficiency
    - 2. Mucosal
      - a. Hereditary lactase deficiency (congenital deficiency is rare)
      - b. Sucrase-isomaltase deficiency
      - c. Glucose-galactose transport deficiency
  - C. Protein malabsorption
    - 1. Pancreatic
      - a. Enterokinase deficiency
      - b. Trypsin deficiency
      - c. Other peptidase deficiencies (asymptomatic)
    - 2. Mucosal
      - a. Hartnup disease, cystinuria, iminoglycinuria, Oasthouse disease, and blue diaper syndrome
- II. Generalized defects
  - A. Pancreatic
    - 1. Cystic fibrosis
    - 2. Schwachman syndrome
    - 3. Chronic or recurrent pancreatitis
  - B. Mucosal
    - 1. Nonspecific biopsy "flat villus lesion"
    - 2. Infections
      - a. Acute and chronic infections
      - b. Bacterial overgrowth, stasis, stagnant loop, and blind loop
      - c. Tropical sprue
    - 3. Allergic or intolerance reactions
      - a. Protein sensitivity (cow milk, soy, human milk, etc.)
      - b. Gluten-sensitivity enteropathy (celiac)
    - 4. Toxic or ischemic reactions
      - a. Radiation, ischemia, and neomycin
    - 5. Malnutrition
      - a. Kwashiorkor
    - 6. Immunodeficiency
    - 7. Specific biopsy
      - a. Eosinophilic gastroenteropathy
      - b. Abetalipoproteinemia, lymphangiectasia, and lymphoma
      - c. *Giardia, Strongyloides, Coccidia*
      - d. Whipple disease
      - e. Collagenous sprue
  - C. Distal mucosal
    - 1. Crohn disease, resection, and necrotizing enterocolitis

Maldigestion is the failure of the intraluminal phase of nutrient processing that results in the fecal excretion of nutrients in excess of the normally expected waste. In general, intraluminal digestion is dependent on normal gastrointestinal motility, pancreatic digestive enzymes (amylase, lipase, colipase, and various peptidases), adequate concentrations of bile salts, and a normal intraluminal pH. Failure of any one of these mechanisms may result in significant maldigestion. It can be diagnosed by demonstrating excessive fecal excretion of nutrients and, at the same time, normal mucosal absorption. Specific disorders of maldigestion are diagnosed most accurately by duodenal intubation and analysis of fluid produced after cholecystokinin-pancreozymin stimulation. However, it is rarely necessary to perform this invasive test because by far the most common pancreatic cause of malabsorption is cystic fibrosis, which can be diagnosed by the sweat test. Also, jaundice will usually implicate cholestasis before it is suggested by malabsorption.

Malabsorption is the failure of the mucosal phase of nutrient processing and also results in excessive fecal excretion of nutrients. Malabsorption may be general, as with celiac disease, or isolated, as with primary lactase deficiency. Specific malabsorption of several micronutrients has been described. Malabsorption can be diagnosed by demonstrating excessive fecal nutrient loss and a mucosal defect.

Diffuse intestinal lesions causing a mucosal defect in absorption will usually produce a low level of serum *d*-xylose 1 hour after the ingestion of a standard dose (0.5 g/kg). In a patient with a low *d*-xylose, specific diagnoses may be defined by the use of peroral small bowel biopsy. Distal ileal lesions are identified by the Schilling test and postprandial serum bile salt evaluation.

Malassimilation usually causes diarrhea, which is a major clue to a gastrointestinal etiology for failure to thrive. Diarrhea results from osmotic forces exerted by the malabsorbed nutrients, principally carbohydrates, and from secretion induced by fatty acids and bile salts. Diarrhea is not uniformly associated with malassimilation, and its absence should not preclude proper investigation.

Several tests assist in the evaluation of maldigested or malabsorbed nutrients. Stool pH and reducing substances will be abnormal in carbohydrate malassimilation. Specific carbohydrate tolerance tests (lactose, sucrose, and glucose) demonstrate the failure of an ingested carbohydrate to appear in the serum. Screening for fat malassimilation can be accomplished using stool spot fat or by the more sensitive 72-hour stool fat test. These tests and the stool tests for carbohydrate malassimilation are meaningless unless an adequate amount of the nutrient is being ingested. Protein malabsorption is more difficult to define. A nitrogen balance study is a useful research tool, and serum albumin and prealbumin, with its shorter half life, provide a clinical measure of protein nutrient status.

Fig. 16-1 is a schematic for evaluation of chronic diarrhea and possible malassimilation in children.

Protein-losing enteropathy

Excessive protein loss into the intestinal lumen is a symptom common to many disorders. The typical clinical presentation in childhood is edema with hypoproteinemia. A child who has these symptoms should be suspected of having protein-losing enteroptathy, especially if other causes of protein loss or reduced synthesis have been excluded.

Protein-*losing* enteropathy is a misnomer; it should be termed *intestinal hypercatabolism of serum protein*. Normally, the intestine is the site of catabolism of 10% of serum albumin, and in the steady state hepatic synthesis equals catabolism by all sources. With excessive loss by any means, the rate of albumin synthesis increases, but the maximum synthetic rate is only about three times the basal rate. In most instances of protein-losing enteropathy, serum proteins are lost into the proximal gut lumen, but the constituent amino acids are reabsorbed after digestion. Excessive fecal nitrogen loss does not occur. The balance between intestinal catabolism and hepatic synthesis determines the level of serum albumin. If the rate of catabolism exceeds the maximum synthetic rate, serum concentration falls.

The loss of serum protein into the gut may occur by several mechanisms: increased mucosal permeability, mucosal ulceration, hypertension of mucosal lymphatics, and local microvascular injury. The diseases causing protein-losing enteropathy produce protein loss by these mechanisms: celiac disease by increased permeability, Crohn disease by ulceration, intestinal lymphangiectasia by hypertension of mucosal lymphatics, measles by microvascular injury, and eosinophilic gastroenteropathy perhaps by a combination of all four mechanisms.

Diagnosis of protein-losing enteropathy depends on documentation of enhanced protein loss into the gut. Circumstantial evidence, such as hypoproteinemia in a child with Crohn disease, may be so strong as to preclude the necessity of specific documentation, but usually it is not. Until recently, excessive enteric catabolism was most accurately documented by demonstrating supernormal fecal loss of ^{51}chromium after intravenous administration of tagged albumin. This test is no longer routinely available, and now the fecal clearance of alpha-1-antitrypsin is used. This protein is similar in size to albumin, but it resists digestion in the gut lumen and is lost in the stool. A timed stool collection and serum concentration give the data to calculate a clearance, which correlates closely with fecal ^{51}chromium loss. It should be remembered that protein-losing enteropathy is not a primary diagnosis but is only a symptom. Therapy depends on the cause and must be individualized.

Hematochezia and melena

The presence of blood in the stool is one of the most sensitive indicators of inflammatory or erosive bowel disease. Grossly apparent blood in the stool, hematochezia, results from bleeding anywhere in the colon. Lesions nearer the anus, especially fissure-in-ano, are evident with less bleeding. Melena, the passage of black, pitchlike stool that is strongly guaiac positive, results from voluminous bleeding anywhere from the esophagus to the ascending colon. Occult blood in the stool tested by guaiac or paper and developer kits results from bleeding from the mouth to the anus. The principal causes of gastrointestinal bleeding are presented on p. 331.

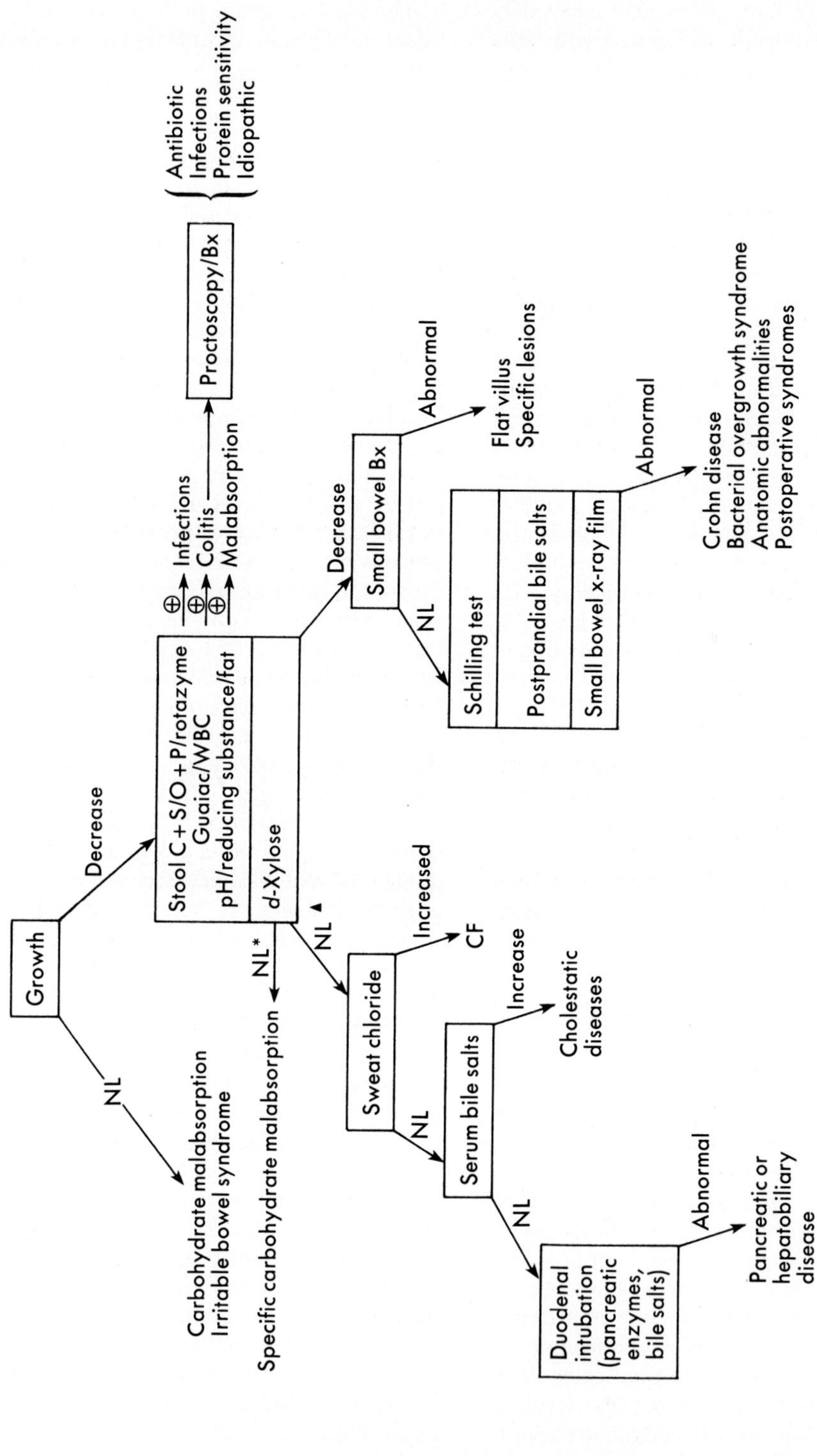

Fig. 16-1. Schematic for evaluating chronic diarrhea in pediatric patients.

Acute infectious enterocolitis

One of the most common problems encountered in pediatric practice is diarrhea and vomiting of acute onset. Such disease in infants and children is indicative of acute infectious gastroenteritis. Epidemics seen in cool months usually have viral etiology, whereas in summertime epidemics are more likely bacterial. Most healthy well-nourished infants and children can be expected to recover quickly, in 48 to 72 hours, with only minimal therapy. All patients with diarrhea and vomiting need careful management with attention to fluid intake and loss because of the possibility of dehydration.

The history is important. Contact with other children with a similar self-limited acute disease suggests viral disease. The presence of pet turtles in the home suggests *Salmonella,* a sick puppy suggests *Campylobacter,* and exposure to chickens or farm animals suggests *Salmonella* and *Campylobacter.*The prior use of antibotics suggests *Clostridium difficile* as a possible etiology. The physical examination in diarrhea is useful to rule out evidence of chronic disease or infection of other systems such as the urinary tract and the central nervous system and to help evaluate the degree of hydration.

A number of viruses have been suspected of causing diarrhea. Some Parvolike agents have been associated with single epidemics, but only human rotavirus has been firmly established as an etiologic agent in human infections. These infections have been recognized on all continents, in all races, and affecting all age groups. The agent has been responsible for 40% to 50% of children admitted with diarrhea in various children's hospitals. The peak incidence is in children below 4 years of age. Rotavirus invades the epithelium of the intestinal tract, usually just the upper intestine but occasionally the entire small bowel and colon.

Clinical manifestations of infection begin with vomiting and fever, followed in a few hours by profuse watery diarrhea. In the usual case, fever and vomiting abate in 24 to 36 hours, and a variable amount of anorexia and lethargy persists for a day or two. The diarrhea gradually diminishes and stops by the end of 5 to 6 days, the entire problem resolving without any serious threat to well-being. There is no specific therapy.

A bacterial cause can be identified in only 10% to 15% of children with severe diarrhea in North America. The incidence of bacterial diarrhea may be higher in the tropics and in populations with less than optimal nutrition. Prolonged diarrhea and presence of blood and pus in the stool suggest a bacterial etiology. *Salmonella, Shigella, Campylobacter, Yersinia,* and certain invasive *E. coli* produce disease by invasion of the mucosa. *Vibrio cholerae* and toxigenic *E. coli* produces toxins that induce diarrhea. Most bacterial infections of the gastrointestinal tract are of short duration, and by the time bacterial confirmation of the diagnosis is available the disease is waning. Gastroenteritis produced by *Campylobacter* is not altered by the use of antibiotics. However, use of erythromycin does shorten the duration of excretion of the organisms. Antibiotics have been shown to be of little help in treating *Salmonella* diarrhea and may be detrimental. In infections caused by *Yersinia, Shigella,* and pathogenic *E. coli,* appropriate antibiotic therapy is indicated.

Most cases of acute gastroenteritis in children do not require laboratory evaluation. If the general status of the patient is good, with only mild to moderate dehydration and acidosis, oral rehydration without extensive laboratory workup beyond blood count and urinalysis is safe and appropriate. Serum electrolytes and blood gases are needed only if there is severe dehydration, acidosis, or seizures. Persistent fever, diarrhea, or blood in the stools dictates that stools be examined and cultures be obtained. Stool examination should include smears for detection of white blood cells, occult blood, and a search for parasites and their ova. In persistent diarrhea suspected to be caused by rotavirus, the Rotazyme test may be useful.

Treatment of diarrhea in children is centered around replacement of fluid and electrolyte deficits and maintenance of fluid, electrolyte, and caloric intake. Children with acute gastroenteritis should be given clear liquids for 24 to 36 hours and then given formula and age-appropriate foods when accepted by the child. The oral rehydrating solution proposed by the World Health Organization (Table 16-1) can be given freely, and fluid and electrolyte deficits are usually corrected in 24 hours without using intravenous fluids. After dehydration is corrected the rehydrating solution may be continued along with water, diluted formula, and soft foods.

Table 16-1. Composition of World Health Organization Oral Rehydration Solution*

Ingredient	Concentration
Na+	90 mEq/L
Cl−	80 mEq/L
K+	20 mEq/L
HCO_3	30 mEq/L
Glucose	2 g/dL

*Powder (1 packet dilutes to 1 liter), cost/qt. ≈ 25¢.

There appears to be no reason to withhold foods for longer than the initial rehydration period. In small infants, avoiding lactose for 48 to 72 hours might be worthwhile because of secondary lactase deficiency following infectious enteritis.

In cases with greater than 10% dehydration (evidence of shock or decreased renal function) rehydration with intravenous fluids will be necessary (see Chapter 10). When shock is corrected and renal function is established, the oral rehydrating solution and water should be started.

Malabsorption syndrome

Malabsorption is the failure of the small intestine's normal absorptive function. Since abnormal fecal losses of nutrients will occur, they should be measured when the diagnosis is considered. Malabsorptive disorders may manifest as weight loss or failure to thrive, usually associated with diarrhea. Depending on the nutrient malabsorbed, stools may be watery, as in carbohydrate malabsorption, or may be foamy and malodorous, as in the generalized malabsorption syndromes. Malabsorptive disorders must be differentiated from maldigestive disorders (see Fig. 16-1), which may have identical symptoms. Another important initial step in their evaluation is the determination of which nutrients are being malabsorbed. These can be determined by measuring stool pH and reducing substances, which will be abnormal in carbohydrate malabsorption, and stool spot fat or 72-hour quantitative stool fat for fat malabsorption.

Isolated carbohydrate malabsorption causes watery, osmotic diarrhea and, rarely, malnutrition or dehydration. *Lactase deficiency* is the most common of the primary intestinal disaccharidase deficiencies. It usually is a primary acquired disorder that is very common in blacks, American Indians, and Eskimos and is present in increasing frequency with increasing age. It is uncommonly encountered as a congenital disease. Lactase deficiency is caused by deficiency of a single enzyme, intestinal lactase, and results in failure to hydrolyse the disaccharide lactose into its component monosaccharides. Symptoms of lactase deficiency are watery diarrhea, abdominal cramping, increased borborygmi, and a full feeling after the ingestion of milk. The diagnosis is established by an abnormal oral lactose tolerance test, enhanced excretion of breath hydrogen after ingestion of lactose, or demonstration of lactase deficiency in a mucosal specimen with normal histology. Treatment, as with all isolated carbohydrate malabsorption syndromes, is avoidance of the offending carbohydrate.

Isolated sucrase-isomaltase deficiency is a congenital defect in the enzyme system necessary for the hydrolysis of sucrose to glucose and fructose. The symptoms are identical to those of lactase deficiency except that they occur when sucrose is ingested, so patients become symptomatic when sucrose-containing formulas or prepared fruits or desserts are introduced into the diet. Establishment of the diagnosis is similar to that of isolated lactase deficiency.

Primary glucose-galactose malabsorption is a severe disorder that is symptomatic in the newborn. Failure of the normal active transport mechanism for glucose and galactose results in malabsorption of most normal dietary sugars.

Isolated *disorders of fat malabsorption* are infrequently encountered, the most common cause being *abetalipoproteinemia,* a disorder of intestinal production of chylomicrons. These patients have symptomatic steatorrhea, liver disease, neurologic disease, and retinitis pigmentosa. A characteristic laboratory finding is acanthocytosis. Many of these symptoms and findings may be caused by malabsorption of fat-soluble vitamins, and this fact has recently suggested a potentially useful therapy. *Intestinal lymphangiectasia* is also a disorder of fat malabsorption, in that lymphatic function is compromised, but it also produces protein-losing enteropathy. Fat malabsorption is also produced by *bile salt deficiency.*

Disorders of amino acid malabsorption are rarely encountered, but investigation of patients with amino acid malabsorption has contributed significantly to our knowledge of the normal mechanisms of nitrogen absorption. Patients with amino acidurias (cystinuria, iminoglycinuria, Hartnup disease, methionine malabsorption, "blue diaper syndrome," and Lowe oculocerebrorenal syndrome) have abnormalities in enterocytes similar to those in their renal tubular cells but do not manifest as problems of protein malabsorption because of functional overlap of peptide absorption.

By far the most common type of malabsorption is generalized malabsorption of multiple nutrients. The most common causes in children are listed below.

- Infectious enteritis (especially rotavirus, miscellaneous viruses, *Giardia*)
- Milk protein sensitivity
- Immunodeficiency syndromes
- Eosinophilic gastroenteropathy
- Malnutrition and kwashiorkor
- Gluten-sensitive enteropathy
- Bacterial overgrowth syndrome

In these generalized malabsorptive syndromes, the degree of malabsorption of the various nutrients is proportional to the amount of mucosal damage. The secondary carbohydrate malabsorption that usually accompanies generalized disorders of intestinal mucosa will first affect lactase because it is the most vulnerable disaccharidase, sucrase-isomaltase and maltase being less severely affected. Acquired monosaccharide malabsorption occurs when injury is very severe. Fat malabsorption also correlates with the degree of injury, untreated celiacs sometimes malabsorbing 100%. The observation of abnormal amounts of microscopic fat droplets on a heated and acidified sample of stool is evidence for mucosal malabsorption of fatty acids in contrast to the fecal neutral fat in maldigestive disorder.

Causes for generalized mucosal malabsorption, which are not discussed elsewhere and will be discussed here, include chronic *Giardia* infections, intractable diarrhea of infancy, celiac disease, bacterial overgrowth syndrome, and surgical short gut syndrome.

Giardia lamblia (duodenalis) (see also p. 770) is a binucleate, flagellate, aerotolerant protozoon parasite and is the most common parasite causing intestinal disease in the United States. *Giardia* cysts may contaminate water or food. Following their ingestion, the acid environment allows excystation, and *Giardia* thrives at the pH present in the upper jejunum. *Giardia* may produce any degree of malabsorption or may be asymptomatic. Possible mechanisms for the malabsorption caused by *Giardia* include competition for nutrients, mechanical obstruction of the villus surface by abundant trophozoites or by the mucus production that they stimulate, or mucosal damage. Examination of stools for the *Giardia* cysts may be diagnostic, but many false negatives occur. Small bowel biopsy or examination of duodenal fluid may sometimes secure a diagnosis when stool examination has not. Quinacrine, metronidazole, or furazolidone may be used in the therapy of *Giardia*.

Intractable diarrhea of infancy is a multifactorial disorder in which a vicious cycle of infectious diarrhea, malabsorption, malnutrition, and immunologic dysfunction combine to produce a chronic, life-threatening malabsorptive disorder. Various infectious causes of diarrhea may initiate or complicate the course of intractable diarrhea of infancy, and formula protein intolerance may be involved as well. Poverty is often a predisposing factor. The disease is more common in underdeveloped countries and in lower socioeconomic groups. Diarrhea lasting longer than 2 weeks, associated with failure to thrive and mucosal malabsorption, fits into this classification.

A period of total parenteral nutrition or careful use of elemental formula will be therapeutic. These patients must be protected from acquiring further infections and from exposure to formulas containing whole protein until their nutrition is more nearly normal. Recovery may be monitored by determining stool pH and reducing substance if an elemental formula is used, or by the *d*-xylose absorption test if parenteral nutrition is used. This disease often takes several weeks to resolve, even with optimal therapy.

Celiac disease or gluten-sensitive enteropathy is a disorder of generalized malabsorption in which the intestinal mucosa reacts with acute and chronic inflammation and epithelial atrophy to the gliadin fraction of gluten that is found in wheat, rye, barley, and oats. This disorder is commonly encountered in parts of Europe and Canada but is infrequent in pediatric practice in the continental United States. Patients with celiac disease show evidence of generalized malabsorption, such as failure to grow, diarrhea, muscle wasting, hypoproteinemia, edema, and anemia. The disease is diagnosed by first proving generalized malabsorption and by demonstrating the typical histologic abnormality in a small bowel biopsy. Because the flat villus lesion found in celiac disease is not specific, the malabsorption and histology must become normal when the patient is placed on a strict gluten-free diet and revert to abnormal when gluten is returned to the diet for a definitive diagnosis. Most patients with celiac disease have a permanent sensitivity to gluten and must be maintained on the gluten-free diet for life, but a small group of infants exhibit transient gluten sensitivity and can ingest gluten safely after a period of time.

Short bowel syndrome most often occurs in pediatric patients after intestinal resection as treatment for necrotizing enterocolitis. It may result in severe generalized malabsorption. Several factors have been determined to affect the amount of malabsorption after small bowel resection. The extent and location of resected bowel are important; it is virtually impossible to survive with less than 15 cm of jejunum or ileum, and 15 to 40 cm of small bowel with an intact ileocecal valve has been reported to support the survival of about 50% of patients. The loss of the ileocecal valve worsens the prognosis. Resection of the ileum is associated with more metabolic consequences than resection of jejunum because of its specialized transport functions. Other intestinal absorptive functions may be assumed by the remaining small bowel by adaptation. The functional capacity of the remaining small bowel, stomach, colon, liver, and pancreas are also important in determining the degree of malabsorption in the short bowel syndrome. When the colon is resected along with part of the small bowel, fluid and electrolyte losses may compound the malabsorptive problem and make enteral nutrition very difficult. Adaptation of the remaining small intestine can compensate for the extensive loss of small intestine. Adaptive changes may require months, so parenteral nutrition is often required. Intralumenal nutrients seem to accelerate the adaptive changes and should be provided in small amounts if possible. Patients who have had more than two thirds of their small intestine removed will often have problematic gastric hypersecretion caused by decrease in gastrin metabolism by the gut.

Bacterial overgrowth syndrome occurs when the levels of normal intestinal bacterial organisms are increased above their usual levels. Normally, the proximal intestine contains streptococci, staphylococci, and diplococci in numbers less than 10^5, and 10^8 with the addition of coliforms, in the distal small intestine. In the colon, anaerobes, especially *bacteroides,* are the predominant organisms, and numbers are greater than 10^9. In the bacterial overgrowth syndrome, normal protective mechanisms are disturbed, and the number of bacteria increase with increasing proportions of anaerobes in the small intestine. Normal protective mechanisms include "barriers" such as gastric acid, bile, the ileocecal valve, distance from the colon, peristalsis, local host defenses such as mucus and antibodies, and bacterial interactions such as reduction-oxidation potential and pH.

Patients become predisposed to bacterial overgrowth syndrome when these normal protective mechanisms are altered. Removal of the normal gastric acid barrier occurs in achlorhydria caused by vagotomy, gastrectomy, or normal neonatal low levels of gastric acid. The ileocecal valve is eliminated in ileocolic resections or enterocolic fistulas. Normal peristalsis is disrupted when stasis occurs because of dysmotility, partial obstruction, or pouches. Local host defenses may be compromised by a lack of antibodies in immunocompromised patients.

In bacterial overgrowth syndrome, bacterial actions include the consumption of nutrients that would otherwise be used by the host, elaboration of enzymes that damage the mucosa, and deconjugation of bile salts that produces malabsorption of fat and fat-soluble vitamins. Generalized malabsorption and diarrhea result. Although diagnosis by colony counts on jejunal fluid is generally recommended, a low D-xylose and an abnormal Schilling test in the presence of a situation predisposing to bacterial overgrowth syndrome is very suggestive. A trial of therapy with an appropriate antibiotic confirms this diagnosis. These patients may need to be on chronic or intermittent antibiotic therapy if the lesion predisposing to bacterial overgrowth syndrome is not cured.

"Allergic" enteropathy (see also p. 694)

Intolerance to food may result from several mechanisms. Some of these, such as carbohydrate malabsorption, are discussed elsewhere in this chapter. Potential allergens are numerous in foods, most often within the protein faction. Intolerance or sensitivity to allergens results in injury to intestinal mucosa. Such intolerance is called food allergy, food sensitivity, protein sensitivity, or, in infants, formula protein intolerance. Although "food allergy" has been blamed for many of the ill-defined symptom complexes that affect children such as colic, crying spells, and abdominal pain, it can be diagnosed infrequently if one follows rigid criteria.

The typical symptoms seen in cases of food sensitivity separate them from usual, mild childhood abdominal complaints. Infants are most often involved. They will exhibit failure to thrive, vomiting, diarrhea, hematochezia, and frequently shock. Older children may fail to grow and have evidence of malabsorption. Some children have a pattern of colitis with hematochezia and polymorphonuclear leukocytes in the stool. Symptoms can all be related to mucosal injury and secondary dysfunction.

Several criteria for diagnosis of food sensitivity have been proposed; they all depend on demonstrating intestinal injury in response to an ingested allergen. Frequently, the diagnosis can be made presumptively if a child has typical symptoms that have recurred with ingestion of the offending allergen and have remitted with exclusion of the food. Simply observing improvement of clinical symptoms while restricting the diet does not constitute an adequate reason for diagnosing food allergy. It must be confirmed by at least one carefully controlled exposure to the allergen. Such exposure may result in extreme distress or shock, so it must be performed under the supervision of a physician. Some objective criteria to define injury should be applied. Small bowel or rectal biopsies before and after challenge are ideal. Measurement of *d*-xylose absorption or evaluation of stool guaiac or WBC's before and after exposure establish injury equally well and are not invasive.

The overwhelming majority of patients with food sensitivity are infants. The reasons for this may involve immaturity of the intestine with excessive absorption of macromolecules, potential allergens. Cow's milk proteins and soy protein, separately or in combination, may be responsible for intestinal injury. Usually, intolerance will resolve by 18 months of age, allowing an unrestricted diet after that age. Transient gluten sensitivity may accompany formula protein intolerance in some infants. Older children have food sensitivity much less frequently, but recent reports indicate that corn, fish, and rice may induce mucosal injury.

Once the diagnosis is established, treatment consists of removing the offending allergen from the diet. In infants, the usual therapy consists of feeding a "hypoallergenic" formula in which the nitrogen source is a hydrolysed protein. Alternative whole proteins, such as soy, lamb, and beef heart, may be the basis for preparation of formulas that are often less expensive than hydrolysates and may be equally effective in some cases. In older children, careful removal of the offending food from the diet is specific therapy. Caution must be exercised because many prepared foods contain additives with "hidden" allergic potential.

Eosinophilic gastroenteropathy

Eosinophilic gastroenteropathy is a disorder of unknown etiology in which eosinophilic infiltration of the intestine is observed. It may result in obstruction, malabsorption, or protein-losing enteropathy. Peripheral blood eosinophilia is often seen in affected patients. Because eosinophils are seen in allergic disease, this disorder has been called "allergic gastroenteropathy." Unfortunately, dietary restriction almost never improves the patient's condition, and systemic corticosteroids or oral cromolyn sodium are often required.

Inflammatory bowel disease

Chronic inflammatory bowel disease in children is conventionally divided into chronic ulcerative colitis and Crohn disease (granulomatous ileocolitis) on the basis of clinical and pathologic findings. However, approximately 10% of patients with chronic colitis cannot definitely be placed into either category, and their condition can be best termed *nonspecific chronic colitis*.

Chronic ulcerative colitis is a disease of unknown etiology that is characterized by acute inflammation of the colonic mucosa and submucosa that progresses over time to fibrous scar formation. Approximately 15% of cases of ulcerative colitis will occur before the age of 16. The annual incidence of this disease in adolescence is approximately 4 per 100,000. It is more common in whites than nonwhites, and more common in Jews than non-Jews.

Initial clinical manifestations usually center about the colon. The most frequent manifestations are bloody diarrhea, abdominal pain, and tenesmus. Occasionally patients will have nonspecific findings, such as anorexia, nausea, fever of undetermined origin, and retarded growth, with no obvious colonic symptomatology. Extraintestinal or systemic manifestations of this disease are common and include skin lesions, such as erythema multiforme, erythema nodosum, and pyoderma gangrenosum, arthralgia, arthritis, conjunctivitis, uveitis, and chronic hepatitis. All of these disorders may be seen before the onset of obvious colonic disease.

Diagnosis of ulcerative colitis is most easily established by proctosigmoidoscopy. Findings of ulcerations, mucosal edema, friability, and mucosal hemorrhage are characteristic although not specific for ulcerative colitis. Since over 95% of chronic ulcerative colitis will involve the rectum, only rarely will patients not exhibit abnormalities at proctosigmoidoscopy. Characteristic histologic findings of acute inflammation of the colonic mucosa, including cryptitis and crypt abscess formation, are usual in ulcerative colitis but also are not specific. Barium enema examination is helpful in determining extent of involvement, which is important in long-term management.

Local complications of chronic ulcerative colitis are infrequent, but may be catastrophic. Free perforations with development of peritonitis occur especially in the setting of toxic megacolon. This latter complication is only rarely seen in children but is associated with a significant mortality. Massive colonic hemorrhage also may occur. The most common and most important complication of chronic ulcerative colitis is growth retardation with associated delayed puberty. Finally, the well-known problem of colonic carcinoma, although not commonly involving the pediatric patient, should be kept in mind with regard to the long-term prognosis. The accumulative cancer risk is 5% after 10 years of disease but rapidly accelerates from that point. As previously mentioned, barium enema examination gives information regarding the extent of colonic involvement, which is important because the patient with involvement of the whole colon is particularly at risk for the development of carcinoma.

Chronic ulcerative colitis is primarily treated with two drugs, prednisone and sulfasalazine (Azulfidine). These drugs are used in concert, prednisone being used to induce remission and sulfasalazine to maintain remission. In addition to these drugs, general supportive care includes a normal diet that should be high in protein and high in calories, hospitalization for acute exacerbations, especially those associated with dehydration and electrolyte imbalance, and surgery, especially for patients who suffer with toxic megacolon or massive colonic hemorrhage. It should be remembered that total colectomy is curative in these patients.

The long-term course and prognosis of these patients is variable. A few patients will have a complete, permanent remission, but the majority will have periods of remission punctuated by acute exacerbations, and a few patients will have chronic continuous colitis.

Crohn disease, a disease that produces noncaseating granulomatous inflammation of the gastrointestinal tract, appears to be increasing in incidence and is now more frequent than ulcerative colitis in the pediatric age group. Approximately 15% of all cases of Crohn disease begin in adolescence or childhood. The etiology is unknown, but there is increasing evidence that a transmissible agent is involved in its genesis, and autoimmune phenomena also may be important.

Unlike ulcerative colitis, Crohn disease may involve any portion of the gastrointestinal tract. The most commonly involved area is the terminal ileum, which appears to be affected in about 70% of cases, either alone or in conjunction with colonic disease. Disease limited to the colon occurs in approximately 10% of cases. Disease limited to the small intestine, including the distal ileum, occurs in 50%. The disease is transmural in nature, and early in its course produces acute inflammation, edema, and deep longitudinal and transverse ulcerations. The serosal surface of the affected bowel is also inflamed, and local lymph nodes are enlarged and may contain granulomata. A characteristic gross finding on the serosal surface of the small bowel affected with Crohn disease is the migration of fat from the mesenteric to the antimesenteric border. Frequently, involvement of the bowel is discontinuous, so that there are areas of actively involved bowel separated by clinically inactive areas, so-called skip areas. The acute edema and inflammation result in thickening of the bowel wall, which may be evident roentgenographically as separation of loops of bowel and which may produce obstruction or partial obstruction of the bowel lumen. This type of obstruction is frequently reversible with appropriate therapy. Late in the course of Crohn disease, full thickness fibrous scarring occurs and may result in irreversible bowel obstruction. The characteristic transmural nature of this disease with serosal inflammation and deep ulceration frequently results in fistula formation, but the intense inflammatory reaction on the serosal surface limits perforation so that spillage of intestinal contents into the peritoneal cavity is rare.

The clinical presentation of Crohn disease in adolescence is variable. In general, its symptoms are similar to those of other systemic inflammatory diseases in adolescents: fever, malaise, growth failure, and anorexia. In addition to these signs, the intestinal signs of abdominal pain and diarrhea are also frequently observed. Occasionally a child will have symptoms of acute appendicitis and, at the time of laparotomy, is found to have acute ileitis. Also, patients may initially have extraintestinal symptoms such as arthritis, skin disease, especially pyoderma gangrenosum, and perianal disease. The difficulty with which Crohn disease is diagnosed is evidenced by the fact that in most series there is a delay of about 2½ years between onset of symptoms and time of diagnosis.

Physical findings often present at the time of diagnosis are evidence of chronic malnutrition and chronic inflammatory disease, such as loss of subcutaneous fat, muscle wasting, short stature, and edema. Careful attention should be given to looking for the extra-abdominal manifestations of Crohn disease, especially a thorough examination of the eyes for evidence of uveitis, of the oral cavity for presence of aphthous ulcers, of the extremities for the possibility of arthritis, of the skin for characteristic lesions, and of the anal area for evidence of fissure or fistula. The abdominal examination may demonstrate tenderness in the area of involved bowel, and frequently thickened loops of bowel or local masses are palpable.

The erythrocyte sedimentation rate is a useful screening test for acute, active Crohn disease, in which it is almost invariably elevated. Definitive diagnosis usually rests in the demonstration of characteristic, radiographic changes in the small bowel or colon (Fig. 16-2). Acute disease produces thickening of the bowel wall, often assuming a nodular or cobblestone appearance, longitudinal and transverse ulcerations, enteroenteric or enterocolic fistulas, and frequently partial obstruction of the bowel. Skip areas and asymmetric involvement of the bowel, especially the colon, help to differentiate Crohn disease from ulcerative colitis. Rectal biopsy is also of importance in diagnosis, since focal acute and chronic inflammation, transmural disease, and especially demonstration of granulomata are characteristic of Crohn disease.

As with ulcerative colitis, the most important complication of adolescent Crohn disease is growth retardation. Occasionally, refractory pyoderma gangrenosum, arthritis, or perianal disease occur. Although the incidence of carcinoma developing late in the course of Crohn disease is much less that that in ulcerative colitis, it is several times higher than the incidence of carcinoma in the general population.

Treatment of adolescent Crohn disease uses nutritional support, adrenal corticosteroids, antibiotics, and, sparingly, surgery. Nutrition is of utmost importance in management, but is frequently hard to deliver because of the anorexia and partial bowel obstruction characteristically observed in the acute stage of this illness. The severely debilitated patient with more severe obstruction will benefit from a course of total parenteral nutrition at the onset of therapy. Chronic enteral drip feedings are also effective in providing nutrition for the severely affected patient. The patient with fewer nutritional problems should be urged to maintain a high-caloric, high-protein intake that may be enhanced with multiple vitamins and caloric supplements, especially at bedtime.

Prednisone is effective in the management of Crohn disease in adolescents. Initially it is administered at 2 mg/kg/day in divided doses. As the disease remits, it is administered once daily in the morning. After a short period of time, the dose is gradually reduced to approximately 1 mg/kg/day. The ultimate goal of prednisone therapy in Crohn disease is to achieve a dose of prednisone on an alternate day schedule that will suppress disease activity yet allow for normal adolescent growth (Fig. 16-3). This can best be achieved by slowly reducing, a few milligrams per week, the alternate-day dose until the patient is receiving 1 mg/kg every other

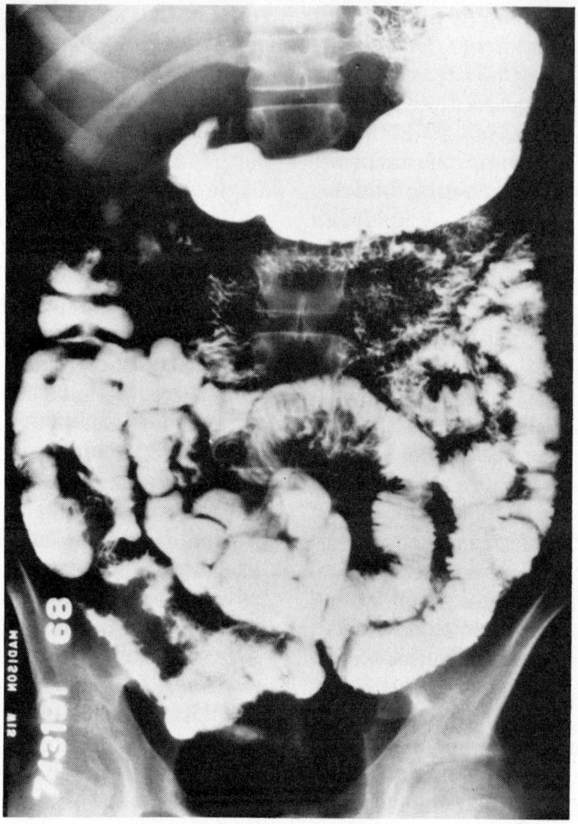

Fig. 16-2. Barium small bowel series in 11-year-old child with Crohn disease. Terminal ileum and ascending colon demonstrate typical changes of thickening, and nodular filling defects, and fissuring.

day. At that time, the every other day dose can slowly be reduced, observing for evidence of reactivation of disease. The usual adolescent can be maintained on 20 to 25 mg of prednisone every other day with little or no symptoms of disease and with normal growth and sexual development.

Antibiotics are sometimes useful in treating Crohn disease, although they can rarely supplant prednisone. Metronidazole is effective in treating perianal complications in some patients. Doses from 250 mg up to 1 g four times daily are administered orally for courses of 6 weeks to 2 months. The expense of such therapy and the occasional side effects preclude its use except in cases with moderate to severe perianal disease. Sulfasalazine (Azulfidine) and tetracycline are occasionally effectively used to reduce the dose of prednisone required to suppress disease activity. Their use must be individualized. Azathioprine (Imuran) likewise has been used to enhance the effectiveness of prednisone therapy.

Surgery should be reserved for patients with unremitting extraintestinal symptoms including severe growth failure, with unresolving intestinal obstruction, or, rarely, with fulminant Crohn disease manifested by massive gastrointestinal hemorrhage or free perforation. It should be remembered that surgery is not curative of Crohn disease, probably since the entire bowel is involved, although subclinically, and surgery may promote extension of disease into areas previously not clinically involved. The long-term prognosis of Crohn disease in adolescence is not known at present. The goal of treatment, however, is to deliver into adulthood an individual of normal stature who has been able to participate in scholastic and social activities and who has minimal anatomic residua

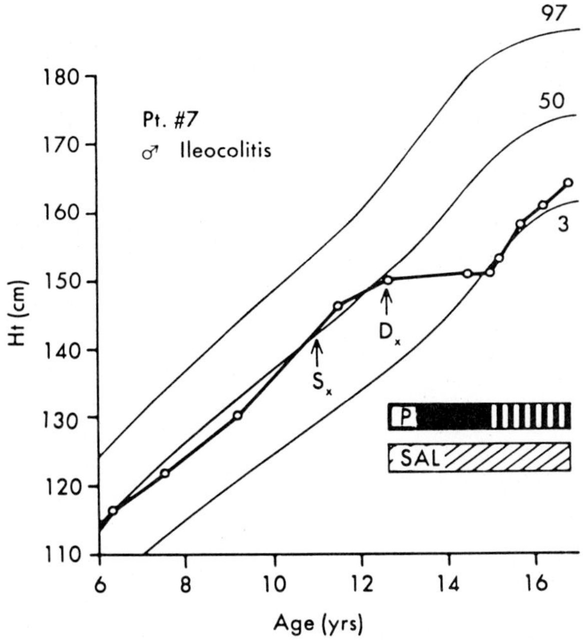

Fig. 16-3. Growth pattern of child with Crohn disease. Reduced growth velocity was observed from time of onset of symptoms *(Sx)* and continued after diagnosis *(Dx)*, while daily prednisone *(P)* and salicylazosulfapyridine *(Sal)* were used to treat active disease. However, when alternate day prednisone therapy *(interrupted bar)* was achieved, catch-up growth was observed.

of disease. These goals can be met in the majority of cases with proper management.

Stooling disorders

Abnormal patterns of stooling are common complaints in the pediatric population. This probably results from two sources. Every child must undergo developmental maturation of stooling, and mothers may interpret normal variations as being abnormal or caused by disease. It is important to distinguish between normal developmental difficulties and stooling disorders because only the latter require therapy.

The "normal" pattern of stooling has not been established. Neither the frequency of stooling nor the difficulty with which stool is passed are indicators of disease, whereas stool consistency and failure to maintain a stooling pattern consistent with general well-being are. Common "normal" complaints are: the newborn who strains, turns red, and grunts while passing a soft, yellow stool, the newborn who passes a soft stool every 2 or 3 days, the toddler who apparently has great difficulty passing a stool when placed on the potty, the school-aged child who stools every third day. These patterns should be recognized as being normal variants, and no therapy is needed. Added dietary bulk and perhaps a stool softener may be prescribed, but laxatives and enemas, if prescribed, may result in a real stooling disorder. Mothers' concerns must be allayed if minimal intervention is to be a success.

Simple constipation, or the passage of hard, usually small stools without progression to more serious problems is a frequent and easily treated condition. It frequently begins around the time of potty training and perhaps represents an imbalance in the retentive aspects of stooling. Therapy should be minimal and designed to repattern stooling. A high-bulk diet, as shown in Table 16-2, is often completely effective. The entire family should be encouraged to participate since the child will be more likely to eat the prescribed foods under this arrangement, and other family members often also have stooling problems. Bulk medication, such as Metamucil, may be used in older children. Infants respond well to Maltsupex. Encouraging the child to spend time on the toilet at a time when

Table 16-2. High fiber diet

Food	Fiber (g/serving)
Fiber content of various foods	
Most vegetables	1 to 3
Corn	5
Baked beans	11
Most fruits (fresh)	1 to 3
Raspberries	5
Dried prunes	8
White bread	2
Whole wheat bread	3
Bran muffins	3
Most cereals	1
Bran cereals	4 to 9
Natural bran (1 tablespoon)	3

Important points

1. Always include a high fiber breakfast cereal (4 g).
2. Substitute whole grain breads for white breads.
3. Use bran cookies or muffins for snacks or desserts.
4. Emphasize fresh fruits and vegetables.

colonic mass movements usually occur, such as after breakfast, may result in the development of a daily stool habit.

Severe constipation and encopresis (see also Chapter 4) represent the most severe of the stooling disorders. In this disease, retention of stool is so severe that a huge fecal mass distends the rectum, producing functional megacolon. The anus becomes effaced, resulting in loss of continence. Leakage of liquid stool around the impacted fecal mass and through the incontinent anus occurs. Fecal soiling is the usual chief complaint in such cases, and is a major social problem for affected children. The differential diagnosis in such cases is very limited, and therapy can safely be initiated with information available from the history and physical examination only.

Therapy of functional megacolon should be directed at reducing the rectal size, since stretching of the wall reduces the effectiveness of peristalsis and possibly impedes the sensation produced by the presence of stool. Ultimately, developing a normal stooling pattern is the goal of therapy. The first phase of treatment is evacuation of the fecal mass, which may be accomplished by frequent enemas of hypertonic phosphate, saline, or mineral oil, singly or in combination. Manual disimpaction is rarely required. We usually rely on daily morning saline or phosphate enemas for 1 or 2 weeks at home rather than intensive inpatient disimpaction. At the same time, stool bulk agents or stool softeners should be initiated. Many authors advocate the use of large doses of mineral oil, but we have found this to be unnecessary and often counterproductive. We prescribe a high fiber diet for the patient and family. Because these patients often need additional assistance early in therapy, a bulk agent and weak stimulant are usually prescribed. We have found Perdiem, which contains seneca and is readily accepted by children, particularly helpful. One or two tablespoons daily are given to older patients until a daily stooling pattern is obtained. Then it is withdrawn in increments as the high fiber diet maintains the stool habit. We have also used intermittent stimulant laxatives with good success. The typical regimen is Senekot granules, 2 teaspoons if the patient has not stooled in the preceeding 3 days. This "cycling" regimen gives the patient an adequate opportunity to stool and does not produce laxative dependency, but prevents the impaction of feces. With reassurance and these treatment measures, successful repatterning of stooling can be accomplished in most cases.

Hirschsprung disease (see also Chapter 33) can be confused with functional megacolon. This disease typically begins in the newborn period, produces marked abdominal distention, often causes growth failure, rarely causes fecal soiling, and usually exhibits an empty rectal vault. Functional megacolon is different in all ways. Barium enema and rectal biopsy will usually be diagnostic.

Atypical Hirschsprung disease may exactly mimic functional megacolon. Here the aganglionic segment is very short or anatomically inapparent. Anorectal tonometry, a technique that measures the myenterically mediated reflex relaxation of the internal anal sphincter, can detect these cases. Biopsy of the rectal wall may confirm a short length of aganglionic colon, or isolated achalasia of the internal anal sphincter may be the sole abnormality. Posterior sphincterotomy is curative in these cases.

Chronic nonspecific infant diarrhea (the irritable colon syndrome of childhood) is probably another simple stooling disorder. These patients, usually toddlers, have several large, loose stools each day. Commonly, the stools are confined to the morning; rarely do such children have nocturnal stooling. The stools almost always contain recognizable food particles. The children are otherwise happy and healthy. Mothers usually complain most about the associated mess. There is a high frequency of irritable colon syndrome in the parents. Evaluation for infection, infestation, and malabsorption are negative. Therapy consists of reassurance and a high fiber diet. Certainly, restrictive anomalous diets should be avoided in such patients because fat deficiency has been implicated in the pathogenesis of the disease. Most cases resolve without sequelae, but some patients have recurrent functional abdominal complaints at an older age.

DISORDERS OF THE LIVER

Neonatal jaundice (see also pp. 309 to 313)

Neonatal jaundice is one of the most frequent disorders confronting the pediatrician. Approximately 15% of a normal newborn population will be visibily jaundiced, having a total serum bilirubin of greater than 7 mg/dl. Of these, only a few will have true pathologic jaundice, whereas the majority will have "physiologic" hyperbilirubinemia. In the outline below the more frequent causes of pathologic jaundice are listed.

- I. Pigment overproduction
  - A. Fetal-maternal blood group incompatibility
  - B. Hereditary spherocytosis
  - C. Nonspherocytic hemolytic anemia
    - 1. G-6-PD deficiency + drug
    - 2. Vitamin K_3-induced hemolysis
  - D. Extravascular blood
  - E. Polycythemia
  - F. Increased enterohepatic circulation
    - 1. Fasting
    - 2. Pyloric stenosis
    - 3. Hirschsprung disease
    - 4. Meconium ileus
- II. Undersecretion of pigment
  - A. Metabolic endocrine disorders
    - 1. Familial nonhemolytic jaundice (Crigler-Najjar syndrome)
    - 2. Hypothyroidism
    - 3. Galactosemia
    - 4. Tyrosinosis
    - 5. Breast milk inhibitors of UDP-bilirubin glucuronyl transferase
    - 6. Prematurity
  - B. Obstructive disorders
    - 1. Biliary atresia – neonatal hepatitis
    - 2. Choledochal cyst
    - 3. Cystic fibrosis
    - 4. Cholestatic syndromes
- III. Mixed disorders
  - A. Sepsis, especially gram negative
  - B. Intrauterine infections
    - 1. Toxoplasmosis
    - 2. Rubella
    - 3. Cytomegalic inclusion disease (CID)
    - 4. Herpes simplex
    - 5. Syphilis
    - 6. Hepatitis B

Generally, an infant who develops visible icterus before 36 hours of age suffers with overproduction of bilirubin usually caused by hemolytic disorders of the newborn. The infant whose total serum bilirubin exceeds 12 mg/dl has pathologic jaundice and, in the absence of hemolytic disease or hepatitis, has an overvigorous enterohepatic circulation of bilirubin, usually because of delayed passage of meconium or gut hypomotility. Jaundice that endures beyond the seventh day of life is also pathologic and is most commonly seen in infants with impaired hepatic excretion of bilirubin. Finally, a direct reacting, conjugated, serum bilirubin of greater than 1 mg/dl is abnormal and is usually associated with systemic infections, hepatitis, either of infectious or metabolic origin, or anatomic biliary obstruction.

Of particular importance in the management of infants with hyperbilirubinemia is the understanding of the relationship between serum bilirubin concentration, the capacity of serum albumin to bind bilirubin, and the development of bilirubin encephalopathy, kernicterus. Unconjugated bilirubin is essentially insoluble in aqueous media at physiologic pH. It is carried in serum bound to albumin, which has two binding sites for bilirubin, a hydrophobic high-affinity site, and a secondary low-affinity site. In most instances, bilirubin is bound exclusively at the high-affinity site; however, when the bilirubin concentration exceeds the concentration of high affinity sites, bilirubin occupies the low-affinity site and can be readily displaced to enter fatty tissue, especially the brain. Therefore, optimal management of neonatal hyperbilirubinemia depends not only on knowledge of the concentration of serum bilirubin but also on the capacity of albumin to bind bilirubin. This depends not only on the concentration of serum albumin but on the presence of competitively bound substances. Several tests are presently available that measure the residual binding capacity of albumin for bilirubin. If one of these tests demonstrates that there is little reserve binding capacity, despite the absolute level of serum bilirubin, active measures should be taken to reduce the level of serum bilirubin. This is best accomplished by exchange transfusion. The absolute criteria for exchange transfusion for neonatal nonconjugated hyperbilirubinemia are (1) a total serum indirect bilirubin of greater than 20 mg/dl in a full-term infant, (2) a total serum indirect bilirubin of greater than 15 mg/dl in a premature infant (very small infants may require transfusion at a lower level of serum bilirubin), (3) critically reduced reserve bilirubin binding capacity, (4) a serum bilirubin of greater than 15 mg/dl for 72 hours in a full-term infant, and (5) a serum bilirubin of greater than 10 mg/dl for greater than 72 hours in a premature infant. The level of serum bilirubin used in these criteria for exchange transfusion is that of nonconjugated bilirubin, but it should be remembered that conjugated bilirubin competes for both high and low affinity binding sites with nonconjugated bilirubin.

The causes of conjugated hyperbilirubinemia in infancy are presented on p. 354. These entities should be considered when serum concentration of direct reacting, conjugated bilirubin exceeds 1 mg/dl. The diagnosis therefore depends on a properly performed analysis of conjugated bilirubin. Many clinical laboratories consistently report concentrations of conjugated bilirubin of greater than 1 mg/dl in the neonatal period, and they should be considered unreliable. A physician encountering a laboratory that reports consistently elevated conjugated bilirubin concentrations should insist on a critical evaluation of the method of analysis.

Portal hypertension

Elevation of pressure in the portal venous system above normal levels of 7 to 10 mm Hg can be the result of any lesion that causes obstruction of flow through the portal vein, through the liver, or out of the liver. Cirrhosis of the liver is the most common lesion causing portal hypertension. Other causes are congenital hepatic fibrosis, thrombosis of the portal vein, and, rarely, obstruction of the hepatic veins (Budd-Chiari syndrome).

Obstruction to the flow of portal blood leads to the development of collateral venous channels. Occasionally, such collateral channels will adequately decompress the portal system and no symptoms will arise. Flow from the portal vein through the coronary (gastric) vein to the vena cava may cause dilation of large mucosal vessels in the gastric fundus and in the esophagus, which frequently rupture and bleed. Reopening of umbilical vein remnants from fetal circulation may cause large dilated veins in the anterior abdominal wall, the caput medusa. Shunting from the portal vein to the hemorrhoidal veins may cause dilation of rectal hemorrhoids.

Portal hypertension should be suspected when there is enlargement of the spleen in conjunction with ascites, a history of previous liver disease, and either hematemesis or melena. Establishment of a firm diagnosis of portal hypertension may require measurement of pressure in the portal system, liver biopsy, x-ray studies or endoscopy of the upper gastrointestinal tract to search for esophageal varices, and proctoscopy to look for hemorrhoids. Arterial portography or splenoportogram may also be helpful in visualizing the portal system.

Treatment of portal hypertension centers around treatment of complications, unless an underlying cause for the liver disease can be found and removed. If cirrhosis is not the cause for the portal hypertension, surgical portal-systemic shunt may be a useful procedure. Portal systemic shunts occasionally lead to hepatic coma because of decreased blood flow through the diseased liver, especially in patients who have cirrhosis.

If the major problem is bleeding from esophageal varices, endoscopic sclerosis of the bleeding varices by injection seems to be the procedure of choice. In the past, the triple-lumen Sengstaken-Blakemore tube was used to tamponade the bleeding vessels. The use of this apparatus has decreased since the advent of sclerotherapy.

Ascites

Free peritoneal fluid, ascites, indicates the presence of an underlying disease that may be renal, cardiac, or hepatic. The most common cause of ascites is portal hypertension secondary to chronic liver disease. Physical findings include a distended abdomen with a fluid wave and flank dullness. Minimal amounts of fluid may be detected by having the patient get on hands and knees and, after a few minutes, finding dullness to percussion in the most dependent portion of the abdomen (the puddle sign). Abdominal x-ray may show generalized haziness, loss of psoas shadows, and obliteration of the hepatic angle. Ultrasound may be used to detect small amounts of fluid. Paracentesis for diagnosis is usually not needed in pediatric patients, but may be helpful in obscure cases or in those patients with persistent fever.

Therapy of ascites obviously should be directed at the underlying disease. When cirrhosis is the cause, low-salt diet, fluid restriction, and diuretics are effective.

Encephalopathy

Central nervous system dysfunction may occur at any time during the course of liver disease. The term *hepatic encephalopathy* has been used to encompass a variety of clinical syndromes that occur under these circumstances. Symptoms manifested by such patients are quite variable and range from subtle personality changes (including loss of drive, irritability, and disturbances of sleep pattern), to confusion, drowsiness, and deep coma. In acute fulminant hepatitis the progress through various stages to coma may be very rapid, whereas in chronic liver disease symptoms may be minimal and changes from normal to abnormal may occur over days. At times, psychologic and neurologic disturbances seen in hepatic encephalopathy may precede recognition of underlying liver disease.

The symptomatology of hepatic encephalopathy may be graded in stages from 1 to 4 on the basis of severity. During stage 1 coma (prodrome), only slight mental disturbance is present. There may be disturbance of sleep pattern, loss of libido, loss of drive, euphoria, occasionally depression, untidiness of habits, and a slight tremor. In stage 2 (impending coma), symptoms are more overt with confusion, drowsiness, euphoria, and inappropriate behavior predominating. Tremor is usually present; so called "liver flap" is characteristic. During this stage, writing ability deteriorates. In stage 3 (stupor), the patient sleeps most of the time, is uncooperative when awake, and demonstrates marked confusion. Tremor is severe and present when the patient is able to cooperate. Electroencephalographic changes are frequently present. In stage 4 (coma), unconsciousness is profound with the patient responding only to painful stimuli. Muscle tone is absent. Tremor is not apparent because of lack of muscle tone. Electroencephalographic changes are usually present.

The etiology of hepatic encephalopathy is not precisely defined, and multiple factors are probably operating simultaneously to produce the clinical picture. Clinical symptomatology can be correlated closely with levels of blood ammonia. One important function of the liver is to clear ammonia from portal blood before returning the blood to the systemic circulation. If portal blood bypasses the liver because of collateral circulation, or if the liver is severely diseased, ammonia removal will not be complete, and blood ammonia levels will increase and in turn may produce encephalopathy. However, the degree of coma does not correlate well with the blood ammonia levels.

Hepatic encephalopathy may be precipitated by a number of factors, among which are dehydration, reduced renal function, alkalosis, potassium deficiency and hypoglycemia. Gastrointestinal hemorrhage, which increases the load of ammonia in portal blood, may precipitate hepatic encephalopathy. Increased intake of dietary protein may lead to hepatic encephalopathy when there is a delicate balance between the protein intake and hepatic ammonia clearance. Infection such as sepsis, or any condition that is stressful to the patient with liver disease, may lead to the production of encephalopathy. Not uncommonly, overzealous medication with diuretics and paracentesis produces coma. Occasionally, sedatives, which are inadequately detoxified by the liver, cause confusion and may lead to coma.

Therapy in hepatic encephalopathy consists of good general supportive care and correction of fluid and electrolyte abnormalities. Particular attention is given to not producing overhydration, avoiding dehydration, and providing adequate vitamin intake, including vitamins B complex and K. Glucose should be given to avoid hypoglycemia. Administration of salt-poor albumin may be used to raise a low serum albumin in specific cases. An effort should be made to decrease ammonia production in the bowel by decreasing protein intake, by giving lactulose, and, at times, by reducing bowel flora with neomycin. Exchange transfusions have been used in the past and at times may be helpful to lower ammonia and correct bleeding problems. Special amino acid mixtures containing branched chain amino acids may offer benefit for reducing the level of encephalopathy. In certain cases of complete liver failure, liver transplant may offer hope.

Cholestasis of the newborn

Direct hyperbilirubinemia in the neonate is always pathologic and usually due to cholestasis. This secretory defect may be at the level of the hepatocyte, canaliculus, or intrahepatic bile ducts (intrahepatic cholestasis), or secondary to obstruction of the extrahepatic biliary tract (extrahepatic cholestasis). The neonatal liver responds to many diverse insults (infections, metabolic, toxic) by the development of cholestasis at the hepatocellular level. Usually the distinction between hepatocellular cholestasis and biliary tract obstruction can be made based on proper evaluation. However, occasionally the patient may have features of both and present a diagnostic dilemma. In general, infants with cholestasis have conjugated hyperbilirubinemia. Other findings include dark urine and acholic stools. Infants with cholestasis secondary to infection or metabolic disease usually appear ill and do not thrive well. In contrast, those with obstructive lesions often appear well and thrive well early in their course. Particular attention should be paid to any extrahepatic signs of systemic illnesses, such as sepsis or congenital viral syndromes, which may affect the liver. Abdominal examinations should include careful evaluation of liver and spleen size and texture, and any masses, such as congenital choledochal cyst, should be noted.

Laboratory studies should include tests of hepatocellular and canalicular integrity and function, including serum total and direct bilirubin, transaminases, gamma glutamyl transeptidase (GGTP), 5′-nucleotidase, and serum bile salts. Infectious etiologies should be sought by means of bacterial and viral cultures, and serologies for syphilis and toxoplasmosis, rubella virus, cytomegalovirus, and herpes simplex viruses (TORCH) should be carried out on both infant and mother. Workup for metabolic causes of cholestasis should include a urine metabolic screen and serum alpha-1-antitrypsin level. A urine specimen of every infant having cholestasis should be immediately checked for the presence of nonglucose reducing substances as a screen for galactosemia. A sweat test for diagnosis of cystic fibrosis may also be considered.

Other valuable studies include ultrasonography to evaluate gallbladder and biliary tract, radionucleotide imaging to document secretion of bile into the gut, and cholangiography (percutaneous or operative) to visualize the biliary tract. Percutaneous liver biopsy is an extremely useful diagnostic tool that can distinguish between hepatocellular and obstructive cholestasis in over 90% of cases.

A list of the causes of neonatal cholestasis appears below.

- I. Acquired
  - A. Infectious
    1. Sepsis, usually gram negative
    2. Other bacterial infections, especially gram-negative urinary tract infection
    3. Syphilis
    4. TORCH, congenital infections
    5. Viral: Coxsackie, hepatitis B (rarely in neonatal period)
  - B. Toxic
    1. Total parenteral nutrition
    2. Drugs
    3. Benign recurrent cholestasis
    4. Byler disease
    5. Inborn errors of bile acid metabolism
    6. Paucity of intrahepatic bile ducts (syndromatic and nonsyndromatic)
- II. Inherited
  - A. Familial
- III. Metabolic
  - A. Galactosemia
  - B. Hereditary fructose intolerance
  - C. Tyrosinemia
  - D. Alpha-1-antitrypsin deficiency
  - E. Cystic fibrosis
  - F. Zellweger syndrome
- IV. Inherited conjugated hyperbilirubinemia without cholestasis
  - A. Dubin-Johnson syndrome
  - B. Rotor syndrome
- V. Anatomic obstruction
  - A. Choledochal cyst and other malformations
  - B. Cholelithasis
- VI. Idiopathic obstructive cholangiopathy
  - A. Biliary atresia
  - B. "Neonatal hepatitis"

Although all should be considered, approximately 70% of patients cannot be specifically diagnosed and fall into the category of idiopathic obstructive cholangiopathy, which encompasses biliary atresia and "neonatal hepatitis."

Biliary atresia accounts for one third of cases of neonatal obstructive jaundice. This disorder is apparently not a static congenital bile duct obstruction as once thought, but an active, progressive process that results in the eventual obliteration of bile ducts. "Neonatal hepatitis," which accounts for one half of infants with prolonged cholestasis, may represent the result of the same insult that causes biliary atresia but is limited and does not involve the ductal tissues. Efforts to identify an infectious or toxic agent as causative of these disorders have so far proved inconclusive, although viral infections have been linked to their etiology.

Treatment of neonatal cholestasis consists of specific medical or surgical therapy in those cases with an identifiable, treatable cause. The majority of infants with idiopathic obstructive cholangiopathy, however, present a problem. Until the introduction of the hepatoportoenterostomy procedure by Kasai as treatment for biliary atresia, the prognosis for these infants was uniformly dismal. Whereas Kasai reported achievement of bile drainage in three fourths of operated infants, results in this country have been poor. Whether this represents technical imperfection or a different disease process in Japanese patients is unsettled at present. Nevertheless, poor surgical outcome and severe postoperative complications, such as ascending cholangitis, have prevented the Kasai procedure from becoming a completely satisfactory treatment. To be most effective, a correct diagnosis must be made early and surgery performed before the child is 6 weeks of age. Infants with "neonatal hepatitis" are treated medically with phenobarbital and cholestyramine, agents that promote bile flow. Scrupulous attention is paid to good nutrition, using medium-chain triglycerides and supplementation with fat-soluble vitamins. Thirty to fifty percent of infants with "neonatal hepatitis" will recover completely, 15% to 25% will develop persistent liver disease or cirrhosis, and 25% will die in the first year of life. Orthotopic liver transplantation in patients with end-stage liver disease of various causes may offer therapy for many infants in the future.

Chronic cholestasis syndromes

Several diseases and syndromes that chronically produce bile retention have been described. Clinical hallmarks of these diseases are that they are chronic or recurrent problems; they cause serum bile salt concentrations to be elevated and very commonly produce pruritis as their principal manifestation; serum bilirubin is unpredictably elevated; serum alkaline phosphatase, 5′-nucleotidase, and gamma glutamyl transpeptidase are usually elevated; abnormal cholesterol metabolism and serum lipoprotein abberrations commonly accompany the cholestasis; and biliary tract obstruction is absent.

Defects in bile salt metabolism may produce chronic cholestasis. Some children with familial chronic cholestasis have been described as having trihydroxycoprostanic acid in their blood. This is the principal bile salt of the American alligator, but evidently its production in humans produces cholestasis and progressive cirrhosis.

Zellweger syndrome counts cholestasis among its manifestations. Defects in mitochondrial bile salt metabolism are present and apparently result in cholestasis. Other children with idiopathic or familial cholestasis have in their systems serum bile salts that are not normally found in mature humans. These may represent the consequences of cholestasis on bile salt metabolism, or they may be the cause of cholestasis.

Byler disease is a chronic cholestasis syndrome described in an Amish kindred. It results in progressive cirrhosis and death. Its cause is unknown.

Syndromic cholestasis with ductular hypoplasia is a group of disorders in which there is a consistent histopathologic finding in the liver of reduced numbers of interlobular bile ducts. This may be associated with peculiar facies, growth retardation, mild mental retardation, vertebral anomalies, and pulmonary artery anomalies (Alagille syndrome) with peripheral lymphedema (Aagenaes syndrome) or with no anomalies (nonsyndromic ductular hypoplasia). These patients suffer with pruritis and many exhibit xanthomata. Progression of disease is variable. It appears to be inheritable.

Benign recurrent cholestasis is a disorder of unknown etiology that results in recurrent and occasionally persistent episodes of cholestasis. Most patients experience the first episode within the first year of life. Pruritis is the major symptom and is occasionally so severe it results in depression and suicide. It usually does not cause progressive or severe liver injury. It is a lifelong problem for affected patients.

Regardless of the cause of chronic cholestasis, treatment is the same and is of limited usefulness. Stimulation of bile flow with phenobarbital occasionally produces significant improvement. Cholestyramine resin may be used to reduce serum bile salts and pruritis. Recently, plasmapheresis and charcoal plasma perfusion have been used in severely affected patients to remove bile salts. All patients should be fed a high-protein, low-fat diet and receive large supplements of fat-soluble vitamins. Vitamin E may be particularly important to prevent neurologic complications. Vitamins K, for clotting factors, and D, to prevent rickets, are also important.

Metabolic liver disease

Liver disease in infants may be caused by inherited metabolic defects. Making an early specific diagnosis is important because these diseases often have specific, effective treatments, and genetic counseling is important.

Galactosemia is an autosomal recessive disorder that occurs in 1 in 20,000 live births and is caused by deficiency of galactose-1-phosphate uridyltransferase activity, resulting in the accumulation of toxic galactose-1-phosphate and galactose and causing brain, kidney, and liver dysfunction. The diagnosis is suggested by finding nonglucose reducing substance in the urine and confirmed by assay of red cell enzyme activity. Treatment consists of dietary galactose elimination.

Hereditary fructose intolerance is an autosomal recessive disorder that occurs in 1 in 20,000 newborns and presents only after the introduction of dietary fructose. Deficient activity of fructose-1-phosphate aldolase activity results in vomiting, hypoglycemia, amino aciduria, and liver disease. Treatment is by dietary exclusion of fruit, vegetables, and sucrose.

The primary metabolic defect in *tyrosinemia,* an autosomal recessive disorder, has not been identified, although *p*-hydroxyphenyl pyruvic acid oxidase deficiency has been noted in the liver. The final result is cirrhosis, hypophasphatemia, rickets, renal tubular dysfunction, and abnormal tyrosine metabolism. Dietary restriction of tyrosine and phenylalanine may be effective in some patients.

Cystic fibrosis results in significant liver disease in relatively few affected infants but this complication increases with age. Steatosis is the most common hepatic lesion, especially in malnourished patients. Focal biliary cirrhosis is also common, and in 2% to 3% of patients may progress to severe multilobular cirrhosis.

Alpha-1-antitrypsin deficiency produces cholestasis in infancy, which may progress to cirrhosis in older children. Three per cent of the population are heterozygotes (PiMZ) and 0.07% are homozygotes (PiZZ); the latter is associated with liver disease. Therefore all children with liver disease should be evaluated for this disorder. No specific therapy is available.

Wilson disease is an autosomal recessive disorder of copper metabolism that results in the accumulation of copper in the cornea, red blood cells, kidneys, and liver. Liver disease is always present and develops before disease of other organ systems. It is rarely diagnosed in children under 6 years of age. Hepatic involvement may be first detected as cirrhosis with portal hypertension, chronic active liver disease, and, less often, acute, severe liver failure. Other clinical signs, usually seen in older children, include neurologic dysfunction and the corneal Kayser-Fleischer ring.

Wilson disease is diagnosed by finding low serum ceruloplasmin and copper levels and increased urinary copper excretion. Treatment consists of copper chelation therapy with *d*-penicillamine and must be started early to be effective.

The glycogen storage diseases (all autosomal recessive) having significant hepatic involvement are:

Type I Glucose-6-phosphatase deficiency. Patients have enlarged liver and kidneys, failure to thrive, hypoglycemia, but normal mental development. Prognosis is fair to good.

Type III Amylo-1.6-glucosidase ("debrancher enzyme") deficiency. These patients have moderate to marked hepatomegaly and occasionally hypotonia and cardiomegaly but without hypoglycemia. Mental development is normal, and the prognosis is fair to good.

Type IV Amylo-1,4—1.6-transglucosidase ("brancher enzyme") deficiency. These patients have severe liver involvement and hepatomegaly progressing to cirrhosis and liver failure. Death occurs in early childhood.

Type VI Hepatic phosphorylase deficiency. Patients have marked hepatomegaly but no hypoglycemia and normal development. The prognosis is good.*

Several disorders of lipid storage have also been described.

In *Wolman disease, hepatic acid-lipase deficiency,* the patients have steatorrhea, hepatosplenomegaly, and jaundice with accumulation of triglyceride and cholesterol ester in the liver, spleen, intestine, and adrenal glands. Death usually occurs within the first year of life.

Although patients with *cholesterol ester storage disease* have the same biochemical abnormality as in Wolman disease, they have only hepatomegaly and hypercholesterolemia with a normal life expectancy.

Abetalipoproteinemia is secondary to defective synthesis of apolipoprotein B by the liver and intestine, resulting in a secretory failure of triglyceride-rich lipoproteins. These patients have steatorrhea, acanthocytosis, retinitis, and neurologic dysfunction. Supplementation of large doses of vitamins A and E may prevent or reverse the retinal and neurologic abnormalities.

Acute hepatitis

Viral hepatitis is a systemic infection with primary involvement of the liver and symptoms related to liver impairment. Three agents are chiefly responsible for such infection: hepatitis A virus, hepatitis B virus, and non-A, non-B hepatitis virus. Liver involvement may occur in other generalized viral infections such as infectious mononucleosis, varicella, cytomegalovirus, coxsackie virus, and enteric cytopathogenic human orphan (ECHO) virus. Hepatitis occurs in all ages, sexes, and races. The incidence of disease is high in undeveloped nations. The spectrum of acute disease is quite broad, ranging from mild asymptomatic anicteric infections to fulminant hepatitis with a high fatality rate. In general, the fatality rate in hepatitis is low, only 0.1% to 0.5% of cases. Acute infection with hepatitis B and non-A, non-B viruses may evolve into a chronic disease state in 5% to 10% of cases, but hepatitis A virus infections do not progress to chronic hepatitis.

*Types II and V have no significant liver involvement.

The clinical syndromes observed in acute hepatitis caused by hepatitis A, hepatitis B, and non-A, non-B are indistinguishable. Serologic testing is necessary for etiologic differentiation. Specific serologic tests are available for hepatitis A and hepatitis B but not for non-A, non-B, this being a diagnosis of exclusion.

Early symptoms of acute hepatitis are similar to symptoms of a viral gastroenteritis with fever, abdominal pain, nausea, and vomiting. Anorexia, weight loss, and malaise are prominent complaints. Some patients notice abnormalities in their sense of smell and taste. Arthralgia, arthritis, and urticaria occur in hepatitis of all three etiologies, but are more common in HB infection. Dark urine and light-colored stools are observed at about the time jaundice appears in icteric cases. Pruritis may accompany jaundice. It is important to remember that a large percentage (possibly as many as 50%) of cases of hepatitis are anicteric. Physical findings include tenderness in the right upper quadrant, jaundice, hepatomegaly, splenomegaly, and occasionally arthritis and skin lesions.

In hepatitis, the SGOT and SGPT begin to rise before jaundice appears and usually exceed 300 U/L. Alkaline phosphatase may be very slightly increased. Serum proteins are usually normal, but albumin may show a slight decrease. Prothrombin time may be prolonged. Just before jaundice becomes apparent, light stools and dark urine are observed, and bile and bilirubin are detectable in urine. Direct reacting serum bilirubin is 8 to 12 mg/dl in usual icteric cases, and elevated to 20 to 30 mg/dl in severely cholestatic cases.

Hepatitis A. Formerly known as infectious hepatitis or short incubation hepatitis, hepatitis A has an incubation time of 3 to 5 weeks and is transmitted usually by fecal contamination of food or water. Infections occur most readily in conditions of crowding and poor sanitary control. Common source outbreaks are frequent and are commonly caused by contaminated food, milk, water, and raw shell fish.

Transmission via blood products, contaminated needles, and oral-anal contact has been recognized. The hepatitis A virus is present in blood for only a short time, but is present in stool for weeks, disasppearing at about the time of onset of jaundice. Viral excretion has stopped by the time the diagnosis is made, so isolation in the home or hospital is not necessary. Gloves should be worn when handling feces, and hand washing after patient contact is encouraged.

Hepatitis A infections are documented by demonstration of specific hepatitis A antibodies in serum. Acute phase IgM antibodies are detectable at onset of symptoms. IgG antibodies indicate either convalescence or past infection.

Immune serum globulin is an effective preventive measure for contacts to prevent clinical disease. Visitors to endemic areas may be given a similar treatment.

Hepatitis B. Hepatitis B was formerly known as serum hepatitis or long incubation hepatitis. Since the discovery of specific serologic markers (HBsAg), core antigen (HBcAg), and e antigen (HBeAg), cases can be specifically identified. Surface antigen has been demonstrated in all body fluids except feces. Transmission is most common via blood by injection or contamination of mucous membranes. Health professionals who work in hemodialysis, oncology, and surgery, laboratory workers who handle blood, parenteral drug users, male homosexuals, and spouses of chronically infected patients are at high risk for hepatitis B infection.

Hepatitis B infection may be suspected if arthritis and urticaria are present in addition to the usual symptoms of hepatitis. Findings suggestive of glomerulonephritis are observed in hepatitis B infections. A papular dermatitis of the cheeks and extensor surfaces of the extremities with hepatitis B constitutes the Gianotti-Crosti syndrome. HBsAg can be demonstrated in the walls of vessels in these skin lesions.

Diagnosis of hepatitis B depends on demonstration of specific antigen and antibodies in blood. HbsAg usually can be demonstrated early in the disease. However, it may disappear before the rise of anti-HBs can be detected, the so-called window of negative serology. Anti-HBc should be detectable during this time and is useful in avoiding misdiagnosis. The anticipated serologic events in hepatitis B are summarized in Table 16-3.

Prevention of the disease requires careful avoidance of contact with blood and body secretions of potentially infectious persons. Gloves should be worn when handling blood and secretions. Masks should be worn when a possibility of aerosolization of body fluids exists, as in dental procedures.

Hyperimmune globulin has been shown to be effective in preventing hepatitis B following exposure, and its use is recommended following needle sticks and mucosal exposure to HBsAg-positive blood. Infants born to mothers with HBsAg-positive blood should receive prophylaxis with 0.5 ml hyperimmune globulin within 24 hours of birth, at 3 months, and at 6 months. It is believed that the use of prophylaxis in the neonate will reduce the overall incidence of the carrier state in the community and may reduce the incidence of hepatoma.

Active immunity against hepatitis B infection may be achieved by use of hepatitis B vaccine, a killed vaccine made from HBsAg taken from infected blood. It has been shown to be both safe and effective in extensive trials. Active immunization is recommended for people at risk because of life-style, for health professionals who may be exposed to infectious blood, and for medical and dental students at the onset of their clinical training.

Non-A, non-B hepatitis. Transmission and incubation studies indicate that non-A, non-B hepatitis is an infection caused by one or more viruses. Incubation time averages 60 days. There are no serologic tests for this disease, and the diagnosis rests on exclusion of hepatitis A

Table 16-3. Serologic events in hepatitis B

Interpretation	HBsAg	HBeAg	DNA-P	Anti-HBc	ALT*	Anti-HBe	Anti-HBs
Very early incubation	+	+	+	−	−	−	
Early incubation	+	+	+	+	−	−	−
Acute hepatitis	+	−	−	+	+	−	−
Early convalescence	−	−	−	+	−	+	−
Late convalescence	−	−	−	−	−	+	+
Early carrier	+	+	+	+	+	−	+
Late carrier	+	−	−	+	−	+	−

*Alanine transaminase.

and hepatitis B by serologic tests. Since the advent of serologic testing of all blood used for transfusions, non-A, non-B has emerged as the most common cause of posttransfusion hepatitis. Transmission of this infection is felt to be the same as in hepatitis B, and high incidence is seen in parenteral drug abusers and male homosexuals. Isolation practices should be the same as for hepatitis B. Maternal-infant transmission has not been observed. Immune serum globulin may be helpful in prophylaxis, but guidelines for use are unclear. In general, this disease is somewhat milder than hepatitis B infection, but as many as 20% to 40% of non-A, non-B hepatitis infections may proceed to chronic hepatitis.

Treatment of acute viral hepatitis.

The treatment of acute viral hepatitis is entirely nonspecific. The management should include bedrest when fatigue dictates, and ambulation when the patient desires exercise. There is no evidence that activity prolongs the disease or causes complications, nor that rest shortens the disease or lessens complications. There is no evidence that manipulation of the diet is beneficial. Meals should be pleasing and appealing to the patient. There has been a proscription of fat during acute hepatitis, but there is no evidence that the intake of fat is detrimental or that the withholding of fat is beneficial. At times there is hypoglycemia during severe acute hepataitis, and the intake of carbohydrates is beneficial during these times. In situations in which acute viral hepatitis is superimposed on severe chronic malnutrition, multivitamin supplementation is recommended. In routine cases, multivitamin supplementation is of no benefit. In general, antiemetics should be avoided. However, if nausea continues longer than 3 or 4 days, metaclopromide in moderate doses may be safely used to promote gastric emptying. There is clear evidence that corticosteroids are of no benefit in acute hepatitis and are likely to be harmful.

Chronic hepatitis

Chronic active hepatitis refers to a specific form of chronic liver disease having multiple etiologies, affecting both sexes and all age groups, and having distinctive liver biopsy findings of inflammation, fibrosis, and piecemeal necrosis. Chronic active hepatitis has the potential to progress to cirrhosis, liver failure, and death. However, many cases wax and wane for years, and many spontaneously improve.

Chronic active hepatitis can be divided into three different etiologic groups: those following hepatitis B infections with positive hepatitis B serology; a group with negative serology but with a history of transfusion or antecedent non-A, non-B hepatitis; and a third large group, known as autoimmune hepatitis, made up preponderantly of young women with amenorrhea, elevated gamma globulin, and a high incidence of autoantibodies and lupus erythematosus cells. Also, they have a predilection to early hepatic failure. Metabolic liver diseases such as Wilson disease, alpha-1-antitrypsin deficiency, and hemochromatosis may mimic chronic active hepatitis by producing chronic liver disease and progressing to cirrhosis. Drugs such as methyldopa, isoniazid, and nitrofurantoin may cause severe chronic liver disease.

Symptoms encountered in chronic active hepatitis are quite variable. Some patients with abnormal liver function tests and liver biopsy are asymptomatic for years, whereas others complain of anorexia, malaise, weight loss, abdominal pain, and diarrhea. Joint pains and urticarial skin rash are common and are frequently the presenting complaints. Amenorrhea is common. Physical findings include hepatosplenomegaly and jaundice. As the disease progresses to cirrhosis, ascites, spider angiomata, palmar erythema, and dilated abdominal veins may be present. Late in the disease hepatic coma may become apparent. At any time during the disease, patients may develop portal hypertension with esophageal varices.

The serum transaminases are always elevated in chronic active hepatitis, usually only to the 200 to 300 U/L range. However, as cirrhosis supervenes, transminases may become normal. Serum bilirubin is elevated in 80% to 90% of cases. Alkaline phosphatase is only slightly elevated. Albumin is decreased and gamma globulin is variably increased, often markedly in autoimmune chronic active hepatitis. In this group, lupus erythematosus cells are found in 10% to 15% of cases and antinuclear and anti–smooth muscle antibodies may be found. Serum bile salts may be mildly to moderately elevated. Serologic markers are positive in chronic active hepatitis following hepatitis B. Usual markers seen are HBsAg, anti-HBc, and

HBeAg. Rarely, surface antigen may be negative or in very low titer, causing diagnostic error. Liver biopsy is necessary for diagnosis and management of chronic active hepatitis.

The therapy for chronic active hepatitis is controversial. Two drugs (prednisone and azathioprine) have been used with possible benefit. In general, chronic active hepatitis does not need to be treated unless the patient is symptomatic, laboratory tests are severely deranged or worsening, or sequential liver biopsies show progression of disease. In chronic active hepatitis caused by hepatitis B, proof of benefit from steroid therapy is lacking, and there may be evidence of an adverse influence. In autoimmune and non-A, non-B virus chronic active hepatitis, there is evidence that prednisone alone or in combination with azathioprine is effective. In addition, patients should be encouraged to exercise moderately to tolerance and eat a regular diet unless ascites dictates sodium restriction. Aspirin should be avoided because of its adverse effect on platelet function and gastric mucosal integrity. Acetaminophen in moderate doses should be harmless.

Cirrhosis

Cirrhosis is a chronic disease of the liver in which there is diffuse parenchymal injury and regeneration, marked increase in connective tissue with severe distortion of the architecture of hepatic lobules, and increased resistance to blood flow through the liver. The symptomatology of cirrhosis is dominated by its two major complications, portal hypertension and hepatic failure. It is believed that to produce cirrhosis hepatic injury must be prolonged and repeated. Some causes of cirrhosis are listed below.

I. Metabolic diseases
  A. Wilson disease
  B. Hemochromatosis
  C. Alpha-1-antitrypsin deficiency
  D. Galactosemia
  E. Hereditary fructose intolerance
  F. Tyrosinosis
  G. Glycogen storage disease types III and IV
II. Biliary obstructions
  A. Biliary atresia
  B. Choledochal duct cyst
  C. Cystic fibrosis
  D. Choledocholithiasis
III. Toxins
  A. Methotrexate
  B. Ethanol
  C. Total parenteral nutrition
IV. Infections
  A. Hepatitis B
  B. Hepatitis non-A, non-B
V. Vascular
  A. Chronic right heart failure
  B. Budd-Chiari syndrome
  C. Veno-occlusive disease
VI. Miscellaneous
  A. Indian childhood cirrhosis
  B. Sarcoidosis
  C. Autoimmune chronic active hepatitis
  D. Intestinal bypass surgery

Cirrhosis may make its presence known in at least three fashions. It may be completely silent during life and be discovered only at autopsy, it may be discovered during the workup of some other unrelated condition, or one of the complications of cirrhosis may lead to its discovery. The symptoms of cirrhosis are nonspecific and include malaise, lethargy, dyspepsia, and bloating. Late in the course of cirrhosis, weight loss, palmar erythema, clubbing of the fingers, and spider nevi are present. Portal hypertension is present in essentially every case of cirrhosis and is responsible for presenting symptoms in many cases. Ascites is also a common finding in cirrhosis. Diffuse hepatic parenchymal injury may give rise to bleeding because of inadequate production of prothrombin, fibrinogen, and factors VII, IX, and X. The etiology of clubbing of the fingers, seen in many children with cirrhosis, is undetermined, but may be caused by the opening of abnormal arteriovenous shunts in the pulmonary circulation. Encephalopathy is frequently seen in advanced cirrhosis.

In some cases of cirrhosis the laboratory findings are minimal. In the usual case there may be a decrease in albumin with an increase in globulin. There may be a decrease in serum sodium and potassium, and a variable degree of anemia, thrombocytopenia, and leukopenia. Serum bilirubin, alkaline phosphatase, transaminases, and gamma glutamyl transpeptidase are frequently normal, but may be variably elevated. Diagnosis requires liver biopsy for histologic confirmation. Liver-spleen scans with 99m technetium sulphur colloid will show a heterogenous uptake pattern with an enlarged spleen. Percutaneous portography by splenic puncture or arteriography may be needed to investigate and delineate obstruction to hepatic blood flow.

There is no specific treatment for cirrhosis. Whenever possible, treatment should be directed at underlying and associated disease. The major therapeutic effort in cirrhosis is the management of complications. Ascites can usually be brought under control by salt restriction. Occasionally, water restriction also is needed. Judicious use of diuretics may be beneficial. The rare case of resistant ascites may require peritoneal-venous shunting (LeVeen shunt) for relief. Bleeding esophageal varices can often be managed with sclerotherapy. In selected cases, portal systemic shunts (splenorenal and portacaval) may be used to relieve portal hypertension and control bleeding. Such shunts are more successful in hepatic fibrosis and less successful in cirrhosis, where shunting frequently precipitates hepatic encephalopathy. When hepatic encephalopathy is present, measures to reduce the load of ammonia may be helpful. Because of their prolonged clearance time in hepatic failure, sedatives should be avoided. Blood glucose should be monitored and glucose should be given to maintain normal levels. Liver transplants may offer reasonable therapy for the future.

Biliary tract disease

In the pediatric population, extrahepatic biliary obstruction is most often caused by anatomic defects, although other causes such as cholelithiasis and tumors should be considered. Extrahepatic obstructive disease should always be quickly and accurately diagnosed because prompt surgical correction can prevent serious and permanent hepatic injury.

In extrahepatic obstruction, transaminases are usually only moderately elevated, whereas the serum direct bilirubin, gamma glutamyl transpeptidase (GGTP), and 5′-nucleotidase are usually markedly elevated. Serum alkaline phosphatase is less useful in children because of the high contribution from growing bone. Serum bile salts are always elevated in cases of extrahepatic obstruction, and the postprandial serum bile salt curve may be completely flat with complete obstruction. Ultrasonography can be very useful in detecting the presence of gallstones and anatomic lesions such as a choledochal cyst. Also, several radiographic and nuclear medicine imaging techniques are used in diagnosis.

After biliary atresia, *choledochal cyst* is the most common malformation of the extrahepatic biliary tract in children, although still relatively rare. There is a definite female preponderance in this disorder. Although patients may have the classic triad of pain, jaundice, and palpable abdominal mass, these findings are inconstant or absent in many patients, especially those less than 1 year of age. There are three distinct morphologic types of choledochal cysts, as shown in Fig. 16-4. True choledochal cyst, or cystic dilation of the common bile duct, is the most common. Histologically, the cyst is not lined by biliary epithelium, but rare foci of epithelial cells may be noted. Diagnosis of congenital choledochal cyst can usually be made by ultraso-

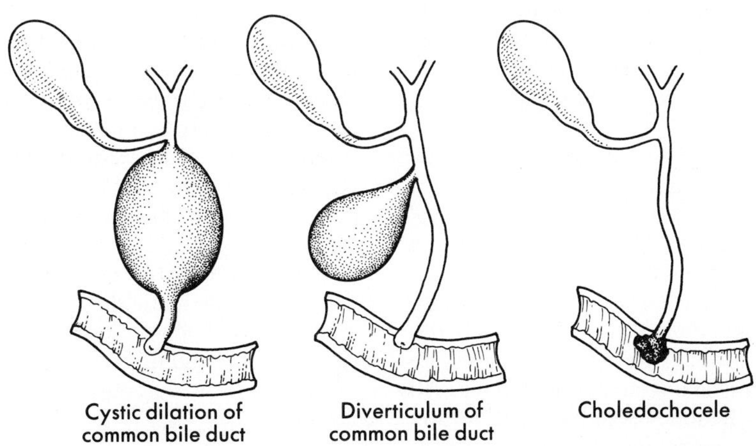

Fig. 16-4. Types of choledochal cyst. (From Barlow, B., et al.: J. Pediatr. **80:**934-940, 1976.)

nography and radiologic techniques. The surgical treatment of choice is total excision of the cyst with a Roux-en-Y jejunal anastomosis. With early surgical intervention, the prognosis is very good.

Rare structural causes of biliary obstruction in children include stenosis of the distal common bile duct, biliary tract duplications, acute hydropic distention of the gallbladder (idiopathic, as associated with Kawasaki disease), biliary tract tumors, and extrinsic compression of the biliary tree.

Gallstones are rare in children unless there is an underlying disorder that predisposes their formation. Chronic hemolytic states such as hereditary spherocytosis or sickle cell disease predispose formation of bilirubin stones. Patients with severe, chronic intrahepatic cholestasis may be at increased risk for stone formation. Other conditions that cause bile stasis, such as an anatomic obstruction in the biliary tree, have been associated with gallstones. Any condition that interrupts the enterohepatic circulation of bile salts, such as ileal resection or severe Crohn ileitis, will lead to the formation of lithogenic bile. Recently, an association has been noted between prolonged total parenteral nutrition and gallstone formation. Finally, it should be kept in mind that in some cases no predisposing conditions can be identified. Hereditary or dietary factors may be important in these cases.

The clinical presentation of cholelithiasis in children may vary greatly. Many cases are detected when the biliary tract is investigated for other reasons. In some cases, gallstones may cause acute obstruction with onset of jaundice and hepatic dysfunction. Biliary colic is rare in children, but its presence should always suggest gallstone disease.

Cholelithiasis may be diagnosed in some cases by a plain radiograph of the abdomen, if the calcium content is high enough. An oral cholecystogram is useful if obstruction is not present. Ultrasonography is also very useful.

Treatment of cholelithiasis in children is surgical. Careful evaluation of the biliary tract with cholangiography should be made at surgery to rule out any predisposing anatomic defects. All children with gallstones should be carefully evaluated for any underlying conditions that predispose them to cholelithiasis.

DISORDERS OF THE PANCREAS

Hyperamylasemia

Acute pancreatitis is not the only condition that causes elevation of the serum amylase concentration. Penetrating or perforated ulcers, intestinal obstruction or infarction, hepatitis, liver trauma, cirrhosis, regional enteritis, ruptured ectopic pregnancy, ovarian cysts and tumors, normal pregnancy, salivary adenitis or trauma, renal failure, and diabetic ketoacidosis may all cause an elevation of the serum amylase. There is evidence that many of the tissues involved in these conditions probably produce isoamylases, and at least seven isozymes of amylase have been detected in serum. The renal amylase and creatinine clearance ratio appears to be a good index of acute pancreatitis, since in this condition renal tubular reabsorption of amylase is decreased. The ratio should be less than 4%, and values greater than 6.5% strongly suggest acute pancreatitis in adults. However, normal values in children have not been firmly established, and false elevations have been reported with severe burns and diabetic ketoacidosis.

Pancreatitis

Pancreatitis in children may be frequently overlooked, because the manifestations may be less severe and even atypical compared to adult patients. Also, whereas adult disease is often secondary to alcoholism and biliary tract disease, these causes are rare in the pediatric patient. However, the diagnosis should always be considered in the child with abdominal trauma, acute or chronic abdominal pain, vomiting, or ascites.

Acute pancreatitis is pathologically divided into interstitial, edematous, and hemorrhagic forms. The latter is the more severe, accounts for about 15% of pediatric cases, and is characterized by widespread necrosis, small vessel thrombosis, and disruption of normal architecture. The major causes of pancreatitis in children are trauma (30%); drugs (30%); infections, especially mumps (15%); and congenital anomalies of the pancreatic duct. Up to 20% of cases may be classified as idiopathic. These and other causes of pancreatitis are listed below.

I. Systemic diseases
   A. Cystic fibrosis
   B. Crohn disease
   C. Diabetes mellitus

D. Henoch-Schönlein purpura
E. Sarcoid
F. Reye syndrome
G. Systemic lupus erythematosus
H. Hyperparathyroidism

II. Trauma
III. Obstruction
A. Biliary tract: choledochal cyst, cholelithiasis
B. Intestinal duplication cyst
C. Duodenal obstruction

IV. Penetrating posterior peptic ulcer
V. Infection
A. *Myocoplasma pneumoniae*
B. Mumps
C. Rubella
D. Influenza
E. Hepatitis A
F. Coxsackievirus B
G. Epstein-Barr virus

VI. Metabolic conditions
A. Alpha-1-antitrypsin deficiency
B. Malnutrition
C. Hyperlipoproteinemia (types I and V)

VII. Toxic substances
A. Ethanol
B. Corticosteroids
C. Tetracycline
D. Valproic acid
E. Sulfasalazine
F. Furosemide
G. Chlorothiazide
H. Oral contraceptives
I. Azathioprine
J. Sulfonamides

VIII. Heriditary pancreatitis
IX. Idiopathic conditions

Although the presentation in older children may be similar to that in adults, with nausea, vomiting, and midepigastric abdominal pain radiating to the back, younger children usually cannot localize the pain well. The history should include inquiries related to trauma, recent infections, drugs, and systemic disease. Physical examination reveals a quiet patient preferring to lie on his side or sit upright. The abdomen is slightly distended and tender in the midepigastric area. Rebound tenderness may be noted in the upper quadrants. Ascites may be present. A mass may indicate a pseudocyst or predisposing choledochal cyst. Bowel sounds are usually reduced. Bluish discoloration around the umbilicus (Cullen sign), or of the flanks (Grey Turner sign), may indicate hemorrhagic pancreatitis.

Important laboratory studies include serum amylase and lipase determinations. Other studies include liver function tests, electrolytes, glucose, calcium, and lipids. Plain abdominal x-ray films may reveal localized ileus or sentinel loop, pancreatic calcifications, or ascitic fluid. Ultrasonography may demonstrate increased size and decreased echo density of the inflamed pancreas or presence of a pseudocyst. Endoscopic retrograde cholangiopancreatography (ERCP) may be useful in delineating predisposing structural abnormalities.

Treatment of pancreatitis should include nasogastric suction in the presence of vomiting or ileus, analgesia with meperidine, reduction of pancreatic exocrine secretion and ductal relaxation with anticholinergic medication, and scrupulous attention to fluids and electrolytes including treatment of hyperglycemia and hypocalcemia when present. Any underlying causes should be identified and treated.

The mortality rate is 18% for acute interstitial edematous pancreatitis and 86% for hemorrhagic pancreatitis. Complications are similar to those seen in adults and include pseudocyst formation and pancreatic insufficiency.

Pancreatic exocrine insufficiency

The pancreas is an extremely important digestive organ. Its exocrine secretions into the duodenum include proteases, lipase, and amylase for the digestion of dietary protein, fat, and carbohydrates, respectively. Pancreatic secretions are also rich in bicarbonate, which neutralizes the acidic fluid reaching the duodenum from the stomach. Steatorrhea and azotorrhea do not develop until there is a 90% reduction in lipase and trypsin secretion, respectively.

Pancreatic exocrine insufficiency may be primary or secondary to another disorder or may involve isolated enzyme deficiencies. Cystic fibrosis is the most important primary cause of pancreatic insufficiency in childhood, comprising 96% of infants and children with pancreatic insufficiency. The incidence is between 1 to 2 per 2,000 live Caucasian births. The extraintestinal manifestations of this disease are discussed elsewhere in this text (Chapter 24).

Schwachman syndrome is the second most common cause of pancreatic insufficiency in children. This syndrome consists of pancreatic insufficiency, neutropenia, and growth retardation. Other features include metaphyseal dysostosis, eczema, and elevated fetal hemoglobin levels. Rarely, diabetes mellitus, Hirschsprung disease, and testicular fibrosis may also be associated. The frequency of this disorder is approximately 1 in 20,000 live births, and girls and boys are equally affected. An autosomal recessive pattern of inheritance is suggested.

The Johanson-Blizzard syndrome is a rare disorder characterized by aplastic nasal alae, microcephaly, deafness, mental retardation, hypothyroidism, absent permanent teeth, and decreased secretion of pancreatic enzymes. There also have been case reports of pancreatic insufficiency associated with an array of congenital malformations. Therefore in any child with multiple congenital anomalies and symptoms of malabsorption, pancreatic insufficiency should be considered.

Secondary causes of pancreatic insufficiency include malnutrition and pancreatitis. In infants with severe protein caloric malnututrition, enzyme output is markedly impaired, but water and bicarbonate secretion are normal. On correction of the malnutrition, enzyme secretion returns to normal. Pancreatitis, especially recurrent episodes, may eventually result in exocrine insufficiency.

Isolated pancreatic enzyme dificiencies have been described for lipase, trypsinogen, enterokinase, and amylase. Deficiency of the cofactor required for lipase, or colipase, has been described in two brothers.

The definitive diagnosis of pancreatic exocrine insufficiency is made by duodenal intubation and collection of pancreatic secretions under basal and stimulated conditions. Measurements of volume, bicarbonate content, and enzyme activities are compared to published normal values.

The treatment of pancreatic insufficiency is aimed at providing adequate caloric intake in a manner that ensures optimal absorption. This involves the use of exogenous pancreatic enzyme replacement, reduction of fat in the diet, increased protein and total calories, and supplementation of fat-soluble vitamins. Treatment should be individualized and monitored closely because much individual variation is noted among patients, and a person's requirements may change over time.

Peter F. Whitington
Gene L. Whitington
Dennis D. Black
Susan R. Orenstein

SELECTED READINGS

Alagille, D., and Odievre, M.: Liver and biliary tract disease in children, New York, 1979, John Wiley & Sons, Inc.

Ament, M.E.: Malabsorption syndromes in infancy and childhood, Part I, J. Pediatr. **81:**685-697, 1972.

Ament, M.E.: Malabsorption syndromes in infancy and childhood, Part II, J. Pediatr. **81:**867-884, 1972.

Andres, J.M., et al.: Liver disease in infants, Part I, J. Pediatr. **90:**686-697, 1977.

Arasu, T.S., et al.: Management of chronic aggressive hepatitis in children and adolescents, J. Pediatr. **95:**514-522, 1979.

Blacklow, A.R., and Cukor, G.: Viral gastroenteritis, New Engl. J. Med. **304:**397-406, 1981.

Burbige, E.J., et al.: Clinical manifestations of Crohn's disease in children and adolescents, Pediatrics **55:**866-871, 1975.

Christie, D.L., and Ament, M.E.: Diagnosis and treatment of duodenal ulcer in infancy and childhood, Pediatr. Ann. **5:**672-677, 1976.

Eastham, E.J., and Walker, W.A.: Adverse effects of milk formula ingestion on the gastrointestinal tract, Gastroenterology **76:**365-374, 1979.

Herbst, J.J.: Gastroesophageal reflux, J. Pediatr. **98:**859-870, 1981.

Jordan, S.C., and Ament, M.E.: Pancreatitis in children and adolescents, J. Pediatr. **91:**211-216, 1977.

Katz, A.J., and Grand, R.J.: All that flattens is not "sprue," Gastroenterology **76:**375-377, 1979.

Lebenthal, E., and Branski, D.: Childhood celiac disease: a reappraisal, J. Pediatr. **98:**681-690, 1981.

Mathis, R.K., et al.: Liver disease in infants, Part II, J. Pediatr. **90:**864-897, 1977.

Olsen, W.A.: A pathophysiologic approach to diagnosis of malabsorption, Am. J. Med. **67:**1007-1013, 1979.

Schiff, L., and Schiff, E.R., editors: Diseases of the liver, Philadelphia, 1982, J B Lippincott Co.

Silverman, A., and Roy, C.C.: Pediatric clinical gastroenterology, ed. 3, St. Louis, 1983, The C.V. Mosby Co.

Sleisenger, M.H., and Fordtran, J.S., editors: Gastrointestinal disease, Philadelphia, 1983, W.B. Saunders Co.

Werlin, S.L., and Grand, R.J.: Severe colitis in children and adolescents: diagnosis, course, and treatment, Gastroenterology **73:**828-832, 1977.

Whitington, P.F., et al.: Medical management of Crohn's disease in adolescence, Gastroenterology **72:**1338-1344, 1977.

17 Respiratory System

Acute illness of the respiratory tract is by far the most common cause of illness in infancy and childhood, accounting for approximately 50% of all illness in children less than 5 years of age and 30% in children between 5 and 12 years of age. Most of these illnesses are caused by acute viral infections, and young children ordinarily have four or five such infections each year. There is a broad spectrum of clinical severity, ranging from trivial and transient to moderate, severe, or even fatal. The introduction of antibacterial agents has resulted in a great decline in death rates and more rapid cure of infections when caused by bacteria. Nonetheless, many deaths still occur, and bacterial diseases and their complications continue to rank high as causes of morbidity and mortality.

The extent to which *chronic* respiratory diseases cripple children in the United States is dramatized by the fact that 1 of every 10 children is handicapped by asthma, cystic fibrosis, bronchopulmonary dysplasia, bronchiectasis, emphysema, or congenital bronchopulmonary disorders. These conditions cause almost half of all childhood chronic diseases.

The incidence of chronic lung disease in the pediatric population is expected to rise as a result of increasing air pollution and cigarette smoking. Throughout the world in the past three decades the concentrations of air pollutants have been rising steadily. Accumulating data suggest that exposure to air pollutants has a significant effect on human health, particularly on the lungs. Clinical experience and experimental studies suggest a strong relationship between cigarette smoking and chronic respiratory disease in adults. Although cigarette smoking is less a problem in chronic respiratory disease in children, all physicians and health professionals who provide care for children and adolescents should take a positive stand to discourage them from smoking. Furthermore, recent studies have indicated that atmospheric pollution with tobacco smoke endangers the health of nonsmokers. In the pediatric population, for example, it has been shown that in the first year of life, exposure to cigarette smoke increases the risk of pneumonia or bronchitis in the infant. If a significant reduction in morbidity and mortality of chronic lung disease is to be effected, major emphasis must be placed on sound measures to prevent air pollution and to discourage cigarette smoking.

Bronchopulmonary embryology. The rudiment of the respiratory tree appears in the fourth week of gestation as a bud from the ventral wall of the pharynx and undergoes progressive bronchial branching in the first weeks of fetal life. Bronchial generations are complete by the sixteenth week. From the sixteenth to the twenty-fourth weeks the solid tubes undergo canalization. At 26 to 28 weeks alveolar ducts and clusters of terminal air spaces appear on the terminal bronchioles and continue until birth. The distensibility of the lung early in gestation is much less than at term. When peak volumes are expressed as milliliters per gram of lung tissue, it is evident that the potential air space is small with respect to lung mass. The ability to retain air at end expiration is not evident until about the twentieth to twenty-fourth week of gestation, the same time at which pulmonary surfactant appears in extracts of lung tissue.

The pulmonary artery arises at 10 weeks from the ventral end of the fourth aortic arch. Capillary proliferation becomes maximal at 26 to 28 weeks of gestation and establishes an intimate relation with the terminal air spaces of the developing lung. At this time the lung becomes the most vascular of all organs of the body. The distensibility of the vascular bed, like that of the lung, increases with fetal age. Little blood flow is possible even at high perfusion pressures in the fetal lung, and the fetal lung is perfused by only 10% to 15% of the cardiac output. Following birth and the onset of pulmonary respiration, the capacity and distensibility of the vascular bed increases, pulmonary vascular resistance drops significantly, and pulmonary blood flow increases fivefold to tenfold to accommodate the whole of cardiac output.

From birth until 8 years of age growth of the lungs results from an increase in numbers of alveoli and dimensions of all the air passages. Further increase in lung size results from expansion of the preexisting alveoli. This in turn results in an increase in surface area of the lungs from 2 to 3 m^2 at birth to about 70 m^2 in the adult.

Supporting structures and respiratory muscles. The human thorax is both a rigid and a pliable structure. It has sufficient rigidity to protect the vital organs it contains, and it provides the pliability that enables it to function as a bellows during the ventilatory cycle. Rigidity results from bony composition of the ribs. Pliability exists because each rib is attached to a resilient cartilage that is fixed to either the sternum or the seventh rib and, in addition, has movable joints at its vertebral and sternal ends. The sternum is held in position by its connection with the ventral ends of the ribs. The increase in chest volume during inspiration occurs because the ribs are elevated as a result of contraction of the scalene and intercostal muscles and the descent of the diaphragm.

The diaphragm is the principal muscle of inspiration. Its contraction increases the volume of the thoracic cage in both its longitudinal and transverse diameters. The increase in transverse diameter occurs because contraction of its fibers moves the lower ribs in an upward and lateral direction. Apart from its function in normal breathing, the diaphragm plays an important role in coughing, sneezing, and, in conjunction with contraction of the abdominal muscles, assists in defecation, vomiting, parturition, and return of venous blood from the abdomen.

Unlike the intercostal muscles, which are innervated from the corresponding thoracic segments of the spinal cord, the diaphragm derives its nerve supply from the third, fourth, and fifth cervical segments by way of the phrenic nerve. Thus the diaphragm continues to function even when the intercostal muscles are paralyzed because of neural injury in the upper thoracic region or the administration of a spinal anesthetic. However, paralysis of both leaves of the diaphragm need not cause serious disability, provided the intercostal muscles are functioning normally and the lungs are healthy.

The muscles of the abdominal wall all arise from surfaces of portions of the lower eight ribs or their cartilages. Because active work is not required for tidal exhalation, these muscles do not normally participate in breathing. However, if a maximum expiration is made voluntarily, they will contract and cause depression of the lower ribs of the chest cage.

The trapezius muscle and the pectoral muscles, although attached to the ribs, are not ordinarily involved in ventilation. However, they do come into play if there is marked hyperventilation. Contraction of the trapezius fixes the shoulder girdle so that the pectoral muscles can elevate the upper ribs.

Lung volumes and capacities. There are four primary lung volumes that do not overlap each other and are essentially anatomic measurements (Fig. 17-1). *Tidal volume* (VT), or depth of breathing, is the volume of gas inspired or expired during each ventilatory cycle. *Inspiratory reserve volume* (IRV) is the maximal amount of gas that can be inspired from the end-inspiratory position. *Expiratory reserve volume* (ERV) is the maximal volume of gas that can be expired from the end-expiratory position. *Residual volume* (RV) is the volume of gas remaining in the lungs at the end of a maximal expiration.

There are four capacities, each of which includes two or more of the primary volumes. *Total lung capacity* (TLC) is the amount of gas contained in the lung at the end of a maximal inspiration. *Vital capacity* (VC) is the maximal volume of gas that can be expelled from the lungs by forceful effort following a maximal inspiration. *Inspiratory capacity* (IC) is the maximal volume of gas that can be inspired from the resting expiratory level. *Functional residual capacity* (FRC) is the volume of gas remaining in the lungs at the resting expiratory level.

Normal values for lung volumes and capacities have been determined for men, women, and children. The standard deviations from the mean show that there is considerable variation even in a homogeneous group. Consequently, deviations from "normal" must be large to be

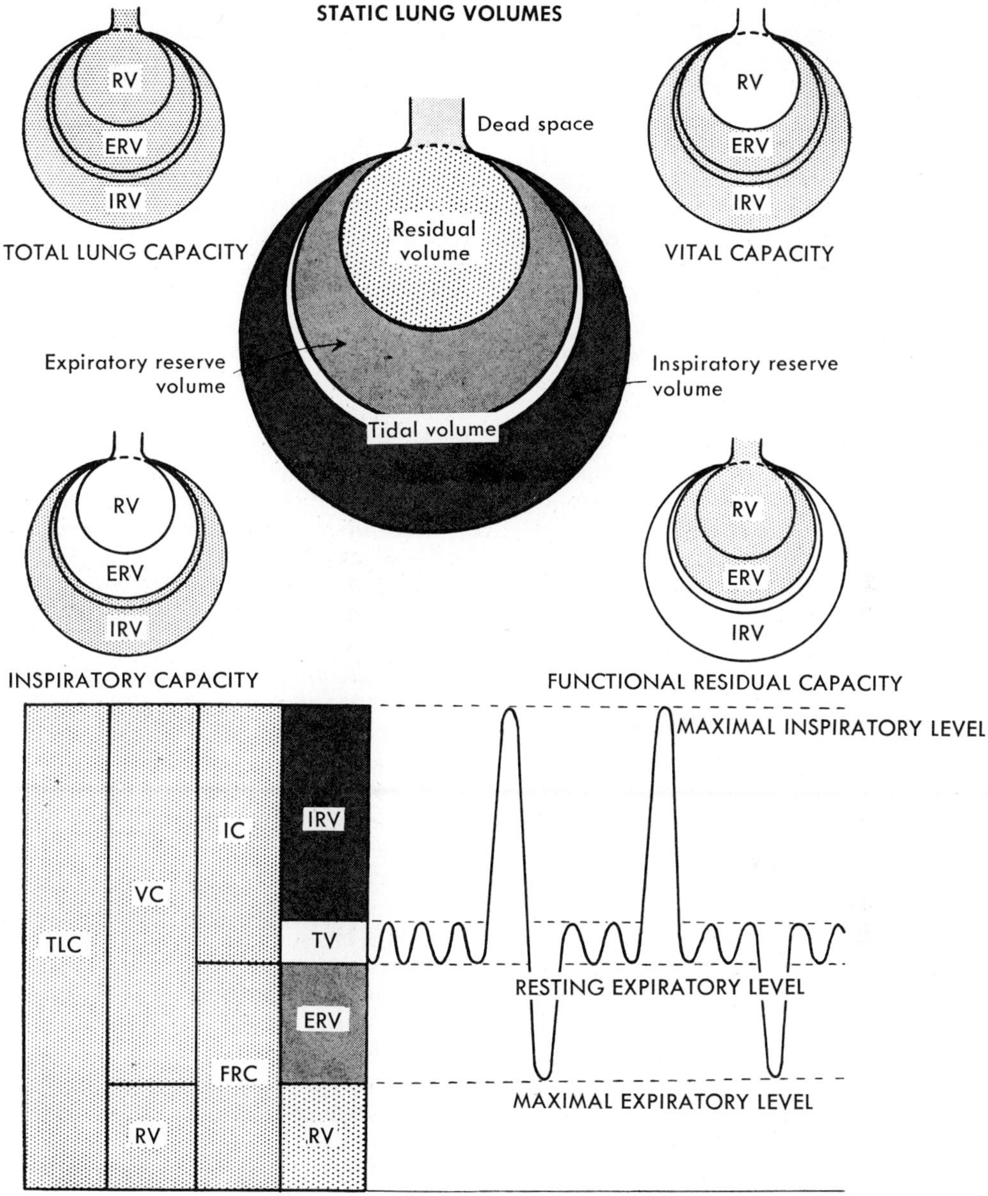

Fig. 17-1. Top, Large central diagram illustrates the four primary lung *volumes* and approximate magnitude. The outermost line indicates the greatest size to which the lung can expand; the innermost circle *(residual volume)*, the volume that remains after all air has been voluntarily squeezed out of the lungs. Surrounding the central diagram are smaller ones; shaded areas in these represent the four lung capacities. The volume of *dead space* gas is included in residual volume, *functional residual capacity* and *total lung capacity* when these are measured by routine techniques. Bottom, Lung volumes as they appear on a spirographic tracing: shading in vertical bar next to tracing corresponds to that in central diagram above. (From Comroe, J.H., Jr., et al.: The lung: clinical physiology and pulmonary function tests, ed. 2. Copyright © 1962 by Year Book Medical Publishers, Inc., Chicago. Reproduced with permission.)

significant. Nevertheless, routine serial determinations of the lung volumes can help in many problems related to diagnosis, therapy, and progression of pulmonary disease.

Control of respiration. Voluntary respiration is governed by the cerebral cortex, and automatic respiration by structures within the brain stem. At 20 to 22 weeks of gestation the central respiratory (medullary) center in the brain stem is sufficiently developed to inherently maintain respiratory rhythmicity and to respond to sensory stimuli and changes in arterial pH, Po_2, and Pco_2. This center acts in concert with the central chemoreceptors located in the brain stem and the peripheral chemoreceptors located in the carotid and aortic bodies to regulate alveolar ventilation and to maintain normal blood gas tensions. The medullary center is also under the influence of the pneumotaxic and apneustic centers located in the pons. The pontine centers are thought to play an auxiliary role in the regulation of respiration. The pneumotaxic center probably functions to tune the respiratory pattern finely by setting the timing of the inspiratory cutoff. However, respiratory rhythmicity can exist without the pneumotaxic center. The apneustic center is thought to be the location of the inspiratory cutoff switch. Thus the phenomena of apneusis (maintained inspiratory activity unrelieved by expiration) arises from inactivation of this inspiratory cutoff mechanism.

The central respiratory center responds reflexly to impulses from the lungs, the skeletal muscles and joints, the peripheral chemoreceptors, and the central chemoreceptors. Proprioceptive impulses from the lungs transmitted by the vagi activate the Hering-Breuer reflex. This reflex results in inhibition of inspiration as the lungs distend and stimulation of inspiration as the lungs deflate. Impulses transmitted by sensory nerves from the muscles and joints also stimulate activity of the respiratory center, producing hyperventilation during exercise.

The peripheral chemoreceptors located in the carotid and aortic bodies are sensitive to certain stimuli. Nerve impulses originating in these structures and traveling to the brain stem by way of the vagus and glossopharyngeal nerves increase in response to (1) hypoxemia, (2) hypercapnia, (3) hypoperfusion of the peripheral chemoreceptors, (4) acidemia, and (5) stimulation by a variety of chemical and pharmaceutical agents. Increased breathing frequency (tachypnea) and tidal volume (hyperpnea) result. However, prolonged and severe hypoxia and hypercapnia will result in central depression of respiration.

Although the peripheral chemoreceptors respond to increasing arterial Pco_2, the brain stem or central chemoreceptor response to alteration in arterial Pco_2 and hydrogen ion concentration (cH^+) is a much more powerful factor in the regulation of breathing. Direct stimulation of this area by increased arterial Pco_2 or cH^+ produces an increase in ventilation. Conversely, a decreased arterial Pco_2 or cH^+ causes a depression of ventilation. The effect of these stimuli on the central chemoreceptors is thought to be mediated by changes in the acid-base composition of the cerebrospinal fluid related to changes in the cerebrospinal fluid cH^+.

Mechanics of breathing. Supplying oxygen to the alveoli and removing carbon dioxide from them are accomplished by the flow of air in and out of the lungs with each breath. This process is a mechanical one for which the muscles of respiration provide the work necessary to overcome the resistive forces to airflow offered by the lung and chest wall during breathing.

Two kinds of resistive forces must be overcome to achieve inflation of the lung. These forces have been characterized as being either static, elastic forces or dynamic, nonelastic, flow-resistive forces. One component of the elastic resistance is called compliance. *Compliance* is a measurement of the distensibility of the lungs and is defined as the volume change produced by a unit pressure change. Its units are liter per centimeter of water. At lung volumes greater than residual volume, lung compliance is 0.2 L/cm H_2O in adults; each cm H_2O pressure applied to the lung forces 200 ml air into the lung. The less the volume change produced by a given pressure change, the "stiffer" or less compliant are the lungs. Conversely, if the volume change for the same pressure change is large, the lungs are highly distensible, or compliant.

The chest wall, like the lung, is a hollow structure with elastic properties and thus also possesses compliance. The compliance of the chest wall is equal to that of the lungs (0.2 L/cm H_2O) in normal subjects. The compliance of the chest, or the total compliance, must necessarily be less than that of either the lung or chest wall. Total compliance is 0.1 L/cm H_2O—

half the compliance of the lung or chest wall individually.

A second component of the elastic resistance of the lungs is caused by the *surface tension forces* created by the air-fluid interface within the alveoli. Reduction of surface tension by surfactant reduces the pressure required to fill the alveoli during inspiration.

Nonelastic resistances, which must be overcome during breathing, consist of airway resistance to airflow and tissue viscous resistance. *Airway resistance* is the result of friction between the flowing gas and the walls of the airways and within the airstream itself. It accounts for approximately 80% of the total nonelastic resistance of the lungs. It varies inversely with the radius of the airway and directly with the volumetric flow rate. At a relatively low flow rate, the flow pattern is laminar. When the respiratory volumetric flow rate exceeds a critical value or when the airway radius decreases, the flow pattern becomes turbulent. Turbulent flow not only increases airway resistance but also greatly increases the work of breathing.

Tissue viscous resistance is a relatively small part of the total nonelastic resistance, accounting for approximately 20%. It is caused by the friction of tissue layers sliding over one another during movement of the lung within the thorax. This resistance factor is relatively constant compared to marked changes in airway resistance that can occur in bronchopulmonary diseases.

In summary, the respiratory muscles must have sufficient work capacity to overcome the elastic and nonelastic resistive forces of the respiratory system. During inspiration active muscular contraction provides the force necessary to overcome (1) elastic recoil of the lungs and chest wall, (2) surface tension forces within the alveoli, (3) frictional resistance to airflow through the tracheobronchial tree, and (4) frictional resistance during movement of the lung and chest wall.

Pulmonary gas exchange. The primary function of the lung is to arterialize the mixed venous blood, which enters the pulmonary artery and perfuses the lungs, by adding oxygen to it and eliminating carbon dioxide from it. This is achieved by pulmonary gas exchange, a function subserved by several processes.

Ventilation is a cyclic process of inspiration and expiration in which fresh air enters the alveoli and then an equal volume of alveolar gas leaves them. Pulmonary ventilation is optimal if the levels of the partial pressure of oxygen and carbon dioxide in the pulmonary alveoli and in the arterial blood are maintained within physiologic limits. Pathologic conditions that interfere with the control of respiration or the mechanics of breathing may impair pulmonary ventilation. Hypoventilation leads to hypoxemia, hypercapnia, and a mixed metabolic-respiratory acidosis. Hyperventilation causes a decrease in arterial P_{CO_2} and respiratory alkalosis.

Even in a healthy subject, however, that part of the tidal volume contained in the conducting airways from the nares to the respiratory bronchioles does not participate in gas exchange with the blood. This fraction of the tidal volume is called the *anatomic dead space* and roughly equals 2.2 ml/kg (1 ml/lb) ideal body weight. That volume of alveolar space ventilated but not perfused by blood is called the *alveolar dead space*. Alveolar dead space is minimal in healthy subjects but may increase greatly in diseased lungs. *Physiologic dead space* is that portion of the tidal volume that does not participate in pulmonary gas exchange. It is the sum of the anatomic and alveolar dead spaces, and in a healthy subject is about 30% of the tidal volume.

The lung is often regarded as a uniform structure in which each alveolus has the same volume, the same distensibility, the same ventilation, the same blood flow, and the same facility for diffusion of gases across its alveolar-capillary membranes. However, the human lung is not uniform, and with an estimated 300 million alveoli the opportunity for *uneven ventilation* is exceedingly great. Uneven ventilation is present to a slight degree in healthy young persons, to a greater extent in healthy older people, and to a significant degree in many pulmonary diseases. Pathologic causes of uneven ventilation include regional changes in elasticity, as in emphysema; regional obstruction, as in asthma; and regional disturbances in expansion, as in pulmonary edema or atelectasis. Uneven ventilation causes hypoxemia but does not necessarily lead to carbon dioxide retention if there is sufficient hyperventilation of the remaining well-ventilated alveoli. It is an inefficient process because minute volume (tidal volume multiplied by the respiratory rate) must increase to compensate for a certain amount of ineffective ventilation.

The functional parts of the pulmonary circulation are the pulmonary capillaries. The right ventricle, pulmonary arteries, and arterioles represent a distributing system and the venules and veins a collecting system. Pulmonary blood flow is approximately equal to systemic blood flow. *Perfusion* of the pulmonary capillary bed, like alveolar ventilation, must be adequate in volume and even in distribution for optimal pulmonary gas exchange.

However, just as there is nonuniformity of gas distribution in healthy persons, there is also some *unevenness of capillary blood flow* in healthy persons. This occurs in large part because of the effect of gravity; thus blood flow is less at the apex than at the base of the upright lung and therefore unevenness of flow is minimized when one is supine or prone and maximal when one is erect. Uneven capillary blood flow occurs in many pathologic conditions affecting the lungs and circulation, such as embolization or thrombosis of parts of the pulmonary circulation, occlusion of the pulmonary artery or arterioles, reduction of the pulmonary vascular bed, and anatomic venous to arterial shunts. The major effect of uneven matching of inspired gas and pulmonary capillary blood flow is to cause incomplete oxygenation of the blood, and ventilation-perfusion mismatching is the most common cause of hypoxemia in clinical medicine.

The *pressure* and *resistance* to flow in the pulmonary capillaries are normally low and must remain so to prevent transudation of fluid into the interstitial spaces or into alveoli. The pressure and resistance to flow in the pulmonary artery and arterioles are also normally low and must remain so to prevent right ventricular strain and hypertrophy and possibly failure, a condition known as cor pulmonale.

Diffusion is a passive physical process that results in the exchange of gases between alveolar air and pulmonary capillary blood. Factors influencing the diffusing capacity of a gas include the pressure gradient of that gas across the alveolar-capillary membrane, the surface area available for diffusion, and the thickness and properties of the diffusion pathway from gas to blood. The latter includes certain characteristics of the alveolar-capillary membrane affecting solubility of the gas in pulmonary tissue and the rate at which the gas passes through the red blood cell membrane and chemically combines with hemoglobin. Exercise increases the pulmonary diffusing capacity of healthy lungs by evening out the distribution of alveolar ventilation while increasing pulmonary capillary perfusion; hence a more uniform match of ventilation to perfusion. Loss of pulmonary diffusing capacity is an uncommon cause of arterial hypoxemia in children. Conditions such as interstitial pulmonary fibrosis, sarcoidosis, pulmonary edema, pulmonary hemosiderosis, and primary pulmonary hypertension with obliteration of pulmonary capillaries may reduce pulmonary diffusing capacity.

Gas transport. The blood carries molecular oxygen in two ways: (1) in loose reversible chemical combination with hemoglobin (Hb) in the erythrocytes as oxyhemoglobin (HbO_2), and (2) as dissolved oxygen (O_2) in physical solution in plasma. By far the larger amount of O_2 in blood is present as HbO_2.

The amount of O_2 dissolved and the amount combined with Hb depend on the partial pressure of O_2 in arterial blood ($Pa{O_2}$), blood temperature, and the solubility coefficient of O_2 in blood. The solubility coefficient of O_2 in blood at 38° C (100° F) is only 0.003 vol%/torr $Pa{O_2}$. Hence at a $Pa{O_2}$ of 100 torr only 0.3 ml O_2 is dissolved in 1 dl blood. Breathing 100% O_2 at sea level increases $Pa{O_2}$ to about 600 torr, while dissolved O_2 rises to about 1.8 ml/dl blood.

Because O_2 requirement of a resting person is about 250 ml/min, the cardiac output would have to be 140 L/min at rest and 800 L/min during moderately strenuous exercise if plasma were the only transporting medium for O_2. Fortunately the gas transport mechanism is whole blood and not just plasma.

Most of the O_2 in blood is carried in erythrocytes in combination with Hb as HbO_2. One gram of Hb is capable of combining chemically with 1.34 ml O_2. With a normal Hb concentration of 15 g/dl, the blood is capable of carrying 20.1 vol% O_2 as HbO_2, in addition to the comparatively small amount carried in the plasma. Although Hb is capable of combining with this amount of O_2, it does not normally do so. The extent to which Hb combines with O_2 is usually expressed as the percent saturation, and in a normal person breathing room air it is about 97%. Incomplete saturation of Hb occurs because approximately 3% of cardiac output bypasses the pulmonary circulation and mixes with oxygenated blood draining from the pulmonary veins into the left side of the heart.

The degree of saturation of Hb with O_2 depends on the PaO_2. This relationship is not linear but rather is defined by a signoid curve known as the *oxyhemoglobin dissociation curve* (OHDC) (Fig. 17-2). From the curve it can be seen that Hb clings to O_2 over a wide range of O_2 tension at the upper end of the scale and releases O_2 readily at lower O_2 tensions. The converse is also true: Hb takes up O_2 very readily at lower O_2 tensions but not at higher tensions.

In addition to the PaO_2, other factors affect the OHDC. These include the arterial carbon dioxide tension ($PaCO_2$), hydrogen ion concentration (cH^+), temperature, level of 2,3-diphosphoglycerate, and type of Hb in the erythrocyte. The concept of P_{50} helps to visualize the relative

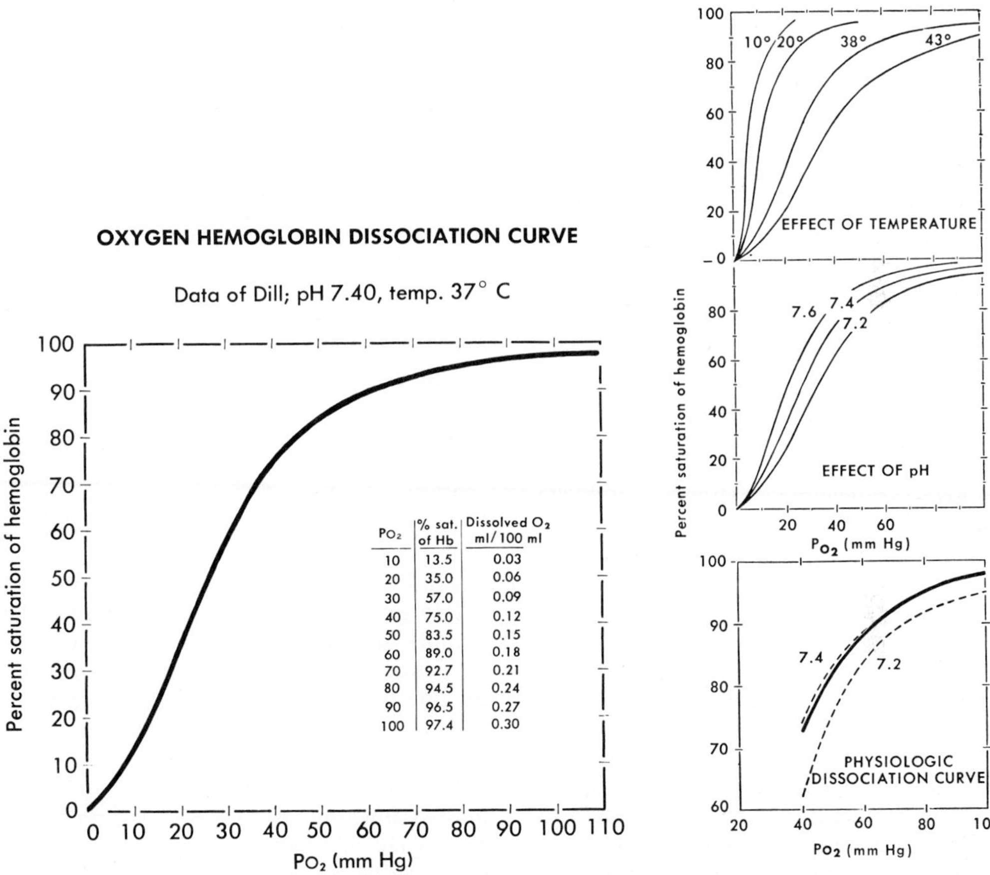

PO_2	% sat. of Hb	Dissolved O_2 ml/100 ml
10	13.5	0.03
20	35.0	0.06
30	57.0	0.09
40	75.0	0.12
50	83.5	0.15
60	89.0	0.18
70	92.7	0.21
80	94.5	0.24
90	96.5	0.27
100	97.4	0.30

Fig. 17-2. Large graph shows a single dissociation curve, applicable when the *pH* of the blood is *7.4* and temperature 37° C (98.6° F). The blood O_2 tension and saturation of patients with CO_2 retention, acidosis, alkalosis, fever, or hypothermia will not fit this curve because the curve "shifts" to the right or left when *temperature,* pH, or PCO_2 is changed. Effects on the O_2-hemoglobin dissociation curve of change in temperature (top right) and in pH (middle right) are shown in the smaller graphs. A small change in blood pH occurs regularly in the body; that is, when mixed venous blood passes through the pulmonary capillaries, PCO_2 decreases from 46 to 40 mm Hg and pH rises from 7.37 to 7.40. During this time, blood changes from a pH 7.37 dissociation curve to a pH 7.40 curve; an approximate "physiological" dissociation curve (solid line, bottom right) has been drawn to describe this change. (From Comroe, J.H., Jr., et al.: The lung: clinical physiology and pulmonary function tests, ed. 2. Copyright © 1962 by Year Book Medical Publishers, Inc., Chicago. Reproduced with permission.)

position of the OHDC curve for a given Hb under various conditions. P_{50} is the PaO_2 at which Hb is 50% saturated with O_2. At any given PaO_2, high-affinity Hb combines with more O_2 than does low-affinity Hb, and the former reaches 50% saturation at a lower PaO_2 than does the latter. Thus the P_{50} of high-affinity Hb is low, reflecting a leftward shift of the OHDC, whereas the P_{50} of low-affinity Hb is high, reflecting a rightward shift of the OHDC. The curve shifts to the right whenever there is a rise in $PaCO_2$, cH^+, body temperature, or an increase in the red cell 2,3-diphosphoglycerate. The OHDC for Hb F is to the left of that for Hb A. Carbon monoxide (CO) competes with O_2 for binding with the iron in Hb. Because its affinity for Hb is 250 times greater than that of O_2, it is firmly bound. CO also increases the affinity of unbound iron atoms for O_2 and thus causes a shift of the OHDC to the left. When methemoglobin is formed as a result of oxidation of an iron atom to the ferric state, the OHDC is altered in a manner similar to the effects of CO.

Carbon dioxide exists in significant amounts in the blood in four different forms: (1) dissolved CO_2, (2) CO_2 combined with protein (carbamino compounds), (3) as bicarbonate ions, and (4) as carbonic acid. Most of the CO_2 in blood exists in the form of bicarbonate ions. Carbon dioxide molecules diffuse from the plasma into the erythrocytes where, under the catalytic influence of carbonic anhydrase, they hydrate to form carbonic acid. Carbonic acid ionizes, forming bicarbonate ion, which diffuses out of the erythrocyte into the plasma and H^+, which is buffered within the erythrocyte by Hb. Relatively few bicarbonate ions form in the plasma because no carbonic anhydrase is there to accelerate the hydration of CO_2. Regulation of plasma bicarbonate ion concentration is one of the many important functions of the kidney.

In a steady state the metabolic production of carbon dioxide by the body is equal to the amount of carbon dioxide being eliminated by the alveoli. Normally the lungs eliminate the carbon dioxide equivalent of 15,000 mEq carbonic acid daily, while the kidneys excrete 60 to 80 mEq in fixed acids. Thus the respiratory system is quantitatively more important than the kidney in regulating the acid-base balance of the body. A decrease in alveolar ventilation at a given metabolic rate will result in an increase in alveolar PCO_2; carbon dioxide is retained excessively in the blood and the arterial PCO_2 increases. Because of the increase in carbon dioxide tension, the ratio between the bicarbonate and dissolved carbon dioxide is less than 20:1. As a result, the pH falls and the patient suffers from a condition called *respiratory acidemia*. If hypercapnia persists, the kidney responds by excreting increased amounts of H^+, retaining increased amounts of bicarbonate ions in the process. This bicarbonate ion retention produces a *compensatory metabolic alkalosis*. Alveolar hyperventilation reduces alveolar and arterial PCO_2. When the arterial PCO_2 falls, the plasma bicarbonate level also falls, but the ratio of bicarbonate to dissolved carbon dioxide is still greater than 20:1. As a result the pH rises, resulting in a condition called *respiratory alkalemia*. If the hypocapnia persists, excess cations and bicarbonate anions are excreted by the kidney, although chloride is conserved.

Probably the most common mixed disturbance of acid-base equilibrium in pediatrics is the mixed respiratory and metabolic acidosis of asphyxia. This is well exemplified in newborn infants who have severe hyaline membrane disease or massive aspiration syndrome. In these instances the low pH is associated with a low PO_2, and a high PCO_2 in arterial blood.

Pulmonary function testing. The quantitative measurement of the many different processes involved in respiration requires a large number of physiologic tests. However, pulmonary function tests are rarely helpful in making specific diagnoses, and it is fortunate that the majority of respiratory illnesses can be successfully diagnosed and managed without recourse to measurements of lung function. Pulmonary function tests are used mainly to assess the degree of functional abnormality and thus the severity of disease, to assess response to therapy, to follow the course of pulmonary illnesses, and to further understanding of the pathogenesis and pathophysiology of chronic childhood respiratory diseases.

Technically, some pulmonary function tests are very simple and may be carried out in the office or clinic. Others require expensive equipment and considerable technical experience and are mainly carried out in a hospital cardiopulmonary laboratory. Still others are research procedures and at present are available only in a few medical centers. In none of the pulmonary function tests has the mechanical adaptation of equipment to pediatric use presented an insurmountable obstacle. Nonetheless, physical limitations, if combined with problems of patient understanding and cooperation, may render some of the tests impractical. Pulmonary function testing in infants is technically more difficult than in children but is by no means impossible. Indeed, in some centers these tests are performed on neonates for investigative as well as clinical purposes.

Results of the measurement of any function must be interpreted on the basis of a set of normal values for that function. Normal values have been determined for the whole age range of pediatrics and correlated with measurable independent variables such as body size, lung volume, or body surface area.

Functionally, pulmonary diseases may be classified into two major groups. The *restrictive group* is caused by diseases of the lung parenchyma and the chest wall and is characterized by limitation of inflation of the lung. The *obstructive group* is caused by conditions that narrow the airways and therefore impede the to-and-fro movement of tidal volume. Some diseases such as cystic fibrosis may have features of both groups, particularly when lung tissue is destroyed.

The term *restrictive* implies an impaired ability of the lung to expand. This may result from reduction in lung volume, as in pneumonia, atelectasis, pleural effusion, and pneumothorax; from decreased distensibility of the lung, as in pulmonary edema and pulmonary fibrosis; or from diseases of the chest wall, as in kyphoscoliosis and neuromuscular conditions. Pulmonary function studies indicate a decreased vital capacity and frequently a stiffer, less compliant lung. There is no impairment in the ability to expire forcibly most of the vital capacity within 1 second following a maximal inspiration (FEV_1).

In contrast, the patient with obstructive disease such as asthma or cystic fibrosis has a reduced vital capacity primarily on the basis of an increase in functional residual capacity. There is a marked reduction in the FEV_1 because of obstruction to airflow. The measurement of vital capacity and timed vital capacity, that is, the percentage of the vital capacity that can be forcibly expired in 1 second, is one of the simplest and most informative tests that can be done.

In addition, all these diseases may result in other physiologic abnormalities, including mismatching of ventilation and perfusion with subsequent hypoxemia; increase in the work of breathing, which increases oxygen consumption and carbon dioxide production; and when severe, hypoventilation with consequent carbon dioxide retention, respiratory acidosis, and hypoxemia.

In practice, the most useful measurement of pulmonary function is the partial pressure of oxygen and carbon dioxide in arterial blood. Of these, the P_{CO_2} is believed to be the more important because it reflects more accurately the adequacy of ventilation. Patients who are hypoventilating will need mechanical assistance when the P_{CO_2} rises to narcotic levels. Carrying out serial determinations of the P_{CO_2} in arterial blood is the most effective way to monitor the efficacy of respirator therapy. Measurement of arterial P_{O_2} is of value in assessing the magnitude of venous admixture resulting from ventilation-perfusion imbalance or anatomic shunts. Serial oxygen measurements are necessary to monitor oxygen therapy to prevent the toxic and lethal effects of hypoxemia and the toxic effects of hyperoxia.

Nongas exchange functions. Recognition that the lung participates in nongas exchange functions has come slowly in the past few years. A number of mechanical, phagocytic, and humoral *defense mechanisms* exist in the respiratory tract to guard against bronchopulmonary infections. Most inhaled airborne particles larger than 10 microns in diameter are trapped in the nose by the hairs, nasal turbinates, and nasal mucociliary blanket. Also, the normal pharyngeal bacterial flora, particularly the alpha hemolytic streptococci, inhibit the growth of many potential respiratory pathogens such as *Streptococcus pneumoniae, Staphylococcus aureus,* and the enteric gram-negative bacilli. The mucociliary clearance mechanism of the lower respiratory tract is of major importance in the defense against inhaled or aspirated pathogens between 1 and 10 microns in size. The critical components of this system include a sol/gel mucus blanket and the coordinated activity of the ciliated epithelium. The latter moves the mucus blanket upwards toward the larynx, from which it is expelled by throat clearing or cough, then either swallowed or expectorated. Inhaled particles deposited beyond the origin of the mucociliary escalator in the proximal respiratory bronchioles are cleared from the distal respiratory bronchioles and alveoli by the alveolar macrophages. Macrophages may enter the lymphatic system and migrate to regional lymph nodes. In the lymph nodes the macrophages present their ingested loads as antigens for processing by the cellular or humoral immune system. Specific immunoglobulins can be secreted into the airways to aid in recognition and phagocytosis of pathogens in addition to their direct microbicidal effect. Secretory IgA appears to be the most important of the immunoglobulins. Cellular immunity is currently thought to play a relatively minor role in clearance of microorganisms from the respiratory tract, but a major role in limiting the activity of pathogens that are not effectively killed by macrophages such as the tubercle bacillus. When the normal clearance mechanisms are overwhelmed by an inoculum of bacteria, the cellular response of the lung is composed primarily of segmented neutrophils mobilized from within the circulation.

The lung is now known to perform important *metabolic* and *endocrine* functions. These include the synthesis, uptake, activation, inactivation, and release of numerous biologically active substances, many of which are vasoactive. The lung is capable of inactivating circulating bradykinin, prostaglandin, serotonin, and histamine. It also contains an enzyme that is responsible for converting angiotensin I to angiotensin II, and it is capable of synthesizing histamine and prostaglandins. Alteration of these metabolic functions may be a factor in causation, perpetuation, or aggravation of certain pulmonary disorders. For example, pulmonary embolism may stimulate the synthesis and release of potent substances that contribute to the pathogenesis of such complications as pulmonary hypertension, systemic hypotension, and bronchial constriction. Although the cellular sites of these metabolic functions are still undetermined, the endothelial cell, in intimate contact with the blood, is a likely candidate.

ACUTE INFECTIONS OF THE RESPIRATORY TRACT

Etiology and pathogenesis. The following factors enter into the etiology and pathogenesis of infections of the respiratory tract: (1) nature of the infectious agent, (2) dose of the infectious agent, (3) age, and (4) host resistance.

Infectious agents. As stated previously, the majority of acute infections of the respiratory tract are caused by viruses. Special studies are required for exact diagnosis, and these are seldom obtained in ordinary practice. Only occasionally can a physician make a clinically presumptive diagnosis of a specific class of virus as the cause of an acute upper respiratory tract infection, examples being herpangina (caused by Coxsackie Group A viruses), pharyngoconjunctival fever (produced by certain types of adenoviruses), herpetic gingivostomatitis, and acute lymphogranular pharyngitis. In view of the self-limited course of viral infections of the respiratory tract and their failure to respond to antibiotic therapy, precise etiologic diagnosis is not required in the usual case. The main thing is to be reasonably certain that one is dealing with a viral, not a bacterial, disease. This opinion is governed by signs, symptoms, often a normal or leukopenic white blood cell count without a relative increase in polymorphonuclear granulocytes, and a negative throat culture.

The second major group of etiologic organisms are the common pathogenic bacteria, of which the Group A beta hemolytic *Streptococcus, Staphylococcus aureus,* pneumococcus, and *Haemophilus influenzae* type B are frequent offenders. By far the most important of these is the beta hemolytic *Streptococcus* because it may cause, in addition to clinically severe upper respiratory tract infection, subsequent acute nephritis or rheumatic fever. Therefore positive identification of this organism as the cause of throat infection constitutes the real crux of the diagnostic problem. Penicillin therapy for a period of 10 days is mandatory for beta hemolytic streptococcal infections to decrease the frequency of subsequent rheumatic fever and acute nephritis. Antibiotic-resistant strains of *S. aureus* constitute fairly common causes of severe infection of the respiratory tract, especially pneumonia.

Size of dose. The larger the dose of an infectious agent, the greater the likelihood of clinically significant infection. Thus the mere presence of potentially pathogenic agents in a throat culture does not imply clinical importance, but a relatively pure culture of them in abundance, indicating increase of dose, does.

Pathogenic bacteria normally harbored in the nose and throat of asymptomatic persons may increase in numbers when such persons contract viral infections. Thus viral infection fosters bacterial invasion, presumably by increasing size of dose and by inflicting damage to the membrane, thereby lowering local defenses against infection.

Age. Age exerts a definite influence on the tendency to acute infections of the respiratory tract. The newborn infant may suffer from pneumonia acquired in utero or may have respiratory infection as a consequence of aspiration, malformations of the respiratory tract, or other condition. During the first months the level of immunoglobulin G (IgG) normally decreases, and if the decrease is exaggerated, this may predispose the infant to infection. Age also governs opportunity for exposure to infectious agents. The limited number of contacts of young infants implies relatively infrequent exposure to infection. On the other hand, children entering nursery school, kindergarten, or grammar school constantly widen their circle of contacts, and an increased frequency of infection results. Age also has an important bearing on the development of immune mechanisms and the acquisition of specific immunities by contact with an ever-increasing variety of infectious agents.

Host resistance. Diminished resistance to infection may result from several factors. Such contributing conditions may be of a general nature, localized to the respiratory tract, or caused by a specific lack of adequate defense against infection. Among general conditions apparently encouraging increased susceptibility to infection or greater clinical severity are malnutrition, anemia, fatigue, and chilling of the body. Of the predisposing conditions in the respiratory tract, allergy (especially allergic rhinitis) is by far the most common. Others are cystic fibrosis of the pancreas, obstructive malformations of the respiratory tract, and immune deficiencies.

Pediatric aspects of acute respiratory tract infections. Young children, especially those between 6 months and 3 years of age, tend to react more severely to acute respiratory tract infection than do older children. The impact of illness on these children often seems far out of proportion to the local manifestations of the disease. The uninitiated are often surprised that such severe manifestations can result from what seems so trivial an infection. Therefore before discussing individual entities, consideration will be given to the special pediatric aspects of acute respiratory tract infections.

Fever. It is characteristic of newborns that infection—even fatal infection—may occur without fever, especially in premature infants. In fact, a subnormal temperature in the neonate may suggest infection, as may fluctuations of temperature. As the months pass the infant tends to develop fever more readily with infection, and this capacity becomes greatest in the age range of 6 months to 3 years. Temperatures of 39.4° to 40.6° C (103° to 105° F) are not uncommon with mild infections. Fever may precede by several hours authentic evidence of infection. A second examination of the child may be required to detect signs of infection that were not evident when fever first developed.

Febrile convulsions. Small children who develop sudden high temperature sometimes have febrile convulsions of a generalized tonic-clonic nature. A more gradual rise in temperature does not elicit a seizure. A third or more of these children have a positive family history for febrile convulsions. Only a small percentage of them later develop epilepsy. Although such febrile convulsions may be repeated at onset of subsequent infections, it is uncommon for them to occur after about 4 years of age.

Meningismus. Abrupt onset of high temperature may cause meningismus in a small child. Meningeal signs are present but not actual infection of the meninges. Lumbar puncture is necessary to exclude meningitis. The cerebrospinal fluid is normal but may be under slightly increased pressure. No treatment is required for this condition. Meningeal signs subside as the temperature drops.

Anorexia. Anorexia almost invariably accompanies acute infections in small children. It frequently precedes fever and signs of infection, thus heralding the onset of illness. When a small child who usually has a good appetite develops an aversion to food, one observes for impending infection. Anorexia persists to a variable degree throughout the febrile phase of the infection and often into convalescence. Resurgence of appetite is a well-known sign that the peak of illness has passed.

Vomiting. Small children often vomit at onset of infection. So true is this that one should immediately think of the advent of infection when a small child vomits for no known reason. In almost all instances the infection will be in the upper respiratory tract. Vomiting may precede by several hours clinical evidence of infection, such as fever and pharyngitis. Although usually occurring only at onset of illness, emesis may continue and become the dominant manifestation of the infection, leading to dehydration and electrolyte imbalance. Thus in a small child with a common respiratory tract infection the fluid and electrolyte problem sometimes outranks in importance the infectious aspects of the illness.

Diarrhea. In small children mild transient diarrhea often accompanies acute respiratory tract infections, especially those of viral etiology. It is sometimes severe, posing more problems than the respiratory tract aspects of the infection.

Abdominal pain. Abdominal pain may be a prominent symptom in acute respiratory tract infections in small children. It may be caused by mesenteric lymphadenitis accompanying throat infection ("Brennemann belly"), in which case differentiation from acute appendicitis may be difficult, if not impossible. Abdominal pain may be associated with the muscular spasm of vomiting. It may have an emotional basis in a tense, nervous child with infection.

Nasal blockade. The small nasal chambers of infants are easily blocked by mucosal swelling and infectious exudate. Because infants are not adept at mouth breathing, this may interfere with respiration sufficiently to cause restlessness. Furthermore, such blockade handicaps nursing, thereby penalizing fluid intake. It also fosters a higher incidence of complications, such as sinusitis and otitis media.

Absence of complaint of sore throat. One of the peculiarities of small children old enough to describe their symptoms is that they often do not complain of sore throat, even when the throat is highly inflamed. Perhaps their tissues are more elastic, and it may be that this results in less pressure on sensitive nerve endings. At any rate, parents are often surprised that throat infection is present without the child having complained of sore throat.

Increased frequency of complications. Partly because of less resistance to infection and partly because of local circumstances (greater degree of nasal and paranasal sinus blockade, relatively large adenoids, etc.), small children have a higher frequency of complications of acute respiratory tract infections. Otitis media and severe cervical adenitis occur much more frequently. Although chronic sinusitis occurs more often in older children, young children have a relatively higher incidence of acute ethmoiditis. Retropharyngeal abscess as a complication of such infections is limited to infants and small children. Furthermore, downward extension of infection to produce laryngitis, tracheobronchitis, bronchiolitis, and pneumonia is much more common in the young child. Septicemia and meningitis are also more frequent complications.

Treatment of upper respiratory tract infections. Because infections of the upper respiratory tract are the most common causes of illness in infancy and childhood, their treatment is of great importance. Complications are fostered by inadequate therapy.

This discussion deals with the overall management of infants and children with such infections. Treatment will be discussed under three headings: (1) general measures, (2) local procedures, and (3) antibacterial therapy when indicated.

General measures. General measures include (1) isolation, (2) rest in bed, (3) diet, (4) fluids, and (5) control of fever.

Isolation. Although often difficult to achieve because of overcrowding or lack of parental cooperation, the sick child should be isolated insofar as is possible. Ideally this should be done at first evidence of illness. Physicians should educate families to remove a sick child from contact with the other children as soon as illness appears.

Parents should avoid the temptation to lie down with the sick child. When a parent, especially the mother, contracts the infection, it is almost impossible to prevent its spread to others.

Rest in bed. There is no acute febrile illness that does not profit by rest. Although rest in bed is more difficult to achieve with young children, parents should be educated to try to train their children to stay in bed when they are sick. If serious efforts to do so are made with each illness, it is surprising how often the child learns to cooperate. Although challenged by some, it is generally held that the acutely ill child should remain in bed until free of fever for at least 1 day. It is believed that rest reduces the frequency of complications. Most importantly, it assists in isolation.

However, the unreasoning small child often forces compromises. Such a child who resists bed rest vigorously and cries excessively may expend more energy than if permitted to play quietly on the floor or in a play pen. Children old enough to be addicted to television may lie more quietly on a couch where they can see their favorite programs. Various other entertainment devices can be employed to humor the child.

Diet. Because (1) anorexia is a characteristic of acute infections, (2) urging food at time of illness may precipitate vomiting or diarrhea, (3) aversion to the feeding situation may arise and carry over into convalescence or later, and (4) the outcome of brief, acute infections does not hinge on normal dietary intake, the sick child should be the judge of how much he eats.

In minor illness and especially when the child retains a good appetite, the usual normal diet may be offered. However, it is generally preferable to restrict the diet to fruit juices, favorite soft drinks in frequent small amounts, soup, broth, soda crackers, toast, gelatin, custard, cooked cereals, and so on. Formula-fed infants sometimes profit by a reduction of milk intake at the beginning of an acute infection.

Fluids. Because of the tendency to dehydration, occasioned by fever, anorexia, and perhaps vomiting and diarrhea, maintenance of fluid intake is important. In most cases this is better accomplished by offering small sips of fluids at frequent intervals than by permitting ingestion of larger amounts less frequently. A cola beverage, fruit juices, or 5% to 10% corn syrup in water may be offered. Normal urinary frequency and a urine properly pale are simple evidences of reasonable hydration. Naturally, when examining the child, the physician observes for signs of dehydration.

There are two common errors in advocating fluid intake: forcing fluids and awakening sleeping children. No sick child should be nagged or harrassed to take more fluids than desired. However, gentle persuasion and the right approach often succeed. The physician should never specify an exact amount of fluid that the child should be made to take, lest the obligation thus imposed on the parents results in undue attempts to fulfill the order. The acutely ill child should not be awakened to take fluids. The fact that the child is asleep indicates that rest is needed and that sleep has temporarily taken precedence over other requirements.

Control of fever. Fever of variable degree accompanies most acute infections in childhood. Frequently it is so mild that it needs no treatment. However, high temperature increases restlessness, accentuates insensible fluid losses from skin and lungs, and may produce meningismus or even precipitate febrile convulsions. Therefore control of fever is advisable when it is upsetting to the child. Although opinions differ, measures are usually taken to reduce the temperature when it exceeds 37.8° C (100° F) orally or 38.3° C (101° F) rectally.

The two chief measures for reduction of temperature are use of antipyretic drugs, usually acetylsalicylic acid (aspirin), and increasing evaporation from the skin. The former is used for moderate fever, and both are employed for high temperature. Acetaminophen (Tempra, Tylenol) is also a useful drug in the control of fever.

The single dose of acetylsalicylic acid for this purpose is 1 grain per year of age, not to exceed 5 grains per dose, given at intervals of not less than 4 hours. Because temperature usually decreases late at night and rises during the day, it is rarely necessary to give more than three or four doses per 24 hours. One should remember that even these doses may result in a cumulative effect. Thus routine administration every 4 hours may cause excessive levels of the drug, especially in young children, particularly when dehydration with consequent impaired renal function is present.

When the infant is less than 1 year of age, particular attention should be paid to dosage. An infant 6 months of age should receive not more than ½ grain per dose. The drug should not be used at all in infants younger than 3 months of age because of immaturity of renal function, which impairs ability to excrete the drug and greatly predisposes to dangerous levels. Physicians should remember that salicylate poisoning is common, may be fatal, and occurs most frequently in young infants. Physicians should keep proper dosages in mind, and they owe it to parents to educate them in the dangers of injudicious frequent administration of aspirin.

Another hazard of the use of aspirin in infants and small children is failure to crush the tablets, leading to aspiration into the larynx or trachea, sometimes causing death.

When the child is vomiting, acetaminophen may be given rectally in the form of suppositories.

Application of rubbing alcohol to the skin (alcohol sponging) results in rapid evaporation with loss of heat. The commercially available 70% preparation is diluted with equal parts of water by some, but it is used undiluted by others. Pouring the alcohol into the cupped palm from time to time, one applies it repeatedly to all parts of the child's body except the face. In a similar but less rapidly effective way, high fever may be reduced by means of repeatedly wrapping the nude child in a sheet wet with cool or tepid water.

In both the alcohol sponging and wet sheet methods one should maintain peripheral circulation by rubbing the skin so that chilling of the skin surface will not result in vasoconstriction with consequent impairment of heat loss.

Local procedures. Local measures may prove helpful in selected cases. Local therapy includes (1) shrinking congested nasal membranes, thus facilitating respiration, promoting comfort, and possibly aiding drainage of paranasal sinuses; (2) suction of abundant mucopurulent nasal secretions for the same reasons; (3) in severe tonsillitis in older cooperative children, throat irrigations for local comfort; (4) hot or cold applications to the neck for acute severe cervical adenitis; and (5) use of a vaporizer to afford moist air to soothe irritated membranes.

Nose drops. Proper use of vasoconstrictive nose drops, isotonic with nasal secretions, may be of benefit. Such drops may be instilled four or five times a day for not more than 5 days. More frequent or prolonged administration may lead to persistent congestion of the nasal membrane.

Technique of instillation should be discussed carefully; it is useful to give printed instructions to ensure proper administration. Unless adequately instructed, the parent tends to hold the small child's head in the crook of the elbow, tilt the head backward, instill the drops into both nostrils, and then hold the child up to comfort him immediately thereafter when he cries and struggles. The drops then run along the floor of the nose and exert little or no action.

The head should be held lower than the body, turned to one side, several drops should be instilled into the lower nostril, cleansing tissue or a handkerchief should be held over the lower eye to prevent irritation should the drops run out of the nose, and after instillation the head should be kept in a low lateral position for at least 1 minute. The procedure is then repeated on the other side.

Oily nose drops should never be employed. If used for a long period, they may be aspirated into the lungs to cause lipoid pneumonia. Antibiotic-containing nose drops cannot reach all infected areas and therefore are of little use. Furthermore, their frequent administration may lead to sensitization.

Vasoconstrictive solutions are available in plastic compressible containers with perforated tops. Pressure on the container at the moment of inspiration produces a nasal spray that has the same effect as nose drops and is more widely dispersed. Such sprays may be preferable in older cooperative children who can time inspiration to coincide with compression of the container.

Nasal suction. When there is abundant mucopurulent exudate, drops or sprays may not come into sufficient contact with nasal membranes, thus being relatively ineffective. Nasal suction by means of an infant nasal aspirator may prove helpful if employed gently not more than four or five times a day. Nose drops or nasal sprays are used afterward.

Throat irrigations. Although rarely needed and seldom used, temporary relief from pain may be afforded older cooperative children with severe tonsillitis by means of a throat irrigation consisting of 1 quart of warm water to which has been added 2 level teaspoonsful of table salt. In a similar way, gargling such a solution may give transient relief to the older child capable of this maneuver.

Hot or cold applications. An ice collar, a hot-water bottle, or a heating pad applied to the neck may decrease the discomfort of painful cervical adenitis in the older child, but these devices are often resisted by the sick infant.

Vaporizer. Moist air from a vaporizer may soothe inflamed membranes and is especially helpful when there is hoarseness or any degree of laryngeal involvement. Electric vaporizers are effective and much safer than use of an open heat source, such as a hot plate. A sheet arranged over the child to form a hood will keep the vapor from dissipating throughout the room. The sheet may be laid over the sides of the crib, or chairs may be placed with backs to the upper part of the bed.

Antibacterial therapy. The crux of the therapeutic problem in infections of the respiratory tract is whether to employ an antibacterial agent. The difficulty arises in making a clinical distinction between bacterial infections, in which such treatment may be indicated, and viral infections, in which it is not. Although cultures are certainly unnecessary in every case of respiratory infection, they are highly indicated when there is a suspicion that Group A beta hemolytic streptococci may be the etiologic agents. An increasing number of physicians are culturing for this organism by simple office laboratory methods. Also, hospitals or local health departments often afford rapid identification of such streptococci by means of fluorescent antibody techniques. Too often the physician, uncertain regarding etiology and wishing to protect against bacterial possibilities, indiscriminately employs antibiotics for almost all these infections. This is perhaps the commonest error in pediatric therapy and, beside being expensive, carries the hazards of immediate adverse reactions to antibiotics, sensitization that may prove troublesome later, and encouragement of growth of resistant bacteria.

A major concern is that the infection may be streptococcal and that failure to detect this fact and to treat adequately with penicillin may set the stage for the subsequent development of rheumatic fever or acute nephritis. Sometimes the streptococcal throat infection is so typical that the physician feels certain of the etiologic diagnosis. However, in many patients with such infections the findings are inconclusive and atypical.

ACUTE PHARYNGITIS AND ACUTE TONSILLITIS

Acute infections of the pharynx or tonsils are among the most common disease syndromes seen in pediatric practice. Acute pharyngitis and tonsillitis may be merely part of a generalized infection of the upper respiratory tract or they may be the dominant clinical manifestations of the acute infection. The pharynx and tonsils may also be inflamed in systemic illnesses, such as infectious mononucleosis and various contagious diseases and in certain viral diseases in which the throat is the portal of entry. Acute infection of the throat may result from lowered defenses, as in agranulocytic angina. Diphtheria and scarlet fever are examples of infections that usually begin in the throat but have widespread toxic effects. The following discussion is limited to bacterial and viral infections of the pharynx or tonsils in which these structures bear the brunt of the invasion and in which their involvement constitutes the outstanding aspect of the infection.

Etiology. As emphasized earlier, the majority of these infections are caused by viruses. The group A beta hemolytic *Streptococcus* is by far the most frequent and important bacterial organism causing tonsillitis and pharyngitis. *Corynebacterium diphtheriae* is a rare cause. Other bacteria occasionally cause tonsillitis and pharyngitis, especially in debilitated patients.

Clinical manifestations. The manner of onset, intensity of local infection, degree of systemic response, and complications vary greatly and to some extent depend on the age of the child and whether the infection is viral or bacterial. In the first year of life the infant does not usually react to these infections in such a severe manner as is likely later on. *In general,* compared to bacterial infections, viral infections begin less abruptly, cause less intense inflammation of the throat, produce a milder degree of illness, are of shorter duration, and produce few complications. The child with acute nasopharyngitis differs from the adult with the same disease in that the child usually has accompanying fever, whereas the adult is usually afebrile. In infancy a frequent presenting sign of acute nasopharyngitis is fever, which may precede by several hours the onset of a serous or seromucoid nasal discharge.

Viral throat infections begin with nonspecific symptoms of fever, loss of appetite, general malaise, and headache. Fever generally lasts only a few days and is usually highest at about the third or fourth day. Complaint of sore throat may be lacking initially and may never be severe. In other instances sore throat appears early and is of greater degree but is seldom as intense as in streptococcal throat infection. Mild hoarseness and slight cough are often present.

Inspection of the throat usually reveals mild to moderate hyperemia, with or without a follicular exudate limited to the posterior pharyngeal wall, the tonsils, or both places. In contradistinction to the follicular exudate of streptococcal throat infection, the follicular exudate of viral infection generally does not coalesce. If group A coxsackievirus is the cause, the syndrome of herpangina is produced, with small grayish vesicles surrounded by reddish areolae or small ulcerated areas, seen on the anterior tonsillar pillars and sometimes on the tonsils, uvula, soft palate, or tongue. In viral throat infections the cervical lymph nodes are usually not enlarged or only slightly so and do not suppurate unless secondary bacterial infection is superimposed. The white blood count is often within normal range, and the differential count is frequently normal. In other instances frank leukopenia occurs. Less often, moderate leukocytosis may be present at onset.

Bacterial throat infections tend to begin more abruptly and to produce a more rapid rise in fever to higher heights than viral infections usually do. Headache, loss of appetite, and general malaise characteristically occur early. There may be no complaint of sore throat the first day or only a feeling of dryness in the pharynx. Later the throat may become extremely painful, even causing difficulty in swallowing.

Inspection of the throat reveals hyperemia of the tonsils and pharynx, which varies from mild congestion to a fiery red edematous appearance, sometimes including, besides the tonsils and the pharynx, the soft palate and uvula. In streptococcal throat infection there is often, but not always, an abundant follicular exudate that spreads to coalesce and covers the tonsils with a pseudomembrane. The cervical glands are characteristically enlarged and tender, and there is a definite tendency to suppuration. Otitis media commonly accompanies streptococcal throat infection.

Bacterial throat infection characteristically causes polymorphonuclear leukocytosis.

Complications. Viral infections of the throat generally cause no complications, except that they may pave the way for secondary bacterial infection. In contrast, streptococcal throat infections may cause not only otitis media and acute cervical adenitis but also acute sinusitis, retropharyngeal abscess in the infant, downward invasion of the lower air passages, and bacteremia with distant localization of infection and may be followed by acute nephritis or an ititial attack or exacerbation of rheumatic fever.

Diagnosis. Despite the fact that certain clinical features help differentiate viral throat infection from bacterial throat infection, often this distinction cannot be made with any degree of confidence. This is so because the manifestations of viral and bacterial infections of the throat may overlap, mild bacterial infections resembling those of viral etiology.

Although the white blood cell count and differential count are often helpful, a throat culture for causative bacteria, especially group A beta hemolytic streptococci, is of great importance.

At present viral diagnostic procedures are too time consuming to be of much help in the diagnosis of the individual case in ordinary practice at the time the information is needed. Some idea of the nature of the infection may be gained from knowledge of what diseases are present in the community at the time the patient is seen, but this is often only a crude guess.

Treatment. Viral throat infections are treated in the manner previously considered in the discussion of treatment of upper respiratory tract infections, with the exception that antibiotic or chemotherapeutic agents are not indicated.

If streptococcal throat infection is present, penicillin should be given in dosage sufficient to control the acute local manifestations of the infection, and a sufficient level of penicillin should be maintained for at least 10 days to eradicate the streptococci that might otherwise cause acute nephritis or an initial attack or exacerbation of rheumatic fever. Such therapy is much more successful in preventing rheumatic fever than acute nephritis.

The surest way to guarantee an adequate level of penicillin for a period of 10 days is to inject benzathine penicillin intramuscularly. The dose is 600,000 units for children under 6 years of age, 900,000 units for children between 6 and 9 years, and 1.2 million units for children more than 9 years of age.

If the patient is not vomiting, if the parents are cooperative, and if added expense is not a factor, acute streptococcal throat infections may be treated satisfactorily with 10 days of oral penicillin therapy. A real danger, however, is that the parents will discontinue the drug within a few days when the child seems clinically well. The oral route should be depended on only when the parents have been thoroughly indoctrinated in the need for a full 10 days of therapy.

Although the oral administration of penicillin V gives higher blood levels than does penicillin G, it has not been proved that these higher levels are necessary, considering the exquisite sensitivity of group A beta hemolytic streptococci to penicillin. Penicillin G is much cheaper. If penicillin G is to be given orally for streptococcal throat infection, the dose is 200,000 units three times a day for 10 days for children weighing less than 22.5 kg (50 pounds) and 400,000 units three times a day for 10 days for those weighing more than 22.5 kg. If the patient is sensitive to penicillin, erythromycin can be given in a dosage of 30 to 50 mg/kg/24 hr for 10 days.

Although sulfonamides are of value in preventing the acquisition of streptococcal infection and are used for this purpose in the prophylactic therapy of penicillin-sensitive children who have had rheumatic fever, they should not be employed in the treatment of known streptococcal infection. They are bacteriostatic, not bactericidal as is penicillin, and they do not eradicate the organisms effectively.

Whether to treat all children with mild throat infections from whom group A beta hemolytic streptococci are cultured has not been settled, but it has been shown that such children with mild throat infection, and especially those without tonsillar exudate, have only a small chance of developing rheumatic fever.

Family and other close contacts of the child with streptococcal throat infection may, of course, contract the infection, but the chances of this are lessened if the child is promptly treated. However, when streptococcal infection does involve one after another of the members of the family, it may be necessary to treat the entire family simultaneously to eradicate the streptococci from the family circle. Also, in concentrated groups, such as in military establishments or in schools, epidemics of streptococcal infection may require mass therapy.

When throat infection is caused by organisms other than group A beta hemolytic streptococci, treatment is best based on culture of the organism and determination of its antibiotic sensitivities.

ACUTE OTITIS MEDIA

Etiology. Infants and young children are predisposed to acute otitis media, the most common complication of upper respiratory tract infection, because (1) their eustachian tubes are relatively short, (2) immunity against the particular organism has not yet been achieved through prior exposure, and (3) tubal blockade is frequently fostered by allergic rhinitis, adenoid enlargement, and infection. The commonest bacterial organism causing acute otitis media in children is the pneumococcus, especially so in children more than 6 years of age. *Haemophilus influenzae* type B is a fairly common cause of acute otitis media in children younger than 6 years old. Group A beta hemolytic streptococci are much less common offenders. At times other types of bacteria are etiologic. Acute otitis media may also be caused by viruses. Because of lack of correlation between organisms in the middle ear and the nasopharynx, nasopharyngeal cultures to identify the organisms causing otitis media are often of little value.

Clinical manifestations. The child usually has signs and symptoms of an acute upper respiratory tract infection in addition to those of otitis media. However, signs of the predisposing infection may have already begun to wane. Fever may be high, moderate, or minimal. In the presence of an upper respiratory infection, persistent low temperature always suggests the complication of otitis media.

The child old enough to describe symptoms complains of earache. The infant gives evidence of such pain by restlessness, irritability, and crying, unrelieved by being held. The infant often makes rolling motions of the head, with or without placing the hand to the head or pulling at the ear. When otitis advances less rapidly, the older child may simply complain of difficulty in hearing, or the parents may have noted this. In some instances, especially in severely debilitated or extremely ill children, purulent drainage from the ear may be the first sign.

Diagnosis. Diagnosis is established by inspection of the eardrums. Earliest evidence consists in loss of the light reflex and hyperemia of the drum. Later, as fluid and exudate accumulate in the middle ear, the drum bulges outward so that landmarks are first obscured, then obliterated. With unchecked infection the drum assumes an angry dusky red color that progresses to a yellow-gray appearance prior to spontaneous rupture or myringotomy. The bulge of the drum is generally in the upper and posterior portions. When the short process of the malleus is no longer seen, the drum is said to be fully bulging.

It must be remembered that red eardrums do not always indicate otitis media. Blockade of eustachian tubes by nasopharyngeal infection, but without otitis, may cause retraction of the drum and hyperemia that may lead the uninitiated to make a false diagnosis of acute purulent otitis media. Also, minimal tympanic hyperemia may be seen when children cry during examination or have a high temperature.

Acute purulent otitis media must be differentiated from serous media, a fairly common condition (p. 383).

Treatment. The *first principle* of successful treatment is early, vigorous antibacterial therapy. When possible, physicians should indoctrinate parents to notify them promptly when the child has an earache. A delay of even a few hours before instituting treatment may make the case more difficult to cure. The *second principle* is to continue antibacterial therapy for a sufficient time and in proper dosage to eradicate the infection completely. The commonest error is to prescribe treatment for only a few days instead of 7 to 10 days—the time usually required to ensure success. The *third principle* is to follow the patient closely enough to observe whether antibacterial therapy is really succeding and to change drugs if it is not. The *fourth principle,* all too frequently violated, is to perform myringotomy if the eardrum continues to bulge despite antibiotic treatment or if the patient has a bulging drum and severe earache.

Identification of the causative organism and determination of its antibiotic sensitivities is, of course, extremely helpful in guiding therapy, but the circumstances of practice do not always permit this; the fact that nasopharyngeal cultures often do not correlate with the organism causing otitis media has already been mentioned. Needle aspiration of the middle ear exudate, with smear and culture, is performed by some physicians to identify the causative organism. Obviously, if the drum has already ruptured, a culture of the discharge is indicated, but there may be contamination by organisms in the ear canal.

Because it is difficult to determine the causative organism for reasons just stated, one usually plays the probabilities in selecting antibacterial agents. In infants and in children less than 6 years of age the commonest organism is the pneumococcus, but *H. influenzae* accounts for about 20% of such infections, and Group A streptococci are sometimes present. In children more than 6 years of age the pneumococcus is by far the most common causative organism, *H. influenzae* is much less often present, and group A streptococci still have to be reckoned with, especially when there is clinical evidence of probable streptococcal throat infection. Ampicillin and amoxicillin are effective against all three of the most commonly encountered organisms, and either may be used for effective treatment. Ampicillin may be given orally in a dosage of 50 to 100 mg/kg/24 hr in four divided doses for a period of 7 days when treatment is started early and for 10 to 14 days when therapy is initiated later, after onset of infection. Antibiotic regimens should therefore be directed against both gram-positive and gram-negative pathogens at any age, unless a single organism has been identified by tympanocentesis or myringotomy. Amoxicillin is given orally in a dosage of 20 mg/kg/24 hr in three divided doses for the same duration of treatment. Amoxicillin has better middle ear penetration than does ampicillin, allowing use of smaller dosages and a diminished incidence of diarrhea and secondary *Candida* (monilial) rash.

For children more than 6 years of age ampicillin may also be employed, or penicillin may be administered, as discussed in consideration of the treatment of streptococcal throat infection (pp. 380 to 381).

If the patient is sensitive to penicillin, a sulfonamide such as sulfisoxazole or erythromycin and a sulfonamide may be administered.

Ideally the child should be reexamined a few days after therapy is initiated to determine whether the ear infection is subsiding. If it is not responding to treatment, a change in therapy to another antibiotic should be considered. If at this time the drum is bulging, myringotomy should be considered. The physician should also examine the child after 10 days of therapy to make certain that the ear infection has fully subsided. Assurance that the infection has really been eradicated is one of the most important aspects of treatment, but one of the most neglected. To this error can be ascribed many of the cases of recurrent otitis media, flaring up a week or so after the first infection seemed to have subsided in patients who did not receive a final examination.

Finally, an increasing number of physicians are obtaining audiograms in their offices to determine the extent of hearing loss the patient may have suffered from an attack of acute otitis media. If a hearing deficit is noted, an otolaryngologist should be consulted.

Pain may be partially relieved by instilling eardrops (Auralgan), by aspirin, mild sedation, or an ice bag placed against the ear.

SEROUS OTITIS MEDIA

Serous otitis media refers to a condition in which a clear, glairy mucoid or viscid secretion collects in the middle ear. There are several alleged causes. It may be caused by blockade of the eustachian tube by the mucosal edema of allergic rhinitis and to a lesser extent by hypertrophied lymphoid tissue (adenoid tissue). It is often ascribed to dysfunction of the eustachian tube. Less often it is caused by inadequate therapy of purulent otitis media. This condition is relatively common and, because it produces no threatening symptoms, is dangerous from the standpoint of causing conduction deafness through organization of the viscid material. Unfortunately the seriousness of this entity is often overlooked.

In addition to the symptoms of allergic rhinitis, present in a high proportion of such children, or those of adenoidal obstruction, there may be no complaint other than impairment of hearing and a feeling of fullness in the middle ear. When there is air in the middle ear above the fluid, motion of the head may cause shifts of the fluid like small waves, and the patient may feel this motion in the ear. Inspection of the eardrum reveals that it is opaque, lackluster, perhaps slightly full. Sometimes a meniscus may be seen through the drum. Pneumatic otoscopy demonstrates decreased mobility of the tympanic membrane as a result of middle ear fluid, a thickened membrane, or both. Tympanometry more precisely quantifies the mobility of the tympanic membrane, and audiometry is extremely valuable in the detection of functional hearing impairment resulting from abnormal air conduction.

Drainage is necessary to avoid hearing loss. This may be done by aspiration or myringotomy. Aspiration may be performed after application of a cotton pledget soaked in a local anesthetic agent. Myringotomy may be performed under local or general anesthesia, the latter carrying the usual hazards. In the initial stages the fluid may be thin enough to permit aspiration, but when it becomes more viscid, it can only be removed satisfactorily by myringotomy and the use of a small suction tip.

In view of the frequency with which conduction hearing loss occurs, children with serous otitis media should be referred to the otologist, who may insert a pressure-equalization tube through the eardrum to facilitate drainage and equilization of air pressure on both sides of the drum.

The most important aspect of long-term management is to relieve the basic cause. This involves an investigation of allergy and treatment along standard lines if allergy is clearly found to be present. If there is evidence of adenoidal obstruction, adenoidectomy may relieve the condition. If the adenoids have already been removed, they may have regrown, sometimes to larger size than formerly. Another adenoidectomy may be indicated.

If the condition is caused by inadequately treated purulent otitis media, myringotomy is indicated. The fluid should be cultured to determine the causative organism and its sensitivities so that an appropriate antibacterial agent may be employed to eradicate the infection.

ACUTE MASTOIDITIS

Acute mastoiditis, formerly a frequent complication of purulent otitis media, is now rare. This has resulted largely from the availability of antibiotics. However, in the untreated child with otitis media, acute mastoiditis still occurs. Furthermore, there is a risk of the development of this complication in the child with ear infection who is treated with inadequate doses of an antibiotic for an insufficient period of time and possibly with an inappropriate drug in the first place. Failure to perform myringotomy when drug therapy does not eradicate middle ear infection is another predisposing factor.

At birth there is a single mastoid cell—the antrum, opening into the middle ear—that is exposed to the infectious agents of otitis media. It undoubtedly participates regularly in such infections but usually clears up as the ear infection recedes. As pneumatization of the temporal bone progresses in the first few years of childhood, intercommunicating mucous membrane–lined air sacs fill the major portion of the mastoid process, extending upward and forward to the zygomatic process and inward into the petrous portion of the temporal bone. This honeycomb arrangement invites extension of infection from inadequately drained and progressively severe purulent mastoiditis.

When pus forms in the mastoid process and cannot escape into the middle ear cavity to drain through a ruptured or incised drum, it seeks another route. In so doing it may involve important structures. The infection may extend medially to reach the meninges. If checked by the dura, it may cause an inflammatory response marked by slightly elevated cell count and protein content of the cerebrospinal fluid but without penetration of organisms—the so-called sympathetic meningitis from contiguous infection. If it breaks through the dura, it may produce purulent meningitis. However, the inflammatory reaction may mat the dura to the surface of the brain, permitting the infectious process to cross the meninges without causing meningitis and to enter the brain to form a temporal lobe abscess. If conditions favor an invasion of the petrous portion of the temporal bone, the infectious process moves medially from air cell to air cell and may eventually break through the bone to produce meningitis or Grandenigo syndrome: ipsilateral orbital pain and paralysis of the sixth cranial nerve with inability to turn the eye outward, associated with purulent discharge from the ear. The infection may extend upward and forward to invade the air cells of the zygomatic process so that mastoiditis is in front of and above the ear. The infection may extend into the lateral venous sinus, producing thrombophlebitis with septicemia. Because young children sometimes have a dehiscence between the bones that form the lateral wall of the mastoid process, the pus may seep through to form a subperiosteal abscess that pushes the ear forward and outward. The area of the mass is fluctuant and tender, and the overlying skin is reddened.

The diagnosis of acute mastoiditis may be difficult when the infection is partially suppressed by antibiotic treatment. Masked by inadequate drug therapy, the infectious process may extend to produce any of the complications mentioned. If the eardrum has ruptured or has been incised, increase in the volume of the aural discharge suggests the development of mastoiditis. Mastoiditis is also suspected when otoscopic examination reveals edematous sagging of the posterior wall of the external auditory canal. In the classic case there is pain over the mastoid process, edema, redness, and tenderness to firm pressure. Radiographs of the affected mastoid, compared to those of the contralateral normal mastoid process, reveal diffuse cloudiness. Thinning or disappearance of the bony septa between the air sacs may be seen.

If an aural discharge is present, it should be cultured, and antibiotic sensitivity tests should be requested to facilitate selection of the proper drug; a blood culture should be obtained. However, vigorous antibiotic treatment should be instituted immediately, rather than waiting for the results of culture and sensitivity tests. The physician evaluates the etiologic probabilities and selects the antibiotic agent along the lines previously discussed in the consideration of therapy of acute otitis media (p. 382). Further antibiotic choice depends on the results of culture and sensitivity tests. Symptomatic treatment consists in control of fever, sedation to allay restlessness, and application of an ice bag to the mastoid process to diminish pain.

Mastoidectomy is indicated if at initial examination a subperiosteal abscess is already evident or if observation of the clinical course during antibiotic therapy fails to show rapid improvement.

ACUTE PYOGENIC CERVICAL ADENITIS

Cervical adenitis of varying degree accompanies many acute infections in the upper respiratory tract. The present discussion is limited to acute pyogenic cervical adenitis in which an infected gland enlarges rapidly and dominates the clinical picture.

The swollen node is tender and at first not fluctuant. As the infection progresses the mass enlarges steadily, the overlying skin becomes hot and red, there is local pain, and the head is tilted toward the shoulder because of muscle spasm. Fever, restlessness, and malaise round out the clinical picture. Fluctuation becomes apparent, and the pus burrows toward the skin, which becomes dusky red and thinned and may rupture spontaneously. In other instances the gland remains large and tender but does not suppurate.

In addition to the usual supportive measures for children with acute infection of the upper respiratory tract, therapy includes treatment with the appropriate penicillin because of the high frequency with which the Group A beta hemolytic streptococcus or *Staphylococcus au-*

reus is the offending organism. Hot, wet saline dressings are applied more or less constantly. Drainage is delayed until the pus is close to the surface. If the physician incises too early, there is danger of spreading the infection to contiguous nodes or of causing cellulitis. Furthermore, incising before the gland has broken down fully may prolong the period of drainage, leading sometimes to an ugly, puckered scar. If one waits too long, however, the overlying skin may have become so devitalized that it sloughs subsequent to incision.

PERITONSILLAR ABSCESS

Peritonsillar abscess is an uncommon infection, rarely occurs in children less than 5 years of age, and is generally caused by a Group A beta hemolytic streptococcus. A common location is the upper pole of the tonsil, the anterior pillar and soft palate being displaced forward and medially and almost obscuring the tonsil. A retrotonsillar abscess pushes the tonsil forward. A parapharyngeal abscess is located laterally to the tonsil and displaces it medially. Displacement of the tonsil and localized swelling may not be apparent during the early stage but soon develop.

The symptoms are severe pain in the throat, worse on the abscessed side, pain in the jaw and neck, difficulty in opening the mouth, impaired swallowing leading to drooling of saliva, muffled voice ("hot potato in the mouth" voice), fever, malaise, and prostration. The head may be pulled down toward the shoulder on the affected side because of muscle spasm.

If detected early and treated vigorously with penicillin, the infection may be eradicated before formation of an abscess. If the infection is unresponsive to antibiotic therapy, incision is indicated when fluctuation occurs. Other aspects of treatment include control of fever, sedation, use of analgesics, application of an ice collar to the neck, liquid diet, and when necessary, parenteral fluid therapy. Irrigations with hot saline solution sometimes offer temporary relief from pain. When the infection has fully subsided, tonsillectomy should be performed.

RETROPHARYNGEAL ABSCESS

Retropharyngeal abscess may occur as a complication of infection of the upper respiratory tract, by perforation of the pharyngeal wall by a foreign body (fish bone, etc.), or rarely by extension of a tuberculous abscess from the cervical spine. This discussion is limited to the form secondary to infection of the upper respiratory tract.

Most of the patients are less than 2 years of age, and the entity is rarely seen after the age of 3 years. The abscess arises from infection of the lymph glands that lie between the posterior pharyngeal wall and the cervical spine. The lesion is dangerous because of the possibility that it may rupture spontaneously to cause aspiration bronchopneumonia or death by asphyxiation, erode a large blood vessel with fatal hemorrhage, or cause septicemia.

The clinical picture is dramatic and diagnostic. Concomitant with or immediately after an acute throat infection the child develops difficulty in swallowing and in breathing. This is caused by the bulging forward of the retropharyngeal mass. The child lies on his side with his head drawn backward to displace the larynx forward of the overhanging mass. Saliva drools from the lower angle of the mouth because of inability to swallow. The cry is husky, and there may be dyspnea. Prostration and fever are present. The cervical glands are enlarged.

If the pharyngeal bulge cannot be seen, the diagnosis may be established by a lateral radiograph of the neck, revealing a widening of the space between the cervical spine and the posterior pharyngeal wall.

Treatment consists in vigorous penicillin therapy, parenteral fluid therapy when the child cannot take adequate amounts of fluid orally, control of fever, mild sedation, placing the child in the prone position with the foot of the bed elevated, and incision when the abscess becomes fluctuant.

ACUTE SINUSITIS

The paranasal sinuses probably participate in all acute infections of the nose, since their mucous membranes and those of the nose are continuous. However, such routine involvement is not designated sinusitis. It is only when the infection in the sinus becomes a dominant part of the clinical picture that this term is employed.

The etiologic organisms are those that have produced the upper respiratory tract infection. Blockade of free flow of sinus secretions through the ostia into the nasal chamber causes localization of infection in a particular sinus. When the ostium of a sinus is occluded by mucosal inflammatory edema, the mucopurulent exudate cannot escape. This condition is called empyema of the sinus. Pus trapped in a sinus seeks to escape. If it cannot gain entry into the nasal chamber, it may burrow elsewhere. In infants this is particularly true of infections of the ethmoid sinus, which tend to extend toward or into the orbit. In older children with frontal sinusitis the infection may extend inward to produce meningitis or brain abscess. Other serious complications of acute sinusitis include septicemia and cavernous sinus thrombosis.

The diagnosis is suspected when, during the course of an infection of the upper respiratory tract, fever and constitutional symptoms increase and there is local evidence of involvement of a particular sinus. Pain is felt in the region of the sinus and may also be referred to distant areas. Sphenoidal sinusitis causes suboccipital pain, anterior ethmoiditis causes pain near the ipsilateral eye and temple, and posterior ethmoiditis causes pain in the tissues overlying the affected sinus and tenderness to deep pressure. Examination of the nose may reveal a profuse mucopurulent discharge pouring from one of the sinal ostia, reappearing as soon as it is wiped away. On the other hand, blockade may be so complete that no discharge is seen.

Although maxillary sinusitis has been noted as early as the newborn period, the sinus most often severely affected during infancy is the ethmoid. The infectious process extends toward the orbit, causing edema, redness, and tenderness near the inner angle of the eye. The eyelids may become swollen to such a degree that the eye is closed. When the infection is located chiefly in the retrobulbar portion of the orbit, it may displace the eyeball anteriorly and at the same time cause optic neuritis.

Diagnosis can be established on clinical grounds. The most definite evidence is the detection of large quantities of pus draining into the nasal chamber through an ostium that is still partially open. Transillumination of sinuses is not very helpful in children. Radiographs often reveal a hazy cloudiness of affected sinuses.

Treatment consists in supportive and symptomatic care, plus vigorous antibiotic therapy and encouragement of drainage. Cultures of the discharge from the affected sinus should be obtained if there is drainage into the nasal chamber. If not, a culture should be taken from the nasopharynx. Sensitivity tests should be obtained to determine the most appropriate antibiotic to employ. Application of a vasoconstrictive agent to the area of the blocked ostium may facilitate drainage. Suction removal of the mucopurulent discharge not only ensures better contact between the vasoconstrictive solution and the mucosa but also may initiate drainage of the sinus. It is seldom necessary to aspirate the sinuses. If pyogenic complications progress, operation may be indicated.

TONSILS AND ADENOIDS (TONSIL AND ADENOID PROBLEM)

One of the commonest problems confronting the pediatrician is the relationship of the tonsils and adenoids to the health of the child. The crux of the problem is to decide when these structures have lost their protective function and have become a menace. This decision is often difficult to make, and there are wide differences of opinion as to indications for operation.

It is generally accepted that the chief function of the tonsils and adenoids is to defend against infection. Because of their strategic location at the entrance to the airway and by virtue of their structure, they are peculiarly adapted to trap invading organisms that have penetrated the mucous membrane. As aggregates of lymphoid tissue they play a role similar to that of lymph nodes anywhere in the body—a filtering effect to check the spread of infection. Furthermore, like other lymphoid tissue they participate in the formation of antibodies.

In former years, tonsils and adenoids were considered to be vestigial structures, of little worth, and best removed if they grew somewhat large in size or participated frequently in infections. In the "summer roundups" of those days, when large numbers of children were being examined for physical fitness before entering school, many were marked for operation merely because of normally hypertrophied tonsils, presence of a few enlarged cervical lymph nodes, or history of several upper respiratory tract infections in the preceding year. In hospitals throughout the nation on "tonsil days" as many children as could be easily accommodated were wheeled to the operating room and subjected to adenotonsillectomy, all in good faith and in the belief that a benefit was being conferred. The more conservative minority who condemned these practices cynically referred to "the mass execution of the tonsils" and to "tonsil parties" and accused those who followed the predominant opinion of the day of believing that "the presence of a pair of intact tonsils represented a duty unfulfilled."

A more critical attitude toward the possible protective function of tonsils and adenoids subsequently developed. It was recognized that perhaps they served a useful purpose. Studies were made of large groups of children, comparing the health of those who had their tonsils and adenoids removed to the health of those who had not. From these observations came better criteria by which to judge the worth of these structures and more definite information concerning advantages and disadvantages of adenotonsillectomy.

The advent of the antibiotic era introduced the next change in concepts. It now became possible to treat tonsillitis and adenoiditis far more effectively so that these structures less commonly became sites of persistent smouldering infection. Armed with antibiotics, the physician became less inclined to remove tonsils and adenoids.

An increased awareness of the role that allergy plays in fostering repeated upper respiratory tract infection changed the situation still further. It was recognized that chronic nasal allergy is frequently responsible for repeated infection, thus taking some of the blame away from the much maligned adenoids and tonsils.

Finally, the epidemiologic applications of virology further clarified the etiology of acute infection of the upper respiratory tract. It was shown that young children have about four or five acute infections in the nose and throat each year, that the majority of these are of viral etiology, and that these infections are exogenously derived and do not come from extension of infection in the tonsils and adenoids. Also, it was established that a relatively durable immunity is achieved to most of the viral agents and to the various types of streptococci that infect the child from time to time. These facts have further diminished the importance attached to the tonsils and adenoids as foci of infection.

Data from studies of growth and development have also been of value in defining more clearly normal variations in tonsillar size at various age levels, emphasizing the normal hypertrophy that occurs in the first few years and the spontaneous decrease in size that generally begins at about the fifth year.

Thus there have developed new concepts concerning the role tonsils and adenoids play in the total drama of upper respiratory tract infection and the general health of the child. A far more conservative attitude has developed with respect to recommending adenotonsillectomy. The physician is now more willing to wait a few weeks, a few months, or longer to observe whether what appear to be bad tonsils now may not then seem normal. In fact, when one does adopt the policy of "watchful waiting," it often becomes apparent within a few months that operation is not indicated after all.

The more conservative viewpoint that has evolved should not, however, lead one to defer operation when a clear reason exists. This is particularly true of the need for adenoidectomy when repeated attacks of otitis media and impairment of hearing are associated with signs of adenoidal enlargement or the need for tonsillectomy in the debilitated child with persistent, significant, cervical lymphadenopathy, failure to gain weight, and anemia. Being too conservative is as bad as being too radical.

Indications for operation. Indications for adenoidectomy and for tonsillectomy differ and will be discussed separately. However, both structures are usually removed at one operation, except in infancy when adenoidectomy alone may be performed. Adenoidectomy may be indicated at any age, including the first year, but tonsillectomy is seldom justified in children less than 3 years of age.

Indications for adenoidectomy. Indications for adenoidectomy are related to obstruction, infection, or both.

Obstruction. Because of the location in the narrow nasopharynx of the child, adenoidal enlargement interferes with the ability of the child to breathe through the nose and often blocks the orifices of the eustachian tubes.

When adenoidal hypertrophy is severe, the child becomes a mouth breather, has a dull facial expression, has difficulty blowing the nose, has a nasal voice, snores at night, and often has broken, fitful sleep. If the posterior nasal air passage is almost completely blocked, the nostrils may be narrower than normal and the palate highly arched, and thoracic deformity may occur if the obstruction persists from early infancy. This apparently results from the increased inspiratory effort necessary to bring air past the nasopharynx. It probably occurs chiefly at night when mouth breathing may be interrupted, as when the child sleeps in the prone position. The xiphoid process may be depressed, and lateral grooves may develop at the level of the diaphragmatic attachment. Chronic upper airway obstruction may result in hypoventilation. This, in turn, results in a decrease in arterial PO_2, an increase in arterial PCO_2, and a respiratory acidosis. Severe pulmonary hypertension and cor pulmonale may result. These can be promptly reversed with relief of the upper airway obstruction.

Obstruction of the orifices of the eustachian tubes causes impairment of hearing. Obstruction without infection can lead to the development of serous otitis media. The fluid in the cavity of the middle ear is initially thin, then mucoid, and then viscid. As it organizes it impairs motion of the ossicles that transmit sound waves from the eardrum to the inner ear. Often otitis media of adenoidal origin is infectious in nature. The child has one attack of purulent otitis media after another as the chronically infected adenoids keep seeding the eustachian tubes with organisms. Once established in the middle ear, the infection tends to persist because of adenoidal obstruction to the tube. Thus the adenoids play a double role: they initiate the infection and handicap its clearing. Progressive hearing loss occurs and may be permanent if the vicious circle is not interrupted by adenoidectomy.

Infection. Repeated attacks of purulent otitis media constitute the most evident complication of adenoidal infection. Opinion differs as to the relationship of chronic adenoiditis to persistent or recurrent sinusitis. In view of the fact that a mucopurulent nasal discharge is associated with adenoiditis, infection of the sinuses does occur and may persist until the adenoidal infection is eliminated. The mucopurulent postnasal drip of adenoiditis may intitiate bronchitis. Of course, cervical adenitis is also a part of the picture, but a minor part as a rule. As with any chronic infection, there may be anorexia, failure to gain weight properly, and anemia.

If characteristic obstructive phenomena are present, the infectious complications such as recurrent or chronic otitis media are clearly related to the adenoids. When obstructive symptoms are less prominent, it is essential to consider whether allergic rhinitis is the true cause of the tendency to repeated infections.

Decision to perform adenoidectomy is based on the facts just presented. If allergic rhinitis has been excluded, operation is clearly indicated when chronic nasal obstruction exists, and particularly so when recurrent or chronic otitis media is a complication, with or without hearing loss, or when cor pulmonale results.

Indications for tonsillectomy. It is more difficult to define the indications for tonsillectomy than to determine when adenoidectomy is advisable. Tonsillar enlargement rarely obstructs respiration or interferes with swallowing. In children of the same age normal tonsils vary greatly in size, and in the individual child tonsillar size changes remarkably. Tonsils that are large during an acute infection may be small when seen a few weeks later. Furthermore, chronic infection of the tonsils does not always imply that they are enlarged; chronically infected tonsils are sometimes small and insignificant in appearance. For these reasons the former belief that greatly enlarged tonsils constitute an indication for operation has been discarded except in the rare instances when greatly enlarged tonsils and adenoids cause cardiac decompensation.

As stated previously, most acute infections of the upper respiratory tract in children are caused by viruses. Therefore the fact that the child has had several sore throats in a given year does not necessarily mean that the tonsils are chronically infected. It is not the number of infections that counts but whether there is evidence that the tonsils themselves are the cause. The chief evidence lies in the response of the cervical lymph nodes at the time of these infections. Viral infections do not usually produce significant, tender enlargement of the cervical nodes, but recurrent tonsillitis does. Therefore when the child has repeated attacks of tonsillitis associated with tender cervical lymphadenopathy, it is likely that chronic tonsillitis exists, and tonsillectomy should be considered. Further observation of the patient over a period of several weeks or months is generally indicated, and vigorous antibacterial therapy should be instituted. If after a period of observation no real improvement occurs, tonsillectomy may be warranted. Persistent, moderate, nontender enlargement of cervical nodes does not in itself constitute an indication for tonsillectomy. Palpable nodes are present for months or even a year to two in many otherwise healthy children.

Peritonsillar abscess is considered to be evidence of deep-seated infection, and tonsillectomy should be performed when the acute infection has subsided.

Tonsillectomy is no longer advocated as a routine procedure in children who have had acute nephritis or rheumatic fever. Indications for tonsillectomy in such children are the same as for those who have not had these diseases.

From the foregoing discussion it is apparent that greater discrimination is now practiced in regard to adenotonsillectomy than was true in former years. Nevertheless, far too many of these operations continue to be performed. In some areas it is still not unusual for two or even three siblings to be subjected to operation on the same day so that the children and the parents may "get it over with" at one time. The operation is still being recommended by some physicians on the basis of one examination of the child. It should be appreciated that there is an element of danger in any operation and in any general anesthesia. It is stated that between 200 and 300 deaths from adenotonsillectomy occur annually in the United States. The causes are cardiac arrest, hemorrhage, lung abscess, pneumonia, and other complications.

LARYNGEAL STRIDOR

The syndrome of laryngeal obstruction with stridor is fairly common in pediatric practice, especially during the first year of life. The pattern varies from children who have merely noisy breathing to those who have an inspiratory crow associated with retraction of the soft tissues in the suprasternal, supraclavicular, intercostal, and subcostal areas. In some patients there is hoarseness or wheezing.

Numerous conditions may produce this syndrome, and some of them are of serious significance. Therefore a precise diagnostic approach is indicated as soon as the condition is noted. This requires skilled laryngoscopy.

Laryngeal stridor appearing within the first days or the first week of life suggests a *congenital cause,* or *trauma to the larynx*. Neonatal laryngeal stridor of traumatic origin is suspected by the history of insertion of a tracheal catheter in resuscitation and is confirmed by laryngoscopic examination. Usually this type of laryngeal stridor disappears within a few days. Treatment consists in placing the infant in a mist-laden atmosphere, such as nebulizing distilled water into the incubator. Tetany of the newborn is now a rare cause of laryngeal stridor.

Laryngeal stridor, beginning in the first week of life and persisting, may be caused by various congenital anomalies. By far the commonest cause is an elongated, floppy epiglottis that falls down over the glottis whenever the child takes a breath. This may be associated with laryngomalacia, a congenital flabbiness of the larynx and supraglottic aperture. The diagnosis of these two conditions is established by laryngoscopy, which should invariably be done as soon as laryngeal stridor is noted. An elongated floppy epiglottis or laryngomalacia is almost harmless, since the child will outgrow both conditions as the larynx grows in length, width, and rigidity. However, they must be distinguished early from the various more serious congenital abnormalities. Laryngeal stridor because of either of these causes usually disappears by 1 year of age and sometimes sooner. There is no specific treatment required, but the certainty that the child will outgrow either condition is of much assurance to parents and physician.

Among the much less common congenital causes of laryngeal stridor are laryngeal webs, retention cysts, rare laryngeal tumors, malformations of laryngeal cartilages, and malformation or duplications of the vocal cords. Diagnosis is established by laryngoscopic examination. Webs, cysts, and the rare tumors can be removed surgically.

Extralaryngeal causes of laryngeal stridor are sometimes present. Micrognathia with a significantly receding mandible may be associated with stridor because the base of the tongue overhangs the supraglottic aperture. Aberrant thyroid tissue at the base of the tongue may also cause stridor. A goiter in early infancy may exert pressure on the larynx and cause stridor. Macroglossia from blood vessel or lymphatic anomalies may be the cause. A double aortic arch or similar anomalies of the great vessels may compress the trachea and give rise to respiratory obstructive manifestations, but there are no laryngeal symptoms such as hoarseness or inspiratory crow.

Acute infections may cause stridor, but they are so dramatic that there is little diagnostic difficulty. These include acute epiglottis, acute laryngitis, laryngeal diphtheria, and acute laryngotracheobronchitis.

Foreign bodies retained or embedded in the larynx may also cause stridor.

As stated previously, the most important aspect of congenital laryngeal stridor is to establish the diagnosis by laryngoscopy as soon as the syndrome is detected to determine whether the cause is potentially serious or not and whether definitive treatment can be afforded. In view of the statistical frequency of an elongated, flabby epiglottis as the cause, the greatest danger is to postpone laryngoscopy in the blind faith that an elongated epiglottis is truly the cause, only to experience later the tragedy of the child with a correctable congenital condition who contracts acute laryngitis and asphyxiates before tracheostomy can be performed.

SPASMODIC CROUP

Spasmodic croup is a common condition in which a small child, usually 1 to 3 years of age, has paroxysmal attacks of laryngeal obstruction occurring chiefly at night. Certain children are peculiarly predisposed, and there may be familial tendency. Some attacks seem to be precipitated by a minor acute upper respiratory tract viral infection and others by sleeping in a cold, overly ventilated room. Allergy seems to be the cause in some instances, and pale watery edema of the subglottic tissues has been seen at laryngoscopy performed during acute episodes.

Clinical manifestations. The child who was put to bed with what seemed to be only a mild cold, or with slight laryngitis and some hoarseness and cough, or was apparently completely well awakens in the night with a croupy, barking cough, hoarseness, dyspnea, and restlessness. He sits up to breathe better, twists and turns, struggles for air, and is apprehensive, frightened, and prostrated. The face is congested, and in severe cases slight cyanosis may be present. Accessory muscles of respiration are utilized to draw air in past the laryngeal obstruction, and inspiratory retractions may occur. After a few hours the attack wears off. The next day the child may appear normal, or the signs of a mild cold, with or without slight hoarseness and fever, may be present. The attack may be repeated one or two nights in succession.

Diagnosis. Although diagnosis is usually easy, the physician must consider simple acute laryngitis, acute epiglottitis, laryngotracheobronchitis, diphtheritic laryngitis, aspiration of a foreign body, and tetany.

Acute laryngitis (pp. 391-393) does not appear suddenly in the night but is of more gradual onset. The child generally has had evidence of an upper respiratory infection, with hoarseness, brassy cough, and perhaps fever. Progression of the process may lead to laryngeal obstruction, in this manner simulating croup.

Acute epiglottitis (p. 391) is a rapidly progressive infection producing high temperature, inflamed throat, prostration, and severe supraglottic obstruction. The diagnosis is established by the appearance of the epiglottis, which is greatly congested, cherry-red, and swollen as seen by depression of the base of the tongue or by swelling of the epiglottis noted on a lateral neck radiograph.

Laryngotracheobronchitis (pp. 393-395) accompanies acute upper respiratory infection. The child is much sicker, more prostrated, has a higher temperature, and presents signs of lower respiratory tract obstruction in addition to those at the laryngeal level. Rales are generally heard, there may be areas of atelectasis or emphysema, and expiratory difficulty may be associated with the inspiratory stridor.

Laryngeal diphtheria (p. 714) is of more gradual onset, there may be a faucial membrane, fever of mild to moderate degree is present, and hoarseness or aphonia has developed over hours or a day or more instead of appearing suddenly in the night. In case of doubt, the physician should resort to direct laryngoscopy to determine whether a laryngeal membrane is present and, if so, to obtain material for culture.

Rarely, acute obstructive laryngeal manifestations appearing suddenly in the night are caused by aspiration of *a foreign body* left in the bed and with which the child has been playing or are caused by aspiration of food particles (peanut, etc.).

Hypocalcemic tetany may produce laryngismus stridulus, which may simulate spasmodic croup. In the age group in which croup is likely to occur, tetany is usually caused by rickets, which has almost vanished from the United States. Therefore laryngismus stridulus is exceptionally rare. The diagnosis would be based on presence of rickets, associated carpopedal spasms and perhaps irritability, tremors, twitchings, and recurrent convulsions. The serum calcium level is low, generally below 7 mg/dl.

Treatment. The condition responds to humidification and subemetic doses of ipecac that can be given in the home. If the child fails to improve, exposure to cool night air en route to the hospital frequently relieves the attack before the hospital is reached. In the emergency room, treatment with an aerosol of racemic epinephrine is usually effective in terminating the attack.

ACUTE EPIGLOTTITIS

Acute epiglottitis is a fulminating inflammation of the epiglottis and neighboring structures, generally caused by *Haemophilus influenzae* type B. It occurs chiefly in children 3 to 7 years of age but may occur in younger children.

Clinical manifestations. The disease appears suddenly, causes moderate to high temperature, severe prostration, and severe supraglottic obstructive manifestations. The throat is red, and the epiglottis is greatly swollen and cherry-red in color. Surrounding tissues are inflamed and edematous. Interference with inspiration appears early and proceeds rapidly, often to alarming degree. The child struggles to breathe, uses accessory muscles of respiration, and suprasternal and infrasternal retractions may be visible. The tongue may be protruded with each inspiratory effort. Interference with adequate oxygenation may produce the sallow complexion of moderate hypoxia or frank cyanosis.

Diagnosis. In view of the characteristic clinical picture and especially the distinctive appearance of the epiglottis, the diagnosis is not difficult. However, as one examines the patient for the characteristically fiery red epiglottis, the child may suddenly have complete respiratory obstruction. This can be fatal; therefore direct examination of the throat is not recommended.

A lateral radiograph of the neck will reveal a swollen epiglottis and is a safer procedure than direct examination of the throat. The child should not be made to lie down for such a radiograph if severe dyspnea is present; sudden respiratory arrest may occur. Other entities to be considered include acute laryngitis, laryngotracheobronchitis, laryngeal diphtheria, spasmodic croup, and foreign body in the larynx or trachea. Differential diagnosis of these entities is discussed elsewhere (p. 390).

Treatment. So severe is the supraglottic obstruction in most of these cases that establishment of an airway is the most urgent immediate need. The disease progresses with such rapidity that death may occur from asphyxia if insertion of an endotracheal tube is delayed. This is usually done in the operating room under general anesthesia. Because the obstruction is supraglottic, immediate relief is obtained.

The child should be placed in a mist tent (Croupette), oxygen should be administered, and vigorous antibiotic therapy should be initiated intravenously as soon as the airway is established. Nasopharyngeal culture and blood culture should be obtained for identification of the organism and determination of its antibiotic sensitivities. The organism is almost always *H influenzae* type B. A combination of ampicillin and chloramphenicol represents logical initial therapy to cover the possibility of infection with *H. influenzae* resistant to ampicillin. When sensitivity to the organism has been determined, the appropriate single drug should be continued. Ampicillin should be given in a dosage of 200 mg/kg/24 hr and chloramphenicol in a dosage of 50 to 100 mg/kg/24 hr. Both drugs should be administered intravenously.

The child should be sustained by parenteral fluid therapy until the peak of illness has passed and should be disturbed for examinations and bedside care only when absolutely necessary. Minimal handling and maximal rest are essential in management. Extubation is usually possible in 48 to 72 hours.

ACUTE LARYNGITIS

Acute laryngitis is a common infectious condition producing hoarseness, brassy cough, and at times respiratory obstruction, usually caused by viral agents. It occurs most commonly between 3 months and 3 years of age.

Etiology. Only a small percentage of cases of acute laryngitis are caused by bacteria. *Haemophilus influenzae* type B and *Corynebacte-*

rium diphtheriae have been incriminated as causes, but there is no conclusive evidence that streptococci, staphylococci, and pneumococci are etiologic. In the majority of cases viral agents can be identified. Parainfluenza viruses are the commonest offenders, and less frequently adenoviruses, influenza viruses, and ECHO and coxsackie viruses. Laryngitis may be a somewhat localized infection, or it may be merely one of the many manifestations of such disease as measles, influenza, or scarlet fever. It may be associated with tracheobronchitis or epiglottis. Inflammation of the larynx may also be the result of inhalation of smoke, noxious fumes, and irritant dusts. The type discussed here is caused by infection.

Pathology. There are usually manifestations of an acute upper respiratory infection, with inflammation, congestion, and discharge from the nasal mucosa. The pharynx is often moderately reddened. The laryngeal membrane and vocal cords are inflamed and edematous, and an exudate, sometimes with pseudomembrane formation, may be present. Subglottic edema is the principal problem in severe cases and may cause variable degrees of obstruction to inspiration.

Clinical manifestations. There is a wide spectrum of severity ranging from mild laryngitis with few symptoms to severe obstructive laryngitis that may be life threatening. The child has generally had a mild upper respiratory infection for a day or two before laryngeal symptoms appear. Evidence that the larynx is affected consists of hoarseness that may progress to almost complete loss of voice, onset of brassy cough, and in severe cases obstruction to inspiration. Stridor, restlessness, irritability, and suprasternal and infrasternal retraction may occur. Fever is usually only of moderate degree. Inflammation of the nasal membranes and pharynx is generally present. If laryngoscopy is performed, the larynx is seen to be reddened and edematous, the vocal cords are swollen, and an exudate may be present. The clinical course usually lasts about a week but may be shorter when the disease is caused by bacteria rapidly responsive to antibiotic therapy.

Diagnosis. Acute laryngitis must be differentiated from epiglottitis, laryngotracheobronchitis, spasmodic croup, laryngeal diphtheria, and presence of a foreign body in the air passages. The distinction between laryngitis as a single entity and laryngitis as part of laryngotracheobronchitis may prove difficult. The latter diagnosis is suggested if, in addition to signs of laryngeal involvement, evidence exists of significant involvement of the lower respiratory passages shown by rales and rhonchi, areas of atelectasis or emphysema, and perhaps some interference with both expiration and inspiration.

Treatment. The child should be placed in an atmosphere of high humidity. If the attack is mild and the child is treated at home, vaporization may be achieved by methods already mentioned (pp. 378 to 379). If the condition is severe enough to merit hospitalization, obstructive symptoms are often of a degree to indicate simultaneous use of oxygen and humidification.

Because acute laryngitis is usually of viral origin, antibiotic therapy is not indicated for the mild uncomplicated case. However, when the disease is moderate to severe in intensity, nasopharyngeal cultures (preferably taken when the child is coughing) should be obtained, and sensitivity tests should be done to guide antibiotic therapy. In severe cases the physician should not wait for results of cultures before instituting treatment. In such severe cases one may give ampicillin intravenously in dosage of 200 mg/kg/24 hr.

The child with severe laryngitis should be disturbed as little as possible. Fluids should be administered intravenously to save the child's strength and to decrease the possibility of vomiting with aspiration. Sedation should not be employed in the usual case because restlessness is caused by hypoxia and sedation may dull the child sufficiently to impair respiration. Also, restlessness is one of the guidelines in estimating the need for tracheostomy. If the child is extremely tense and agitated, sedation may be employed cautiously, using phenobarbital or chloral hydrate.

No benefit is derived from use of antihistamines, expectorants, or bronchodilators. Atropine should not be employed because it dries secretions and makes them more difficult to expel by coughing. The use of adrenal corticosteroids to diminish inflammatory reaction and thereby improve respiration is controversial. Some authors state that corticosteroids are valueless in this situation. Others administer corticosteroids intravenously in the hope that tracheostomy may be avoided.

Intubation is seldom required in acute laryngitis. If, despite supportive measures, serial blood gas analyses point to hypoxemia unresponsive to supplemental oxygen and progressive carbon dioxide retention, an artificial airway and mechanical ventilation may be necessary.

ACUTE LARYNGOTRACHEOBRONCHITIS

Acute laryngotracheobronchitis is a common infection of infants and small children in which the larynx, trachea, and bronchi are the seat of intense inflammation and obstruction to respiration tends to be severe. Use of the term is justified only when clinically significant signs of laryngeal infection are associated with inflammatory obstructive phenomena in the lower respiratory tract.

Etiology. In the majority of instances the disease is of viral origin. Many viruses are capable of causing this syndrome, and etiologic diagnosis can be achieved only by special studies. In other cases pathogenic bacteria are present, either primarily or as secondary invaders.

Pathology. A variable degree of inflammation of the upper respiratory passages is generally present. The larynx is greatly inflamed and edematous, the vocal cords are red and swollen, and subglottic edema is often severe. Acute inflammation, usually intense, affects the mucosa of the trachea and bronchi. A thick, tenacious, gummy, crusting exudate is frequently present and accounts for the high frequency of partial or complete obstruction of bronchi. In severe cases areas of atelectasis are present, varying in size from small and patchy to segmental or lobar. Likewise, when obstruction is partial, hyperaeration may be present to a variable degree, involving segments of lobes or entire lobes. Peribronchial inflammation is commonly present, and bronchopneumonia may be an extension of the process.

Clinical manifestations. At first the illness appears to be a simple acute upper respiratory infection, with rhinitis and pharyngitis, mild to moderate fever, and little or no prostration. The infection then rapidly descends, first producing laryngeal symptoms of hoarseness, brassy cough, and stridor. Fever and prostration increase. Inspiratory dyspnea may result from subglottic edema, with suprasternal and substernal retraction. The lower respiratory findings swiftly ensue. Various types of rales are heard, ranging from coarse and bubbling to fine and sticky; these may vary with coughing. Now, in addition to inspiratory dyspnea from subglottic edema, expiratory dyspnea may occur. Inadequate oxygenation of blood results in loss of the normal ruddy complexion and the advent of pallor or cyanosis. The hypoxic child becomes irritable and restless, twists and turns, sits up to breathe better, uses accessory muscles of respiration, and struggles for breath. If the condition is not relieved, inflammatory edema and obstructive crusts progressively occlude the trachea, bronchi, and bronchioles. The patient dies of exhaustion, asphyxiation, bronchopneumonia, septicemia, or combinations of these.

Physical findings in the chest are of great interest. Inspection reveals suprasternal and substernal retraction and use of accessory muscles of respiration, and there is ordinarily more dyspnea than tachypnea. If large areas of atelectasis or emphysema are present, motion of the overlying chest wall may be impaired. Palpation may reveal displacement of the cardiac apical beat toward an area of massive atelectasis or away from an area of lobar emphysema. Percussion often reveals areas of dullness, which may represent large zones of coalescent bronchopneumonic consolidation, but more frequently signify lobar atelectasis.

Auscultation may be obscured by stridor and frequent brassy cough. Tachycardia and weak heart sounds are common. Rales of various types may be heard. Breath sounds may be absent over emphysematous areas. Bronchial breathing may be heard over large zones of bronchopneumonia or atelectasis. Obstructive emphysema, which may be present, is seldom generalized and ordinarily does not displace the diaphragm downward to a significant degree. Therefore the spleen is usually not felt, and the liver does not seem enlarged, as is often the case in acute bronchiolitis.

Laboratory findings are not specific and are more helpful in the management of the patient than in the diagnosis. The total white blood cell count may be normal or shifted slightly to the left in the more severely affected patient. Most patients will have a low arterial P_{O_2}. Initially the arterial P_{CO_2} is normal or low, resulting from increased ventilation in response to hypoxemia. However, the increased effort of breathing fatigues these patients, and respirations become shallow as they tire. Ventilation is thus impaired and the arterial P_{CO_2} rises. The resulting hypercapnia aggravates the hypoxemia, and respiratory failure may ensue.

Diagnosis. Laryngotracheobronchitis must be differentiated from (1) acute epiglottitis, (2) simple acute laryngitis, (3) laryngeal diphtheria, (4) bronchiolitis, (5) bronchopneumonia, (6) bronchial asthma, and (7) foreign body in the air passages, especially food particles that may set up an intense inflammatory response.

Epiglottitis is distinguished by the greatly swollen reddened epiglottis and by swelling of the epiglottis noted on neck radiograph. There is no obstruction of the lower air passages, and dramatic findings in the lungs are lacking.

Simple acute laryngitis is probably always associated with a degree of tracheal and bronchial inflammation, but the diagnosis is established by evidence of laryngeal involvement without marked lower respiratory manifestations.

Diphtheria is currently extremely rare. A history of adequate immunization practically excludes this possibility. Laryngeal diphtheria may be associated with a faucial membrane, which facilitates diagnosis.

Bronchiolitis is easily differentiated by findings of generalized obstructive emphysema. It generally occurs at an earlier age than does laryngotracheobronchitis, usually causes little or no fever, and ordinarily does not produce marked leukocytosis. Although differentiation from bronchiolitis should be simple, mistakes are made. The most serious result is to perform tracheostomy when the patient actually has bronchiolitis. Because in the latter condition the obstructed areas are far below the level of the tracheostomy, no benefit is obtained from this procedure, and in fact much harm can be done.

Simple bronchopneumonia is easily differentiated by the fact that there is rapid respiration but ordinarily less dyspnea from obstruction to respiration in the larger air passages. Laryngeal symptoms of hoarseness and brassy cough are usually lacking. Radiographs of the chest may reveal bronchopneumonic consolidations without evidence of atelectasis or emphysema.

An attack of bronchial asthma in an infant or small child may be triggered by a mild acute upper respiratory infection, and the combination of obstructive manifestations associated with evidence of respiratory tract inflammation may simulate laryngotracheobronchitis. This is especially true when one is dealing with the first attack of asthma in an infant. Generally, expiratory distress is greater than inspiratory distress, hoarseness and stridor are usually lacking, the temperature is lower, and the child appears less prostrated. A therapeutic trial of epinephrine ordinarily results in rapid improvement of the asthmatic child but does little for the one with laryngotracheobronchitis.

A foreign body in the air passages, especially one of vegetal origin, may closely mock acute laryngotracheobronchitis, provided that the initial choking and obstruction to breathing have passed unnoticed. If the child aspirates food, usually a peanut but sometimes meat or other substances, the resulting inflammatory reaction may cause symptoms almost identical with those of laryngotracheobronchitis. If the diagnosis is not suspected when the child is first seen, eventually it is suspected when signs of obstruction persist after those of inflammation subside. Fluoroscopy (or chest radiographs on full inspiration and full expiration) and bronchoscopy are the routes to proper diagnosis.

Treatment. The child with laryngotracheobronchitis should be immediately hospitalized where facilities for intubation are present and preferably where a skilled otolaryngologist is available.

The child should be placed in an atmosphere of high humidity and oxygen concentration, usually best achieved by nebulization of plain water into an oxygen tent. It is important to realize that when oxygen is used in a tent the concentration at the child's face varies and may be inadequate. Therefore it is important to monitor oxygen concentration and arterial blood gases at frequent intervals.

Nasopharyngeal and blood cultures should be obtained, and sensitivity tests should be requested to guide subsequent antibiotic therapy if a pathogenic bacterial agent is identified. Racemic epinephrine may produce clinical improvement, but the improvement is usually transient. Additionally, the arterial Po_2 is not affected, and the degree of hypoxemia is unchanged. Corticosteroid therapy is not recommended.

The patient should be evaluated immediately as to the need for intubation. Patients with mild or moderate laryngotracheobronchitis may often be managed successfully without this procedure. Repeated determinations of arterial blood gases afford objective criteria to determine the need for an artificial airway. In general, intubation should be performed when (1) hypoxemia persists despite supplemental oxygen and (2) there is a progressive increase in carbon dioxide retention. Excessive secretions not removed by coughing may be another indication.

Besides an atmosphere of high humidity and oxygen concentration, supportive care of the patient requires adequate fluid intake, best achieved by intravenous fluid therapy. Proper hydration should be ensured to minimize drying of secretions. Children less severely affected may be able to take adequate amounts of fluids orally if offered repeatedly in small amounts. Excessively high temperature should be controlled by antipyretics, alcohol sponging, or wet packs.

Unless the clinician is experienced with this disease and knows its pitfalls, it is good to avoid sedation. Parents sometimes press the physician to take measures to allay the irritability and restlessness of these children. However, it should be remembered that survival depends on adequate oxygenation and that a child lulled into deep slumber by heavy sedation may quietly stop up his air passages without ability to respond to the stimulus of hypoxia with increased respiratory effort. Atropine or similar preparations should not be used because they tend to dry secretions that are already too dry. Furthermore, expectorants are of no avail.

ACUTE BRONCHIOLITIS

Bronchiolitis is an acute infectious disease with maximum impact at the bronchiolar level that produces generalized obstructive emphysema. It occurs chiefly in the winter and spring and is rare after 2 years of age; most patients are less than 6 months old.

Etiology. Acute bronchiolitis is a clinical syndrome produced by viral agents, of which the respiratory syncytial virus is by far the commonest offender. This virus is estimated to cause more than half the cases. Adenoviruses and parainfluenza viruses may also cause acute bronchiolitis. There is suggestive evidence that *Mycoplasma pneumoniae* (Eaton agent) may cause this disease. It has also been suggested that *H. influenzae* plays a causative role, possibly in combination with a virus. It is probable that bronchiolitis is simply a reaction pattern that may be produced by various agents. Indeed, a similar clinical picture may be produced by asthma in infancy.

Pathology. Pathologic changes fall into two categories: infectious and mechanical. There is usually evidence of a diffuse respiratory tract infection, but the reaction is most severe in the bronchioles. Bronchiolar lumens are filled with exudate and mucus, the mucosa is swollen, the walls of the bronchi and bronchioles are infiltrated with inflammatory cells, and peribronchiolar interstitial pneumonitis is present.

Bronchioles are partially or completely obstructed because of intraluminal exudate, mucosal swelling, and inflammatory thickening of walls. Variable degrees of obstruction are present in smaller air passages, leading to hyperinflation or patchy areas of atelectasis. The principal finding is generalized obstructive emphysema from partial obstruction. On inspiration, with dilatation there is sufficient space to permit ingress of air. However, on expiration, egress of air is prevented by expiratory narrowing. Thus air is trapped distally to the obstruction, and both lungs become progressively overinflated. In severe disease this leads to hypoxemia, hypercapnia, and a mixed metabolic-respiratory acidosis. In less severe disease arterial hypoxemia develops as a result of mismatching of pulmonary ventilation and perfusion, but the arterial Pco_2 and pH are variable. Also, the overinflated alveoli increase resistance in the lesser circulation, imposing a strain on the right heart.

Clinical manifestations. The disease usually begins like a simple cold. There may be rhinorrhea and a slight cough but usually no fever. Then evidence of lower respiratory tract infection ensues, with progressive dyspnea and rapid, shallow respiration. The cough may become so paroxysmal that it simulates that of pertussis. Vomiting may be associated with bouts of coughing. Fever is variable. In most cases there is little or no fever, whereas in others it is moderately high. When so extensive as to interfere with gaseous exchange, hypoxia may cause a sallow complexion or definite cyanosis, and the child becomes restless. The infant is so busy breathing that he has little time for nursing, and fluid and food intake may thus be handicapped. With improvement, dyspnea and tachypnea gradually disappear, the color comes back to the cheeks, the child is no longer restless, and cough and fever subside.

Physical examination reveals an infant of the appearance and behavior just described, evidence of mild upper respiratory infection, and dramatic signs referable to the lungs. In moderate to severe cases the chest appears overinflated (barrel chest). Respiratory excursions are usually shallow and rapid. Accessory muscles may be used. Characteristically, inspiration is associated with an indrawing at the lower costal margins where the diaphragm inserts.

Palpation confirms the fact that the chest is moving only slightly with respiration. The apical beat of the heart may not be felt because of overinflated lungs crowding in front of the heart. Because the voluminous lungs push the diaphragm downward, the spleen may be felt, and the liver may seem to be enlarged.

Percussion of the chest produces marked hyperresonance everywhere, even in the precordial area.

The chief diagnostic finding on auscultation is great reduction in breath sounds—as if the child were not really breathing. This is caused by decreased flow of air into and out of the smaller air passages and the dampening effect of the overlying emphysematous lungs. Sticky inspiratory rales, like the distant crackling of cellophane, may be heard and at times coarser rales or expiratory wheezes are present. It may be difficult to hear the heart sounds.

Laboratory findings. The white blood cell count is often normal, but there may be polymorphonuclear leukocytosis when secondary bacterial invasion is present. The electrocardiogram may show evidence of right heart strain. In severe disease there is decreased arterial P_{O_2}, increased P_{CO_2}, and a low pH.

Radiographic findings. Because of generalized emphysema, the ribs appear more horizontal than normal, the intercostal spaces are somewhat widened, the lung fields are extremely radiolucent, the diaphragm is depressed and flattened (best seen in the lateral view), and the heart may appear narrowed. In the central lung fields patchy areas of atelectasis are often noted.

Diagnosis. The disease is so typical that it can hardly be mistaken for anything else. However, bronchial asthma, which sometimes occurs in early infancy, must be excluded. Injection of a small dose of epinephrine may help make this distinction. It rarely helps the bronchiolitis patient but may cause improvement in the asthmatic patient. Additionally, serum IgE is elevated in approximately 80% of infants with asthma. Occasionally, cardiac decompensation may be mistaken for bronchiolitis.

Treatment. The chief points of treatment are (1) an atmosphere of high humidity, (2) oxygen in moderate to severe cases, (3) adequate fluid intake, (4) possible administration of a broad-spectrum antibiotic in some instances, (5) therapeutic test of epinephrine when bronchial asthma is suspected, (6) the controversial question of steroid therapy, and (7) digitalization in some instances.

High humidity loosens tenacious secretions and results in less vapor loss from the lungs, thereby helping prevent dehydration. Best results are obtained by placing the child in a plastic tent. A nebulizer that delivers a mist of small particle size is preferred.

Oxygen should be administered when there is more than mild dyspnea, when the complexion is sallow, when cyanosis is present, or preferably when arterial blood gas analysis indicates hypoxemia. The child usually needs humidification for a longer period than oxygen administration. As breathing improves and the child becomes obviously better, brief trial periods outside the tent may be attempted. In this way it may be shown that the child maintains adequate oxygenation although mild dyspnea persists and humidification is still indicated. Thus treatment shifts from combined use of oxygen and humidification to humidification alone.

Adequate fluid intake should be ensured to prevent dehydration, which would make tenacious secretions even more so and would handicap renal function necessary to combat respiratory acidosis.

Because of weakness, dyspnea, and tachypnea the child may be unable to take fluids well by mouth. It is usually preferable to give fluids intravenously until the crisis of the disease has passed.

Antibiotic therapy is a highly controversial

issue. General opinion is that antibiotics should not be employed routinely. However, occasionally bacteria are present as secondary invaders. If the white blood cell count is high or if a nasopharyngeal culture reveals a pathogenic organism, a broad-spectrum antibiotic such as ampicillin may be employed.

Steroid therapy has been advocated in severe cases, but such treatment has not been proved to be of value.

Digitalization is indicated when cardiac decompensation from cor pulmonale is present. It is sometimes difficult to know when decompensation has occurred because the patient is already dyspneic, rales may be present, and the liver, displaced downward by emphysema, may seem enlarged. It is important to note the degree to which the liver is palpable when the child is first admitted to the hospital and to follow closely whether its edge descends lower during the course of the illness. If it does, it would be strong evidence of cardiac failure and would indicate need for digitalization.

Approximately 3% of infants and young children hospitalized with bronchiolitis require intubation and mechanical ventilation because of progressive hypercapnia or persisting hypoxemia, despite supplemental oxygen administration. This should be monitored by serial arterial blood gas studies and requires hospitalization in an intensive care unit.

BRONCHIECTASIS

Bronchiectasis is a chronic, progressive, suppurative process that causes cylindric, fusiform, or saccular dilations of bronchi. Emphasis should be placed on prevention or early detection at a time when medical management may check its progress or in rare cases permit full recovery. Once the disease becomes well established, surgical excision of the affected area is the only cure.

Etiology. Although rarely congenital in origin, bronchiectasis is generally acquired—most often during infancy and the early years. It usually results from bronchial obstruction (pp. 408 to 409), but it may be caused by repeated bacterial invasion or unusually severe destructive changes in an acute infection.

Pathology. Dilation of bronchi results from (1) weakening of the walls through loss of muscular and elastic tissue; (2) increase in intraluminal pressure from paroxysms of coughing or from the pressure of accumulated secretions distal to a point of obstruction; (3) traction on the walls from peribronchial fibrosis; (4) loss of the cushioning effect the normally inflated alveoli would have when atelectasis is present; and (5) increased negative pressure on the side of large areas of atelectasis.

Inflammation of the ciliated columnar epithelium of the bronchi is followed by loss of the membrane and replacement by cuboidal or squamous epithelium, which does not produce mucus and has no cilia. More severe infection leads to ulceration and production of granulation tissue that may bleed, causing hemoptysis. Spread of infection to the wall itself results in loss of elastic and muscular tissue and replacement fibrosis. Peribronchial chronic inflammation, fibrosis, and atelectasis are commonly present. The rigidly dilated bronchi contain exudate consisting of bacteria (usually a mixed flora), pus, and cellular debris.

Bronchiectasis may be limited to a portion of one lobe or may involve one or more lobes. Lower portions of the lungs are more commonly affected. Bronchiectasis that began in one area may spread to another by overflow of infected material or by blocking with granulation tissue the bronchial orifice of another lobe or segment.

Bronchiectatic cavities may drain from time to time, but these periods of improvement are often followed by renewed blockade, frequently with resultant massive atelectasis that is often mistaken for pneumonia. This is why the physician should always suspect bronchiectasis when a patient has "pneumonia" repeatedly in one area.

Prolonged suppuration may cause malnutrition, anemia, clubbing of the fingers, amyloidosis, or even metastatic brain abscess.

Clinical manifestations. Minimal bronchiectasis may produce few distinctive symptoms. In the usual case persistent cough, often paroxysmal in nature, is the commonest symptom. In moderate to severe cases large amounts of sputum, sometimes foul smelling, are produced in the bronchiectatic cavities and may be coughed up and expectorated or coughed up and swallowed. Characteristically, coughing is initiated by changes in position, such as lying down, rolling over, sitting up, and so on. Such maneuvers cause spillage of abundant exudate from the dilated cavities into relatively healthy bronchi that have retained their sensitive nerve endings. The paroxysms of coughing may be severe enough to cause vomiting.

Hemoptysis may occur from bleeding granulation tissue or ulcerations. In childhood, hemoptysis is more often caused by bronchiectasis than by tuberculosis.

Extensive bronchiectasis associated with severe pulmonary fibrosis, as well as with bronchitis of the nonbronchiectatic areas, may produce shortness of breath, easy fatigability, and clubbing of the fingers.

The persistent infection may lead to anemia, debility, fatigability, anorexia, malnutrition, and in long-standing cases to stunting of growth. Brain abscess may result from septic emboli from the lungs.

Characteristically there are periods in which the cavities drain relatively well, and the child improves in a general sense. But these interludes are interrupted by exacerbations in which the cavities are blocked off again, infection and toxemia increase, fever mounts, and the child appears to have pneumonia. Administration of antibacterial agents may result in temporary improvement, but the underlying basic bronchiectasis remains.

Physical findings depend on the duration and severity of the chronic process, the extent of bronchiectasis (lobes affected), and whether an acute exacerbation is present. When major lobes are involved, there is generally some increase in respiratory rate, lack of adequate expansion of the chest in the area affected, dullness to percussion, diminished breath sounds, and moist or bubbling rales heard best after the patient has coughed. When extensive unilateral atelectasis coexists, the heart and mediastinum may be shifted toward the affected side. When exacerbations occur, physical findings may resemble those of lobar pneumonia, with the exception of mediastinal shift when atelectasis is present.

Diagnosis. The diagnosis may be suspected by clinical manifestations and findings and by plain chest radiographs that show atelectatic areas with a honeycomb appearance or merely heavy bronchial markings to the lower lobes. However, final proof rests on bronchograms (Fig. 17-3). The entire bronchial tree is mapped out by bronchography to determine whether bronchiectasis is present, to determine its distribution, and to delineate the normal bronchi. The importance of evaluating the entire bronchial tree rests on the fact that surgical extirpation should not be attempted until the extent of normal tissue is known.

Bronchoscopy should be employed to obtain bronchograms for the following reasons: (1) bronchoscopy may reveal the cause of the bronchiectasis, as when a foreign body, granulation tissue, or area of narrowing is found to be the obstructive cause; (2) aspiration of secretions through the bronchoscope permits better filling of bronchi for the bronchogram, furnishes sputum for bacterial culture and sensitivity tests, and is therapeutically beneficial; and (3) by use of the bronchoscope it is possible to instill the contrast medium exactly where desired.

In addition to bronchograms, the workup includes examination for contributing factors, such as chronic sinusitis, chronic tonsillitis and adenoiditis, allergy, and cystic fibrosis.

Treatment. Minimal early bronchiectasis may yield to medical management, but surgical extirpation of the diseased areas is the only cure for well-advanced bronchiectasis. Medical management may be employed in the following circumstances: (1) when the process is early, minimal, and potentially reversible; (2) when the child's condition is such that a major surgical procedure cannot be tolerated; and (3) in preoperative preparation.

Medical management. The following procedures may prove useful:

1. Deep cough sputum cultures to determine predominant organisms, antibiotic sensitivity tests, and full therapeutic dosage of the appropriate antibiotic(s) are helpful. Orally administered or parenterally injected antibiotics may not be able to penetrate into the bronchiectatic cavities because of fibrosis, but they take action against peribronchial inflammation and the frequently present paranasal sinusitis.
2. Antibiotics by aerosol therapy, as well as inhalations of mucolytic agents such as acetylcysteine and brochodilators can be administered. Such aerosol therapy results in high concentrations of the agents in the bronchi and cavities. The aerosol may be administered three or four times a day.
3. Postural drainage, in which the child assumes the position productive of the most coughing and raising of large quantities of sputum, is often helpful. Such drainage can be used

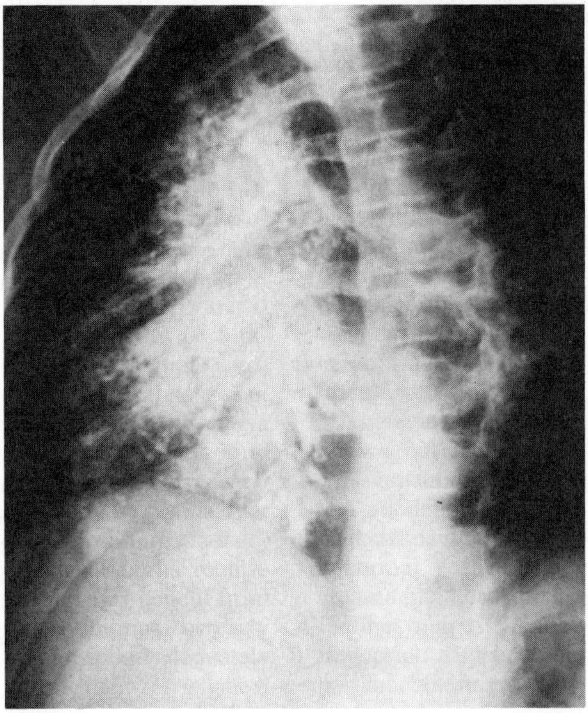

Fig. 17-3. Bronchogram, left anterior oblique view, showing right lower lobe bronchiectasis. (Courtesy Dr. W. Webster Riggs, Le Bonheur Children's Medical Center, Memphis.)

several times a day for periods of several minutes. Better drainage of bronchiectatic cavities may be achieved by combining postural drainage with physical therapy—clapping the cupped hand against the chest wall over the affected area, followed immediately by vibrating the hand against the chest wall.

4. Investigation of a possible allergic contributing factor should be carried out, and then hyposensitizing injections should be given or the allergen should be avoided when possible.

5. When chronic tonsillitis and adenoiditis are present, adenotonsillectomy may prove beneficial. Treatment of chronically infected paranasal sinuses may also help.

6. A high-calorie diet, adequate in proteins and vitamins, is advisable.

7. Anemia should be corrected.

8. Because bacterial resistance may emerge, periodic cultures and sensitivity tests should be performed, preferably on sputum obtained by bronchoscopy.

All in all, medical management is laborious and frequently does not suffice to hold the disease in check, and reactions may occur to use of the various drugs. Therefore a thoracic surgeon may need to be consulted.

Success of surgical management depends on excising all the diseased areas. This implies the necessity for accurate bronchograms of the entire bronchial tree. The operative mortality is extremely low in competent hands.

IMMOTILE CILIA SYNDROME

Immotility of the cilia in the respiratory tract has recently been described in persons with chronic respiratory disease. Ultrastructural studies of the cilia from these persons reveal changes in their normal configuration. These include absent dynein arms, absent radial spokes, transposition of ciliary microtubules, and loss of parallelism of the plane of arrangement of the central pairs of microtubules in adjacent cilia. Absence of dynein arms is classically found in patients with Kartagener syndrome (sinusitis, bronchiectasis, situs inversus). Dynein arms contain the ciliary adenosine triphosphatase protein, dynein. Adenosine triphosphate induces active sliding of adjacent microtubular doublets, resulting in ciliary movement.

Impairment of mucociliary clearance is the most common problem associated with immotile cilia. As a result, thick mucopurulent secretions are retained in the nose, paranasal sinuses, middle ear, and bronchi. Recurrent episodes of rhinitis, nasal polyposis, sinusitis, otitis media, bronchitis with segmental atelectasis, bronchiectasis, and pneumonia have all been noted in patients with ciliary dysfunction. Male patients may also have immotile spermatozoa and are usually sterile.

The diagnosis is made by direct examination of cilia obtained by nasal scrapings or by nasal or bronchial mucosal biopsies. Motility may be assessed by light microscopy using wet preparations of nasal scrapings. Changes in ciliary structure are observable by electron microscopy.

Treatment is the same as for chronic sinusitis and bronchiectasis. Ciliary immotility is compatible with a reasonably normal life and, with proper continuous prophylactic bronchopulmonary drainage and intermittent antibiotic therapy for acute exacerbations, a fairly normal life span. Chronic bronchitis, however, eventually leads to obstructive changes in the airways.

PNEUMONIA

Pneumonia is one of the commonest diseases of childhood. It may be the major illness or a complication of other infections or debilitating conditions. It occurs most often during the newborn period, infancy, and early childhood. The common practice of prescribing antibiotics for most upper respiratory tract infections has undoubtedly reduced the incidence of bacterial pneumonia, especially pneumococcal pneumonia.

Because proper treatment depends on knowledge of the causative organism, an etiologic classification has more rationale than one based on types of pathologic changes. Thus the clinical approach is in terms of identification of the organism and determination of its sensitivity to antibiotics and less in terms of whether the pathologic changes are of lobar, lobular, interstitial, or bronchopneumonic types.

Many organisms may cause pneumonia including bacteria, viruses, and fungi. Pneumonia may also be caused by aspiration of various substances or by circulatory congestion in the lungs (hypostatic pneumonia). Pyogenic bacteria causing pneumonia include pneumococcus, *Staphylococcus, Streptococcus, Haemophilus influenzae, and Klebsiella.* Tuberculous or syphilitic pneumonia may also occur, the latter rarely. Viruses may also cause pneumonia, usually interstitial. Less often, pneumonia is caused by fungi, as in histoplasmosis and coccidioidomycosis. Infrequently pneumonia may occur as part of the clinical picture of blastomycosis, cryptococcosis, mucormycosis, nocardiosis, sporotrichosis, and thrush. Pneumonia may result from aspiration of infected amniotic fluid or food (usually milk). Less often the cause is aspiration of foreign bodies or irritating substances such as kerosene. The incidence of lipoid pneumonia has decreased since mineral oil, oily nose drops, and cod liver oil have been virtually abandoned in pediatric therapy.

In the following discussion only four types of bacterial pneumonia will be considered: pneumococcal, staphylococcal, streptococcal, and *H. influenzae*.

Pneumococcal pneumonia

The incidence and severity of pneumococcal pneumonia have greatly diminished since the availability of antimicrobial therapy. The pneumococci are extremely vulnerable organisms and yield readily to antibacterial agents. Such treatment of pneumococcal upper respiratory tract infection eliminates the organisms before they infect the lungs. Moreover, even if pneumonia has occurred, rapid cure is the usual result.

Etiology and epidemiology. Pneumococcal pneumonia occurs more commonly in the winter and early spring, the peak season of respiratory tract infections. The organisms are transmitted by droplet infection, a hazard that is increased by overcrowding.

Pathologic findings. In the child who has not been given antibacterial therapy the changes to be described are characteristic. However, treatment has so modified the disease process that numerous variations from this picture now occur.

Pneumococcal pneumonia is usually lobar in distribution but may be lobular. It progresses through four stages: (1) engorgement, (2) red hepatization, (3) gray hepatization, and (4) resolution. In the stage of *engorgement* the affected lobe is congested, heavy, and dark but not solidified. Interalveolar capillaries are congested, and there is an effusion of blood and serum into the alveoli. In the stage of *red hepatization* the lobe is solid, dark red, and airless, and the alveoli contain fibrin, serum, red cells, neutrophils, and pneumococci. In the stage of *gray hepatization* the lobe is larger than normal, firm, and gray, and the pleural surface is dull in appearance. Cellular elements in the alveoli have now decreased, bacteria have almost disappeared, and much fibrin is present. In the stage of *resolution* the pneumonic exudate is progressively liquefied and absorbed, and the tissues become normal again.

Clinical manifestations. Because antibiotics (especially penicillin) are so rapidly effective against the pneumococcus, the patient treated soon after onset may not exhibit all the manifestations to be discussed.

Pneumonia may start abruptly or may follow what seemed to be a minor upper respiratory tract infection. The child is restless and prostrated. At onset of illness there may be vomiting or brief diarrhea. Early and throughout the severe phase of the illness, anorexia is profound. Temperature rises rapidly, perhaps producing a febrile convulsion or meningismus. Chills rarely occur in young children but may be present in older ones. The pulse rate is rapid. A weak pulse or a slow pulse is a bad sign. Respiration is rapid and shallow, and in severe cases inspiratory retraction may be observed. Characteristically, there is flaring of the alae nasi. A dry, hacking cough that causes pleural pain is often present early in the disease; later, as resolution occurs, it becomes looser and more productive. The child may lie on the affected side to reduce thoracic excursions that accentuate pleural pain. The pain may be referred to the abdomen, at times simulating that of appendicitis. Abdominal distention may occur. Cyanosis may be present because of widespread pulmonary involvement or may be secondary to circulatory failure. Jaundice is occasionally present.

Physical findings are largely limited to the chest. These depend on the stage and extent of involvement. At onset typical signs may be absent, and the pneumonia may be missed by physical examination but detected by a chest radiograph. When full consolidation is present, findings are more characteristic. The abnormal signs revert to normal as resolution progresses.

Inspection reveals rapid, shallow respiration, perhaps with splinting of the affected side.

Palpation usually reveals no abnormality, but inspiratory lag of the chest wall over large affected areas (lobar or greater) may be detected by laying the fingertips lightly on the chest. Palpation also confirms the location of the apex of the heart. The apex is not displaced in uncomplicated pneumonia. It is displaced toward an area of massive atelectasis that might be confused with pneumonia and is displaced away from a large collection of pleural fluid. Percussion may be normal at onset, but later if areas of consolidation are large enough, *percussion* reveals a dull note. If pleurisy with effusion or empyema fluid is present, the percussion note is flat.

In early stages, *auscultation* may reveal decreased breath sounds and crepitant rales. When consolidation appears, bronchial breathing and egophony may be heard. Occasionally, a pleural friction rub is detected. As resolution progresses, rales are looser and may have a bubbling quality.

Radiographic findings. Chest radiographs reveal the area(s) of consolidation, which becomes more definite as consolidation advances. Pneumococcal pneumonia in young children is more often patchy than truly lobar in distribution. Small areas of pneumonia located posterior to the heart may escape radiographic detection unless, in addition to anteroposterior films, lateral views are obtained. As resolution progresses, shadows become less homogenous and less distinct.

Laboratory findings. Usually there is polymorphonuclear leukocytosis, with a total white cell count varying from 15,000 to 40,000/mm_3. Counts below 10,000/mm_3 may indicate a worse prognosis. If the disease is rapidly treated, anemia may not occur, but if the disease progresses unchecked by therapy, anemia does occur. The sedimentation rate is accelerated. The urine is concentrated, reduced in amount, dark yellow, and contains an excess of urates and often moderate amounts of albumin, hyaline casts, and acetone bodies. Early in the disease the blood culture is often positive for the pneumococcus.

Nasopharyngeal cultures may also be positive. Serologic typing of the organism is now rarely done because of rapid response to antibiotics, regardless of type of organism.

Differential diagnosis. Lobar pneumonia offers few diagnostic difficulties if the disease is suspected and if radiographs are obtained. It is distinguished from atelactasis by displacement of the heart toward the atelectatic side and by the appearance of the radiograph. Atelectasis causes shrinking of the affected area, whereas pneumonia does not. Sometimes pleural effusion proves confusing, but presence of a flat percussion note, shifting of the heart toward the opposite side, and general haziness and obscurity of the affected side of the chest on the film help differentiate this condition from pneumonia. At onset, meningismus or febrile convulsions may make differentiation from meningitis important. Examination of the spinal fluid settles this point. Pleuritic pain referred to the abdomen sometimes suggests appendicitis, but physical findings of pneumonia, chest radiographs, and close observation for abdominal signs of inflammation make the distinction fairly easy. In pneumonia, fever and leukocytosis are both generally higher than in appendicitis. Gastroenteritis may be suggested by vomiting and diarrhea, but these are usually transient, and evidence of pneumonia can be obtained if suspected.

Complications. Fibrinous pleurisy is commonly present and usually mild. A small amount of serous effusion in the pleural space is also frequent. Empyema, formerly so common, is now a much less frequent complication. Purulent pericarditis is also rare. Early therapy usually prevents bacteremic complications of peritonitis, meningitis, arthritis, and osteomyelitis. Likewise, the complications of parotitis, nephritis, endocarditis, and myocarditis have been almost eliminated by modern therapy. At times atelectasis follows pneumonia. Abdominal distention from paralytic ileus, formerly frequent, is now rare because of more effective treatment and resultant decreased disturbance of fluid and electrolyte balances. It is probable that this complication is caused by hypokalemia, rather than toxicity, as formerly thought. Otitis media is sometimes present but today rarely progresses to mastoiditis or lateral sinus thrombosis.

Prognosis. When pneumococcal pneumonia in the otherwise normal child is diagnosed early and treated promptly, the mortality rate is less than 1%. The rate is higher in malnourished or debilitated children and those treated late in the course of the disease.

Treatment. Treatment consists of antibacterial therapy, supportive care, and management of complications if they occur.

Penicillin is the most effective antibiotic. It is given in full therapeutic dosages by the intravenous or intramuscular route to guarantee retention. It should be continued for 4 or 5 days after the temperature is normal and the chest radiograph demonstrates clearing. The response is usually so rapid that the patient is afebrile within 24 to 48 hours. Erythromycin or a cephalosporin may be used if the patient is sensitive to penicillin.

Humidified oxygen is beneficial if hypoxia occurs and is definitely indicated in the presence of cyanosis. It is also employed when dyspnea is severe or if circulatory failure ensues.

Fever is controlled by antipyretic drugs, alcohol sponging, or tepid packs.

The diet should be liquid at first and then soft and bland. Return to a normal diet should be according to the patient's appetite.

If vomiting is a problem, a brief period of fasting (but with administration of parenteral fluids) may suffice to check it. Mild sedation, as by a barbiturate-containing suppository, may also control emesis. Injection of a tranquilizer is rarely needed for this purpose in children with pneumonia.

Adequate fluid intake should be maintained to overcome dehydration caused by high temperature, vomiting, anorexia, and sometimes diarrhea. Offering the sick child small sips of fluid at frequent intervals usually suffices, but parenteral fluid therapy should be instituted when oral intake is inadequate.

Control of restlessness and pain from pleural inflammation can be achieved by cautious use of sedative agents or codeine, being careful not to depress the respiratory effort.

Bed rest, instituted at onset, should be continued for at least several days after the temperature has become normal.

Staphylococcal pneumonia

The innate virulence of staphylococci and their remarkable capacity to develop resistance to antibiotics account for the fact that staphylococcal pneumonia is such a serious pulmonary infection of childhood. Although it may occur at any age, its greatest incidence is in the first 2 years of life, especially the first year.

Etiology and epidemiology. The causative organisms are coagulase-positive staphylococci whose specific identity can be determined by bacteriophage typing. From a therapeutic viewpoint they can be divided into two groups: those sensitive to penicillin G and those resistant to it. The latter pose the principal problem. The rapidity with which staphylococci mutate and their inherent adaptability to antibiotics account for the emergence of resistant organisms under hospital circumstances. Indiscriminate administration of antibiotics thus eliminates the weak and favors the strong.

Furthermore, these organisms are not only resistant but also persistent. They establish themselves in the nasal passages of nurses, physicians, attendants, and other personnel or infect them in the form of furuncles or paronychiae. They contaminate the floors, furniture, mattresses, blankets, and bed linen. Cross infection is common, not only in nurseries but also in wards and private pavilions. When the patients or personnel who are persistent nasal carriers go home or make their way about the community in their daily lives, they may transmit the resistant staphylococci to others. In this manner persons who have not been in hospitals become infected with "hospital staphylococci." What began as a hospital problem is now a community problem.

Staphylococcal pneumonia is usually contracted as a primary respiratory infection, but it may arise as a result of septicemia from impetiginous lesions, furuncles, or other foci of staphylococcal infection. Newborn and young infants are easily invaded. Debilitation occasioned by many diseases also fosters infection.

Pathologic findings. Whereas a localized abscess is the characteristic lesion of staphylococcal infection in older children and adults, infection in infants tends to be more diffuse and results more often in septicemia. In the infant the pneumonic process may be at first diffuse, but it soon progresses to the formation of multiple abscesses. The mucous membrane of the bronchi is subjected to the necrotizing exotoxin of the staphylococci and may slough.

The principal complications are based on the tissue necrosis that characterizes staphylococcal infection. Abscesses contiguous to bronchi erode bronchial walls and discharge their contents into the lumen. Air then enters the abscess cavity on inspiration (perhaps because inspiratory dilation and elongation of bronchi enlarge the opening in the bronchial wall) but has difficulty egressing (perhaps because expiratory collapse of bronchi narrows the aperture). This progressive inflation of the area of the abscess in the interstitial tissue causes pneumatoceles that are visible on radiographs and are virtually pathognomonic of staphylococcal pneumonia. Several such lesions may develop, some of only moderate size but others enlarging progressively. Fluctuations in size occur, but the pneumatoceles disappear within a few weeks to a few months. Epithelization of the wall of the pneumatocele may occur. Occasionally a pneumatocele ruptures into the pleural cavity and causes pneumothorax—often sudden life-threatening tension pneumothorax. Abscesses in the periphery of the lung often break through the pleura to cause empyema or pyopneumothorax. Any child less than 2 years of age who develops empyema has staphylococcal pneumonia until proved otherwise. Abscesses may also erode toward the heart and cause purulent pericarditis. Septicemia may occur in severe infections with extensive pulmonary involvement.

Clinical manifestations. Upper respiratory tract manifestations usually precede those related to pulmonary involvement. The child develops fever, listlessness, irritability, anorexia, nasal discharge, cough, grunting respiration, and progressively severe dyspnea that may be associated with subcostal retraction. The respiratory rate becomes rapid, and cyanosis may ensue. Clinical manifestations related to the complications just discussed may occur, such as those caused by pneumothorax, empyema, pericarditis, septicemia, and so on.

Diagnosis. Pneumonia in a child who already has visible evidence of staphylococcal infection, such as furunculosis, impetigo, omphalitis, or mastitis, is assumed to be staphylococcal in etiology. If a newborn infant contracts pneumonia in a nursery where other cases of staphylococcal infection have occurred, it is probable that the same organism is infecting the infant. The characteristic complications of staphylococcal pneumonia also help identify it. Thus when an infant has a pneumonic process accompanied by pneumatoceles, pneumothorax, pyopneumothorax, or pericarditis, it is almost certain that he has staphylococcal pneumonia. The initial radiograph may reveal a picture similar to that of pneumococcal pneumonia, but the pneumococcal infection clears rapidly with treatment, whereas staphylococcal pneumonia does not.

Treatment. The child with staphylococcal pneumonia should be hospitalized immediately, isolated from other patients because of the possibility of spreading an antibiotic-resistant staphylococcal strain to them, and given comprehensive supportive therapy. This includes oxygen if necessary, parenteral fluid therapy in the acute stage of the disease, control of fever, and judicious sedation when needed. Transfusions of blood are sometimes required.

Cultures should be obtained immediately from the nasopharynx and blood, and the antibiotic sensitivity of organisms identified should be determined. If pleural fluid is present, a diagnostic paracentesis should be performed to obtain material for culture and sensitivity tests.

A high percentage of these patients, especially infants with staphylococcal pneumonia, develop empyema or pyopneumothorax, and sometimes tension pneumothorax. When any of these three is noted, a chest surgeon should be consulted immediately, a tube should be inserted into the pleural cavity, and closed underwater drainage should be instituted. In some patients more than one tube is needed.

Because staphylococcal pneumonia is a rapidly necrotizing process with abscess formation, it is essential to initiate vigorous antibiotic therapy as soon as cultures have been taken, not delaying until the results are known. Because many patients with staphylococcal pneumonia are infected with penicillinase-producing staphylococci (penicillin G—resistant staphylococci), one of the semisynthetic penicillins should be employed parenterally in high dosage. Examples are nafcillin, oxacillin, and methicillin.

If cultures from blood or pleural fluid indicate that the staphylococcus is sensitive to penicillin G, it should be started using the aqueous form intravenously in a dosage of 100,000 to 400,000 units/kg/24 hr. The semisynthetic penicillin is discontinued.

The cephalosporins or clindamycin may be used in patients with serious infections who are allergic to penicillin. Five to ten percent of patients who react to penicillin will also react to the cephalosporins. Vancomycin may be used in patients allergic to both penicillin and the cephalosporins.

Therapy should be continued until all evidence of disease has disappeared and the chest radiograph has returned to normal. In view of the tendency for staphylococci to persist in microabscesses and to cause recurrence of infection after therapy has ceased, it is advisable to treat staphylococcal pneumonia for at least 4 weeks and often longer. Each case must be individualized, but failures will result if one depends on short courses of therapy.

Streptococcal pneumonia

Streptococcal pneumonia occurs more often as a complication of measles and influenza than as a primary infection. Young children are more susceptible. It may appear without other evidence of illness, may follow a streptococcal infection of the upper respiratory tract, or may occur as a complication of a contagious disease.

The infectious process extends swiftly through the lymphatics of the lungs and may initiate empyema early. The child is prostrated and has a high temperature. Physical findings initially consist of rales only, but signs of consolidation soon appear. There is a large amount of fluid in the pleural space when empyema occurs, and the heart and mediastinal structures are displaced to the opposite side. Respirations become shallow and rapid, and cyanosis may appear.

Diagnosis is suggested by appearance of signs of pneumonia as a complication of measles or influenza and by early onset of empyema. The thin purulent nature of the empyema fluid also indicates probable streptococcal infection. Cultures of pleural fluid, blood, and nasopharyngeal secretions substantiate the diagnosis.

Penicillin G is the antibiotic of choice and is highly effective. It is given intravenously in a dosage of 30,000 to 50,000 units/kg/24 hr in newborn infants and from 500,000 to 1 million units/24 hr in children. If sufficient empyema fluid collects to warrant aspiration, penicillin should be instilled into the pleural cavity. Aspiration and instillation of penicillin are repeated daily until the need for these procedures disappears.

Haemophilus influenzae pneumonia

Haemophilus influenzae type B is one of the more frequent causes of serious bacterial infection of the respiratory tract in infants and children. The incidence of pneumonia caused by *H. influenzae* in infants and children appears to be increasing, and may be related to lower levels of circulating anti–*H. influenzae* antibody in the adult population.

H. influenzae pneumonia is usually lobar in distribution, although segmental pneumonia does occur and diffuse miliary bronchopneumonia has been described. Microscopic pathology reveals circumscribed areas of consolidation, with heavy infiltration of polymorphonuclear leukocytes, fibrin, edema fluid, and red blood cells filling the alveoli. The edema may be striking and often extends into the interstitial spaces. The mucosa of the bronchi and bronchioles usually shows extensive destructive changes.

The clinical features of *H. influenzae* pneumonia do not differentiate it from pneumonia caused by other bacteria, especially the pneumococcus. However, there is a tendency to a more insidious onset and a clinical course that is less acute, sometimes prolonged over several weeks. At the outset the bronchopneumonia variety may mimic acute bronchiolitis. Pneumatoceles have also been described.

Diagnosis is established by culturing *H. influenzae* from blood, empyema fluid, or lung aspirate. Predominant growth of the organism from nasopharyngeal cultures is suggestive. Countercurrent immunoelectrophoresis, when available, confirms the diagnosis quickly and precisely.

When *H. influenzae* infection is suspected but not proved, initial antimicrobial treatment consists of the simultaneous administration of ampicillin and chloramphenicol in the event of the occurrence of an ampicillin-resistant strain of the organism. If an organism is isolated and its sensitivity determined, the appropriate drug may then be continued. Both drugs should be given by the parenteral route until clinical improvement occurs, and oral preparations may be used. Supportive therapy and the treatment of complications are as described for pneumococcal and staphylococcal pneumonias.

Mycoplasmal pneumonia

Mycoplasma pneumoniae, one of the smallest free-living organisms, is a pleuropneumonia-like organism responsible for approximately 10% to 20% of hospital admissions of infants and children with pneumonia. It is the single most frequent cause of pneumonia in school-aged children.

Etiology and epidemiology. The organism is transmitted from person to person by droplet spread. The incubation period is approximately 7 to 14 days. Although mycoplasmal pneumonia occurs chiefly in an endemic manner, with predilection for the early fall and winter months, limited epidemics have been reported in groups living under crowded circumstances, such as in military barracks, orphanages, and so on.

Pathologic findings. Interstitial round cell infiltration and edema of alveolar septa are found, as well as inflammation, necrosis, and ulceration of the lining mucosa of bronchi and bronchioles. Inflammatory areas may be large or small and vary greatly in distribution. Areas of consolidation are present, as well as areas of emphysema and atelectasis from obstruction of terminal bronchioles. The pleural surface is usually normal but sometimes has patchy areas of fibrinous exudate. As a rule, healing occurs without residual lung damage.

Clinical manifestations. The onset may be insidious or abrupt. Constitutional symptoms appear first, such as fever, chills in older children and adults, headache, malaise, anorexia, and myalgia. Rhinitis and sore throat may then appear, followed by a dry, hacking cough. At first there is little or no sputum, but then the cough produces seromucoid sputum, which may later become mucopurulent or blood streaked. Dyspnea is uncommon. The fever usually lasts several days to 2 weeks.

Physical examination may reveal no abnormalities at the beginning of illness, or only mild pharyngeal hyperemia and slight enlargement of cervical lymph nodes may be noted. Later fine crepitant rales are heard over various areas of the lung fields, but signs of consolidation usually cannot be demonstrated.

Radiographic findings. The chest radiograph reveals abnormalities out of proportion to the paucity of physical findings. Poorly defined areas of hazy or fluffy infiltrate radiating out from the hilar regions are commonly present. Such infiltrates may affect only one or several lobes. Lower lobes are most commonly involved.

Laboratory findings. The white blood cell count is usually normal. The causative organism can be recovered from the pharynx and sputum by special techniques. Specific serologic tests, including immunofluorescent techniques and complement-fixation and hemagglutination tests, are sometimes available for diagnosis. In more than half the patients there is a rise in cold agglutinins, usually within 7 to 10 days after infection, but this is a nonspecific response to *M. pneumoniae* infection, not being limited to infection with this organism. A single cold agglutination titer of 1:32 is suggestive, but a fourfold rise in titer is more convincing. Agglutinins for the MG strain of nonhemolytic streptococci may also develop, but again this test is nonspecific.

Diagnosis. On clinical grounds alone, pneumonia resulting from *M. pneumoniae* cannot be distinguished from pneumonias resulting from viruses or rickettsiae. Definitive diagnosis rests on recovery of the organism or demonstration of rise in titer of specific antibodies.

Treatment. Most patients do well with only symptomatic management and recover from the acute illness in 7 to 10 days, followed by a brief convalescent period of about a week. Erythromycin is the preferred antimicrobial agent in children less than 9 years old. Tetracycline is also effective and may be used in older children.

Viral pneumonia

Many viruses may produce pneumonia, including those of influenza, parainfluenza viruses, measles, respiratory syncytial virus, rhinoviruses, and adenoviruses. Pathologic changes are interstitial pneumonitis, inflammation of the mucosa and walls of bronchi and bronchioles, and at times secondary bacterial infection. Complications are infrequent. Symptoms vary, ranging from mild fever, slight cough, and some malaise to high fever, prostration, and severe cough. A slight upper respiratory infection is often present. Physical findings in the chest are frequently normal or minimally abnormal. The radiograph reveals diffuse infiltration extending from one or both hilar areas usually associated with a patchy bronchopneumonia. The white cell count is usually normal, but slight leukocytosis may be present. Viral pneumonias are treated symptomatically, antibiotics being employed only if bacterial complications ensue.

DISEASES OF THE PLEURA

Pleural effusions. The pleural space and the fluid within it are not under static conditions. During each ventilatory cycle the pleural pressures fluctuate widely. Fluid constantly moves into and out of the pleural space. In health a dynamic equilibrium is reached where there is a small amount of pleural fluid, and fluid formation equals fluid absorption. Many disease states may alter the dynamics of the pleural space so that pleural fluid accumulates.

Pleural effusions have classically been divided into transudates and exudates. A *transudate* occurs when the systemic factors influencing the formation or absorption of pleural fluid are altered. Decreased plasma colloid–osmotic pressure or elevated hydrostatic pressure in the systemic or pulmonary circulation are alterations that produce transudates. In these situations the pleural surfaces are not involved by the primary pathologic process. In contrast, an *exudate* results from disease of the pleural surface. The two main mechanisms by which pleural disease leads to pleural fluid accumulation are increased capillary permeability for protein and lymphatic obstruction.

A pleural fluid is classified as an exudate when the protein levels exceed 3 g/dl or its specific gravity exceeds 1.016. If the effusion is a transudate, no further diagnostic procedures are necessary, and therapy is directed toward the underlying systemic disease. If the effusion proves to be an exudate, more extensive diagnostic procedures are necessary to establish its precise cause. Following is a list of causes of pleural effusions.

- Transudative pleural effusions
  - Congestive heart failure
  - Cirrhosis
  - Acute glomerulonephritis
  - Nephrotic syndrome
  - Hypoproteinemia
- Exudative pleural effusions

- Infectious diseases
  - Tuberculosis
  - Bacterial infections
  - Viral infections
  - Fungus infections
  - Parasitic infections
- Neoplastic diseases
  - Metastatic disease
  - Mesothelioma
- Collagen vascular diseases
  - Systemic lupus erythematosus
  - Rheumatoid arthritis
- Pulmonary infarction
- Gastrointestinal diseases
  - Esophageal rupture
  - Pancreatitis
  - Subphrenic abscess
  - Hepatic abscess
- Uremia
- Trauma
  - Hemothorax
  - Chylothorax

The most distinctive symptom of pleural disease is pain. Pleuritic pain is typically sharp and aggravated by respiration. The pain may be located over the area of pleural irritation, or it may be referred to the shoulder or abdominal wall when the diaphragmatic pleura is involved. The pleural friction rub is the salient physical finding associated with acute pleuritic pain. Additionally, when pleural disease is associated with large effusions, the trachea is deviated to the contralateral side, and over the involved area are found diminished movement, a flat percussion note, absent tactile fremitus, and absent breath sounds.

The chest x-ray film will show evidence of the pleural effusion, with obliteration of the diaphragmatic contour and an opacity rising laterally along the chest wall. Decubitus radiographs will demonstrate whether the fluid is free or loculated and can detect smaller amounts of fluid than can the standard films. A diagnostic thoracentesis should be performed on all patients with pleural effusion from whom pleural fluid can be easily obtained. If the fluid is a transudate (hydrothorax), no further diagnostic procedures need be directed toward the pleura. If the fluid is an exudate, the diagnosis will frequently be made by cytologic, biochemical, or microbiologic study of the fluid.

Empyema. Empyema refers to the presence of purulent material in the pleural space. It is the result of extension of infection from a contiguous structure such as the lung, esophagus, or abdomen. The primary inflammatory process may be pneumonia, lung abscess, subdiaphragmatic abscess, or perforation of the esophagus.

The incidence has been greatly reduced by the effective treatment of bacterial pneumonias, and pneumococcal and streptococcal empyemas are now uncommon. The incidence is highest in infancy. The majority of infections are caused by the staphylococcus, and less frequently *H. influenzae* and various other gram-negative bacilli. Anaerobic pleuropulmonary infections are seen in increased incidence in patients who manifest periodontal infections and who have altered consciousness and dysphagia, which leads to aspiration of oropharyngeal secretions in the presence of disturbed clearing mechanisms.

The diagnosis is established at thoracentesis when pus is aspirated from the pleural space. If it is putrid, anaerobic infection is likely. Gram stain and culture of the aspirated material identify the causative organisms in most cases. Countercurrent immunoelectrophoresis has recently proved useful for the diagnosis of certain bacterial antigens in the body fluids, including pleural fluid. Antimicrobial therapy should be initiated on the strength of a positive Gram stain or grossly purulent fluid. Initial choice of antimicrobial agent(s) is based on a consideration of the clinical data. Dosage must be adequate, and administration initially should be by the intravenous route. Changes in antimicrobial therapy are guided by results of culture and sensitivity tests. Needle aspiration may be adequate for prompt relief of dyspnea, but a moderate to severe effusion, especially in the presence of overwhelming toxicity, indicates either intercostal tube placement or open thoracotomy for continuous drainage.

Hemothorax. Hemothorax is usually the result of trauma (accidental or nonaccidental), but it may occur from erosion of a blood vessel in association with an inflammatory process or from neoplastic pleural disease, and occasionally as a result of blood dyscrasia. Rupture of an aortic aneurysm is unlikely in childhood. The diagnosis is established at thoracentesis. A chest catheter should be inserted to remove the blood, assess the rate of bleeding, and ensure expansion of the lung. Transfusion is necessary when loss of blood is excessive. Persistent bleeding, usually from a tear in a systemic artery such as an intercostal or internal mammary vessel, requires open thoracotomy for treatment. If bleeding into the pleural space is extensive and the blood is not adequately removed, fibrin deposition and subsequent fibrous organization may occur. This will result in restriction of lung function and may require decortication with removal of the fibrous peel.

Chylothorax. Chylothorax results from abnormality involving the thoracic duct. The duct ascends to the right of the midline in the lower part of the chest so that injury at this site tends to produce a right-sided effusion. The duct gradually crosses to the left of the midline in the upper part of the chest so that injury in this region results in a left-sided effusion. Rarely, a chylothorax may be caused by congenital anomalies of the thoracic duct system, metastatic malignancy, lymphoma, or trauma or may be a postoperative complication of chest surgery. It is diagnosed on the basis of the gross appearance of the pleural fluid and the finding of a fat concentration greater than 400 mg/dl in the fluid. Treatment depends on the cause. Radiation therapy may control chylothorax that is caused by malignancy. Traumatic chylothorax may respond to multiple thoracenteses or intercostal catheter drainage. However, if it does not respond, surgical ligation of the thoracic duct below the point of rupture is indicated.

Fibrothorax. Extensive fibrosis of the pleural space may occur after pyogenic empyema, tuberculous empyema, or traumatic hemothorax. The diffuse fibrosis may encase the lung and result in restricted function. The diagnosis can be established on the basis of the clinical history, pulmonary function tests, and x-ray demonstration of the fibrous peel. Evidence of calcification within the thickened pleura may be noted on the chest film. Selected patients may be improved by surgical decortication of the lung.

Pneumothorax. Pneumothorax refers to the presence of air in the pleural space. A pneumothorax may be associated with either a serous or a purulent effusion; it is then termed *hydropneumothorax* or *pyopneumothorax*, respectively. Beyond the neonatal period, pneumothorax usually occurs as a complication of other respiratory diseases, especially asthma and cystic fibrosis; as a result of trauma; as a complication of resuscitation or mechanical ventilation; and spontaneously in persons without known underlying pulmonary disease. Additionally, a *pneumomediastinum* may be associated with a pneumothorax. This occurs when a pressure gradient exists between the alveolus and the interstitial tissue, usually as a result of a check valve obstruction or high inspiratory pressures. In this situation the air escaping from the ruptured alveoli tracks along the sheaths of the perivascular structures, causing pulmonary interstitial emphysema. The interstitial air may track either peripherally toward the pleural surface or medially toward the mediastinum. In either case, rupture of the visceral or mediastinal pleura results in pneumothorax or pneumomediastinum.

The major clinical symptoms of pneumothorax are pain and dyspnea. The pain may be sharp and severe or mild and dull. The severity of the dyspnea depends on the degree of collapse of the affected lung and the functional state of the unaffected lung. Physical examination reveals tracheal deviation to the opposite side. The affected side exhibits diminished movement, hyperresonance on percussion, absent tactile fremitus, and absent breath sounds. The chest radiograph establishes the diagnosis by demonstrating the hyperlucent area with an absence of lung markings. A film taken in expiration may be helpful in demonstrating a small pneumothorax by increasing the contrast between the lung and the air in the pleural space.

The therapeutic approach to spontaneous pneumothorax is usually conservative. If the pneumothorax is small and the patient is relatively asymptomatic, observation alone is sufficient. When there is a large collection of pleural air, thoracentesis is indicated, and as much air is removed as possible. If air reaccumulates or if a tension pneumothorax develops, reexpansion of the lung is achieved by placement of an intercostal chest tube and application of negative pressure. Once the lung is reexpanded, the treatment is continued for 24 to 48 hours in hope that the pleural leak will seal and that pleural adhesions will prevent recurrence.

BRONCHIAL OBSTRUCTION

The airways are involved in most pulmonary diseases. Even when the disease affects primarily the lung parenchyma, the lumen of the bronchus draining the diseased area may be narrowed by mucosal swelling or inflammatory exudate, and air movement into and out of the alveoli and drainage of secretions are impaired.

There are three mechanisms by which a bronchial lumen may be narrowed. *Extrabronchial lesions* result in extrinsic compression of the bronchus. Enlarged mediastinal lymph nodes compressing the right middle lobe bronchus is an example. *Mural lesions* such as mucosal edema or a bronchial adenoma projecting into the lumen of the bronchus may also cause airway narrowing. *Intraluminal causes* of bronchial obstruction include inhaled foreign bodies or thick or inspissated bronchial secretions.

Bronchial obstruction may be either partial or complete. Lesions producing a partial obstruction act either as a bypass valve or a check valve, depending on the degree of narrowing of the bronchial lumen and the nature of the lesion. A bypass obstruction only slightly narrows the lumen of the bronchus. Although airflow resistance is increased, air is still able to move in and out past the site of obstruction. Overdistention of the lung parenchyma distal to the obstruction results because as the airways narrow during expiration the resistance to flow is higher than it is during inspiration, leading to incomplete emptying of the lung. A check valve type of bronchial obstruction completely occludes the bronchial lumen during expiration so that egress of air is prevented. During inspiration the bronchial lumen widens so that air is able to pass over the obstruction. However, expiratory narrowing of the bronchial lumen completely occludes it. Air is then trapped in the lung and the alveoli become overdistended. If a large portion of the lung is involved in partial obstruction, the mediastinum is shifted toward the opposite side and movement is diminished, the percussion note is hyperresonant, and the intensity of the breath sounds is reduced over the affected area.

In complete bronchial obstruction, gas cannot move into or out of the lung distal to the obstruction. The consequence of this type of obstruction is atelectasis, which results from absorption of the alveolar gas into the circulating blood and collapse of the alveoli. The affected part of the chest may appear retracted, the ribs are close together, and there is retraction of the intercostal spaces. The trachea and the apex beat of the heart are shifted to the affected side. Chest movement is diminished, the percussion note dull, and vocal fremitus and breath sounds reduced or absent over the affected area.

If obstruction of a large bronchus develops gradually, there may be no symptoms except cough. If the obstruction develops abruptly, intense dyspnea is usually experienced. A cough is almost always associated with all types of bronchial obstruction. As the degree of obstruction increases, so does the cough. Interference with bronchial drainage is a predictable consequence of bronchial obstruction, and because bacteria grow very easily in retained secretions, infection frequently develops in the affected area of the lung. This creates a vicious cycle with the production of more cough, more secretions, and more obstruction.

The cause of bronchial obstruction can be determined by bronchoscopic examination and, in the case of foreign body or inspissated mucus plugs, can be relieved by extraction at the time of bronchoscopy. Oxygen therapy is indicated when there is dyspnea. In other forms of bronchial obstruction the treatment is that of the underlying condition.

EMPHYSEMA AND ALPHA-1-ANTITRYPSIN DEFICIENCY

Emphysema is defined pathologically as dilation of distal air spaces accompanied by disruption of alveolar walls, resulting in *permanent* overdistention of the respiratory portion of the lung beyond the terminal bronchioles. *Reversible* overaeration of the lung is best termed *hyperinflation*.

Two major forms of emphysema have been described. The more common centrilobular variety, which involves predominantly the respiratory bronchioles, usually occurs in adult males and is often associated with chronic bronchitis and cigarette smoking. Panlobular emphysema involves the acinus uniformly. It is as common in women as in men and is not usually associated with chronic bronchitis or cigarette smoking. Panlobular emphysema is highly characteristic of alpha-1-antitrypsin deficiency, which occurs in persons homozygous for a mutant gene.

To date, only a small number of infants and children with alpha-1-antitrypsin deficiency have been reported in the world literature. However, the common occurrence of the genes responsible for the deficiency in many populations suggests that the deficiency may be more frequent than is currently appreciated.

Alpha-1-antitrypsin deficiency in association with chronic obstructive lung disease, with onset in young adult life, was first reported in 1963. It was not until 1971 that this deficiency was first reported in association with emphysema in a child. However, in 1969 alpha-1-antitrypsin deficiency was described in neonates with liver disease, often progressing to cirrhosis in early life, and since 1973 several instances of cirrhosis in association with emphysema in young children have been reported.

Alpha-1-antitrypsin is the major alpha-1-globulin in serum and is responsible for over 90% of its trypsin-inhibitory capacity. Its major protective function is inhibition of tissue enzymes, particularly one or more elastases released under normal circumstances from polymorphonuclear leukocytes, to prevent the damage of tissue, particularly elastin. In its absence, uninhibited leukocyte elastase results in elastic tissue destruction and dilation of the distal air spaces. Disruption of the alveolar walls results. It is thought that any infection or toxic injury to the lung that might increase the number of granulocytes in pulmonary tissue could enhance the release of elastase and hasten the progression of elastin destruction in deficient persons.

The onset is insidious. Dyspnea is usually the earliest symptom and is generally progressive. Cough and sputum production are not common in the early stages. The chest is in a position of hyperinflation. The diaphragm is depressed, movement of the chest cage is diminished, and heart sounds are distant. Chest radiographs demonstrate increasing hyperinflation of both lungs. Pulmonary function tests reveal progression of irreversible chronic obstructive pulmonary disease and reduced diffusing capacity. Arterial hypoxemia is present, and in advanced disease the carbon dioxide tension of arterial blood is frequently elevated. A presumptive diagnosis can be made if serum protein electrophoresis reveals a missing alpha-1-globulin band. The diagnosis is confirmed by quantitative measurement of alpha-1-antitrypsin function and concentration.

No specific treatment is available, although low blood levels of alpha-1-antitrypsin rose to normal in one patient who underwent liver transplantation. In this and all other cases, however, there has not been any reversal of lung damage, and a downhill course is to be expected.

ACUTE RESPIRATORY FAILURE

Respiratory failure is best defined in terms of primary functions of the respiratory system, which are to deliver oxygen to the pulmonary circulation and to remove carbon dioxide from it. If the respiratory system is thought of as the total integrative system dealing with respiration, including the central nervous system medullary centers, the chest bellows, and the airways and lungs, then respiratory failure is defined as an abnormally high P_{CO_2} or abnormally low P_{O_2} in the arterial blood when caused by any defect in the system. In most clinical situations—at sea level breathing room air—an arterial P_{O_2} less than 60 torr, an arterial P_{CO_2} greater than 50 torr, or both are considered indicative of respiratory failure. Thus two types of respiratory failure can be recognized. One is manifested by a low P_{O_2} and normal or low P_{CO_2}. The other is manifested by low P_{O_2} and high P_{CO_2}. It is apparent that a decreased arterial P_{O_2} is present in all cases of respiratory failure. The designation "acute" implies that development of the failure has been so rapid that the patient has had inadequate time for compensation and may be experiencing a serious alteration in acid-base balance. Acute respiratory failure may develop de novo in persons with normal lungs, as in severe barbiturate intoxication, or it may be superimposed on chronic respiratory failure in patients with long-standing pulmonary disease or impairment of any component of the integrated respiratory system.

Respiratory failure may result from a variety of diseases and dysfunctions of the respiratory system. Management of blood gas and acid-base abnormalities and specific treatment of the underlying disease and the reversible precipitating factors depend on an understanding of the etiology and pathophysiology in any given case. Many of the commonly encountered causes of acute respiratory failure are listed below. They are classified* according to the components of the respiratory system that are primarily involved.

A. Diseases of the lung and airways
  1. Causing obstructive ventilatory impairment
    a. Asthma
    b. Chronic bronchitis
    c. Bronchiolitis
    d. Obstructive emphysema
    e. Cystic fibrosis
    f. Upper airway obstruction
  2. Causing restrictive ventilatory impairment
    a. Interstitial or alveolar infiltration or fibrosis
    b. Surgical resection of pulmonary parenchyma
  3. Altering alveolar-capillary gas exchange, primarily for oxygen
    a. Diffuse interstitial pneumonitis or fibrosis
    b. Pulmonary embolization
    c. Pulmonary edema
B. Diseases impairing the chest bellows
  1. Altering the mobility of the thoracic cage and diaphragm
    a. Kyphoscoliosis
    b. Trauma: flail chest
    c. Thoracoplasty
    d. Disease of pleura
    e. Extreme obesity, ascites, postsurgical abdominal distention
  2. Causing neuromuscular impairment
    a. Affecting the spinal cord and medulla
      (1) Bulbospinal poliomyelitis
      (2) Guillain-Barré syndrome
      (3) Cervical cordotomy
      (4) Trauma to cervical cord
      (5) Werdnig-Hoffman disease
    b. Affecting the myoneural junction
      (1) Myasthenia gravis
      (2) Curariform drugs
      (3) Neuromuscular blockade caused by certain antibiotics
    c. Affecting muscles of respiration
      (1) Polymyositis
      (2) Muscular dystrophy
C. Respiratory center depression or dysfunction
  1. Narcotic or sedative overdosage
  2. Organic lesions of the respiratory center
  3. Central or primary alveolar hypoventilation

Inadequate oxygenation of tissues may be a consequence of low arterial oxygen tension and oxygen content in patients with severe pulmonary disease. This may result from diffusion defects, venous to arterial shunts, unequal ventilation-perfusion ratios, alveolar hypoventilation, or any combination of these abnormalities. *Hypercapnia* develops whenever alveolar ventilation is inadequate in relation to the level of metabolic carbon dioxide production. Because alveolar hypoventilation results in inadequate oxygen exchange and inadequate carbon dioxide elimination, the hypercapnia is always accompanied by hypoxemia unless the patient is breathing an oxygen-enriched mixture. The work of breathing is particularly important in the genesis of alveolar hypoventilation. The cost of an increase in ventilation in patients with increased mechanical resistances to breathing is much higher than in healthy subjects, and in some patients the oxygen consumption of the respiratory muscles is as high as 50% of the total oxygen consumption. Thus increased work of breathing contributes to hypoxemia and hypercapnia by increasing oxygen consumption and carbon dioxide production. Alveolar hypoventilation results when, in patients with pulmonary insufficiency, a proportionate increase in alveolar ventilation cannot be achieved.

The manifestations of altered blood gas tensions vary considerably and depend largely on their severity and duration. The central nervous system is particularly vulnerable to hypoxia and hypercapnia, and neurologic manifestations usually predominate. These include headache, lassitude, slurred speech, incoordination, restlessness, irritability, tremors, and mood fluctuations such as anxiety, depression, and euphoria. Some of the mental changes may be related to the increase in cerebral blood flow and the elevated cerebrospinal fluid pressure that occur when arterial carbon dioxide tension rises. Tachycardia, hyperpnea, dyspnea, and cyanosis may be additional dominant features.

Heart failure is a frequent manifestation of severe respiratory insufficiency. Acute hypoxemia and acidosis increase pulmonary vascular resistance and may precipitate acute right ventricular failure. Left ventricular function is compromised because catecholamine release results in tachycardia and systemic hypertension and because hypoxemia and acidemia depress myocardial function. The resultant pulmonary edema in turn further increases the work of breathing and aggravates the hypoxemia so that gross right and left heart failure may be present.

Clinical assessment of the adequacy of oxy-

*Modified from classification of Davis, H.L.: Acute respiratory insufficiency, Adv. Intern. Med. **19**:213-238, 1974.

genation and ventilation has been shown to be unreliable. Therefore determination of arterial blood gases and pH is necessary to confirm the presence of acute respiratory failure. The definitive diagnosis depends on the demonstration of hypoxemia, with or without carbon dioxide retention, by analysis of arterial blood.

The development of acute respiratory failure represents a medical emergency that clearly requires immediate therapy. Management is designed to reverse the physiologic disturbances that are present.

Hypoxemia is the single most lethal consequence of acute respiratory failure and should be dealt with immediately. When hypoxemia results from hypoventilation, provision of an adequate aveolar ventilation will restore the arterial Po_2 to normal levels. However, in most instances oxygen enrichment of the inspired air is required to correct the hypoxemia resulting from ventilation and perfusion imbalance caused by respiratory disease. In all patients receiving oxygen therapy, the lowest inspired oxygen concentration that will result in an arterial Po_2 between 80 and 100 torr should be administered. The administration of oxygen may result in cellular toxicity if given in too high a concentration for more than 48 to 72 hours. In addition to retrolental fibroplasia, which may be precipitated by high oxygen concentrations in the newborn infant, pulmonary edema, atelectasis, and alveolar exudates have followed administration of high concentrations of oxygen to children and adults. In addition, the inhalation of oxygen in high concentrations leads to a washout of nitrogen from the lungs. If airway obstruction develops in this situation, gas is rapidly absorbed from the distal alveoli. A fall in arterial Po_2 despite continued inhalation of a constant concentration of oxygen may signal the development of focal areas of atelectasis that may still be perfused.

Measures to reduce the work of breathing should be started as soon as possible. Reduction of the mechanical resistances to breathing will lower the oxygen uptake and carbon dioxide production of the respiratory apparatus. This is achieved through relief of airway obstruction and pulmonary edema if they are present.

Airway obstruction is usually increased because of accumulation of bronchial secretions or bronchoconstriction. Reduction of the production of secretions requires elimination of all irritants and eradication of infection. Improved elimination of secretions is facilitated by efforts to reduce their viscosity. This requires provision of adequate hydration, humidification of the inspired air, chest physiotherapy, and endotracheal suction. When bronchospasm is present, the administration of nebulized or intravenous bronchodilating agents will result in a marked reduction in airflow resistance. In patients with severe bronchial obstruction, particularly those in status asthmaticus, it may be necessary to administer high doses of corticosteroids. Pulmonary edema, if present, further increases the work of breathing and aggravates the disturbances of gas exchange. Reduced fluid intake and the administration of diuretics, digitalis, and a salt-free diet frequently result in improvement in ventilatory function and arterial blood gas tensions.

In order to ensure adequate alveolar ventilation it is essential that a patent airway be maintained. Insertion of an endotracheal tube is frequently lifesaving in patients with laryngeal or tracheal obstruction. In the seriously ill patient with generalized airway obstruction who is comatose, an artificial airway is also indicated when it is obvious that a safe and patent airway will be difficult to maintain otherwise. This allows oxygenation and provision of assisted or controlled ventilation, if it is required, and facilitates the aspiration of secretions. If it is decided that the acute situation will be prolonged, a tracheostomy is preferred over an endotracheal tube.

A mechanical ventilator may be necessary to manage patients with acute respiratory failure when there is (1) persistent marked alveolar hypoventilation despite intensive therapy directed at reducing the work of breathing, (2) excessive fatigue on the part of the patient, (3) severe progressive hypoxemia refractory to conservative therapy, and (4) need for internal fixation of a flail chest.

The therapy of acute respiratory failure is directed at the *immediate* provision of oxygenation and the *gradual* reduction of the arterial Pco_2. The effect of therapy is assessed by monitoring arterial blood gas tensions and pH at regular intervals. In patients with carbon dioxide retention, the arterial Pco_2 should be lowered slowly to maintain the pH between 7.35

and 7.50. If the Pco_2 is reduced rapidly to normal levels by artificial ventilation in patients with compensated chronic hypercapnia and an elevated plasma bicarbonate, severe alkalemia may result, and the patient may develop convulsions or coma. The management of respiratory failure should not be directed at the arterial Pco_2 but rather at the arterial Po_2 and any associated hydrogen ion disturbance.

Successful treatment of the underlying pathology and the factors that precipitated respiratory failure will allow a patient to be weaned from a ventilator. Patient fatigue is common in the early stages of weaning, and it is therefore best to employ short periods off the ventilator at increasingly frequent intervals, rather than long periods off the ventilator at infrequent intervals. Blood gases should be monitored repeatedly during the weaning period, and, when possible, tidal volume and vital capacity should be assessed at intervals. Short periods of spontaneous ventilation can usually be tolerated if the patient has an adequate tidal volume and vital capacity roughly twice the tidal volume.

SUDDEN INFANT DEATH SYNDROME

Since biblical times it has been known that seemingly healthy infants often die within the first year of life for no apparent reason. During the twentieth century, for lack of an understanding of the tragedy, the condition has become known as sudden infant death syndrome.

The sudden and unexpected deaths of apparently thriving infants represent an appalling tragedy to families of victims and are a major cause of infant mortality. Approximately 10,000 unexplained infant deaths occur each year. This condition is the leading cause of death between 1 month and 1 year of age, accounting for 50% of deaths in this age group.

Sudden infant death syndrome, or SIDS, is defined as the sudden and unexpected death of an apparently healthy infant or young child on whom a thorough autopsy fails to demonstrate an adequate cause of death. The term "near-miss" SIDS is applied to those infants who are found under circumstances that suggest that they have died of SIDS but who, after vigorous resuscitative efforts, survive.

Certain biologic characteristics and environmental features common to victims of SIDS have been identified. These include death at a peak age of 3 to 4 months (50% in 3 months, 90% in 6 months), occurring invariably during sleep and without an audible cry. There is a higher incidence in males, premature births, nonwhites, lower socioeconomic classes, winter season, and in subsequent siblings of SIDS victims.

Until the present decade investigators had proposed and then discarded over 100 hypotheses in an attempt to explain sudden death for which no cause could be found at autopsy. Although most authorities agree that there may be multiple causes of death in these infants, in the past 10 years a major focus of research has been on factors that contribute to the regulation of respiratory and cardiovascular function.

The most important discovery that has permitted investigation of these abnormalities in function was that not all infants at risk of SIDS die with their first episode. These near-miss infants have been the subject of intense investigation, and it is primarily from study of them that mechanisms have been identified that explain their spells. It is presumed that similar mechanisms account for death in those cases diagnosed as SIDS.

The most consistent abnormality noted in these infants during long-term study has been the presence of frequent episodes of cessation of breathing during sleep for as little as 3 seconds and for longer than 20 seconds. This is thought to result either from impaired regulation of breathing because the brain fails to respond to rising carbon dioxide levels in the blood during sleep or because of impaired regulation of the tone of the muscles surrounding the upper airway that permit them to relax during sleep. This allows the tongue and other upper airway muscles to collapse, thus causing total respiratory obstruction.

The second most consistent group of abnormalities found related to impairment of control of the heart beat. Disturbances in heart rate, both tachycardia and bradycardia, as well as abnormal heart rhythms were identified.

Many infants who appear to be near-miss SIDS victims have other illnesses that need to be diagnosed and treated. These include seizure disorders; sepsis, pneumonia, meningitis, and other severe infections; hypoglycemia, hypocalcemia, and other metabolic disorders; severe anemia; and gastroesophageal reflux.

Therefore it is imperative that infants suspected of having suffered a near-miss SIDS spell be studied to exclude other diagnosable and treatable conditions. This usually involves admission to a hospital where a pneumocardiogram can be recorded and studied for irregularities in respiratory and cardiac rates and rhythms. Other tests usually done include an electroencephalogram, electrocardiogram, selected chemical determinations of the blood, arterial blood gases, radiographs of the chest, skull, and upper gastrointestinal tract, and perhaps other tests depending on the individual patient's history and physical examination.

Once immediately treatable causes have been identified, there still remains a population of infants who by medical history had a near-death spell but for whom there is no obvious cause. These infants can be effectivly treated at home in a way that significantly reduces the risks of SIDS.

Home management involves training the parents to detect and to respond to their infant's respiratory or cardiovascular problem. Before the infant is discharged from the hospital, the parents are taught to use an electronic device that continuously monitors the infant's breathing and heart beat and sounds an alarm when irregularities occur. They are also taught to evaluate their baby when an alarm sounds and to perform cardiopulmonary resuscitation when needed. With the use of home monitoring of these infants and parents trained in cardiopulmonary resuscitation the survival rate of near-miss SIDS infants is 95%. Theophylline reduces the number of episodes of abnormal breathing in some infants.

In the majority of infants the spells become progressively less frequent, so that usually within 6 months of the first episode monitoring is no longer necessary.

There continues to be a serious question about the negative psychologic impact of monitoring on the family, but for the majority of parents it is a positive experience if they receive the appropriate education and support of medical personnel. Most families consider the use of an electronic monitor far preferable to the anxiety of wondering if their infant will have another spell and the resultant loss of sleep from frequent or even continuous nighttime observation of their infant. Most parents have been found to cope best with this situation if they have not only medical and technical support but also support from other parents whose infants have been or are still being monitored.

Phillip George
James G. Hughes

SELECTED READINGS

Comroe, J.H., Jr., et al.: The lung; clinical physiology and pulmonary function tests, Chicago, 1962. Year Book Medical Publishers, Inc.

Kendig, E.L., Jr., and Chernick, V.: Disorders of the respiratory tract in children, ed. 4, Philadelphia, 1983, W.B. Saunders Co.

Polgar, G., and Promadhat, V.: Pulmonary function testing in children, Philadelphia, 1971, W.B. Saunders Co.

Scarpelli, E.M., and Auld, P.A.M.: Pulmonary physiology of the fetus, newborn, and child, Philadelphia, 1975, Lea & Febiger.

Slonim, N.B., et al.: Pediatric respiratory therapy, Sarasota, Fla., 1974, Glenn Educational Medical Services, Inc.

18 Pediatric Cardiology

Developments in the field of pediatric cardiology during the past two decades have been impressive. In prior years, infants born with major congenital cardiovascular defects were viewed with a certain degree of understandable pessimism by the pediatrician and cardiologist alike. Improved understanding of the pathophysiology of the various cardiac defects, a more skilled aggressive approach toward the diagnosis and medical management of these patients, and advances in diagnostic instrumentation have made possible the surgical palliation or functional correction of more than 90% of congenital cardiovascular defects. New and improved surgical techniques and postoperative care have likewise contributed greatly to this more optimistic outlook. For many infants with congenital heart disease, however, successful application of these advances must depend on early recognition and referral by the practicing physician.

The mortality of infants born with congenital cardiovascular disease is clearly greatest in the first few months of life, with most deaths occurring during the first month. Because this infant group could potentially benefit most from early diagnosis and treatment, the importance of awareness of the signs and symptoms of heart disease peculiar to this age period has been emphasized. Physicians concerned with the care of infants and children have a responsibility to be alert to the possibility of hemodynamically important heart disease in the pediatric age group because it is only through their efforts that early referral can be made to centers having appropriate diagnostic and therapeutic capabilities.

CLINICAL EVALUATION

The infant or child suspected of having heart disease should be subjected to a careful pediatric history and physical examination because clues to the presence of heart disease are often subtle, particularly in the young infant.

History. The antenatal history is often unrewarding, but a history of possible exposure to known teratogens, for example, radiography, infections, or drugs, should be sought. Rubella is the most important infection known to be related to the production of congenital cardiovascular malformations. The incidence of affected offspring of infected mothers varies with the gestational age of the fetus at the time infection occurs. By far the most common cardiovascular malformations are patent ductus arteriosus and pulmonary stenosis, alone or in combination. Although less well documented, there is evidence suggesting the possible etiologic role of other viral agents in the production of congenital cardiac lesions, notably coxsackie B virus. Maternal diabetes is clearly associated with a higher-than-average incidence of congenital malformations, although cardiac abnormalities are less frequent than abnormalities of other organ systems.

A family history of prior congenital heart defects is important because the risk of subsequent occurrence is increased approximately threefold. In general, lesions occurring in siblings are of similar type. Identical twins, however, usually are discordant for the occurrence of heart disease; that is, only one is affected. Familial occurrence of several common lesions has been reported (atrial septal defect, patent ductus arteriosus, ventricular septal defect, tetralogy of Fallot, aortic stenosis, endocardial fibroelastosis). In most instances this is thought to be a result of multifactorial inheritance: polygenic factors interacting with environmental conditions.

Methods of eliciting information bearing on cardiovascular function in children will, of necessity, vary with age of the patient. For example, exercise tolerance in the infant is best assessed by carefully evaluating his feeding pattern, particularly regarding nursing or bottle feeding. The infant who appears hungry at feeding time but requires frequent rest periods, taking an inordinately long time to consume an amount of formula often less than expected for his age, is suspected of having compromised cardiac function. This suspicion is heightened by a history of respiratory distress or diaphoresis, at rest or with feeding. A detailed record of height and weight gain is invaluable because poor growth, especially involving weight, is a common manifestation of chronic congestive failure, severe hypoxemia, or large left-to-right shunt.

In the older child the questions become a little more straightforward, but the examiner must be careful when assessing exercise tolerance to delineate the child's entire activity pattern, especially in relation to peers. In this manner, overemphasis of symptoms that actually result from a preference for a sedentary life-style or the mother's overconcern may be avoided. Complaints of chest pain are common during adolescence but are rarely related to cardiovascular disease. The nature and location of the pain, as well as its radiation and precipitating factors, should be interpreted in the same manner as one would approach angina in the adult. Brief, stabbing, localized pain that may be anywhere over the precordium and not related to exercise is typical of the benign idiopathic discomfort seen so often at this age, and the finding of a normal cardiovascular examination makes further investigation unnecessary. Syncope or presyncopal equivalents (lightheadedness, vertigo, blurred vision) may be present as symptoms of arrhythmia and, less commonly, of severe semilunar valvular stenosis.

Physical examination. In every patient in the pediatric age group the possibility of primary heart disease should be considered in the presence of any of the following: (1) cyanosis, (2) murmur, (3) cardiomegaly, (4) arrhythmias, (5) abnormal situs, (6) growth failure, and (7) congestive heart failure.

Cyanosis. The clinical detection of cyanosis, one of the more obvious manifestations of congenital heart disease, is influenced by skin coloring, hemoglobin level, lighting conditions, and experience of the observer. Unless severe, cyanosis is seldom noted by the parents. Although in older infants and children persistent cyanosis usually is related to congenital heart disease with right-to-left shunt, in the neonate extracardiac causes are more often responsible. Acrocyanosis is common at this age and is of peripheral origin because of vasomotor instability, capillary stasis, and the high hematocrit normally present. It is recognized by the characteristic mottling of the skin, particularly of the distal extremities, with normally pink oral mucosa, and is precipitated most often by a cool environment. Although transient, it may recur during the first few weeks of life.

Other extracardiac causes for cyanosis in the neonate include diseases of the respiratory system (respiratory distress syndrome, airway obstruction, persistent atelectasis), central nervous system (with secondary hypoventilation), and hematologic system (hyperviscosity syndrome, methemoglobinemia). Hypoglycemia from any cause also may be associated with significant cyanosis. In most of these instances increased inspired oxygen concentration will significantly improve arterial oxygen saturation.

True central cynosis implies the presence of at least 5 g/dl reduced hemoglobin circulating in the systemic arterial circuit. In this instance, cyanosis is apparent both peripherally (nail beds, skin) and in the oral mucosa and often is not significantly improved by oxygen administration. A *precyanotic state* often may be recognized in patients with central right-to-left shunts. This is characterized by an outstanding reddish appearance of highly vascular areas such as the terminal digits, earlobes, and mucous membranes and is related to the polycythemia of mild arterial unsaturation. It may be mistaken for a healthy, ruddy appearance.

It should be noted that cyanosis is difficult to evaluate by clinical appearance alone. The patient with a PaO_2 of 35 torr may appear no more cyanotic than the patient with a PaO_2 of 60 torr, although the former instance is obviously a more critical situation. The oxyhemoglobin dissociation curve is shifted to the left in newborn infants because of the presence of fetal hemoglobin, resulting in a greater percent of saturation at a given PaO_2 and therefore less cyanosis.

Low levels of circulating hemoglobin tend to obscure the clinical detection of cyanosis because a greater degree of unsaturation is required to produce 5 g/dl reduced hemoglobin. This fact may be responsible for delayed recognition of cyanosis in some instances. The importance of obtaining arterial blood gases in any patient, particularly infants, suspected clinically of having cyanosis cannot be emphasized too strongly. Visual estimation of the degree of hypoxemia is unreliable and may be seriously detrimental to the patient's care.

Measurement of the partial pressure of arterial oxygen is most urgent in newborn infants in whom the circulatory status is notoriously unstable. Many infants with cyanosis in the immediate newborn period have critical obstruction to pulmonary blood flow and depend on persistent patency of the ductus arteriosus in order to oxygenate. Spontaneous closure of the ductus arteriosus is the rule rather than the exception in such situations, and the infant may progress from mild to severe hypoxemia within a short period of time with resultant respiratory distress, metabolic acidosis, and eventually death. Although cyanosis at any age is of concern and warrants thorough investigation, the slightest hint of cyanosis in the newborn mandates immediate measurement of arterial gases and, if hypoxemia is present, prompt and thorough diagnostic evaluation.

Murmur. A murmur representing audible turbulence in blood flow may be the first indication of a cardiac defect. When a murmur is detected the examiner should describe the murmur in terms of all of the following parameters:

1. Intensity
2. Maximal location
3. Radiation
4. Timing
5. Duration
6. Contour
7. Quality
8. Pitch
9. Changes with physiologic or pharmacologic maneuvers

Intensity of a murmur is graded on a scale from I to VI, with a grade I murmur being the faintest and audible usually only after careful auscultation under optimal listening conditions. A grade II murmur is also faint but is easily audible even by relatively inexperienced examiners and does not tend to radiate widely. A grade III murmur is moderately loud and should be easily heard even under suboptimal conditions. It frequently radiates widely but is not accompanied by a thrill. When the murmur is palpable (i.e., a thrill is present) the murmur is of grade IV intensity or greater. If the murmur can be heard only when the stethoscope chest piece is in complete contact with the chest, it is classified as grade IV. A grade V murmur can be heard with the chest piece incompletely contacting the skin and a grade VI murmur with the chest piece 1 cm removed from the skin.

It is generally easy to determine the area in which the murmur is heard maximally. Radiation of the murmur away from that point may occur in one of two ways. Most important from a diagnostic standpoint is the radiation following the lines of turbulent blood flow, such as the radiation of the murmur of aortic stenosis from the upper right sternal border preferentially to the carotid arteries. This type of radiation is generally unidirectional, in that it clearly is best heard along one pathway, and is of importance because it carries with it diagnostic significance as to the cause of the murmur. Omnidirectional radiation spreading out virtually equally in a circumferential manner around the primary location is generally simply related to the intensity of the murmur. Obviously, both forms of radiation are almost always present, but with careful attention to detail the examiner can learn to differentiate.

Although it is usually easy to tell whether a murmur is systolic, diastolic, or both, sometimes the inexperienced examiner may become confused and accordingly it is best to get in the habit of timing audible cardiac events with a peripheral pulse. Having established the primary phase of the cardiac cycle occupied by the murmur the examiner should then define the duration, i.e., the portion of either systole or diastole occupied by the murmur and its position within that phase of the cycle. Thus one attempts to roughly quantitate the length of systole or diastole occupied by the murmur and to describe whether it is an early, mid-, or late-cycle murmur. Although there are technically slight differences between the terms *holosystolic* and *pansystolic*, in common usage they are interchangeable. Specifically they refer to a murmur that occupies all of systole extending from S_1 up to at least the aortic component of S_2 with no periods of silence at either end. This has nothing to do with other parameters such as the contour of the murmur and should not be confused. The term *contour* refers to changes in the amplitude of the murmur over its total length. A plateau-type murmur is one in which the intensity remains constant throughout, whereas the diamond-shaped murmur increases in intensity to a peak and then decreases until it is inaudible. The crescendo and descrescendo phases need not be of equal duration. Pitch is largely self-explanatory. Most pediatric murmurs consist of a mixture of midrange and low frequencies, although occasionally murmurs at the extremes of the audible range may be present. The quality of the murmur refers largely to the presence or absence of vibrations. When many vibrations are present the murmur assumes a rough or harsh quality; when absent, the murmur is usually described as "blowing." Finally, it is useful to assess the behavior of the murmur with certain physiologic or pharmacologic alterations. Some murmurs may be heard only when a certain body position is assumed, and such changes with position should be carefully described. Alterations of the murmur with the Valsalva maneuver are also extremely beneficial. A fairly good Valsalva maneuver will usually be performed by the child in the 4- to 8-year-old range if he is asked to hold his feet the distance of about 8 to 10 inches off the table while the examiner listens to his heart. He will usually take a deep breath and bear down in an effort to maintain this position. In a somewhat older child an even better effort is achieved if the examiner places his hand on the child's abdomen and presses in gently, instructing the child to take a deep breath, hold it, and push his abdomen back hard against the examiner's hand. Although frequent use is made of pharmacologic manipulation such as an inhalation of amyl nitrite, we have found this to be of much less help in pediatrics in differentiating the etiology of murmurs. In addition, children often find this offensive.

Although the detection of a heart murmur may signify the presence of a cardiac lesion, innocent or functional, murmurs are exceedingly common throughout infancy and childhood. Differentiation of innocent from organic murmurs is important, even though the latter may be of minor hemodynamic importance, because an organic lesion requires antibiotic prophylaxis at times of potential bacteremia to prevent bacterial endocarditis. Common innocent murmurs heard in children are the venous hum, systolic ejection murmurs, vibratory murmur of Still, carotid bruit, and cardiorespiratory murmur. All have in common the lack of associated evidence of significant heart disease by symptomatology, physical examination, electrocardiogram, or chest x-ray film.

The *venous hum* is outstanding for its continuous quality and its great variability. This murmur has its origin in turbulent flow in the neck veins. Most commonly it is heard best in the neck or high along the sternal margin beneath the sternoclavicular junction. It may be bilateral and occasionally is present only on the left side, where it may be confused with the murmur of patent ductus arteriosus. In contrast to the ductus murmur, however, the intensity and duration of the venous hum may be altered considerably by simple maneuvers. In the supine position the venous hum may be absent, faint, or exhibit only a late systolic component. The hum may only appear or its intensity and duration may be enhanced in the upright position. Commonly, a late systolic crescendo is noted, with maximum intensity occurring in early diastole. Slight accentuation with inspiration is often noted. Hyperextension of the neck may produce or intensify this murmur, whereas flexion may cause disappearance or diminution. Rotation of the head toward the opposite side enhances the noise, whereas firm pressure over the neck veins may obliterate it. Conditions that increase the rate of blood flow (anemia, fever, excitement) will promote prominence of this murmur, which is one of the most frequent innocent murmurs of childhood.

The *systolic ejection murmur* is related to the rapid phase of systolic ejection across the pulmonary or aortic outflow tract. This murmur has a short, soft, blowing quality, with a distinct crescendo-decrescendo pattern terminating within the first two thirds of systole. Intracardiac phonocardiography has demonstrated this murmur both in the main pulmonary artery or its proximal branches and in the aortic root in children and adults alike. The thin chest wall and more rapid circulation of the child probably account for its more frequent detection in this age group. The intensity of this murmur is usually grade 2, but it may achieve grade 3 in children with thin chest walls or high output states. It may be detected first during a febrile state. The purely auscultatory characteristics of this murmur may be difficult to distinguish from those of the murmurs of secundum atrial septal defect and mild pulmonary valvular stenosis. Attention to other auscultatory features, however, and absence of other abnormal findings usually establish the benign character of this murmur. Important among these are physiologic splitting of the second sound, normal intensity of the pulmonary component, and absence of ejection click, thrill, or abnormal right ventricular impulse.

A closely related murmur, especially in the newborn, is an early systolic ejection murmur, usually of grade 2 intensity, heard best at both upper sternal borders but radiating to the entire anterior, posterior, and lateral thorax. We prefer to call this murmur the "physiologic pulmonary flow murmur of the newborn" and have detected it more commonly in premature infants, although not only in this group. It may be impossible to differentiate from the murmur of peripheral pulmonary stenosis except by virtue of its eventual disappearance over the first few months of life. The reason for this similarity is evident in the presumed origin of the innocent flow murmur. The branch pulmonary arteries are small in the fetus because of the low pulmonary blood flow. This *physiologic hypoplasia* may result in turbulence, and in fact, small gradients have been demonstrated at the junction of these vessels and the main pulmonary artery. Increased pulmonary flow in the postnatal state results in gradual enlargement of pulmonary arteries and decrease in the murmur.

The innocent *vibratory murmur* (Still murmur) is identified by its characteristic tonal quality. This murmur is predominantly a single-frequency vibration lacking the harmonic overtones of most murmurs. Maximum intensity is at the midsternal and lower left sternal border or medial to the apex, and it is best heard with the bell of the stethoscope. The Still murmur is often well heard over the entire precordium but does not usually radiate significantly beyond the heart borders. Phonocardiographically this murmur has a crescendo-decrescendo configuration ending at two thirds of systole. It has often been described as a "twanging string," "moaning," or "groaning" sound. Intracardiac phonocardiography has suggested the origin of this murmur to be in the left ventricular outflow tract. It is most commonly heard in the early school-age child and seems to disappear uniformly after puberty.

The *supraclavicular carotid arterial bruit* is a common murmur heard in children and young adults. This murmur characteristically is of short duration, clearly separated from both first and second heart sounds, and occupying less than one half of total systole. A distinct crescendo-decrescendo pattern can be noted. Maximum intensity is greatest over the neck, and it is more often present on the right side. The more intense bruits may radiate to the upper sternal margins, suggesting aortic or pulmonary stenosis. However, the shorter duration, delayed onset, maximum intensity in the neck, and effect of arterial compression should make the distinction clear. Hyperextension of arms with elbows flexed at a 90-degree angle frequently results in diminution or total disappearance. The mechanism of production of this murmur is not certain, but evidence suggests that it is related to turbulence at the origin of the brachiocephalic vessels.

The *cardiorespiratory murmur* is perhaps the least common of the group of innocent murmurs. It is usually heard best near the apex of the heart or along the left cardiac border. What appears to be a blowing, mid- to late systolic murmur is heard with marked respiratory variation. With careful attention to detail the examiner will recognize that the murmur is heard only during inspiration, disappearing completely during expiration or with held respiration. In fact, this is not a murmur at all but appears to be a breath sound occurring in a segment of lung positioned anterior to the cardiac apex so that the lung is compressed partially during systole, altering the breath sound characteristics.

Cardiomegaly. Cardiomegaly may be indicated during physical examination by observation and palpation of abnormal precordial activity. A prominent lower left parasternal and xiphoid systolic impulse outside the early infancy period is evidence of right ventricular enlargement. At any age a laterally and downward-displaced apex impulse is evidence of left ventricular enlargement. Cardiomegaly suspected by physical examination clearly indicates the need for a chest radiograph in posteroanterior and lateral views. This permits confirmation of heart size and allows evaluation for specific chamber enlargement, pulmonary vascularity, and state of the pulmonary parenchyma. Cardiomegaly usually indicates a state of altered cardiac function, although not necessarily of primary cardiac etiology (e.g., anemia, hypertension). When present, however, cardiomegaly should suggest underlying heart disease until proved otherwise.

Arrhythmias. Rhythm disturbances are common in pediatrics, and at times may present serious problems because of significant interference with normal cardiac function. Arrhythmias may occur as disorders in an apparently structurally normal heart or may occur in association with certain congenital cardiac defects. Although the presence of rhythm abnormalities should raise the possibility of an underlying cardiac defect, it should be noted that normal newborn infants, especially the premature ones, may exhibit transient supraventricular rhythm disturbances (ectopic atrial or junctional activity) of no clinical significance, and premature beats may be seen at any age, usually unassociated with cardiac disease. Specific arrhythmias are discussed later. (See pp. 468 to 474.)

Abnormal situs. Terminology regarding the cardiac malpositions is confusing and lacking in general agreement. The simplest concept is to consider dextrocardia to be any heart positioned predominantly in the right hemithorax, regardless of other features present. Levocardia indicates a heart in the left chest, which is of course the normal position, but the term is usually reserved for a left-sided heart associated with abdominal situs inversus. Abnormal cardiac situs may be associated with cardiovascular anomalies. Persons having situs inversus of both abdominal and thoracic viscera (*mirror image* dextrocardia) uncommonly have an intrinsic cardiac defect. Dextrocardia associated with abdominal situs solitus or levocardia with abdominal situs inversus frequently is associated with complex cardiovascular malformations.

CONGESTIVE HEART FAILURE

Congestive heart failure occurs when the cardiac output is inadequate to meet the metabolic needs of the body and results in accumulation of excessive blood volume in the pulmonary or systemic venous systems. Approximately 90% of all cases of congestive heart failure in children occur in the first year of life, primarily because of congenital heart disease. Heart failure occurs in 20% of all cases of congenital cardiovascular defects. Much of the mortality in the young infant with heart disease is caused by lack of early recognition of signs and symptoms of heart failure peculiar to the infant age group. Heart failure in the infant most often begins as left ventricular failure with subtle manifestations. Right heart failure is usually a later development, although certain forms of congenital heart disease may result in pure right heart failure. Notable among these are critical pulmonary valve stenosis with intact ventricular septum, congenital tricuspid insufficiency, Ebstein's malformation of the tricuspid valve, and congenital absence of the pulmonary valve.

Heart failure may be related to (1) primary depression of the contractile (inotropic) state of the myocardium, as seen in primary endomyocardial diseases, myocarditis, severe hypoxemia, or certain metabolic and endocrinologic disturbances; (2) volume overloading of one or both ventricles, as in left-to-right shunts; or (3) pressure overloading, as occurs in severe obstructive lesions or hypertension. It must be borne in mind, however, that the signs and symptoms of congestive heart failure may be produced by factors not affecting myocardial performance. Thus findings of left heart failure may be caused by a straightforward mechanical obstruction such as mitral stenosis, and right heart failure may be produced by factors that restrict cardiac filling, such as tricuspid stenosis, pericardial tamponade, or constrictive pericarditis. In addition, significant abnormalities of rhythm may result in some of the manifestations of heart failure listed below, but have nothing to do with changes in the inotropic state. High output states such as severe anemia or thyrotoxicosis, although actually producing cardiac hyperfunction, may result in manifestations of failure because of inability to meet tissue metabolic demands. Careful analysis of the nature of the pathophysiologic alteration is crucial, as treatment may vary significantly depending on location of the problem.

Clinical manifestations of congestive failure

in the infant may be peculiarly nonspecific for the cardiovascular system and often suggest disease in other organ systems—respiratory system, central nervous system, or gastrointestinal system.

In the absence of pulmonary infection or metabolic acidosis, a persistent resting respiratory rate exceeding 60 respirations/min should signal the possibility of heart disease because tachypnea is perhaps the most common manifestation of left ventricular failure at this age. Initially only the rate is increased, respirations appearing rapid and shallow, but dyspnea may soon become apparent. Wheezing is a common finding, and there may be an expiratory grunt. A nonproductive irritative cough may be present. Because these symptoms suggest pulmonary disease, a diagnosis of recurrent respiratory tract infection is common. In contrast to the older patient, the infant with pulmonary edema usually does not manifest audible pulmonary rales except late in the development of left heart failure. The absence of rales therefore should not preclude congestive heart failure from consideration. Tachycardia at rest is also a common finding. Resting pulse rates exceeding 160 beats/min are often present in infants with left ventricular failure, and rates of 200 beats/min or slightly above are occasionally seen.

Failure to thrive is often noted in infants with left ventricular failure of significant duration. The increased work of breathing increases energy expenditure and caloric requirements, whereas the effort of feeding induces fatigue and dyspnea, thereby limiting the infant's caloric intake. Weight gain may plateau, or weight loss may even occur. Irritability at feeding time may result from the infant's frustrating inability to satisfy hunger. Tachypnea and dyspnea during feeding may result in excessive air swallowing. These symptoms may suggest colic or formula intolerance; a history of frequent formula changes is common.

Hepatomegaly, a feature of right heart failure, is absent in the infant with early left ventricular failure—a fact sometimes not appreciated. Apparent hepatomegaly may occur, however, because of hyperinflation of the lungs with depression of the diaphragm. Pallor and excessive sweating are often prominent features related to the increased labor of breathing and increased catecholamine secretion, a compensatory mechanism to maintain cardiac output. The very young infant in failure may exhibit decreased motor activity, and periods of apnea may be noted. Older infants are likely to be extremely irritable when disturbed. These symptoms, plus apparent slow neuromotor development, may arouse suspicion of central nervous system disease.

Depending on the underlying cause of failure, a heart murmur may or may not be present. Nonspecific systolic murmurs of functional quality may be associated with cardiac dilation alone. Murmurs related to specific defects may assume a highly uncharacteristic quality or even disappear in the presence of severe failure. A protodiastolic (summation) gallop sound is commonly present. In left heart failure the pulmonary component of the second sound may exhibit increased intensity. The peripheral pulse is often rapid and weak, and in severe left ventricular failure, pulsus alternans is sometimes present.

Isolated right heart failure results in peripheral signs of elevation of systemic venous pressure and fluid retention. Respiratory symptomatology is often minimal. Neck vein distention, a common feature in older children and adults, is difficult to evaluate in infants. Hepatomegaly with hepatojugular reflux and tenderness indicate liver engorgement. Obvious peripheral edema is uncommon in the infant, except in the periorbital region, but may be apparent in the child.

Older children exhibit signs and symptoms of congestive heart failure similar to those seen in adults. Fatigue, exertional dyspnea, and malaise are noted initially. Hacking cough, orthopnea, and nocturia develop as failure progresses, and anorexia, abdominal distention, and swelling of feet and ankles may appear.

Biochemical changes accompanying heart failure in infants and children are similar to those occurring in adults, that is, dilutional hyponatremia, hypochloremia, hyperkalemia, increased blood volume, and prerenal azotemia. In addition, biochemical manifestations of respiratory insufficiency commonly occur in the infant with left ventricular failure. Respiratory insufficiency at this age is related to several factors, including reduced lung compliance, edema of the smaller air passages and capillary bed, reduced lung volume caused by cardiac enlargement and atelectasis, and often superimposed pulmonary infection. Impaired ventilatory efficiency is indicated by hypoxemia and respiratory acidosis, which frequently is compounded by the metabolic acidosis associated with hypoxemia and poor tissue perfusion.

Treatment of congestive heart failure is aimed at improving cardiac output, chiefly by pharmacologic means with certain adjunctive supportive measures. Digitalis continues to be the mainstay of therapy. The pharmacologic effects of digitalis are well known. Numerous preparations of this drug are available, but digoxin is the preparation of choice for use in pediatrics because of its rapid onset of action, relatively short duration (an important consideration in the event of toxicity), and convenient dosage forms available. Two facts to be emphasized are (1) that digitalization should be tailored to the needs of the individual patient and (2) that often in the critically ill infant with congenital heart disease, digitalization and other aspects of medical management, although extremely important, must be considered only temporizing measures in anticipation of prompt surgical intervention.

Digitalization usually is accomplished by administration of a calculated total digitalizing dose over a relatively short period of time. This loading dose, based on body weight, is designed to achieve promptly a therapeutic blood level in the average patient. The route and rapidity of administration of this dose must be tempered by the urgency of the situation and the patient's response. The physician should always keep in mind that the aim of digitalization is to give enough to achieve a satisfactory clinical response while avoiding toxicity. Dosage guidelines for routine digitalization by the oral route are shown in Table 18-1. Full-term neonates and premature infants in particular require less medication because of reduced renal excretion at this age. If parenteral administration is anticipated, the oral dosage should be reduced by approximately one third to compensate for the more complete absorption by this route. Dosage reduction is also indicated in acute myocarditis (because of possible increased myocardial sensitivity to the glycoside), as well as in the presence of significant renal disease.

In most instances, digitalization over a 24-hour period is satisfactory and safe. The calculated total digitalizing dose based on weight and age group may be administered as follows: Half the total dose is given initially, followed by one-fourth the total dose in 9 to 12 hours. The remaining fourth is given in another 8- to 12-hours. This dosage schedule may be followed for all routes of administration. An electrocardiographic recording of the cardiac rate and rhythm should be obtained before completion of digitalization, and careful attention should be paid to the P-R interval and presence of arrhythmias. Significant P-R prolongation may indicate early toxicity. In general, the oral route is perferred. In severe failure in which gastrointestinal absorption may be erratic, the intravenous route obviously is advantageous. The intramuscular route has the disadvantage of pain and irritation to tissues and of an unpredictable rate of absorption in the patient with poor tissue perfusion. This route is generally to be avoided.

Table 18-1. Routine digitalization for congestive heart failure

Drug and route of administration	Dosage mg/kg
Digoxin (Lanoxin)	
Oral loading dose (see text)	
Newborn	0.03-0.05
Infant (2 wk-2 yr)	0.05-0.08
Child (>2 year)	0.04-0.06
Intravenous loading dose	⅔-¾ of above doses
Maintenance	¼ of loading dose daily

A maintenance dose is necessary to replenish daily losses of the drug, primarily through renal excretion. This is usually 20% to 30% of the total digitalizing dose. An initial daily maintenance dose of one fourth of the total digitalizing dose, given in two divided doses, is usually satisfactory. Maintenance requirements may need to be adjusted according to clinical response and subsequently in keeping with the patient's weight gain.

If the patient demonstrates a satisfactory clinical response to digitalization with no signs of toxicity, measurement of the serum digoxin level may not be necessary. However, the level should be determined if the infant shows any possible signs of toxicity or if response is not as good as desired. The blood sample should be drawn no less than 6 hours after the preceding dose and may be obtained as late as immediately

Table 18-2. Commonly used diuretic agents

Drug	Route of administration	Dosage
Furosemide	Intravenous	1 mg/kg/dose
	Oral	1-3 mg/kg/24 hr
Chlorothiazide	Oral	20-40 mg/kg/24 hr in 2 doses
Hydrochloro-thiazide	Oral	2-4 mg/kg/24 hr in 2 doses
Spironolactone	Oral	1-2 mg/kg/24 hr in 2-3 doses

before the next dose (trough level).

Diuretics are a valuable adjunct in the treatment of congestive heart failure for the relief of symptoms of fluid retention, such as pulmonary or peripheral edema. The more potent and rapidly acting diuretics such as furosemide have currently almost entirely supplanted the mercurial diuretics in the acute phase of management. Table 18-2 outlines dosages of commonly used diuretic agents. The chlorothiazide preparations are useful for long-term intermittent therapy, and spironolactone is especially beneficial in the presence of right heart failure with secondary hyperaldosteronism. Excessive use of diuretics may lead to volume depletion and serious electrolyte imbalance. Therefore intermittent therapy is preferred if possible. Electrolyte imbalance may be especially serious in the digitalized patient in whom potassium depletion may result in signs of digitalis toxicity. The risk of this complication can be minimized by careful monitoring of serum electrolytes and administration of supplemental potassium (1 to 1.5 mEq/kg/24 hr) when indicated. Potassium administration, however, is not needed or recommended when spironolactone is used because this drug causes potassium retention.

If maximum obtainable improvement in myocardial contractility and fluid retention has been achieved through the use of digoxin and diuretics, and yet the overall clinical response remains unsatisfactory, one may consider attempting to reduce impedance to left ventricular emptying in an effort to improve cardiac output. A number of systemic arterial vasodilators have been employed in an effort to make it easier for the diseased myocardium to function. Experience with this approach in children is modest to date, but there is clear evidence that at least temporary improvement may be achieved in many instances. There is no clear choice among the fairly large number of agents in this group. Sodium nitroprusside probably represents a prototype that is both an arterial and a venodilator. The latter property increases systemic venous capacitance and may ameliorate some of the effects of systemic venous congestion and pulmonary edema. Chronic oral therapy in children has been most often instituted using either prazosin, which like nitroprusside is a mixed arterial and venodilator, or hydralazine, which is a pure arterial dilator. Some workers have preferred the combination of hydralazine and nitroglycerine, the latter being used for its venodilating properties. A word of caution is in order when this therapeutic approach is being considered. The indication for *after-load reduction,* as this approach is termed, is severe myocardial failure (primarily left ventricular) unresponsive to more conventional treatment. Primary benefit has been in the group of primary endomyocardial diseases (q.v.). For the most part, congenital structural abnormalities with recalcitrant failure are better treated surgically rather than by attempting after-load reduction.

PATHOPHYSIOLOGY

Understanding the hemodynamic alterations produced by congenital heart defects is greatly simplified by the recognition of broad areas of similarity that relate anatomically dissimilar lesions. The nature and magnitude of these alterations are determined almost entirely by two factors: the resistance opposing blood flow through a portion of the circulation and the presence of abnormal pathways of flow. The volume of blood flowing through any pathway within the circulatory system is defined by the following relation: Flow = Pressure/Resistance.

In the process of adaptation to extrauterine existence the newborn infant changes his circulation from one in which the two major vascular beds (pulmonic and systemic) are in parallel to one in which they are in series. This transition is brought about by the elimination of certain pathways of flow (foramen ovale, ductus arteriosus, ductus venosus, placenta), together with changes in the resistance to flow in the two vascular beds. Pulmonary vascular resistance (PVR), which is higher than systemic vascular resistance (SVR) in the fetus, decreases rapidly (first because of reduction in vasomotor tone after the initiation of respiration and then more gradually as a result of reduction of medial muscle in the small muscular pulmonary arteries), whereas systemic vascular resistance increases because of elimination of the low resistance placenta. Thus the relationship is established wherein the right ventricle is able to perfuse the pulmonary vascular bed at a much lower pressure against a lower resistance than is true of the systemic circulation.

Left-to-right shunts. If there is an anatomic communication between the two major circulations (e.g., ventricular septal defect or patent ductus arteriosus), the direction of blood flow through that communication is determined by the pressure relationship between the connecting cardiac chambers or vessels and the resistance to flow in the two vascular beds. To illustrate this more clearly, the ventricular septal defect (VSD) will be examined in some detail.

Because the right ventricular pressure and the resistance opposing its emptying (PVR) are lower than on the left side, the usual direction of blood flow through a VSD is from left ventricle to right ventricle and thence into the pulmonary circulation. This is referred to as a left-to-right shunt. Left ventricular pressure is the propelling force for the shunt; this pressure remains in the normal range. Thus larger shunts are not the result of higher left ventricular pressure in the isolated VSD of a given size. Rather, the volume of the shunt is determined by the resistance opposing the flow. In the case of the VSD, resistance may occur at two points: the defect itself and the pulmonary vascular bed.

If the VSD is small, the resistance that it exerts in opposition to blood flow is high and the left-to-right shunt is small. A large amount of energy is expended in overcoming this resistance, and this is reflected by a large drop in pressure across the defect. Thus left ventricular pressure is not transmitted into the right heart, and pressure in the pulmonary circulation remains normal. The pressure gradient across the VSD exists from the time of atrioventricular valve closure until the closure of the semilunar valves; thus the murmur resulting from flow across the defect is holosystolic and generally loud because of the turbulence caused by high-velocity flow between chambers of widely disparate pressure.

As the size of the VSD increases, the resistance it produces decreases until the defect area exceeds 1 cm^2/m^2 body surface area, at which point its resistance becomes negligible, and for all practical purposes the only opposition to blood flow is caused by the PVR. If this is low in relation to SVR, a large shunt results. The left ventricle must maintain normal blood flow to the body, whereas a large portion of its output is lost by way of the shunt. The left ventricular output is the sum of these two flows; thus there is a large volume overload on that chamber. If the shunt is so large that systemic output cannot be maintained, congestive heart failure results.

Because there is little resistance to flow across the large VSD, left ventricular pressure is freely transmitted to the right ventricle and main pulmonary artery, and pulmonary hypertension is the result. This type of pulmonary hypertension occurring with a large left-to-right shunt is referred to as "hyperkinetic" or "dynamic" pulmonary hypertension. Because of the small pressure difference between the two ventricles, the murmur is generally less intense than that seen with small defects and may be less than holosystolic.

In some patients with a large VSD the PVR may be elevated to a variable degree, either because of failure of involution of the fetal pulmonary vessels or because of secondary increase in thickness of the vessel wall and decrease in the lumen size (pulmonary vascular obstructive disease). In this case the PVR limits the shunt volume. If PVR is sufficiently elevated (i.e., equal to or greater than SVR), there may be reversal of this shunt to a right-to-left direction (Eisenmenger physiology). As with any large VSD, right and left ventricular pressures are usually at the same level, and when the shunt is small, the dominant hemodynamic stress is the pressure overload of the right ventricle.

All lesions with a communication between ventricles or great arteries share hemodynamic behavior similar to that just outlined. Thus a left-to-right shunt through a patent ductus arteriosus is a function of the size of the ductus and the PVR. The only difference is the presence of a pressure gradient between the aorta and the main pulmonary artery throughout systole and diastole if the communication is not large; therefore the murmur is continuous rather than limited to systole.

Factors influencing shunting at the atrial level, that is, in atrial septal defects, are more complicated. Pressure gradients between the atria are small regardless of the size of the defect. The left-to-right shunt appears to occur during two phases of the cycle rather than being limited to systole, as with the VSD. During the latter part of atrial filling (ventricular systole), left atrial pressure rises faster than right atrial pressure and there is a shunt at that time. This is, of course, influenced by the resistance caused by the size of the defect. Because the right ventricle has a thinner wall than the left ventricle, it distends more rapidly and thus poses less resistance to the emptying of the atria. The major left-to-right shunt occurs during diastole and is governed by the relative ventricular compliances. As the atria contract to complete ventricular filling, left atrial pressure rises more than right atrial pressure, and the left-to-right shunt is accentuated. Pulmonary hypertension is, of course, not induced by transmission of left atrial pressure into the right atrium across the defect, as was true of the large VSD. Elevation of PVR caused by pulmonary vascular obstructive disease is rare in childhood. As long as the tricuspid valve is competent, elevated PVR would have no effect on atrial left-to-right shunts until thickening of the right ventricular wall develops sufficiently to interfere with filling of the ventricle.

Cyanotic lesions. Cyanotic congenital heart defects are characterized by an anatomic abnormality that produces obligatory shunting of unsaturated systemic venous blood back into the systemic circulation without passing through the lungs. From a pathophysiologic standpoint these defects can be grouped into the following categories:

1. Admixture lesions—those in which there is almost complete mixing of the systemic and pulmonary venous streams in either an atrium, ventricle, or great vessel because of anatomic pathways of flow that bring the two streams together (as opposed to mixing caused by altered function such as occurs in the ventricular septal defect with severely elevated pulmonary vascular resistance)
2. Pulmonary hypoperfusion lesions—those with reduced pulmonary blood flow
3. Transposition of the great arteries—those in which the systemic and pulmonary circulations are separated and do not connect either directly or through a capillary bed

This separation is useful in understanding the hemodynamic alterations, but it is somewhat arbitrary; overlap between groups frequently occurs.

Examples of group 1 would include (1) tricuspid atresia, total anaomalous pulmonary venous drainage, and hypoplastic left ventricle syndrome (atrial mixing); (2) single ventricle (ventricular mixing); and (3) truncus arteriosus (arterial mixing), as well as several other lesions. Except in total anomalous pulmonary venous drainage, the mixed venous streams enter either one ventricle or one great artery, and subsequent distribution to pulmonary and systemic arterial beds are determined by the resistance to flow into or through these two areas, as was the case of the large VSD discussed previously. Stenosis of the pulmonary outflow tract may exist with almost any of the lesions in this group, in which case pulmonary blood flow is reduced and the hemodynamic characteristics are those of group 2. In the absence of such stenosis, systolic pressure in the two circulations is the same. The typical early picture is one of relatively low PVR with high pulmonary blood flow and significant diastolic overload of one ventricle. Cardiomegaly and pulmonary vascular congestion are characteristic radiographic findings, and congestive heart failure is common. Cyanosis is usually mild, and systemic oxygen saturation may occasionally be as high as 90%, varying directly with the pulmonary blood flow. If the PVR is elevated, the increase in pulmonary flow is less, or pulmonary flow may even be less than systemic flow in extreme cases.

When severe obstruction to pulmonary flow coexists with a large (nonobstructive) VSD, as in tetralogy of Fallot (a group 2 lesion), right ventricular output will be divided between the pulmonary and systemic vascular beds. If the pulmonary stenosis is severe, a large portion of the right ventricular output will be directed to the aorta as a right-to-left shunt. Reduced pulmonary blood flow and significant arterial hypoxemia will result. Ventricular pressures are generally identical, and pulmonary artery pressure is low. The primary hemodynamic stress on the myocardium is the increased pressure work required of the right ventricle. Hypertrophy of the right ventricle occurs in the absence of severe dilation. Because the right ventricle is in free communication with the aorta, right ventricular pressure cannot exceed that necessary to perfuse the systemic vascular bed. This limits right ventricular pressure work, and congestive heart failure in the uncomplicated case is rare in childhood. A similar hemodynamic picture may be seen in other lesions such as truncus arteriosus with stenosis of the pulmonary arteries, single ventricle with pulmonary stenosis, and some forms of tricuspid atresia.

In complete transposition of the great arteries (group 3) the aorta arises from the right ventricle, and the main pulmonary artery arises from the left ventricle. Thus parallel circulations result, with systemic blood flow returning to the right atrium, right ventricle, and aorta without passing through the lungs. Likewise pulmonary blood flow is returned to the lungs without reaching the body. In the absence of associated defects there is severe systemic arterial hypoxemia, and pulmonary arterial blood is fully saturated. For survival of any duration there must be a communication between the two circulations so that mixing may occur (that is, pulmonary venous blood must reach the aorta and systemic venous blood must reach the pulmonary artery). This may occur by way of an ASD, VSD, or PDA. The best mixing and therefore the best arterial saturation occurs with a large VSD. If the PVR is low, pulmonary blood flow may be large with resultant congestive failure. The right ventricle is also working against SVR and thus must generate systemic pressure, which generally presents no problem in childhood. Pulmonary vascular obstructive disease occurs frequently in the first to second year of life and may progress rapidly to levels that preclude surgical correction.

Obstructive lesions. Semilunar valve stenosis produces resistance to ejection from the associated ventricle, which then must generate a higher systolic pressure if normal cardiac output is to be maintained. Energy is expended across the obstruction, and there is a systolic gradient from ventricle to great artery. This gradient is present during the ejection phase of systole, and the turbulent flow produced during that period is responsible for the typical ejection murmur. If critical pulmonic stenosis exists in utero, systemic venous return may be directed to a greater degree into the left heart by way of the foramen ovale, bypassing the right ventricle, with resultant hypoplasia of that chamber. Likewise, in severe aortic stenosis pulmonary venous return may shunt to the right heart, with underdevelopment of the left ventricle and perfusion of the entire systemic circulation by way of the patent ductus arteriosus. The course with ventricular hypoplasia is generally fulminant in the newborn period.

When the ventricular septum is intact, the ventricle proximal to the obstruction can increase its systolic work (i.e., pressure) several times and thus can maintain a normal output in the face of severe obstruction. This is in part brought about by the development of ventricular hypertrophy. In the case of pulmonary stenosis, this increase in pressure work is in contrast to tetralogy of Fallot, in which the presence of a VSD provides a path of less resistance to ventricular ejection and pulmonary blood flow is reduced. Infants are occasionally seen with normally developed ventricles in the face of critical aortic or pulmonic stenosis, but in whom the magnitude of the systolic work required cannot be maintained for a sufficient period of time after birth for hypertrophy to develop. Thus severe congestive heart failure may be seen in the first few months of life. Failure is uncommonly seen in the older child once hypertrophy is present.

The most common lesion associated with pulmonary venous obstruction is total anomalous pulmonary venous drainage, particularly of the infradiaphragmatic type. Mechanical obstruction to pulmonary venous return may vary from nonexistent to complete, and the degree to which the clinical presentation resembles one of the cyanotic admixture lesions, as discussed above, or pure pulmonary venous obstruction will vary accordingly.

CONGENITAL HEART DISEASE

Congenital cardiovascular anomalies are the major cause of heart disease in the pediatric age group. A large number of congenital defects, both simple and complex, have been reported; however, relatively few anomalies account for the majority of the problems encountered in the average pediatric practice. These more common defects are discussed below.

Atrial septal defects

Atrial septal defects (ASD), representing about 10% of all congenital heart defects, include secundum defect, ostium primum defect,

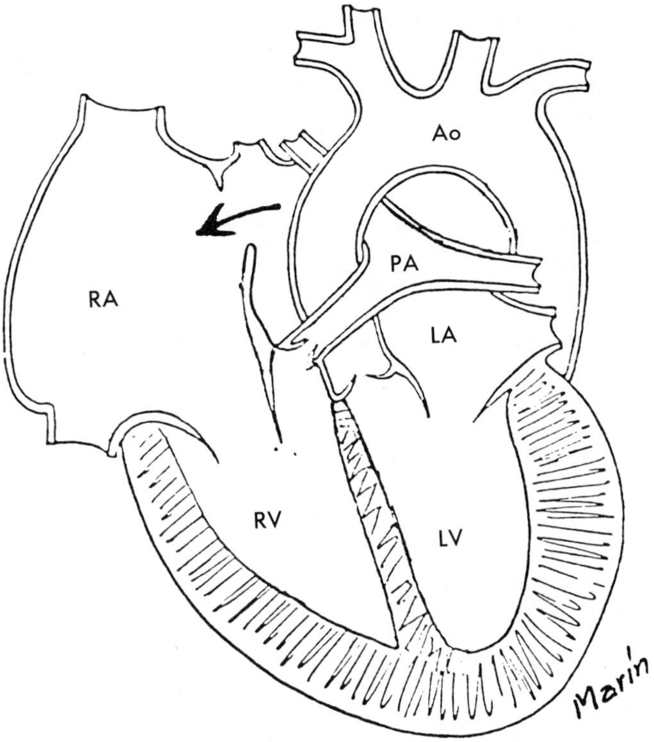

Fig. 18-1. Atrial septal defect, ostium secundum type. *RA,* Right atrium; *RV,* right ventricle; *LA,* left atrium; *LV,* left ventricle; *PA,* pulmonary artery; *Ao,* aorta.

patent foramen ovale, and sinus venosus defect. The secundum defects, resulting from inadequate embryonic development of the septum secundum, are the most commonly encountered and are found most often in the midatrial septum (Fig. 18-1). The defect is twice as common in females as in males, and familial instances have been observed. It may be present in association with upper extremity abnormalities in the Holt-Oram syndrome.

The ASD is usually of sufficient size to allow unrestricted flow between the atria. Its pathophysiology and hemodynamics have been previously discussed (p. 425). The left-to-right shunt results in volume overloading of the right ventricle and pulmonary vascular beds.

The child with an ASD is usually asymptomatic, although infants occasionally develop congestive heart failure and older children may complain of exertional fatigue and dyspnea. A history of recurrent respiratory tract infections is sometimes obtained. The usual presenting feature of ASD is the detection of a cardiac murmur. A right ventricular tap is noted in most patients; however, a systolic thrill occurs in less than 25% of cases. The second heart sound characteristically exhibits abnormally wide splitting without phasic variation (fixed splitting). This is perhaps the most typical auscultatory feature of ASD, although it may not be detected in the presence of a small shunt. The systolic murmur is an ejection type and is caused by increased blood flow across the pulmonary valve. It has no features to distinguish it from the functional pulmonary systolic ejection murmur. At times wide radiation over both sides of the chest may resemble a murmur of peripheral pulmonary stenosis. A diastolic rumble is also commonly noted at the lower left sternal border. This murmur, which occurs at the time of the third heart sound, is caused by increased blood volume flow across the tricuspid valve.

The electrocardiogram typically shows right ventricular hypertrophy, manifested by prominent terminal rightward forces producing a rsR′ complex in lead aVR and right precordial leads with broad deep S waves in lead I and left precordial leads. The chest radiograph may show cardiac enlargement, primarily right ventricular, with increased pulmonary vascularity. Two-dimensional echocardiography may confirm the diagnosis. Cardiac catheterization and angiography are useful techniques for the exclusion of associated anomalies.

Small shunts are tolerated well, and most patients remain asymptomatic. Congestive heart failure and pulmonary vascular obstruction are uncommon in childhood, and bacterial endocarditis is rare. Surgical correction under direct vision during cardiopulmonary bypass is indicated for all defects with significant left-to-right shunt. Operative mortality in uncomplicated cases is less than 1%.

Ventricular septal defect

Ventricular septal defect (VSD) is the most common congenital cardiac lesion, accounting for at least 20% of all cases of congenital heart disease. In addition, it is frequently associated with other defects as part of a complex of lesions. Although defects in the ventricular septum occur at various sites, approximately 70% are located in the membranous portion lying beneath the aortic valve in the left ventricular outflow tract and between the supraventricular crest and tricuspid valve on the right ventricular side (Fig. 18-2). The size of the defect may vary from pinpoint to virtual absence of the septum. Multiple openings of varied size are occasionally present.

The clinical signs of ventricular septal defect were first defined by Roger in 1879, and the term *maladie de Roger* is often used to indicate a small asymptomatic VSD. Eisenmenger in 1897 described the postmortem findings in a cyanotic patient with a large VSD, and the term *Eisenmenger complex* commonly indicates a VSD associated with pulmonary hypertension caused by greatly increased PVR and right-to-left shunt. The term *Eisenmenger syndrome* or *physiology* refers to any freely communicating defect between the pulmonary and systemic cir-

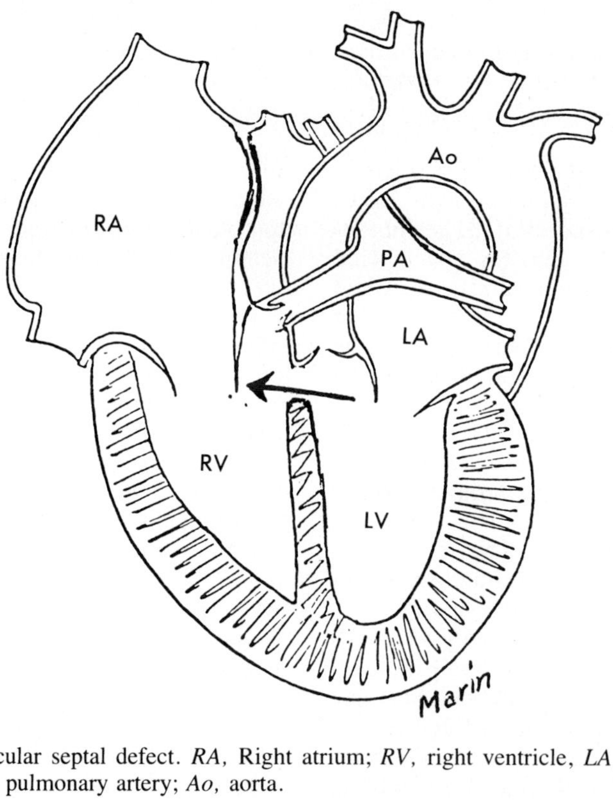

Fig. 18-2. Ventricular septal defect. *RA*, Right atrium; *RV*, right ventricle, *LA*, left atrium; *LV*, left ventricle; *PA*, pulmonary artery; *Ao*, aorta.

cuits with pulmonary vascular obstruction and predominant right-to-left shunt.

Physiologically the clinical manifestations of VSD are related to the size of the defect and the relationship between resistance in the pulmonary and systemic circuits. Defect size may measure from 1 to 25 mm or more. Detailed clinical, hemodynamic, and pathologic studies have clarified the relationship between defect size, PVR, and pathophysiologic changes. These have been previously discussed (p. 424). The response of the pulmonary vascular bed to a left-to-right shunt at any site varies, defect size and shunt volume interacting with certain as yet ill-defined individual peculiarities. The net result in some patients produces a large left-to-right shunt with evidence of volume overload and congestive heart failure. In others high PVR develops, leading to the Eisenmenger physiology.

VSD does not usually become clinically manifest early in the neonatal period because the normally high pulmonary vascular resistance at this age prevents significant shunting. A murmur is absent or atypical at this time.

In the infant with a small VSD the decline in PVR proceeds normally. A left-to-right shunt begins as normal adult pressure relationships are reached within the first week of life. The presence of the defect becomes clinically apparent during this time by the appearance of a systolic murmur along the middle and lower left sternal margin. This murmur is often not quite pansystolic. A faint systolic thrill may or may not be present. Signs of congestive heart failure are absent, and both electrocardiogram and radiograph may reveal no specific abnormality. This course is more likely to occur in the premature infant. Most infants, however, show somewhat slower than normal decline in PVR, with shunt volume peaking between the third and sixth week of life. Congestive heart failure is therefore most common at this time in infants with isolated VSD of significant size.

The symptomatic infant is irritable, nurses fretfully with obvious poor weight gain, and exhibits diaphoresis, tachypnea, and pallor. Pulmonary rales are infrequent, except in profound pulmonary edema. The heart is obviously enlarged, with a hyperactive precordium. A systolic thrill at the lower left sternal edge is present. Abnormal right and left ventricular impulses are usually found. Auscultation reveals a loud first sound and a variably split second sound with prominent pulmonary component. Most striking is a harsh, loud, pansystolic murmur maximal along the middle and lower left sternal margin, with radiation to the right. A middiastolic inflow rumble at the apex is often audible and generally implies a large shunt volume. If heart failure is well developed, an apical gallop is noted. The liver may be enlarged. Peripheral edema is seldom observed in the infant. However, when present it is usually manifested as periorbital and facial puffiness. Pulses are rapid and of small or normal volume. Cyanosis is absent, although infants with congestive heart failure may exhibit a dusky appearance.

The chest radiograph reveals hyperinflated lungs with depressed diaphragms. Pulmonary vascularity is increased. The pulmonary artery segment may appear full, and the aorta is small. Left atrial enlargement may be indicated by an upwardly displaced left main bronchus and occasionally by a double atrial density in the frontal view. The heart size is increased, often with evidence of enlargement of both ventricular chambers. The electrocardiogram may demonstrate a normal axis, with left ventricular and left atrial enlargement. Hyperkinetic pulmonary hypertension produces evidence of right ventricular hypertrophy as well.

The infant with a large defect and systemic pressure in the right ventricle who survives the first year of life may begin to improve clinically during the second year. Congestive heart failure may disappear, with accompanying improvement in growth pattern and exercise tolerance. Such a course may falsely suggest a decrease in the defect size with lessening shunt and improved hemodynamics when in reality it may be associated with the development of pulmonary vascular obstructive disease of an irreversible nature. Several changes may be observed during this period. Tachypnea, exertional fatigue, and dyspnea gradually disappear. A significant improvement in growth and weight gain may develop, and respiratory infections may diminish in severity and frequency. Cyanosis with exertion, and later at rest, is gradually observed. The precordium becomes less hyperactive, with increasing intensity of the right ventricular impulse and diminished left ventricular impulse. The thrill disappears, whereas the pulmonary closure impulse becomes increasingly prominent. Auscultation reveals decreased intensity and harshness of the systolic murmur, which becomes shorter, exhibits more ejection quality, and may even disappear. There is early disappearance of the diastolic apical filling murmur as shunt volume diminishes. The pulmonary component of the second sound becomes increasingly loud, a manifestation of the rising pulmonary vascular resistance.

Chest radiographs demonstrate a gradual decrease in heart size while right ventricular prominence develops. The pulmonary vascularity becomes diminished peripherally, but the hilar branches and main pulmonary artery segment may become prominent. Rapid tapering *(pruning)* of the hilar branches may be noted. Evidence of left atrial and left ventricular enlargement disappear. Electrocardiographically, progressive right axis deviation and right ventricular hypertrophy occur, with loss of evidence of left atrial and left ventricular enlargement.

Other patients may follow a similar clinical course, resulting from true physiologic improvement caused by actual or relative decrease in defect size or to acquisition of pulmonary infundibular stenosis. In the latter situation, right ventricular outflow obstruction represents a point of resistance imposed between the shunt site and the pulmonary vascular bed. This exerts a limiting influence on the magnitude and direction of shunt flow, a limitation that may become more significant with age. The deleterious effects of large shunt volume and transmission of systemic pressure into the pulmonary vessels may thereby be reduced. Eventually such patients may progress to balanced ventricular pressures and bidirectional or dominant right-to-left shunt with cyanosis (i.e., physiology similar to that of tetralogy of Fallot).

Spontaneous closure of the defect has been repeatedly documented both clinically (serial catheterizations) and at autopsy. Spontaneous closure is estimated to occur in 20% to 50% of children, even including infants with large defects who initially present with congestive heart failure. When closure takes place, it is more likely to occur early than late (approximately 60% by 3 years of age and 90% by 8 years), but closure in adulthood may occur. Closure is accomplished by muscular or fibrous encroachment or by adherence of the septal leaflet of the tricuspid valve. In addition, partial closure may take place in about one half of the large defects, resulting in improved prognosis.

The clinical findings in the patient with a small VSD are usually typical enough to permit a diagnosis without cardiac catheterization. The patient with clinical evidence of significant left-to-right shunt, pulmonary hypertension, or atypical features requires cardiac catheterization to establish the diagnosis, to assess the hemodynamic state, and to detect unsuspected associated defects. Catheterization is a prerequisite for surgical management.

Medical management of symptomatic infants primarily concerns maintenance of optimum general health, routine bacterial endocarditis prophylaxis (pp. 467-468), maximum control of congestive heart failure, and careful frequent clinical evaluation of the hemodynamic status.

Two surgical approaches are now available. Palliation may be achieved by producing artificial pulmonary stenosis (banding of the main pulmonary artery). The procedure, however, carries significant risk and has the disadvantage of necessitating two thoracotomies because subsequent repair of the defect and removal of the band must be anticipated. Therefore, current emphasis has been directed at primary repair, utilizing cardiopulmonary bypass even in infants under 6 months of age. Results have been encouraging and will certainly improve with future experience and improved techniques.

Endocardial cushion defects

Failure of fusion of the endocardial cushions yields a spectrum of cardiac malformations of the atrioventricular valves and the atrial and ventricular septa. In the complete form of endocardial cushion defect (common atrioventricular canal), large atrial and ventricular septal defects are incompletely separated by a single atrioventricular valve ring, with deformed leaflets forming a functionally incompetent, five-leaflet, common atrioventricular valve. In its partial form (ostium primum defect) there is a large interatrial communication with its inferior margin formed by the atrioventricular valve ring. There is almost invariably an associated deformity of the anterior mitral leaflet, which is cleft, thickened, and has abnormal chordae tendineae, resulting in varying degrees of mitral insufficiency. Transitional forms also occur. Pulmonary stenosis is the commonest associated cardiac lesion.

In the absence of mitral insufficiency, the partial form of endocardial cushion defect is indistinguishable from ostium secundum atrial septal defect by clinical and radiographic examination. The characteristic electrocardiogram (discussed in the next paragraph) is the principal clue to diagnosis. A complete endocardial cushion defect is seen in approximately one third of patients with Down syndrome. The presenting clinical picture is usually that of a large ventricular septal defect with hyperdynamic pulmonary hypertension. Again, the major clue to diagnosis lies in the electrocardiogram.

The electrocardiographic abnormalities are related on the one hand to an abnormal pattern of atrioventricular conduction referable to the malformation itself and on the other hand to the hemodynamic abnormalities resulting therefrom. Typically there is prolongation of the P-R interval, with left axis deviation greater than − 30 degrees, associated with right or combined ventricular hypertrophy. The right ventricular hypertrophy, as in secundum ASD, is usually manifested by prominent terminal rightward forces. The vectorcardiogram demonstrates a superiorly oriented, counterclockwise loop in the frontal plane. Specific P wave abnormalities are generally not identified. Rhythm disturbances are uncommon. The diagnosis can be established by two-dimensional echocardiography and confirmed by cardiac catheterization and cineangiocardiography. The latter shows a typical deformity of the left ventricular outflow tract related to the abnormal anatomy and motion of the cleft anterior mitral leaflet.

The hemodynamic abnormalities of endocardial cushion defects are those of the underlying lesions. Severe mitral regurgitation in the presence of an ostium primum ASD adds significantly to the left-to-right atrial shunt and therefore is associated with a slightly higher incidence of congestive heart failure and pulmonary vascular changes in children than is seen in the secundum form of ASD. In the absence of pulmonary stenosis, patients with complete endocardial cushion defects have pulmonary hypertension at or near systemic level. It is usually the hyperdynamic type but may rapidly progress to development of pulmonary vascular obstructive disease during early childhood.

Surgical treatment is available for all forms of endocardial cushion defect prior to the development of pulmonary vascular obstruction, although the surgical morbidity and mortality are somewhat higher than in the less complicated forms of ASD and VSD. Complete repair is accomplished by closure of the atrial or ventricular septal defects and simultaneous repair of the atrioventricular valve abnormalities with cardiopulmonary bypass. Mitral valve replacement is frequently indicated in patients with severe valve deformity. Because of the nature of the malformation and the course of the conduction system, extreme care is required to avoid complete heart block at the time of surgery. The long-term prognosis is favorable for those patients whose defects can be successfully treated. Repair of this and of all congenital cardiac defects in patients with Down syndrome and with all other forms of severe mental retardation should be undertaken only after the parents have been carefully counseled regarding the natural history of the disease and of the underlying mental retardation syndrome.

Patent ductus arteriosus

Patent ductus arteriosus (PDA) ranks as the second or third most common congenital cardiac malformation and is one of the most frequent cardiovascular defects associated with the congenital rebella syndrome. Except in the rubella syndrome, the lesion is two or three times more frequent in females. The defect results from persistence of the fetal channel connecting the pulmonary artery to the descending aorta, causing direct communication between the high pressure systemic circulation and the pulmonary circuit (Fig. 18-3). The incidence of persistent patency and of delayed closure is higher in the premature infant probably because of a poorly developed ductal muscular wall, decreased responsiveness to stimuli normally inducing constriction, or neonatal respiratory distress and hypoxemia. Recent clinical experience suggests a higher incidence of PDA in distressed neonates requiring ventilatory assistance.

Pathophysiologic changes associated with PDA are similar to those of ventricular septal defect and have been previously discussed (p. 424). A wide pulse pressure indicated by bounding pulses is related to increased left ven-

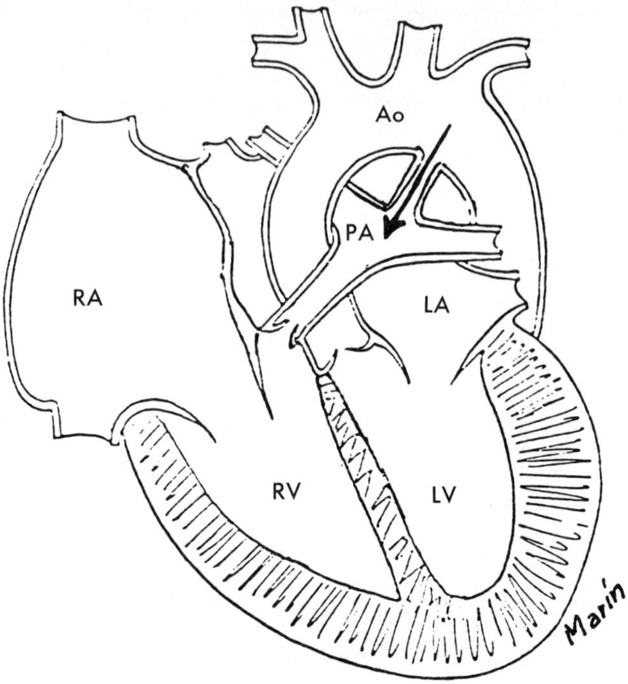

Fig. 18-3. Patent ductus arteriosus. *RA,* Right atrium; *RV,* right ventricle; *LA,* left atrium; *LV,* left ventricle; *PA,* pulmonary artery; *Ao,* aorta.

tricular stroke output and a low diastolic pressure caused by rapid runoff into the pulmonary artery and decreased systemic resistance.

The small PDA may be identified only by the presence of a faint late systolic crescendo murmur of high frequency, with or without a diastolic component. Significantly, the second heart sound is normal, and pulses are not bounding. The chest radiograph and electrocardiogram may reveal no abnormalities.

The symptomatic infant with a large left-to-right shunt may present with manifestations of left ventricular failure. Cyanosis is absent. The precordium is hyperdynamic with evidence of left ventricular enlargement. A systolic thrill may be palpable at the upper left sternal margin and in the suprasternal notch, where prominent arterial pulsations may be observed. Peripheral pulses are bounding even in the presence of congestive heart failure. The first sound is normal, whereas the second sound, occurring near the peak intensity of the murmur, may be narrowly split, paradoxically split (because of prolonged left ventricular ejection), or obscured. Auscultation is dominated by a continuous murmur of grade 3 or greater intensity at the upper left sternal border or atypically at the third to fourth interspace. In many instances an uneven rasping or clanging character gives the continuous murmur the so-called machinery quality. A low-frequency apical diastolic mitral inflow rumble often is heard. Electrocardiography demonstrates a normal QRS axis, left ventricular hypertrophy, and often left atrial enlargement. The chest radiograph reveals pulmonary hypervascularity, a full pulmonary artery segment, dilated ascending aorta and arch, and left ventricular and left atrial enlargement. The lungs may appear overexpanded with depressed diaphragms.

The other extreme of the clinical spectrum is represented by the patient with a large PDA, pulmonary hypertension caused by severe elevation of pulmonary vascular resistance, and a right-to-left shunt across the ductus, producing a variable degree of unsaturation in the distal aortic compartment. Pulmonary blood flow is decreased, and there is no longer volume overload of the left heart chambers. The right ventricle, however, hypertrophies because of increased pressure work. True shunt reversal usually occurs as a late complication of the large PDA.

Symptoms are minimal, consisting of mild exertional dyspnea and fatigue. Congestive right heart failure is a late development. Cyanosis, of variable and transient nature early, may be limited distinctly to the part of the body below the pelvic brim (differential cyanosis). The precordium is less hyperdynamic, but a prominent right ventricular impulse and palpable pulmonic closure may be present. Thrills are absent. Auscultation is dominated by the loud, resonant pulmonary component of the second sound, indicating severe pulmonary hypertension. Murmurs are absent, or a short midsystolic ejection murmur may be heard at the pulmonic area. Peripheral pulses are normal. Chest radiograph reveals normal or slightly increased cardiac size with a contour of right ventricular enlargement. Most striking are the dilated pulmonary artery segment, prominent hilar vessels, and absence of pulmonary plethora peripherally. The aorta appears normal or small. Right axis deviation and isolated right ventricular hypertrophy are present on the electrocardiogram.

Many infants exhibit an intermediate clinical spectrum related to coexistent hyperkinetic pulmonary hypertension and moderate elevation of pulmonary vascular resistance. Clinical features are primarily those of a significant left-to-right shunt. However, biventricular enlargement may be apparent, together with hepatomegaly. Pulses are bounding. Auscultatory features include an abbreviated continuous murmur and a significantly increased pulmonic component of the second sound. Biventricular hypertrophy is present on the electrocardiogram, and the chest radiograph reveals prominence of both ventricles, pulmonary artery, and aorta.

Diagnosis of the typical PDA can be made on the basis of clinical features alone. Cardiac catheterization to exclude possible associated defects is warranted in all young infants and in all patients with clinical evidence of pulmonary hypertension or atypical features. Surgical closure by ligation or division is the treatment of choice and can be accomplished with minimal risk even in ill neonates. Specific contraindications are the presence of severe obstructive pulmonary hypertension and complex malformations in which the ductus is an obligatory component. In premature or distressed neonates complete spontaneous closure of the ductus may be delayed up to 6 months of age, and in the absence of symptoms these infants can be safely observed for this period of time. However, in an ill premature neonate with hyaline membrane disease and PDA medical closure with indomethacin or surgical ligation is often necessary.

Aortic stenosis

Aortic stenosis (AS) may occur at any of three anatomic sites. The most frequent form is related to a stenotic congenital unicuspid or bicuspid valve. The obstruction to the left ventricular outflow may also occur in the subvalvular region in the form of either an isolated fibrous ring or muscular hypertrophy (Fig. 18-4, *A*). The third type of AS occurs in the ascending aorta and is termed supravalvular AS (Fig. 18-4, *B*). The latter type may be seen in children either with idiopathic hypercalcemia of infancy or with a familial history. Regardless of the site of obstruction, the hemodynamic consequences are similar because the left ventricular pressure must rise in order to maintain a normal cardiac output. As a result, left ventricular hypertrophy develops.

In 5% of cases of isolated AS, congestive cardiac failure develops in the first year of life. In this group severe aortic valve stenosis with hypoplastic aortic valve ring is usually present. The symptomatic infant is tachypneic and has the dusky pallor characteristic of the low output state. Blood pressure is low, and pulses are weak and rapid. When present, the murmur is the ejection type; it begins after a pause following the first heart sound and extends to the aortic valve closure. The location is atypical and is most prominent along the left sternal border. Commonly, no murmur is audible until myocardial contractility is improved by medical therapy. Provided the valve is mobile, an apical systolic ejection click may be present—a helpful auscultatory clue. The electrocardiogram usually demonstrates abnormal left ventricular forces but may suggest combined or right ventricular hypertrophy if pulmonary hypertension from elevated pulmonary venous pressure is present. Chest radiograph reveals left or combined ventricular enlargement, with signs of pulmonary venous congestion.

The symptomatic infant with congenital AS should be considered a medical emergency. Medical therapy alone frequently provides only

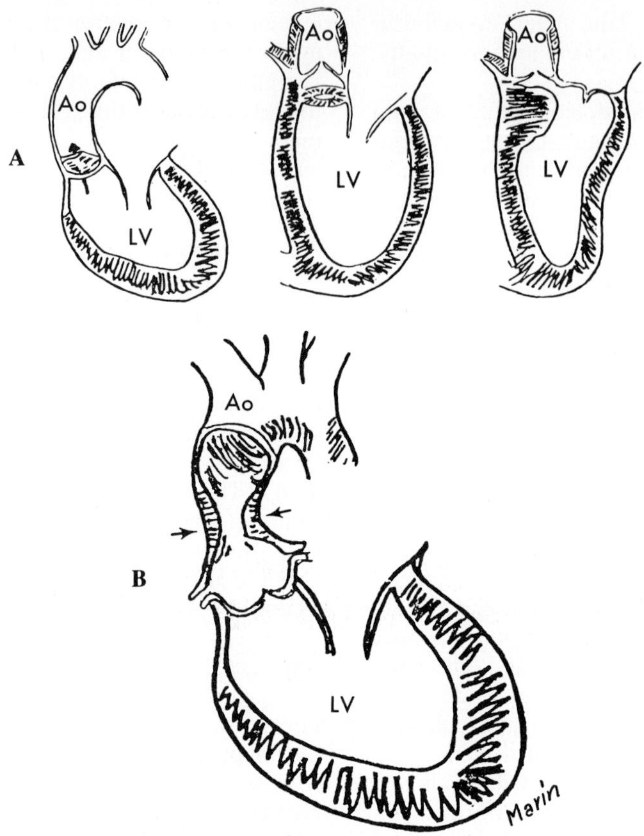

Fig. 18-4. Aortic stenosis. **A,** Valvular, discrete subvalvular, and muscular. **B,** Supravalvular (arrows).

transient improvement, followed by progressive congestive heart failure and death. Prompt cardiac catheterization should be undertaken for definitive diagnosis, including detection of possible associated lesions that may require surgical correction or palliation. The operative procedure of choice is valvotomy by direct vision under cardiopulmonary bypass. On the other hand, in moderately severe forms of stenosis, children may be asymptomatic throughout the period of childhood. Chest pain with characteristics of angina may develop in some children as they approach adolescence. Cardiac evaluation commonly is sought because of the presence of a heart murmur. Sudden death, probably caused by myocardial ischemia and dysrhythmia, is a potential hazard. Children with AS should be discouraged from strenuous physical exertion, and competitive team sports in particular are inadvisable. The absence of symptoms should not be construed to indicate mild disease. Numerous reports attest to the inconsistent correlation between measured hemodynamic severity and the clinical manifestations of this potentially lethal lesion.

There are several clinical findings that suggest the diagnosis of AS. In severe stenotic lesions the pulse pressure is narrow so that the quality of the peripheral pulse is weak. A sustained left ventricular lift is usually present. A thrill in the aortic area or along the upper sternal border, with radiation into the suprasternal notch and neck, is frequently present. The first sound is usually followed by an apical systolic ejection click, related in most instances to an aortic opening snap. This sound marks the onset of the murmur and implies a degree of valve mobility generally associated with mild to moderate stenosis. A harsh systolic crescendo-decrescendo murmur is present with maximal intensity at the base, radiating into the carotids and toward the apex. In up to 35% of patients a faint, early descrescendo diastolic murmur of aortic valve insufficiency is present. Prolonged left ventricular ejection results in a delayed aortic valve closure sound, producing a narrowly split or single second sound. Occasionally, extreme delay of aortic valve closure results in paradoxical splitting of the second sound. A prominent third sound is common, and an audible fourth sound suggests severe stenosis. The carotid pulse may be diminished and slow rising.

The electrocardiogram generally reveals a normal axis. Left ventricular hypertrophy is typically present if the obstruction is significant. It is usually manifested by deep S waves in lead V_1 and normal R waves in V_6. Attention should be directed to serial changes in the S-T segment and T wave in precordial leads V_5 and V_6. The inversion of T waves and alterations of the S-T segment are evidence for significant left ventricular hypertrophy and left ventricular strain. The presence of the latter should be a warning to the physician, since the children with AS who die suddenly usually manifest these electrocardiographic findings.

Cardiomegaly is usually absent on chest radiograph, and only dilation of the ascending aorta is often seen. Gross cardiac enlargement suggests severe obstruction with cardiac dilation, a manifestation of beginning decompensation. Left atrial enlargement and signs of pulmonary venous hypertension may be noted. In general, the x-ray examination is not as valuable as the electrocardiogram in following the course of AS.

Estimation of the severity of AS by clinical means has not been completely satisfactory. Echocardiography has become an important adjunct in the evaluation of patients with this disease. Serial evaluation of left ventricular wall and septal thickness, chamber dimensions, and indices of left ventricular function may be useful in evaluating the progression of AS.

All patients with definite or suggestive symptomatology should have hemodynamic assessment by cardiac catheterization. In the presence of a normal cardiac output, a resting peak systolic gradient exceeding 75 mmHg across the aortic valve or a calculated aortic valve area less than 0.7 cm^2/m^2 body surface area are generally indications for surgical consideration. Aortic valvotomy under direct vision during cardiopulmonary bypass is the procedure of choice. Surgery does not produce an anatomically or functionally normal valve, and eventual recurrent stenosis is to be anticipated. Aortic regurgitation of variable degree is a common complication of surgery. Postoperative patients therefore deserve the same careful clinical follow-up and periodic hemodynamic evaluation as does the unoperated patient with AS.

The natural history in the unoperated state is one of progressive obstruction, although a critical degree of stenosis may not be reached until adolescence or later. A similar course holds for the bicuspid aortic valve, which may be of no hemodynamic significance in childhood, yet creates severe obstruction in adult life because of fibrotic and calcific changes. Eventual aortic valve replacement can be anticipated, therefore, in almost all patients with this lesion.

Supravalvular AS is a congenital narrowing of the ascending aorta above the level of the coronary vessels at the upper margin of the sinuses of Valsalva. The obstruction may be localized or diffuse. There is no sex predilection. This obstruction most commonly occurs as part of the supravalvular AS syndrome, which may be associated with idiopathic infantile hypercalcemia, a disease suspected to result from deranged vitamin D metabolism in the mother or fetus during pregnancy. Experimentally the aortic lesions may be reproduced in the offspring of pregnant rabbits with induced hypervitaminosis D. The other clinical features include "elfin facies," mental retardation, strabismus, dental abnormalities, and peripheral pulmonary stenosis. Affected patients have a striking facial resemblance to each other. Supravalvular AS also occurs in a familial form, which is transmitted as an autosomal dominant with variable expressivity, and in a sporadic form. In neither of these are the other features of the syndrome associated.

The clinical, electrocardiographic, and radiographic findings are those commonly associated with valvular AS. Exceptions are that the aortic valve closure sound may be unusually prominent because of the high pressure in the aortic root, and that there is sometimes a significant difference in blood pressure between the arms, the pressure in the right arm being higher. Poststenotic dilation of the ascending aorta is not commonly seen. If cardiac catheterization reveals hemodynamically significant obstruction, surgical treatment is indicated but is technically more difficult than that for valvular AS.

Discrete subaortic stenosis consists of a fibrous ring or diaphragm encircling the left ventricular outflow tract just beneath the aortic annulus. This form of obstruction is less common than valvular AS and, like the valvular lesion, is more common in males (2:1). The clinical manifestations are those common to left ventricular outflow obstruction, although symptoms in early infancy occur much less commonly than with the valvular lesion. Physical examination cannot reliably differentiate this lesion from valvular stenosis, but certain differences may be noted. A systolic ejection click is rarely present in subaortic stenosis. The murmur of aortic regurgitation, however, is more common because of trauma to the valve by the high velocity ejection stream through the subvalvular diaphragm. Differentiation at catheterization can be made by withdrawal pressure recording (as the catheter tip is withdrawn), which demonstrates a subvalvular pressure gradient, and by angiocardiography, which outlines the subvalvular level of obstruction. Indications for surgery are similar to those for valvular stenosis. Excision of the fibrous ring or diaphragm under cardiopulmonary bypass is curative in most cases, although incomplete excision and recurrent obstruction may occur. Aortic regurgitation, when present preoperatively, may persist.

Pulmonary stenosis

Right ventricular outflow obstruction can occur at the supravalvular, valvular, or subvalvular level. Infundibular pulmonary stenosis (PS) as an isolated lesion is uncommon. Isolated supravalvular stenosis or stenosis of the individual pulmonary arteries is also uncommon and is usually associated with the rubella syndrome. In the majority of cases the obstruction is at the level of the pulmonary valve. Anatomically the stenotic pulmonary valve is dome shaped and has a narrowed central orifice. Because of the obstruction, the right ventricular pressure must increase in order to maintain a normal cardiac output. With the elevation of the right ventricular pressure, right ventricular hypertrophy and occasionally right atrial enlargement develop. Infundibular PS as a consequence of right ventricular hypertrophy may occur. Also, the combination of elevated right atrial pressure and right atrial enlargement may stretch the foramen ovale open, and a right-to-left shunt may develop at the atrial level. Clinical manifestations are related to the severity of obstruction. Patients with mild stenosis are asymptomatic. Those with significant obstruction may develop symptomatology after 2 to 3 years of age. Exertional fatigue and dyspnea from moderate exercise are the initial complaints, but severe stenosis may produce chest pain, exertional dizziness, or syncope. However, up to 25% of patients with severe stenosis claim no disability. Although cyanosis and clubbing are seen in one third of patients with severe stenosis, squatting is not characteristic. Cyanosis, usually related to venoarterial shunting at the atrial level, may be of peripheral origin in patients with low cardiac output. Occasionally, severe PS in the young infant produces profound right heart failure accompanied by cyanosis.

As a rule, patients with PS have normal growth and development. Prominent "a" waves in the jugular venous pulse may accompany severe obstruction. A systolic thrill is almost always present at the pulmonic area and frequently also in the suprasternal notch. A left parasternal impulse of right ventricular origin is prominent, but the apex impulse is seldom displaced. An ejection-type systolic murmur, heard along the upper left sternal border and below the clavicle, is transmitted to the left upper back. In milder degrees of PS the murmur is louder and longer than in more severe stenosis. The quality and characteristics of the second heart sound may also give an indication of the severity of the stenosis. In severe stenosis the pulmonary valve closure may be soft, and the second sound appears single. A systolic ejection click may also be heard. This finding is usually present in mild to moderate PS, and may be absent in severe PS in which an audible right-sided fourth sound may appear.

The electrocardiogram may be normal in 30% to 40% of patients with mild PS and 10% of those with moderate obstruction. The frontal plane axis is usually normal or deviated moderately to the right, and mild right ventricular hypertrophy may be evident. Severe PS almost always results in prominent right axis deviation and severe right ventricular hypertrophy, often with right atrial enlargement. In contrast to aortic stenosis, electrocardiographic changes correlate more closely with severity of obstruction. An R wave in lead V_1 exceeding 20 mm in amplitude suggests at least systemic pressure in the right ventricle, and if associated with significant S-T segment depression and sharply inverted T waves in the right precordial leads, a ventricular pressure of 150 torr or more is often present. The cardiothoracic ratio is usually normal on chest radiograph in the absence of right ventricular decompensation. The rounded, elevated apex is typical of right ventricular prominence. Poststenotic dilation of the pulmonary artery is common. The peripheral pulmonary vascular pattern is normal unless diminished by venoarterial shunting or right ventricular failure.

Although in most cases accurate clinical assessment is possible, cardiac catheterization is indicated in all patients in whom surgical therapy is anticipated. Cardiac catheterization will permit localization of the site of obstruction and its severity. Pressure recordings as the catheter tip is withdrawn from the pulmonary artery to the right ventricle show the systolic pressure gradient at the pulmonary artery branch, valvular, or infundibular levels. Right ventricular angiography will confirm the diagnosis (Fig. 18-5). Surgical treatment is indicated in all patients with severe stenosis. Commissurotomy under direct vision with cardiopulmonary bypass is the surgical technique of choice. Extremely dysplastic valves may require complete valve excision, and widening of the valve annulus by a patch is required occasionally. The resulting pulmonic regurgitation is usually well tolerated.

Pulmonary atresia

Pulmonary valve atresia with intact ventricular septum represents the extreme degree of pulmonic outflow obstruction, typically presenting in the newborn period. Occasionally the main pulmonary artery is also atretic, and varying degrees of right ventricular hypoplasia are present. An obligatory right-to-left shunt across

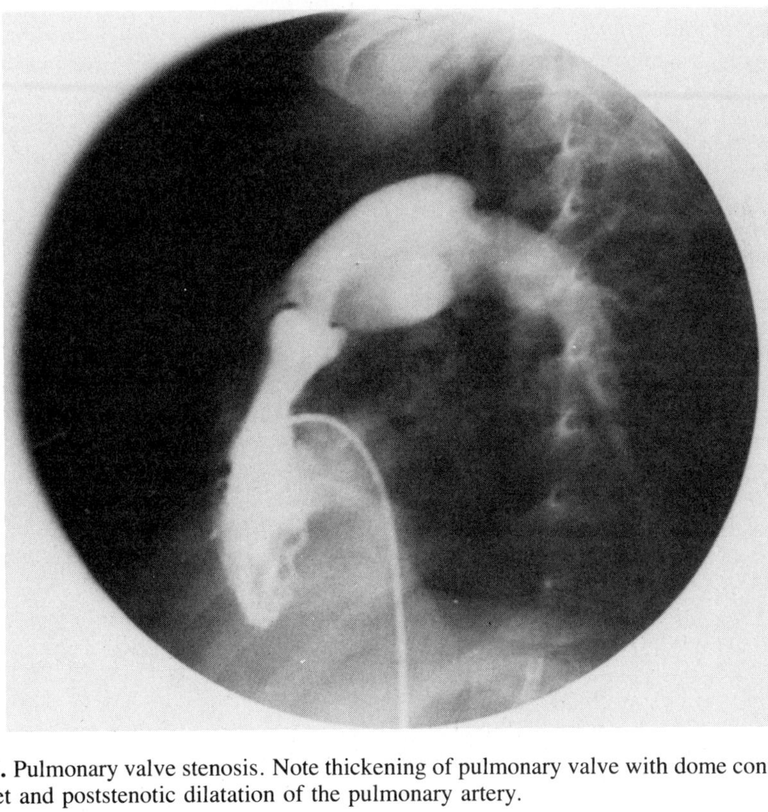

Fig. 18-5. Pulmonary valve stenosis. Note thickening of pulmonary valve with dome configuration. Centric jet and poststenotic dilatation of the pulmonary artery.

the atrial septum exists, and pulmonary blood flow is solely dependent on the ductus arteriosus (Fig. 18-6).

Progressive neonatal cyanosis with tachypnea and signs of congestive heart failure are the clinical features. The cardiovascular examination may be rather unremarkable except for signs of hypoxemia. Murmurs may be absent, but a continuous murmur caused by ductal flow or a systolic murmur of tricuspid regurgitation may be heard. The second sound is single. Right atrial and left ventricular hypertrophy are the electrocardiographic features, although right or combined ventricular hypertrophy is seen occasionally. The frontal plane QRS axis is usually within the normal range and may be helpful in differentiating this defect from tricuspid atresia, in which a left superior axis is characteristic. On chest radiograph the heart and lungs may appear normal initially, but cardiomegaly and reduced vascularity soon become apparent.

Diagnosis can be established by two-dimensional echocardiography, but cardiac catheterization and cineangiocardiography is still required preoperatively for a more precise delineation of the size of the right ventricular cavity and pulmonary branches. Without surgery, most infants with pulmonary atresia die within the first few weeks of life. Rapid deterioration may follow spontaneous closure of the ductus arteriosus. Surgical palliation in the form of a systemic-pulmonary shunt often results in prompt clinical improvement with relief of hypoxemia. The Waterston procedure (right pulmonary artery to ascending aorta anastomosis) has been employed widely in this defect. In selected cases with less extreme degrees of right ventricular hypoplasia, pulmonary valvotomy has proved to be beneficial. By allowing forward flow through the right ventricle and pulmonary artery, further growth of these structures may be stimulated and the prognosis significantly improved.

Coarctation of the aorta

Coarctation of the aorta consists of an obstruction of the aortic lumen that usually occurs at the junction of the arch and descending aorta, near the point of attachment of the ligamentum arteriosum. It is a common malformation, accounting for approximately 7% of congenital heart disease, and is two to four times more frequent in males than females. Although the lesion generally can be readily diagnosed clin-

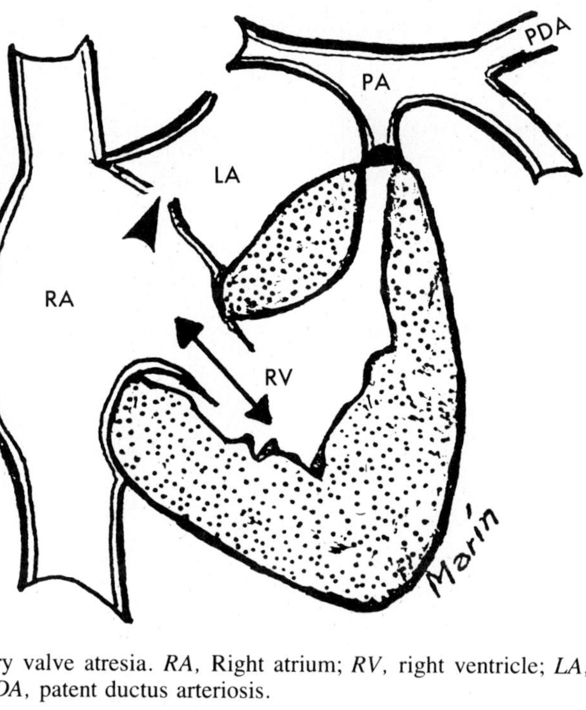

Fig. 18-6. Pulmonary valve atresia. *RA*, Right atrium; *RV*, right ventricle; *LA*, left atrium; *PA*, pulmonary artery; *PDA*, patent ductus arteriosis.

ically, it is often missed because of failure to perform a thorough physical examination—specifically, failure to measure blood pressure in the leg or to palpate simultaneous pulses in upper and lower extremities.

The relative positions of the coarctation and the ductus arteriosus vary. In general, two major positions for coarctation are identified: the postductal type and the preductal type (Fig. 18-7). In the postductal type collateral arterial vessels bypassing the obstruction develop before birth and overcome the obstruction after birth. In the preductal type the fetal circulation is little disturbed by the aortic obstruction, and collateral vessels do not develop before birth. Frequently associated defects include patent ductus arteriosus, ventricular septal defect, and tubular hypoplasia of the aortic arch. A bicuspid aortic valve is seen in about 50% of the cases.

The major hemodynamic problem imposed by coarctation of the aorta is maintenance of adequate distal aortic blood pressure and flow. To this end three main compensatory mechanisms are active: (1) peripheral vasoconstriction to maintain a higher level of diastolic pressure in the aorta, (2) increased blood pressure in the proximal aortic compartment, and, most importantly, (3) development of extensive collateral arterial pathways to bypass the site of obstruction. These pathways involve primarily the intercostal arteries, branches of the subclavian arteries, and anterior spinal arteries. The major hemodynamic burden is borne by the left ventricle, which must eject against increased resistance. Additionally, left ventricular volume overload may occur in patients with left-to-right shunts. The obstruction to pulsatile flow and the circuitous collateral pathway result in damping of the peak systolic pressure in the distal aortic segment, with narrow pulse pressure and weak delayed pulses in the lower extremities.

Clinical manifestations relate to the severity of obstruction, presence of associated defects, and adequacy of compensatory mechanisms. From the second week through the end of the first month of life coarctation is the leading cause of congestive heart failure, but most affected infants have associated defects that add to the hemodynamic burden. Many patients are asymptomatic during infancy. Those surviving the first 6 months of life without symptoms are likely to progress well. Symptomatic infants exhibit tachypnea, dyspnea, poor feeding, and slow weight gain as manifestations of left ventricular failure. The most significant clue to diagnosis is the presence of weak or absent femoral pulses and a significant gradient of blood pressure between the upper and lower extremities. Infrequently the right or left subclavian artery arises at or below the coarctation, resulting in low pressure in the corresponding arm. The importance of evaluation of pulse and

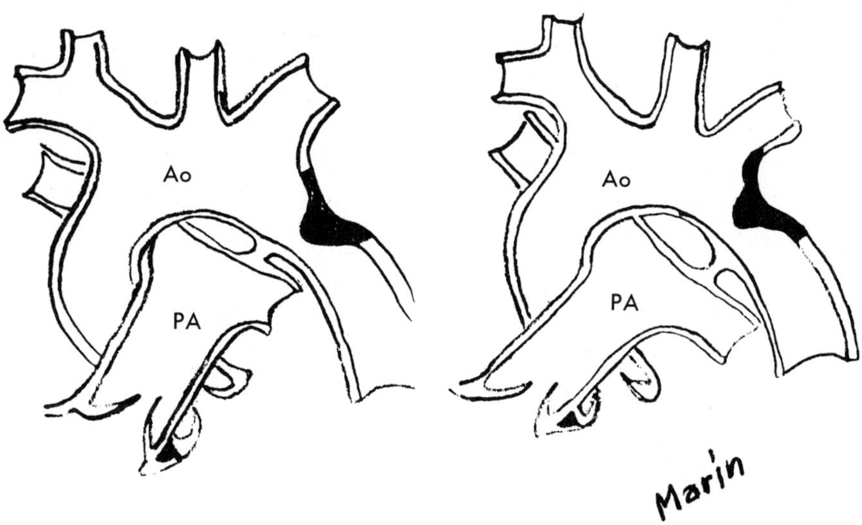

Fig. 18-7. Coarctation of the aorta. *Ao,* Aorta; *PA,* pulmonary artery.

blood pressure in both arms is therefore obvious. Prominent suprasternal notch pulsations and thrill are common. A heart murmur may be absent when congestive failure is present but is usually best heard at the second and third left intercostal spaces near the sternal edge. It may be of equal or greater intensity in the back along the upper left border of the spine, particularly in the older patient. Murmurs associated with coarctation arise from turbulence at the site of the lesion and flow through arterial collateral pathways or they arise from associated defects that may produce a dominant murmur (e.g., ventricular septal defect). Collateral flow may produce a soft systolic, occasionally continuous, arterial bruit of superficial quality, usually heard widely around the left scapular area. The murmur arising from the coarctation site is delayed in onset, with a late peaking ejection quality; rarely is it continuous. The second sound is narrowly split, and the aortic component is prominent.

Coarctation in the older child is usually detected because of a murmur or hypertension. It should be emphasized that significant absolute hypertension is not consistently found in patients with coarctation. Rather, it is the disparity between pressure in the upper and lower extremities that is most important. Hypertension increases in frequency with age and contributes both to the morbidity and mortality of coarctation. The etiology of this hypertension is not clearly defined but is probably related to both mechanical and humoral factors.

The electrocardiographic changes are variable, commonly showing right or combined ventricular hypertrophy in infants under 6 months of age and left ventricular hypertrophy in older patients. The chest radiograph in the infant may reveal nonspecific changes consisting of cardiomegaly, increased vascularity, or pulmonary venous congestion. In older patients the heart may appear normal or slightly enlarged, with a prominent ascending aorta and arch. An indentation of the descending aorta may result in a "figure 3" deformity, whereas barium esophagram may reveal a double indentation of the coarcted site (reversed figure 3). Rib notching, related to rib erosion by the tortuous and dilated intercostal arteries, is uncommon in young patients but frequent (75%) in adults. Notching is usually confined to the middle one third of the fourth through eighth ribs posteriorly in an asymmetric manner. Although characteristic, rib notching is not pathognomonic for coarctation.

Except for congestive heart failure in early infancy, the major complications of coarctation of the aorta usually appear in the second and third decades and include increasing incidence and severity of hypertension, cerebral aneurysm formation and hemorrhage, rupture of the aorta, and bacterial endocarditis. Congestive heart failure also appears with increasing frequency after age 30. The average age of death in untreated patients is 35 years.

Surgical resection with end-to-end anastomosis is indicated for the uncomplicated coarctation, including significant hemodynamic obstruction. The optimum age for elective surgical correction is 4 to 6 years. Correction in infancy may be indicated for those not responding well to medical management. Restenosis at the anastomotic site may occur, the incidence being highest in the infant age group.

Aortic arch anomalies

A large number of congenital anatomic variants are included in this group, many of which are of no clinical importance. However, there are several structural aberrations that may produce symptoms varying from mild to life-threatening because of pressure on the trachea, esophagus, or both. Most of these fall into the category of *vascular rings* because they encircle the mediastinal structures. All vascular rings result from abnormal persistence or regression of various portions of the primitive system of aortic arches and dorsal and ventral aortae. The most serious of these is the double aortic arch, in which there are two complete arches, one on either side of the trachea and esophagus, that join posteriorly to form the descending aorta. The right arch is generally larger than the left. Severe obstruction of the upper airway with inspiratory stridor occurs in most patients, usually starting in early infancy. Because of esophageal compression, swallowing may be difficult, and passage of the bolus of food may compress the trachea, further worsening the respiratory difficulty. Congenital heart disease is uncommonly associated.

The other forms of vascular ring have a unilateral aortic arch and are divided according to the side on which the arch is located. In the majority of patients the arch is on the right. If the right arch is associated with a mirror image arrangement of the brachiocephalic vessels (i.e., left innominate artery, right carotid artery, and right subclavian artery in order from anterior to posterior), the ligamentum arteriosum usually connects the innominate and left pulmonary arteries and a ring is not formed. There is a high incidence of associated congenital heart disease. Rarely, the ligamentum passes behind the esophagus from distal arch to left pulmonary artery, creating a ring. The left subclavian artery may also arise separately as a fourth vessel from the right arch and pass behind the esophagus to reach the left arm. The ligamentum arteriosum then arises from the base of the left subclavian artery and courses anteriorly to the pulmonary artery. Thus the mediastinal structures are completely encircled, and the incidence of symptoms depends on the length of the ligamentum. Approximately 20% of these patients are symptomatic. Associated congenital heart disease is less common in this group.

An arrangement that is the mirror image of the foregoing may be seen in patients with a left arch, but these vascular rings are extremely uncommon. A left arch with an aberrant right subclavian artery is seen frequently as an incidental finding on chest radiographs with barium in the esophagus (taken for other reasons) and rarely produces symptoms when the ligamentum is in the normal location.

The most important element in the approach to this group of lesions is suspicion of their presence. Although not a common cause of stridor or respiratory embarrassment, vascular rings should be considered in the presence of these findings, especially when the distress is persistent.

All forms of vascular rings can be detected on a good quality barium esophagram. A filling defect on the posterior aspect of the esophagus is seen (Fig. 18-8). It may be small and oblique in the case of an isolated aberrant right subclavian artery or large if the arch is the posterior element. The side of the major arch can usually be identified. More complicated studies such as bronchoscopy, bronchography, and aortography generally add little and may carry a significant element of risk; they are rarely necessary. If respiratory embarrassment or feeding difficulty is great, surgical division of the ring is indicated. The smaller arch is divided in the case of a double arch, generally where there is enough length to avoid injury to the brachiocephalic vessels. In other forms of vascular ring, only division of the ligamentum and mobilization of the ring are necessary. Because of the presence of tracheomalacia involving the segments compressed by the ring, some degree of noisy respiration may persist for months after successful surgery.

Hypoplastic left heart syndrome

Hypoplastic left heart syndrome is a term that refers to a group of closely related anomalies characterized by underdevelopment of the left cardiac chambers. Aortic valve atresia or pinpoint stenosis, mitral atresia or stenosis, and hypoplasia or atresia of the aortic arch may occur alone or in combination. The complex is the commonest cause of congestive heart failure in the first week of life. A slight male preponderance (3:2) is noted.

In the most common form of hypoplastic left heart syndrome there is aortic valve atresia with hypoplasia of the annulus and ascending aorta. The pulmonary artery is enlarged and communicates with the descending aorta by way of a large patent ductus arteriosus. The mitral valve annulus is small, and the valve is hypoplastic or atretic. A small left atrium communicates with the right atrium through a stretched and prolapsed foramen ovale. The left ventricle is thick walled, with a tiny cavity or only a potential cavity. Left atrial and pulmonary venous hypertension are present. Aortic flow is dependent on the patent ductus arteriosus. Coronary flow may be compromised in the presence of hypoplasia of the ascending aorta.

Typically, an infant previously considered normal develops signs of distress within 48 to 72 hours of birth, with rapid deterioration. Tachypnea, often unrecognized, is usually present from birth. Cyanosis is initially minimal but becomes more pronounced with the onset of congestive heart failure, when the former appears as the dusky pallor characteristic of poor peripheral perfusion. Profound right heart failure develops rapidly and progresses relentlessly in spite of vigorous treatment. The most striking feature of the physical examination is the weakness of all peripheral pulses, including the ca-

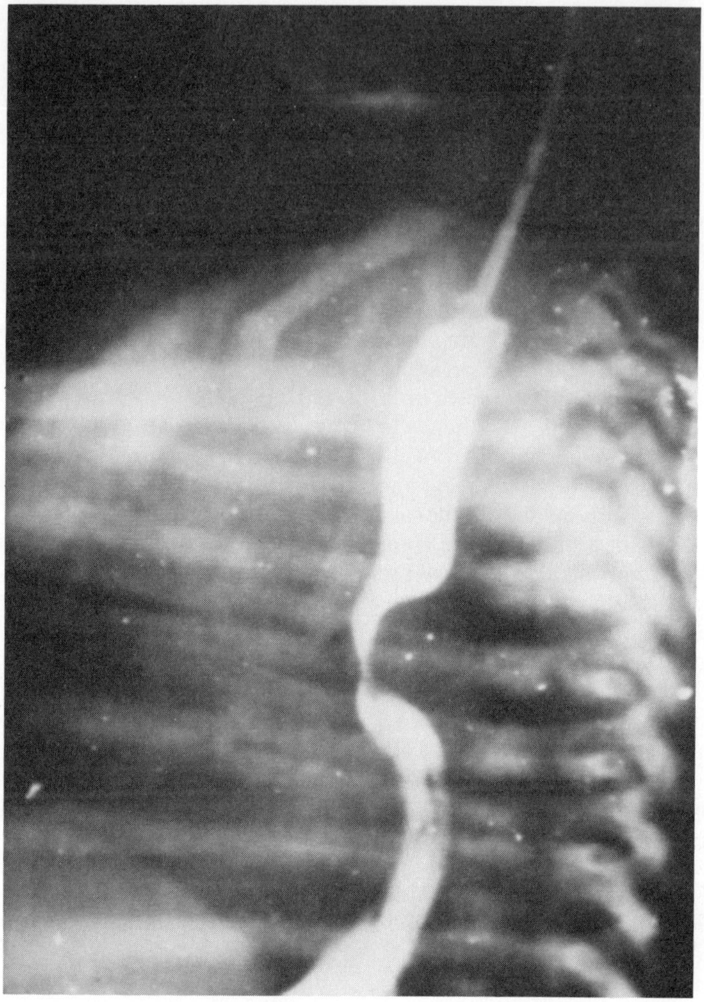

Fig. 18-8. Left lateral projection barium esophagogram of infant with double aortic arch. There is large posterior indentation on esophagus caused by posterior element of ring.

rotids. Right ventricular tap is present, and the second heart sound is loud and single. A nonspecific systolic ejection murmur is noted in most cases. The chest radiograph demonstrates generalized cardiomegaly with pulmonary venous engorgement. Right ventricular hypertrophy and right atrial enlargement are typical electrocardiographic findings. Septal q waves are commonly absent. Echocardiographic findings include a very small or absent left ventricle, small aortic root with or without recognizable aortic cusps echoes, and small or absent mitral valve. Although M-mode echocardiography is relatively reliable, two-dimensional echocardiography is superior, especially if one is planning to avoid cardiac catheterization.

The prognosis is uniformly poor. Most infants die within 48 hours of the onset of symptoms, the average age of death being 5 days. Survival beyond 1 month is rare. At present the lesion is not amenable to surgical correction. Palliation has been attempted, but results have not been encouraging.

Tetralogy of Fallot

Tetralogy of Fallot is the classic prototype of cyanotic congenital heart disease and traditionally consists of four anatomic features: ventricular septal defect (VSD), pulmonary stenosis, overriding aorta, and right ventricular hypertrophy. The VSD is large, approximating the size of the aortic orifice, and is more anterior in position than the usual isolated VSD. The aortic root appears to override to a variable degree the interventricular septum partly because of the location of the VSD and partly because of the exaggerated anterior rotation of the aortic root in this defect.

Although anatomic variations are common, recent concepts emphasize that pulmonic stenosis in the classic tetralogy is always partially or totally subvalvular (infundibular) because of underdevelopment and narrowing of the infundibulum, with displaced and hypertrophied septal and parietal bands of the crista supraventricularis. The pulmonary valve may be variably stenotic, often with a small annulus. In extreme cases the valve is atretic, and pulmonary blood flow is only by way of the ductus arteriosus. Rarely, the leaflets are aplastic (congenital absence of the pulmonary valve). In some cases, hypoplasia of the main pulmonary artery and its branches is seen, whereas in others segmental stenosis of the origin of one or both pulmonary branches is present. Rarely, tetralogy is associated with congenital absence of the left pulmonary branch. The right ventricular cavity size is slightly increased, with a thick wall and heavy trabeculations—a reflection of the increased right ventricular pressure work. The aorta, which receives output from both ventricles, is dilated, and a right aortic arch is present in 25% of patients.

Physiologically the important components of the complex are the large nonrestrictive ventricular septal defect and the pulmonary outflow obstruction. Ventricular pressures are usually equal, since the right ventricle need only to generate sufficient pressure to eject into the aorta. The magnitude and direction of the shunt are thus a function of the ratio of the overflow tract resistances, plus the phasic differences in the development of pressure in the two ventricles. Therefore the degree of pulmonary stenosis is the major determinant of clinical severity in this lesion.

Tetralogy of Fallot accounts for approximately 15% of congenital heart defects in patients past 2 years of age and is the most common cyanotic lesion seen in children beyond infancy. The clinical picture is dominated by manifestations of hypoxemia. In infants with severe pulmonary stenosis, cyanosis is apparent at or soon after birth and becomes striking with crying or straining. These infants develop increasingly severe signs of hypoxemia within the first few months of life and usually require surgical intervention within the first year of life.

More typical is the neonate who appears acyanotic early but develops obvious cyanosis later in the first year of life. The initial sign of hypoxemia may be only minimal tachypnea. Exertional fatigue, dyspnea, and hyperpnea become more pronounced with age. The child old enough to walk commonly exhibits the phenomenon of squatting because of early recognition that this position promptly improves his physiologic state. Hemodynamic studies suggest that several physiologic benefits derive from this posture. Basically, a reduction in systemic venous return of blood of low PO_2, high PCO_2, and elevated lactate and an increase in systemic arterial resistance result in decreased right-to-left shunt and increased pulmonary blood flow. The net result is an increased systemic arterial saturation.

A more serious manifestation of hypoxemia is the occurrence of acute episodes of profound cyanosis and hyperpnea. These have been variously described as hypoxic spells, hypercyanotic spells, anoxic attacks, or paroxysmal hyperpnea. Such attacks classically occur in tetralogy of Fallot, but they may also be seen in other forms of cyanotic heart disease. They are characterized by uncontrollable crying, followed by severe dyspnea, hyperpnea, and progressively intense cyanosis, which may terminate in unconsciousness, convulsions, or even death. Metabolic acidosis is a common accompaniment of the severe hypoxemia experienced during these attacks. Typically, the spells occur after a period of rest, but at times they appear to be precipitated by straining or exertion. Their duration varies from a few minutes to several hours. They are more frequent in the younger age group but seldom occur before 3 or 4 months of age. In infants the irritability and restlessness associated with milder attacks are sometimes mistaken for colic. Once apparent, spells tend to increase progressively in frequency and duration.

The precise mechanism responsible for these

episodes is not clearly defined, but several theories have been offered, including acute infundibular spasm and variations in respiratory center sensitivity leading to severe hyperpnea. Regardless of the precipitating mechanism, it is clear that during these episodes pulmonary blood flow is further reduced and right-to-left shunting is increased, resulting in a more profound hypoxic state. Urgent treatment of such spells is indicated. Oxygen should be administered promptly and the patient should be placed in the knee-chest position. If the spell is not quickly terminated by this maneuver, morphine should be administered subcutaneously in a dose of 0.1 mg/pound body weight. Some patients require the administration of vasopressor agents, and if the spells are prolonged, metabolic acidosis must be counteracted.

Clubbing is a common finding in the cyanotic patient with tetralogy of Fallot but is not limited to this lesion. Clubbing is poorly developed in early infancy but often is apparent by 2 to 3 months of age. Cardiac examination reveals a right ventricular impulse at the lower sternal margin, but the heart is neither hyperdynamic nor grossly enlarged. The first heart sound is prominent. The second heart sound is usually single (aortic component), but occasionally a faint pulmonic component can be detected. A cardiac murmur directly reflects the major anatomic feature of the tetralogy of Fallot. It originates from blood flow through the stenotic right ventricular outflow tract and not from blood flow through the ventricular septal defect. Thus it is a pulmonary ejection murmur, and its intensity varies inversely with the severity of the stenosis. In more severe pulmonary outflow obstruction, less flow occurs through the stenotic area. In extreme cases (pulmonary atresia) murmurs are absent. The murmur may likewise diminish or disappear during a hypoxic spell. Signs of congestive heart failure are rarely seen in the absence of complicating factors such as severe anemia, bacterial endocarditis, or profound hypoxia. Chest roentgenograms reveal normal heart size, with a rounded uplifted apex characteristic of right ventricular hypertrophy. The pulmonary artery segment is deficient, and the pulmonary vascular pattern is decreased. A right aortic arch, present in 25% of patients, may be recognized by the rightward bowing of the superior vena cava shadow with leftward displacement of the tracheal air column. Electrocardiography reveals right axis deviation, right ventricular hypertrophy, and less commonly right atrial enlargement. In patients with less severe pulmonary stenosis and significant left-to-right shunt, biventricular hypertrophy may be present. Echocardiography provides a method to evaluate the relation between the aorta and the interventricular septum (overriding) and the presence of right ventricular outflow obstruction.

Medical management of the patient with tetralogy of Fallot is limited to maintenance of an optimum hemoglobin level, bacterial endocarditis prophylaxis, observation for signs of increasing hypoxemia, and treatment of acute hypoxic spells.

Maintenance of optimum hemoglobin levels is important because relative anemia results in less total oxygen-carrying capacity of the blood and may contribute to hypoxic symptoms. The hypoxic stimulus to the bone marrow results in increased iron requirements, often leading to iron deficiency. A prompt rise in hemoglobin and hematocrit levels may result from increased iron intake, with amelioration of the severity of the patient's symptomatology. On the other hand, an excessively high hematocrit level (more than 70 vol%) is undesirable because the great increase in the blood viscosity can be hemodynamically detrimental and may result in serious thrombotic accidents. An excessively high hematocrit level can be acutely alleviated by plasmapheresis but is generally an indication for surgical intervention to prevent recurrences.

Bacterial endocarditis is more common in tetralogy of Fallot than in other cyanotic heart defects. It most often occurs in patients with functioning systemic-pulmonary artery shunts. The indications for endocarditis prophylaxis are outlined elsewhere (pp. 467-468).

Young infants in particular should be observed closely for evidence of increasing hypoxemia. Past the infancy age, the clinical course may be relatively stable, with only gradually developing symptomatology. The development of an excessive hematocrit level, significant limitation of exercise tolerance with frequent squatting, and in particular the occurrence of episodes of paroxysmal hyperpnea are indications for surgical intervention.

Cardiac catheterization and angiocardiogra-

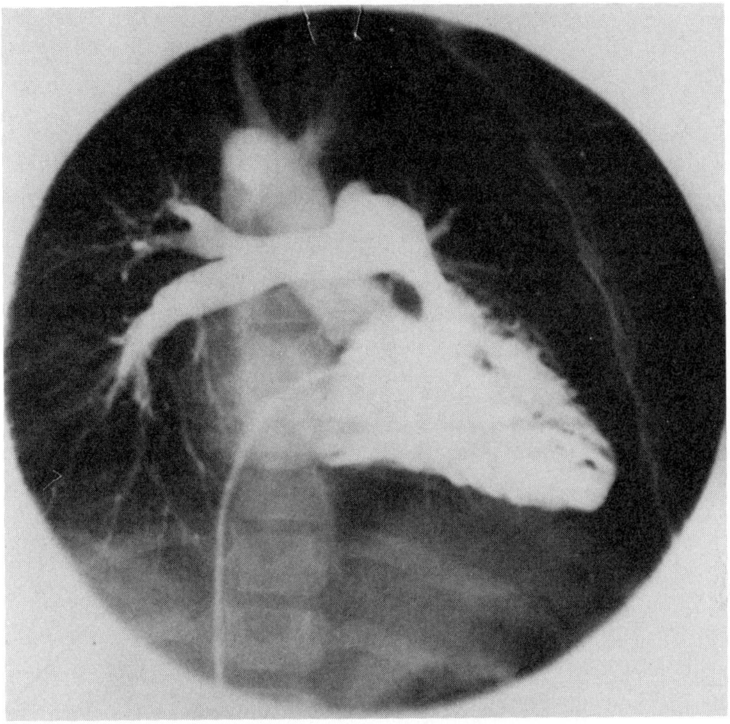

Fig. 18-9. Tetralogy of Fallot. Note infundibular narrowing. Opacification of pulmonary artery and aorta following right ventricular angiogram. Right aortic arch.

phy are essential for adequate surgical treatment. These techniques permit confirmation of the diagnosis and specifically define the anatomy of the right ventricular outflow tract obstruction, a feature of particular importance in the selection of the proper surgical approach (Fig. 18-9).

Operative treatment may be palliative or corrective. Palliative procedures are directed at relief of hypoxemia by increasing pulmonary blood flow with some form of systemic-pulmonary arterial anastomosis. The Blalock-Taussig operation (subclavian artery to pulmonary artery anastomosis) is commonly used when palliation is the preferred approach. With improved techniques for cardiopulmonary bypass, primary total correction of tetralogy of Fallot can now be achieved in most patients, even in infants under 1 year of age.

Transposition of the great arteries

Transposition of the great arteries is a cyanotic congenital cardiac defect of major importance, accounting for most fatalities from congenital heart disease in the first 2 months of life. Once considered inoperable, the prognosis for this serious malformation has improved significantly with the advent of palliative procedures and the possibility of surgical functional correction. Transposition complexes encompass a broad spectrum of anatomic variants that are of interest embryologically as well as clinically. Only the most common form, *d*-transposition, (complete transposition), which accounts for 80% of the group, is discussed here.

The lesion basically consists of reversal of the relationships of the great vessels, resulting in origin of the aorta anteriorly from the right ventricle, the pulmonary trunk arising posteriorly from the left ventricle (Fig. 18-10). This results in parallel and independent pulmonary and systemic circulations. Significantly, the coronary circulation is perfused with blood of low oxygen content. Mixing between the major circuits is essential if the patient is to survive. Shunting may occur by way of intra-cardiac (atrial or

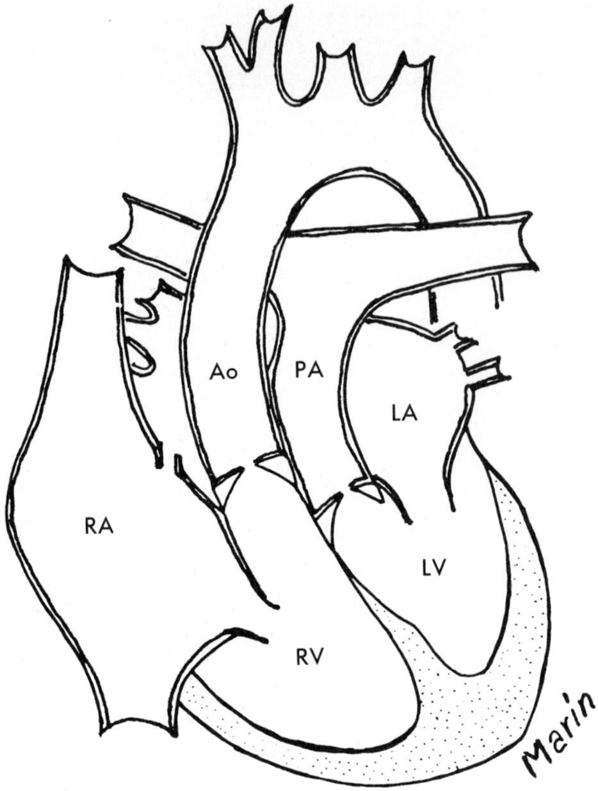

Fig. 18-10. Transposition of the great arteries. Right atrium, RA; right ventricle, RV; left atrium, LA; left ventricle, LV; pulmonary artery, PA; aorta, Ao.

ventricular septal defect) or extracardiac (ductus arteriosus, bronchopulmonary collaterals) communications. Approximately one half of patients have a ventricular septal defect, and roughly one third of these have associated pulmonary stenosis. Those with an intact ventricular septum infrequently have pulmonary stenosis, and most shunt at the atrial level (atrial septal defect, patent foramen ovale) or by way of the ductus arteriosus. Although often delayed, ductus closure occurs in most infants with transposition. The adequacy of mixing and the presence or absence of pulmonary stenosis govern the clinical picture, which is characterized by cyanosis and congestive heart failure in the first 2 months of life.

Cyanosis appears in the first week of life in about 90% of patients, usually by the third day. The intensity of cyanosis is determined by the degree of mixing and the volume of pulmonary blood flow. The more intensely cyanotic infants are more likely to have intact interventricular septum or severe pulmonary stenosis and to exhibit signs and symptoms related to severe hypoxemia. Systemic oxygen tension often is in the range of 20 to 40 torr, resulting in anaerobic metabolism and severe metabolic acidosis. Hypoxic myocardial depression leads to congestive heart failure, the second most common manifestation of this lesion.

The infant with an intact ventricular septum appears grossly cyanotic, with variable degrees of tachypnea and dyspnea. The precordium is hyperdynamic with a dominant right ventricular impulse. Hepatomegaly is usual if congestive heart failure is present. The pulses are often full. Cardiac auscultation reveals a prominent first sound and a loud single or narrowly split second sound. Murmurs are absent in one third of patients, whereas an apparently nonsignificant ejection murmur at the base is present in a like number. The chest radiograph may appear normal in the neonate, but pulmonary plethora and cardiomegaly, with the characteristic "egg-shaped" contour and narrow base, are often apparent within the first week of life. The aorta amd main pulmonary artery are not readily seen, although the aortic arch is generally on the left. The electrocardiogram may also exhibit a normal pattern initially, becoming abnormal by the second week of life. Right axis deviation and right ventricular hypertrophy are characteristic. Right ventricular hypertrophy may be suggested initially only by abnormal persistence of upright T waves in the right precordial leads.

Infants who have transposition with ventricular septal defect but not pulmonary stenosis generally have cyanosis of a lesser degree than do those with an intact septum, and it appears slightly later. Although appearing by the end of the first week in some patients, cyanosis is present in nearly all patients by the fourth week of life, but may be relatively mild. Right and left ventricular impulses and hyperdynamic precordium are present. Auscultation reveals a systolic murmur of grade 3/6 or greater intensity, maximal along the lower left sternal border, often radiating well toward the apex and left axilla. A low-frequency, mid-diastolic apical filling murmur is commonly present. The chest radiograph demonstrates cardiomegaly with the characteristic narrow base, egg-shaped contour, and more pronounced pulmonary plethora. The electrocardiogram reveals right or combined ventricular hypertrophy, with an axis usually in the normal range. Two-dimensional echocardiography shows both semilunar valves in a typical anterior-posterior relationship on the short axis view.

If pulmonary stenosis is present in the infant with transposition and ventricular septal defect, the clinical picture frequently resembles tetralogy of Fallot. Congestive heart failure is not a feature of these infants. Cyanosis is usually present at birth or soon after. Cardiomegaly is less impressive, and the precordium is seldom hyperdynamic. Auscultation reveals a systolic ejection murmur along the midleft sternal border that, in contrast to the usual murmur of pulmonary stenosis, radiates toward the right upper sternal border and infraclavicular area.

The possibility of transposition should be suspected in any infant who presents with tachypnea and cyanosis, particularly if congestive heart failure is present.

Untreated, over 50% of infants with transposition of the great arteries die within the first month, and 90% die by the end of the first year of life. Death results from the effects of severe hypoxemia or congestive heart failure, with the accompanying serious metabolic derangement characteristic of this malformation. Medical management of these infants is an extremely important aspect of their care, but it should be considered only as temporizing. Medical treatment is directed at optimum supportive care, including administration of oxygen, maintenance of normothermia, monitoring of arterial blood gases, and correction of the metabolic acidosis usually present in these patients. Hypoglycemia, a frequent occurrence in stressed infants, should be avoided by attention to blood glucose levels. Digitalization and diuresis should be accomplished in the routine manner when congestive failure is present (pp. 422 and 423).

Most patients require improved intracardiac mixing, which can be accomplished nonsurgically or surgically. Nonsurgical creation of an atrial septal defect by balloon septostomy, originally described by Rashkind and Miller in 1966, has proved an important emergency procedure that avoids the risks of thoracotomy in a critically ill infant. The procedure basically consists of positioning a balloon-tipped catheter across the atrial septum in the left atrium, inflating the balloon with contrast solution, and rapidly withdrawing the inflated balloon across the septum to the right atrium (Fig. 18-11). The entire procedure is performed during fluoroscopic monitoring. This maneuver tears the atrial septum, permitting free communication between the atrial chambers, and results in two beneficial effects: (1) improved systemic arterial saturation as left atrial blood shunts toward the systemic circuit and (2) lessening of the tachypnea and dyspnea as left atrial and pulmonary venous pressures decline. Although immediate results are usually obvious, long-term results of this procedure frequently are less satisfactory. Surgical creation of an atrial septal defect (Blalock-Hanlon procedure) is often necessary in the weeks or months after the balloon procedure and in those infants in whom attempted balloon septostomy is unsuccessful.

In individual cases other palliative procedures are sometimes indicated. These include banding of the pulmonary artery to limit excessive pul-

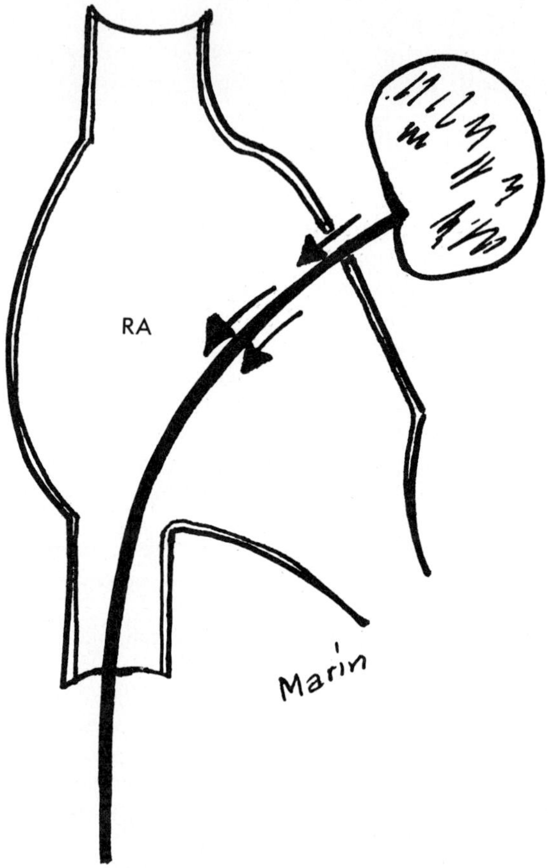

Fig. 18-11. Balloon-type catheter. *RA*, Right artery.

monary blood flow in patients with large ventricular septal defect or creation of a pulmonary artery–systemic artery anastomosis (Waterston or Blalock-Taussig shunt) to increase pulmonary blood flow in patients with severe pulmonary stenosis.

Functional surgical correction of this defect by the Mustard or Senning techniques is now possible in most cases. These procedures redirect venous input in such a manner that pulmonary venous blood is directed across the tricuspid valve to the right ventricle and aorta, and systemic venous blood is directed to the mitral valve, left ventricle, and pulmonary artery. Best results are obtained in simple transposition with intact ventricular septum, a procedure in which the mortality rate in experienced hands approximates 10%. Results are less satisfactory if a ventricular septal defect is present, and they are least satisfactory if pulmonary stenosis is present.

Truncus arteriosus

Truncus arteriosus is a malformation in which a single arterial trunk arises from the heart and supplies systemic, pulmonary, and coronary circulations. The lesion most often presents in the first few weeks of life. It is of increasing importance because in many patients it is now amenable to complete surgical correction.

Four anatomic types have been described, depending on the origins of the vessels supplying the pulmonary circulation. In type I a common pulmonary artery arises from the base of the truncus and divides into right and left pulmonary branches (Fig. 18-12). In types II and III the pulmonary arteries arise singly and in close proximity from the dorsal wall or independently

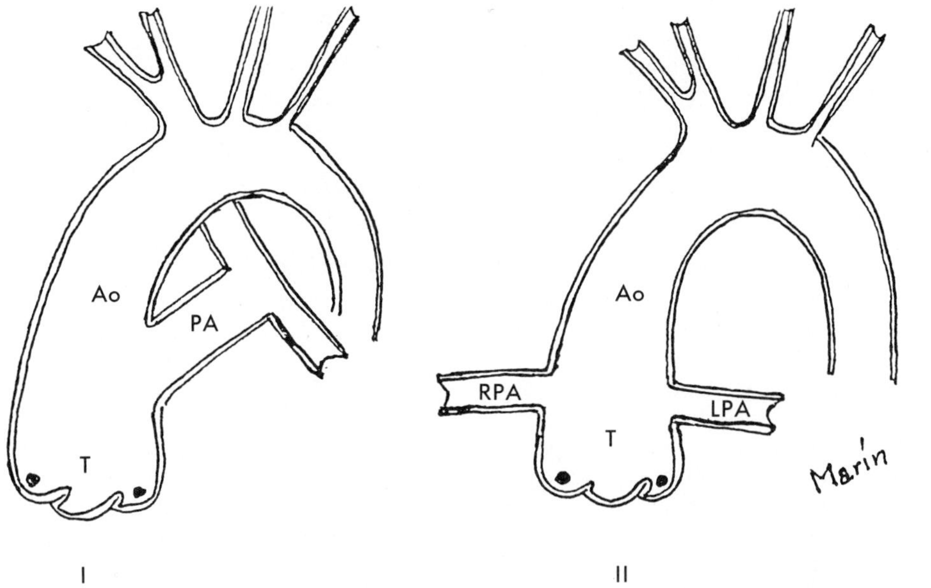

Fig. 18-12. Truncus arteriosus. *Ao,* Aorta; *PA,* pulmonary artery; *T,* truncus; *RPA,* right pulmonary artery; *LPA,* left pulmonary artery.

from either side of the truncus. In type IV no true pulmonary arteries are present, and the arterial supply to the lungs is by way of large bronchial arteries from the descending aorta. Clinically similar to type IV truncus arteriosus is pulmonary atresia with ventricular septal defect (so-called pseudotruncus), which is, however, generally considered an extreme variant of tetralogy of Fallot. In 25% of cases the aortic arch is on the right. A large ventricular septal defect is always present, and both ventricles eject with equal pressure into the common truncus. The number of truncal valve leaflets varies, but usually there are three. The valve is frequently incompetent. The status of the pulmonary arteries is variable; both vessels may be large, or one or both may be diffusely small or stenotic at their origins from the truncus. It is this variability that determines the clinical features of the defect.

Blood is ejected from both ventricles into the common truncus, where mixing occurs. The level of saturation is therefore essentially equal in all three circulations supplied by the truncus and is dependent on the ratio of pulmonary to systemic blood flow. If the pulmonary arteries are large and the pulmonary blood flow is increased, the level of saturation may be correspondingly high. If pulmonary blood flow is restricted because of small pulmonary vessels or pulmonary vascular obstruction, saturation will be low.

The lesion results in the appearance of cyanosis, a cardiac murmur, or signs of congestive heart failure. Most patients exhibit cyanosis early, but its degree is variable, depending on the volume of pulmonary blood flow. Tachypnea, dyspnea, and fatigue appear early. Heart murmurs are noted in about 70% of cases within the first month of life. A harsh systolic murmur, often with thrill, is usually present at the third and fourth left interspaces. Approximately one half of patients will have an apical, diastolic rumble. The first sound is normal, but a systolic ejection sound is sometimes present near the apex. The second sound is loud and single, and an early decrescendo diastolic murmur of truncal valve insufficiency is sometimes present.

A rightward axis is usually seen on the electrocardiogram, with a pattern of left or combined ventricular hypertrophy in the great majority of cases. Isolated right ventricular hypertrophy is relatively uncommon. The chest radiograph shows gross cardiomegaly in three fourths of patients. Pulmonary vasculature is prominent, except in those with severe pulmonary stenosis. The main pulmonary segment is small or absent in most patients. The left pulmonary artery exits from the mediastinum at a higher than usual level, curving up and out into the lung—a feature that is fairly common and may suggest the diagnosis. A right aortic arch is frequently noted. The echocardiographic diagnosis of persistent truncus arteriosus is based on the presence of a large arterial trunk overriding the interventricular septum and demonstration of the origin of both the aorta and the pulmonary artery (or arteries) from this arterial trunk.

With medical management, perhaps 30% of patients will survive early infancy, but survival to adulthood is uncommon. Palliative surgical procedures are available to increase pulmonary blood flow (shunt procedures) in those patients with restricted flow and to decrease flow (banding of the pulmonary arteries) in those having excessive flow. Since 1967, surgical correction has been successfully achieved in selected cases by means of the Rastelli procedure. In this operation the ventricular septal defect is closed, incorporating the truncal root into the left ventricle. An outflow tract is constructed from the right ventricle with a conduit made of Dacron or Teflon and an incorporated porcine valve. The pulmonary arteries are disconnected from the truncus and anastomosed to the distal end of the conduit. Early surgical results have been encouraging.

Tricuspid atresia

In tricuspid atresia there is failure of development of the tricuspid valve and thus no direct communication between the right atrium and right ventricle. Although uncommon, it should always be considered in the differential diagnosis of cyanotic heart disease in infants and children.

Because the right atrium does not communicate with the right ventricle, an obligatory atrial right-to-left shunt exists by way of an atrial septal defect or, more commonly, a patent foramen ovale (Fig. 18-13). The ventricular septum may be intact or open, with a variable degree of under-development of the right ventric-

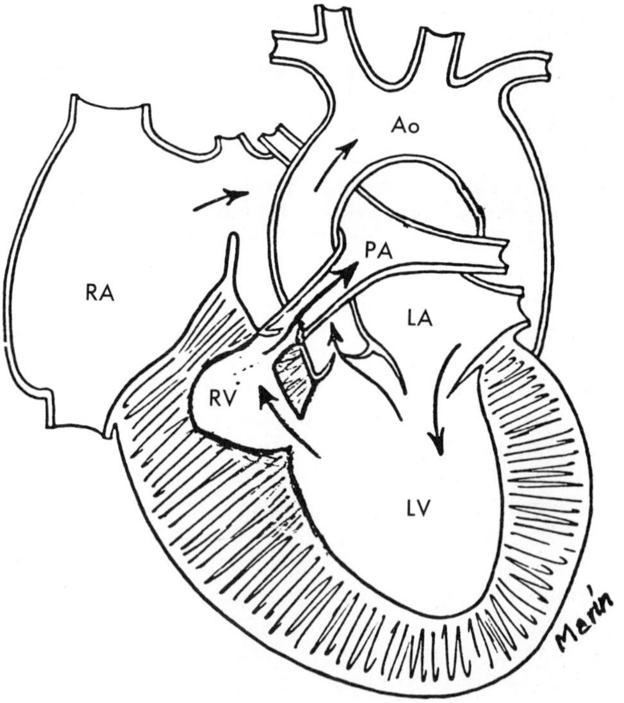

Fig. 18-13. Tricuspid artresia. *RA*, Right atrium; *RV*, right ventricle; *LA*, left atrium; *LV*, left ventricle; *PA*, pulmonary artery; *Ao*, aorta.

ular chamber. Pulmonary atresia, pulmonary valvular or subvalvular stenosis, or hypoplasia of the pulmonary artery may be present, and transposition of the great arteries occurs in approximately 30% of the cases. These associated defects form the basis of an anatomic classification and account for the varied clinical features of the lesion. The admixture of pulmonary and systemic venous blood in the left heart results in peripheral arterial desaturation in every case. Left ventricular output is distributed to both systemic and pulmonary circuits, the latter by one or a combination of possible routes—a patent ductus arteriosus, ventricular septal defect (in the absence of pulmonary atresia), or bronchial arterial collateral flow. The severity of cyanosis depends on the volume of pulmonary blood flow.

The most frequently encountered of all anatomic types (60% to 70%) is that associated with normally related great arteries, a small ventricular defect, a diminutive right ventricle, subpulmonary stenosis, and moderate hypoplasia of the pulmonary artery and valve annulus. Restriction of pulmonary blood flow is the rule. In the presence of transposition of the great arteries the pulmonary trunk is most often normal or large and arises from the left ventricle, whereas the aorta arises from a relatively hypoplastic right ventricle. Increased pulmonary blood flow is characteristic of this type.

Neonates with restricted pulmonary blood flow develop cyanosis early, with moderate tachypnea, dyspnea, and if severely hypoxemic, congestive heart failure. Attacks of acute paroxysmal hyperpnea may occur. At times prominent "a" waves are present in the venous pulse, and a presystolic hepatic pulsation may be detected—findings frequently associated with an inadequate interatrial communication. The precordium is usually not hyperdynamic, but occasionally a thrill related to a ventricular septal defect may be palpated. Murmurs are also variable, depending on the presence of associated malformations. The first heart sound is normal, and the second sound often is single or has a diminished pulmonic component.

The chest radiograph reveals suggestive but nondiagnostic features. Pulmonary vascular volume is typically diminished, and the heart size is normal to moderately large, usually with a concave pulmonary artery segment. The superior vena cava may appear prominent. Right atrial enlargement may be suspected, but the normal right atrial convexity at times may be absent, the atrial border appearing to overlay the vertebral column. Oblique views may suggest a small right ventricle.

In the presence of large pulmonary blood flow, cyanosis may be minimal, and the clinical picture is dominated by congestive heart failure, usually appearing beyond the neonatal period. Tachypnea, dyspnea, and pulsatile hepatomegaly may be noted, with peripheral edema in older patients. The precordial impulse is hyperactive, and the apex laterally displaced. A well-split second sound and blowing harsh systolic murmur at the lower left sternal border are present in over one half of the cases. The radiographic findings in this group are characterized by hypervascularity, a prominent pulmonary artery segment, and a greater degree of cardiomegaly.

The electrocardiogram is always abnormal—a valuable asset of clinical diagnosis. In 80% to 90% of patients the mean QRS frontal plane axis is leftward and usually superior, ranging between +15 degrees and −60 degrees even in the newborn period. The more uncommon normal or right axis deviation generally occurs in the presence of transposition and increased pulmonary blood flow. Left ventricular hypertrophy is almost always present; rarely, associated right ventricular hypertrophy is seen. Right atrial enlargement is seen in over one half of patients, and combined atrial enlargement is common in older infants and children. Thus the clinical findings of cyanosis and an electrocardiographic pattern of left axis deviation, left ventricular hypertrophy, and right or combined atrial enlargement should suggest the diagnosis of tricuspid atresia. The diagnosis will be confirmed by two-dimensional echocardiography and subsequently by preoperative cineangiocardiograms.

Treatment of tricuspid atresia is primarily with surgical palliation directed at increasing pulmonary blood flow by shunt procedures in patients having serious hypoxemia or at reduction of pulmonary circulation by banding the pulmonary artery in those with excessive flow. Creation of an atrial septal defect surgically or by balloon septostomy may be indicated if the interatrial communication is obstructive. In selected patients the Glenn procedure (anastomosis of right pulmonary artery to superior vena cava) is the operation of choice, although a systemic-to-pulmonary artery shunt may also be used. Recently a procedure directed toward more physiologic correction has been devised (Fontan operation). This technique basically is to connect the pulmonary artery to the right atrium by means of a conduit graft. The atrial septum is closed. The systemic venous return thus bypasses the right ventricle to perfuse the pulmonary circulation. In selected cases this operation has given satisfactory results.

Total anomalous pulmonary venous drainage

All the pulmonary veins in total anomalous pulmonary venous drainage (TAPVD) are connected to the systemic venous circuit instead of to the left atrium. The site of this connection varies, providing a basis for anatomic classification as follows:

- Supracardiac site—connection to the superior vena cava directly or by way of a persistent left vertical vein
- Cardiac site—connection to the right atrium or coronary sinus
- Infracardiac site—connection to the portal vein, ductus venosus, or other subdiaphragmatic site
- Mixed site—combinations of the foregoing

In the commonest type of connection (supracardiac) the pulmonary veins connect to the right heart by way of a persistent left vertical vein, the left innominate vein, and the superior vena cava (Fig. 18-14). The second most common site of connection is into the coronary sinus.

A right-to-left atrial shunt is an integral part of the lesion because pulmonary venous blood must have access to the systemic circulation.

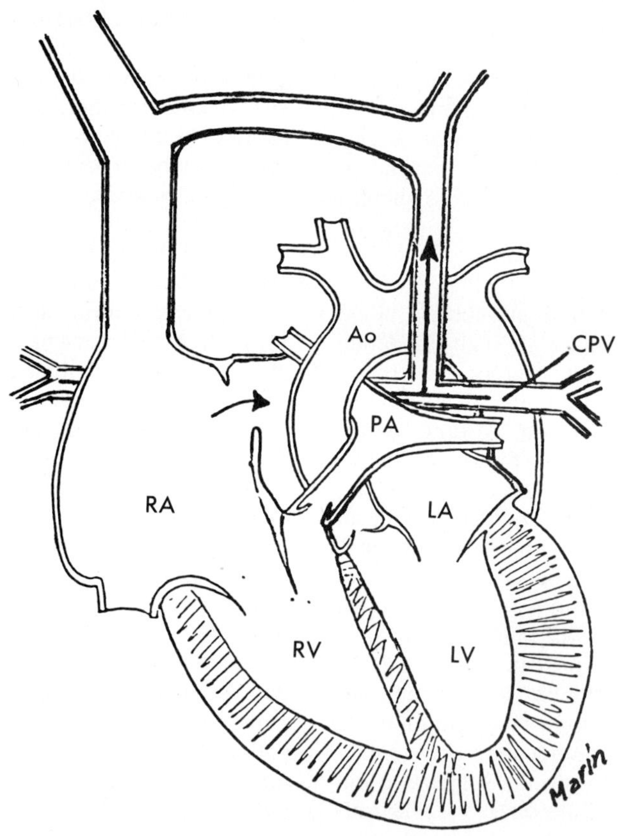

Fig. 18-14. Total anomalous pulmonary venous drainage. *RA*, Right atrium; *RV*, right ventricle; *LA*, left atrium; *LV*, left ventricle; *PA*, pulmonary artery; *Ao*, aorta; *CPV*, common pulmonary vein.

The adequacy of the interatrial communication, the site of drainage, and the presence or absence of pulmonary venous obstruction influence the clinical picture. The latter may be related to the course, length, and size of the common pulmonary venous channel, to stenosis at its site of connection, or to an inadequate interatrial communication.

Three clinical pictures of this disease can be defined. Infants with signs of pulmonary venous obstruction usually have infradiaphragmatic connections and present in the neonatal period with tachypnea and cyanosis unrelieved by oxygen administration. A normal or hyperkinetic right ventricular impulse may be present, and clinical cardiomegaly is not noted. Murmurs are absent or insignificant. The second heart sound is narrowly split, with a loud pulmonic component. Clinical signs of right heart failure are not present initially, although hepatomegaly is frequently noted. The chest radiograph suggests the diagnosis by demonstrating evidence of severe pulmonary venous congestion in the absence of significant cardiac enlargement.

Infants without venous obstruction present slightly later with tachypnea and a cardiac murmur, often with rapid progression to congestive heart failure at 6 to 8 weeks of age. Pulmonary blood flow is excessive, and cyanosis is therefore minimal or absent. The heart is hyperdynamic from volume overwork. The second sound is widely split, with accentuation of the pulmonic component. A pulmonary systolic ejection murmur and a mid-diastolic tricuspid flow rumble are typically present.

Patients with an adequate interatrial communication, absence of pulmonary venous obstruction, and normal pulmonary vascular resistance may present in late infancy, childhood, or adult life with a clinical picture mimicking atrial septal defect. Because of the large pulmonary blood flow, these patients are rarely cyanotic clinically. The chest radiograph may suggest the diagnosis if there is supracardiac drainage because dilation of the vertical vein and superior vena cava may result in a rounded shadow, which combines with the cardiac silhouette to produce a *figure eight,* or *snowman,* configuration. This picture is rarely present before 4 months of age.

All patients with TAPVD have electrocardiographic evidence of right ventricular hypertrophy, usually with a qR pattern in the right chest leads. Right axis deviation and right atrial enlargement are the rule. Cardiac catheterization and angiography are necessary to define the type of anomalous connection and any associated hemodynamic abnormalities.

Infants with pulmonary venous obstruction or early onset of congestive heart failure have a grim prognosis without surgical treatment. Although surgical mortality is high, correction should be attempted during infancy in all these patients. The surgical prognosis in older infants, children, and adults with normal or minimally elevated pulmonary vascular resistance is generally excellent.

Ebstein malformation of the tricuspid valve

Ebstein malformation is an uncommon defect consisting of abnormal attachment and redundancy of the posterior and septal leaflets of the tricuspid valve. The site of attachment of these leaflets appears to be displaced into the right ventricle, away from the true annulus of the valve (Fig. 18-15). The anterior leaflet is attached more or less normally. A portion of the right ventricular myocardium is thus incorporated within the right atrium above the functional (false) tricuspid valve annulus. This "atrialized" right ventricular myocardium is often abnormally thin, sometimes aneurysmal. The tricuspid valve is usually redundant and incompetent and may be severely so; stenosis is less frequent, and atresia has been rarely reported. The right ventricular outflow tract is often underdeveloped, and there is generally an atrial septal defect or patent foramen ovale. Other associated cardiac defects are relatively uncommon.

The clinical spectrum of this lesion is broad, a feature related to the great variability of its anatomy. Symptoms may be absent throughout a normal life span, or death from congestive heart failure may occur in early infancy. Most infants, however, are asymptomatic. Cyanosis may be present early but disappears gradually during the first few weeks or months of life as right-to-left shunting across the atrial septum diminishes with the normal decrease of pulmonary vascular resistance. Subsequent symptoms may be gradual in onset, becoming apparent in later childhood or adolescence. Symp-

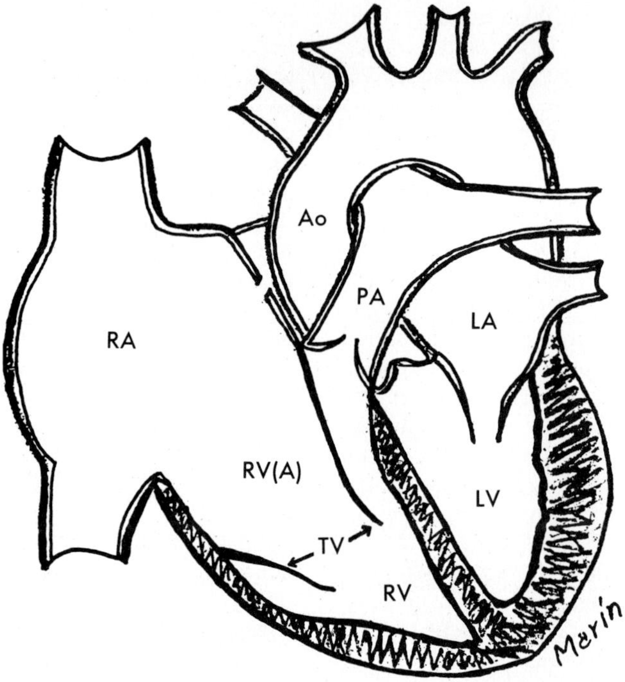

Fig. 18-15. Ebstein malformation of the tricuspid valve. Right atrium, RA; right ventricle, RV; atrialized right ventricle, RV(A); left atrium, LA; left ventricle, LV; pulmonary artery, PA; and aorta, Ao.

toms are generally related to manifestations of right heart failure and to the occurrence of paroxysmal tachyarrhythmias, to which these patients are predisposed. Such paroxysms may result in syncopal attacks.

Cyanosis, usually of mild degree, may be noted at physical examination. A left precordial deformity may be present. The cardiac impulse is generally feeble and diffuse, with a rippling quality from the lower left sternal border to the apex. A systolic thrill may be noted at the left sternal border. There is generally a pansystolic murmur of tricuspid regurgitation in this same area. A scratchy diastolic murmur frequently produces a to-and-fro murmur at this site. A systolic ejection murmur suggesting pulmonary stenosis may also be heard. The heart sounds are notable for the presence of a triple or quadruple rhythm, sometimes associated with a tricuspid opening snap. This complex of sounds is produced by delayed vibrations of the tricuspid valve, a single or narrowly split second sound, and prominent third or fourth heart sounds.

In most cases there is cardiomegaly, which varies from moderate to severe. The right atrium may appear enlarged radiographically, and a prominent bulge high along the left border may be produced by a displaced or dilated right ventricular outflow tract. The size and contour of the cardiac silhouette may at times suggest pericardial effusion. Pulmonary vasculature usually appears reduced. In milder cases the radiograph may demonstrate minimal or no abnormality. The electrocardiogram typically shows a prolonged P-R interval, right atrial enlargement, and a right bundle branch block pattern, with low voltage and polyphasic ventricular complexes in the right precordial leads. P wave amplitude may equal or exceed that of the splintered QRS complexes. Various rhythm and conduction disturbances and ventricular preexcitation (Wolff-Parkinson-White, type B) are commonly seen.

Two-dimensional echocardiography can provide identification of the abnormally displaced tricuspid valve and cardiac catheterization and cineangiocardiography will confirm the diagnosis. The recording of an intracardiac electrocardiogram, with simultaneous pressure waveform during cardiac catheterization, is helpful in confirming the displacement of the tricuspid valve. Angiocardiography is useful in demonstrating the abnormal position of the tricuspid valve with tricuspid regurgitation, the abnormal and paradoxical motion of the atrialized portion of the right ventricular myocardium, intracardiac shunting across the atrial septum, and possibly associated defects.

The course and prognosis for this lesion are variable. Occasionally deaths occur in infancy and childhood, but patients with typical clinical features often survive until the third or fourth decade. Death usually results from congestive heart failure, although fatal dysrhythmia may occur. Tricuspid valve replacement is the surgical procedure of choice for the severely symptomatic patient, but it should be reserved only for those whose condition is refractory to intensive medical management. Symptomatic cyanotic patients without congestive heart failure may benefit from a superior vena cava–pulmonary artery anastomosis.

PRIMARY ENDOMYOCARDIAL DISEASES

Primary endomyocardial diseases comprise a heterogenous group of disorders that includes a large number of congenital, inflammatory, metabolic, and idiopathic cardiac abnormalities with similar clinical manifestations. They have in common decreased myocardial contractility in the absence of significant anatomic abnormalities.

Children having primary endomyocardial diseases usually present in infancy or early childhood with congestive heart failure, unexplained cardiomegaly, failure to thrive, or rhythm disturbances. Because cardiac failure in this group of diseases is predominantly left ventricular failure, an initial impression of bronchiolitis, pneumonia, or other respiratory disorders is not uncommon. Respiratory tract infections may also complicate or antedate the onset of cardiac failure. Atelectasis of the left lower lobe is a frequent complication of the massive cardiac enlargement often seen in these patients.

Tachypnea and tachycardia are the principal presenting manifestations. The precordium may be hyperdynamic or quiet, depending on the type of abnormality, with a dominant left ventricular impulse. The first heart sound is normal to diminished in intensity and often introduces a soft, high-pitched murmur of mitral regurgitation. Pulmonary hypertension caused by left ventricular failure may lead to accentuation of the second heart sound. Gallop sounds are generally noted, but diastolic murmurs are uncommon. Respiratory distress with rales or wheezing is noted in most patients. Hepatomegaly and edema may be seen if right ventricular failure has supervened.

In most cases of primary endomyocardial disease the electrocardiogram shows left ventricular hypertrophy, frequently with left atrial enlargement. Rhythm disturbances, low voltage, and nonspecific S-T segment and T wave abnormalities are common, particularly in patients with myocarditis. The chest radiograph usually demonstrates generalized cardiac enlargement associated with varying degrees of pulmonary venous congestion.

The most important disorders in this group of diseases are endocardial fibroelastosis, idiopathic cardiomyopathy, acute myocarditis, and anomalous origin of the left coronary artery from the pulmonary artery.

Endocardial fibroelastosis

Endocardial fibroelastosis (EFE) is a disease of uncertain etiology characterized by fibroelastic thickening of the endocardium, especially of the left heart chambers. It may occur in the absence of coexisting cardiac malformations (primary EFE) or in association with congenital cardiac defects (secondary EFE). The latter group includes patients with obstructive lesions of the left heart (coarctation of the aorta, aortic stenosis, hypoplastic left heart syndrome) and patients with anomalous origin of the left coronary artery from the pulmonary artery. When the disorder occurs in siblings, the pattern of inheritance is inconstant.

The pathology consists of an abnormal proliferation of fibroelastic tissue in and beneath the endocardium, with extension of fibrous bands into the myocardium. The papillary muscle and chordae become embedded in this process, resulting in distortion of the mitral valve apparatus. Aortic valve and right heart involvement occur less commonly. Microscopically there is evidence of a perivascular inflammatory

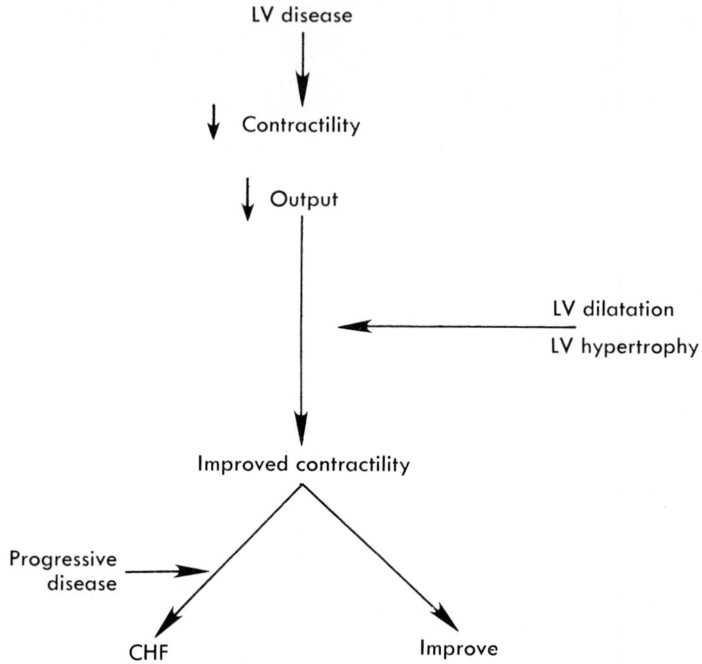

Fig. 18-16. Pathophysiology of endomyocardial disease. (From Anthony, C.L., et al.: Pediatric cardiology, Medical Outline Series, Flushing, N.Y., 1979, Medical Examination Publishing Co., Inc.)

process, with areas of fibrosis and muscle necrosis. The cause of this disease is not clear. One current theory is that this represents an intrauterine pancarditis related to coxsackie B virus infection. The diffuse left ventricular myocardial disease results in diminished left ventricular contractility, which leads to hypertrophy and dilation (Fig. 18-16). Volume overloading secondary to mitral regurgitation contributes only minimally to the dilated, poorly contracting left ventricle with diminished stroke volume and decreased cardiac output.

Physical examination and radiographic findings do not permit differentiation of EFE from other disorders in the primary endomyocardial disease group. The electrocardiogram characteristically shows severe left ventricular hypertrophy, often with a *strain* pattern. Deep Q waves are frequently seen in leads I, aVL, aVF, and V_5 and V_6. Patterns suggesting myocardial infarction have also been reported. In contrast to acute myocarditis, low voltage conduction disturbances and dysrhythmias are uncommon. The electrocardiographic pattern is highly suggestive of the diagnosis of EFE, especially when seen in the context of severe heart failure in an infant less than 6 months old who has no findings of congenital heart disease. The chest radiograph shows massive enlargement of the cardiac silhouette mainly attributed to left atrial and left ventricular dilation. Evidence of left heart failure, such as wet fissures and interstitial edema, is usually present (Fig. 18-17). Cardiac catheterization and angiocardiography may be necessary to exclude anomalous origin of the left coronary artery from the pulmonary artery.

Treatment of EFE is the management of congestive heart failure as outlined in the previous section. Digoxin is the cornerstone on which this therapeutic program is built, and prompt careful digitalization has significantly improved the outcome, especially as far as early mortality is concerned. The clinical course after initiation of appropriate therapy is extremely varied and difficult to predict. We have seen patients whose failure was so fulminant as to result in death within 12 hours of the onset of symptoms despite vigorous treatment. A small

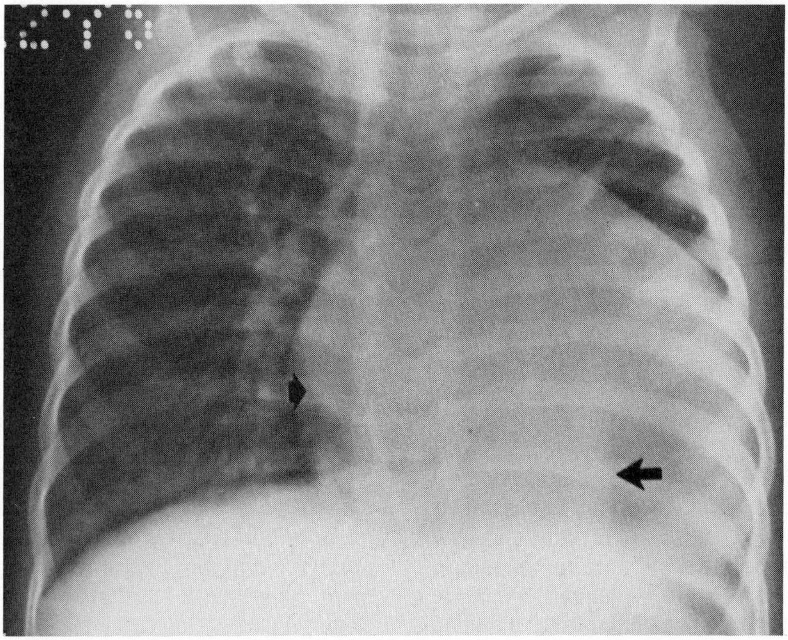

Fig. 18-17. Three-month-old with endocardial fibroelastosis. There is diffuse cardiomegaly with evidence of left atrial enlargement *(small arrow)* and left lower lobe atelectasis *(large arrow)*. Pulmonary vascular markings are hazy, suggestive of pulmonary edema. (From Anthony, C.L., et al.: Pediatric cardiology, Medical Outline Series, Flushing, N.Y., 1979, Medical Examination Publishing Co., Inc.)

but significant number of patients may show rapid improvement on therapy, then 5 to 10 years later may show no signs whatever of cardiac malfunction even when evaluated by such relatively sophisticated modalities as echocardiography and exercise testing. The majority of patients, however, seem to improve somewhat initially but retain considerable cardiomegaly and evidence of left ventricular dysfunction, thereby following a course consistent with a chronic cardiomyopathy. Occasionally, such a patient may progress to apparent clinical recovery, but the majority eventually show deterioration and death in either childhood or adolescence. The reason for the wide spectrum of clinical courses is not clear; neither is it clear whether EFE is one single disease or rather a group of distinct but closely related clinical entities. Perhaps the best prognostic indicator is the degree of improvement in congestive failure and cardiac size after initial digitalization. Although the use of diuretics can be initiated or discontinued as clinically indicated, digoxin is continued for many years, as premature discontinuation may result in recurrence of congestive failure, which at that point may be unremitting and unresponsive to further intervention. Digoxin should be continued at least until all manifestations of myocardial dysfunction have completely disappeared.

An uncommon form of EFE results in a small contracted left ventricle. In these patients the clinical presentation is pulmonary venous congestion with right ventricular hypertrophy. Heart size and configuration are often normal radiographically. The differential diagnosis of this form of the disease principally includes obstructive lesions of the left atrium and pulmonary veins.

Idiopathic cardiomyopathy

The term *idiopathic cardiomyopathy* clearly includes a heterogeneous group of entities having in common the presence of myocardial dysfunction. These are all diseases seen more commonly in adults, and in the pediatric age group are for the most part restricted to later childhood and adolescence. There are many ways of classifying the idiopathic cardiomyopathies, and a detailed discussion is beyond the scope of this presentation. Perhaps the easiest way to look at this group is to consider that most forms can be classified as either dilated (or congestive) or hypertrophic. Idiopathic congestive cardiomyopathy presents in a manner virtually identical to EFE but at a much later stage of life. The clinical manifestations are the same; at times, differentiation from myocarditis may be difficult and there is considerable overlap between these groups. Those patients classified as having idiopathic congestive cardiomyopathy typically demonstrate severe left ventricular hypertrophy on the electrocardiogram, a phenomenon not generally seen in myocarditis. Sporadic cases exist, and this type of presentation may also secondarily accompany some of the generalized systemic diseases, such as Duchenne muscular dystrophy. There is also a definite familial incidence, with autosomal dominant inheritance. It appears that the course may be far more fulminant in the familial form. Treatment modalities employed have also been previously discussed under EFE. If clinical condition deteriorates despite vigorous medical therapy, myocardial biopsy may be considered, as a few such patients show evidence of chronic myocardial inflammation and may respond to therapy with steroids and immunosuppressive agents. For the most part the clinical course is unfavorable, with gradual deterioration.

Hypertrophic cardiomyopathy is a genetically transmitted disease of the heart muscle, characterized by disproportionate thickening of the septum compared with the left ventricular wall. It is more common in adults but has been reported as early as the neonatal period. The clinical manifestations are variable and relate to the presence or absence of left ventricular outflow obstruction. In patients in whom outflow obstruction is absent, there are bizarre hypertrophied muscle cells throughout the myocardium, whereas these cells are limited to the ventricular septum in the obstructive form of the disease. In the obstructive form there is midsystolic and late systolic obstruction of the left ventricular outflow tract caused by abnormal mitral valve motion or outflow tract hypertrophy.

There is considerable disagreement among investigators in this field as to whether the outflow tract obstruction is the primary hemodynamic alteration or whether it is simply the result of disordered ventricular contraction. There is a considerable body of evidence indicating that many, if not most, of the manifestations may result from abnormal diastolic function, that is, poor ventricular compliance with abnormally high left ventricular filling pressure.

The usual presenting symptoms are fatigue, palpitations, and effort dyspnea. Syncope and angina pectoris may also occur, but congestive heart failure is a less frequent and usually late manifestation. A familial history of sudden death is sometimes elicited. Physical signs may include pulsus bisferiens, a prominent fourth heart sound, a double apical impulse, and an apical or lower left sternal border systolic ejection murmur that is accentuated by the Valsalva maneuver. A superimposed mitral regurgitant murmur may also be heard. Clinical and radiographic evidence of significant cardiac enlargement occurs only late in the course of the disease.

Electrocardiographic changes are similar to those seen in endocardial fibroelastosis. The Wolff-Parkinson-White syndrome is often present in familial cases.

Inotropic agents are contraindicated in patients with obstructive cardiomyopathy because they may aggravate the outflow obstruction. Some patients with the obstructive form of the disease do respond to therapy with beta-adrenergic blocking agents, which reduce or abolish the outflow obstruction by decreasing the intensity of muscular contraction. Calcium channel blockers, such as verapamil, also decrease myocardial contractility and have been used in a limited number of cases; there is some evidence to suggest that diastolic function may also be improved. Arrhythmias, particularly ventricular ectopy, are frequently present. Beta-adrenergic blockade may produce improvement, but when such an approach is unsuccessful, other antiarrhythmic agents may be tried. The general prognosis in this group of patients is also unfavorable. Surgical treatment of obstructive cardiomyopathy has had variable success and should be attempted only in patients who fail to respond to intensive medical treatment.

In the nonobstructive form of hypertrophic cardiomyopathy, the patient may present with manifestations of congestive failure resembling dilated cardiomyopathy or alternatively may simply show cardiomegaly with ventricular arrhythmias. Antiarrhythmic therapy is used when indicated; control of other manifestations would depend on a careful evaluation of whether the myocardial dysfunction is primarily systolic or diastolic.

Acute myocarditis

Acute myocarditis is an inflammatory disease of the heart, characterized pathologically by interstitial infiltrations of lymphocytes, plasma cells, and occasionally polymorphonuclear leukocytes. Varying degrees of interstitial edema and myocardial necrosis are also noted. Grossly, the heart is dilated and pale, but it may appear normal in isolated cases. Coxsackie B viruses are the cause of most instances of myocarditis in children and may be responsible for a syndrome of encephalitis, hepatitis, and myocarditis in the neonate. Most of the other common viruses have also been identified as causative agents of myocarditis in at least a few cases. Other rarer types of myocarditis include toxic myocarditis caused by diphtheria endotoxin or chemotherapeutic agents such as doxorubicin hydrochloride (Adriamycin); myocarditis caused by bacteria, fungi, and parasites; and myocarditis of the various multisystem diseases.

Acute myocarditis is one cause of sudden unexplained death in infancy. In the typical patient, however, respiratory illness, low-grade fever, cough, and tachypnea are the principal manifestations. Also, poor heart tones are characteristic. Congestive heart failure is identified by the presence of tachycardia, gallop rhythm, pulmonary congestion, hepatomegaly, and occasionally peripheral edema. Cardiogenic shock may be present. The electrocardiogram usually shows only low voltage, sinus tachycardia, nonspecific S-T segment, and T-wave abnormalities. Arrhythmias and conduction abnormalities, including complete heart block, are also seen. Chest radiographs demonstrate diffuse cardiac enlargement with evidence of pulmonary venous congestion.

Treatment of acute myocarditis is directed toward control of congestive cardiac failure and arrhythmias, as well as reversal of cardiogenic shock, if present. Digitalization should be accomplished cautiously because some patients show increased sensitivity to cardiac glycosides. Oxygen, morphine, and intravenously administered diuretics are frequently indicated. Arrhythmias should be controlled with appropriate pharmacologic agents, and transvenous pacing should be promptly instituted in the presence of complete heart block. Monitoring of the central venous or pulmonary wedge pressure is mandatory in patients with cardiogenic shock.

The response to therapy is variable and probably dependent on the extent of myocardial necrosis. Most patients improve with careful medical management, although convalescence is prolonged for some, and all require long-term digitalis therapy. Some children die after a rapidly or relentlessly deteriorating clinical course. Cardiogenic shock and complete heart block are particularly ominous signs but do not preclude complete recovery. After recovery the electrocardiogram and chest radiograph usually return to normal, and the patient shows no signs of residual cardiac dysfunction. Even children with complete atrioventricular block during the acute illness may show a return to normal sinus rhythm and normal atrioventricular conduction.

Anomalous origin of the left coronary artery

Anomalous origin of the left coronary artery from the pulmonary trunk is relatively uncommon. When it occurs, the right coronary artery system has a normal aortic origin and distribution. The basic physiologic handicap in this anomaly is inadequate perfusion pressure in the left coronary artery. Of relatively minor significance is the lower level of oxygen saturation in that vessel.

During fetal life equal pressures and oxygen saturations in the pulmonary artery and aorta ensure adequate perfusion of the left ventricular myocardium. Postnatally the normal reduction in pulmonary arterial pressure results in a pressure insufficient to overcome left ventricular intramyocardial resistance. Maintenance of adequate myocardial blood flow then becomes dependent on development of intercoronary anastomosis, which permits retrograde perfusion of the left coronary artery from the right. The direction of flow is thus from the aorta to the pulmonary artery by way of the coronary system. Although uncommon, the anomaly is important because it enters into the differential diagnosis of the primary endomyocardial diseases and because a surgical approach is feasible.

Symptoms usually appear in the infant between 2 and 6 months of age. Episodes of fretfulness, pallor, diaphoresis, tachycardia, and tachypnea may represent anginal attacks. They are often precipitated by the exertion of feeding, and a history of poor dietary intake is common. The irritability and discomfort associated with feeding may lead to the erroneous diagnosis of colic. Between such episodes the infant may appear well. Other infants or older children present with unexplained cardiomegaly or cardiac murmurs. Infants may also present with respiratory symptoms such as tachypnea, wheezing, and dyspnea as manifestations of left ventricular failure.

Physical examination usually reveals a laterally displaced apical impulse, but the precordium may not be hyperdynamic. Murmurs are more common in older patients than in infants. The most characteristic type is a pansystolic murmur of mitral insufficiency related to papillary muscle dysfunction or superimposed endocardial fibroelastosis. Less commonly, one hears a continuous murmur related to the presence of extensive collateral flow shunting into the pulmonary artery.

Generalized cardiomegaly is noted radiographically. Pulmonary vascularity is usually normal. At times a localized bulge of the left ventricle may be noted. The electrocardiogram and vectorcardiogram are extremely helpful in diagnosis, showing a pattern of anterior or anterolateral myocardial infarction. Diagnosis is established with certainty only by cardiac catheterization and angiocardiography. The latter demonstrates only a large single right coronary artery arising from the aortic root, with extensive collateral flow and retrograde filling of the left coronary artery system and pulmonary artery. In patients with inadequate collateral flow, injection of contrast into the main pulmonary artery may permit visualization of the origin of the left coronary artery.

The clinical course is variable. Symptomatic infants with inadequate collateral flow have angina-like attacks and early onset of congestive heart failure, generally pursuing a rather stormy course that terminates in early death. Patients with more abundant collateral flow present in later infancy or childhood with minimal or no symptoms. An intermediate course is followed by some patients.

Medical treatment of congestive heart failure should be vigorous. When cardiac catheterization demonstrates the presence of adequate intercoronary collaterals with retrograde filling of the left coronary system, a conservative approach may be adopted, at least initially, if there is significant improvement in ventricular function and freedom from signs of on-going myocardial ischemia. The long-term prognosis, however, is generally unfavorable and there have been several reports in the literature of sudden death even in completely asymptomatic adults who are not previously known to have the anomaly. For this reason, the treatment of anomalous origin of the left coronary artery from the pulmonary artery is ultimately surgical. There have been several approaches, including direct replantation of the left coronary into the ascending aorta, creation of an aorticopulmonary window together with creation of an intrapulmonary arterial tunnel between the window and the left coronary artery, and end-to-end anastomosis of the left coronary artery and left subclavian artery. Early surgical intervention is mandatory in the presence of persistent left ventricular dysfunction and in infants with poor collaterals who have evidence of significant ischemia. Surgical mortality is high in the latter group, but mortality with medical management alone approaches 100%. Long-term data dealing with the effect of early surgery on ultimate myocardial performance are lacking.

ACUTE RHEUMATIC FEVER

Acute rheumatic fever (ARF) is one of the most important systemic inflammatory diseases of the pediatric age group. Although its exact pathogenesis remains uncertain, its relationship to antecedent infection with certain strains of group A beta hemolytic streptococcus ("throat strains") has been clearly established. In about one half of the clinically recognized instances a history of such an infection is elicited, and precedes the symptoms of ARF by a period of 2 to 3 weeks. Fortunately, less than 0.5% of children with an untreated streptococcal infection will develop clinical ARF, although the attack rate may be considerably higher (2% to 3%) during epidemics of streptococcal disease in closed military populations. ARF has the same age-incidence epidemiologic curve as does scarlet fever, the classic streptococcal disease of childhood. The disease is most prevalent among schoolchildren, with its peak incidence at 6 or 7 years of age. It rarely occurs during the first 2 years of life and is uncommonly seen before 5 years or after 25 years of age.

It is currently accepted that rheumatic fever represents a peculiar host response to *Streptococcus*. The M protein (*Streptococcus* M antigen) present in the cell capsule crossreacts with human myocardium and was therefore thought to be the causative agent. However, ultrapurified M protein does not seem to cause host sensitivity.

The pathognomonic lesion of rheumatic fever is the Aschoff body. Detailed investigation of this lesion since its first description in 1904, however, has not clarified its relationship to rheumatic activity.

The acute illness may take the form of a mild respiratory or systemic infection, or it may present the cardinal features of the disease. In the former case the diagnosis cannot be established, and an acute attack of rheumatic fever can only be inferred after the diagnosis of chronic rheumatic valvular disease in later childhood, adolescence, or adult life.

The revised and modified criteria of T. Duckett Jones serve as the most useful guideline for the diagnosis of ARF at any age. Various clinical and laboratory manifestations of the disease have been classified as major and minor manifestations and serve as the foundation for the diagnosis of ARF in the appropriate clinical situation.

Major manifestations
- Polyarthritis
- Carditis
- Chorea
- Subcutaneous nodules
- Erythema marginatum

Minor manifestations
- Clinical
  - Fever
  - Arthralgia
  - Previous rheumatic fever or rheumatic heart disease
- Laboratory
  - Acute phase reactants: erythrocyte sedimentation rate, C-reactive protein, leukocytosis
  - Prolonged P-R interval

Plus supporting evidence of preceding streptococcal infection, with the exception of patients presenting with smouldering carditis or chorea

With these guidelines one may entertain the diagnosis of possible ARF if the patient's illness presents two major criteria or one major and two minor criteria, along with substantial evidence of a recent, antecedent group A beta hemolytic streptococcal infection. The latter may be absent in patients having Sydenham's chorea or long-standing carditis because of the remote nature of the streptococcal infection. It should be emphasized that the modified Jones criteria are merely a guideline to diagnosis. Fulfillment of these cirteria neither includes all cases of acute rheumatic fever nor excludes all other diagnoses. A patient may, for example, present with migratory polyarthritis, fever, elevated sedimentation rate, and a high antistreptolysin O (ASO) titer, only to be proved to have juvenile rheumatoid arthritis associated with a recent, and incidental, streptococcal infection. Viral myocarditis and a host of other diseases may similarly fulfill the Jones criteria, yet not be ARF. To further confuse the issue, as noted earlier, ARF may occur in a subclinical form or may present as a minor illness, perhaps merely with arthralgia.

Major manifestations. *Migratory polyarthritis* is the classic presenting symptom of acute rheumatic fever. The joints are exquisitely tender, perhaps more so than in any illness other than acute septic arthritis. The knees, ankles, elbows, and wrists are characteristically affected. Several joints are involved simultaneously or in succession, and the involvement is typically asymmetric. The hips and shoulders are less commonly involved, and the small joints of the extremities, neck, and back as well as the temporomandibular joints are rarely affected. In spite of its apparent severity, the arthritis of ARF is self-limiting and does not result in permanent joint dysfunction. There appears to be some degree of inverse relationship between severity of the arthritis and extent of the cardiac involvement. Arthralgia is a minor manifestation no matter how many joints are affected.

Acute rheumatic *carditis* is an inflammatory process that involves all layers of the heart. Myocarditis is noted but with somewhat less of an inflammatory reaction than is seen in the usual case of infectious myocarditis. Pericarditis is common, although significant pericardial effusion occurs infrequently. The classic endocardial lesion is the MacCallum patch, seen in the left atrium at the base of the posterior mitral leaflet. The valves may be involved by an inflammatory reaction of both leaflets and chordae tendineae, affecting mitral and aortic valves most frequently. Tricuspid involvement is uncommon, and pulmonary valvulitis extremely rare. Scarring with valve stenosis does not occur acutely. The acute disease is nearly always associated with a significant cardiac murmur.

Other manifestations of carditis, which may occur alone or in combination with a significant murmur, are unequivocal cardiac enlargement in a person without previously known heart disease, pericarditis, or congestive heart failure appearing de novo and with no other clearly identifiable cause. The cardiac murmurs associated with ARF are the apical high-pitched pansystolic murmur of mitral regurgitation, the basal blowing decrescendo diastolic murmur of aortic regurgitation, and the early and mid-diastolic apical rumble associated with acute valvulitis or large volume regurgitation (Carey-Coombs murmur). The murmur of mitral insufficiency generally appears early in the course of the disease, but may be delayed until the second or third week. If mitral insufficiency is severe, the Carey-Coombs murmur is soon detectable and indicates a less favorable prognosis from the standpoint of residual heart disease. The murmur of aortic insufficiency may also occur early in the course of the acute illness, with or without signs of associated mitral disease.

In a person with preexisting rheumatic heart disease, the appearance of a new significant murmur or a significant change in a previously noted murmur is an important finding.

Long-term follow-up evaluation reveals that the murmur of mitral regurgitation eventually disappears in more than 60% of patients if it is the only murmur noted during the acute illness. Aortic insufficiency generally indicates a more severe carditis in which the eventual disappearance of this murmur is less common. The healing of the valves occurs only if there are no recurrences of the disease.

Sydenham chorea is almost pathognomonic of rheumatic fever. It may also be seen in a benign familial form and has been reported as an occasional complication of Henoch-Schönlein purpura, systemic lupus erythematosis, and several other uncommon diseases. This acute neurologic disturbance is most often seen in the preadolescent female. It is characterized by the gradual or abrupt appearance of involuntary purposeless movements involving all parts of the body. Emotional lability is a common accompaniment and may be the presenting symptom. Dysarthria, severe gait disturbances, and deterioration of handwriting are characteristic. Hemichorea occurs occasionally. In the more severe cases the patient may be bedfast and may require restraint or protective measures to prevent body harm. The purposeless movements disappear with sleep.

Rheumatic *subcutaneous nodules* are uncommonly seen, but when they occur, they generally indicate severe carditis. They are freely movable, nontender lesions that are symmetrically localized over bony prominences such as the occiput and the extensor surfaces of the extremities, usually of the elbows.

Erythema marginatum is a macular, circinate, erythematous rash that involves the trunk and proximal portions of the extremities but spares the face. Although nonspecific for rheumatic fever, it is most commonly seen in association with this disease. It is rarely, if ever, the sole major manifestation of ARF. It generally appears late in the course of the acute episode and may occur intermittently over a period of many months, in which case its appearance and disappearance cannot be correlated with other signs of rheumatic activity.

Minor manifestations. The minor manifestations of rheumatic fever are subdivided into clinical and laboratory manifestations.

Clinical manifestations include a history of rheumatic fever or the presence of preexisting rheumatic heart disease, arthralgia, and fever. A history of rheumatic fever should be well documented, and the evidence of preexisting heart disease should be unequivocal. Arthralgia may be considered a minor manifestation only in patients without arthritis. Fever is defined as a rectal temperature in excess of 38° C (100.4° F) occurring at least twice in a 24-hour period.

Laboratory manifestations include elevation of acute phase reactants, which provide confirmatory evidence of a nonspecific inflammatory reaction; leukocytosis, which is also nonspecific; and prolongation of the P-R interval. The latter should not be considered evidence of carditis because it has been clearly documented in patients without acute or long-term cardiac involvement and because it may, in some cases, be totally unrelated to the rheumatic process.

In recent years studies of the body's immunologic response in acute rheumatic fever have demonstrated some very interesting findings. Although not considered as part of the Jones criteria, heart-reactive antibodies have been found in the majority of patients with acute rheumatic carditis. In some large series there have been no instances of false positive findings. These antibodies differ from heart-reactive antibodies that are seen in other conditions such as postpericardiotomy syndrome by virtue of the fact that the antibodies present in acute rheumatic fever may be absorbed both by cardiac sarcolemmal sheaths and streptococcal cell membranes. Antineuronal antibodies have been demonstrated in nearly half of patients with rheumatic chorea. Antibodies against valvular glycoproteins have also been detected. Heart-reactive antibodies may be particularly useful in the uncertain case.

Other clinical features of acute rheumatic fever that are not considered major or minor manifestations of the disease include abdominal pain, tachycardia, malaise, anemia, and epistaxis. Some patients may show episodes of sinus bradycardia in the second or third week of illness.

Evidence of streptococcal infection. The most reliable evidence of an antecedent streptococcal infection is an elevated, or preferably rising, streptococcal antibody titer. The ASO titer is most commonly used. A single titer of 333 Todd units, or a titer rising by two or more tube dilutions, is generally considered significant. Antihyaluronidase, antideoxyribonuclease B, and antistreptokinase titers are available in specialized laboratories and may be used when the ASO titer is nondiagnostic (15% to 20% of cases). Recently, a rapid slide test that detects antibodies to all five streptococcal antigens has become available and is more reliable. As a rule, when the streptozyme titer is less than 1:150, the ASO Todd units are less than 250. A well-documented history of recent scarlet fever is considered acceptable evidence of preceding streptococcal infection. A positive throat culture for group A beta hemolytic streptococcus is helpful but not diagnostic because of the presence of a streptococcal carrier state in some persons.

Treatment. There is no well-documented evidence that drug treatment of any type in any way alters the long-term prognosis of rheumatic fever. Several well-controlled studies have shown no statistical difference in the incidence of residual heart disease in patients receiving salicylates or adrenal corticosteroids in varying dosages for varying periods of time or no medication at all. However, there is evidence that steroids may favorably affect the acute cardiac complications of ARF and that they may be lifesaving in some patients.

All patients with reasonably well-documented attacks of ARF should be placed at bed rest, and a program of gradual mobilization should precede the resumption of unrestricted physical activity. This traditional approach is based on the assumption that there is some relationship between the workload imposed on an inflamed heart and the development and degree of residual cardiac damage. The absence of clear evidence of such a relationship and the difficulty encountered in determining when the acute inflammatory process has actually subsided makes determination of the duration of these stages difficult and at times arbitrary. The interval of bed rest may be as short as 2 weeks in the patient without carditis and as long as 3 to 6 months in the patient with evidence of severe carditis.

Anti-inflammatory agents are generally indicated in the acute stage for relief of symptoms and lysis of fever. In the absence of clinical carditis or in mild carditis without cardiomegaly, aspirin is used in a dose of 100 mg/kg/24 hr for the first 48 hours, with reduction to 60 to 75 mg/kg/24 hr thereafter. Aspirin therapy should be monitored by salicylate levels, striving for a blood level of 20 to 25 mg/dl. Treatment should be continued for 2 to 4 weeks in patients without carditis and for 6 to 8 weeks in those with mild carditis. The patient having severe carditis and cardiomegaly, with or without congestive heart failure, should receive prednisone in a dose of 2 mg/kg/24 hr for a period of 2 to 4 weeks. During the last week of prednisone therapy, administration of salicylates is begun as steroids are tapered and is continued for 6 to 12 weeks, depending on the severity of involvement and the response.

There is a dramatic lysis of fever and disappearance of joint inflammation after institution of anti-inflammatory therapy—to such a great extent that a *therapeutic trial* of aspirin may help to influence the physician's diagnosis in borderline cases. The patient who has mild carditis and no arthritic manifestations or fever does not require any medication. This is based on the evidence that treatment during the acute phase of the disease does not affect the ultimate outcome of residual heart disease. The response to therapy merely reflects suppression of the disease manifestations, and treatment does not shorten the clinical course when compared to the untreated attack. It is suggested that suppressive therapy may, in fact, slightly prolong the total duration of the acute illness.

Rebounds occur sometimes after reduction or discontinuation of anti-inflammatory therapy. These consist of a recurrence of clinical or laboratory signs of rheumatic activity, which may be mild or severe, depending on the severity of the initial attack and the abruptness of discontinuation or reduction of therapy. The exact mechanism of production of these rebounds is uncertain, but it is clear that they are not recurrences of ARF. Mild rebounds subside spontaneously; more severe rebounds respond to reinstitution of salicylate therapy.

Prevention of recurrences. Once affected, the patient seems predisposed to recurrent episodes of rheumatic fever. Of greatest importance in determining this predisposition are the proximity of the most recent acute attack, the age of the patient, the severity of cardiac involvement, and the number of previous attacks. At greatest risk is the young child with a recent, recurrent attack of rheumatic fever who has severe cardiac involvement. At least risk is the adult patient with a remote single attack and no evidence of cardiac involvement. Recurrent attacks tend to be mimetic in approximately two thirds of cases. Thus a patient without carditis in the initial attack will probably not have carditis if rheumatic fever recurs. However, since this mimetic feature of the disease is not invariable, it should not influence the physician's approach to prophylaxis.

Prevention of recurrent attacks of rheumatic fever is achieved by the regular administration of prophylactic penicillin. The perferred form of therapy is intramuscular benzathine penicillin G, 900,000 or 1.2 million units every 28 days, depending on the patient's weight. Alternatively, penicillin V or G may be administered orally in a dose of 125 mg twice daily. Oral sulfadiazine is the preferred method of prophylaxis in those patients who are allergic to pencillin. It is given in a dose of 250 mg twice daily in patients weighing less than 27 kg (60 pounds) and 500 mg twice daily in those weighing more than 27kg. Erythromycin may be used by patients who are sensitive to both penicillin and sulfadiazine. It must be emphasized however, that parenteral medication is definitely superior in preventing recurrences of the disease.

On the basis of current knowledge, continuous prophylaxis should be used throughout the childhood years, probably well into adult life. Exceptions must never be made for persons at high risk of exposure to streptococcal infections, such as young children or parents of young children, nurses, schoolteachers, and military personnel. When indicated, additional prophylaxis should be used for prevention of infective endocarditis.

PERICARDITIS

Pericarditis is uncommon as a primary disease in childhood. Its occurrence should alert the pediatrician to the possible presence of a systemic illness. In the past a vast majority of cases of pericarditis were a result of acute rheumatic fever. This is probably not true in recent years with the declining incidence of that disease. Other common etiologic causes are (1) pyogenic infection, (2) acute viral pericarditis, (3) rheumatoid arthritis, (4) lupus erythematosus, and (5) uremia. Less common causes are tuberculosis, histoplasmosis, and constrictive pericarditis.

Physiology. Pericardial tamponade is the major clinical feature of acute pericarditis because compression of the heart by pericardial fluid compromises cardiac filling and eventually cardiac output. Impairment of diastolic filling leads to compensatory elevation of systemic and pulmonary venous pressures and to increasing tachycardia. If restriction to diastolic filling progresses because of increasing intrapericardial pressure, these compensatory mechanisms eventually fail, and signs of cardiac decompensation ensue. Further impairment of function results in a progressive hypotension, syncope, and eventually death. Similar extrinsic cardiac compression by fibrosis is present with constrictive pericarditis, although it is a more slowly progressive mechanism. The signs most commonly identified with pericardial tamponade, such as increased venous pressure, increased pulse rate, and narrow pulse pressure, are compensatory mechanisms and should not be "corrected." For this reason the sole effective treatment of pericardial tamponade, or constriction, is removal of the effusion by pericardiocentesis, surgical drainage, or removal of the membrane by pericardiectomy. The administration of cardiac glycosides is contraindicated in pericarditis because slowing of the heart rate may remove the patient's sole effective means of maintaining cardiac output.

Clinical picture. Chest pain, the characteristic clinical symptom of pericarditis, is seldom seen in children. When present, however, it is typically severe and is often aggravated by movement and respiration. It is also exaggerated by lying down and relieved by sitting up. This is probably a result of involvement of the diaphragm and pleura because there are no sensory nerves in the pericardium proper. Fever is commonly present as a nonspecific sign. Attention is usually drawn to the pericardium as the possible site of inflammatory disease by the discovery of a pericardial friction rub or by the presence of an enlarged cardiac silhouette on the chest radiograph.

The pericardial friction rub is not limited to any part of the cardiac cycle and may be evanescent. Cardiac tamponade manifests itself in distention of the neck veins, enlarged liver, and a tachypneic and anxious-looking patient. The systolic blood pressure is low, with a low pulse pressure. Pulsus paradoxus is usually present and consists of a drop in systolic pressure of more than 10 mmHg at the end of deep inspiration. The recognition of pericardial tamponade constitutes a medical emergency.

When sizable pericardial effusion is present, it manifests itself in the chest radiograph by an enlarged cardiac silhouette, the so-called water bottle shape. The diagnosis is confirmed by the demonstration of pericardial effusion by noninvasive techniques (echocardiogram, cardiac scan) and by the occurrence of typical electrocardiographic changes consisting of diffuse S-T segment elevation early, followed by T-wave inversion. Aspiration of the pericardium (pericardiocentesis) should be performed only after the presence of an effusion has been confirmed, except in immediately life-threatening situations.

Specific pericardial disease entities. As previously mentioned, acute rheumatic fever is the most common cause of pericarditis in children. It is invariably accompanied by other manifestations of acute rheumatic fever and evidence of pericarditis. Steroid treatment and decongestive measures are mandatory.

In this era of open heart surgery a common and perhaps most readily recognized form of pericarditis is that associated with the postpericardiotomy syndrome. This complication of cardiac surgery or pericardial trauma is apparently an autoimmune response to myocardial injury, with evidence of high titers of antiheart antibodies. Postoperative fever, chest pain, pericardial effusion, pleural effusion, and water retention are the cardinal manifestations of the disease. Electrocardiographic changes and a pericardial friction rub are less helpful in the diagnosis because they are present in many postsurgical patients. Pericardial tamponade may occur in the course of the disease but is uncommon. The syndrome is self-limiting but may be recurrent. Patients usually respond promptly to therapeutic doses of aspirin and diuretics.

The most serious form of pericarditis in the pediatric patient is septic, or purulent, pericarditis. It may be seen in any age group but occurs most frequently in children less than 2 years of age. The usual infecting agents are *Staphylococcus aureus,* group B *Haemophilus influenzae,* and the meningococcus. This is a particularly treacherous illness because pyogenic infection of the pericardium almost invariably occurs as a complication of a more evident serious infection, for example, pneumonia, meningitis, osteomyelitis, or overwhelming sepsis. In such a situation the pericarditis may be occult and is identified only by maintaining a high index of suspicion. Open surgical drainage is indicated both for relief of pericardial compression and as an adjunct to appropriate antibiotic therapy. Acute or subacute constriction may occur in occasional cases.

Viral or acute nonspecific pericarditis is also seen with some frequency in older children. It usually follows an upper respiratory illness. The causative virus may be coxsackie B, echovirus, or adenovirus. The disease is generally a self-limiting illness. Treatment with bed rest and aspirin is indicated until signs of inflammation have subsided. Pericardial drainage by pericardiocentesis or catheter is indicated in the presence of tamponade. The disease may be recurrent in some cases.

Uremic pericarditis also deserves special mention because its incidence is rising with the increasing survival of uremic children through the use of chronic hemodialysis. The pericardial inflammation and effusion generally respond to improvement in the degree of azotemia. Some patients with a severe illness are effectively treated by pericardiectomy.

INFECTIVE ENDOCARDITIS

A congenital cardiac defect is the usual substrate for infective endocarditis in children. Less frequently, a valve deformed by rheumatic heart disease or a prosthetic valve, patch, or suture line is the site of the infection. Rarely, normal valves are affected, as in the tricuspid and pulmonary valve involvement seen in drug addicts. In a recent series, tetralogy of Fallot was the most common underlying lesion, followed by aortic valvular stenosis and ventricular septal defect.

Many questions regarding the pathogenesis of infective endocarditis remain unanswered. Particularly enigmatic is the low incidence of the infection, even though transient bacteremia is a day-to-day occurrence in the normal population. The localization of lesions has been convincingly explained by Rodbard's theory that high-velocity flow through a narrow orifice predisposes to distal or "downstream" infection. Interference with endothelial integrity and nonlaminar flow with accumulation of microorganisms in the "stagnant" area distally appear to be the responsible mechanism.

Microorganisms can become implanted in previously damaged endocardial surfaces. Vegetations form as small granular masses that can become large and friable and may account for continuous seeding of the bloodstream.

Oral surgical procedures are the most common preventable source of bloodstream invasion. Other described causes are tonsillectomy, reduction of open fractures, and extensive burns.

The commonest infecting organisms are alpha-hemolytic streptococci, accounting for approximately 50% of the cases. The enterococcus group of streptococci is relatively common in the adult, but rarely is it a causative agent in children. Coagulase-positive *Staphylococcus aureus* accounts for approximately 40%. Other bacteria and fungi, as well as coxsackie B viruses, have been described.

Manifestations. Fever, anemia, and cardiac murmur should always suggest endocarditis, especially if associated with petechiae (Fig. 18-18). The clinical picture, however, is not as clearly defined as one would like. Fever is present in nearly all patients but may be relapsing in nature and to some degree is dependent on

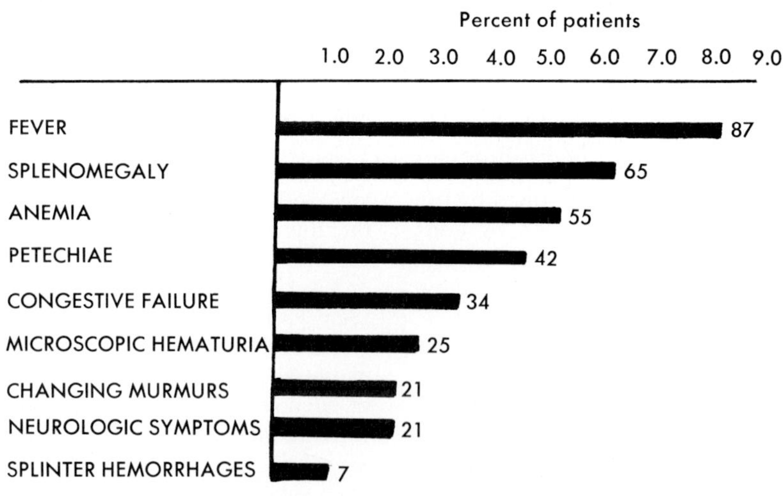

Fig. 18-18. Admission findings in 149 episodes of infective endocarditis.

the virulence of the organism. The classically described hallmarks of the disease, such as Osler nodes, Janeway lesions, splinter hemorrhages, and Roth spots are either rare or occur late and are nonspecific. The occurrence of neurologic symptoms such as sudden hemiplegia, subarachnoid hemorrhage, or meningitis and gangrene, visceral (splenic, renal) infarction, or hematuria should alert the astute clinician to the possibility of endocarditis. Arthralgia is a common symptom, and septic arthritis is occasionally seen. Cardiac manifestations include new organic murmurs (not merely a change of a preexisting murmur) and sudden appearance of congestive heart failure in a previously compensated patient. Suspicion remains, however, the most important factor in diagnosis.

Blood cultures are positive in 85% to 90% of cases, but the existence of patients with repeatedly negative cultures requires emphasis. The percentage yield of positive cultures diminishes rapidly after the third blood culture, and more than six cultures are rarely indicated. There is no advantage to be obtained from arterial cultures or from timing cultures with temperature spikes. Once the diagnosis is seriously considered, three to six blood cultures should be drawn over a period of several hours and therapy instituted.

Treatment should be instituted promptly once the diagnosis is suggested and appropriate cultures obtained. Details of antibiotic selection are summarized in Table 18-3. Basic principles of treatment of endocarditis include the following: (1) bactericidal agents must be used, (2) high blood levels of antibiotic should be achieved, (3) the drugs used must penetrate fibrin, (4) intravenous therapy should be used, and (5) treatment must be continued for a sufficiently long time to effect a cure. With prompt diagnosis and effective therapy a favorable response may be anticipated in more than 80% of patients.

Endocarditis after open heart surgery, especially after insertion of a prosthetic material, is a serious disease. It may resist antimicrobial treatment and requires surgical replacement of the prosthetic material without delay.

Prevention of bacterial endocarditis in patients with congenital heart disease is imperative. It is now recommended that patients with congenital or acquired heart defects should receive antibiotic prophylaxis during periods of potential significant bacteremia. Such procedures include tooth extraction, oral surgery and periodontal procedures, tonsillectomy and adenoidectomy, bronchoscopy, and instrumentation of an infected genitourinary tract. Surgery and instrumentation of the lower gastrointestinal tract may also be associated with bacteremia. The indiscriminate use of antibiotics during febrile episodes in children who have heart disease is unwarranted. Penicillin is the drug of choice for use with upper respiratory tract and oral procedures. Erythromycin is used if there is a history of penicillin allergy. Coverage for gram-negative organisms is also indicated for procedures involving the genitourinary or lower gastrointestinal tracts. Prophylaxis for infective endocarditis in patients undergoing oropharyngeal manipulations is presented on p. 468.

Table 18-3. Antibiotic treatment in endocarditis

Organism	Antibiotic	Dose/kg/day	Doses per day	Duration
Streptococcus viridans	Penicillin	250,000 u I.V.	4-6	4 weeks
Staphylococcus aureus	Methicillin	300 mgm I.V.	4-6	6 weeks*
	Nafcillin	200-300 mg I.V.	4-6	6 weeks*
	Oxacillin	200-300 mg I.V.	4-6	6 weeks*
	Vancomycin†	30-40 mg I.V.	3	6 weeks*
Enterococcus	Pencillin G	250,000 u I.V.	4-6	4-6 weeks*
	Streptomycin	20 mg I.M. (max. 500 mg)	2	2 weeks
	Ampicillin	300 mg I.V.	6	4-6 weeks*
	Gentamycin‡	4.5-7.5 mg I.V.	3	4-6 weeks*

*Intravenous therapy for 4 weeks; the latter 2 weeks could be given intramuscularly or orally.
†For patients allergic to penicillin.
‡Gentamycin dose is modified according to the patient's age and renal function.

PROPHYLAXIS OF INFECTIVE ENDOCARDITIS IN PATIENTS UNDERGOING OROPHARYNGEAL MANIPULATIONS

Regimen A

For most congenital heart disease, rheumatic fever and acquired valvular disease, mitral valve prolapse syndrome with mitral insufficiency

Penicillin

1. *Parenteral-oral combined*
   600,000 units procaine penicillin G mixed with 30,000 units/kg crystalline penicillin G (not to exceed 1 million units) intramuscularly 1 hour before the procedure, followed by 250 mg penicillin orally every 6 hours for eight doses. For children over 27 kg (60 pounds), 500 mg penicillin V is substituted
2. *Oral*
   1 g penicillin V 1 hour before the procedure and then 250 mg every 6 hours for eight doses; for children above 27 kg, 2 g penicillin an hour before the procedure and then 500 mg orally every 6 hours for eight doses

For patients suspected to be allergic to penicillin or for those receiving continual oral penicillin for rheumatic fever prophylaxis who may harbor penicillin-resistant streptococci

Erythromycin

Oral

For small children 20 mg/kg orally 1 ½ hours before the procedure and then 10 mg/kg every 6 hours for eight doses (Maximum: 1.0 g initially and 500 mg every 6 hours)

Regimen B

For patients with prosthetic heart valves or for gastrointestinal or genitourinary manipulation

Penicillin

Follow recommendation in Regimen A

OR

Erythromycin

Follow recommendation in Regimen A

PLUS

Streptomycin

Intramuscular

20 mg/kg (not to exceed 1 g) 1 hour before the procedure, then every 12 hours for 2 doses, or gentamycin 2 mg/kg 1 hour before the procedure, then every 8 hours for 2 doses

Modified from Anthony, C.L., et al.: Pediatric cardiology, Medical Outline Series, Flushing, N.Y., 1979, Medical Examination Publishing Co., Inc.

CARDIAC ARRHYTHMIAS

Rhythm disturbances are encountered less frequently in children than in adults. Nevertheless, they are sufficiently common that the clinician who cares for children must at least be familiar with the more frequent forms and their treatment. It is not possible in this book to catalog all arrhythmias that have been reported in childhood, and this discussion will include the more common, spontaneously occurring problems.

Sinus arrhythmia. Sinus arrhythmia is a normal variant characterized by a phasic increase in heart rate generally related to inspiration. Electrocardiographically it is manifested by the association of one normally directed P wave with each QRS complex and a nonvarying P-R interval (Fig. 18-19). The irregularity of rate is caused by variation in the discharge of the sinoatrial node, as manifested by a change in interval between P waves. It is of no clinical concern except that its presence indicates normal

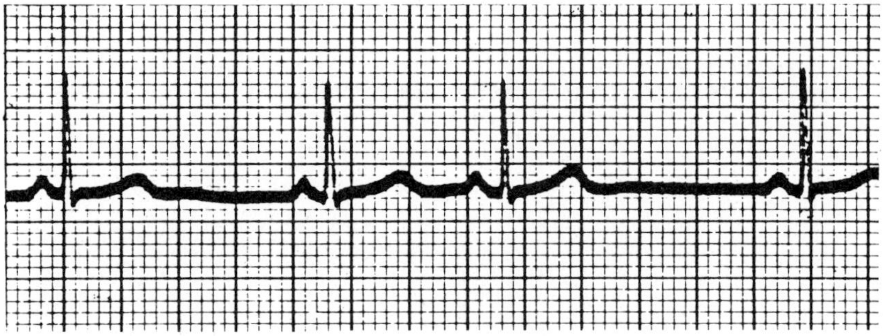

Fig. 18-19. Sinus arrhythmia. Note the 1:1 P-QRS relationship with a nonvarying P-R interval and P wave configuration. (From Anthony, C.L., et al.: Pediatric cardiology, Medical Outline Series, Flushing, N.Y., 1979, Medical Examination Publishing Co., Inc.)

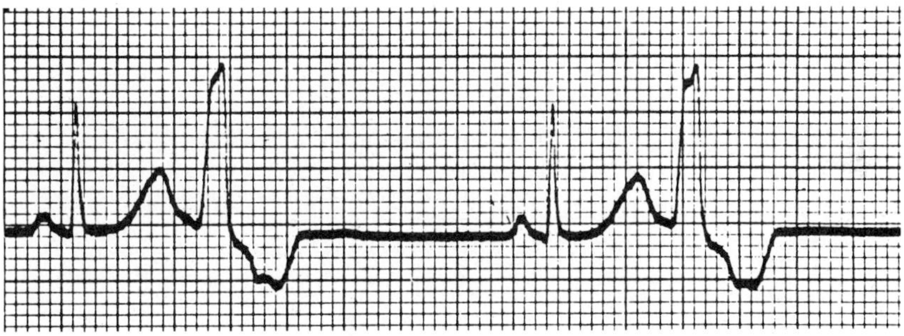

Fig. 18-20. Premature ventricular depolarization occurring in a bigeminal rhythm is an asymptomatic 9-year-old girl. The deformity at the bottom of the inverted T wave following the PVC is caused by an atrial depolarization of sinus node origin that is not conducted to the ventricles because of the premature beat. (From Anthony, C.L., et al.: Pediatric cardiology, Medical Outline Series, Flushing, N.Y., 1979, Medical Examination Publishing Co., Inc.)

neuroregulatory control and therefore usually a good cardiac reserve.

Premature beats. Premature beats are not uncommonly seen in children with a normal heart but they may also be caused by specific causes such as digitalis toxicity, myocarditis including acute rheumatic fever, and acid-base disturbances. Thus a careful search for an underlying etiology is indicated. Premature beats may originate at any level: atrial, atrioventricular junctional, or ventricular. Atrial premature beats are generally recognized by the normal QRS configuration and duration and also by the presence of a preceding P wave, although the latter may be hard to identify if superimposed on the T wave. The P wave may be normal or abnormal in direction, depending on the exact location of the ectopic focus. The pause after an atrial ectopic beat is usually not fully compensatory (i.e., less than twice the sinus R-R interval). Atrioventricular junctional premature beats (i.e., nodal or His bundle) resemble atrial premature beats, except that the P wave is superiorly directed and either precedes the QRS complex closely, follows it, or may be superimposed on it and thus not visualized. Ventricular premature beats are wide and slurred, appearing bizarre in relation to the normal QRS complex and without associated P waves (Fig. 18-20). The T wave is usually directed opposite to the QRS complex, and the pause after the premature beat is generally fully compensatory. Premature beats, regardless of focus of origin, can generally be abolished by exercise if they originate from a normal heart. If premature beats are unusually frequent, seem multifocal, or occur in couplets, or if there are any associated symptoms, 24-hour ambulatory ECG monitor-

Table 18-4. Drugs used in treatment of paroxysmal tachycardia

Drug and route of administration	Dosage
Digoxin (Lanoxin)	See Table 18-1
Propranolol (Inderal)	
Intravenous*	0.01-0.05 mg/kg given slowly; may be repeated in 10 min
Oral	0.2-1 mg/kg/24 hr
Verapamil	
Intravenous	0.1-0.2 mg/kg given slowly over 2 min
Lidocaine (Xylocaine)	
Intravenous*†	0.5-1 mg/kg stat dose; may be repeated after 5 min, not to exceed 3 mg/kg in 1 hr
Intravenous infusion*	0.02-0.05 mg/kg/min as a 0.1% solution in 5% D/W
Procainamide (Pronestyl)	
Intravenous*	2 mg/kg diluted in 5% D/W given slowly
Oral	40-60 mg/kg/24 hr in 4 divided doses
Quinidine	
Oral	20-50 mg/kg per day of quinidine base, divided into 4-6 doses. Quinidine sulfate is 80% quinidine base and quinidine gluconate is 60% base.
Phenytoin, or diphenylhydantoin (Dilantin)	
Intravenous*	2-4 mg/kg slowly; may repeat every 20 min to maximum of 10 mg/kg total
Oral	5-7 mg/kg/24 hr
Edrophonium (Tensilon)	
Intravenous*	0.1-0.2 mg/kg; maximum dose 10 mg

*Monitor electrocardiogram and blood pressure during intravenous administration.
†Use only the cardiac preparation of lidocaine.

ing (Holter monitoring) or exercise electrocardiography should be performed to evaluate the possibility of a more serious rhythm disturbance, such as unrecognized ventricular tachycardia.

If the cardiovascular system is normal and there is no other underlying cause, treatment is not indicated unless awareness of the beats is sufficiently disturbing to the child. The problem often disappears spontaneously in adolescence. If necessary, the treatment of choice for supraventricular beats is digoxin, and for ventricular beats propranolol, procainamide, or quinidine (Table 18-4).

Tachyarrhythmias. The commonest arrhythmia of clinical significance in childhood is *paroxysmal supraventricular tachycardia* (PSVT). It occurs most often in infants 1 to 3 months of age but may have its onset in utero or at any age. Although this arrhythmia may be associated with congenital heart disease, infection, myocardial tumors, drugs, or Wolff-Parkinson-White syndrome, no specific etiology is found in about 50% of patients. The cardiac rate is variable, depending on age, and usually ranges from 250 to 300 beats /min in the young infant to 160 to 200 beats/min in the older child and adults. Although the infant with PSVT may appear well for a surprising period of time, congestive heart failure eventually develops, and the infant's condition may become critical in an extremely short period of time. Approximately 50% of infants develop congestive heart failure within 48 hours of the onset of the paroxysm. Electrocardiographically, the typical picture is normal-appearing QRS complexes occurring at a rapid rate; P waves are often difficult or impossible to identify (Fig. 18-21). Rarely, there may be aberrant conduction of the action potential through the His-Purkinje system with widening and slurring of the QRS complexes, resembling ventricular tachycardia. Differentiation may be difficult and is beyond the scope of this discussion.

Digoxin remains the drug of choice for PSVT (Table 18-1). Almost all patients respond dramatically by an abrupt return of the heart rate to normal, often within a few hours of starting the drug. Vagal maneuvers such as carotid massage may be effective after digoxin has been given but rarely before. Once sinus rhythm is restored, administration of maintenance digoxin

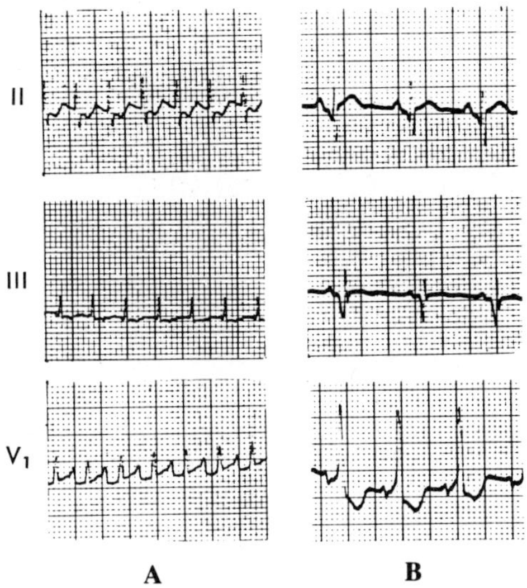

Fig. 18-21. A, Paroxysmal supraventricular tachycardia at a rate of 290 beats/min in an infant. Although P waves are not clearly identified because of the rapid rate, the presence of narrow QRS complexes identifies this rhythm as being supraventricular in origin. **B,** Following conversion to normal sinus rhythm, the electrocardiogram revealed a short P-R interval with a wide QRS complex and slurring of the initial portion of the QRS (delta wave), characteristic of the Wolff-Parkinson-White type of preexcitation. These features are seen best in lead V_1. (From Anthony, C.L., et al.: Pediatric cardiology, Medical Outline Series, Flushing, N.Y., 1979, Medical Examination Publishing Co., Inc.)

should be continued for at least 6 months because of the high rate of recurrence.

Verapamil administered intravenously has also proven extremely useful in rapidly terminating paroxysms of supraventricular tachycardia (Table 18-4). If this drug is used to restore normal sinus rhythm, it should be followed by digitalization to prevent recurrences. If congestive heart failure is already present when the child is first seen, the therapeutic plan is dominated by the principle of restoring normal sinus rhythm as rapidly as possible because the child's condition may otherwise deteriorate rapidly. When skilled personnel and proper equipment are available, synchronized direct current (DC) cardioversion is the method of choice. Verapamil may also be used, but this drug depresses myocardial contractility and may further worsen the hemodynamic status. Digoxin is not particularly useful in the presence of failure because the time required to restore normal sinus rhythm would be expected to be greater than could be tolerated by an infant in this critical state. DC cardioversion in a fully digitalized patient theoretically carries some risk of inducing severe digitalis toxic arrhythmias, which is another reason for not selecting this drug as a first choice when failure has occurred. Rapidly pacing the atrium for a brief period of time, using an intracardiac electrode catheter inserted transvenously, is another effective method of terminating the tachycardia; this may be used in digitalized patients. Regardless of the method chosen, the patient is digitalized once normal sinus rhythm is restored for prophylaxis against future recurrences.

The above modalities will terminate virtually all paroxysms of supra-ventricular tachycardia, and other drugs or maneuvers should be rarely necessary. Immersion of the face in ice water for a few seconds has been reported to achieve a high degree of success. This is obviously applicable only to infants, but may be useful particularly in the hands of someone not experienced in treating this problem. In the presence of congestive failure, sympathetic tone and circulating catecholamines are generally elevated so that such vagal stimulating maneuvers are much less likely to be effective. Intravenous edrophonium has also been successful in a number of patients. A variety of alpha adrenergic stimulating agents, such as phenylephrine, have been infused to elevate the blood pressure and provoke a reflex parasympathetic discharge. Careful monitoring of blood pressure is essential. This method carries a significant hazard in young infants and its use should probably be restricted to older children.

Although digoxin alone will prevent recurrences in the majority of patients, some will break through repetitively even when adequate serum levels of digoxin are present. The addition of a second drug is then indicated. Propranolol has been the drug of choice for this purpose in most centers, and the combination with digoxin has been highly effective. Verapamil has been recently released for oral administration and should also prove to be of value. In the presence of the Wolff-Parkinson-White syndrome, failure to control the tachycardia using digoxin or propranolol to slow conduction through the AV junction may indicate the need to use a drug that will block the bypass tract. Quinidine, pro-

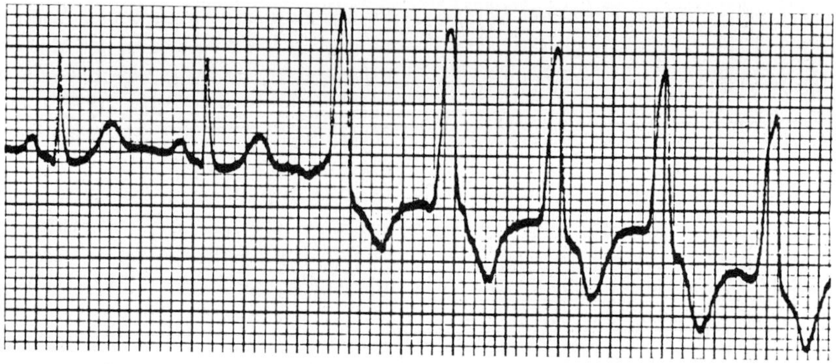

Fig. 18-22. Postexercise rhythm strip in the same patient as in Fig. 18-21. There is a wide QRS tachycardia at approximately 150 beats/min with no evidence of associated atrial activity. This pattern is characteristic of ventricular tachycardia. (From Anthony, C.L., et al.: Pediatric cardiology, Medical Outline Series, Flushing, N.Y., 1979, Medical Examination Publishing Co., Inc.)

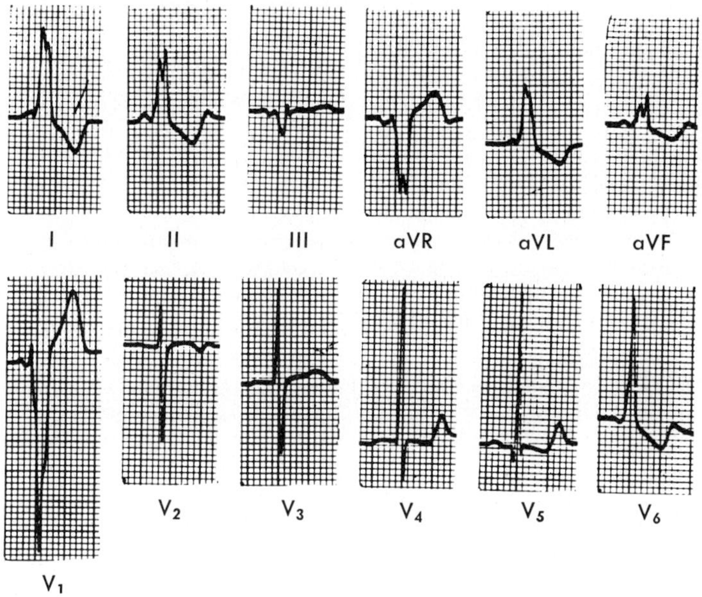

Fig. 18-23. Wolff-Parkinson-White type of preexcitation in a 7-year-old boy with a history of paroxysmal supraventricular tachycardia. The short P-R interval and wide QRS complex are readily noted. There is slurring of the upstroke of the QRS complex, best seen in lead V_6. Leads V_2 through V_5 demonstrate a transient return to normal conduction with disappearance of the preexcitation. (From Anthony, C.L., et al.: Pediatric cardiology, Medical Outline Series, Flushing, N.Y., 1979, Medical Examination Publishing Co., Inc.)

cainamide, and disopyramide have been used for this purpose.

Ventricular tachycardia as a spontaneous arrhythmia is fortunately rare in childhood but is more serious than the supraventricular form because of its greater deleterious effect on cardiac output and because it may be followed by ventricular fibrillation. The rate is usually slower than in paroxysmal supraventricular tachycardia, and the electrocardiogram reveals wide, slurred QRS complexes, often with no associated P waves (Fig. 18-22). As just mentioned, differentiation from paroxysmal supraventricular tachycardia with aberrant conduction may be difficult. Intravenous lidocaine or procainamide (Table 18-4) will often produce reversion to normal sinus rhythm. The former is preferred because of its shorter duration of action. Cardioversion is also highly effective. If arrhythmia is recurrent, oral procainamide, phenytoin, quindine, or propranolol may be used.

Preexcitation. Preexcitation is a term covering a group of disorders that have as a common denominator premature activation of ventricular myocardium from the atria, generally by a pathway that bypasses the atrioventricular node. In the commonest form, the electrocardiogram shows a short P-R interval and a QRS complex that is widened by the presence of slowing of its initial portion (so-called delta wave) (Figs. 18-21 and 18-23). This is referred to as the Wolff-Parkinson-White (WPW) pattern and has been subdivided according to the direction of the delta wave.

Depolarization of ventricular myocardium occurs over two pathways: The AV node–His bundle–Purkinje fiber path and the bypass tract. The proportion of ventricular myocardium activated over the individual pathways may vary, and thus at times the QRS complex may appear nearly normal when the majority of depolarization is occurring over the normal pathway. At other times the typical widened QRS is present, coincident with the majority of the depolarization wave passing over the bypass tract. These patients are likely to develop paroxysmal tachycardia, especially the supraventricular form. WPW is the underlying basis for PSVT in most infants less than 4 months of age; preexcitation usually disappears within a few months. The electrocardiographic pattern is also seen in certain congenital heart defects, especially Ebstein anomaly of the tricuspid valve. The WPW pattern alone requires no treatment. If tachyarrhythmias occur, they are treated in the usual manner.

Atrioventicular block. Atrioventicular block is characterized by delay or failure of conduction of the electrical impulse through the atrioventricular junction. *First-degree atrioventricular block* is simply a slowing of conduction manifested by a prolonged P-R interval, whereas *second-degree block* is manifested by conduction of some but not all beats. The commonest variety of second-degree ventricular block is the Wenckebach phenomenon (Mobitz type I), wherein progressively delayed conduction is manifested by lengthening of the P-R interval until a QRS complex is dropped because of complete failure of impulse transmission (Fig. 18-24).

This sequence then recurs, although the cycle length may vary. It would appear that the location of the block is most commonly in the AV node. Second-degree block with a constant PR interval is referred to as Mobitz Type II. When the block is high-grade (i.e., most of the P waves are not conducted) the block is usually caused by extensive disease of the distal specialized conducting tissue; this is primarily seen in adults. Also seen occasionally in children is second-degree block with a P wave: QRS complex ratio of 2:1; it is difficult to be sure of the exact mechanism with this variant. First- and second-degree atrioventricular block may occur congenitally, with or without underlying heart disease, or either block may be a manifestation of acute rheumatic fever or other forms of myocarditis.

The most serious form of heart block is *third-degree (or complete) atrioventricular block,* in which there is total failure of conduction through the atrioventricular junction, the atria and ventricles beating independently. In children this is usually a congenital arrhythmia, sometimes associated with congenital heart disease, but it also occurs as an occasional complication of open heart surgery. P waves and QRS complexes occur independently, with the ventricular rate being slower than the atrial rate (Fig. 18-25). In most congenital cases the pacemaker driving the ventricles is located in the atrioventricular junction, in constrast to the situation in adults; after surgery it is usually located in the ventricles. In the former instance the QRS complexes are of normal duration, and the ventricular rate is slightly more rapid, generally varying between 40 and 70 beats/min. The junctional pacemaker may also accelerate somewhat with exercise. Most of these children are asymptomatic, with a slow heart rate being noted only incidentally. Cardiomegaly and basal ejection murmur are common because of the increased diastolic filling. Although the course is benign in most patients with congenital heart block, increasing exertional fatigue or syncope (Stokes-Adams attacks) may occur. Congestive heart failure is uncommon but may be seen in the

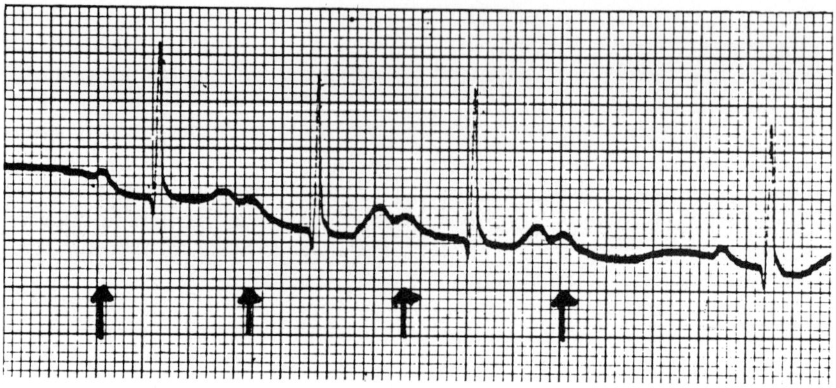

Fig. 18-24. Mobitz type I second-degree atrioventricular block. P waves are indicated by arrows. Note the progressive lengthening of the P-R interval following the first three P waves. The fourth P wave is blocked at the AV junction and is not followed by a QRS complex, giving rise to a 4:3 periodicity. After this the cycle resumes. (From Anthony, C.L., et al.: Pediatric cardiology, Medical Outline Series, Flushing, N.Y., 1979, Medical Examination Publishing Co., Inc.)

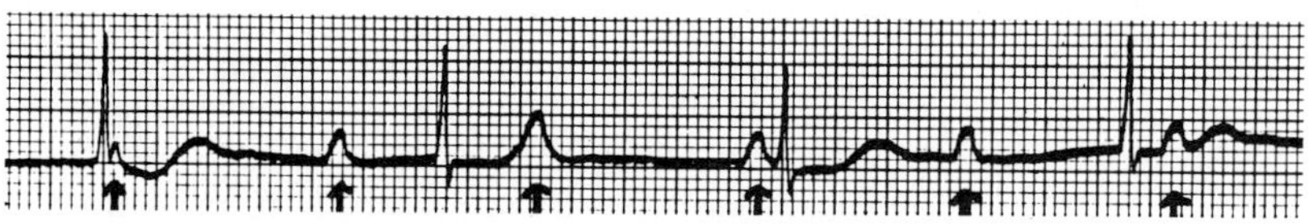

Fig. 18-25. Third-degree (complete) atrioventricular block. P waves are indicated by arrows. Note the absence of any relationship between P waves and QRS complexes. This tracing was from an asymptomatic 8-year-old girl. (From Anthony, C.L., et al.: Pediatric cardiology, Medical Outline Series, Flushing, N.Y., 1979, Medical Examination Publishing Co., Inc.)

newborn infant with or without congenital heart disease. When the pacemaker is below the atrioventricular junction, the prognosis is often poor. The asymptomatic patient with congenital complete block requires no treatment. Infants with congestive heart failure should have a temporary transvenous electronic pacemaker inserted and should be treated with diuretics and even digoxin if necessary, although the latter must be used cautiously. Implantation of a permanent pacemaker is usually indicated in such infants and is almost invariably required in patients with Stokes-Adams attacks and in those whose block occurs as a complication of surgery.

Courtney L. Anthony, Jr.
José Marín-García

SELECTED READINGS

Anthony, C.L., et al.: Pediatric cardiology, Medical Outline Series, Flushing, N.Y., 1979, Medical Examination Publishing Co., Inc.

Goldberg, S.J., et al.: Pediatric and adolescent echocardiography, ed. 2, Chicago, 1980, Year Book Medical Publishers, Inc.

Markowitz, M., and Gordis, L.: Rheumatic fever, Philadelphia, 1972, W.B. Saunders Co.

Moss, A.J., et al.: Heart disease in infants, children and adolescents, ed. 2, Baltimore, 1977, the Williams & Wilkins Co.

Nadas, A.S., and Fyler, D.C.: Pediatric cardiology, ed. 3, Philadelphia, 1972, W.B. Saunders Co.

Park, M.K., and Guntheroth, W.G.: How to read pediatric ECG's, Chicago, 1981, Year Book Medical Publishers, Inc.

Roberts, N.K., and Gelband, H.: Cardiac arrhythmias in the neonate, infant and child, New York, 1977, Appleton-Century-Crofts.

Rudolph, A.M.: Congenital diseases of the heart, Chicago, 1974, Year Book Medical Publishers, Inc.

19 Arthritis in Childhood

Musculoskeletal symptoms are fairly common in children. They may be a reflection of systemic illness, including connective tissue diseases, infections, and blood dyscrasias, or may represent local problems, such as traumatic arthritis and epiphyseal dysplasias. Clinical features and management of the most common conditions will be reviewed.

JUVENILE RHEUMATOID ARTHRITIS

Juvenile rheumatoid arthritis (JRA) is a chronic illness of unknown etiology and is one of the leading causes of disability in childhood. About three fourths of children with a major generalized rheumatic disease have JRA. By definition its onset occurs before the age of 16 years. It differs in a number of ways from adult rheumatoid arthritis: (1) systemic features such as high fever, rash, uveitis, and pericarditis are common, (2) the rheumatoid factor test is usually negative, (3) the patient is less likely to complain of joint pain, and (4) the prognosis for remission is excellent. Three major clinical patterns have been described: oligoarticular, polyarticular, and systemic. Features of these subsets are outlined in Table 19-1. These categories relate to the signs and symptoms during the early months of the illness. However, there is a tendency for some children with the oligoarticular and systemic forms to develop polyarticular involvement during the extended course of JRA.

Onset before the age of 6 months is very rare. The peak incidence is between 1 and 3 years, but onset can occur at any time during childhood. Overall, girls are affected twice as often as boys, but the sex incidence in the systemic form is about equal. In some cases the illness appears to be precipitated by physical or emotional trauma, but in the majority of cases no contributing factor can be identified.

Oligoarticular arthritis. This variety, also called pauciarticular, is the most common and also the most benign subset of JRA. The large joints such as the knees, ankles, and wrists are usually involved, but the knee is by far most frequently affected. About half of affected children have a monoarthritis at onset, but signs may appear in other joints later. The hips are usually spared; a monoarthritis in the hip is seldom, if ever, caused by JRA. Isolated involvement in one or two small joints in the hands and feet may occur but is uncommon. These children usually have considerable swelling in the affected joints, although half of them have little or no pain. Frequently, the child will be seen by a physician because of swelling noted by a parent or because the child is observed to walk with a limp, particularly in the morning. The

Table 19-1. Clinical categories of JRA at onset

	Systemic	Oligoarticular	Polyarticular
Percent of total patients	20%-30%	35%-45%	30%-40%
Sex ratio (female to male)	1:1	2:1	2:1
Age	<10	Variable	Variable
Number of joints	Variable	<5	≥5
Positive rheumatoid factor	Rare	Rare	10%
Positive antinuclear antibody	10%	25%-50%	20%-40%
Systemic features	Marked	Mild	Mild
Uveitis	<5%	20%	5%
Prognosis	40% deformity	Excellent	25% deformity

onset may be insidious or abrupt, the latter often suggesting the possibility of septic or traumatic arthritis. The joints may be warm, tender, and painful on motion but seldom show erythema of the overlying skin. Large effusions are often present. Most of these children feel well in general, although a few have mild systemic symptoms such as low-grade fever and malaise.

The natural history of oligoarticular arthritis is usually one of smoldering synovitis over a period of several years. There are frequent remissions and exacerbations, the latter often related to excessive physical activity or trauma. About a third of cases evolve into the polyarticular form. Complications of articular disease include the development of flexion contractures, instability with resulting valgus deviation or subluxation of the knee, and leg length discrepancy caused by overgrowth in the affected limb. Accelerated epiphyseal growth may be the result of increased vascularity because of the local inflammatory process. A functionally significant leg length discrepancy of several centimeters may develop.

Although the oligoarticular group appears homogeneous from the clinical point of view, there are important subsets that have recently been identified. Uveitis, or iridocyclitis, is far more frequent than in the other groups, particularly in girls with positive tests for antinuclear antibody. These patients usually have onset before age 10, and may have very mild arthritis. Boys who have onset after age 10 must be suspected of having juvenile ankylosing spondylitis. They usually have synovitis in the knees and later complain of hip pain. The histocompatibility type (HLA) B27 is present in these patients, as it is in adult-onset ankylosing spondylitis. During the childhood years low back pain is seldom a major complaint.

Polyarticular arthritis. Polyarticular arthritis has the closest resemblance to adult-onset rheumatoid arthritis. The joint disease usually overshadows generalized symptoms, but some patients have malaise, low-grade fever, fatigue, anorexia, weight loss, and other features noted in the systemic form. Most patients have morning stiffness, but it is seldom reported as such. Sluggish behavior may be observed by the parents and, although many children have little or

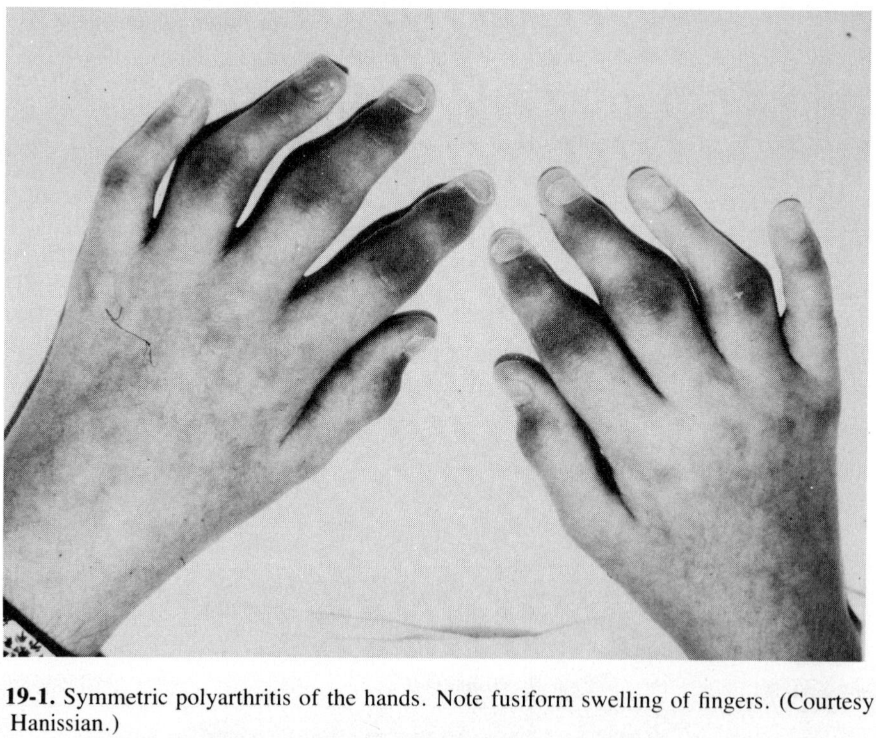

Fig. 19-1. Symmetric polyarthritis of the hands. Note fusiform swelling of fingers. (Courtesy Dr. A.S. Hanissian.)

no pain, pain is more likely to be experienced in the morning. Joint involvement, including tenderness and soft tissue swelling, is present in both large and small joints and is often symmetric in distribution (Fig. 19-1). Arthritis in the cervical spine may present as painless neck stiffness, but there may occasionally be severe pain and torticollis. Temporomandibular joint involvement is common, leading to impaired bite, decreased mouth opening, and in later stages shortening of the mandible (micrognathia). Over a period of several years most children will develop some limitation of joint motion and deformity, most commonly flexion contractures of hips, knees, and elbows, impaired dorsiflexion of the wrists, and hand deformities. Ulnar deviation, which occurs frequently in adults, is rare in JRA; in fact, radial deviation at the metacarpophalangeal joints is more common. Many children develop flexion contractures of the proximal finger joints, weakness of grip, and inability to make a fist. Females with onset after age 10 may represent a subset with a more serious prognosis. In these older girls more of the features of adult-onset disease may occur, including a positive test for rheumatoid factor, rheumatoid nodules, and a lesser tendency toward spontaneous remission.

Systemic onset (Still's disease)

In some children systemic manifestations, such as fever and rash, accompany or precede the onset of arthritis. Joint swelling for 6 weeks or more must be present to make a definite diagnosis of JRA. Therefore many alternative causes of persistent fever must be considered during this interval in which systemic features predominate. Extensive investigations are often performed to rule out conditions such as chronic infections, malignancies, rheumatic fever, and other collagen-vascular diseases. Many weeks or months may elapse before the appearance of joint swelling, which allows a definite diagnosis.

Typically the fever pattern is remitting, with daily or occasionally twice-daily elevations of 39° to 40° C (102.2° to 104.0° F), most often in late afternoon or evening. In contrast to rheumatic fever, temperature usually returns to normal in the morning. Shaking chills are unusual. The child may appear acutely ill during fever spikes and surprisingly well when the fever remits.

A characteristic rash often accompanies the fever, with pink macular skin lesions most often noted on the trunk and proximal extremities (Fig. 19-2). The rash is evanescent and migra-

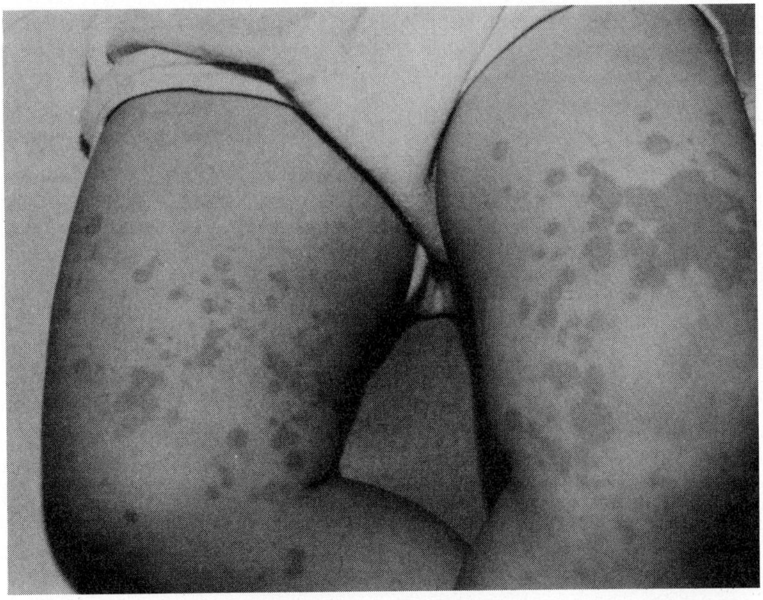

Fig. 19-2. Juvenile rheumatoid rash. (Courtesy Dr. A.S. Hanissian.)

tory, and there is little or no itching. Therefore a careful examination must be made during fever spikes to identify it. A macule may be surrounded by a ring of pale skin, and some lesions may show central clearing. Lesions may extend or appear after scratching or rubbing the skin or after a hot bath.

Other extra-articular manifestations may also be seen, including pericarditis, lymphadenopathy, and hepatosplenomegaly, and rarely myocarditis and pulmonary infiltrations. Pericarditis is usually asymptomatic, but some children have chest pains, pericardial friction rub, and tachycardia disproportionate to fever, anemia, and other factors. Pericardial tamponade is very rare. Pericarditis is usually suspected because of an enlarged cardiac silhouette on the chest radiograph.

When joint swelling appears the patient usually follows the course of polyarticular JRA, but fever and rash may recur intermittently.

Uveitis (iritis, iridocyclitis). Involvement of the anterior uveal tract is particularly common in girls with early-onset oligoarticular JRA. Since blindness is common, even with treatment, early diagnosis is essential. Frequently there will be insidious visual loss with no symptoms or abnormalities on gross examination. For this reason routine slit lamp examinations by an ophthalmologist at intervals of 4 to 6 months are recommended for all children with JRA. Secondary complications include band keratopathy, cataracts, and glaucoma. Local corticosteroid therapy is usually used, but some patients require systemic treatment. In the past, blindness resulted in more than half of patients with uveitis, but in a recent report only 21% of involved eyes had visual loss.

Laboratory studies

In the systemic form leukocytosis is common, often with WBC counts of 15,000 to 20,000/mm^3. More modest elevations occur in active polyarticular JRA. A normochromic or hypochromic anemia is frequent, and also relates to disease activity, as does thrombocytosis. The erythrocyte sedimentation rate (ESR) is markedly elevated in children with systemic disease and active polyarthritis, but is normal in a minority of children with oligoarticular JRA. It is the most convenient laboratory marker for monitoring the inflammatory process, but other acute phase reactants such as C-reactive protein may also be used and have the advantage of being unaffected by anemia. Complement levels are often elevated, and protein electrophoresis shows elevated alpha globulins. Immunoglobulins may be increased in chronic JRA. Congenital IgA deficiency is present in about 5% of JRA patients, more frequent than would be predicted by chance, but there are no differences in the clinical course of these patients. Children with other immunodeficiency states such as common variable immunodeficiency, X-linked agammaglobulinemia, and C2 complement deficiency may have arthritis similar to JRA, but usually mild and nondeforming.

Rheumatoid factor is found in about 20% of all JRA patients but is very rare when the disease onset is below 9 years of age. Thereafter, the proportion of seropositive cases increases progressively and is highest in older females. When rheumatoid factor is found in young children a false-positive test, often caused by chronic infection, must be suspected. In early-onset disease seropositivity does not develop with increasing age regardless of the severity of arthritis. The antinuclear antibody test is positive in about 40% of cases overall. It does not correlate with disease severity but is more likely to be found in females, particularly those with uveitis. It is not a specific diagnostic test and is positive in almost all patients with systemic lupus erythematosus (SLE) and in most with scleroderma. In contrast to SLE, antibodies to native DNA do not occur and LE cells are very rare in JRA. Antistreptolysin-0 may be found in about one fourth of JRA patients, and elevations may be persistent. The reason for this is unknown but the finding may add confusion to the differential diagnosis between JRA and rheumatic fever.

Abnormal liver function tests, particularly the transaminases, are commonly present. In most cases the abnormality is unassociated with clinical signs of liver disease and may be attributed to salicylate therapy. However, enzyme elevations may be seen occasionally in untreated patients presumably related to hepatic involvement. Liver biopsies on such patients reveal minimal, nonspecific changes or may be entirely normal.

Synovial fluid should be examined mainly to rule out other conditions, such as infections.

This is most important in patients with monoarthritis or high fever. In JRA, the WBC falls within a broad range (2,000 to 60,000 white cells/mm^3). Infectious arthritis must be strongly suspected when WBCs exceed this range, even when cultures are negative. The proportion of neutrophils increases in relationship to the total WBC and often exceeds 90%. The mucin clot is usually fair or poor. Determinations of complement, total protein, glucose, or rheumatoid factor rarely provide clinically useful information.

Urinalysis is usually normal in JRA. Mild proteinuria may accompany high fever. Marked proteinuria should provoke consideration of alternative diagnoses such as SLE. In chronic cases secondary amyloidosis may be the explanation. Intermittent microscopic hematuria may indicate focal glomerulitis associated with JRA but more often may be associated with hypercalciuria, probably because of skeletal demineralization and resulting in intermittent passage of small calcium stones.

Pathology. Synovial histology shows characteristic but nonspecific chronic inflammatory cell infiltration and synovial lining cell hyperplasia. A biopsy is seldom required for diagnosis but may be obtained when there is suspicion of an alternative disorder such as synovial tumor or tuberculosis. Biopsy of the characteristic rash shows only mild round cell infiltration around capillaries and venules. Lymph nodes, which may be biopsied in children with fever and prominent lymphadenopathy to rule out lymphoma, show follicular hyperplasia.

Radiographic findings. Soft tissue swelling, periarticular osteoporosis, and periosteal new bone formation are frequently noted during the first year of disease. Marginal erosions and joint space narrowing develop in polyarticular JRA, but seldom before 2 or 3 years have elapsed. Therefore x-ray films are seldom of value in the early diagnosis. Characteristic late changes include cervical fusions, particularly between C2 and C3, and intercarpal and carpal-metacarpal fusions. These changes are most common in children with systemic onset and may allow a retrospective diagnosis even after remission has occurred. In young children, ossification centers and epiphyses may develop prematurely but may have an abnormal appearance because of destructive changes. This may result in premature epiphyseal closure and local growth disturbances, such as brachydactyly, usually caused by metacarpal shortening. With active synovitis in the knee the epiphyses may be abnormally large and the patella may have a squared appearance on lateral view.

Treatment. The aims of treatment are to preserve function, prevent deformity, and ameliorate discomfort in a condition that is eventually likely to remit spontaneously. In most cases it is conservative and does not involve the use of hazardous drugs. Aspirin is used initially and is given four or five times daily in a total dose that varies with the severity of disease and the treatment setting. For acutely ill inpatients, 100 mg/kg/day is given, and dose adjustments are made to avoid constant tinnitus and other side effects, attempting to achieve blood levels between 20 and 30 mg/dl. For outpatients, smaller doses are used (60 to 80 mg/kg). Gastrointestinal symptoms may be avoided by giving aspirin with milk or meals, using buffered or enteric coated preparations, or nonacetylated salicylates such as salsalate or choline magnesium trisalicylate, which is available in a liquid preparation. Gastrointestinal bleeding from salicylate therapy in children appears to be less common than in adults. A mild hepatotoxicity caused by salicylates has been noted frequently in children with JRA, SLE, and rheumatic fever but rarely in normal children. This is seldom symptomatic and is manifested mainly by liver enzyme elevations. The liver dysfunction may disappear spontaneously if salicylates are continued, and it is seldom necessary to discontinue therapy. However, it may be prudent to stop salicylates temporarily and resume in smaller doses if the SGOT level rises above four times the upper limit of normal. Salicylates are given on a regular basis as long as there are signs of inflammation such as joint swelling and ESR elevation.

In children who do not tolerate salicylates or show no benefit, other nonsteroidal anti-inflammatory drugs are available, but these are seldom effective when a full salicylate dose has failed. Many nonsteroidal anti-inflammatory drugs have been used in JRA, but tolmetin and naproxen have FDA approval and the most extensive therapeutic background.

More potent and hazardous agents are reserved for a small minority of children with severe progressive polyarthritis and deformity that is resistant to conservative measures. These include gold salt injections, antimalarials, penicillamine, and immunosuppressive drugs, all of which are used to treat adult-onset disease. Their use in children is not approved and should be undertaken only by physicians who have considerable experience in their use.

Corticosteroids are often used in JRA, particularly for children with systemic disease who fail to respond to salicylates. Large doses are usually required to suppress fever and other systemic manifestations. Side effects are inevitable, and there is no evidence that the course of the disease in terms of joint destruction or deformity is modified. Moreover, because of recurrent inflammation, it is extremely difficult to discontinue steroids. Therefore it is best to avoid initiation of this treatment if at all possible by taking advantage of all conservative measures, including hospitalization if necessary. Systemic steroids may be indicated in refractory uveitis and in a few children with rampant refractory extra-articular disease, including high fever, severe anemia, inanition, weight loss, and carditis. Intra-articular steroid injections may be used sparingly in unusually symptomatic joints. For instance, an impending knee flexion contracture may be aborted by a steroid injection, which will often suppress synovitis temporarily, allowing the more effective application of conservative measures such as active exercise and splinting. Repeated injections may accelerate the destructive process, because steroids suppress articular cartilage matrix synthesis. Activity should be limited for several days afterward to avoid overuse of a joint in which pain has been reduced.

Other conservative measures are as important as drug therapy in reaching a favorable end result. A physical therapy program should be instituted in every case. Various heat modalities, particularly moist heat, give temporary relief of pain and stiffness and allow the child to exercise more effectively. Muscle groups near inflamed joints should be strengthened to avoid atrophy and contractures. Weight bearing should be minimized when there is marked synovitis in the lower extremities. Crutches or other devices to avoid full weight-bearing force may be necessary. A balanced program of rest and exercise should be tailored to the individual case with the aim of achieving maximal levels of active exercise but avoiding fatigue. Play and sporting activities that result in sudden impact on inflamed joints, such as contact sports, gymnastics, and basketball, must be avoided in some children. Other activities may be substituted, such as bicycle riding and swimming. The latter is particularly efficacious since it involves active use of most muscle groups against mild resistance and avoidance of weight-bearing force. Splinting is often used for wrists, hands, and knees to avoid flexion contractures and reduce synovitis. With hip involvement, a daily period of prone lying combined with active gluteal exercise is appropriate. If knee flexion contractures have developed, correction with serial casting may be attempted. Severe neck pain may be ameliorated with a cervical collar.

Reconstructive surgery plays an important role in rehabilitation of severely disabled children. Useful procedures include total hip and knee replacement, which are generally performed after growth is complete. Correction of hand deformities is indicated if there is a reasonable chance that function will be improved. Synovectomy of the knee or wrist is seldom indicated because JRA has a good prognosis with medical treatment, but is occasionally justified for refractory disabling synovitis as a measure to prevent further joint destruction.

Natural history and prognosis

A satisfactory functional result is achieved in most cases of JRA. About 20% to 30% have significant disability in adulthood, although much of this can be addressed with reconstructive surgical procedures. Continuing synovitis during the adult years is rare. Occasional flare-ups may occur in the third decade, but most disease progression is related to a continuing secondary degenerative process in severely damaged joints. Short stature may be caused by severe epiphyseal erosion with failure of longitudinal growth but is seen most often as a result of long-term steroid therapy. Very little growth occurs with daily-dose steroids, and an alternate day program that permits limited growth is seldom tolerated. Additional steroid-related side effects include cataracts, osteoporosis resulting in fractures and vertebral collapse, diabetes, hypertension, and muscle atrophy. The impact of chronic steroid use may therefore continue well beyond the period of active synovitis. Total discontinuation may be difficult because of hypoadrenalism. Death occurs in 2% to 4% of children with JRA. The most common cause is infection, which in turn is related to steroid therapy, or a bedridden status conducive to pneumonia, skin ulceration, and bacteremia. A few die from other steroid complications, adrenal insufficiency, or heart failure. Secondary amyloidosis is rare in American series but has been reported more frequently in Europe. It usually includes a nephrotic syndrome and progressive renal failure.

RHEUMATOID VARIANTS IN CHILDHOOD

Juvenile ankylosing spondylitis. Juvenile ankylosing spondylitis usually occurs in teenaged boys, but at onset may be indistinguishable from oligoarticular JRA. There is often a family history of spine stiffening in young male relatives. Individuals with histocompatibility type HLA-B27 are susceptible to this disorder. HLA-B27 has a prevalence of about 8% in the general population but over 90% in ankylosing spondylitis patients. The early clinical picture in these children includes acute intermittent attacks of pain and swelling in many joints, often suggesting a diagnosis of rheumatic fever. However, fever is rare. Heel pain is frequent. Hip and low back pain with typical morning stiffness become more prominent with the passage of time. Acute anterior uveitis is common, differing from the insidious, slowly progressive visual loss of JRA-associated uveitis. This usually responds promptly to treatment and seldom leads to blindness. Most cases respond well to nonsteroidal anti-inflammatory drugs. Indomethacin is the most commonly used agent in teenagers and young adults. Juvenile spondylitis may go into natural remission or may progress during adulthood, leading to extensive spinal ankylosis and hip limitation. Characteristic sacroiliac joint radiographic abnormalities cannot be detected until age 17 or older because the joint is not fully developed during childhood.

Reiter syndrome. The triad of urethritis, conjunctivitis, and inflammatory arthritis, mainly in the lower extremities, is also most common in young adult males but is seen occasionally in the late teens. Over 90% have the HLA-B27 tissue type. The clinical manifestations often overlap with those of ankylosing spondylitis, and treatment is similar.

HLA-B27–positive individuals are also predisposed to developing a reactive arthritis after various bowel infections caused by *Yersinia, Campylobacter, Salmonella,* and *Shigella* organisms. This acute polyarthritis generally remits spontaneously after several weeks.

Psoriatic arthritis. Although psoriasis is rare in children, a minority of patients develop the varieties of arthropathy seen in adults. These include polyarthritis and sacroiliitis. The distal finger joints are particularly susceptible.

Arthritis of inflammatory bowel disease. A nondeforming inflammatory arthritis, particularly in the knees, may occur in 5% to 10% of patients with ulcerative colitis or Crohn disease. It is likely to be intermittent, corresponding to periods of active bowel disease.

Benign rheumatoid nodules. Subcutaneous nodules occur in about 10% of patients with JRA, usually those with more severe polyarthritis and a positive test for rheumatoid factor. However, nodules with similar histology, a core of central necrosis surrounded by palisaded histocytes, are sometimes found in healthy children without arthritis and with negative rheumatoid factor tests. These may be found in various locations but frequently appear over the anterior tibia, an unusual location in arthritic children. They are usually asymptomatic, require no treatment, and disappear after several years. On extended follow-up these children do not develop arthritis.

SYSTEMIC LUPUS ERYTHEMATOSUS

About 20% of systemic lupus erythematosus (SLE) patients have onset before age 16. SLE is about 10 times less frequent than JRA. The disorder is three to five times more frequent in girls, even more in postpubertal children, and is more common and severe in blacks. The clinical manifestations and prognosis are very similar to the findings in adults. Common early features include rash, fever, malaise, arthritis, pleuritis, Raynaud's phenomenon, alopecia, and buccal ulcerations. More serious visceral involvement may accompany these manifestations or may develop later. These include nephritis, encephalopathy, carditis, and vasculitis.

The characteristic erythematosus rash is found in light-exposed areas, particularly over the ma-

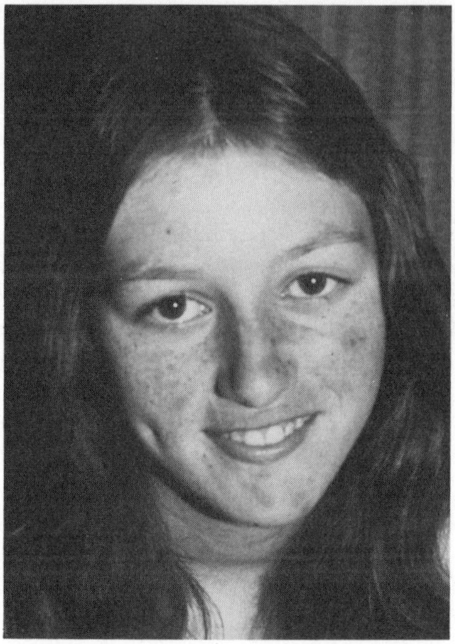

Fig. 19-3. Typical "butterfly" rash of systemic lupus erythematosus. (Courtesy Dr. A.S. Hanissian.)

lar area in a "butterfly" distribution (Fig. 19-3). Isolated skin involvement (discoid lupus) is uncommon in children. Arthralgia or arthritis tends to involve small joints in an intermittent fashion. In some patients arthritis is the main feature, and differentiation from JRA is difficult until other systemic involvement occurs; laboratory abnormalities may facilitate the diagnosis in these cases. Articular destruction does not occur in SLE. Musculoskeletal discomfort may also occur from myositis, usually accompanied by proximal muscle weakness. Pericarditis is the most common cardiac manifestation, occasionally causing severe chest pain or tamponade. Myocarditis and valvulitis may also occur. About half of the patients have some type of neurologic disease. Seizures, psychosis, and diffuse encephalopathy are the most frequent, but virtually any neurologic syndrome may be simulated by SLE. Presently chorea is more frequently caused by SLE than by rheumatic fever. Strokes, aseptic meningitis, subarachnoid hemorrhage, and transverse myelitis are infrequent. Vasculitis may cause necrotic skin lesions, neuropathy or an acute abdominal crisis with vascular insufficiency, infarction, or ileus of the bowel.

The most seriously affected organ is the kidney. Three basic forms of nephritis may be seen. The most benign is focal nephritis, presenting with microscopic hematuria, minimal proteinuria, and good renal function. Most of these patients do well, particularly the mesangial subset, but a few (with focal proliferative glomerulitis) evolve into more extensive renal involvement. Membranous nephritis is the least common variety but these patients also form a good prognostic group. It presents with marked proteinuria; some children have edema and other signs of the nephrotic syndrome. Unfortunately, about half of the children with renal disease, up to 70% in some series, have diffuse proliferative glomerulonephritis, characterized by microscopic hematuria, proteinuria, and progressive renal failure. Most authorities recommend renal biopsy as a guide to prognosis and therapy; however, a minority opinion that has gathered momentum in recent years focuses on the likelihood that biopsy findings are predictable on clinical grounds and that progressive renal disease will be treated vigorously with corticosteroids or immunosuppressive drugs even in the absence of biopsy data. A reasonable approach is to perform biopsies when the resulting information is likely to lead to a major alteration in therapy.

Laboratory features. Almost all SLE patients have hematologic abnormalities at some time during their illness. Leukopenia is present in more than half of children with SLE. The differential count is often normal, indicating an absolute decrease in both neutrophils and lymphocytes, the latter being in part related to the presence of antilymphocyte antibodies. Severe anemia is often caused by hemolysis and is usually associated with a positive Coombs test, but Coombs positivity occurs in 40%, often without significant anemia. Other patients appear to have anemia typical of chronic disease. Thrombocytopenia (less than 150,000 platelets/mm^3) occurs in a third and when severe is associated with purpura. Circulating anticoagulants may cause clotting abnormalities in about a quarter of children, but this seldom results in significant bleeding.

A broad spectrum of autoantibodies is characteristic of SLE. The most sensitive test, for antinuclear antibody, is positive in 99% of patients and may be used for screening purposes.

However, it lacks specificity because it is often positive in JRA, other collagen-vascular diseases, chronic liver disease, and a variety of chronic infections. Thus more specific tests are required to confirm the diagnosis. The LE cell test was formerly used for this purpose. It is rarely positive in JRA; "false positives" occur in drug-induced lupus and chronic hepatitis. Because it is not quantitative, requires a great deal of technician time, and is undependable in the presence of severe leukopenia, the LE cell test has been largely supplanted by tests for antibodies against native or double-stranded DNA. This is a quantitative determination that gives abnormal values in about 50% of SLE patients, particularly those with renal involvement. Another specific test detects antibodies against an antigenic determinant in ribonucleoprotein; anti-Sm, so named for a patient (Smith) in whom it was first detected, is not found more frequently in any particular SLE subset. Many other autoantibodies against nuclear or cytoplasmic determinants may be identified in SLE patients but are less useful in diagnosis because of low specificity. A biologic false positive test for syphilis is present in 10% to 15% of patients and is directed against a lipoprotein antigen. Many cases of SLE have been identified after investigation of such biologic false positive reactions in blood obtained on premarital examinations or on routine hospital admissions. However, only a minority of biologic false positive reactors develop SLE on extended follow-up studies.

The pathogenesis of SLE involves the deposition of circulating immune complexes in tissue and in the walls of small vessels. Such deposition may be demonstrated in the glomeruli and on the epidermal basement membrane ("lupus band test"). Serum complement levels are frequently low in SLE, including total hemolytic complement (CH50) and components (C3 and C4). The depression of complement is related to disease activity, particularly that of the renal disease. For this reason, complement and anti-DNA are often used to monitor activity and predict impending exacerbations.

Diagnostic criteria. The American Rheumatism Association criteria have been revised recently and are listed below. For the diagnosis of lupus, four or more of the criteria must be present, serially or simultaneously, during any interval of observation.

Malar rash
Discoid rash
Photosensitivity
Oral ulcers
Arthritis
Serositis (pleuritis or pericarditis)
Renal disorder (persistent proteinuria greater than 0.5 g/day, or cellular casts)
Neurologic disorder (seizures or psychosis)
Hematologic disorder (hemolytic anemia, leukopenia, or thrombocytopenia)
Immunologic disorder (positive LE cells, anti-DNA, anti-Sm or biologic false positive test)
Antinuclear antibody

Treatment. There is no standard treatment for SLE because curative therapy is unavailable and patients vary greatly in type and severity of organ involvement. Arthritis may be managed with salicylates and nonsteroidal anti-inflammatory drugs. Antimalarials are often effective for rash and arthritis that does not respond to anti-inflammatory agents. Long-term use of these drugs occasionally results in retinal damage, and regular monitoring by an ophthalmologist is a necessary precaution. Corticosteroids are the standard therapy for persistent or refractory serositis, fever, and hematologic, neurologic, cardiac, and renal disease. Large doses are often necessary. An alternate-day schedule is preferred to minimize side effects, but this is often not possible in patients with severe arthritis, fever, and serositis. Large intravenous pulses of steroids, for example, 500 to 1000 mg of methylprednisone on 3 consecutive days, may be used in patients with rapidly progressive renal failure. Immunosuppressive agents such as azathioprine and cyclophosphamide and plasmapheresis have also been used in steroid-unresponsive nephritis, but their value has not yet been confirmed in controlled trials. Standard therapy for seizures and psychosis are used when appropriate. Patients with light-sensitive rash must avoid direct sun exposure and use sunscreens, but strict avoidance of sun for those without rash is not emphasized as it was in the past.

Prognosis. There has been progressive improvement in survival of reported series of SLE patients. For all patients 5-year survival is well over 90%. Diffuse proliferative nephritis may progress to terminal renal failure, but death may be avoided with dialysis and transplantation. Infection is the main cause of death and is often caused by unusual organisms such as fungi,

Pneumocystis, and rare bacteria in immunosuppressed children. Spontaneous remissions are uncommon, but extended survival in patients without renal disease is commonplace, particularly if high-dose steroid therapy can be avoided.

Neonatal lupus. Because antinuclear antibodies are usually in the IgG class, transplacental passage occurs, resulting in positive tests in the infant. However, clinical illness is rare. Transient leukopenia and thrombocytopenia has been reported. Some infants have discoid skin lesions that disappear within a few months. Maternal lupus is a common cause of congenital heart block. About half of such cases have mothers with clinical or serologic findings suggestive of SLE. The mechanism of injury to the cardiac conducting system is unclear.

Drug-induced lupus. Adults often develop a lupus-like syndrome related to the use of hydralazine and procainamide, drugs that are seldom used in children. Anticonvulsants are the most common provoking agents in children. Since seizures may be manifestation of SLE, it is often difficult to differentiate drug-induced LE from idiopathic disease, unless remission occurs after drug withdrawal or substitution of another agent. Several drugs, including isoniazid, methyldopa, and phenothiazines, may induce positive antinuclear antibody tests in the absence of any clinical illness.

DERMATOMYOSITIS

Inflammatory myopathy of unknown cause affecting skeletal muscle occurs in the form of dermatomyositis (DM) with associated inflammatory skin lesions or polymyositis (PM). PM is the most common variety in adults but is rare in children. Myositis may also occur as a part of generalized connective tissue diseases such as SLE, JRA, and scleroderma. In childhood DM, an immune complex vasculopathy probably plays an important role in some cases. Diagnosis depends on the clinical finding of prox-

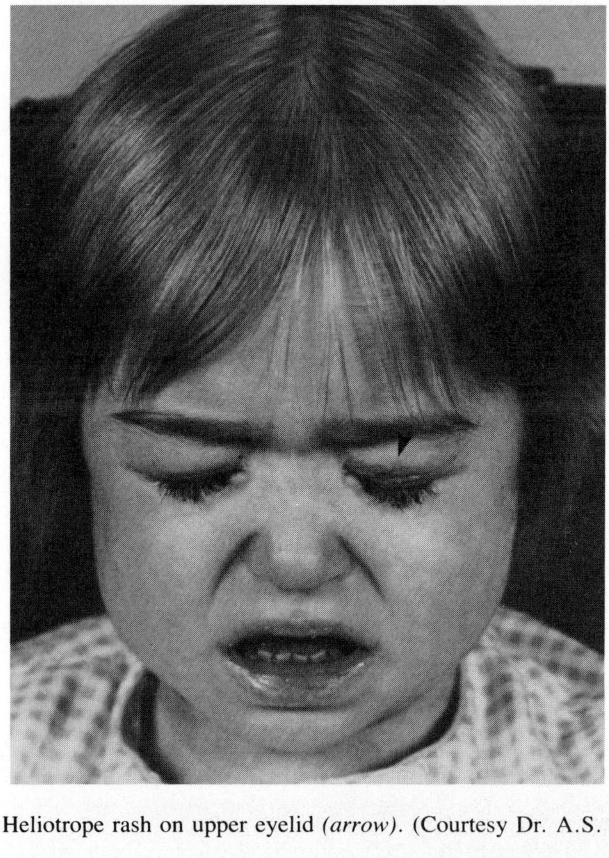

Fig. 19-4. Heliotrope rash on upper eyelid *(arrow)*. (Courtesy Dr. A.S. Hanissian.)

imal muscle weakness, which may have acute or insidious onset. The child may experience difficulty in rising from the floor, climbing stairs, raising the arms overhead, or combing hair. Dysphagia and dysphonia occur when pharyngeal and laryngeal muscles are involved. Many but not all patients have significant muscle pain and tenderness. An associated acute arthritis may also contribute to pain in about a quarter of cases. The skin lesions are quite characteristic, and may precede muscle weakness by weeks or months. There is a diffuse erythematous rash on the face, neck, and upper chest, particularly in light-exposed areas. Periorbital edema is common, with a dusky lilac hue on the upper lids, sometimes referred to as a "heliotrope eruption" (Fig. 19-4). Erythema also occurs over bony prominences on the extensor surfaces such as the knees, elbows, knuckles, and malleoli (Fig. 19-5). Many children are acutely ill with fever, anorexia, weight loss, tachycardia, and dyspnea. Others feel generally well except for muscle weakness.

A few children may have life-threatening vascular occlusions caused by necrotizing arteritis. The abdominal vessels are affected most frequently, leading to gastrointestinal hemorrhage or perforation.

Laboratory studies are most notable for elevations in muscle-derived enzymes, such as creatine kinase, aldolase, serum glutamic oxaloacetic transaminase (SGOT), and lactic dehydrogenase (LDH). The ESR may be elevated but is often normal and does not serve as a good indicator of disease activity. Only a few patients have autoantibodies such as rheumatoid factor and antinuclear antibody.

Electromyography shows changes typical of myopathy in more than 90% of cases. However, these abnormalities are nonspecific and may also occur in muscular dystrophy and other primary muscle disorders. They include low-amplitude polyphasic potentials, fibrillations, and irritability on needle insertion.

Muscle biopsy will demonstrate fiber necrosis and infiltration of inflammatory cells in most cases (Fig. 19-6). Vasculitis may be demonstrated on light microscopy (Fig. 19-7) but is

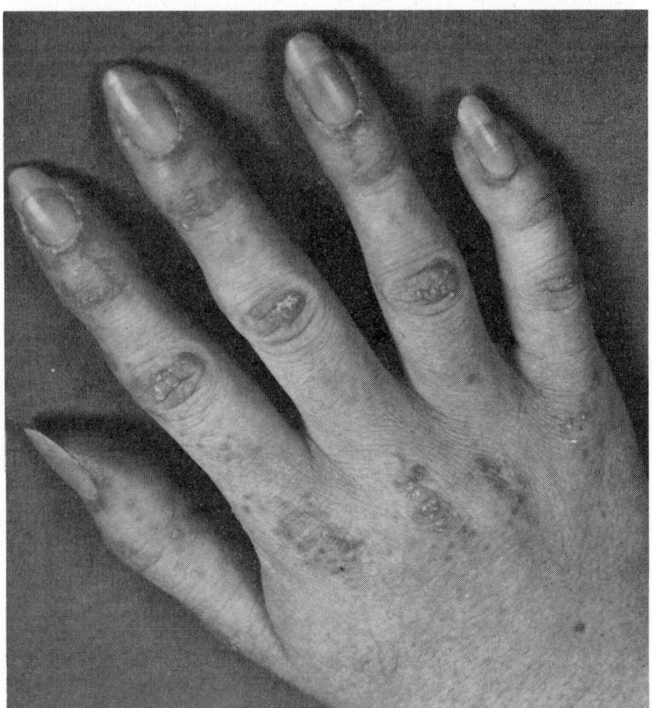

Fig. 19-5. Typical rash of dermatomyositis on extensor surface of fingers. (Courtesy Dr. A.S. Hanissian.)

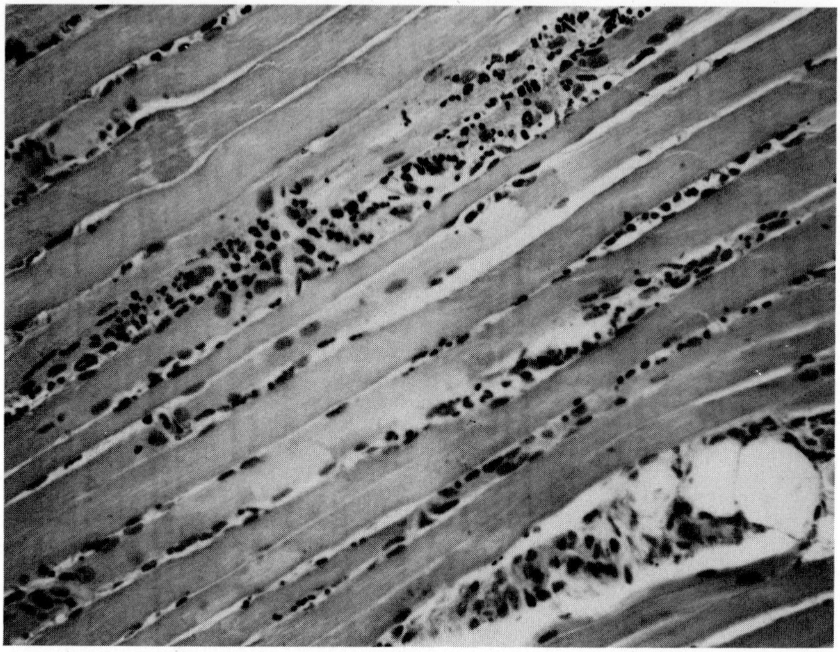

Fig. 19-6. Degeneration of muscle fibers with polymorphonuclear infiltration. (Courtesy Dr. A.S. Hanissian.)

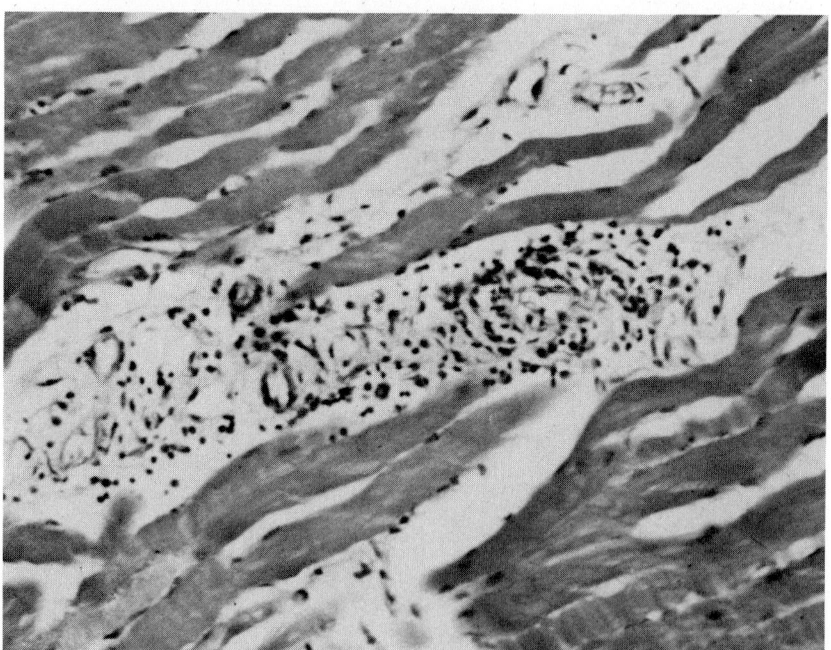

Fig. 19-7. Perivascular infiltration with inflammatory cells denoting a vasculitis component to dermatomyositis of childhood. (Courtesy Dr. A.S. Hanissian.)

A

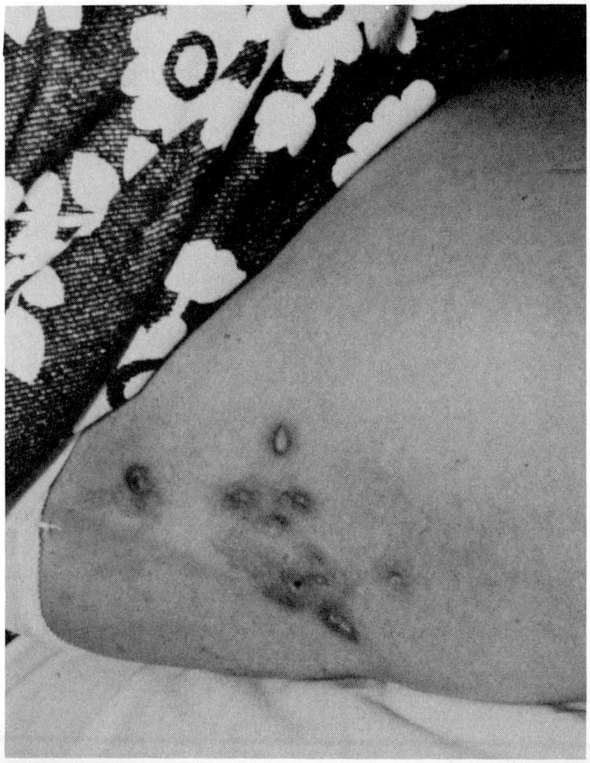

B

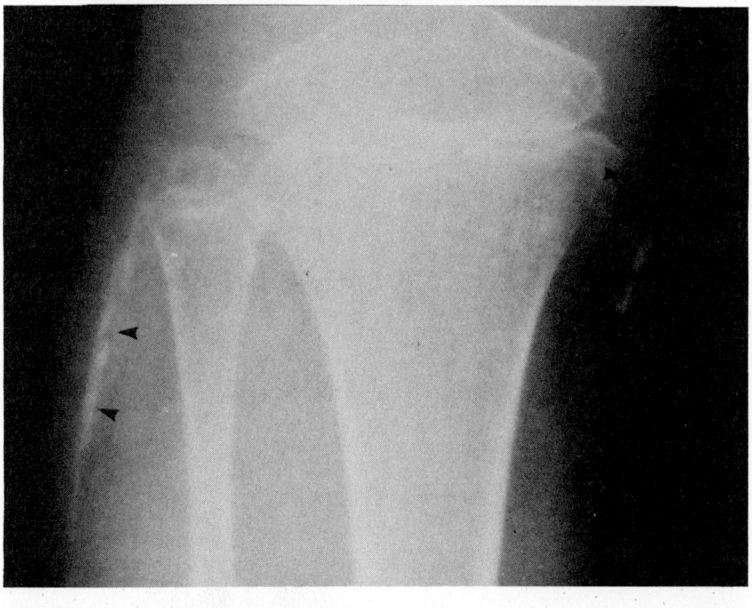

Fig. 19-8. A, Subcutaneous calcifications on upper thigh. **B,** Subcutaneous calcifications in upper leg *(arrows)*. (Courtesy Dr. A.S. Hanissian.)

more readily identified with immunofluorescent techniques. A moderately weak proximal muscle such as the deltoid or triceps is the best choice for biopsy. Gastrocnemius biopsies may not show the expected findings. In various series 5% to 20% of biopsies have been normal on light microscopy, but the diagnosis may still be made if other features are typical. Biopsy in a different area may be positive, but this should not be a requirement for initiation of therapy.

If untreated, DM usually leads to progressive weakness, muscle atrophy, and contracture. Respiratory muscle impairment may lead to ventilatory problems and pneumonia. Dystrophic calcification in muscles and skin is a late finding (Fig. 19-8). There is a tendency for the inflammatory process to remit spontaneously after several years, but, in the absence of treatment, residual contractures and muscle atrophy are very frequent.

Treatment. Corticosteroids are required in most cases, with a starting daily dose equivalent to prednisone 1 to 2 mg/kg/day. Within a week or two systemic toxicity diminishes, but significantly improved muscle power may not be noted for several weeks. The rash is often surprisingly refractory to steroid therapy. When muscle enzymes approach the normal range the steroid dose is lowered in stepwise fashion. Both enzyme levels and muscle strength are used to monitor steroid dose. In a minority of children who have not responded at least partially after 3 or 4 months, immunosuppressive drugs including cyclophosphamide, azathioprine, and methotrexate have been used, with benefit in about half of the cases. Recent reports on the use of plasmapheresis in refractory cases have been encouraging, but the basis for this treatment is unclear since circulating immune complexes are rarely present in DM.

Most DM patients survive and eventually achieve a reasonable functional level, but about 5% die of infection, vasculitis, or respiratory failure.

SCLERODERMA

In contrast to SLE, in which disease localized to the skin is rare in childhood, most children with scleroderma have cutaneous involvement only, without the life-threatening visceral disease frequently seen in adults. The cutaneous lesions are focal and are seen as thickening of skin, which is bound down to underlying muscle and fascia. The most common and benign variety is morphea (Fig. 19-9). These are single or multiple plaque-like lesions, surrounded by

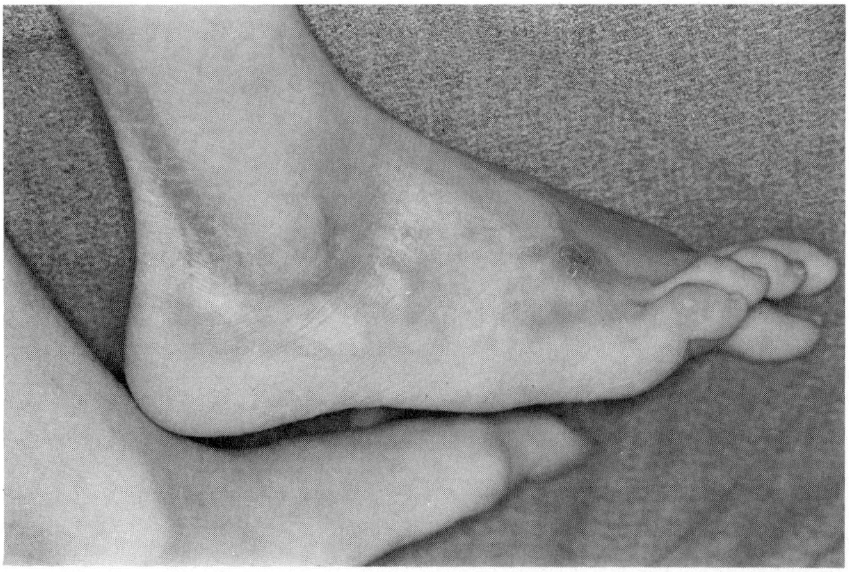

Fig. 19-9. Morphea on extensor surface of foot with atrophy of subcutaneous tissues. (Courtesy Dr. A.S. Hanissian.)

a violaceous halo, that enlarge centrifugally. Rarely there are many confluent lesions (generalized morphea), but generally morphea represents a cosmetic problem that does not compromise function. Linear scleroderma is a more significant problem. There is a linear streak of skin induration on one or more extremities, often extending into muscle. Muscle contractures and atrophy and impaired growth of the limb may cause serious functional impairment, including gross leg length discrepancies. Partial or complete spontaneous remissions may occur after several years. No medical therapy has proved to be effective. A very rare form, hemiatrophy, usually involves the face and cranium, resulting in profound disfiguration.

The adult variety of systemic sclerosis is quite rare in children. Most patients have Raynaud's phenomenon, skin tightening most prominent in the distal upper extremities, and progressive fibrotic changes in the heart, lungs, and gastrointestinal tract. Renovascular disease is a frequent cause of death. No specific treatment has proved to be effective, but *d*-penicillamine therapy has shown promise in open trials.

MIXED CONNECTIVE TISSUE DISEASE

Mixed connective tissue disease (MCTD) is an overlap syndrome that most often occurs in young adult females but has also been seen in older children. It combines clinical features of several connective tissue diseases, including Raynaud's phenomenon, arthritis, myositis, serositis, esophageal dysmotility, anemia, and leukopenia. Many autoantibodies may be present, but the hallmark of the illness is a high titer of antibodies directed against ribonucleoprotein. These antibodies may also be found in SLE, but in MCTD the specific antibodies found in SLE, anti-DNA and anti-Sm, are absent. Also, in contrast with SLE, renal and central nervous system involvement are rare. Corticosteroid therapy is generally successful. In some patients MCTD evolves into a pattern more characteristic of scleroderma or SLE.

SYSTEMIC VASCULITIS

Periarteritis nodosa

Potentially lethal systemic vasculitis is rare in childhood. In most cases the cause is unknown. However, increasing numbers of cases related to hepatitis B virus antigenemia have been reported in young adults but very rarely in children. These cases are clinically identical to idiopathic disease except that most have symptomatic or subclinical hepatitis. Immune complexes containing hepatitis B virus antigen and antibody can be demonstrated in the serum and in certain target tissues. Presumably many of the idiopathic cases have a similar infectious etiology. Fever, abdominal pain, necrotizing skin lesions, inflammatory arthritis, and neuropathy are common presenting features. Occlusion of major vessels may result in myocardial, cerebral, renal, and mesenteric infarctions. Coronary artery vasculitis with nodular aneurysmal dilation has been described in infants. Most patients succumb to the illness, often with terminal renal failure.

The diagnosis may be confirmed by biopsy of skin, muscle, or visceral organs if laparotomy is performed. Angiography may demonstrate multiple small aneurysms in the mesenteric, renal, or coronary arteries (Fig. 19-10). This procedure has resulted in a greater proportion of diagnoses during life and provides an opportunity for vigorous therapy in early cases. Large doses of steroids are used, often combined with immunosuppressive drugs such as azathioprine and cyclophosphamide. Preliminary results with plasmapheresis are encouraging.

Anaphylactoid purpura (Henoch-Schönlein purpura)

This is the most common type of systemic vasculitis in childhood. It may occur at any age, with a peak between 4 and 7, and is somewhat more common in boys. It is a vasculitis of capillaries, arterioles, and venules and has very selective organ involvement, usually affecting skin, joints, gastrointestinal tract, and kidneys. Most cases are preceded by an upper respiratory infection, presumably viral in origin, but no specific organisms have been identified. A few cases have been precipitated by drugs, foods, immunizations, and insect bites. The most obvious clinical feature is a purpuric rash, more prominent on the lower extremities and buttocks (Fig. 19-11). A pink maculopapular lesion appears first, later developing a purpuric center. Multiple lesions may become confluent. During their resolution, which may take about 2 weeks, the lesions turn brown and heal without scarring. IgA may be demonstrated in lesions in the skin and kidney by immunofluorescent techniques and may also be found in circulating immune

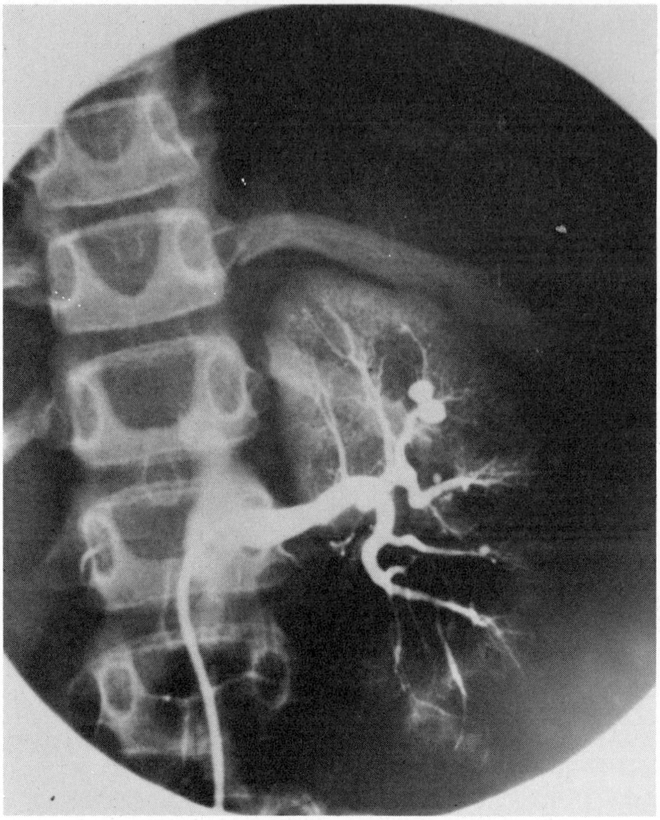

Fig. 19-10. Note aneurysms of intrarenal arteries. (Courtesy Dr. A.S. Hanissian.)

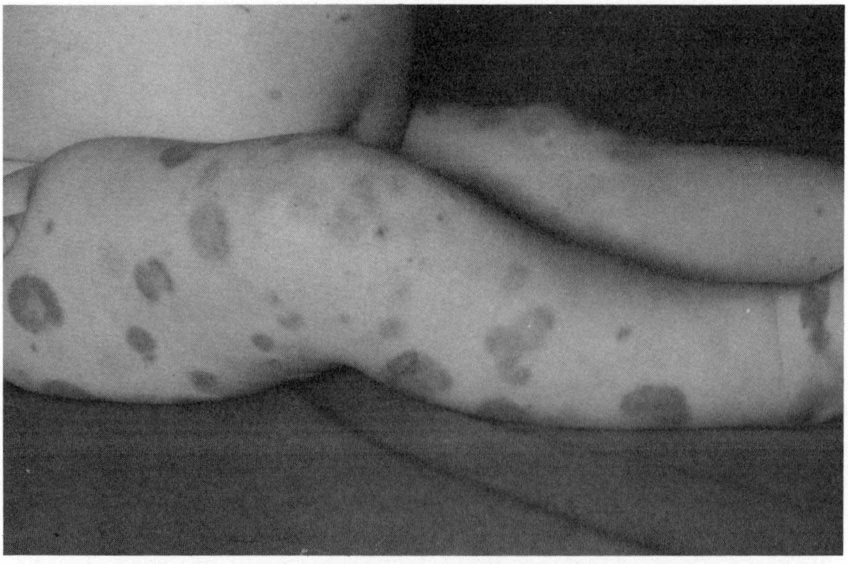

Fig. 19-11. Purpuric rash seen in anaphylactoid purpura. (Courtesy Dr. A.S. Hanissian.)

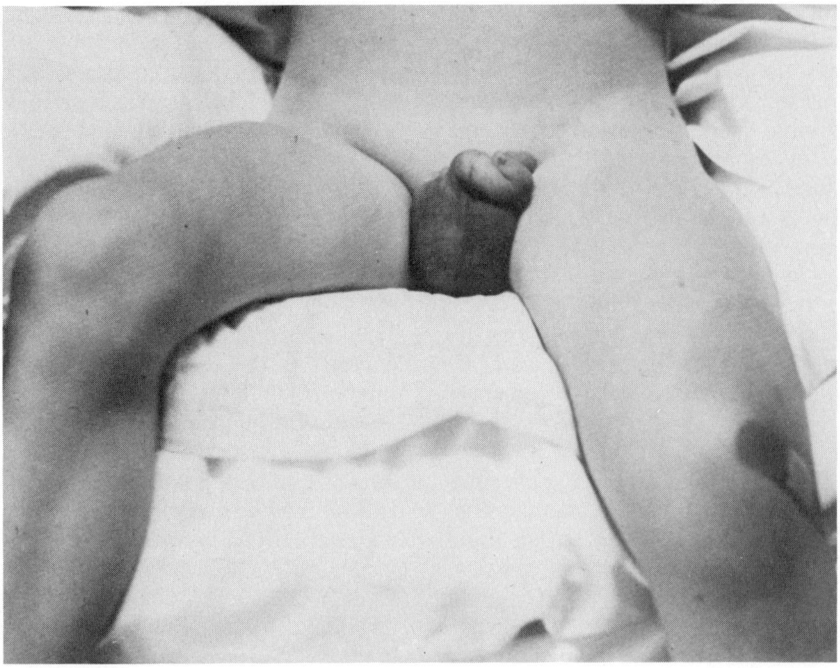

Fig. 19-12. Note edema of penis and scrotal hemorrhage. Also, patient has a swollen left knee. (Courtesy Dr. A.S. Hanissian.)

complexes. Moreover, C3 and properdin factor B can be demonstrated in the absence of the early components of the complement pathway, suggesting that activation of the alternate complement pathway may be important in pathogenesis.

Joint pain and swelling may be migratory or additive, with involvement of knees, ankles, wrists, and elbows in descending order of frequency. Purpuric bowel lesions cause abdominal pain, nausea, vomiting, and blood loss in most cases. Major hemorrhage requiring transfusion occurs in 5% of cases. Rarely, intussusception or bowel perforation requires surgical intervention. Renal involvement occurs in half of the cases and is usually a mild focal nephritis with hematuria and minimal proteinuria (pp. 545-546). It generally resolves without therapy. Progressive nephritis and renal failure are rare. A peculiar localized edema is present in a third of the cases, more frequently in infants, usually appearing on the scalp, face, scrotum, neck, hands, or feet (Fig. 19-12). Other organs are seldom involved. Intracranial hemorrhage is a rare but serious complication. Laboratory studies show a mild leukocytosis and normal platelet count. About a third have an elevated ESR. Elevated immunoglobulins, especially IgA, are found in half the cases.

Anaphylactoid purpura usually resolves spontaneously without treatment, and treatment usually consists of supportive care. Corticosteroid therapy may reduce local edema and suppress arthritis and perhaps gastrointestinal symptoms, but there is no evidence that the course of disease is altered. Aspirin is usually avoided for fear of increasing the risk of bleeding.

MUCOCUTANEOUS LYMPH NODE SYNDROME (KAWASAKI DISEASE)

Mucocutaneous lymph node syndrome (MLNS) is an acute disorder mainly occurring in children less than 8 years of age. It was first reported in Japan and is much more frequent there than in other countries. The first American reports were from Hawaii where MLNS was found with much greater frequency in children of Japanese ancestry. However, in recent years groups of children, both white and black, have been reported from various areas in the continental United States. The clinical picture suggests an infectious etiology, but efforts to identify an etiologic agent have been unsuccessful. Virtually all patients have fever for several days up to 3 weeks, generally with spontaneous resolution during the second week. Most patients have a confluent, generalized exanthem without vesiculation accompanied by erythema of the palms and soles. This leads to a characteristic desquamation later in the illness, usually beginning at the fingertips. Erythema of the tongue, buccal mucosa, and conjunctivae and lymphadenopathy, most prominent in the cervical area, are the other typical findings. A minority of patients have other manifestations. Arthritis or arthralgia occur in 20%; joint involvement is usually transient and may be oligoarticular or polyarticular. Myositis may be responsible for severe discomfort in the extremities. Other relatively common findings include pneumonitis, diarrhea, tympanitis, aseptic meningitis, and urethritis. Cardiac involvement is the most serious complication. Coronary vasculitis with aneurysm formation may result in myocardial infarction. Some children have myocarditis or valvular lesions, which may also lead to congestive heart failure. If coronary disease is strongly suspected, two-dimensional echocardiography or angiography may confirm the presence of aneurysms.

Laboratory studies show leukocytosis and elevated erythrocyte sedimentation rate in most cases but are generally not helpful in diagnosis, which is made largely on clinical grounds. In the differential diagnosis are JRA, Stevens-Johnson syndrome, and various acute infectious diseases, including Rocky Mountain spotted fever, meningococcemia, scarlet fever, viral exanthems and, in older girls, the toxic shock syndrome, many of which may be ruled out by appropriate studies.

The treatment is supportive and symptomatic. The fever does not respond well to antipyretics. Corticosteroids have been used in more severe cases, but there is no evidence that the course of the illness or the mortality is altered. Despite the rather frightening toxic appearance of children with MLNS, mortality is only 2% and is mainly related to cardiac involvement or vasculitis in other organs.

ACUTE RHEUMATIC FEVER

Rheumatic fever is discussed in Chapter 18. This section will deal with the joint manifestations and differentiation of acute rheumatic fever (ARF) from other rheumatic disorders, particularly the systemic form of JRA. Joint involvement is more frequent in older children. In contrast with JRA, ARF is rare below age 3. Younger patients are more likely to have carditis with little or no arthritis. The characteristic pattern is a migratory arthritis. Large joints are more likely to be involved than small joints of the hands and feet. The spine and temporomandibular joints are spared. A single joint may be inflamed for only a few days. Severe pain and erythema are more prominent than swelling, in contrast to the usual picture in JRA. Several joints are often involved simultaneously and inflammation may return to a joint in which synovitis had resolved several days previously. In JRA this migrating pattern is seldom seen. Fever in ARF may be high or low, but the high spiking pattern of JRA, with return to normal levels in the morning, is seldom seen. The response of fever to high-dose salicylates is often helpful in differential diagnosis. In ARF there is a dramatic suppression of fever and arthritis within 48 hours. Only a modest effect on fever is observed in JRA, and although joint pain may diminish, swelling is usually minimally affected during the first few days of therapy.

Erythema marginatum (Fig. 19-13) can usually be distinguished from the rash of JRA, but it has been found in only a small minority of ARF patients in recent years. Subcutaneous nodules have also been seen infrequently in the modern era (Fig. 19-14). They are usually found in patients with carditis located over pressure points, but histologically they cannot be clearly differentiated from JRA nodules.

Laboratory studies in ARF always show marked elevation of ESR and other acute-phase reactants such as C-reactive protein. Leukocytosis seldom reaches the high levels seen in JRA. Rheumatoid factor and antinuclear antibody tests are negative. Streptococcal antibodies are elevated in more than 95%, but, as previously noted, a few JRA patients may also show modest elevations. Joint fluid cell counts are similar in the two disorders, but the mucin clot is seldom poor in ARF as it is in most JRA cases.

The Jones criteria cannot be used to differentiate ARF and JRA, because many children with the latter disorder will satisfy the requirements. The distinction is sometimes difficult when a brief episode of JRA remits temporarily on salicylate therapy, but since JRA is a chronic,

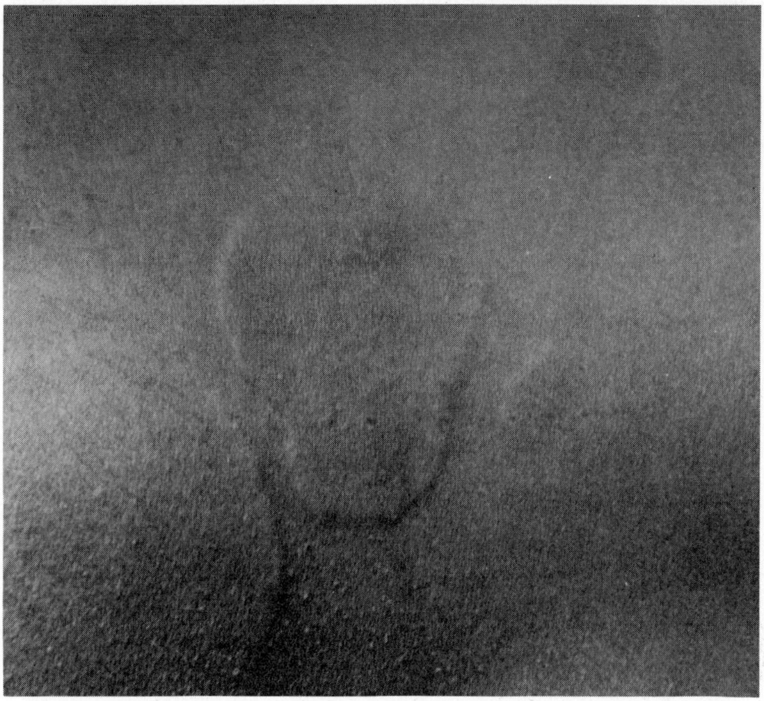

Fig. 19-13. Erythema marginatum in acute rheumatic fever. (Courtesy Dr. A.S. Hanissian.)

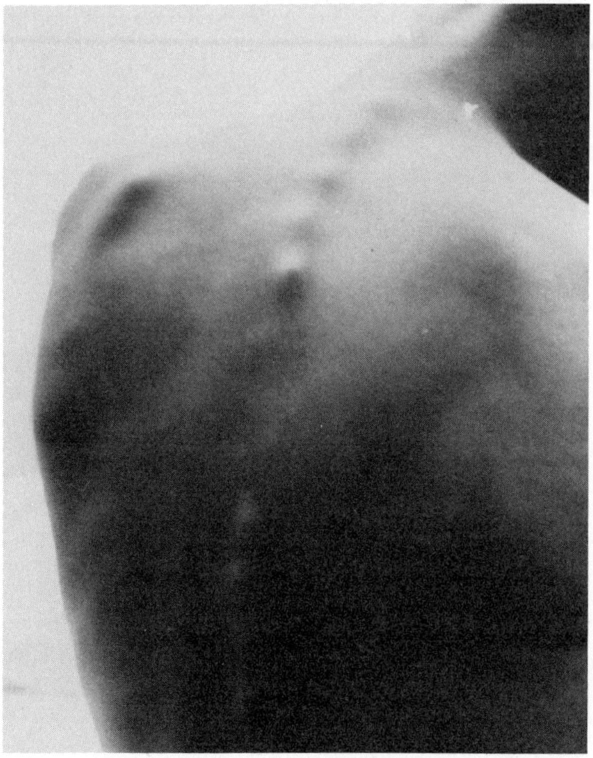

Fig. 19-14. Subcutaneous nodules overlying spinous processes of vertebrae and scapula. (Courtesy Dr. A.S. Hanissian.)

recurring illness, the subsequent course will clarify the diagnosis.

SEPTIC ARTHRITIS

Septic arthritis is still a fairly common occurrence in childhood despite the widespread use of antibiotics. Patients with chronic illness and immunodeficiency states are predisposed. Any local infection resulting in bacteremia may result in articular localization and, in a few cases, direct seeding may occur from puncture wounds or intra-articular injections. A history of preceding trauma is obtained in a third of cases, presumably because the resulting hyperemia increases the chance that organisms will be entrapped by the synovial membranes. A primary focus of infection, usually skin, respiratory, or genitourinary tracts, may be identified in about half the cases. *Staphylococcus aureus* is the most frequent organism. *H. influenzae* is common in children less that 5 years of age (especially less than 2 years old). Other important organisms are streptococci, meningococci, gonococci, and less commonly other gram-negative and gram-positive organisms.

With the exception of neisserial sepsis, most patients have monoarticular involvement, most frequently involving the knee, followed by the ankle and elbow. Hip infection is common in infants.

The onset is usually acute, with chills, high fever, and marked pain in the affected joints. There is usually swelling, effusion, warmth, and redness. With lower extremity involvement the child may be unable to walk.

Laboratory studies reveal leukocytosis and elevated ESR. The blood culture is positive in 40%, and joint fluid culture is positive in 70% of patients. Joint fluid white cell counts usually exceed 50,000/mm^3 with over 90% polymorphonuclear leukocytes, except in cases with neisserial infection. Joint fluid glucose is normally about 10 to 15 mg/dl lower than blood glucose, but in septic arthritis the difference is often 50 mg/dl or more.

Gonococcal arthritis may occur at any age but is more common in older children. Characteristically there is a migratory arthritis for several days, later stabilizing in one or more joints. Painful vesicular or pustular skin lesions on an erythematous base are often found on the extremities in patients with gonococcemia. More than half the cases have negative joint fluid cultures, and the diagnosis must be established by urethral, vaginal, throat, or rectal cultures, all of which require special Thayer-Martin media.

Meningococcal arthritis has a similar clinical pattern, with negative synovial fluid cultures and positive blood cultures. Some patients develop sterile inflammatory arthritis within a week or 2 after having meningococcal meningitis. This may represent an immune reaction to meningococcal antigen; the synovitis resolves spontaneously without specific treatment even if the course of antibiotic therapy has been completed.

Tuberculous arthritis is now quite rare in American children. It generally presents as an indolent, monoarticular, inflammatory arthritis resembling oligoarticular JRA. A tuberculin test should be performed on all such children. Synovial fluid cultures are negative in half of the cases, and a biopsy may be necessary to establish the diagnosis.

Joint sepsis must be identified and treated promptly because the outcome is largely related to the time elapsed before treatment. Broad-spectrum antibiotic therapy is appropriate until the organism is identified. Intravenous therapy is given for about 2 weeks and may be followed by oral antibiotics, depending on the characteristics of the organism and the clinical response. Joint fluid should be aspirated daily, or as often as it reaccumulates, to minimize articular damage from proteolytic enzymes in the purulent exudate. Surgical drainage is indicated if fever and swelling fail to improve within 3 or 4 days, or if cultures remain positive despite antibiotic therapy during this interval. The hip is more susceptible to damage because of its precarious blood supply and is difficult to aspirate adequately. Therefore surgical drainage is indicated immediately in most cases. With septic arthritis in the lower extremity, the patient should be kept in bed until swelling has subsided. Splints and traction are used in more severe cases. Isometric exercises are used to minimize muscle atrophy and range of motion exercise is instituted during the recovery phase.

Gonococcal arthritis responds dramatically to penicillin, which may be given intravenously in severe cases and intramuscularly in milder ones. Repeated aspirations and surgical drainage are seldom required.

VIRAL ARTHRITIS

Arthralgia and myalgia often accompany viral infections, but true viral synovitis is rare. The main causes in the United States are rubella, both natural and vaccine-induced, and hepatitis B virus, and both occur more frequently in young adults than in children. Rarely, arthritis occurs in mumps, varicella, infectious mononucleosis, erythema infectiosum, and adenovirus and enterovirus infections.

The incidence of arthritis after natural rubella infection in children is less than 1% overall, and postpubertal girls are more frequently affected. Arthritis appears after the exanthem has disappeared, usually affecting the hands, wrists, and knees. There is often morning stiffness and occasionally a positive rheumatoid factor test. Therefore confusion with rheumatoid arthritis is possible, but remission takes place within a few weeks. Rubella virus has been isolated from joint fluid. The effusion contains 500 to 5000 white cells/mm^3, mostly mononuclear cells. Vaccine-induced arthritis was quite frequent before the early arthritogenic vaccines were withdrawn, but is now uncommon. Joint symptoms develop at about the time circulating rubella antibodies appear. Most patients have arthralgia without actual joint swelling, with most frequent involvement of the knees. Duration of symptoms seldom exceeds 2 weeks.

Hepatitis B viremia may cause polyarthritis, often accompanied by an urticarial rash as a prodrome to the development of symptomatic liver disease and jaundice. This may occur in adolescents but has not been seen in younger children. Pathogenetically, it resembles a serum sickness-like illness, with circulating antigen-antibody complexes and activation of the complement system.

LYME ARTHRITIS

Named for a Connecticut coastal town where it was first described, Lyme arthritis is a subacute inflammatory arthritis that appears to be transmitted by an arthropod vector, probably a tick, and is presumed to be an infectious disorder. Recently a spirochete recovered from the tick vector reproduced the disease in rabbits. The illness is most common in children and young adults. The peak incidence of new cases is in the summer and early fall. Most reported cases have been from southern New England coastal areas, but a few typical patients have been seen in other areas of the United States, corresponding to the distribution of the putative tick vector *(Ixodes dammini)*. The first manifestation is often an unusual skin lesion, erythema chronicum migrans, which begins as a red macule and expands, often with central clearing, to a large irregular ring several inches in diameter. This lesion may last for several weeks and others may appear. Within a few months about half of the patients develop an oligoarthritis very similar to JRA. Fever may accompany the skin lesion and the arthritis. Some patients have neurologic manifestations such as Bell's palsy, aseptic meningitis, and cerebellar ataxia. Cardiac conduction abnormalities have also been reported. Circulating immune complexes have been demonstrated, but their role in pathogenesis is uncertain.

The course of the illness is often episodic, similar to JRA. Remission may occur after variable periods, ranging from months to more than 2 years. Treatment of Lyme arthritis is symptomatic, but there is some recent evidence that penicillin and tetracycline may attenuate the illness.

ARTHRITIS ASSOCIATED WITH HEMATOLOGIC DISORDERS

Sickle cell disease. Sickle cell crises result in localized skeletal pain caused by ischemia and infarction. Less commonly, sickling in synovial vessels causes joint pain and effusion. The arthritis usually attacks suddenly and may involve one or more large joints. Despite local signs suggesting inflammation, the joint fluid usually does not show elevated white cell counts. The attack generally ends spontaneously within several days. Microvascular obstruction in the synovium is the presumed mechanism. Although hyperuricemia is common in sickle cell disease, attacks of gout are rare. Septic arthritis occurs occasionally but osteomyelitis, particularly caused by *Salmonella*, is more common. Avascular necrosis of the hips may lead to a chronic degenerative arthritis for which total hip replacement may be necessary.

Arthritis in leukemia. Children with lymphocytic leukemia may have musculoskeletal pain. This is usually bone pain, but some patients have palpable joint swelling related to leukemic infiltration of the synovium or hemorrhage into joints or periarticular structures. In contrast to JRA, pain is usually disproportionate to physical signs. In most cases examination of peripheral blood or bone marrow will establish the diagnosis.

Hemophilic arthropathy. Recurrent hemarthrosis is one of the principal clinical features of hemophilia. Single or multiple joints may be involved in individual episodes. Permanent joint damage often results from recurrent synovial and subchondral bleeding. Deformities and radiographic changes resemble those of JRA. Administration of factor VIII is the mainstay of therapy. Analgesics may be used, but aspirin is avoided because of its interference with platelet aggregation. There is some evidence that short-term corticosteroid therapy may accelerate recovery from acute attacks and retard development of chronic arthropathy, but this approach is not widely accepted.

TOXIC SYNOVITIS

Toxic synovitis is a transient synovitis of the hip that occurs in young children, causing hip pain that disappears spontaneously in 2 to 6 weeks. Joint fluid is often obtained to rule out septic arthritis but is sterile and shows evidence of a mild inflammatory reaction. The cause of toxic synovitis is unknown. Treatment consists of analgesics, traction, and avoidance of weight bearing until pain disappears. Attempts to identify viral infection have been unsuccessful.

JUVENILE DIABETES

Painless flexion contractures of the proximal finger joints have been reported in 20% of children with diabetes. Thickening and tightening of the skin of the fingers and dorsum of the hand, resembling the changes in scleroderma, have been reported in about 33%. Both features are believed to be related to increased glycosylation and cross-linking of collagen in the skin and joint capsules. Signs of inflammation are absent, and there is little or no functional impairment.

BENIGN ARTHRALGIA

Transient, unexplained musculoskeletal pain is fairly common in childhood. Often these episodes are referred to as "growing pains." They are most common in the lower extremities, not necessarily localized to joints, and are most frequent late in the day or at night. In contrast to JRA, the child is generally well in the morning and has no objective evidence of joint disease such as soft tissue swelling. Sometimes there is an association with unusual exertion or emotional stress. The cause is unknown. Various local and systemic conditions must be ruled out by careful examination and simple studies such as the ESR. The symptoms usually respond to measures such as heat, massage, and analgesics.

Robert S. Pinals

REFERENCES

Brewer, E.J., et al.: Juvenile rheumatoid arthritis, ed. 2, Philadelphia, 1982, W.B. Saunders Co.

Cassidy, J.T.: Juvenile rheumatoid arthritis. In Kelley, W.N., et al.: Pediatric rheumatology for the practitioner, New York, 1982, Springer-Verlag New York, Inc.

Ruddy, S., and Sledge, C.B., editors: Textbook of rheumatology, Philadelphia, 1981, W.B. Saunders Co.

Williams, G.F.: Children with chronic arthritis: a primer for patients and parents, Littleton, Mass., 1981, John Wright-PSG, Inc.

SELECTED READINGS

Juvenile rheumatoid arthritis

Baum, J.: Juvenile arthritis, Am. J. Dis. Child. **135:**557, 1981.

Brewer, E.J., and Giannini, E.H.: Methodology and studies of children with juvenile rheumatoid arthritis: the pediatric rheumatology collaborative study group, J. Rheumatol. **9:**107, 1982.

Brewer, E.J., et al.: Juvenile rheumatoid arthritis, ed. 2, Philadelphia, 1982, W.B. Saunders Co.

Calabro, J.J., et al.: Juvenile rheumatoid arthritis: a general review and report of 100 patients observed for 15 years, Semin. Arthritis Rheum. **5:**257, 1976.

Miller, J.J.: Juvenile rheumatoid arthritis, Littleton, Mass., 1979, John Wright-PSG Inc.

JRA variants

Arnett, F.C., et al.: Juvenile-onset chronic arthritis: clinical and roentgenographic features of a unique HLA-B27 subset, Am. J. Med. **69:**369, 1980.

Jacobs, J.C., et al.: HLA-B27 associated spondyloarthritis and enthesopathy in childhood: clinical, pathologic, and radiographic observations in 58 patients, J. Pediatr. **100:**521, 1982.

Systemic lupus erythematosus

Caeiro, F., et al.: Systemic lupus erythematosus in childhood, Ann. Rheum. Dis. **40:**325, 1981.

King, K.K., et al.: The clinical spectrum of systemic lupus erythematosus in childhood, Arthritis Rheum. **20** (suppl.):287, 1977.

Singsen, B.H., et al.: Antinuclear antibodies and lupuslike syndrome in children receiving anticonvulsants, Pediatrics **57:**529, 1976.

Wallace, C., et al.: Prospective study of childhood systemic lupus erythematosus, Arthritis Rheum. **21:**599, 1978.

Dermatomyositis and polymyositis

Goel, K.M., and Shanks, R.A.: Dermatomyositis in childhood: review of 8 cases, Arch. Dis. Child. **51:**501, 1976.

Hanissian, A.S., et al.: Polymyositis and dermatomyositis in children: an epidemiologic and clinical comparative analysis, J. Rheumatol. **9:**390, 1982.

Sullivan, D.B., et al.: Dermatomyositis in the pediatric patient, Arthritis Rheum. **20**(suppl.):327, 1977.

Scleroderma

Cassidy, J.T., et al.: Scleroderma in children, Arthritis Rheum. **20:**351, 1977.

Kornreich, H.K., et al.: Scleroderma in childhood, Arthritis Rheum. **20:**343, 1977.

Fleischmajer, R., and Nedwich, A.: Generalized morphea, Arch. Derm. **106:**509, 1972.

Mixed connective tissue disease

Singsen, B.H., et al.: Mixed connective tissue disease in childhood, J. Pediatr. **90:**893, 1977.

Systemic vasculitis

Ettlinger, R.E., et al.: Polyarteritis nodosa in childhood, Arthritis Rheum. **22:**820, 1979.

Fink, C.W.: Polyarteritis and other diseases with necrotizing vasculitis in childhood, Arthritis Rheum. **20:**378, 1977.

Glanz, S., et al.: Regression of coronary-artery aneurysms in infantile polyarteritis nodosa, New Engl. J. Med. **294:**939, 1976.

Mucocutaneous lymph node syndrome

Calabro, J.J., et al.: Kawasaki syndrome, N. Engl. J. Med. **306:**237, 1982.

Melish, M.E., et al.: Mucocutaneous lymph node syndrome in the United States, Am. J. Dis. Child **130:** 599, 1976.

Yanagihara, R., and Todd, J.K.: Acute febrile mucocutaneous lymph node syndrome, Am. J. Dis. Child. **134:**603, 1980.

Acute rheumatic fever

Stollerman, G.H.: Rheumatic fever. In Kelley, W.N., et al., editors: Textbook of rheumatology, Philadelphia, 1981, W.B. Saunders Co.

Taranta, A.: Rheumatic fever. In McCarty, D.J., Jr., editor: Arthritis and allied conditions, ed. 9, Philadelphia, 1979, Lea & Febiger.

Septic arthritis

Fink, C.W.: Gonococcal arthritis in children, JAMA **194:**123, 1965.

Granoff, D.M., and Nankervis, G.A.: Infectious arthritis in the neonate caused by *Haemophilus influenzae,* Am. J. Dis. Child. **129:**730, 1975.

Morrey, B.F., et al.: Septic arthritis in children, Orthop. Clin. North Am. **6:**923, 1975.

Nelson, J.D.: The bacterial etiology and antibiotic management of septic arthritis in infants and children, Pediatrics **50:**437, 1972.

Viral arthritis

Phillips, P.E.: Viral arthritis in children, Arthritis Rheum. **20**(suppl.):584, 1977.

Malawista, S.E., and Steere, A.C.: Viral arthritis. In Kelley, W.N., et al., editors: Textbook of rheumatology, Philadelphia, 1981, W.B. Saunders Co.

Lyme arthritis

Burgdofer, W., et al.: Lyme disease—a tickborne spirochetosis?, Science **216:**1317, 1982.

Steere, A.C., et al.: Chronic Lyme arthritis, Ann. Intern. Med. **90:**896, 1979.

Steere, A.C., and Malawista, S.E.: Cases of Lyme disease in the United States: locations correlated with distribution of *lxodes dammini,* Ann. Intern. Med. **91:**730, 1979.

Arthritis associated with hematologic disorders

Espinoza, L.R., et al.: Joint manifestations of sickle cell disease, Medicine **53:**295, 1974.

Mainardi, C.L., and Levine, P.H.: Hemophilia and arthritis. In Kelley, W.N., et al., editors: Textbook of rheumatology, Philadelphia, 1981, W.B. Saunders Co.

Schaller, J.: Arthritis as a presenting manifestation of malignancy in children, J. Pediatr. **81:**793, 1972.

Toxic synovitis

Jacobs, B.W.: Synovitis of the hip in children and its significance, Pediatrics **47:**558, 1971.

Juvenile diabetes

Sherry, D.D., et al.: Joint contractures preceding insulin-dependent diabetes mellitus, Arthritis Rheum. **25:**1362, 1982.

Siebold, J.R.: Digital sclerosis in children with insulin-dependent diabetes mellitus, Arthritis Rheum. **25:**1357, 1982.

20 Pediatric Hematology

Blood is a multipurpose fluid composed of formed elements and plasma. Its primary function is to transport oxygen, nutrients, and regulatory substances to tissues. It also serves to bring waste substances from tissues to excretory sites such as the kidney and lung. The blood acts as a pathway for lymphocytes, granulocytes, and monocytes to travel from the site of origin to the place of function. The tissue is provided with a system of hemostasis that includes the blood platelets as well as plasma factors. This system has the capability of promptly stopping blood loss from the vascular system following injury.

Since the blood is involved in so many of the body's functions, it is understandable that diseases of various tissues are frequently reflected in changes in blood components. These characteristic changes are frequently of great help in the diagnosis of a variety of conditions. Blood is easily available for study, and its analysis has become one of the most routine parts of the diagnostic studies of patients. Since the blood also performs essential functions for the body, primary diseases of this tissue may have consequences for other areas of health. A knowledge of hematology is therefore an important part of a physician's background. In this chapter focus is on nonmalignant primary and secondary changes in blood. It is important to begin a consideration of blood with an appreciation of the average normal values for age, which are given in Table 20-1.

ORIGIN OF FORMED ELEMENTS

The cells in the blood are formed by differentiation from stem cells within the bone marrow. A schematic representation of this formation is shown in Fig. 20-1. It is likely that all the blood cells are derived from a common undifferentiated stem cell. Definitive proof for that relationship is not yet available, but both

Table 20-1. Average normal blood values at different age levels

	At birth	At 2 days	At 14 days	At 3 mo	At 6 mo	At 1 yr	At 2 yr	At 4 yr	At 8 to 12 yr
Red cells/mm^3 (in millions)	5.1	5.3	5.0	4.3	4.6	4.7	4.8	4.8	5.1
Hemoglobin (g/dl)	17.6	18.0	17.0	11.4	11.5	12.2	12.9	13.1	14.1
Packed cell volume (%)	54	54	50	35	35	36	37	38	40
Platelets/mm^3 (in thousands)	350.0	400.0	300.0	260.0	250.0	250.0	250.0	250.0	250.0
White cells/mm^3 (in thousands)	15.0	21.0	11.0	9.5	9.2	9.0	8.5	8.0	8.0
Differential count (%)									
Polymorphonuclear neutrophils	45	55	36	35	40	40	40	50	60
Eosinophils and basophils	3	5	3	3	3	2	2	2	2
Lymphocytes	30	20	53	55	51	53	50	40	30
Monocytes	12	15	8	7	6	5	8	8	8
Immature white cells	10	5	—	—	—	—	—	—	—
Percentage of nucleated red cells in total nucleated cells	1 to 5	2	—	—	—	—	—	—	—
Percentage of reticulocytes in total red cells	2	3	1	0.5	0.8	1	1	1	1

Modified from Smith, N.J., et al.: In Nelson, W.E., editor: Textbook of pediatrics, ed. 7, Philadelphia, 1959, W.B. Saunders Co.

experimental and clinical evidence to date support the concept of a common precursor cell for all blood cells.

Differentiation is associated with the progressive development of the cytoplasmic characteristics of the mature functioning cell. Early differentiating cells retain the capacity for cell division, thus providing for amplification of cell production of that specific line. Erythrocytes and platelets function in the blood without nuclei. The platelets are formed from the cytoplasm of the megakaryocyte within the bone marrow and released into the blood. The nucleus of the normoblast is extruded from the cell before the resulting erythrocyte is released to the blood. The mature granulocytes retain their nucleus but are no longer capable of cell division. Lymphocytes and probably monocytes still retain the capability for further cell division at the time of their release from the marrow. Both erythrocytes and platelets undergo further development after leaving the marrow, before the final functional state is achieved.

Blood cell production by the bone marrow is carefully regulated. In the well person, production is adjusted to match the rate with which each cell line needs replacement in blood. This regulatory system is also capable of responding to accelerated needs caused by stress such as blood loss or a pyogenic infection. Complete details of this marrow regulatory system are still to be worked out. The most important regulatory role is currently assigned to substances specific for each cell line capable of inducing differentiation and proliferation.

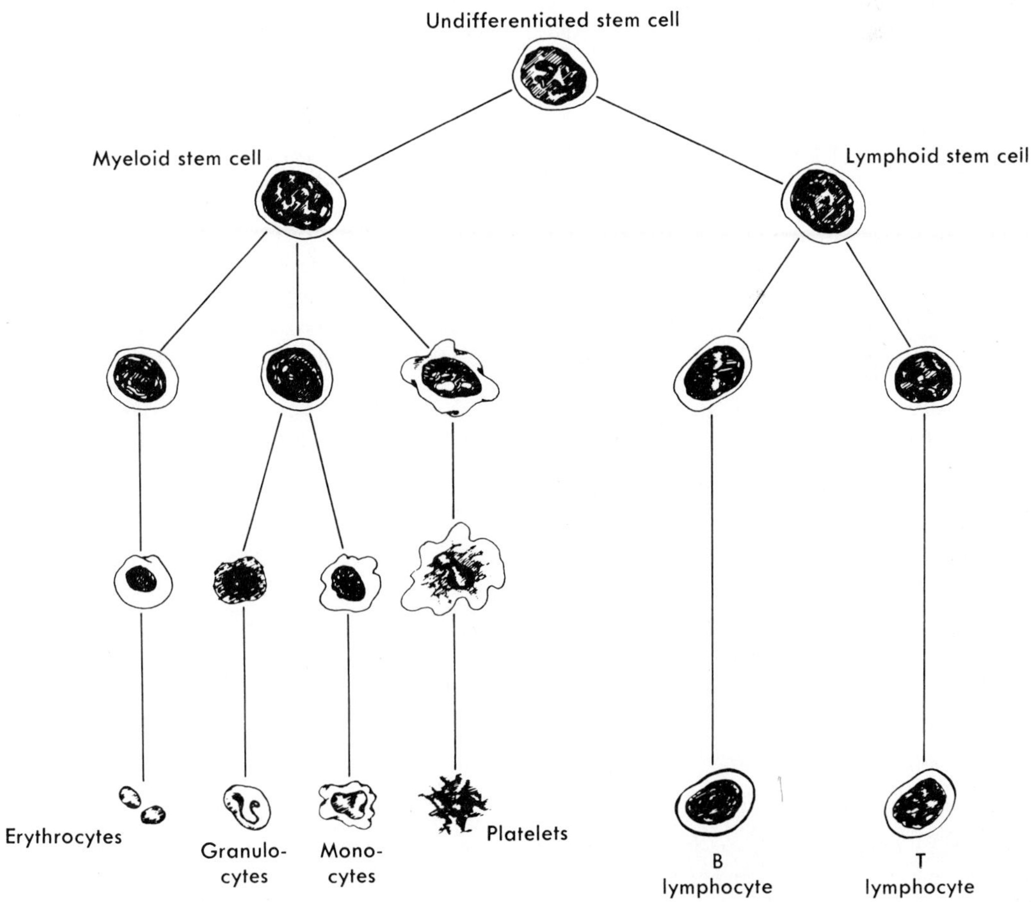

Fig. 20-1. Schematic representation of blood cell formation.

ERYTHROCYTES

The mature human erythrocyte is a nonnucleated cell with the primary function of oxygen and carbon dioxide transport. About one third of the content of this cell is the oxygen-carrying protein hemoglobin. The cell normally has the shape of a biconcave disc about 7 μm in diameter. It is elastic enough to traverse small capillaries with ease.

In fetal life the site of erythrogenesis is first in the mesenchymal tissues and then moves to liver, spleen, lymphatic tissue, and the bone marrow during the later months of gestation. The extramedullary portion of hematopoiesis normally ceases within the first 4 days of extrauterine life. Erythropoiesis is regulated by the humoral substance erythropoietin. The production of this substance is primarily in the kidney under the control of some sensing mechanism involving tissue oxygen levels. As oxygen levels decrease in the tissues, for whatever reason, the production of erythropoietin is increased, resulting in increased production of erythrocytes by the bone marrow.

Production of erythrocytes requires the availability of specific metabolic precursors. The most important of these from the clinical standpoint are iron, protein, and the vitamins B_{12} and folic acid. Other minerals and vitamins, as well as the full range of nutrients, are also necessary but clinically less important. However, deficiencies of copper and pyridoxine have occasionally produced abnormal erythropoiesis.

With respect to function, the most important content of the erythrocyte is hemoglobin. Hemoglobin is composed of a protein structure called globin with the addition of four heme moieties that are produced from protoporphyrin and iron. These heme moieties are responsible for the oxygen-carrying capabilities of this protein. The metabolism of glucose by anaerobic glycolysis provides the major energy source for the red cell. Glycogen cannot be stored by the erythrocytes, and therefore glucose must be continually available for use. Glycolysis is necessary for the generation of adenosine triphosphate (ATP) for energy and the production of NADPH and NADP to function as redox systems. These redox systems are particularly important to protect the hemoglobin from oxidation. Another important function of glycolysis is to produce 2,3-diphosphoglycerate (2,3-DPG). This production is an important mechanism to rapidly compensate for hypoxia. Increasing the levels of 2,3-DPG within the red cell increases oxygen delivery from hemoglobin to the tissues.

The normal survival of the erythrocytes in blood is 120 days. Removal of the senile cell is through phagocytosis by macrophages, primarily in the spleen but also in the liver and bone marrow. Once in the macrophage, the cell is rapidly digested. The amino acids are returned to the body pool for further use. The most important result of this digestion is the conservation of the iron from hemoglobin. The iron is released by the macrophage to the serum-transport protein transferrin and returned to the bone marrow, where it is reused for the synthesis of new hemoglobin. The protoporphyrin portion of the heme is converted to a water-insoluble form of bilirubin, which is carried to the liver bound to albumin. Binding proteins in the hepatocytes allow for conjugation of bilirubin to a water-soluble diglucuronide, which is then excreted into the gut for further conversion to the urobilinogens. Some of the urobilinogens are reabsorbed for subsequent excretion in the urine. It is possible to determine roughly the rate of red cell breakdown by the daily amount of urobilinogen excreted in the feces.

In a normal person about 0.8% of the erythrocytes die each day. The red cell production in the bone marrow must balance this removal to maintain a normal red cell mass. If red cell destruction is accelerated for any reason, or if the bone marrow is unable to produce sufficient numbers of red cells for replacement, anemia results.

ANEMIA

The concentration of erythrocytes in blood can be determined by measuring the packed cell volume (PCV), the hemoglobin concentration, or the number of erythrocytes. As a single determination the measurement of the PCV by a microhematocrit is the least expensive and the most accurate. Today most clinical laboratories use an electronic particle counter that simultaneously determines the PCV, hemoglobin concentration, and number of erythrocytes. With these three values it is possible to calculate the mean corpuscular volume (MCV), mean corpuscular hemoglobulin (MCH), and mean corpuscular hemoglobin concentration (MCHC). In

Table 20-2. Morphologic classification of anemia

Type of anemia	MCV (μm^3)	MCH ($\mu\mu g$)	MCHC (%)
Macrocytic	97-160	35-40	32-36
Normocytic	80-96	26-34	32-36
Microcytic, hypochromic	50-79	12-29	24-31

assessing the presence of anemia in a child it is important to take into consideration the expected normal values for age, as shown in Table 20-1. Further studies to determine the cause of anemia are greatly assisted by classifying the erythrocytes according to structure—normocytic, macrocytic, or microcytic and hypochromic. The assignment of the erythrocyte to one of these morphologic groups can be accomplished from the results of the electronic blood-counting machine test and confirmed by the inspection of a blood smear under a microscope. The values for MCV, MCH, and MCHC for these three morphologic classifications are shown in Table 20-2.

The finding of anemia must be regarded as an important sign of some underlying disease. A careful history and physical examination are important beginning steps and frequently will indicate the proper diagnosis. The importance of an inspection of the blood smear for diagnosis cannot be overemphasized. There are many specific morphologic alterations of red cells associated with various kinds of anemia that can be pathognomonic. A simplified classification for the consideration of the causes of anemia can be designed, based on whether the fault lies primarily with decreased erythrocyte production or accelerated cell loss. Following is an outline based on that system. This will be the basis for considering anemias of childhood in this section.

- I. Decreased erythrocyte production
  - A. Nutritional deficiency
    - 1. Microcytic hypochromic erythrocytes
      - a. Iron
      - b. Pyridoxine
    - 2. Macrocytic erythrocytes
      - a. Folic acid
      - b. Vitamin B_{12}
  - B. Marrow failure
    - 1. Acquired
      - a. Aplastic anemia
      - b. Transient hypoplasia
      - c. Inflammatory diseases
      - d. Organ failure (liver, kidney)
    - 2. Congenital
      - a. Diamond-Blackfan syndrome (erythrogenesis imperfecta)
      - b. Fanconi syndrome (constitutional marrow failure)
- II. Accelerated erythrocyte loss
  - A. Hemolysis
    - 1. Acquired
      - a. Immunohemolytic anemia
      - b. Infections
      - c. Chemicals
      - d. Microangiopathic conditions
    - 2. Congenital
      - a. Membrane related
        - 1. Hereditary spherocytosis
        - 2. Ovalocytosis
        - 3. Stomatocytosis
      - b. Enzyme related
        - 1. Glucose-6-phosphate dehydrogenase
        - 2. Pyruvate kinase
      - c. Hemoglobinopathy
        - 1. Sickle cell disease
        - 2. Hemoglobin C disease
        - 3. Double heterozygotes (S-thalassemia, SC)
        - 4. Thalassemia (alpha and beta chain)
  - B. Blood loss
    - 1. External (gastrointestinal)
    - 2. Internal (pulmonary)

Anemias caused by decreased erythrocyte production

Nutritional anemias

By far the most common cause of anemias in children is related to a deficiency of the nutritional factors essential to erythrocyte production. The most typical of these nutritional deficiencies concerns iron. Currently in the United States deficiency of folic acid is uncommon, and anemias caused by a deficiency of vitamin B_{12} are almost always related to an abnormality of absorption. Pyridoxine deficiency is a rare cause of anemia and is almost always related to a congenital metabolic abnormality. Severe protein calorie malnutrition, fortunately rare in the United States, is associated with an anemia of complex origin. Copper deficiency has been reported as a potential cause of anemia but is of no real consideration as an etiologic factor in the United States.

Nutritional anemias with microcytosis and hypochromia

Iron deficiency anemia. During gestation the fetus receives iron from the mother. This process is so efficient that the infant's iron stores at birth are unaffected by maternal iron stores. The full-term infant at birth has a total body iron content of 78 mg/kg body weight, about three fourths of which is in circulating hemoglobin. By the age of 1 year the infant has doubled the circulating erythrocyte mass, which means that during this time an additional 150 mg of iron is necessary for hemoglobin synthesis. The only source of iron for the infant is in the diet, and therefore about 0.5 mg/24 hr must be absorbed to provide an adequate erythrocyte mass. The infant who is small at birth or who for some reason has depleted iron stores is in even greater jeopardy of developing iron deficiency during this first year of growth.

It is important that all infants have an adequate source of iron during the initial period of rapid growth. Cow's milk has only 1 mg of iron per liter and therefore by itself is inadequate as a source of iron, since the infant can only absorb about 10% to 20% of dietary iron. Most proprietary formulas have iron supplemented in the amount of 8 to 15 mg/L. Iron can also be provided in the form of supplemental liquid concentrates in the amount of 10 to 15 mg/24 hours. Solid foods, which are preferably begun at about 4 to 6 months of age, contain variable amounts of iron. The prepared cereals are generally fortified with iron, but other commercially available foods for infants vary widely in their iron content. Therefore the pediatrician must be careful about dietary recommendations for the developing infant. Fortunately, breast-fed infants fare well with respect to iron absorption and with adequate solid food supplementation during the latter half of the first year should be at no particular risk, unless there has been a reason for decreased iron stores from birth.

Another period of risk for iron deficiency is during the second decade of life. The preadolescent growth spurt puts demands on iron stores for the necessary increase in red cell mass as well as the expansion of lean body mass. Some studies have shown that as many as one fourth of persons during the second half of the second decade have iron deficiency, with some actually having a degree of anemia. Because of their greater proportional increase in lean body mass and also because their red cell mass is greater, boys are at a greater risk than girls for the development of iron deficiency.

Iron deficiency on a nutritional basis is unusual after 4 and before 12 years of age. Therefore any patient who develops iron deficiency anemia during these years should be examined for some cause other than a nutritional deficiency. The usual cause is blood loss; if there is no immediately evident source of blood loss, bleeding into the gastrointestinal tract should be considered and appropriate studies carried out.

The early phases of iron deficiency are frequently unattended by any clear-cut signs or symptoms. The parents may even be unaware of the presence of anemia, even in a child in whom the hemoglobin value has already decreased to 7 or 8 g/dl. The anemia may be noted as an incidental finding on a routine office visit or on admission to the hospital for some other condition. It should therefore be routine for the physician to establish a hemoglobin or hematocrit value on all infants at about the first year of age because of the likelihood of iron deficiency anemia during that period.

If the anemia becomes increasingly severe, the infant will begin to demonstrate the characteristic findings of lethargy, easy fatigability, and irritability. If the hemoglobin value decreases below 3 g/dl, the infant may show the features of congestive cardiac failure.

The physical examination will generally show only the pallor of the patient. The possibility of this feature must be investigated carefully because it is frequently missed. A useful clinical rule is that at a hemoglobin value of around 7 g/dl the characteristic red color of the palmar creases disappears. If signs of congestive cardiac failure are present, then there will be hepatomegaly, tachycardia, and tachypnea. In some patients the spleen may be palpably enlarged, but it is unusual for it to be much below the left costal margin. In an anemic patient a cardiac murmur is usual and cannot be evaluated for significance until the anemia has been corrected.

The diagnosis is usually established by the history. Specific features of importance are the birth history, the diet, and the age of the child. After age 4 a careful history for blood loss must be taken. Again, during adolescence a dietary history is of great importance.

The laboratory features are those of a microcytic hypochromic anemia, as demonstrated by the electronic blood counter and inspection of the blood smear. In a typical patient no further studies are actually necessary to complete the diagnosis of iron deficiency anemia.

In a more difficult diagnostic situation it is important to recognize the characteristic events leading to iron deficiency anemia. The most sensitive indicators of iron depletion are the absence of stainable iron in the marrow and a decrease in the number of siderocytes (stainable iron in the cytoplasm of normoblasts). With an even greater degree of iron depletion the saturation of the iron-binding protein transferrin decreases below 20% (normal serum iron value is 100 μg/dl, with an iron-binding capacity of 300 μg/dl). With further iron depletion the saturation decreases below 15%, and at this level anemia generally becomes evident. Also, there is a demonstrable increase in the free erythrocyte protoporphyrin, since insufficient iron is present during hemoglobin synthesis to completely use this compound for heme. In the final stages the anemia becomes microcytic and hypochromic, usually about the time that the hemoglobin value decreases below 10 g/dl. By this time the saturation of the iron-binding capacity is usually less than 10%.

If the development of iron deficiency has not been prevented by a good diet, then therapy at the time of diagnosis should begin with daily administration of iron in a dosage of 6 mg of elemental iron per kilogram of body weight for a period of 2 to 3 months. This duration of therapy is necessary so that not only will the hemoglobin value be returned to normal, but also iron stores will be created. An effective and less expensive form of iron medication is ferrous sulfate, which is available in many forms. Other easily absorbable iron compounds are ferrous gluconate, ferrous fumarate, and ferrous succinate, but these compounds are generally more expensive than the equally effective ferrous sulfate. Other iron compounds are to be avoided because they are less easily absorbable and also frequently more expensive. There is no reason for multicomponent hematinics for the treatment of iron deficiency anemia. Parenteral iron medications are also available but rarely indicated. The response to parenteral iron compounds is neither faster nor more complete than with orally administered ferrous sulfate.

Response to the iron is indicated by reticulocytosis beginning within the first week and reaching a peak after the second week of therapy. Thereafter the reticulocyte count decreases, while the hemoglobin value continues to increase toward normal. Although the treatment of the iron deficiency anemia by medication is essential, equally important is the counseling of the parents about nutrition for the infant or child. The presence of iron deficiency should only be regarded as a symptom of inadequate nutrition, and the physician should take the opportunity for a full counseling session about this matter.

If the infant is severely anemic at diagnosis and in particular if there is the stress of an infectious process, transfusion therapy must be considered. In general, the infant will not have difficulty if the hemoglobin value is greater than 5 or 6 g/dl, but below that level there must be a consideration of transfusion with additional stress. If the hemoglobin value is less than 2 or 3 g/dl, the infant must be considered at risk for congestive cardiac failure. For these infants it is important not to precipitously increase the blood volume, and therefore it is judicious to administer the blood by doing a modified exchange transfusion by removing 10 to 20 ml aliquots of the patient's blood and replacing immediately with 10 to 20 ml aliquots of packed red blood cells until the monitored hemoglobin value reaches 10 g/dl or more. Such a procedure will provide the patient with the margin of safety necessary to prevent the development of congestive cardiac failure. Transfusion may also be indicated for the patient who is anemic and who requires an immediate surgical procedure with anesthesia. In this situation packed erythrocytes should be given to increase the hemoglobin value greater than 10 g/dl.

Pyridoxine-responsive anemia. Pyridoxine is essential to the production of protoporphyrin. Therefore its deficiency or abnormalities of metabolism will lead to the development of inadequate heme formation and a consequent microcytic hypochromic anemia. A dietary deficiency of pyridoxine is rare today. Pyridoxine-responsive anemias are therefore almost always seen in patients with an abnormality of pyridoxine metabolism. In children this abnormality may lead to the development of microcytic hypochromic anemia during the first years of life. On blood smear there are considerable anisocytosis and poikilocytosis of the erythrocytes. The serum iron concentration is increased, and there is abundant iron in the bone marrow as well as the presence of an increased number of sideroblasts. There is erythroid hyperplasia on bone marrow examination. A characteristic abnormality of tryptophan metabolism can be demonstrated by a loading dose of this amino acid, with the subsequent demonstration of excessive excretion of xanthurenic acid, kynurenine, and kynurenic acid. The final demonstration of the nature of this anemia is the response, which may be only partial to the administration of pyridoxine. For these patients the requirement for pyridoxine administration persists.

Nutritional anemias with macrocytosis. Macrocytic anemias on a nutritional basis are unusual in children in the United States. A deficiency of either folic acid or vitamin B_{12} can result in macrocytic anemias, which in the severe state can also be associated with neutropenia and thrombocytopenia. The characteristics of the blood and bone marrow are identical for both these nutritional deficiencies. On blood smear there is anisocytosis and poikilocytosis of the erythrocytes, with many large red cells well filled with hemoglobin. In the neutrophils there is a tendency to an increased number of nuclear lobes, so that a characteristic feature is the presence of hypersegmented, large, neutrophilic granulocytes. Platelets do not have any significant morphologic characteristics but may be decreased in number. Occasionally on blood smear a megaloblastic normoblast is found.

The bone marrow is pathognomonic of a megaloblastic anemia. The marrow is hypercellular, with asynchrony between nuclear and cytoplasmic maturation in the erythroid series. The cytoplasmic maturation continues without retardation, but the nucleus remains large with poor nuclear chromatin condensation. The myeloid series are also involved, with poorly condensed nuclear chromatin. The hypersegmented, large, mature neutrophils are also seen in the bone marrow.

Having defined the macrocytic anemia as megaloblastic in character from blood and bone marrow findings, the next essential step is to determine if the anemia is caused by a deficiency of folic acid or vitamin B_{12}. This step is essential because therapy must be specific. Even though a patient with vitamin B_{12} deficiency will respond transiently to the administration of folic acid, the patient is put at great risk for the possible development of accelerated neurologic deficits characteristic of vitamin B_{12} deficiency.

Folic acid deficiency. In children this is the most common cause of megaloblastic anemia in the world. In the United States, however, the deficiency on a dietary basis is most unusual. Whole cow's milk and the vitamin-supplemented proprietary formulas contain adequate amounts of folic acid. If the milk is boiled, however, there is a risk of reducing the available folic acid to the infant. Goat's milk, on the other hand, has little folic acid content, and a diet from this source alone provides a risk of folic acid deficiency. Breast milk, of course, has adequate folic acid content.

The typical cause of folic acid deficiency in the United States is a problem of gastrointestinal malabsorption. Diseases such as nontropical sprue and celiac disease or other causes of malabsorption are the usual instigating factors in folic acid deficiency. The usual findings in affected infants and children are therefore the consequences of intestinal malabsorption. Weight loss or poor weight gain, irritability, and lethargy have been reported. A history of abnormal stools, characteristic of malabsorption, may be obtained. On physical examination the infants demonstrate malnutrition and usually have the potbelly characteristic of intestinal malabsorption. Pallor increases with the severity of the anemia, and if thrombocytopenia is significant, there may be petechiae. In some patients minimal hepatosplenomegaly can be found.

The diagnosis may be suspected from history and physical examination. Further confirmation is found in the presence of a macrocytic anemia with megaloblastic bone marrow changes. Confirmation comes by demonstrating a decreased serum folate level (normal values, 5 ± 1 ng/ml; mean $\pm$ 1 SD). Also, there can be confirmation from the demonstration of a response of the megaloblastic bone marrow appearance to the administration of a dose of 50 μg folic acid as a test for response.

Therapy should be directed toward the primary disease unless a true dietary deficiency of folic acid can be demonstrated by history. The patients should receive from 5 to 10 mg of folic acid daily by mouth until all evidence of folic acid deficiency has disappeared. If the malabsorption persists, folic acid supplementation should be continued.

The metabolism of folic acid can also be interfered with by the administration of certain drugs. This interference is deliberate with the administration of methotrexate for the treatment of childhood malignancy. However, the anticonvulsant drugs—phenytoin, primidone, and phenobarbital—can also interfere with folic acid metabolism. Patients being treated with these drugs who have a marginal diet of folic acid may develop macrocytic megaloblastic anemia. In these patients supplemental folic acid should be administered.

Vitamin B_{12} deficiency. The deficiency of this vitamin in the diet is rare in the United States, with one exception. The infant breast-fed from a mother who is a strict vegetarian runs the risk of vitamin B_{12} deficiency because of inadequate amounts in maternal milk. Vegetarian mothers who prefer to breast-feed should give their infants supplements of vitamin B_{12}.

The usual cause of this rare vitamin deficiency in children is a selective or generalized problem of malabsorption (Table 20-3).

Vitamin B_{12} requires for absorption a gastric intrinsic factor and a functional distal portion of the ileum. Therefore any condition that alters intrinsic factor production or interferes with normal intestinal function in the area of the terminal ileum can reduce the availability of vitamin B_{12} for the body. There are several situations in which this problem might arise.

There may be a congenital deficiency of intrinsic factor with the onset of a megaloblastic anemia generally within the first 2 or 3 years of life. The gastric mucosa is normal in function with the exception of an inability to produce intrinsic factor.

Acquired deficiencies of intrinsic factor may occur in three situations generally seen late in the first decade or into the second decade of life. The absence of intrinsic factor can be specific without other gastric abnormalities, can be associated with gastric atrophy and antibodies to parietal cells, or can be associated in addition with antibodies directed against other endocrine organs with the development of a multiple endocrinopathy. There may be selective or generalized intestinal malabsorption in patients who have a normal production of intrinsic factor.

In all these situations the patient shows evidence of vitamin B_{12} deficiency. There is macrocytic anemia associated with megaloblastic bone marrow. In patients with more advanced deficiency states there may be alterations of the oral mucosa and the development of a smooth, shiny tongue. Mucosal abnormalities in the remainder of the gastrointestinal tract can lead to diarrhea and weight loss. The neurologic abnormalities characteristic of adult pernicious anemia are uncommon in children.

The diagnosis may be suspected by history and confirmed by the demonstration of normal folic acid levels and decreased vitamin B_{12} levels in the serum. The mechanism for abnormal absorption of vitamin B_{12} can then be demonstrated by the Schilling test. In this test, absorption of radioactive vitamin B_{12} is determined with and without administered intrinsic factor. By this means the abnormality of absorption can be ascribed to an absence of intrinsic factor production by the stomach or the malabsorption of the vitamin by the terminal ileum. From the standpoint of therapy and prognosis it is important to determine the specific cause of the vitamin B_{12} deficiency.

Treatment for vitamin B_{12} deficiency megaloblastic anemia should be initially a dosage of 1000 μg of vitamin B_{12} followed by 100 μg of

Table 20-3. Vitamin B_{12} deficiency in childhood

Type	Usual age of onset	Gastric intrinsic factor	HCL	Schilling test (intrinsic factor)	
				Without	With
Congenital	Under 2½ yr	Absent	Present	Decreased	Normal
Acquired					
Simple	Second decade	Absent	Present	Decreased	Normal
Adult	Second decade	Absent	Absent	Decreased	Normal
Multiple gland involvement	Second decade	Absent	Absent	Decreased	Normal
Selective malabsorption	Infancy	Present	Present	Decreased	Decreased
Generalized malabsorption	Any age	Present	Present	Decreased	Decreased
Acquired intestinal lesions	Any age	Present	Present	Decreased	Decreased

the vitamin given monthly. If it is anticipated that the deficiency state is permanent, then this medication will be required for life.

Megaloblastic anemia may also be seen in a rare hereditary disorder—orotic aciduria. The disease is of particular interest because it is the only genetic disorder so far described of pyrimidine or purine nucleotide synthesis. The disease is caused by a defect involving the conversion of orotic acid to uridine 5-monophosphate. It is an autosomal recessive disorder and is associated with symptoms beginning within the first month of life. The anemia is usually present by 6 months of age and has all the characteristics of megaloblastic anemia. It is unresponsive to folic acid or vitamin B_{12} therapy but does respond to the administration of pyrimidines beyond the demonstrated block in orotic acid metabolism. The urine of these infants contains abundant amounts of orotic acid.

Marrow failure

The bone marrow must continually replace the red cells that are normally removed by the aging process. Thus, if there is a decreased rate of production of erythrocytes by the bone marrow, anemia develops. In some situations there is a combination of events associated with a shortened erythrocyte survival time, as well as a relative inability of the bone marrow to compensate with increased erythrocyte production. Normally the bone marrow can increase its production of red blood cells about seven times the normal value. If for one of several reasons this increased production is not an adequate response to shortening of the red cell survival time, then anemia out of proportion to what might be expected will be the consequence. In all cases the hallmark of decreased erythrocyte production is an inappropriately low percent of reticulocytes in the blood for the degree of anemia. In the bone marrow a relative paucity of erythroid precursors is found. In some of the anemias to be discussed in the following sections there is also reduced production of white cells and thrombocytes. Therefore the anemia is accompanied by associated pancytopenia. In all cases the first step in arriving at a diagnosis is the determination of blood counts and the inspection of the blood smear. A reduced number of reticulocytes and a lack of appropriate polychromatophilia in the red blood cells on the blood smear should lead to a consideration of those anemias associated with decreased marrow production.

Acquired marrow failure. The reduced erythroid production can be associated with many diseases. In the initial studies the physician should pay careful attention to history and physical examination, looking for any primary diseases that are characteristically associated with a failure of marrow cell production.

Aplastic anemia. Aplastic anemia is relatively uncommon in children, occurring with the frequency of about 1 patient with acquired aplastic anemia to about 10 patients with acute leukemia. This proportion is important because the initial findings may be similar for both diseases. In both cases there is a failure of marrow production for red cells, platelets, and normal white blood cells. The initial findings in both instances can be the bleeding manifestations of thrombocytopenia, the pallor and other consequences of anemia, and the predisposition to bacterial infections of neutropenia.

The initial symptoms in a patient with aplastic anemia usually relate to the disappearance of one of the three elements of the blood. Anemia is characterized by progressive weakness, fatigability, and associated pallor. Thrombocytopenia produces a history of excessive bruisability, petechiae, especially in dependent areas, and bleeding, especially from mucous membranes such as the gums and the nose. The patients may also have fever caused by an infection resulting from the decrease in normal blood granulocytes. Although there might be evidence of cellulitis, there frequently is an unexpected absence of pus formation because of decreased numbers of the necessary neutrophils. This triad of bleeding, infection, and anemia should immediately alert the physician to the possibility of bone marrow failure.

The history in about one half of these patients will indicate a possible causative mechanism. There are several drugs, such as chloramphenicol, some sulfonamides, a variety of anticonvulsants, and antithyroid medications, that can produce selective or complete marrow failure. Additionally, there is a variety of chemicals used in industry as well as around the home that can cause suppression of marrow cell production. The physician should first obtain a complete exposure history and then review the various drugs and chemicals involved to determine the likelihood of their liability for aplastic anemia. This review is essential because, in general, patients with drug-related aplastic anemia have a better opportunity for bone marrow recovery once exposure to the agent has been discontinued.

Additionally, there are some viral infections, specifically viral hepatitis, that can be associated with the development of aplastic anemia. Recently there has been the implication of a cellular immune response producing lymphocytotoxic suppression of marrow cell production. This mechanism is yet to be completely defined and validated. There are also some congenital diseases associated with marrow failure that are discussed later. The physician should therefore request a careful family history for similar diseases and conduct a scrupulous physical examination.

On physical examination the physician usually finds pallor, manifestations of bleeding, and sometimes the presence of an infectious process. If the anemia has progressed to the point of congestive cardiac failure, these findings also will be present. Generally, the liver and spleen are not palpable, but, if there is associated viral hepatitis, the organs may not only be palpably enlarged but also tender. In a small proportion of patients the spleen may be just palpable at the left costal margin. Generally, lymphadenopathy is not significant, and there is no associated bone tenderness. Examination of the nose and mouth might indicate mucous membrane bleeding. Sometimes hemorrhages can also be found on fundoscopy.

The diagnosis is confirmed by finding pancytopenia, on the examination of the blood, associated with hypocellular bone marrow. If an adequate specimen cannot be obtained, a bone marrow biopsy is sometimes necessary, preferably with the Jamshidi needle, so that the paucity of normal marrow elements can be confirmed. At times patients with acute leukemia can also have inadequate marrow aspirate specimens, and thus this disease must be ruled out by a bone marrow biopsy examination.

Treatment is primarily supportive. Patients require blood transfusions and at times of active bleeding transfusions of platelets as well. In some patients transfusions of granulocytes can tide them over a period of severe overwhelming bacterial infection. The best hope for these patients is the transplantation of bone marrow from an HLA-matched sibling. From recent studies it is evident that this is best done before blood transfusions are given, to avoid the risk of sensitization to a variety of non-HLA antigens. Certainly, in patients in whom it is possible that an HLA-matched sibling is available, all transfusions, especially from family members, should be avoided until the transplantation can take place. For those patients who do not have an HLA-matched sibling, supportive therapy for anemia, bleeding, and infection has been the only treatment available until at least some degree of spontaneous bone marrow cell production begins.

Recently, improvement in some patients with aplastic anemia has been described with the administration of antithymocyte globulin. It is presumed that the responsive patients have a mechanism for marrow failure involving immune suppression. More experience with this form of therapy will be needed to determine its role in treatment. In the past the use of testosterone or other steroid agents has been proposed, but recent studies do not indicate that these agents have any value whatsoever for acquired aplastic anemia. Without the availability of a matched sibling for transplantation, the mortality is about 50%. There is a particularly poor prognosis for patients in whom a specific etiologic agent cannot be identified and in whom the greatest degree of marrow failure is present at diagnosis.

Transient hypoplasia. Transient reduction in red cell production is a common association with a variety of bacterial and viral infections. Since these infectious processes are short-lived, the whole period of hypoplasia generally lasts only a few days. Red cell life span is normally 4 months; therefore this absence of red cell production for a few days is not reflected in a blood count. As will be discussed later, patients with either acquired or congenital hemolytic anemias may have significant decreases in hemoglobin concentration with even relatively brief periods of marrow hypoplasia. There are a few children in whom the period of erythroid hypoplasia in the bone marrow lasts for several weeks and can be associated with the development of significant anemia. This process is referred to as transient erythroblastopenia of childhood (TEC).

The cause of this hypoplastic process is unknown, but it is assumed that it is an extension of the usual consequences of a viral infection. In some patients there is evidence of antibody-mediated immune suppression. Frequently a history of such an infection cannot be elicited, and the patient primarily has pallor and the findings of anemia, such as weakness and easy fatigability. The white blood cell and platelet counts are generally normal, and on blood smear the erythrocytes are normocytic and normochromic. There is no polychromatophilia, and the reticulocyte count is not increased. On bone marrow examination pronormoblasts are present, but there is little evidence of differentiation of the erythroid series, although the other marrow elements are generally normal in numbers and appearance. The physical examination generally demonstrates only the features associated with the degree of anemia. The age of the patient varies, but generally this anemia occurs sometime during the middle part of the first decade of life. The only possible problem of differentiation is a drug-related suppression of red cell production or the infrequent possibility of an immunologic process. A drug history should be carefully reviewed, and screening procedures for immunoglobulin and inappropriate antibodies should be done. If no primary disease can be found, corticosteroids in a dosage of 2 mg/kg body weight/24 hours of prednisone may sometimes be effective in returning erythroid production to normal. In other patients it may be necessary to wait a period of several weeks or months before normal erythroid production begins.

Inflammatory diseases. Almost all inflammatory processes are associated with some reduction in erythroid production. Formerly these were most often the inflammation of chronic infection. With current antibiotic therapy, that is less frequently the case, and now the usual causes are chronic inflammatory diseases such as rheumatoid arthritis or other noninfectious inflammatory processes. In some patients the suppression of erythroid production may be associated with an accelerated red cell destruction, as in patients with rheumatoid arthritis and splenomegaly. The diagnosis is relatively simple, with the features of the primary disease being predominant. In general, the anemia is not severe, and the usual hemoglobin values will be in the 7 to 10 g/dl range. There is rarely any indication for specific treatment of the anemia, except for an occasional patient in whom a surgical procedure with anesthesia is necessary. In these patients blood transfusions should be given to increase the hemoglobin value to a level greater than 10 g/dl to avoid excessive anesthetic risk.

Organ failure. Several of the body organs are essential to normal marrow function. Of these, three that are particularly important are the kidney, the liver, and the thyroid. Failure of any of these three organs will result in the development of anemia. The kidney is an essential organ because of its production of erythropoietin; therefore in renal failure anemia develops because of decreased erythropoietin production. This anemia is generally normocytic and normochromic, associated with inappropriately low reticulocytosis and a relatively hypocellular bone marrow. In some patients with renal disease there also may be associated accelerated red cell destruction, and in these patients there is an inappropriately low response by the bone marrow to the anemia. The liver also is important because it is the site of metabolism for many of the necessary precursors of red cell production. With advancing liver failure there is the likelihood of developing anemia. In some patients with liver failure the anemia may be somewhat macrocytic, and a characteristic morphologic change on the blood smear is the development of target cells among the erythrocytes. The thyroid regulates the rate of metabolism in the body, and with failure of this gland the demand for oxygen may decrease with decreasing metabolic rate. The level of hemoglobin may decrease to a value commensurate with the need to deliver oxygen to tissues with this lessened demand for oxygen. The diagnosis in all these patients is related to the findings associated with the primary disease.

Congenital anemia. The two forms of congenital anemia are Diamond-Blackfan syndrome, the failure of red cell production as a selective process (erythrogenesis imperfecta), and Fanconi anemia, a constitutional marrow failure associated with progressive pancytopenia. In both cases the genetic process is presumed to be an autosomal recessive one.

Diamond-Blackfan syndrome (erythrogenesis imperfecta). The cause of this inherited defect in erythroid production is obscure and, in fact, may be multiple. In a few patients a chromosome abnormality has been described, and in others a defect involving tryptophan metabolism has been reported. In most patients, however, no specific features that would explain the failure of red cell production can be demonstrated.

In many patients with this condition the failure of red cell production becomes evident during the first months of life, with the development of progressive pallor. In almost all patients the failure of red cell production is complete during the first year of life. There are no symptoms other than those associated with progressive anemia, such as increasing lethargy, irritability, anorexia, and finally the features of congestive cardiac failure. On physical examination the infant is found to be pale, but there are no other specific features unless congestive cardiac failure has occurred. Examination of the blood indicates anemia, but all other blood cells are normal in number and structure. Blood smear shows no polychromasia, and the reticulocyte count is not increased. The erythroid series may contain some pronormoblasts but virtually no other differentiated cells of this line. The other cells, however, are normal in proportion and structure.

About half these patients will respond to the administration of corticosteroids with an increase in red cell production, which may subsequently continue even after steroids are stopped or be dependent on the continued administration of steroids. In the other half no response is evident, and these patients become dependent on transfusions to maintain their red cell level. For these patients a late consequence is the progressive development of hemosiderosis, with its impairment of liver, pancreas, and heart function. The value of a bone marrow transplantation for those patients who have an HLA-matched sibling has not been clearly defined but may be another approach in some patients to the treatment of this disease.

Fanconi anemia (constitutional marrow failure). This form of congenital anemia was described by Fanconi in 1927. It is an autosomal recessive disorder associated with a specific chromosomal abnormality in which karyotypes are found to have excessive breaks and recombinations. These chromosomal abnormalities are not isolated to the bone marrow cells but can be found in all the cells of the patient.

The onset of clinical symptoms usually occurs between 4 and 6 years of age, although in some patients findings may be delayed until the second decade of life. The first symptoms and signs are usually related to the onset of anemia, although in some patients the consequences of thrombocytopenia may be the first indications of this disease. Certainly the first cells to show the influence of marrow failure are the platelets, followed by decreased production of red cells and finally granulocytes. During the course of treatment the usual problems are anemia and bleeding; infections caused by neutropenia are a much less common problem.

The physical findings are typically helpful because there are a variety of associated abnormalities, which follow:

Anomaly	Percent frequency
Abnormal skin pigmentation	51
Skeletal deformation	40
Thumb	28
Decreased ossification centers in wrist	17
Aplasia of first metacarpal	7
Aplasia of radius	7
Others	5
Retarded growth	38
Microcephaly	29
Renal anomalies	19
Strabismus	18
Mental retardation	14
Hypogenitalism	15

The diagnosis can be presumed in a child who develops evidence of marrow failure during the first half of the first decade of life and in whom the associated physical findings can be demonstrated. On blood smear, pancytopenia is found and the bone marrow is hypocellular. The fetal hemoglobin concentration is increased, and the chromosome analysis will demonstrate the characteristic karyotypic findings. The family history may be helpful if other siblings have also been affected.

Administration of testosterone to these patients can effect a temporary improvement in marrow cell production. This improvement may last for months or years. Eventually the patients become refractory to testosterone. Also, significant liver disease resulting from androgens, such as the development of peliosis hepatis or even the evolution of hepatic tumors, can occur. These hepatic consequences are generally indications to stop androgen therapy. If an HLA-matched sibling is available, bone marrow transplantation may be tried. There are too few patients in whom this situation has occurred for an adequate analysis of the effectiveness of this treatment. Supportive therapy with blood transfusions, platelets, and, when necessary, granulocytes can tide patients over specific periods of stress. Some of these patients will develop malignancies, the most common of which is monoblastic leukemia. However, other tumors, including the liver tumors already mentioned, have been described in patients with Fanconi anemia.

Accelerated erythrocyte loss

Hemolysis

Accelerated erythrocyte destruction can be caused by extracorpuscular (acquired) factors or intracorpuscular (hereditary) factors. Following are the features of a hemolytic process of whatever cause:

- I. Increased erythrocyte destruction
  - A. Anemia
  - B. Decreased serum haptoglobin
  - C. Increased serum bilirubin
  - D. Increased urobilinogen
  - E. Anisocytosis and poikilocytosis (may be specific)
- II. Increased erythrocyte production
  - A. Polychromasia
  - B. Reticulocytosis
  - C. Nucleated red blood cells on smear
  - D. Bone marrow erythroid hyperplasia
  - E. Basophilic stippling

Not all these features are necessarily found in each patient with a hemolytic process, and the degree of severity will vary, depending on the rate of hemolysis and the effectiveness of the bone marrow response by increased red cell production.

It is important to establish whether the process has been long standing or of recent onset. The family history must be carefully reviewed and the recent history of illness or drug and toxicant exposure gone over in detail. The physical examination is frequently helpful in determining if the process is acquired or congenital. The patient with recent onset of anemia may not have had time for compensatory mechanisms to respond, and the patient will therefore show a greater degree of weakness, fatigability, and perhaps even early findings of congestive heart failure. On the other hand, a patient who has had anemia for a long period of time may be well compensated and even with relatively severe anemia have little in the way of symptoms and signs. The spleen is an organ in which much of the erythrocyte removal takes place. With a long-standing hemolytic process splenic enlargement takes place, but with recent onset of hemolysis little if any splenic enlargement occurs.

Inspection of the blood smear is an important part of the beginning study. The erythrocytes will have the polychromasia and basophilic stippling indicative of a compensatory bone marrow response. The most important feature, however, is erythrocyte structure because frequently the appearance of the red cell will be the determining factor for the diagnosis. Many of the erythrocytic features of the congenital hemolytic anemias are discussed under the individual sections. For most children with a hemolytic anemia the diagnosis can be established from history, physical examination, and a blood smear. Further laboratory studies are frequently only confirmatory.

Acquired hemolytic anemias

Immunohemolytic anemias. Hemolytic anemias that result from the formation of antibodies against the erythrocytes are uncommon in children. Hemolytic disease of the newborn results from isoimmunization of the mother against erythrocyte antigens of the infant. This condition is discussed on pp. 303 to 305. Immunohemolytic anemias caused by autoimmunization may result from infections, drugs, and primary diseases affecting the immune system; at times they are idiopathic.

The patient with an immunohemolytic anemia generally has symptoms of recent onset. Severity of the symptoms depends on the degree and rapidity of onset of the anemia. Symptoms may range from weakness and fatigability to shortness of breath and edema resulting from congestive heart failure. Physical examination will indicate pallor, usually scleral icterus, and sometimes a minimally enlarged spleen. There may also be evidence of a specific underlying disease process.

A careful history should be obtained, with emphasis on evidence of a recent infection such as infectious mononucleosis or symptoms suggesting a nonspecific upper respiratory tract infection. A careful history for drug exposure should also be obtained. Likewise, a search should be made for the findings associated with disease processes such as lupus erythematosus.

The laboratory work should include a complete blood count to indicate the severity of the anemia. On blood smear there will be polychromasia associated with reticulocytosis, and sometimes some spherocytes may be seen. The Coombs test will be positive, indicating coating of the erythrocytes with the antibody. It is important to determine the nature of the antibody because it is sometimes helpful in establishing the cause of the immunohemolytic anemia. A Donath-Landsteiner antibody is usually associated with an infection, a cold agglutinin with infectious mononucleosis or other viral and mycoplasm infections, and a warm 7S, IgG incomplete antibody with underlying diseases such as lupus erythematosus. Although these associations are not absolute, they are certainly frequent enough to be helpful in establishing the cause of the immunohemolytic anemia.

Some of the immunolytic anemias are self-limiting, such as postinfectious episodes associated with the Donath-Landsteiner antibody. Others can persist for weeks and be sufficiently severe to require corticosteroid therapy. Blood transfusions are rarely indicated but when necessary may require careful matching of donor cells to find the most nearly compatible unit of blood. Splenectomy may be required in severe persistent immunohemolytic anemia, although this procedure is not always successful in alleviating the process. Rarely, other immunosuppressive regimens with drugs such as cyclophosphamide or azathioprine (Imuran) are required.

Infections. A variety of infectious diseases can produce an associated hemolytic anemia. In the newborn period congenital infections such as cytomegalic inclusion disease, toxoplasmosis, and syphilis can be associated with a moderately severe hemolytic anemia. Bacterial sepsis during infancy may be associated with some hemolysis, but generally this is minimal. If the sepsis is associated with disseminated intravascular coagulation, more severe hemolysis might be found. Gram-negative infections during infancy and childhood, particularly of the urinary tract, may cause a brisk, sudden, hemolytic process called Lederer anemia. These anemias associated with bacterial sepsis respond to treatment of the infection and rarely require specific measures such as blood transfusions.

Chemicals. Chemical exposure is a rare cause of hemolysis in children. There are certain toxic venoms of snakes and insects such as the brown recluse spider that may produce hemolytic anemia through direct chemical damage of the erythrocyte membrane. The local effects of the bite are clearly evident, and there should be no diagnostic problem in identifying the cause of the hemolysis.

Microangiopathic hemolysis. In certain diseases there is damage to the small blood vessels, which results in subsequent mechanical damage to the erythrocytes. Such diseases include chronic renal disease, severe hypertension, and the hemolytic uremic syndrome (pp. 544-545). In these patients the underlying disease is evident, and the hallmark of the hemolysis is the presence of fragmented erythrocytes on blood smear. Another source for mechanical erythrocyte damage with fragmentation is defective artificial heart valves. Fragmented erythrocytes are also found in patients with disseminated intravascular coagulation and those with large hemangiomas that are associated with thrombocytopenia and sometimes localized intravascular coagulation.

Congenital hemolytic anemias

Membrane-related causes. In this group of diseases specific membrane defects involving abnormalities of structural proteins have been described for several of the disorders. Much remains to be learned, however, concerning the causes of membrane dysfunction and their relationship to the hemolytic anemias that result.

Hereditary spherocytosis. Hereditary spherocytosis is the most frequent of the membrane-related congenital hemolytic anemias. It may occur during the newborn period as neonatal icterus, and at times these infants require exchange transfusions to prevent kernicterus. During infancy and childhood the patient may have icterus that periodically becomes more noticeable. Pallor is generally minimal, and frequently the patients are unaware of any specific symptoms. With greater degrees of anemia they may have easy fatigability and lethargy. Later in life the continuing hemolytic process can produce bilirubin stones in the gallbladder with symptoms of cholelithiasis. These patients have a requirement for increased marrow production of erythrocytes. If they have even temporary periods of decreased production associated with infections, they may become severely anemic within a few days. In some patients such an episode of hypoplastic crisis may be the first indication of the underlying congenital hemolytic anemia.

Physical examination may reveal minimal findings. The patient may have evident scleral icterus and frequently will have a palpably enlarged spleen 2 to 3 cm below the left costal margin.

On laboratory examination the anemia is usually minimal, with hemoglobin values in the 9 to 11 g/dl range. Reticulocytosis is evident, and there is polychromasia of the erythrocytes on blood smear. The hallmark of this anemia is the presence of many spherocytes on the smear. The defect can be further identified by the finding of increased osmotic fragility on specific testing.

It is important to study family members as well. The disease is most often inherited as an autosomal dominant condition. Since it is so mild, history and even physical examination may fail to indicate other family members who have hereditary spherocytosis. Appropriate family members should therefore have blood counts and blood smears to screen for this disease.

Treatment should be splenectomy, which results in complete alleviation of the anemia and reduction of the reticulocyte count to normal. The characteristic spherocytes on smear, however, persist. The splenectomy should not be done before 2 years of age because of the excessive risk of subsequent pneumococcal sepsis. It is preferably done sometime during childhood to prevent episodes of hypoplastic crisis and also to avoid the later risk of cholelithiasis.

Ovalocytosis. Ovalocytosis is also inherited as an autosomal dominant disease. Symptoms present during the newborn period are neonatal icterus and hemolysis. In later life it is generally mild, and few patients have sufficiently severe anemia to warrant specific treatment. During the neonatal period the erythrocyte structure on blood smear features many bizarre forms, fragmentation, and some elongated shapes or ovalocytes. During the first months of life the characteristic ovalocytosis of the erythrocytes on blood smear appears. There may be minimal reticulocytosis and usually no icterus. The patients may have a palpably enlarged spleen, but frequently the physical examination is completely normal. Splenectomy should be reserved for those patients with a symptomatic degree of anemia.

Stomatocytosis. Stomatocytosis is the rarest of all the membrane-associated hemolytic anemias. The shape of the erythrocytes resembles a mouth—hence the name. Reticulocytosis and splenomegaly are present. If the anemia is severe, splenectomy is likely to be of help.

Enzyme-related hemolysis. There is a variety of congenital nonspherocytic hemolytic anemias associated with specific erythrocyte enzyme defects. Only two of these are of sufficient frequency to warrant discussion—glucose-6-phosphate dehydrogenase deficiency and pyruvate kinase deficiency.

Glucose-6-phosphate dehydrogenase (G-6-PD) deficiency. G-6-PD deficiency is the most frequent enzyme deficiency found throughout the world. There are many varieties of G-6-PD deficiency, but the most common is found in Africa and is associated with an enzyme that rapidly deteriorates in the newly formed erythrocyte. In the second most frequent form, found in the Mediterranean area and in Southeast Asia, the enzyme deficiency is severe in the erythrocytes from the beginning of their life span. Other forms of G-6-PD deficiency range from a severe, continuing, nonspherocytic hemolytic anemia to those with such minimal disturbances of erythrocyte metabolism that no hemolysis occurs.

Patients with either the African or Mediterranean varieties of G-6-PD deficiency have no anemia unless challenged by specific drugs or chemicals. These drugs include sulfonamides, nitrofuranes, antipyretics such as phenacetin, and compounds such as methylene blue, naphthalene, and vitamin K. Individuals with the Mediterranean variety also have a sensitivity to the fava bean. All these chemicals are capable of producing oxidation. In the G-6-PD–deficient erythrocyte there is no mechanism for protecting the hemoglobin by the generation of reduced glutathione. The hemoglobin is therefore oxidized to an insoluble form, leading to Heinz body production and removal of the affected erythrocytes by the spleen.

The usual clinical course for a patient in whom the appropriate drug exposure has occurred is a lapse of 2 to 4 days, followed by the onset of a brisk hemolytic process and rapid development of anemia. During this period icterus may develop, and the patient may become weak and even demonstrate findings of early congestive cardiac failure. Splenomegaly is uncommonly found. On blood smear, during the development of the anemia there is considerable fragmentation of the erythrocytes, and with supravital staining with brilliant cresyl violet, Heinz bodies can be demonstrated. After 3 or 4 days of hemolysis a brisk reticulocytosis will occur, and polychromasia is also seen on the blood smear. The diagnosis can be confirmed by testing for erythrocyte G-6-PD activity. It is advisable to remember that in the African form of G-6-PD deficiency newly formed erythrocytes have near normal levels of the enzyme. Thus, during the period of reticulocytosis, simple screening studies for G-6-PD deficiency may not be positive, and it will be necessary to repeat them when the patient has completely recovered.

The enzyme defect is inherited in an X-linked recessive fashion. In the United States about 10% of black males have the defect and about 1% to 2% of black females are homozygous for the abnormal X-linked gene. A much smaller proportion of Americans of Mediterranean ancestry will have that variety of G-6-PD deficiency. These individuals are susceptible to hemolysis on exposure to drugs capable of producing oxidation. Routine screening should be done for G-6-PD deficiency in American blacks. Those with the defects should be provided with a list of drugs to avoid.

Pyruvate kinase (PK) deficiency. PK deficiency is inherited in an autosomal recessive fashion. Although it is the second most frequent of the congenital nonspherocytic hemolytic anemias, it is a rare disorder. The defect in PK causes inadequate generation of adenosine triphosphate, resulting in excessive red cell destruction in the spleen. The reticulocyte, with its greater metabolic activity, is particularly at risk for destruction. Thus in these patients there is a paradoxical finding of a hemolytic anemia with an inappropriately low reticulocytosis. The severity of the hemolysis is variable. In the most severe forms it may be evident during the newborn period and result in significant anemia in infancy. The anemia is chronic and may be associated with considerable splenomegaly. On blood smear the cells may be somewhat macrocytic, and there are also some small dense speculated cells. One of the special features on blood smear is the relative lack of polychromasia consistent with the degree of anemia. The diagnosis may be suspected in a patient with chronic nonspherocytic hemolytic anemia with this kind of blood smear, in whom splenomegaly is present. It must be confirmed by specific erythrocyte enzyme levels of pyruvate kinase. If the patient is severely affected with moderate to marked anemia, splenectomy will be helpful in increasing the hemoglobin levels. Splenectomy will also result in a striking increase in reticulocytes and some increase in abnormalities of red cell structure.

Hemoglobinopathies. Hemoglobin makes up about one third of the content of the red cell. The hemoglobin molecule is formed by two pairs of polypeptide chains, each of which contains an oxygen-carrying heme moiety. There are three major normal hemoglobins—F (fetal), A (adult), and A_2. The polypeptide chain designated α is common to all three of these major normal hemoglobins. The remainder of A hemoglobin consists of β chains, F hemoglobin γ chains, and the A_2 hemoglobin δ chains.

During fetal life the principal hemoglobin molecule formed is F. Beginning at about 36 weeks' gestation an increasing proportion of A hemoglobin is formed. The average F hemoglobin concentration at birth is about 80%, and this decreases gradually in the first weeks of life until the expected adult values of 2% or less are reached between ages 3 and 6 months. The normal concentrations thereafter are 95% hemoglobin A, less that 2% hemoglobin F, and less than 3% hemoglobin A_2.

Amino acid substitutions with or without alteration of hemoglobin function have been described for all the polypeptide chains. The substitutions of greatest frequency and significance have occurred in the β chain. Disease states are also associated with the abnormalities involving rates of production of these chains, leading to the hypochromic anemias associated with the thalassemias. These two forms of hemoglobinopathy are discussed separately.

Hemoglobinopathies caused by amino acid substitutions. There are many varieties of hemoglobin that have been produced by genetically determined amino acid substitutions. These abnormal hemoglobins are associated with various clinical syndromes, depending on

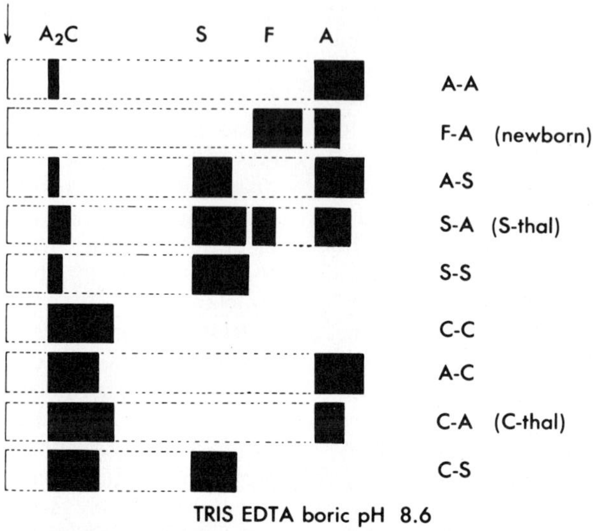

Fig. 20-2. Schematic diagram of the electrophoretic mobility of most common hemoglobins. Starch gel electrophoresis. Arrow indicates point of origin.

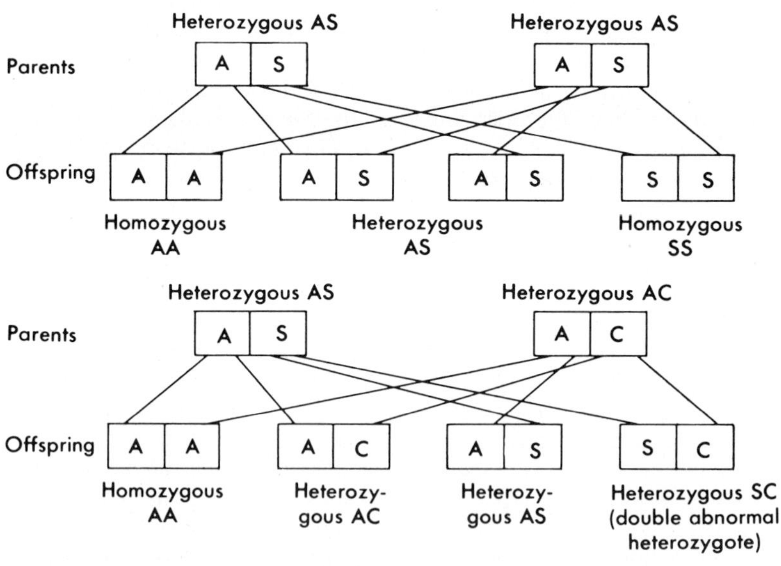

Fig. 20-3. Inheritance of abnormal heterozygous, homozygous, and double abnormal heterozygous hemoglobin types.

the nature and site of the substitution in the polypeptide chain. As would be expected, α chain substitutions are clinically evident from birth, whereas β chain substitutions are usually not evident until ages 3 to 6 months or later. Some hemoglobin abnormalities can be associated with alterations in oxygen affinity. Those with a high affinity for oxygen result in polycythemia, and those with a low affinity result in a decreased hemoglobin concentration. Some abnormal hemoglobins favor the formation of methemoglobin, with the clinical picture resembling mild cyanosis. Other abnormal hemoglobins are unstable and precipitate as Heinz bodies, leading to a clinical picture similar to the Heinz body hemolytic anemia of G-6-PD deficiency.

There are many techniques for studying hemoglobins, but the one used most frequently for specific diagnosis of a hemoglobin abnormality is electrophoresis. Schematic diagrams of the electrophoretic characteristics of the most common hemoglobins are shown in Fig. 20-2.

Hemoglobin abnormalities are inherited. If a single defective gene is present, there may be only minimal signs of disease in this heterozygous state. If two defective genes, either for the same hemoglobin abnormality or for two different hemoglobin abnormalities, are inherited, then the homozygous or doubly heterozygous state is usually associated with moderate to severe clinical disease. The patterns of inheritance of abnormal hemoglobins are shown in Fig. 20-3.

The two more common hemoglobin abnormalities in the United States are hemoglobin S and hemoglobin C. They are discussed as clinical entities in more detail.

SICKLE CELL DISEASE. The principal defect of homozygous sickle hemoglobin is the formation of rigid, intracellular tactoids that leads to a distorted sickle-shaped erythrocyte. These rigid cells clog small blood vessels in a logjam fashion, leading to ischemia and infarction of distal tissue. Sickling can be promoted by hypoxia and acidosis. Clinically, therefore, intravascular sickling can be fostered in the affected individual by diseases associated with fever, dehydration, vascular stasis, or acidosis.

Clinical complications of sickle cell disease are caused by chronic anemia, repeated thrombotic episodes in various tissues, and hypoplastic crises caused by transient marrow failure during an infectious episode. Hemoglobin values are usually about 7 g/dl, and although this anemia is generally well tolerated there is an associated reduction in exercise tolerance and usually some growth retardation.

The thrombotic episodes can occur in any tissue and are frequently associated with the sudden onset of pain in that area. Depending on the organ involved, there may be additional clinical consequences. Cerebrovascular accidents, pulmonary infarction, and bone infarction can mimic stroke, pneumonia, and osteomyelitis, respectively. An intra-abdominal thrombosis may cause severe pain. Many times the thrombotic episode is in soft tissues and produces severe local pain. These episodes of painful crisis are treated by pain relief, reduction of fever, if present, and careful attention to hydration. If the thrombosis has occurred in a critical area, then transfusions with packed red cells are given to dilute the sickled cells and reduce the likelihood of extension of the thrombosis.

A possible long-term consequence of sickle cell anemia is progressive myocardial damage leading to chronic congestive failure. Also, renal damage may be associated with nephrosis or progressive renal failure. Infarcts of the neck of the femur can result in aseptic necrosis, with pain and progressive deformity of that bone.

These patients must maintain active erythropoiesis to replace the red blood cells that have a shortened survival time. Transient marrow failure can result in precipitous decreases in hemoglobin concentrations, resulting in congestive cardiac failure and death. Any patient who has developed increasing pallor should have a blood smear done. If the blood smear does not have the expected polychromasia and nucleated red cells and the reticulocyte count is below 2%, blood transfusions may be necessary to tide them over the pariod of marrow hypoplasia, which usually lasts from 4 to 6 days.

From early in life these patients have functional asplenia. Although during the first decade the spleen may be palpable, the blood passes through the tissue without significant emptying into the sinusoids. Therefore the sudden onset of a febrile episode must be regarded as pneumococcal sepsis until proved otherwise. Any patient with sickle cell disease having unexplained fever should be treated with penicillin until the blood cultures have been determined to be negative.

The onset of clinical symptoms usually does not begin until the second 6 months of life or even during the first years of childhood. During infancy a peculiar hand-foot syndrome can be present, resulting from infarction of the phalanges of the hands and feet.

Sickle cell hemoglobin is present almost exclusively in blacks, and about 10% of American blacks are heterozygous for this hemoglobin. All black patients should be screened for sickle cell disease by solubility testing or preferably hemoglobin electrophoresis. A homozygous patient will have evident sickling on the blood smear, but the heterozygous patient will only form sickled cells on special testing.

Although there are currently studies underway to determine methods of prevention of sickling, none has yet been successful. Patients must be cared for symptomatically during crises and the parents cautioned about precipitating factors.

Individuals who are heterozygous for sickle cell trait have hemoglobin values near normal and little, if any, evidence of disability. Under special circumstances, such as exposure to hypoxia, they can undergo infarction, usually of the spleen. Other than avoiding situations in which hypoxia might occur, these patients need no special counseling or care.

HEMOGLOBIN C DISEASE. In the United States hemoglobin C disease is also found primarily in blacks. The heterozygous state is found in about 2% of American blacks; the homozygous state is extremely rare. The heterozygous state is completely asymptomatic, and even the homozygous state is quite mild. Growth is normal, and there is no shortening of the expected life span. There may be splenomegaly on physical examination and symptomatically they may occasionally have episodes of pain. On blood smear the characteristic of the homozygous state is the presence of target-shaped red cells. The hemoglobin values may be near normal.

DOUBLE HETEROZYGOTES. Combinations of S and C hemoglobin or S and β thalassemia trait can result in clinical pictures resembling sickle cell disease. The S-C heterozygote tends to be milder than sickle cell disease, but splenomegaly is more prominent and pulmonary infarctions a more frequent clinical complication. S thalassemia, on the other hand, may be fully as severe as sickle cell disease and may also be associated with considerable splenomegaly. Specific diagnosis of these syndromes can be made on hemoglobin electrophoresis and examination of the parents.

Hemoglobinopathies caused by reduced polypeptide chain synthesis (thalassemic syndrome). Defective synthesis of the α or β chain can result from abnormal gene function, causing inadequate messenger RNA production for that polypeptide. Reduction in synthesis can be partial or complete, depending on the severity of the lesion. The thalassemic syndromes can be inherited as a heterozygous, homozygous, or doubly heterozygous condition. In general, the heterozygous conditions are asymptomatic, but the homozygous and doubly heterozygous states can be associated with moderate to severe hypochromic anemias.

α THALASSEMIA. There are four gene loci that code for the RNAs responsible for α chain production, two loci on each chromosome inherited from the parents. Deletion of the function of all four of these gene loci is incompatible with life because the α chain is required for synthesis of all hemoglobin molecules. The affected infant is either stillborn or dies shortly after birth with a syndrome resembling erythroblastosis fetalis. Deletion of the function of three α chain gene loci results in the clinical picture called hemoglobin H disease. Tetramers of β chains form the hemoglobin H, which is unstable and causes a hemolytic anemia associated with hypochromia. Deletion of one or two gene sites results in an asymptomatic condition associated with only a slight microcytic hypochromic anemia. The usual hemoglobin values are in the 10 to 12 range, the blood smear shows only the minimal findings of microcytosis and hypochromia. At birth the heterozygous state can be demonstrated by the presence of tetramers of γ chains called Bart hemoglobin. Deletion of α chain genes is found mostly in people from Southeast Asia, the Mediterranean region, and parts of Africa.

β THALASSEMIA. Genes associated with reduced or absent production of the β chain cause the most common symptomatic form of thalassemia. These genes have been found in all the world's populations but most frequently around the Mediterranean area and in Africa. The gene associated with completely absent production of β chain is most frequent in the Mediterranean

bacterial infections from the first months of life. The total leukocyte count may be normal, but the absolute neutrophil count is usually below 200/mm^3. The bone marrow examination indicates a cellular marrow but few neutrophils beyond the promyelocyte stage. In another form of congenital marrow failure there is a characteristic cyclic neutropenia. Because the cycles are about 21 days, these patients typically have periodic episodes of fever, aphthous stomatitis, and bacterial infections. The blood counts indicate neutropenia at those times, lasting about a week. Subsequently the neutrophil count returns to normal, with the episode being repeated with typical periodicity. In any patient with recurrent bacterial infections, blood counts should be done to determine if a congenital neutropenia is the underlying cause. A rare form of neutropenia is associated with exocrine pancreatic dysfunction. These patients, from the first weeks of life, have failure to thrive and recurrent bacterial infections and on blood counts are usually found to have some degree of pancytopenia. Their marrows are generally hypocellular.

Recurrent bacterial infections can also be caused by functional abnormalities of granulocytes. Among these rare conditions the most frequent is chronic granulomatous disease, which is usually inherited as an autosomal recessive disorder. From early life these patients have recurrent deep infections and frequently lymphadenitis, leading to open draining wounds. They typically respond poorly to antibiotics. The usual infecting organism is *Staphylococcus aureus*. Their leukocyte counts are normal or increased with infection, and they form abundant pus. In a patient with a history of such recurrent, severe, purulent infections, granulocyte function studies should be done. The neutrophils from these patients can phagocytize but not kill bacteria. The cells are incapable of generating hydrogen peroxide and do not have the usual metablic oxidative activity following phagocytosis.

There are a number of hereditary morphologic abnormalities, some of which have no functional significance. Pelger-Huët anomaly is associated with altered segmentation of the nucleus, so that only two lobes are formed. Hereditary hypersegmentation of neutrophils, on the other hand, is associated with an excessive formation of nuclear lobes. Alder anomaly is characterized by abnormally heavy cytoplasmic granulation and may be found in patients with Hurler's disease. All these cell types, however, function normally. A finding in Chédiak-Higashi syndrome, an autosomal recessive disease, is neutrophils with large, bizarre, cytoplasmic granules. This abnormality of granulation is also found in melanocytes, and affected individuals have hypopigmentation of the skin, hair, and iris. They may have periodic episodes of neutropenia and an increased susceptibility to infection. Intermittent episodes of severe unexplained fever may be associated with hepatosplenomegaly.

Eosinophils

The eosinophils also have a phagocytic function but interact with special immunoglobulins, primarily in allergic reactions. They may be increased in the blood of patients with asthma, hay fever, and vasomotor rhinitis. An increase may also be seen in systemic diseases such as dermatitis herpetiformis, ulcerative colitis, Hodgkin disease, and periarteritis nodosa. Pulmonary infiltrate with eosinophilia (PIE) syndrome is a condition of unknown cause that is generally benign and self-limiting. In some patients, however, it is severe, with fever, weakness, and cough. In some of these patients there may also be eosinophilic pericarditis. Corticosteroids are useful in treatment.

In the United States the usual cause of extreme eosinophilia in children is visceral larva migrans. The eosinophilia may even be as great as 100,000 white blood cells per cubic millimeter. In the acute phase there may be associated fever, hepatosplenomegaly, and cough. The eosinophilia will persist for weeks and even months after the acute episode is over. Eosinophilia may be seen in other parasitic infections, especially during the phase when pulmonary migration takes place. Trichinosis is currently uncommon in the United States, but in the affected patient there generally will be eosinophilia.

Basophils

The basophil is an infrequent cell in blood, usually 1% or less. It may be increased slightly following resolution of a bacterial infection. It is found to be increased in absolute numbers in patients with chronic myelocytic leukemia. Other than these conditions there are no characteristic changes of basophils of any importance.

Lymphocytes

A great deal of knowledge has been gained about the nature of lymphocytes. There are two major classes of lymphocytes arising from a common stem cell. The thymic-dependent lymphocyte (T-lymphocyte) is conditioned by the thymus to function in cellular immunity; T-lymphocytes also have helper and suppressor cell activity with respect to immunoglobulin formation. The lymphocytes conditioned by a mammalian equivalent of the avian bursa of Fabricius are called B-lymphocytes. The fetal liver may condition this class of cells to be responsible for the synthesis of immunoglobulins, regulated at least in part by the specialized T-lymphocytes. The mature B-lymphocyte is the plasma cell that synthesizes specific immunoglobulin.

In normal children there is a relative increase in blood lymphocytes in comparison with adult values, as shown in Table 20-1. Increases in normal-appearing lymphocytes can be seen in infections such as pertussis, parapertussis, and infectious lymphocytosis. Viral infections may cause atypical lymphocytes characterized by a larger size with a greater degree of basophilic cytoplasm and a more irregular nucleus with finer nuclear chromatin. Infectious mononucleosis at the height of clinical symptoms is usually characterized by greater than 20% of the total leukocyte count being atypical lymphocytes.

Monocytes

Much knowledge has been gained in recent years concerning the function and life cycle of the monocyte. The monocyte is derived from the same stem line as the myeloid cells in the bone marrow. After 4 to 6 days of maturation and differentiation it is released into the blood. Subsequently these cells are distributed to various body sites where there are tissue or vascular macrophages, such as the Kupffer cells of the liver, the alveolar macrophages of the lung, and the splenic sinusoid macrophages. These cells also follow a neutrophilic infiltration of an inflammatory site within 12 to 18 hours and become tissue macrophages. They are the principal component of the inflammatory process for chronic infections such as tuberculosis and histoplasmosis. The monocyte in the blood is a relatively undifferentiated cell that does, however, have the capability of phagocytosis and bactericidal activity. As it reaches its tissue or vascular site of function, the cell progressively undergoes changes to the fully differentiated macrophage characteristic of that site. It is a flexible cell and assumes the functional characteristics necessary for a particular job. Since it is responding primarily to its phagocytic function, this cell is a direct result of what it eats. The monocyte also has an important function in antigen processing and modulating the cellular and humoral immune responses.

Monocytosis is typical of chronic inflammatory processes and the recovery phase of acute infections. A characteristic vacuolated monocyte can be seen in long-standing sepsis, such as in subacute bacterial endocarditis. Following

Table 20-4. Laboratory tests used in investigating hemostatic disorders

Disorder	Test
Vascular defects	Bleeding time (BT)
	Capillary fragility
	Skin biopsy
	Vitamin C levels
Platelet defects	Blood smear, bone marrow
	Bleeding time
	Platelet count
	Clot retraction (CR)
	Prothrombin consumption (PC)
	Platelet aggregation, adhesion tests
	Platelet activity in thromboplastin generation test (TGT)
	Plasma recalcification time (PRT)
Plasmatic defects	General (nonspecific)
	Partial thromboplastin time (PTT) (normal in platelet and factor VII deficiencies)
	Plasma recalcification time (PRT)
	Clotting time (may be normal in moderate deficiencies)
	First stage
	Specific factor assays
	Prothrombin consumption
	Thromboplastin generation test
	Second stage
	One-stage and two-stage "prothrombin" time
	Specific factor assays
	Stypven time
	Third stage
	Fibrinogen determination
	Thrombin time
	Anticoagulants: partial thromboplastin time, one-stage prothrombin time in mixtures of control's and patient's plasma
	Fibrinolysis: observation of whole blood clot, plasmatic clot, euglobulin lysis, or degree of lysis in fibrin plates

bone marrow suppression by chemotherapy, the first cell to make its reappearance in the blood is the monocyte. Thus monocytosis in a neutropenic patient is a harbinger of subsequent neutrophil recovery. In patients with chronic neutropenia there is usually a reactive monocytosis, apparently as a compensatory mechanism.

HEMOSTASIS

There are three aspects to the mechanisms for maintaining an intact vascular system. These are the blood vessels, the platelets, and the hemostatic plasma factors. After vessel injury an immediate mechanism of vasoconstriction occurs to reduce blood flow through the injured site. Exposure of the platelets in blood to the underlying collagen induces platelet adhesion and the release of platelet factors that are important contributors to subsequent events. The release of adenosine 5′-diphosphate (ADP) promotes platelet aggregation and helps form a mechanical plug in the damaged vessel wall. Serotonin release provides for further vasoconstriction. The platelet phospholipids interact with the plasma hemostatic factors to begin the process of clot formation. In addition to the induction of the intrinsic coagulation process, beginning with factor XII, the exposure of plasma to tissues allows for the interaction of tissue thromboplastin with factor VII, which begins the extrinsic coagulation process through factor X. As a final result thrombin is formed, which enzymatically acts on fibrinogen to convert it to fibrin. The fibrin strands are then interconnected by the enzyme factor XIII to form a stable clot. The platelets are enmeshed in this fibrin network and on retraction complete the process of filling the damaged vessel wall with a tight, effective, mechanical plug. Subsequently the activation of plasminogen to plasmin begins the final process of clot lysis and allows for repair of the damaged vessel. This clot lysis is associated with the release of fibrin-split products into the plasma.

A bleeding diathesis can result from defects in any of the three areas of the hemostatic mechanisms. Laboratory tests of value in demonstrating the specific defect involved in a patient with a bleeding problem are shown in Table 20-4. Some characteristics of the plasma hemostatic factors are shown in Table 20-5. The diagnostic application of the available laboratory studies to the diagnosis of specific bleeding disorders is shown in Table 20-6.

Vascular disorders

Petechial lesions indicative of capillary fragility can be seen with various viral infections or associated with bacterial sepsis. These lesions may be most common in areas of increased capillary pressure, such as in the head and neck area of a crying child. Occasionally the petechial lesions of infections such as meningococcemia may be associated with disseminated intravascular coagulation, as will be discussed shortly. The petechial skin lesions of scurvy and anaphylactoid purpura are discussed on pp. 173 and 489, respectively.

Table 20-5. Coagulation factors

International number	Synonym	Comments*
I	Fibrinogen	b, c, e
II	Prothrombin	a, c, f, g
III	Platelet factor	c
IV	Calcium	
V	Proaccelerin, labile factor	b, c, f
VI	Not assigned	
VII	Stable factor, proconvertin	a, d, e, g
VIII	Antihemophilic factor (AHF) or globulin (AHG)	b, c, f
IX	Plasma thromboplastin component, PTC, or Christmas factor	a, d, e, g
X	Stuart-Prower factor	a, d, e, g
XI	Plasma thromboplastin antecedent (PTA)	b, d, e
XII	Hageman factor	b, d, e
XIII	Fibrin-stabilizing factor	

*Key: *a*, adsorbed by $BaSO_4$; *b*, not adsorbed by $BaSO_4$; *c*, consumed in the process of coagulation; *d*, remains in serum after coagulation; *e*, stable; *f*, labile; *g*, vitamin K dependent.

Table 20-6. Laboratory findings in various bleeding disorders

Factor deficiency	I	II	Platelets		V	VII	VIII	IX	X	XI	XII
			Quantity	Quality							
Tests*											
Bleeding time	N†	N	A	A	N	N	N	N	N	N	N
Capillary fragility	N	N	A	A	N	N	N	N	N	N	N
Platelet count	N	N	A	N	N	N	N	N	N	N	N
Platelet function	N	N	N	A	N	N	N	N	N	N	N
Clot retraction	A	N	A	±A	N	N	N	N	N	N	N
Clotting	A	N	N	N	N	N	A	A	A	N	A
Plasma recalcification time	A	A	A	±A	A	A	A	A	A	A	A
Partial thromboplastin time	A	A	N	N	A	N	A	A	A	A	A
One-stage prothrombin time	A	A	N	N	A	A	N	N	A	N	N
Prothrombin consumption		N	A	±A	A	N	A	A	A	A	A
Thromboplastin generation test		N	A	A	A	N	A	A	A	A	A
Thrombin time	A	N	N	N	N	N	N	N	N	N	N

Modified from Abildgaard and Schulman. In Barnett, H., editor: Pediatrics, ed. 14, New York, 1968, Appleton-Century-Crofts.
*Some of these tests may be normal in mild deficiencies.
†KEY: *N,* normal; *A,* abnormal; ±, variable.

Hereditary hemorrhagic telangiectasia

Hereditary hemorrhagic telangiectasia, also known as Rendu-Osler-Weber disease, is not typically a problem during childhood. Beginning during the second decade of life, the characteristic telangiectasias appear and can be seen on skin and mucous membranes. They may bleed, particularly when located in mucosa or gut epithelium. Thus these patients may have epistaxis and gastrointestinal bleeding. All hemostatic studies are normal.

Platelet disorders

Platelets (thrombocytes) are formed from megakaryocytes in the bone marrow. The megakaryocytes come from the same common stem cell as do the granulocytes and erythrocytes. The platelets are formed from the cytoplasm of the megakaryocytes and are released into the blood. Normally there are from 200,000 to 400,000 platelets per cubic millimeter, and there is no variation according to age as there is for granulocytes and erythrocytes. Platelets are essential to maintain hemostasis, not only because of their ability to form a plug in a damaged blood vessel but also because of their release of platelet factors during this process, which contributes to the formation of a clot, and their subsequent contribution to clot retraction, providing for a stable compact plug. Deficiencies in number or function of platelets result in clinical problems with bleeding. The hallmark of this type of bleeding problem are the petechiae. There is also characteristically bleeding from mucous membranes and excessive bruisability with trauma. There may be gastrointestinal bleeding and, uncommonly, intracranial hemorrhage. Usually good hemostasis is maintained by platelet counts greater than 50,000/mm^3. Platelet counts less than 20,000/mm^3 are almost always associated with some bleeding manifestations. In addition to the platelet count, the functional bleeding abnormalities associated with platelet defects can be demonstrated by prolonged capillary bleeding times, poor clot retraction, and, for qualitative defects, abnormal platelet aggregation studies.

Qualitative platelet disorders

Hereditary qualitative platelet defects, such as Glanzmann's disease or Bernard-Soulier disease, are rare. Platelet numbers are normal, but all the typical bleeding manifestations involving platelet defects are present. The bleeding time and clot retraction are abnormal. Recently it has been possible to demonstrate in these disorders that there are specific defects in platelet membrane proteins. Platelet aggregation studies are abnormal and provide the definitive diagnosis. Acquired platelet defects may be found in patients with uremia and in persons taking some medications, the most common of which is aspirin. These two situations rarely pose clinically significant problems.

Abnormalities of platelet number

Thrombocytosis. Increased numbers of blood platelets can be associated with iron deficiency anemia; this disorder is seen in some children with the adult form of chronic myelocytic leukemia. After splenectomy for conditions such as hereditary spherocytosis or traumatic rupture there will be a transient increase in blood platelets. These values may reach levels greater than 1 million/mm^3 but in children are associated with no additional clinical features. Within weeks of the splenectomy the platelet count returns to normal and there is no specific therapy indicated.

Thrombocytopenia. The most frequent form of thrombocytopenia in children is associated with infections. Although their disease is generally referred to as idiopathic thrombocytopenic purpura (ITP), most of these children have had a viral infection within the previous week that has instigated the subsequent episode of thrombocytopenia. Sometimes the viral infections can be specifically identified, such as rubella or varicella, but most frequently the nature of the precipitating infection cannot be identified by specific clinical features.

The onset of ITP is sudden and occurs during childhood, with a median age of 7 years. The parents can usually identify the specific day or even hour that the bleeding manifestations were noted. Typically there are petechiae and excessive bruisability. There may be bleeding from mucous membranes such as the nose or gums, and hematuria may be present. Petechiae in the skin are most frequently seen in dependent areas or in the head and neck area if there has been crying. With the presence of petechiae there is no need to confirm the capillary fragility by doing a tourniquet test.

The more serious complications of ITP, fortunately rare, are gastrointestinal bleeding and intracranial hemorrhage. The usual course of ITP is relatively brief, with about 50% of the patients having spontaneously returned their platelet counts to normal within 1 or 2 months. The remainder will improve within 6 months to a year, with less than 10% of these patients running a more chronic course. Bleeding manifestations are usually most severe during the first week or so, and there is clinical improvement subsequently, even though platelet counts may remain reduced for a longer period of time. The other aspects of the blood counts are normal unless sufficient bleeding has occurred so that anemia develops. A bone marrow examination is not essential for the diagnosis unless some clinical feature suggests another disease. On bone marrow examination a cellular specimen is found, with generally increased numbers of megakaryocytes.

Therapy is not indicated, nor is it helpful. Corticosteroids have not proved effective in alleviating the bleeding manifestations or shortening the course of disease. Platelet transfusions are entirely ineffective because the infused platelets are destroyed as rapidly in ITP as the patient's own cells. If there are severe or life-threatening bleeding manifestations, splenectomy will usually result in prompt return of platelet counts to normal. The major indication for a splenectomy in these patients is the prevention or treatment of intracranial hemorrhage. There is a greater risk for this rare complication in patients who have severe mucous membrane bleeding and who have retinal hemorrhages.

Chronic idiopathic thrombocytopenic purpura is unusual in children and is more frequently seen during the second decade of life. Chronic ITP may be the first indication of an underlying disease such as lupus erythematosus. It may also be associated with other evidence of immunologic disease, such as Coombs positive immunohemolytic anemia. The onset is generally insidious, and there may be a history of petechiae or easy bruisability for several months. The condition is caused by antibody formation against platelets. Sometimes this antibody formation is instigated by drugs such as quinidine. In patients with chronic ITP a careful history and physical examination should be done for the presence of a specific underlying disease. Certainly, these patients should have laboratory studies such as immunoglobulin and antinuclear antibody tests as a routine part of their diagnostic work-up. The bone marrow examination in these patients typically indicates hypercellularity with an increased number of megakaryocytes. These patients may show response to corticosteroid administration, and, in fact, some of them may be steroid-dependent to maintain normal counts. For some patients splenectomy is effective in improving the thrombocytopenia.

Neonatal thrombocytopenia is usually associated with an infectious disease such as cytomegalovirus infection, toxoplasmosis, or even bacterial sepsis. In a few infants, however, neonatal thrombocytopenia may be associated with the formation of a maternal antibody directed against an antigen on the infant's platelets, much like erythroblastosis fetalis. The affected newborns will have petechiae but generally no serious bleeding manifestations. These infants spontaneously improve during the first weeks of life as the maternal immunoglobulin disappears from their plasma. For those infants who do have severe bleeding during the first days of life, an exchange transfusion reduces the maternal immunoglobulin and can increase the infant's platelet count. Corticosteroids may be of some value on a temporary basis.

Thrombocytopenia may be associated with infections. Intrauterine infections such as rubella, cytomegalovirus, toxoplasmosis, or syphilis can produce a thrombocytopenic newborn infant. Bacterial sepsis, particularly during infancy, also can be associated with thrombocytopenia. Many times infections producing thrombocytopenia also produce disseminated intravascular coagulation, which is discussed later. Infections associated with large spleens, such as disseminated histoplasmosis, can also cause thrombocytopenia. Large spleens related to other causes, such as portal hypertension or storage diseases, may cause thrombocytopenia because of splenic trapping of platelets. Any disease process associated with bone marrow failure will cause decreased numbers of blood platelets.

The hemolytic uremic syndrome is frequently accompanied by thrombocytopenia early in the course of disease, which may produce symptomatic bleeding. Thrombotic thrombocytopenic purpura is a rare disease in children. The thrombocytopenia is associated with microangiopathic hemolytic anemia as well, and the abnormal vasculature of this disease can produce thrombotic episodes in various organs of the body, most seriously in the central nervous system.

Amegakaryocytic thrombocytopenia. Congenital thrombocytopenia may be inherited as an autosomal dominant, autosomal recessive, or X-linked recessive disease. It may also occur sporadically. In some infants the congenital thrombocytopenia is associated with specific skeletal abnormalities involving absence of the radius—thrombocytopenia–absent radius syndrome (TAR). In some infants the skeletal abnormalities may be more severe and result in phocomelia of the upper extremities. The bone marrow in all patients with these forms of congenital thrombocytopenia is of normal cellularity with reduced numbers or absence of megakaryocytes.

Plasma factor deficiencies

Deficiencies of plasma factors leading to bleeding disorders are either congenital or acquired. Because the approach to diagnosis and treatment for these two types of lesions is different, they will be considered separately. From the standpoint of patient care the treatment of a child with a congenital bleeding disorder requires the development of a comprehensive program that will be lifelong. Although congenital bleeding disorders are unusual, they will be considered first because of their implications for the involved child and family. About 90% of the congenital bleeding disorders of plasma factor deficiency are accounted for by factors VIII and IX. These two factor deficiencies are inherited in an X-linked recessive pattern; therefore most children with congenital bleeding disorders are boys.

Congenital plasma factor deficiencies

Factor VIII deficiency. Factor VIII deficiency is also known as hemophilia A, or classic hemophilia. This deficiency results from the production of an abnormal factor VIII molecule that is functionally deficient although present in its abnormal form in the usual concentration in plasma. In these patients, by means of specific antibodies, the concentration of factor VIII can be demonstrated to be normal as an antigen but functionally deficient in clotting studies. This functional deficiency results in defective thromboplastin production and clot formation. As mentioned previously, the disease is inherited as an X-linked recessive gene. In a few patients there appears to have been spontaneous mutation. The mother of a patient in whom it has been inherited as an X-linked recessive can be demonstrated to have a greater amount of factor VIII antigen present in plasma than there is factor VIII activity. In this manner carriers of this disease can be identified. Rarely, a girl has been identified as having factor VIII deficiency because of a spontaneous mutation, or she is the daughter of a factor VIII deficiency carrier woman and a factor VIII–deficient man.

Bleeding may be evident early in life. During the neonatal period there may be hemorrhage from circumcision or from the umbilical stump. The absence of bleeding from circumcision, however, does not rule out factor VIII deficiency. Most often evidence of the disease appears when the child begins to walk, at which time an increased risk of trauma is present. The usual early finding is a tendency toward excessive bruisability from trauma. Furthermore, the bruises are found in atypical places, such as on the trunk and upper arms, rather than usual places such as the legs below the knees. Another early finding is bleeding from the mouth with trauma. As the toddler begins to move about, there is the risk of bumping his gums or biting his tongue. These traumatized areas then continue to bleed. The presence of fibrinolysin in saliva accentuates the problem of forming an adequate clot, and significant blood loss may occur. As the child becomes older and heavier, bleeding into the joints becomes a characteristic finding. The knees, ankles, and elbows are most frequently involved. The affected joints are first painful and then become swollen and hot because of the associated inflammatory change. There may be significant bleeding into the joint cavity, and fluctuation of the joint space can be demonstrated.

Treatment should be designed to detect the hemarthrosis at the earliest possible phase, before the swelling becomes evident. If treatment is not given, the painful joint may develop destruction of the joint space because of the inflammatory process. Furthermore, within a matter of a few days significant fixed contraction of a joint may occur, necessitating subsequent orthopedic relief by gradually returning the joint to full range of motion.

There may be bleeding from minor surgical procedures, particularly dental extractions. Epistaxis and other mucous membrane bleeding are uncommon without trauma. Hematuria may occur. There may also be the serious complication of intracranial hemorrhage, especially with head trauma. During the second decade of life gastrointestinal bleeding may occur as a significant complicating factor, although this is unusual during the first decade.

The diagnosis should be expected in a boy with excessive bruisability, prolonged bleeding from surgical trauma, or prolonged bleeding from mucous membrane trauma. The family history should be carefully taken, but it may be negative. The results expected in the laboratory studies are shown in Table 20-6. Of greatest importance is the prolonged partial thromboplastin time, with the subsequent demonstration of the deficiency in factor VIII by specific factor assay.

The prognosis for these patients varies considerably with the severity of the disease, the experience of trauma during life, and the availability of good clinical care. It must be remembered that these patients are facing a limitation of their life's activities, and there must be considerable counseling and preparation of both the patients and the family to help them adjust to this circumstance. Psychologic support is an extremely important part of the overall care pattern. The treatment is designed to provide for prevention when possible and prompt, early treatment if bleeding occurs. In talking with the parents the physician must be careful to stress methods of prevention that provide the child with protection from trauma without limiting his activities so significantly that development is impaired.

With trauma or evidence of spontaneous bleeding there should be prompt administration of factor VIII as replacement. Factor VIII is present in fresh plasma and fresh frozen plasma, but currently the usual preparations given are cryoprecipitate fraction of fresh plasma and the commercially available lyophilized concentrates that can be stored in a refrigerator. These two forms of concentrate provide the opportunity for adequate replacement with small volumes. The factor VIII activity of fresh plasma, which assays at 100% of the normal average, is arbitrarily assigned as having 1 activity unit/ml. The factor VIII activity in a single bag of cryoprecipitate is about 100 units/ml but there can be significant variation. The factor VIII activity of the lyophilized concentrates is stated on the label, which presents a distinct advantage.

Factor VIII has a short life span in the circulation. The transfusion of one factor VIII unit per kilogram of body weight increases the circulating activity level 2%, with a subsequent half disappearance time of 8 hours and a second half disappearance time by 24 hours. As an example, if 200 activity units are transfused into a boy weighing 10 kg there will be an initial level of 40%, which decreases to 20% by 8 hours and to 10% by 24 hours.

The usual types of bleeding, such as acute hemarthrosis and muscle hematomas, can be treated successfully with a single infusion of factor VIII calculated to increase the initial level from 20% to 40%. Greater blood levels for longer periods are necessary during severe hemorrhage, prophylaxis for surgical procedures, or bleeding into vital structures such as the central nervous system.

Control of hemarthrosis is a most important aspect of the management of these patients. Unless bleeding is promptly treated, progressive and eventually irreversible damage to joints can take place. This is particularly important in weight-bearing surfaces such as the knees and ankles. To prevent more serious hemorrhage, factor VIII should be administered as soon as pain and swelling appear. For treatment of the pain propoxyphene and acetaminophen are recommended, since aspirin may enhance bleeding because of its effect on platelets. Prolonged immobilization of the painful joint is not recommended because of the rather rapid development of contractures. Aspiration of the joint space is not indicated unless control is not being achieved by the administration of factor VIII. Short-term administration of corticosteroids may be helpful in reducing the inflammatory component.

Physiotherapy for the affected joint is an important part of rehabilitation. If a good program can be maintained, muscle and tendon strength around joints will be increased, and there will be a greater resistance to traumatic hemarthrosis. The physiotherapy should be undertaken by an experienced individual in conjunction with the physician.

In the care of these patients, medical trauma such as venipunctures into jugular and femoral veins should be avoided. Routine immunization schedules should be followed, of course, with a subcutaneous route in the anterolateral thigh. A 25-gauge needle should be used, and subsequent application of pressure and cold packs helps minimize hematoma formation. A good time for the administration of immunizations is when the child is receiving factor VIII concentrate for some other purpose.

Dental care should be meticulous, and great effort should be made to provide prophylaxis in the prevention of cavities. If teeth are to be extracted, the procedure should be done with extreme care. Prophylactic coverage with factor VIII may be necessary. Similar prophylaxis will be needed if other surgical procedures are necessary.

Some patients with hemophilia develop an antibody against factor VIII that is not necessarily related to the number of factor VIII transfusions they have had. The antibody has the characteristic of a circulating anticoagulant. For bleeding episodes in these patients, exchange transfusions with massive replacement therapy and corticosteroids have been used. They are of temporary value only but may tide the patient over an episode of severe bleeding.

Factor IX deficiency. Factor IX deficiency is also known as hemophilia B, PTC deficiency, and Christmas disease. It also is transmitted as an X-linked recessive. The clinical features are indistinguishable from factor VIII deficiency. It also is caused by the production of normal amounts of an abnormally functioning factor. The diagnosis can be established by finding a prolonged partial thromboplastin generation time in the patient, followed by the demonstration of decreased levels of factor IX on specific factor assay.

The general principles of treatment are similar to those recommended for factor VIII deficiency. Fresh plasma or fresh frozen plasma is effective for correcting factor IX levels. For these patients a loading dose of 16 ml of plasma per kilogram of body weight, followed by 8 ml/kg at 12-hour intervals, controls most bleeding problems. This regimen can be maintained for 2 or 3 days for the usual bleeding problem. Longer periods of control with greater amounts of plasma may be necessary for major surgical procedures or serious trauma. Recently a plasma product containing factors IX, VII, II, and X in a concentrated lyophilized form has been made available and provides satisfactory results. There is a somewhat greater risk of serum hepatitis with the use of this product.

Other congenital deficiencies with abnormal thromboplastin generation time

There are three other congenital abnormalities that can result in a prolonged partial thromboplastin generation time with a normal plasma prothrombin time. They are all inherited as an autosomal dominant. Factor XI deficiency is associated with mild bleeding manifestations, apparent usually at the time of surgery or major trauma. The demonstration of a prolonged partial thromboplastin generation time, followed by the specific factor assay, provides a definitive diagnosis. Bleeding manifestations may be corrected by the administration of fresh frozen plasma. The half-life of the infused factor XI is long; therefore a single infusion of plasma is frequently all that is necessary. Factor XII deficiency, also known as Hageman factor deficiency, frequently is clinically asymptomatic even in the face of severe surgical trauma such as tonsillectomy. The condition is inherited as an autosomal recessive trait and may be demonstrated by the finding of a prolonged clotting time on routine testing. Therapy is not indicated.

Von Willebrand disease, or vascular hemophilia, is inherited as an autosomal dominant trait. The bleeding manifestations are generally mild but can be severe in some patients. The laboratory characteristics are a prolonged bleeding time and a prolonged partial thromboplastin generation time. Factor assay levels for factor VIII are found to be decreased, both on functional studies and in the presence of factor VIII antigen. Abnormal platelet aggregation can be demonstrated in some of the patients. Treatment with fresh or fresh frozen plasma, as well as a plasma cryoprecipitate, can be effective.

Congenital factor deficiencies associated with a prolonged prothrombin time

There is a small group of patients with deficiencies of the second phase of coagulation. In these patients both the partial thromboplastin generation time and the prothrombin time are prolonged, thus identifying them as belonging in the second phase of clotting. Defects of factor I, or fibrinogen, may result from abnormal protein or absolute deficiencies. In these patients the thrombin time is also found to be prolonged. In patients with abnormal fibrinogen, immunoassay for fibrinogen is found to be normal. These patients rarely have difficulty except from trauma. Deficiencies of factor II, or prothrombin, are exceedingly rare and are associated only with excessive bleeding after severe trauma. Similarly, deficiencies of factor V are rare and generally mild and respond to correction with frozen plasma. The deficiency for factor VII is associated with a normal partial thromboplastin time but an abnormally prolonged plasma prothrombin time. The definitive diagnosis is based on specific factor assay. The severity of the clinical picture is variable but can be corrected by the administration of plasma. The deficiency of factor X, or Stuart-Prower factor, is inherited as an autosomal trait; only homozygotes have severe bleeding disease. Specific factor assay is necessary for definitive diagnosis. If bleeding should be a problem, the administration of plasma, either fresh or fresh frozen, is effective.

Factor XIII deficiency. Factor XIII, or fibrin-stabilizing factor, deficiency is a rare cause of bleeding disorder. It is inherited as an autosomal recessive trait. It may appear during the neonatal period as excessive bleeding when the umbilical cord separates. A moderately severe bleeding disorder clinically, it resembles factor VIII deficiency. All routine coagulation studies are within the normal range in spite of the severe bleeding disorder. The defect can be demonstrated by the finding of a faulty clot with dissolution by a solution of urea of monochloroacetic acid. Treatment of bleeding episodes or prophylaxis for surgery can be accomplished by the infusion of fresh frozen plasma.

Acquired plasma factor deficiency

Hemorrhagic disease of the newborn. This condition occurs in the immediate postnatal period as the result of a deficiency of vitamin K. Vitamin K is not produced by the infant and therefore must be absorbed from the gastrointestinal tract, where it is made by enteric bacteria or absorbed from available food sources. Immediately after birth the infant's diet may not contain adequate vitamin K, and there is not yet the establishment of enteric bacteria for spontaneous production. The period of greatest risk from bleeding, caused by a deficiency of vitamin K, is between the second and seventh day of life. It can be completely prevented by the prophylactic administration of vitamin K at birth. The appearance of bruising or spontaneous bleeding in an infant during the first week of life should prompt consideration of this condition. The partial thromboplastin time and prothrombin time are found to be prolonged. It should be determined if the infant was given vitamin K at birth; if this was not the case, it should be immediately provided in a dosage of 1 mg. Correction of the bleeding disorder should be expected within 4 to 6 hours. Serious bleeding can be treated immediately by plasma infusion.

Vitamin K deficiency. Vitamin K deficiency may also result in a bleeding problem later in life. Vitamin K is a fat-soluble vitamin, and any problem of malabsorption may be associated with its deficiency. Suppression of intestinal bacteria by antibiotics, especially in the newborn period, can also result in its deficiency. The absorption of fat-soluble vitamins is promoted by bile acids. Therefore biliary obstruction leads to deficient absorption. Some drugs, such as coumarin, can inhibit the effect of vitamin K in the liver. The drugs are used in prolonging clotting time in patients with thrombosis and may sometimes be accidentally ingested by children. Large amounts of salicylates, such as aspirin, taken over prolonged periods also can inhibit vitamin K effect in the liver and be associated with prolonged prothrombin times.

Vitamin K is essential to the formation of factors II, VII, IX, and X. In vitamin K deficiency factors VII and X are most sensitive and therefore are found to be decreased earliest and most severely. An important point in the differential diagnosis of this condition is that all these factors are made in the liver and are dependent on vitamin K. Factor V is also made in the liver but is not dependent on vitamin K; therefore in differentiating liver disease from vitamin K deficiency the presence of normal factor V levels supports the diagnosis of vitamin K deficiency.

The acquired bleeding manifestations of vitamin K deficiency are similar to those of other plasma factors. A careful history and physical examination will usually indicate the reason for the deficiency. Laboratory determinations indicate a prolonged partial thromboplastin time and plasma prothrombin time but normal thrombin time. If a patient has the appropriate history, the administration of vitamin K in a dosage of 1 mg should return these values to normal within a period of 4 to 6 hours. If the bleeding manifestations are severe, the administration of vitamin K–dependent factor concentrate may promptly restore normal clotting activity.

Liver disease. Since several important clotting factors are made in the liver, any severe liver disease may be associated with bleeding problems. There will be deficiency in formation of factors II, V, VII, IX, and X. If liver disease is severe enough to cause hemorrhagic difficulties, the cause is always evident clinically. As mentioned previously, the presence of factor V deficiency clearly implicates the liver as the source of a problem, rather than vitamin K deficiency.

Disseminated intravascular coagulation. There can be several causes of disseminated intravascular coagulation. They all involve activation of the first stage of clotting, with subsequent consequences of uncontrolled intravascular promotion of coagulation. There may be the deposition of fibrin in small capillaries in organs of the body leading to specific organ dysfunction. The usual problem, however, is the depletion of clotting factors, causing what appears to be the paradoxical consequences of excessive bleeding. Not only are the labile plasma factors such as fibrinogen II, V, and VIII decreased on concentration, but platelets are also consumed in the process. Thus the laboratory findings indicate prolongation of the partial thromboplastin time, the prothrombin time, and the thrombin time, as well as decreased concentration, but platelets are also consumed in the process.

The formation of intravascular fibrin meshes leads to mechanical damage of erythrocytes, and the finding of fragmented red cells on the blood smear is characteristic. The deposition of fibrin activates the plasminogen system, leading to fibrinolysis. Fibrin-split products are usually present and can lead to a further prolongation of the thrombin time, out of proportion to the fibrinogen level in plasma. On specific factor assay the fibrinogen, as well as factors V and VIII, is decreased. In some situations it is important to demonstrate the decrease in factor VIII to rule out the possible contributing factor of liver disease in the clinical bleeding syndrome.

The conditions that can produce disseminated intravascular coagulation include gram-negative bacterial sepsis, meningococcemia, some severe viral infections (especially in the newborn period), promyelocytic leukemia, brain trauma, and acute promyelocytic leukemia. The list of described associated diseases is long, and disseminated intravascular coagulation may be anticipated in patients who have conditions leading to shock. If excessive, especially spontaneous, bruising and bleeding from mucous membrane surfaces appears during the course of an illness, this condition should be suspected. An examination of the blood smear will be helpful in suggesting the diagnosis, and specific coagulation studies may be confirmatory.

In general, treatment of the underlying condition associated with disseminated intravascular coagulation will be sufficient. Once the disease process is under control, the clotting problem spontaneously resolves. In patients for whom primary disease control cannot be achieved promptly, heparinization may be effective but it must be carried out under carefully controlled conditions by experienced individuals. Attempts to replace the clotting factors or blood platelets without control of the clotting problem will only enhance bleeding by providing replacement factors for continuation of the process. If such treatment is necessary, the patient should be given heparin before replacement is begun. The administration of heparin should only be for that period of time necessary to cover effective treatment of the primary underlying disease.

Excessive fibrinolysis. Hemorrhagic disorders resulting from increased fibrinolysis are rarely encountered in children. Plasminogen activators are present in the liver and may be released in some severe liver diseases. Surgical procedures on the lung and uterus, likewise, can cause plasminogen activation. As mentioned previously, disseminated intravascular coagulation will activate the fibrinolytic system, but only as a secondary feature. Fibrinolysis will lead to digestion of fibrinogen as well as fibrin and result in decreased fibrinogen levels. There will be prolongation of the partial thromboplastin time, the plasma prothrombin time, and the thrombin time. The increased values of plasmin can be demonstrated by appropriate tests for fibrinolysis. Since this condition rarely exists as an isolated problem in children, treatment is almost never necessary and should only be begun under experienced supervision.

Alvin M. Mauer

SELECTED READINGS

Iron deficiency anemia

Charlton, R.W., and Bothwell, T.H.: Iron deficiency anemia, Semin. Hematol. **7:**67, 1970.

Pollitt, E., and Leibel, R.L.: Iron deficiency and behavior, J. Pediatr. **88:**372, 1976.

Woodruff, C.W., et al.: Iron nutrition in the breast-fed infant, J. Pediatr. **90:**36, 1977.

Aplastic anemia

Li, F.P., et al.: The mortality of acquired aplastic anemia in children, Blood **40:**153, 1972.

Storb, R., et al.: Aplastic anemia treated by allogeneic bone marrow transplantation: a report on 49 new cases from Seattle, Blood **48:**817, 1976.

Hypoplastic anemia

Wang, W.C., and Mentzer, W.C.: Differentiation of transient erythroblastopenia of childhood from congenital hypoplastic anemia, J. Pediatr. **88:**784, 1976.

Fanconi anemia

Nilsson, L.R.: Chronic pancytopenia with multiple congenital abnormalities, Acta Paediatr. (Suppl.) **49:**518, 1960.

Immunohemolytic anemia

Habibi, B., et al.: Autoimmune hemolytic anemia in children: a review of 80 cases, Am. J. Med. **56:**61, 1974.

Congenital spherocytosis

MacKinney, A.A., Jr.: Hereditary spherocytosis, Arch. Intern. Med. **116:**257, 1965.

Schilling, R.F.: Hereditary spherocytosis: a study of splenectomized persons, Semin. Hematol. **13:**169, 1976.

Congenital nonspherocytic hemolytic anemia

Beutler, E., et al.: Biochemical variants of glucose-6-phosphate dehydrogenase giving rise to congenital nonspherocytic hemolytic disease, Blood **31:**131, 1968.

Tanaka, K.R., and Paglia, D.E.: Pyruvate kinase deficiency, Semin. Hematol. **8:**367, 1971.

Sickle cell disease

Kumar, S., et al.: Anxiety, self-concept, and personal and social adjustments in children with sickle cell anemia, J. Pediatr. **88:**859, 1963.

Lindsay, J., Jr., et al.: The cardiovascular manifestations of sickle cell disease, Arch, Intern. Med. **133:**643, 1974.

Portnoy, B.A., and Herion, J.C.: Neurological manifestations in sickle-cell disease, Ann. Intern. Med. **76:**643, 1972.

Powars, D.R.: Natural history of sickle cell disease—the first ten years, Semin. Hematol. **12:**267, 1975.

Rucknagel, D.L.: The genetics of sickle cell anemia and related syndromes, Arch. Intern. Med. **133:**595, 1974.

Sears, D.A.: The morbidity of sickle cell trait, Am. J. Med. **64:**1021, 1978.

Thalassemia

Graziano, J.H., and Cerami, A.: Chelation therapy for the treatment of thalassemia, Semin. Hematol. **14:**127, 1977.

Mazza, U., et al.: Clinical and haematological data in 254 cases of beta-thalassemia trait in Italy, Br. J. Haematol. **33:**91, 1976.

Schwartz, E.: Abnormal globin synthesis in thalassemic red cells, Semin. Hematol. **11:**549, 1974.

Leukocyte disorders

Howard, M.W., et al.: Infections in patients with neutropenia, Am. J. Dis. Child. **131:**788, 1977.

Johnston, R.B., Jr., and Baehner, R.L.: Chronic granulomatous disease: correlation between pathogenesis and clinical findings, Pediatrics **48:**730, 1971.

Joyce, R.A., et al.: Neutrophil kinetics in hereditary and congenital neutropenias, N. Engl. J. Med. **295:**1385, 1976.

Kauder, E., and Mauer, A.M.: Neutropenias of childhood, J. Pediatr. **69:**147, 1966.

Marsh, W.L., et al.: Chronic granulomatous disease and the Kell blood groups. Br. J. Haematol. **29:**247, 1975.

Platelet disorders

Lightsey, A.L., et al.: Childhood idiopathic thrombocytopenic purpura: aggressive management of life-threatening complications, JAMA **232:**734, 1975.

McClure, P.D.: Idiopathic thrombocytopenic purpura in children: diagnosis and management, Pediatrics **55:**68, 1975.

McClure, P.D.: Idiopathic thrombocytopenic purpura in children, Am. J. Dis. Child. **131:**357, 1977.

Simons, S.M., et al.: Idiopathic thrombocytopenic purpura in children, J. Pediatr. **87:**16, 1975.

Coagulation disorders

Biggs, R.: Haemophilia treatment in the United Kingdom from 1969 to 1974, Br. J. Haematol. **35:**487, 1977.

Hamilton, P.J., et al.: Disseminated intravascular coagulation: a review, J. Clin. Pathol. **31:**609, 1978.

Jones, P.: Developments and problems in the management of hemophilia, Semin. Hematol. **14:**375, 1977.

Pitney, W.R.: Disseminated intravascular coagulation, Semin. Hematol. **8:**65, 1971.

Ratnoff, O.D., and Jones, P.K.: The laboratory diagnosis of the carrier state for classic hemophilia, Ann. Intern. Med. **86:**521, 1977.

Strawczynski, H., et al.: Delivery of care to hemophilic children: home care versus hospitalization, Pediatrics **51:**986, 1973.

21 Nephrology

DEVELOPMENT OF RENAL STRUCTURE AND FUNCTION

Nephrogenesis begins during the second month of embryonic life and continues until the fetus reaches a weight of 2100 to 2500 g, a length of 46 to 49 cm, or a gestational age of 34 weeks, with the final number of nephrons being approximately 1 million per kidney. Infants born before achieving this size continue to form new nephrons postnatally until a conceptional age (gestational age + postnatal age) of 34 weeks is reached. The first glomeruli formed are positioned in the juxtamedullary region of the renal cortex, and they are larger and functionally more mature at birth than the younger population of glomeruli formed later in embryonic life and situated more superficially in the cortex. The tubules are short at birth, with an incomplete differentiation of their subcellular structures, and the loops of Henle of 20% of nephrons are still within the cortex. Increments in kidney size occur by the enlargement of existing nephrons; however, tubular growth accounts for most of the increase in renal mass, which parallels body growth.

Congenital abnormalities of the renal parenchyma result in hypoplasia when the formation of any structure fails to occur and in dysplasia when the development of any structure does not proceed along set patterns. Combinations of hypoplasia-dysplasia may result in any number of renal structural abnormalities. The cause of cystic diseases of the kidney is vague but is most likely a developmental abnormality that can be produced experimentally by obstruction of the fetal collecting system.

Urine is first formed by the human fetal kidney during the third month of gestation. Regulatory function provided by the kidney after birth is assumed by the placenta during fetal life. Birth results in abrupt functional demands on the neonatal kidney. Glomerular filtration rate (GFR) remains approximately 0.5 ml/min before a conceptional age of 34 weeks, but it increases thereafter in a linear fashion with age to 125 ml/min at a time during adolescence when adult height has been reached. Correction of absolute values of GFR for body surface area to compare with values for the normal adult is not a reliable calculation before 6 months of age; therefore one has to refer to a table of normal values for age in the neonate and young infant to determine whether or not GFR in an individual infant is normal.

Reabsorptive mechanisms of the neonatal renal tubule differ quantitatively from the mature nephron, but their functions are comparable in that both reabsorb about 99% of the sodium and water presented to them. The proximal tubule provides quantitative passive reabsorption of sodium chloride and water (about 70% of the filtered load), the loop of Henle reabsorbs another portion of sodium (15%), and the fine regulatory control of sodium and water balance (10% to 15%) occurs in the distal tubule and collecting duct. When proximal tubular reabsorption of sodium is decreased for any reason, the distal tubule in the neonate has the unique capacity to reabsorb up to 50% of the filtered sodium.

A sodium load (greater than 20 mEq/kg/24 hr) is not excreted in the infant as it is in the child or adult, and retention of saline results in volume expansion and even edema formation. Ingestion of salt in excess of 50 mEq/kg/24 hr, as in formula improperly diluted, results in hypernatremia and often is corrected only by peritoneal or extracorporeal dialysis. The apparent inability of the newborn kidney to excrete a sodium load must be interpreted with regard to the fact that sodium is distributed in the extracellular fluid and only that which circulates to the kidney in plasma can be excreted. Because plasma represents only 25% of extracellular fluid, only 25% of the sodium load would be excreted. Moreover, plasma renin activity and plasma aldosterone levels are high at birth and decrease with age and may account further for increased tubular reabsorption of sodium even when total body sodium is greater than normal. In the experimental animal, sodium excretion is related directly to arterial blood pressure, which in turn is dependent on the dynamic relationship in vasoactive hormones—prostaglandins and angiotensin.

Nearly all filtered potassium is actively reabsorbed in the proximal tubule and secreted into the distal tubular fluid. Active reabsorption by specific carrier-mediated transport mechanisms occurs in the proximal tubule only for substances such as amino acids, glucose, and perhaps uric acid. Tubular reabsorption of phosphate is within the range of adult normal values, that is, 85% even in premature infants before the introduction of oral feedings. Serum phosphate levels increase with dietary phosphorus, and renal phosphate excretion increases appropriately. In addition to filtration, there is active tubular secretion of organic acids such as creatinine, para-aminohippurate, penicillin, guanidine, choline, and histamine. Tubular transport capacity for both reabsorption and secretion of substances is quantitatively low at birth and increases appropriately with tubular growth and glomerular filtration.

Although functionally appropriate for meeting normal excretory and regulatory demands, extremes in either direction are not easily compensated for by the newborn kidney. The ability of the mature kidney to excrete a water load rapidly, lowering the urine osmolality to 50 mOsm/L, is paralleled by the newborn kidney but occurs over a period four to five times longer. A decrease in plasma osmolality or increase in intravascular pressure inhibits the release of antidiuretic hormone (ADH) and renders the collecting duct impermeable to water. At the other extreme, the ability of the kidney to concentrate urine is dependent on the medullary gradient established by concentrations of sodium and urea, as well as by the release of and response to ADH. The infant's anabolic state provides little excretory urea necessary for establishing a maximal gradient, in spite of normal amounts of ADH in the circulation and normal responsiveness of the neonatal collecting duct to vasopressin. These factors limit the ability of the infant's kidneys to concentrate urine to more than 700 mOsm/L, whereas kidneys of the older child and adult concentrate urine to 1200 mOsm/L; therefore water deprivation is not tolerated for long periods in the infant. Hence periods of fasting before surgical and diagnostic procedures are shortened from the usual 8 hours for the adult to 4 hours for the infant.

The normal ratio of bicarbonate to carbonic acid as a buffer system depends in part on the renal reabsorption of bicarbonate and the ability of the lungs to control concentrations of carbonic acid. The daily metabolic hydrogen ion load of 50 to 80 mEq/1.73 m^2 is secreted by the renal tubule to effect the reabsorption, and thus conservation, of bicarbonate. Hydrogen ion in excess of that required to reabsorb sufficient bicarbonate is excreted with filtered phosphate and creatinine as titratable acid and with ammonia, synthesized by the tubular epithelial cell from glutamine, as ammonium. The normal full-term newborn infant has an arterial blood pH of 7.40, whereas the premature infant has a more acid value, which is related to a decreased plasma concentration of bicarbonate and is associated with a reduced bicarbonate threshold. The renal threshold for bicarbonate increases with age; therefore the normal plasma level for bicarbonate in the infant is 21.5 to 22.5 mmol/L; in the child, 23 to 25 mmol/L; and in the adult, 25 to 27 mmol/L. The ability to excrete hydrogen ion as titratable acid depends partly on the amount of phosphate in the diet; therefore the infant fed cow's milk, which is relatively high in phosphorus, has a greater capacity to form titratable acid than does the infant fed breast milk, whose hydrogen ion is excreted mostly as ammonium. Just as in regulating salt and water balance, the developing kidney is able to maintain a normal acid-base status within a narrow range, but the imposition of extremes, such as an acid load when ammonium chloride is given, indicates that the young kidney has functional limitations.

CLINICAL EVALUATION OF RENAL FUNCTION

Urinalysis

The single most important test of renal function remains the routine urinalysis. The convenient use of color changes in segmented areas of strips impregnated with specific reactants gives highly sensitive, but occasionally false positive, semiquantitative tests for glucose, protein, blood and pH to profile the character of the final product of glomerular and tubular function. When an abnormal finding is noted by this method, documentation is required by a more specific chemical method to quantify the abnormal presence of the substance in the urine. These determinations, complemented by measurement of urine-specific gravity or osmolality, and the microscopic examination of the centrifuged urine sediment serve as indicators of the status of renal function.

The normal color of the urine varies from dark amber under conditions of thirst and maximal water conservation by the kidney, when pigments normally found in the urine are in greatest concentration, to pale yellow, and to nearly colorless during water diuresis. The color of urine becomes red when it contains fresh blood, and it assumes a brownish hue as red blood cells are hemolyzed and hemoglobin is released into the urine. There are many drugs and food dyes, in addition to the excessive production of body pigments, normally excreted through the kidney, any of which may alter significantly the color of the final urine. The clarity and odor of the urine is usually associated with insoluble amorphous materials and ammonia production by urea-splitting organisms when the urine is retained in the bladder or allowed to remain in a container for extended periods. The characteristic odor of a freshly voided, acid urine is not offensive.

The specific gravity or osmolality of urine varies with the body's need to conserve water, and thus for screening purposes it may be noted to vary from 1.001 to 1.040 (50 to 1200 mOsm/L). Any value equal to or greater than 1.017 on routine screening is considered to be an indication of adequate but not maximal concentrating ability by the kidney. A persistently low urine specific gravity of less than 1.005, in the absence of water diuresis, suggests an inability of the nephron to conserve water properly: an inherently defective renal tubule as in juvenile nephrophthisis, end-stage renal parenchymal disease, obstructive uropathy, unresponsiveness of the distal tubule and collecting duct to antidiuretic hormone as in nephrogenic diabetes insipidus, or inadequate production of ADH by the posterior pituitary. A specific gravity in the range of 1.036 to 1.040 is considered maximal for the human kidney and never exceeds these limits unless the final osmolality of the urine is increased by protein, glucose, or radiographic contrast material.

Within the range of normal blood glucose levels of 60 to 120 mg/dl, and even postprandially when blood glucose concentration is greatest, the normal renal threshold for glucose (200 mg/dl) is not exceeded. Nearly all glucose filtered by the glomerulus is reabsorbed by the active transport mechanism of the proximal tubule, and the quantity of glucose in the final urine is less than 20 mg/dl, an amount undetectable even by glucose-specific screening methods in which the trace reaction compares with a glucose concentration of 125 mg/dl. When the renal threshold for glucose is exceeded, either during the intravenous infusion of glucose-containing fluids in the poorly controlled diabetic patient or because the nephron's capacity to reabsorb glucose is reduced congenitally or through injury, glucose appears in the final urine in increasing amounts. Screening tests for total reducing substance in the urine (Clinitest) rather than glucose-specific methods (Clinistix) may give false-positive reactions when other sugars or certain interfering drugs are present.

Proteinuria must be considered an abnormal finding on routine urinalysis. Except in instances of gross hematuria, protein found in the final urine is filtered by the glomerulus and indicates abnormal structure or function at that level. The urine most likely to be protein free is that first voided on arising from a prolonged supine position in that any orthostatic component to the proteinuria is minimized. In any event, the quantity of protein excretion must be established.

The pH of the urine varies with the time since formation, with intervals after meals following alkaline tide, and with the kidney's ability to reabsorb bicarbonate and excrete hydrogen ion. The range of pH expected in screening samples of urine varies from 4.5 to 8.0.

Microscopic examination of the urine sediment is important. It is imperative that the urine examined be freshly voided, cleanly obtained, and promptly examined to ensure meaningful results. Urine that is allowed to remain in the container unexamined for a long period of time will become alkaline as a result of ammonia production by urea-splitting organisms. In an alkaline medium the important elements of the urine sediment will be physically altered. Urine collected after inadequate cleansing of the female perineum or urine that has been allowed to flow over contaminated areas of the genitalia will likely produce an abnormal finding of cells, cellular debris, and bacteria when the urine sediment is examined. Equally misleading will be the urine sediment of the catheterized specimen collected after improper cleansing or introduction of a bladder catheter that has become contaminated before insertion. Urine obtained by suprapubic aspiration of the bladder will likely contain fresh red blood cells secondary to the procedure, but no other cellular element or culture should be affected by this means of urine collection. Suprapubic aspiration is the preferred method of collecting urine for culture when there is difficulty in collecting a clean, midstream specimen.

Although pyuria is a nonspecific finding, the presence of more than five polymorphonuclear leukocytes per high-power field is considered abnormal in any centrifuged urine specimen and should prompt further investigation. Differentiation between lymphocytes and renal tubular cells from polymorphonuclear leukocytes is important when examining the unstained urine sediment. Renal tubular cells are commonly noted and do not necessarily indicate tubular disease, but the appearance of lymphocytes in the urine is indeed a rare finding, most often associated with the rejection of a renal allograft, tuberculosis of the genitourinary tract, and malignancy. Polymorphonuclear leukocytes, on the other hand, may be seen with almost any genitourinary inflammatory process and also in association with intra-abdominal abscess, peritonitis, or periureteral irritation, even when the urine is sterile.

The presence of blood in the urine in any quantity should alert the clinician to disease. The finding of gross blood is indicated by casual inspection of the voided urine and may be associated with glomerular disease, intrarenal arteriovenous fistula, coagulopathy, tubular injury, renal trauma, prolonged exercise, urolithiasis, intrarenal hematoma, or neoplasm. The finding of more than three red blood cells per high-power field in the centrifuged urine sediment is considered abnormal. The presence of microscopic hematuria in association with proteinuria can only occur at the glomerular level; therefore renal biopsy is more likely to provide definitive diagnostic information that any other procedure.

Urinary casts are formed within the renal tubules and collecting ducts and are indications of the prolonged transit of fluid through the tubule, during which time cells or cellular debris may be trapped within a protein matrix. If red blood cells are present within the intrarenal collecting system, a red blood cell cast may be found in the urine and is considered pathognomonic of glomerulitis. Likewise, polymorphonuclear leukocytes, associated with inflammatory disease, may be noted within casts. In the absence of identifiable cells only the cast matrix may be noted in the sediment. Noncellular casts are seen often in the urine of a patient recovering from an episode of dehydration, when renal perfusion is reduced, but they do not necessarily indicate renal pathology.

Crystals may be noted in the urine sediment and are usually nonspecific findings. Crystals are more prominent when the urine pH renders them less soluble; that is, uric acid crystals are seen in an acid urine but disappear when the urine becomes alkaline.

Addis count

The Addis count is a laboratory method designed to reflect more accurately quantitative renal excretory function. This means of urinalysis begins most conveniently by requiring the patient to thirst after 2 PM, offering a dry evening meal, and having the patient empty the bladder completely at bedtime, discarding the urine and noting the time. All urine voided during the night and the first urine of the morning is collected, and the time of the final specimen is noted. An aliquot of urine, representing the volume of urine formed in 20 minutes, is centrifuged and the sediment resuspended in a volume of 1 ml. A standard 0.9 mm^3 counting chamber is used to count the cells and casts of the urine sediment in all 9 squares; the results multiplied by 40,000 represent the 12-hour excretion rate for each element. A normal Addis count for a child should contain up to 240,000 red blood cells, 1 million white blood cells, and 5000 noncellular casts. The pH, specific gravity or osmolality, and quantitative protein content of the urine are determined to complete the examination. If properly executed, the specific gravity or osmolality measured should document the maximal renal concentrating ability, the range for normal infants and children being a specific gravity of 1.024 to 1.036 or 800 to 1300 mOsm/L. More often than not, this portion of the test is the least accurate, resulting from poor patient cooperation usually fostered by a failure to understand the importance of this test. Total protein level is measured and should ideally be zero, but the amount should not exceed 4 mg/m^2/hr in any child. In the presence of proteinuria an orthostatic component can be demonstrated. The patient voids in the early morning, while still supine after overnight bed rest, and that urine is discarded. The patient remains supine until it is possible to void again, reflecting urine formed only after assuming a supine position. Then the patient assumes a lordotic posture for 30 minutes or engages in physical exercise, such as running in place or climbing stairs for 10 minutes, and voids once more. An increase in protein content from the first to the second urine collection is proof of at least an orthostatic component to the proteinuria.

Glomerular filtration rate

Serum creatinine concentration is a reliable and reproducible reflection of renal function. The normal value for the infant is 0.3 mg/dl, and increments above that level correlate well with increased lean body mass to the adult normal of 1 mg/dl. Creatinine is an end product of protein metabolism in muscle, is freely filtered at the glomerulus, and in addition is secreted by the renal tubular cells. Renal excretion of creatinine varies little from day to day in any given individual, and plasma levels are not affected significantly by diet or hydration. The renal clearance of creatinine is calculated by the standard formula UV/P where U is the concentration of urine creatinine expressed in milligrams per milliliter, V is the rate of urine flow in milliliters per minutes, and P is the plasma concentration of creatinine in milligrams per milliliters. When the collection is complete and accurately timed, the results reflect the GFR and compare favorably with the clearance of inulin, which is performed simultaneously within the normal range of renal function (125 ml/min/1.73 m^2). The clearance of creatinine is the most useful clinical estimation of GFR. As GFR decreases and the portion of urine creatinine added by tubular secretion becomes a more significant portion of the total creatinine excreted, the clearance of creatinine becomes less an estimate of GFR and more a reflection of increased plasma creatinine and of tubular secretion. Therefore at lower levels of GFR (less than 20 ml/min/1.73 m^2) the clearance of creatinine overestimates true GFR by 18%.

Another screening method, though not a consistent indicator of renal function, is the chemical determination of BUN, the normal value of which is less than 20 mg/dl. Urea is freely filtered by the glomerulus and is passively reabsorbed with water in the renal tubule. The blood level of urea is dependent also on the dietary intake of protein, liver function, and the state of hydration. Therefore the BUN level may be normal or possibly low, even in the face of impaired renal function, when there is a low dietary intake of protein, liver failure, or overhydration, whereas the level may be increased in the converse situation of increased protein intake, normal liver function, and dehydration.

The renal mechanism whereby an acid urine is formed depends on the ability of the renal tubular cell to secrete hydrogen ion to first conserve filtered bicarbonate and then generate new bicarbonate as is necessary. After bicarbonate is reabsorbed in sufficient amounts, any additional hydrogen ion is excreted in the form of titratable acid and ammonium. To evaluate this renal mechanism, 5 mEq/kg ammonium chloride can be given in divided doses to the patient over the period of 1 hour and the urine collected at frequent intervals for determination of its pH. The response to the acid loading is noted when, after several hours, the urine reaches its lowest pH, which normally is at least less than 5.5 but usually less than 5.0. If urine collections are timed, titratable acidity and ammonium measured, and the GFR determined, the renal ability to excrete hydrogen ion as titratable acid (range of normal for the infant is 43 to 111 μEq/min/1.73 m^2 and for the child is 33 to 71 μEq/min/1.73 m^2) and ammonium (42 to 79 μEq/min/1.73 m^2 and 46 to 100 μEq/min/1.73 m^2) can be calculated.

GLOMERULOPATHIES

Several renal diseases of known or unknown etiology directly affect the renal glomeruli and produce pathologic changes that may aid the clinician in establishing an exact diagnosis. The obtaining of renal tissue by percutaneous needle biopsy of the kidney has greatly improved the knowledge of pathologic changes but has also led to confusing terminology and classification of glomerulopathies. In this section several of the more commonly observed glomerulopathies in children are discussed.

Poststreptococcal acute glomerulonephritis

Acute glomerulonephritis that follows an infection with a nephritogenic strain of group A beta-hemolytic stretococci (PS-AGN) is the commonest form of renal parenchymal disease in childhood. A favorable outcome can be anticipated in most patients, and the associated morbidity of the early stages of the disease is of little consequence when acute complications respond to currently recommended forms of therapy.

Etiology. Acute glomerulonephritis may follow an infection with one of the few nephritogenic strains of group A beta-hemolytic streptococci. Tonsillitis, pharyngitis, sinusitis, and otitis precede 75% to 80% of the cases of PS-AGN reported in the United States. As many as 70% of cases in the South follow skin infections. Cases that occur after pyoderma are usually seen in the summer and early fall, and the peak incidence lags approximately a month behind that of pyoderma. A latent period of 7 to 10 days occurs between streptococcal infections of the upper respiratory tract and the onset of clinical manifestations of PS-AGN.

Poststreptococcal acute glomerulonephritis closely resembles acute "one-shot" serum sickness in which animals develop glomerulonephritis 7 to 10 days after the single injection of a foreign protein. Circulating immune complexes have been found in 60% to 80% of patients with PS-AGN, especially during the first 2 weeks of the disease. Additional evidence of the immune complex nature of PS-AGN include elevated serum IgG and IgM concentrations, decreased serum complement values, and deposition of complement and IgG along the glomerular basement membrane. Traditionally, streptococcal antigens have been considered to be the exogenous antigen stimulating–antigen-antibody circulating immune complexes that are subsequently deposited along the glomerular basement membrane. It has been recently suggested that nephritogenic streptococci modify native IgG so that altered autologous IgG would then act as an endogenous neoantigen that would produce antibody-antibody circulating immune complexes. Anti-IgG antibodies have been identified in sera and have been found in glomeruli of patients with PS-AGN. Nephritogenic streptococci might antigenically alter IgG by decreasing its sialic acid content through the action of the extracellular product nuramidase, which has been shown to be increased in sera of patients with PS-AGN.

Incidence. PS-AGN occurs with greatest frequency among children and young adults. Seventy percent of patients are children between 2 and 8 years of age. PS-AGN is rarely observed during the first year of life, but up to 10% of cases have been reported to occur after 50 years of age. The actual incidence of subclinical cases of PS-AGN is undetermined, as has been noted in a study of sibling contacts of known nephritics. Although a 2:1 preponderance of males is reported, it is our experience that PS-AGN affects the sexes equally.

Clinical manifestations

History. The onset of the clinical picture of PS-AGN may vary from a coincidental finding of hematuria in an otherwise asymptomatic child to common constitutional symptoms such as malaise, fatigue, anorexia, lethargy, and weakness. Nausea, vomiting, and abdominal pain are not uncommon. Over 70% of patients with PS-AGN will have periorbital edema or hematuria as presenting complaints, and 30% of patients will notice a decrease in urine volume. More seriously ill children will present with cardiovascular symptoms such as tachypnea or dyspnea or with central nervous system symptoms such as headache, somnolence, or seizure activity.

Physical examination. Early in the clinical course of PS-AGN or when the disease is mild, typical physical findings may be absent. If the latent period is sufficiently short, the evidence of active streptococcal upper respiratory tract infection or pyoderma may be noted. Edema, manifested usually by periorbital puffiness and rarely by anasarca, is a consistent finding in 75% of cases. Hypertension is noted in more than one half of hospitalized patients and may appear abruptly at any time during the initial phase of the disease.

From 20% to 60% of patients with PS-AGN have findings related to the cardiovascular system. Cardiac decompensation caused by increased extracellular fluid volume is associated with tachypnea, dyspnea, arrhythmia, gallop rhythm, venous engorgement, hepatomegaly, or cardiomegaly.

Signs of encephalopathy can be expected in approximately 20% of patients. These may vary from nausea, vomiting, and severe headache to changes in visual acuity, diplopia, focal or generalized seizure activity, or coma. Vascular spasm and retinal edema, described as preretinal sheen, are noted on funduscopic examination. Hemorrhages, exudates, or papilledema are rarely noted because of the abrupt onset of symptoms in patients with encephalopathy caused by PS-AGN.

Laboratory evaluation

Urine studies. Careful examination of freshly voided urine is critical to the diagnosis of PS-AGN. Early in the course of the disease, pyuria may be the only abnormality of the urinary sediment because PS-AGN represents a nonsuppurative inflammatory reaction within the renal parenchyma. When glomerular damage has occurred, red blood cells appear in the urine in microscopic or gross quantities at one time or another in all patients. Red blood cell casts, the specific indicator of acute glomerulonephritis, should be searched for when hematuria is present. The upper limits of normal cellular excretion (Addis count) are exceeded for red blood cells in all patients, for white blood cells in 90% of patients, and for cellular casts in 80% of patients. Proteinuria of more than 100 mg/24 hr, resulting from glomerular or tubular damage, is noted in 60% of patients with PS-AGN.

Hematology. A mild to moderate anemia, secondary to hemodilution rather than blood loss, is common at the outset of PS-AGN and may persist until diuresis occurs. Leukocytosis with a shift to less mature forms is noted in those patients who present during or soon after a streptococcal infection. The erythrocyte sedimentation rate is almost always elevated in PS-AGN.

Blood chemistry. The BUN concentration is elevated in 75% of patients and may result from a reduction in GFR and from prerenal factors such as cardiac decompensation and continued dietary intake of protein. The serum creatinine concentration, a more reliable indicator of renal function, is abnormal in more than one half of the patients with PS-AGN. Hyponatremia may be noted as an effect of hemodilution. Hyperkalemia, hypocalcemia, and metabolic acidosis are seen only in patients with the most severe forms of PS-AGN. Hypoalbuminemia of less than 2.5 g/dl is seen only in the 5% of patients who have an associated nephrotic syndrome.

Renal function studies. Almost every hospitalized patient with PS-AGN has some impairment of renal function from the onset of the disease (endogenous creatinine clearance less than 95 ml/min/1.73 m^2). In patients with more severe renal involvement a reproducible estimate of renal function, such as the endogenous creatinine clearance, is an indispensable aid in the follow-up care of the patient. Renal plasma flow in most patients with PS-AGN is normal. Therefore, with a reduced GFR and normal renal plasma flow, the filtration fraction is characteristically low, reflecting that the primary functional alteration in PS-AGN is in the glomerulus. The ability of the kidney to concentrate urine maximally under circumstances of water deprivation is preserved in about 50% of patients with PS-AGN. Mechanisms of urine acidification remain intact.

Serology. Streptozyme is a commercially available rapid slide agglutination test that will detect a rise in any one of five streptococcal antibodies (antistreptolysin O, antihyaluronidase, anti-DPNase, anti-DNase B, and antistreptokinase). This test has replaced the ASO titer in many clinical laboratories and is abnormal in a titer of greater than 1:100. A rising or falling titer should be documented by repeating the titer during the recovery phase of the disease.

The beta-1-C globulin (C′3) fraction of complement is decreased (less than 80 mg/dl) in 96% of patients with PS-AGN and returns to normal within 6 to 8 weeks. Further investigation including a renal biopsy is indicated if the beta-1-C globulin does not return to normal.

Bacteriology. About 20% of patients with pharyngitis-associated PS-AGN will have positive throat cultures for beta-hemolytic streptococci, whereas more than 50% of patients with pyoderma-related PS-AGN will have positive skin cultures for streptococci. Appropriately collected urine for culture may be necessary to exclude bacteriuria in patients with pyuria.

Other studies. Radiographic examination of the chest may demonstrate pulmonary congestion and pleural effusion, even in the absence of associated symptoms. Cardiac size is normal except in the presence of pending or actual heart failure, in which case generalized cardiomegaly is found. Routine intravenous pyelography is not indicated in patients with PS-AGN. Electrocardiographic findings include flattened or inverted T waves, prolongation of the QRS and Q-T segments, and lengthening of the P-R interval. In patients with severely impaired renal function the T-wave changes that occur in hyperkalemia may be noted.

Renal histology. A renal biopsy is indicated in patients with PS-AGN who have a normal beta-1-C globulin, who have a persistently low beta 1-C globulin 6 to 8 weeks after disease onset, or who have a rapidly progressive or otherwise atypical course.

Fig. 21-1 illustrates the light, immunofluorescence, and electron microscopic findings in PS-AGN. Light microscopy shows diffuse proliferation of mesangial and endothelial cells and prominent infiltration of polymorphonuclear leukocytes. Peripheral coarsely granular deposits of beta-1-C globulin and IgG are evident by immunofluorescence microscopy. Characteristic subepithelial dense deposits with overlying obliteration of epithelial foot processes are seen by electron microscopy.

Pathophysiology. The pathophysiology of PS-AGN follows the pathway outlined in the following diagram:

Early in the course of PS-AGN a statistically insignificant increase in plasma volume, red blood cell mass, and total blood volume has been demonstrated by us in a study of 10 patients. Extracellular fluid volume was significantly increased in these 10 patients during the acute phase of their illness and returned to normal after diuresis.

Management. Because no therapy is specifically directed toward reversing or preventing the immune complex reactions that damage glomeruli, the management of PS-AGN consists of general supportive care and early recognition and prompt treatment of complications such as hypertension, cardiac decompensation, and encephalopathy.

General measures. It is essential that even the mildest case of PS-AGN have serial measurements of vital signs, body weight, and fluid balance to detect complications that might appear abruptly at any time during the acute phase of the disease. Noncomplicated cases require only a short period of hospitalization, and prolonged hospital stays are necessary only for those patients with severe impairment of renal function.

Bed rest is recommended only during the acute phase of the disease. Ambulation is allowed after diuresis has occurred, when complications have subsided, and when there is significant improvement in the urinary sediment. A rebound phenomenon characterized by a transient elevation of the BUN concentration and increase in hematuria or proteinuria may be noted when ambulation is allowed, but further bed rest is unnecessary. In the patient whose renal impairment is severe and prolonged, ambulation should be limited to quiet activity until renal function returns toward normal or plateaus

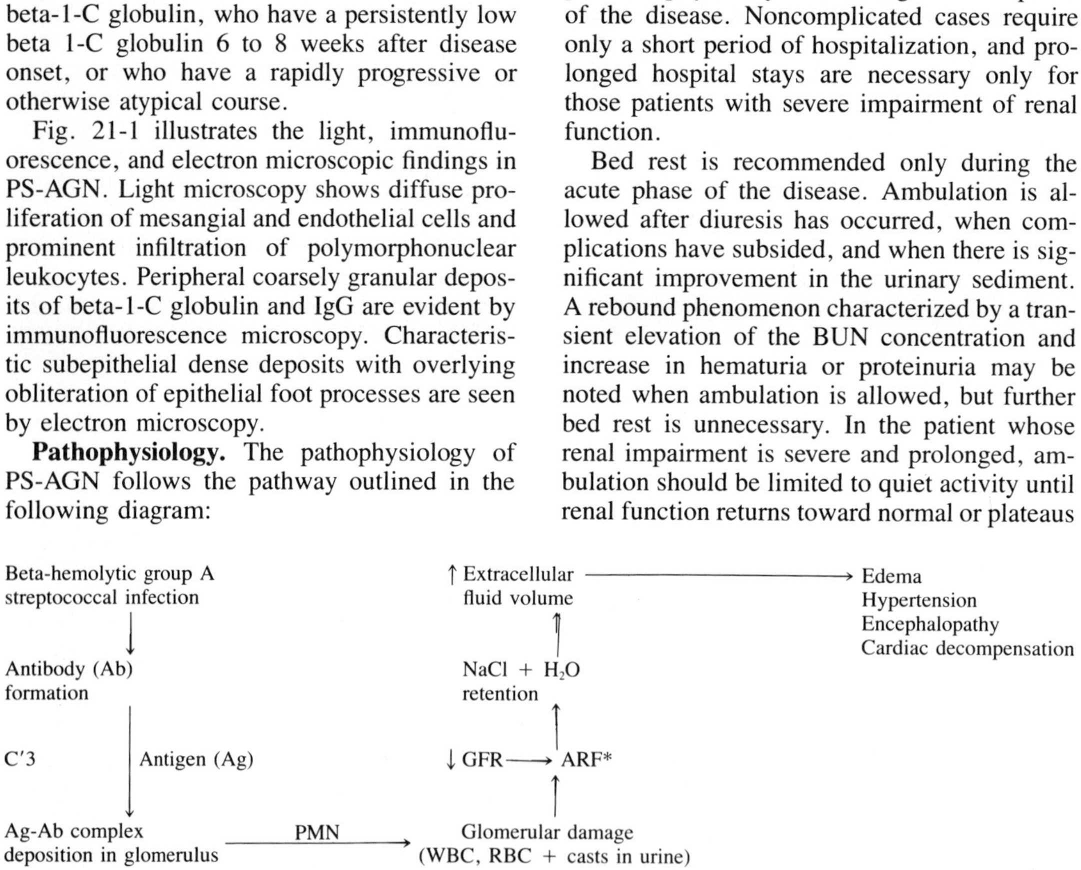

*Acute renal failure.

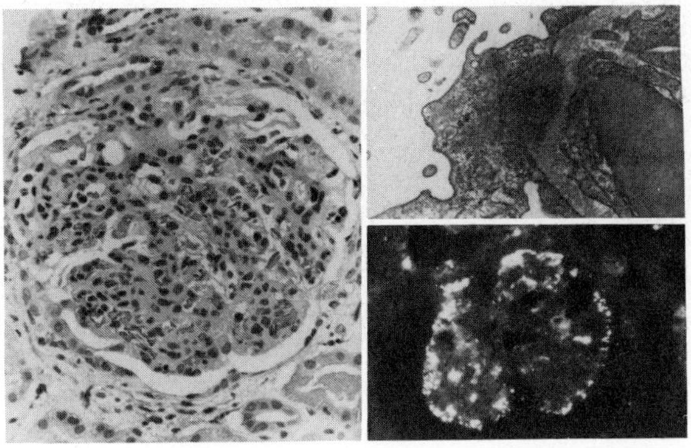

Fig. 21-1. Findings in patients with PS-AGN. **A,** Light microscopy. **B,** Electron microscopy. **C,** Immunofluorescence.

at the level compatible with normal activity.

A regular diet is permissible in uncomplicated cases. Salt restriction is necessary only while the patient is edematous or hypertensive or while in heart failure or renal failure. Protein intake is restricted in severely oliguric and anuric patients, but a return to normal protein intake is permitted once recovery begins.

Fluid intake should be restricted in patients with edema to a volume equal to the insensible water loss (300 to 500 ml/m^2/24 hr), plus a portion of the daily urinary volume. Further progression of salt and water retention may be minimized if this regimen of fluid restriction is applied to every patient with PS-AGN during the acute phase of the disease.

Antibiotic therapy is indicated only for the patient who has evidence of persisting streptococcal infection demonstrated by a positive culture. A 10-day course of antimicrobial therapy is indicated to ensure eradication of the streptococcus, which may be transmitted to susceptible persons. Throat and skin lesion cultures and urinalyses are indicated for sibling contacts of patients with PS-AGN because 20% to 50% of sibling contacts have been reported to have unsuspected glomerulonephritis. Prophylactic use of penicillin in these contacts is not recommended unless streptococci are cultured.

Treatment of complications

Hypertension. Guidelines have been established for the upper limit of normal blood pressure for children of various ages (Report of Task Force, 1977) (p. 560). Blood pressures above the 95th percentile for age should be treated.

Hypertension in PS-AGN is primarily the result of an expanded extracellular fluid volume resulting from salt and water retention. Restriction of salt and water intake is mandatory in the management of each child with PS-AGN from the time the diagnosis is suspected. Fluids are not given to the hypertensive child until the blood pressure is brought under control. Thereafter, 300 ml/m^2/24 hr can be allowed until the patient's dry weight is reached, assuming the blood pressure remains normal.

Furosemide, 1 mg/kg intravenously or 2 mg/kg orally, will usually produce a brisk diuresis and can be repeated at 6- to 8-hour intervals until the desired diuresis is obtained.

Patients with hypertensive encephalopathy and seizure activity constitute a medical emergency. Diazoxide, a potent vasodilator, in a dose of from 3 to 5 mg/kg intravenously as a rapid bolus injection, will lower the mean arterial pressure by 25% within a few seconds of its administration. If no hypotensive effect is observed after the initial dose of diazoxide, the same dose can be repeated in 15 to 30 minutes. The hypotensive effect of diazoxide may last up to 8 hours, permitting sufficient time for antihypertensives with a slower onset and longer duration of action to be administered.

Hydralazine, which has a prompt arteriolar vasodilatory effect, can be given intravenously or intramuscularly in a dose of 0.1 to 0.15 mg/kg. The peak action of intravenous hydralazine can be expected in approximately 20 minutes, and the duration of action is up to 4 to 6 hours. The dose of hydralazine can be doubled every

4 to 6 hours until the desired hypotensive effect is achieved or until the side effects of headache, chest pain, flushing, or tachycardia occur.

It is infrequent for hypertension to last more than a few days except in the most severe cases of PS-AGN. Oral antihypertensive therapy is recommended in these patients. (See the discussion on hypertension, pp. 559-562.)

Extracellular fluid volume expansion. Mild to moderate degrees of expansion of the extracellular fluid volume will respond to the previously outlined fluid and salt restriction, in addition to intravenous furosemide, 1 mg/kg/dose, or oral furosemide, 2 mg/kg/dose. Extreme volume expansion causing pulmonary edema or cardiac decompensation requires emergency measures such as phlebotomy, rotating tourniquets, oxygen, morphine, digitalis, and peritoneal or hemodialysis.

Clinical course. A typical clinical course can be anticipated in most children with PS-AGN. Evidence of the acute phase of the disease diminishes significantly by 10 days after the diagnosis is made in all patients with the exception of those few with the most severe renal damage. Death from PS-AGN is rare and when it occurs early it is attributable to acute renal failure and its inherent complications that fail to respond to adequate treatment. Currently recommended forms of therapy give reasonable assurance that sepsis, hypertension, and volume overload can be managed effectively, and peritoneal dialysis as a procedure for reversing renal failure should be available in every hospital setting.

The resolving phase of PS-AGN is initiated by a brisk diuresis and return of blood pressure to normal limits. The average duration of hypertension is 3 days. Many patients' blood pressure returns to normal in a few hours and requires minimal therapy. Rarely, hypertension will persist for 10 to 14 days. Persistent hypertension beyond this period should alert the clinician to the possibility of some other cause of glomerulonephritis.

A decreasing BUN or creatinine concentration, an increase of the serum complement level, and a quantitative decrease in protein, cellular, and cylindric elements of the urine indicate a resolving phase of PS-AGN. Red blood cells and casts may remain for 6 to 12 months after onset of PS-AGN without other evidence of progressive renal disease. The best documentation of improvement is provided by a rising level of renal function, measured most conveniently by the endogenous creatinine clearance. Persistent hematuria, cylinduria, and proteinuria associated with a failure in the return of renal function toward normal may define only the most severe glomerular lesions with epithelial proliferation and crescents and do not eliminate the possibility of complete recovery. These findings demand close observation for evidence of deterioration in renal function. When renal function returns to a nearly normal level after the acute phase of the disease, any subsequent deterioration of renal function is associated with progressive disease.

Our long-term follow-up study in 35 children with PS-AGN (Roy et al., 1976) demonstrated no evidence of progressive glomerulonephritis over the 12 years of the study. Cumulative morphologic healing occurred in 20% of the children at 24 months, in 46% at 48 months, 77% at 60 months, 94% at 120 months, and 97% in 144 months. One patient was unhealed at 49 months and was subsequently lost to follow-up.

Second attacks of PS-AGN have been reported (Roy et al., 1969) and in our experience do not preclude eventual recovery from the disease.

Because the ultimate outcome is favorable for most children with PS-AGN, and because the clinical courses of acute glomerulonephritis from other causes are more formidable, it is imperative that the diagnosis of PS-AGN be documented by bacteriologic or serologic evidence of a recent streptococcal infection as well as a low serum level of beta-1-C globulin. If the beta-1-C globulin is normal, a renal biopsy is recommended for histologic documentation and for demonstration of immunofluorescent staining of the specimen for beta-1-C globulin and gamma globulin in a granular deposition along the glomerular basement membrane.

A definitive evaluation of every patient with suspected PS-AGN is necessary to prevent further confusion in assessing the prognosis and natural history of this disease.

Idiopathic nephrotic syndrome

The nephrotic syndrome is characterized by proteinuria (greater than 40 mg/m^2/hr), hypoalbuminemia (less than 2.5 g/dl), hypercholesterolemia, and edema. The nephrotic syndrome in children generally occurs in the absence of recognizable systemic disease or preexisting renal disease so that approximately 80% of children with the nephrotic syndrome are categorized as idiopathic. Rarely, the nephrotic syndrome in children may occur during the course of systemic diseases such as lupus erythematosus, Henoch-Schönlein purpura, malaria, syphilis, sickle cell disease, cyanotic congenital heart disease, diabetes mellitus, tuberculosis, and amyloidosis; in association with infected ventriculojugular shunts; after renal vein thrombosis; or as a result of toxicity to drugs such as trimethadione (Tridione), mercurials, gold salts, penicillamine, tolbutamide, and bismuth. The nephrotic syndrome may also occur secondary to renal parenchymal diseases such as acute poststreptococcal glomerulonephritis, rapidly progressive glomerulonephritis, membranous nephropathy, and membranoproliferative glomerulonephritis. A congenital form of the nephrotic syndrome may be recognized soon after birth and is generally fatal.

Incidence. Estimates of the incidence of the nephrotic syndrome in children in the United States range from 2 to 3 cases per 100,000 white children below the age of 10 years. The peak age of onset is between 2 and 3 years of age, with 60% of the patients being males.

Pathophysiology. Abnormal permeability of the glomerular capillary basement membrane to normal plasma proteins is accepted as the cause for the proteinuria of the nephrotic syndrome. The nature of the glomerular lesion is unknown.

Increased rates of catabolism of protein and protein loss through the gastrointestinal tract also contribute to the observed hypoproteinemia. Serum albumin is generally decreased, alpha-1 globulin is normal or decreased, alpha-2 and beta globulins are increased, and gamma globulin is decreased. Serum cholesterol, phospholipids, and triglycerides are all elevated, but the cause of the hyperlipidemia remains obscure.

Hypoalbuminemia results in a reduction in colloid oncotic pressure of the plasma, permitting a shift in plasma water into the interstitial space with resultant decrease in plasma volume and edema formation. Increased tubular absorption of sodium chloride and water leads to continued increase in edema. This increase in tubular reabsorption of sodium has been attributed to both increases in aldosterone excretion and nonadrenal mechanisms. Antidiuretic hormone release in response to vascular volume contraction contributes to water retention. Decreased renal plasma flow and glomerular filtration rate occur in a few patients and may contribute to sodium and water retention.

Clinical manifestations. Even though proteinuria may have been present for days or weeks, edema is usually the symptom that prompts medical evaluation of the child. Periorbital edema that is apparent on arising in the morning and subsides during the day may be present for weeks before gradual or rapid increase in generalized edema occurs. Abdominal swelling from ascites, respiratory embarrassment from pleural effusion, and labial or scrotal swelling are usually present. Extreme skin pallor and diarrhea are frequent, and the latter has been attributed to edema of the intestinal mucosa.

During periods of edema, a tendency to develop peritonitis, sepsis, or cellulitis occurs. Pneumococcal infection was common in the past, but infections with gram-negative organisms such as *Escherichia coli* are now more common.

Laboratory manifestations. During the active stage of the disease, urine protein excretion may reach levels of 15 to 20 g/24 hr. Hyaline casts and oval fat bodies can be found in most patients' urine. Microscopic hematuria is relatively frequent early in the disease, but gross hematuria is seldom observed. Total serum protein concentrations range from 3 to 5 g/dl with serum albumin concentrations of 0.5 to 2.5 g/dl. Cholesterol concentrations range from slightly above normal to well over 1 g/dl.

Beta-1-C globulin concentrations are generally normal. Serum calcium concentrations are reduced to as low as 6 mg/dl, but the reduction is primarily in the protein-bound fraction so that the risk of tetany is low.

Renal pathology. Of 521 patients with the primary nephrotic syndrome reported by the International Study of Kidney Disease in Children (ISKDC report, 1978), 76.4% had minimal changes (MCNS) by renal biopsy, 7.5% had membranoproliferative glomerulonephritis (MPGN), and 6.9% had focal segmental glomerulosclerosis (FSGS). Membranous nephropathy and various forms of proliferative

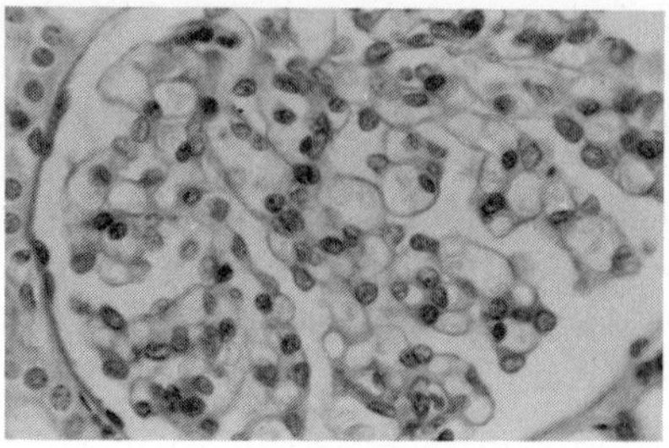

Fig. 21-2. Minimal changes. No pathologic changes by light microscopy. (H & E; ×400.)

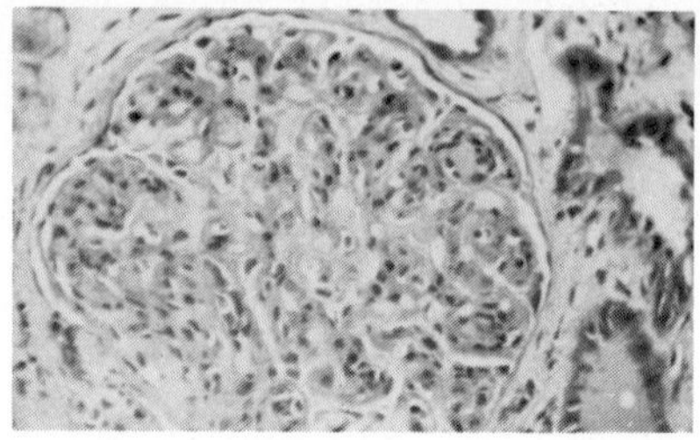

Fig. 21-3. Membranoproliferative glomerulonephritis. Enlarged glomerulus with hyperplasia of mesangial cells and compression of capillary loops. (H & E; ×250.)

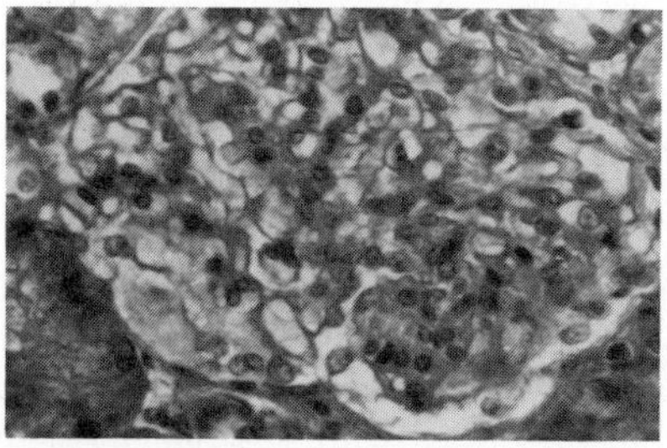

Fig. 21-4. Focal segmental glomerulosclerosis. Sclerosis and hypercellularity of the right lower segment of the glomerulus. (H & E; ×400.)

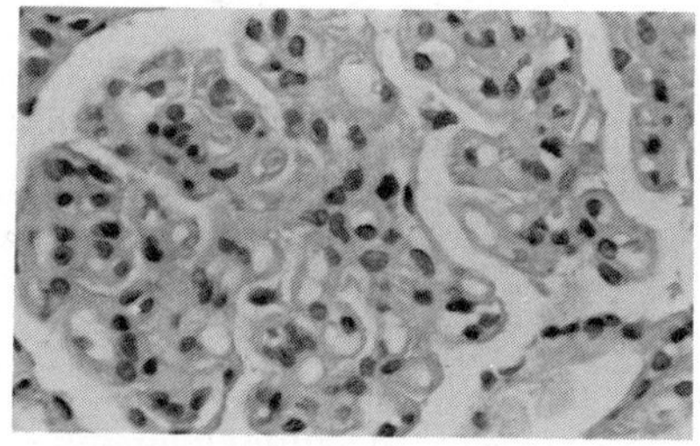

Fig. 21-5. Membranous nephropathy. Diffuse thickening of capillary walls. (H & E; ×400.)

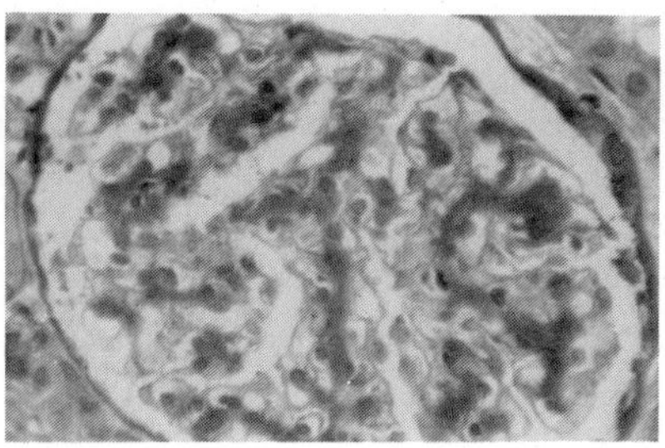

Fig. 21-6. Mesangial proliferation. Diffuse mesangial hypercellularity. (H & E; ×400.)

glomerulonephritis constitute the remaining 9.2% of the histologic types.

The histologic types are illustrated in Figs. 21-2 through 21-6.

Treatment

General measures. A regular diet is suitable for the nephrotic child who is in remission. During periods of massive edema, salt must be restricted. Activity is not restricted. Kindergarten and regular school classes are continued. Playmates with obvious infections should be excluded from contact with the nephrotic child. Intercurrent infections are treated with appropriate antibiotics, but continuous prophylactic antibiotics are not recommended.

Steroid therapy. Elimination of proteinuria is the primary goal of therapy in managing children with the nephrotic syndrome. The following regimen is recommended and followed by the ISKDC. Parents are instructed to test the child's first urine specimen each morning for protein concentration, using either 10% sulfosalicylic acid or Albustix. The presence or absence of proteinuria is the best indicator of disease activity, and changes in therapy are based on these test results.

Initial therapy. Prednisone, 60 mg/m^2/24 hr in three divided doses is given orally for 28 days once the diagnosis has been confirmed. The maximum prednisone dose should not exceed 80 mg/24 hr. The daily therapy for 1 month is followed by intermittent therapy, 40 mg/m^2, in three divided doses given 3 consecutive days out of 7 for an additional 28 days. Most steroid-responsive patients will clear their proteinuria during the 56 days of prednisone therapy. Prednisone is then discontinued abruptly, and the patient's urine is monitored for evidence of recurrent proteinuria.

Treatment of relapses. A relapse is defined by a recurrence of proteinuria of 2+ or greater on 3 consecutive days. Prednisone, 60 mg/m^2, is given in three divided doses daily until the urine is protein free for 3 consecutive days. This is followed by 4 weeks of intermittent prednisone, 40 mg/m^2, on 3 consecutive days out of 7. Prednisone is again discontinued abruptly and the patient observed for future relapses. A patient who relapses more than twice in a 6-month period of time is classified as a frequent relapser.

Immunosuppressant therapy. Either cyclophosphamide or chlorambucil is recommended for patients who are steroid responsive but have frequent relapses and for those children who have unacceptable steroid side effects such as growth failure, obesity, and osteoporosis. Either of these drugs may induce a prolonged remission. In a controlled study, relapses occurred in 48% of a cyclophosphamide-prednisone–treated group with minimal change frequently relapsing disease, whereas 88% of the prednisone-treated control group relapsed. The subsequent relapse rate was also lower in the cyclophosphamide-treated group. Chlorambucil has also been shown to prolong the length of remission in a similar but smaller controlled trial (Grupe et al., 1976). Because of the experimental nature of these latter two drugs in this disease, patients who are candidates for immunosuppressant drugs should be managed by or in consultation with investigators in this field of clinical research. Several untoward side effects of these drugs have been recognized and reported and preclude their use on a wider scale.

Diuretic therapy. Diuretic therapy is generally not indicated in patients with mild or moderate edema. The use of diuretics is considered in children who are uncomfortable from edema, who are infected, and in whom steroid therapy must be delayed or is contraindicated. Diuresis is initially attempted by administering 2 mg/kg hydrochlorothiazide orally, followed by 1 mg/kg furosemide intramuscularly or intravenously 3 hours later. When effective, this regimen will produce a brisk diuresis lasting at least 4 hours.

In patients whose edema is refractory to diuretic therapy alone, the infusion of salt-poor human albumin, plus the previously mentioned diuretics, is usually effective. Hydrochlorothiazide, 2 mg/kg, is given orally before the albumin infusion. From 0.5 to 1 g/kg human albumin is then infused over 1 to 1.5 hours. After a 1-hour equilibration time, 1 mg/kg furosemide is given intravenously. The diuresis is usually short lived because the infused albumin is rapidly lost into the urine. The albumin infusion followed by furosemide can be repeated at 4- to 6-hour intervals, depending on the diuretic response.

Course and prognosis. Approximately 93% of children with minimal change idiopathic nephrotic syndrome (MCNS) attain a remission during therapy with prednisone. About 35% will not relapse during the first 10 months of their disease, 18% will have infrequent relapses, and 40% will relapse frequently.

Recent studies have shown that a favorable response to initial prednisone therapy accurately predicts the presence of minimal changes histologically. However, almost 50% of children less than 6 years of age, who are resistant to steroid therapy, may still have MCNS histologically. Prognosis for these patients must be withheld until a renal biopsy identifies the histopathologic variant present. The initial steroid response rate in patients with glomerular lesions other than MCNS is approximately 28%.

After several years of protein-free urine without steroid therapy, patients may be considered in permanent remission. We have observed relapses, however, in some patients who have been in remission and not receiving prednisone therapy for periods of time of up to 5 years.

Lupus nephritis

Lupus nephritis is another example of immune-complex renal disease. Several nucleoproteins serve as antigens and can be demonstrated in the circulation associated with antinuclear antibody in the form of soluble immune complexes. These complexes, along with complement, have been demonstrated in the glomeruli of patients with lupus nephritis.

Children with systemic lupus erythematosus (SLE) may present insidiously with joint involvement and fever, with skin manifestations, or with neurologic symptomatology. At times asymptomatic proteinuria or hematuria will be the presenting complaint. More often the diagnosis of SLE is apparent by the time renal involvement is recognized. Two thirds or more of the children with SLE will manifest renal disease, and the nephrotic syndrome is usually seen at some point in the course of their disease.

The diagnosis of SLE nephritis may be confirmed in a child with SLE by the demonstration of hematuria, proteinuria, red blood cell casts, azotemia, reduced creatinine clearance, and serum complement or beta-1-C globulin depression. Additional features of the nephrotic syndrome, such as hypoalbuminemia and hypercholesterolemia, may be present. In other instances a clinical picture of acute or rapidly progressive glomerulonephritis may be seen.

A renal biopsy is clinically important in estimating the prognosis and planning treatment for patients with lupus nephritis. It is helpful clinically to divide the nephritis of SLE into the following histologic categories: (1) focal glomerulonephritis, (2) membranous glomerulonephritis, and (3) diffuse proliferative glomerulonephritis. Patients with focal changes have a uniformly good prognosis and seldom develop renal insufficiency. The nephrotic syndrome is seen in most patients with membranous changes. They have a poorer prognosis and frequently develop septicemia after high-dose steroid therapy. Patients with diffuse proliferative nephritis appear to have a progressive disease leading to renal insufficiency and a uremic death.

A growing body of evidence suggests that patients with lupus nephritis may benefit from adrenocortical steroids alone or in combination with azathioprine or cyclophosphamide. Improvement in renal function and renal histology, as well as suppression of clinical and laboratory manifestations of the disease, are observed. Most centers recommend initial treatment with steroids alone. If severe steroid toxicity develops or the disease is not completely controlled, azathioprine or cyclophosphamide is added.

Serial determinations of complement and antinuclear antibody titers aid in determining the presence of active disease. Low complement and high antinuclear antibody titers are nearly always associated with active disease, whereas normal values for these tests indicate inactive disease. A 50% fall in serum complement level usually accompanies or precedes the onset of active nephritis.

Familial nephritis or nephropathy

Familial nephritis has been described under a variety of names. The condition was initially described by Guthrie and later by Alport who noted nerve deafness and ocular defects. Familial nephritis most likely includes a variety of different conditions with varying etiologic and pathophysiologic mechanisms.

Familial nephritis with nerve deafness (Alport syndrome) appears to be transmitted as an autosomal dominant trait with variable and incomplete penetrance. The disease characteristically progresses to uremia and bilateral nerve deafness and is usually most severe in the male. Features of both glomerular and interstitial disease are generally present in renal biopsy material. By electron microscopy glomerular capillary basement membranes appear split and have nonosmophilic material deposited between their layers, resulting in a layered appearance.

Several other familial forms of nephropathy have been recognized. Associated with the renal disease are either thrombocytopenia, osteolysis, nail-patella dysplasia, retinitis pigmentosa, or partial or generalized lipodystrophy. Familial distribution may also be observed in a syndrome of benign hematuria that does not appear to be progressive. A familial form of the nephrotic syndrome has also been described.

Hemolytic-uremic syndrome

The hemolytic-uremic syndrome is characterized clinically by acute renal failure, hemolytic anemia, thrombocytopenia, and bleeding manifestations. It is characterized pathologically by thrombotic microangiopathy in the kidney and renal cortical necrosis.

The condition is frequently preceded by several days of acute gastroenteritis in a previously well infant or young child. Clinical features of acute glomerulonephritis develop in association with a severe hemolytic anemia and thrombocytopenia. Neurologic manifestations such as irritability, convulsions, and coma are frequently observed.

Some patients develop renal cortical necrosis, whereas others show a severe form of glomerulitis. Fibrinoid necrosis and thrombosis of arterioles and glomeruli are seen in both pathologic forms. Endothelial and mesangial swelling are the predominant glomerular changes associated with thrombotic microangiopathy.

Therapy consists of blood transfusions for acute hemolytic anemia and management of acute renal failure and its complications. The role of heparin in this condition has not been adequately defined through controlled trials.

Benign recurrent or persistent hematuria

A syndrome of recurrent or persistent hematuria not associated with hypertension, edema, or significant proteinuria is relatively common in children. An episode of gross or microscopic hematuria frequently follows a mild respiratory illness by 2 to 5 days and does not usually progress to more serious renal involvement. Abdominal or flank pain may be present during the episode of gross hematuria. Hematuria may subside between the acute attacks of gross hematuria or may persist microscopically. Renal biopsy specimens may be normal or show areas of focal hypercellularity or focal sclerosis.

Berger has described a distinct subgroup known as IgA/IgG nephropathy. Mesangial deposits of IgA, IgG, and occasionally beta-1-C globulin have been demonstrated by immunofluorescence microscopy. A recent multicenter clinicopathologic study (Southwest Pediatric Nephrology Study Group) of 63 children with IgA nephropathy revealed a direct correlation between proteinuria and damage of peripheral glomerular capillary walls and an association between decreased glomerular filtration rate and tubulointerstitial damage. One patient in this study progressed to end-stage renal failure.

Hematuria and hypercalciuria

Recently, isolated hematuria (gross and microscopic) has been associated with idiopathic hypercalciuria without detectable urinary calculi (Roy et al., 1981). Initially, it was noted that hematuria in hypercalciuric children occurred months, and even years, before calculi developed. Subsequently, over 25% of children referred for isolated hematuria (without urolithiasis) have demonstrated increased urinary calcium loss.

In these patients, hematuria may be microscopic or gross, but is usually painless. Red blood cell casts are rare, and hematuria may be found in bilateral ureteral urine samples. A family history of renal stones is present in most patients; the pattern of inheritance appears to be autosomal dominant.

The mechanism by which increased urinary calcium produces hematuria is unknown. Renal biopsy specimens demonstrate no glomerular, tubular, or interstitial abnormalities. Furthermore, increased urinary calcium loss is not present in either acute or chronic glomerulonephritis. Disappearance of hematuria occurs when urinary calcium excretion is reduced by hydrochlorothiazide therapy.

Because the relative risk for subsequent calculus formation in these patients is unknown, specific anticalciuric drug therapy cannot be recommended. On the other hand, measurement of urinary calcium excretion should be included in the routine evaluation of children with hematuria, especially if there is a family history of urolithiasis.

Henoch-Schönlein nephritis (anaphylactoid purpura with nephritis)

Anaphylactoid purpura (see also pp. 489-491) occurs more commonly in children than in adults and has a peak incidence between 3 and 5 years of age. Preceding upper respiratory tract infections are common, but their relationship to the disease is unproved.

The frequency of renal involvement varies considerably, depending on diagnostic criteria. Probably 25% to 50% of children manifest signs of renal involvement. This is noted within a few days to a few weeks after the onset of skin, joint, and gastrointestinal manifestations. Severity of the renal disease may vary from minimal urinary abnormalities to a severe, rapidly progressive glomerulonephritis with or without an associated nephrotic syndrome. A consistently normal serum beta-1-C globulin concentration serves to differentiate this disease from acute poststreptococcal glomerulonephritis.

Focal proliferative glomerular lesions are most commonly seen in renal biopsy specimens from patients with mild renal involvement. Epithelial cellular crescents and progressive glomerular hyalinization occur in more severely affected patients. Fibrin, IgG, and beta-1-C globulin deposits are demonstrated in glomeruli by immunofluorescent techniques.

Most patients with renal involvement follow a self-limiting course of gradual recovery over a period of a few weeks to a few months. A chronic course with repeated remissions and exacerbations may occur with progression to renal insufficiency.

Although steroid therapy causes a prompt remission of extrarenal manifestations of the disease, a beneficial effect on the renal manifestations has not been demonstrated. A controlled trial of cyclophosphamide therapy in children with significant histologic changes and laboratory manifestations of nephritis is ongoing at the present time.

Disorders of renal tubular function

Disorders of renal tubular function are conditions in which there are one or more permanent or transient abnormalities in specific mechanisms of tubular transport or reabsorption, not associated with altered glomerular function at the onset, but which may over a given period of time predispose to renal parenchymal alteration, glomerular destruction, and ultimately renal failure. Still other disorders such as renal glycosuria are often incidental findings that never affect overall renal function. Tubular dysfunctions may originate as primary disorders in the proximal or distal tubule (renal tubular acidosis), or they may arise as a secondary effect of metabolic disease (cystinosis) or from circulating toxins. In addition, tubular dysfunctions may be secondary functional abnormalities that may be reversible when the primary cause is removed, such as the concentrating defect found in potassium depletion. Renal tubular disorders may have a characteristic pattern of genetic transmission, may occur sporadically in the general population, or may be noted as an acquired defect, with or without a specific cause. Defects may be manifested early in life, in particular the genetic disorders that behave in a predictable fashion, or may present at any time after birth as a secondary or acquired abnormality. Inherited disorders associated with renal tubular abnormalities are listed in the following outline:

- Aminoacidurias
  - Beta-aminoisobutyric aciduria
  - Cystinuria
  - Dibasic aminoaciduria
  - Familial iminoglycinuria
  - Glucoglycinuria
  - Hartnup disease
  - Hereditary glycinuria
  - Vitamin D–resistant rickets with hyperglycinemia
  - Nonspecific disorders of tubular function with generalized aminaociduria
    - Cogenital lactose intolerance
    - Galactosemia
    - Heavy metal poisoning
    - Hereditary fructose intolerance
    - Malnutrition
    - Vitamin D–resistant rickets
    - Wilson disease
- Glycosurias
  - Type A—reduced threshold and transport maximum
  - Type B—reduced threshold
- Idiopathic hypercalciuria
- Disorders of phosphate transport
  - Hereditary hypophosphatemia
  - Pseudohypoparathyroidism
- Renal tubular acidosis
  - Distal (type 1)
    - Primary, idiopathic
    - Secondary
  - Proximal (type 2)
    - Primary, idiopathic
    - Secondary
- Fanconi syndrome
  - Primary
    - Idiopathic Fanconi syndrome
    - Oculocerebrorenal (Lowe) syndrome
    - Luder-Sheldon syndrome
  - Secondary
    - Cystinosis
    - Exogeneous toxins
    - Galactosemia
    - Glycogen-storage disease
    - Hereditary fructose intolerance
    - Nephrotic syndrome
    - Tyrosinemia
    - Wilson disease
- Potassium-losing disorders
  - Bartter syndrome
  - Pseudohyperaldosteronism (Liddle syndrome)
- Sodium-losing disorders
  - Chronic pyelonephritis
  - Fanconi syndrome
  - Hypoplasia-dysplasia
  - Interstitial nephritis
  - Medullary cystic disease
  - Obstructive uropathy
  - Nephrophthisis
  - Polycystic disease
  - Pseudohypoaldosteronism
- Disorders of concentrating mechanisms
  - Hypokalemia
  - Nephrogenic diabetes insipidus

Aminoaciduria. Amino acids filtered by the glomerulus are almost completely reabsorbed in the proximal tubule by one of several transport mechanisms specific for dibasic, acidic, and neutral amino acids. In addition, amino acids and beta-amino compounds have identifiable transport mechanisms. Increased amounts of amino acids excreted in the urine result from (1) an overflow type of aminoaciduria, in which the tubular transport mechanism is saturated when an increased plasma level of the amino acid results in an increased filtered load and the transport capacity is exceeded; (2) a combined aminoaciduria, in which competition exists between amino acids sharing a common transport mechanism when the plasma level of one or both is increased; (3) a specific renal aminoaciduria, in which there is a defect in selective reabsorption of one group of amino acids; or (4) a nonspecific renal aminoaciduria, in which generalized tubular dysfunction results in aminoaciduria. For the most part, aminoacidurias are inborn errors of metabolism and are considered in detail in another section of this book (pp. 645 to 655).

Renal glycosuria. As with reabsorption of amino acids, essentially all glucose found in the glomerular filtrate is reabsorbed in the proximal tubule by a specific transport mechanism. Even at normal levels of blood glucose some glucose appears in the final urine of all persons, but in quantities less than 20 mg/dl—a level not detectably by routine semiquantitative screening methods. The normal renal plasma threshold for glucose is considered to be 180 to 200 mg/dl, above which level glucose appears in the urine in increasing amounts. The maximal tubular transport capacity for glucose (T_mG) has been determined to be 375 mg/min in the adult male and 300 mg/min in the adult female. Deviations from normal patterns may be detected when the renal threshold for glucose is reduced below normal or when the transport mechanism is defective, as in a congenital disorder or as a result of an acquired tubular injury.

Type A renal glycosuria, in which both the renal plasma threshold and the T_mG are low, is inherited as an autosomal dominant trait and is present at birth, but it usually is undetected for many years. This is a benign condition, and only rarely does the patient have symptomatic hypoglycemia. This type of renal glycosuria most often results from generalized tubular dysfunction such as the Fanconi syndrome.

Type B, or "pseudorenal diabetes," is seen only as a reduction in the renal plasma threshold for glucose and a significant splay in the glucose titration curve, most likely representing increased nephron heterogeneity. T_mG is normal in this condition. Neither form of renal glycosuria requires specific treatment.

Disorders of phosphate transport. Under normal circumstances 85% to 95% of filtered phosphate is reabsorbed in the proximal tubule, but this function of tubular transport varies inversely with the levels of parathyroid hormone and with intravascular volume, while varying directly with 1,25-dihydroxyvitamin D_3. The tubular reabsorption of phosphate may be maximal during the period of high phosphate demands for the growing child, whereas lower levels of reabsorption are seen in the infant with multiple defects of tubular function, such as Fanconi syndrome. Vitamin D–resistant or renal rickets is the result of impaired ability of the kidney either to produce or respond to 1,25-dihydroxyvitamin D_3 or parathyroid hormone or both. Familial hypophosphatemic rickets is an inherited metabolic defect associated with target organ unresponsiveness to normal levels of active vitamin D metabolites. Pseudohyperparathyroidism is a congenital disorder in which the proximal tubule is unresponsive to parathyroid hormone.

Renal tubular acidosis. Renal tubular acidosis (RTA) is a clinical condition of systemic metabolic acidosis in which the hydrogen ion content of the urine is expectedly maximal but the pH of the urine is inappropriately alkaline. The role of the kidney in maintaining acid-base homeostasis consists primarily of its ability to secrete hydrogen ion into the tubular fluid, in order to first reabsorb and conserve bicarbonate filtered by the glomerulus—largely a function of the proximal tubule, and then to excrete hydrogen ion excess from the body as titratable acidity and ammonium—a distal tubular mechanism. An abnormality of either bicarbonate reabsorption or hydrogen ion secretion, whether congenital or acquired, results in RTA. If the abnormality is in bicarbonate reabsorption, the RTA is said to be the proximal type, whereas an inability to secrete hydrogen ion, and thus form an acid urine, is referred to as the distal type of RTA. The latter is occasionally referred to also as type 1 RTA in that it was the first disorder classically described; therefore proximal RTA may be mentioned as type 2. When the defect is isolated and idiopathic, it is said to represent a primary form of the disorder, but when the abnormality is associated with other dysfunctions of the renal tubule or follows tubular injury from any cause, it is designated as a secondary form of RTA. Heavy metal poisoning and renal transplantation are two of several clinical situations in which both proximal and distal tubular functions may be affected, and a combined form of RTA has been reported.

Distal (type 1) renal tubular acidosis. The primary form of RTA that is referred to as distal, or type 1, RTA occurs in families as a dominant trait with incomplete penetrance. It characteristically affects females in a ratio of 7:3, who present after 2 years of age with growth failure. Often the history of vomiting, polyuria, and dehydration is obtained in the younger patient, and occasionally urolithiasis is noted in older children and adults.

When there is an inability to secrete hydrogen ion from the distal tubule, accumulation of hydrogen ion occurs within the body, which soon depletes the available bicarbonate buffer, and acidosis is sustained. Acidemia retards normal body growth, and hypercalcemia develops as bone salts are mobilized to buffer excessive hydrogen ion. Increased circulating levels of both calcium and phosphorus predispose to nephrocalcinosis, and with increased amounts of each being excreted into an alkaline urine, urolithiasis may occur. Although glomerular function is normal at birth, calcium deposition in the kidney results in an interstitial nephritis, which eventually destroys renal parenchyma, and renal function is impaired. In an effort by distal tubular mechanisms to conserve sodium, excessive potassium is secreted because the basic defect of distal RTA prevents hydrogen ion from participating in the distal mechanism of sodium reabsorption. Total body potassium is reduced and renders the kidney unable to concentrate the urine maximally. Hyponatremia stimulates the production of increased amounts of aldosterone, which further aggravates potassium depletion. Hypokalemia may be associated with periodic paralysis in some persons. As bicarbonate is depleted, volume contraction occurs so that more sodium chloride is reabsorbed from the proximal tubule, and hyperchloremia results.

When the patient with distal RTA is given an acid load, bicarbonaturia continues, even when blood pH is low, and the pH of urine never decreases below 6.0. The renal bicarbonate threshold and the tubular reabsorption of bicarbonate are normal in these patients; however, serum bicarbonate levels are lowered in the effort to buffer accumulated hydrogen ion.

The defect of primary distal RTA is a permanent one, but in the child who is diagnosed and treated early, the outlook is favorable.

Bicarbonate replacement therapy in the infant is necessary to promote growth, normalize the glomerular filtration rate, heal rickets if present, and prevent nephrocalcinosis. Recent data in infants with distal RTA (Rodriquez-Soriano, et al.) indicate that renal bicarbonate wasting, present during the first few years of life, requires a replacement bicarbonate dosage of 3.9 to 10.0 mEq/kg/day, decreasing to approximately 1 to 3 mEq/kg/day after 6 years of age. Hypokalemia may not resolve with sodium bicarbonate therapy and thus should be corrected. The recommended form of alkali therapy is sodium bicarbonate, which can be prepared as a 1 mEq/ml solution by dissolving an 8-ounce box of baking soda in 2.88 liters of distilled water. Bicitra (1 mEq/ml) is a commercially prepared alkali preparation that also may be used. These solutions can be administered either undiluted or mixed with a small amount of milk or formula.

Distal RTA occurs secondarily in malnutrition, hyperparathyroidism, hyperthyroidism, vitamin D intoxication, drug nephropathy, hypergammaglobulinemic states, hepatic cirrhosis, medullary sponge kidney, acute tubular necrosis, and renal transplantation. When the primary disorder is amenable to therapy. RTA is transient in most cases.

Proximal (type 2) renal tubular acidosis. Proximal RTA is a defect in bicarbonate reabsorption, the mechanism of which is unknown. The renal threshold for bicarbonate is reduced to 18 to 19 mM/L from the normal of 21.5 to 22.5 mM/L in the infant and 23 to 25 mM/L in the child. The distal tubular mechanism for hydrogen ion secretion is intact in the individual with proximal RTA, as evidenced by an appropriately acid urine when systemic acidosis is pronounced or by the formation of normal titratable acid and ammonium after an acid load.

The primary, idiopathic form of the proximal

disorder is a transient phenomenon and occurs sporadically in males almost without exception; however, the diagnosis has been made recently in at least two females. Growth failure is almost always the presenting feature of this defect, and complications are rare.

Glomerular filtration rate may be slightly decreased in the untreated patient, but with adequate bicarbonate replacement, glomerular function returns to normal and the linear growth pattern of the child shows a dramatic response. Therapy is decided on an individual basis. Because large quantities of bicarbonate are lost into the urine, replacement of up to 10 to 15 mEq/kg/24 hr of bicarbonate is not unusual; even more may be required at frequent intervals during the day and night to produce the desired effect of a relatively constant blood bicarbonate level.

The secondary form of proximal RTA is seen in association with other disorders of tubular function, such as Fanconi syndrome, toxic nephropathies, and renal transplantation.

The syndrome previously described by Lightwood and considered a transient form of distal RTA is now placed in the category of secondary proximal RTA, in that his patients were mostly male infants whose defects were transient, who responded well to bicarbonate replacement, and who evidenced no complications associated with distal RTA, particularly rickets and nephrocalcinosis. Furthermore, the condition described by Lightwood occurred during a limited period of time in Great Britain, and because it was a transient defect, it may have been associated with vitamin D intoxication.

In summary, the clinical distinctions between the proximal and distal forms of renal tubular acidosis are several. The primary proximal type affects males who present in infancy with a transient defect in bicarbonate reabsorption and a normal ability to secrete hydrogen ion, requiring large quantities of replacement therapy. The primary distal type, however, occurs predominantly in females who present during childhood with complications arising from the inability to acidify the urine—nephrocalcinosis, urolithiasis, growth failure, and rickets—and in whom bicarbonate reabsorption and the renal threshold for bicarbonate is normal. These latter patients, except during infancy, require only small amounts of replacement therapy.

Fanconi syndrome. Multiple disorders of proximal tubular function, including abnormal transport mechanisms in the reabsorption of amino acids, glucose, bicarbonate, and phosphate, are designated Fanconi syndrome. Moreover, wasting of sodium and potassium and an inability to conserve water normally may be noted in the same patient.

The primary forms of Fanconi syndrome include the *idiopathic type*, which exhibits multiple abnormalities of tubular function but, in contradistinction to cystinosis, without impairment of glomerular function; therefore it may be seen well into adult life. The *oculocerebrorenal* syndrome, described by Lowe, is the association of Fanconi syndrome with mental retardation and abnormalities of the eye, characteristically cataracts and frequently glaucoma.

The secondary forms of Fanconi syndrome include *cystinosis*, the only one to be discussed here. It is an inborn error of metabolism, inherited as an autosomal recessive trait, in which there is excessive intracellular accumulation of cystine within lysosomes of up to a hundred times normal when the plasma level of cystine is normal. Although there is a less severe form of cystinosis, the onset of which occurs during adolescence or even adult life, persons affected with the infantile form of the disease have a distinctive clinical course. At the outset glomerular function is normal, but as cellular levels of cystine increase, multiple abnormalities of tubular transport may be detected: first as aminoaciduria and glycosuria, then as a limited ability to concentrate the urine, which results in polyuria, polydipsia, and frequent episodes of dehydration. At some time during the course of the disease renal tubular acidosis of the secondary proximal type develops. Therefore all the tubular abnormalities of the Fanconi syndrome are identifiable and are secondary to the effect of accumulated intracellular cystine. As tubular function deteriorates, so does the function of its associated glomerulus, resulting in a slowly progressive impairment of renal function with the onset of uremia, usually before the age of 10 years.

The diagnosis of cystinosis is suspected in any patient with Fanconi syndrome and is documented by slit-lamp identification of amino acid crystals in the corneas and by increased content of cystine within fibroblasts grown in cell culture. This latter technique is especially useful in the intrauterine diagnosis of cystinosis and in genetic counseling. Therapy of this disorder is directed at replacing bicarbonate, maintaining electrolyte balance, preventing dehydration, treating rickets, and managing renal failure as it develops. Hemodialysis and transplantation in this disorder have been successful for the limited number of patients offered this form of therapy to date. The general metabolic defect of cystinosis persists, but in the transplanted kidney no intracellular accumulation of cystine has been noted in the follow-up of patients biopsied and reported as long as 5 years later; however, cystine crystals are found in the interstitium.

Potassium-losing disorders. The associated findings of juxtaglomerular hyperplasia, secondary hyperaldosteronism, hypokalemic alkalosis, and normal blood pressure despite high levels of plasma renin and aldosterone is referred to as Bartter syndrome. Early symptoms are polyuria, polydipsia, intermittent vomiting, constipation, and episodes of dehydration. Growth retardation has been noted in each patient reported. Although a rise in blood pressure is produced by the intravenous infusion of angiotensin II, the response is blunted when compared to the normal. The pathophysiologic mechanism producing this syndrome remains undefined; however, an important relationship may exist between prostaglandin synthesis and the renal tubular defect. Bartter proposed originally that there was a vascular unresponsiveness to angiotensin and that the resulting hyperaldosteronism resulted in potassium loss. It has been suggested that there is a defect in the distal tubular reabsorption of sodium associated with elevated renal prostaglandin synthesis. More recently, however, it has been suggested that active tubular reabsorption of chloride in the thick ascending limb of the loop of Henle is defective in this syndrome. Because of impaired chloride transport, sodium and potassium chloride are lost in the urine. Hypovolemia, hyperreninemia, hyperaldosteronism, and hypokalemia are the inevitable results.

Impairment of renal function is not a constant feature of the syndrome, although glomerular insufficiency and even death from renal failure have been reported. Response to therapy is unpredictable, with hypokalemia being the most difficult to correct. Administration of inhibitors of prostaglandin synthetase, such as aspirin and indomethacin, have been associated in Bartter syndrome with improvement that is often dramatic. Potassium-sparing diuretics—triamterene and spironolactone—have not been of significant value in the management of these patients.

Pseudohyperaldosteronism, or Liddle syndrome, is characterized by hypertension and hypokalemic alkalosis in the absence of hyperaldosteronism. Seemingly, there is an increased tendency for the kidney to reabsorb sodium and thereby excrete potassium from the distal tubule, just as if increased amounts of aldosterone were present. Therapy is directed at inhibiting distal tubular sodium reabsorption with triamterene and providing supplementary potassium chloride.

Sodium-losing disorders. The inability to conserve sodium when its intake is restricted characterizes all sodium-losing disorders. Any destructive renal parenchymal disease at some time in its course will result in the tubular inability of the nephron to reabsorb adequate sodium to maintain balance. *Pseudohypoaldosteronism,* a congenital failure of the distal nephron to respond to aldosterone, is inherited as a sex-linked trait in that all reported cases have been males. This defect results in the excessive loss of sodium in the urine so that hyponatremia and hyperkalemia develop. Symptoms are first manifested in the newborn infant by a failure to thrive, episodes of dehydration, and vascular collapse. Large quantities of sodium continue to be excreted in the urine in spite of dehydration, hyponatremia, and volume contraction. Aldosterone secretion rates are abnormally high. Supplemental sodium chloride, in a quantity sufficient to maintain positive sodium balance, usually effects a decrease in symptomatology and a growth response.

Disorders of concentrating mechanisms. *Diabetes insipidus,* in which there is a deficiency of ADH, is discussed on pp. 571 and 572. *Nephrogenic diabetes insipidus* (NDI) is characterized by an insensitivity of the tubule to ADH. It is inherited as an X-linked recessive disorder, expressed in males whose mothers are carriers, and may exhibit a mild defect in their urine-concentrating abilities. This disorder is manifested during the newborn period, when the infant presents with vomiting, unexplained fever, recurrent dehydration, and failure to thrive. Serum electrolytes and BUN concentration may be elevated, and the urine specific gravity is always less than 1.005, except during periods of severe dehydration when urine osmolality may increase slightly. There is no response to administration of even large amounts of vasopressin. An intravenous pyelogram may be considered abnormal and may reveal findings compatible with obstructive uropathy, such as megaloureter and hydronephrosis, but these findings are associated with the high rate of urine flow and are not considered abnormal in the patient with NDI. Glomerular filtration rate is normal when hydration is adequate. The mechanism of this tubular defect is thought to be the result of an abnormality in the adenylcyclase system. Therapy is successful, and the ultimate prognosis is favorable when the diagnosis is made early in life and water replacement is given in sufficient amounts to compensate for urinary loss. In that most of the infant's and young child's time is spent drinking water, adequate caloric intake becomes problematic and growth is retarded. Psychomotor retardation is apparent as an effect of hyperelectrolytemia and dehydration, whereas the constant need for water replacement leaves little time for normal handling and stimulation of the child by the parent. The use of chlorothiazide diuretics has greatly enhanced the management of these patients, often making it unnecessary for the parent to offer fluid replacement hourly throughout the day and night. When the diuretic effect results in sodium depletion, there is increased proximal reabsorption of sodium and water, with decreased delivery of tubular fluid to the distal nephron, hence a decrease in free water clearance and urine volume.

Persistent *hypokalemia* is associated with an inability of the kidney to concentrate the urine maximally. For the most part, this is considered a reversible phenomenon when total body potassium is restored to normal. Hypokalemia may result from gastrointestinal losses and from a disorder of the renal tubule in which potassium wasting is a feature. The exact mechanism whereby potassium depletion interferes with the concentrating ability of the kidney is unclear; however, most evidence suggests an abnormality in the countercurrent concentrating mechanism or in a decreased permeability of the collecting duct to water.

Urolithiasis (see also pp. 945 to 948)

Compared to adults, children in the United States are afflicted by urinary calculi relatively infrequently. In the South, urinary stones account for 1 in 1000 pediatric hospital admissions. There is a predilection for boys, particularly those less than 2 years of age. In children, urinary calculi often occur early in life, reflecting the frequent association of calculi with urinary obstruction.

Urinary tract infections, with or without obstruction, account for 30% to 50% of renal calculi. *Proteus* and other urea-splitting bacteria produce an alkaline urine in which dramatic stone growth may occur. When immobilization and its attendent hypercalciuria accompany a urinary infection, a particularly hospitable environment is prepared for the development of a calculus. Children with spinal dysraphism frequently have urolithiasis, presumably from this association.

Metabolic abnormalities that increase the urinary concentration of crystalloids are the most common causes of urolithiasis in children. Increased urinary calcium excretion (hypercalciuria) is now recognized as the most frequent metabolic abnormality in children with urolithiasis (Stapleton et al., 1982) and may be the result of hypercalcemia, renal calcium wasting, increased gastrointestinal calcium absorption or, rarely, hyperparathyroidism. Uric acid stones are uncommon in the United States and are usually found in children with malignancies or enzymatic defects in purine metabolism. Calcium oxalate calculi are found in primary oxalosis, either type 1 or type 2. Increased urinary excretion of oxalate also occurs with excessive intake of ascorbic acid or oxalate-rich foods such as rhubarb and in association with inflammatory bowel disease. Increased cystine excretion is the hallmark of cystinuria.

Children with urolithiasis most often seek medical evaluation for painless microscopic or gross hematuria. Renal calculi have even been responsible for the presumptive diagnosis of "exercise-induced hematuria" in some children. Renal colic may accompany childhood urolithiasis; however, pain is a less-frequent complaint in children. Other symptoms include

Table 21-1. Normal values for urinary crystalloids important in the genesis of urolithiasis

Crystalloid	Normal values
Calcium	Less than 4 mg/kg/24 hr Less than 0.21 mg/mg creatinine in a random fasting urine
Uric acid	Less than 800 mg/1.73/m^2/24 hr Less than 0.6 mg/dl creatinine clearance
Oxalate	Less than 50 mg/1.73/m^2/24 hr
Cystine	Less than 0.07 mg/mg creatinine

urinary retention, dysuria, vague abdominal pain, fever, and anorexia. The complaint of passing a calculus, or the presence of a stone in the bladder or urethra, may occasionally represent factitious disease. For this and other reasons, crystallographic analysis of urinary calculi is essential in the diagnostic evaluation of childhood urolithiasis.

In some instances, analysis of the stone will allow definitive diagnosis. A careful history is also important in evaluating children with urolithiasis. Essential historical information includes: dietary history, including medications and vitamins, family history of urinary stones, and a history of infections or urologic symptoms. Laboratory evaluation should document renal function with a creatinine clearance and 24-hour excretion of calcium, uric acid, oxalate, and cystine (Table 21-1). Xanthine excretion should be measured if hypouricemia is present. When hypercalciuria is identified, an oral calcium-loading test will allow further characterization of hypercalciuric states (Stapleton et al., 1982). Measurement of serum concentrations of calcium, phosphorus, uric acid, and bicarbonate is indicated. Roentgenograms of the abdomen and excretory urography are required. Computerized axial tomography may be helpful in identifying small calculi. Medical therapy for urinary stones includes a generous fluid intake and specific pharmacologic agents designed to reduce urinary excretion of responsible crystalloids. Surgical intervention is warranted when stones obstruct the urinary tract.

ACUTE RENAL FAILURE

Any given patient whose urine output falls below 15 ml/kg/24 hr (400 ml/m^2/24 hr) is considered to be oliguric and must be managed in principle as one with acute renal failure.

Causes

Prerenal failure

The normal kidney responds appropriately by conserving water in the face of dehydration that is obvious and untreated or when the fluid loss has been underestimated. A high urine specific gravity will persist in either instance. When in doubt as to the prerenal origin of oliguria and azotemia, such as in dehydration, a useful diagnostic procedure is the administration of 10 to 15 ml/kg intravenous fluid over 1 to 2 hours, which should be followed promptly by an accelerated rate of urine flow. Azotemia and urine specific gravity will not decrease, however, until fluid replacement is adequate. Other causes of prerenal failure, more obvious to the clinician, are those with impaired circulation and hypotension when renal blood flow is reduced.

Urinary retention

The patient with acute urinary retention presents with a history of diminished urinary output and perhaps a history of no micturition for more than 24 hours. Azotemia is an unlikely finding in this situation. The physical examination should reveal a palpable abdominal mass rising out of the pelvis in the midline. Introduction of a catheter into the urinary bladder is not only diagnostic but also remedial in most cases. This clinical condition may arise as a result of an overdistended bladder from any cause such as dysuria, voluntary urine holding, priapism, balanitis, or drug therapy, but it is rarely associated with mechanical obstruction, as with a foreign body or tumor. When no cause for retention can be demonstrated, recurrence of this condition is unusual.

Obstructive uropathy

Obstructive uropathy as a cause of acute renal failure is less easily diagnosed or managed than are the previously mentioned causes. Obstruction at any point along the urinary tract will retard the rate of urine flow and on occasion may be the etiologic basis for oliguria; if allowed to continue over sufficient time, the obstruction will also result in azotemia. An intravenous pyelogram and occasionally a voiding cystourethrogram are all that are generally needed to localize the site of obstruction.

Renal parenchymal disease

Acute renal failure from renal parenchymal damage occurs with relative infrequency in the pediatric age group and may be transient, as in the child having acute glomerulonephritis of poststreptococcal etiology, with mild acute tubular or cortical necrosis, or in some cases of hemolytic-uremic syndrome. More severe renal parenchymal damage requires temporarily specialized care for peritoneal or extracorporeal dialysis. Acute but obviously progressive renal disease from which recovery of function is unlikely is seen most often in children as a rapidly progressive form of glomerulonephritis. Glomerulonephropathies are discussed in detail on pp. 535-544.

Treatment

Fluid and electrolytes. Whatever the cause, the treatment of acute renal failure is similar. Fluid balance is achieved by limiting intake from all sources to insensible loss (300 to 500 ml/m^2/24 hr), plus the volume of the patient's urinary output, including the rate of metabolic water formation and that amount given to ingest medications. Body weight, determined at the outset and at frequent intervals thereafter, serves as the most accurate indicator of fluid balance. Daily sodium intake is restricted to sodium loss, most conveniently measured as that excreted in the urine. A decrease in serum sodium level more likely represents the effect of water retention than of sodium loss. Because potassium excess, evidenced by a serum potassium level of greater than 6 mEq/ L and by characteristic changes in the electrocardiogram, represents imminent danger to cardiac function, particular attention should be paid to limiting potassium intake and to monitoring serum potassium levels. Specific therapy for hyperkalemia may be instituted in the form of a sodium-potassium cation exchange resin such as polysterene sodium sulfonate (Kayexalate) at 0.5 to 1.5 g/kg given either orally or as a retention enema.This treatment may be repeated as often as is necessary to maintain serum potassium levels within a safe range. Administration of sodium bicarbonate (1 to 2 mEq/kg) intravenously or hypertonic glucose and insulin (1 unit regular insulin/4 g carbohydrate) in amounts sufficient to move potassium into the cell without producing hypoglycemia may be effective. In the event these methods fail, dialysis must be introduced. Acidosis is treated with sodium bicarbonate in an amount sufficient to buffer hydrogen ion excess, but the quantity of sodium administered must not produce a sodium excess, which will further aggravate the overall management of the patient.

Diet. Dietary management should be directed toward limiting the daily intakes of protein, sodium, potassium, and water, whereas a high carbohydrate and fat intake is provided for caloric requirements to minimize breakdown of body protein stores during renal failure.

Peritoneal dialysis. Prolonged renal failure, with BUN levels in excess of 100 mg/dl, particularly when problems of hyperkalemia, volume expansion, or acidosis are constant, should be treated by dialysis.

Peritoneal dialysis can be performed successfully by most physicians, even those practicing outside large medical centers. The availability of appropriately sized, disposable catheters for pediatric use has greatly facilitated the ease with which this procedure is carried out. Commercially prepared dialysate can be safely introduced into the peritoneal cavity through a large-bore hypodermic needle, preferably of the plastic catheter type. Once the peritoneal cavity has been distended with a volume of dialysate sufficient to produce slight discomfort, but short of compromising pulmonary function, an appropriate-sized dialysis catheter can be inserted under local anesthesia into the abdomen in the midline halfway between the symphysis pubis and umbilicus. When there is fluid in the dependent portion of the peritoneal cavity, the bowel floats upward and out of the way of the catheter site. Besides rare intestinal perforation, the only other technical hazard associated with this procedure is damage to the bladder; therefore the bladder should be emptied before this procedure. Any discomfort resulting from fluid dissecting along the mesentery may be minimized by adding a small quantity of local anesthetic (1 ml of a 1% procaine hydrochloride solution) to the first volume of dialysate. Heparin (250 units/L) is frequently added to the dialysate during the first days of dialysis to prevent clotting and obstruction of the catheter.

Although dialysate preparations are available as potassium-free solutions, the osmolality of which is altered by varying the glucose content in 1.5%, 4%, and 7% concentrations, it is recommended that only 1.5% and 4% solutions be used and that the latter concentration be used only to remove fluid; otherwise the 1.5% solution is adequate for the removal of abnormal concentrations of electrolyte and metabolic waste products. Potassium is added to the dialysate in the final concentration desired, usually 2 mEq/L, depending on the need for removing potassium from the plasma. The volume of fluid for each exchange is 45 to 50 ml/kg for the child, with a maximally efficient exchange volume being 2000 ml in the adult-sized patient. Smaller volumes are used at the initiation of dialysis to avoid leakage of dialysate. A standard protocol recommends that 1-hour exchanges be done by allowing fluid to infuse over 10 minutes, to remain in the peritoneal cavity for 40 minutes, and to drain over a 10-minute period. The net fluid balance is tabulated as the difference between fluid infused and that recovered.

Effective therapy usually requires continuation of dialysis for about 48 hours, but in selected cases 72 hours may be necessary. Accurate weight monitoring becomes increasingly important in the smaller patient. Removal of large quantities of albumin in the ascitic fluid of the nephrotic patient may result in hypovolemia and shock; therefore albumin may be given intravenously from the beginning of the dialysis. Prolonged courses of peritoneal dialysis may significantly reduce the serum calcium level; therefore the addition of calcium to the regimen is recommended when a fall in the serum calcium level is noted. In addition to the treatment of renal failure, peritoneal dialysis may be used in the removal of certain poisons and abused drugs, in the rapid removal of fluid from a patient in congestive heart failure, and in the correction of gross electrolyte imbalances in life-threatening situations. The routine use of antibiotics during peritoneal dialysis is not recommended; however, aseptic techniques should be adhered to throughout the procedure, and cultures of both blood and peritoneal fluid should be done initially and at the termination of dialysis as a precautionary measure.

Recovery. During recovery after acute renal failure, the patient should be observed for a diuretic phase in which urine output of sodium and water may rapidly exceed the restricted sodium and fluid allowances. Appropriate advancement, as indicated, of both salt and water intakes is important to prevent hyponatremia, contraction of the vascular volume, hypotension, and diminished renal blood flow.

The duration of acute renal failure and the continued need for dialysis in each case is never predetermined but is best estimated by the nature and severity of the renal disease. As examples, a patient with acute glomerulonephritis of post-streptococcal cause may require only one course of dialysis before recovery is evident, and a patient with acute tubular necrosis may need several dialyses over the approximate 2-week period of renal failure characteristic of that condition. For the person with rapidly progressive glomerulonephritis whose recovery of renal function is unlikely, peritoneal dialysis is employed as a temporary measure while preparations are made for hemodialysis.

CHRONIC RENAL FAILURE

Chronic renal failure may be the end result of any clinical condition in which renal function has been permanently and irreversibly compromised to the point that the remaining nephrons are unable to support life. It is estimated that as many as 40 persons in 1 million population present annually as candidates for a program of maintenance hemodialysis or transplantation, and, of these, less than 10% are of pediatric age.

From birth to 6 years of age the major causes of chronic renal failure fall within the categories of developmental defects and bilateral Wilms tumor. In older children and adults, however, chronic glomerulonephritis accounts for the largest single group of renal failure patients. Obstructive uropathy that is present at birth, affects both kidneys, and continues undetected for months or even years will eventually result in renal failure. This is a preventable cause of renal failure and is discovered only when alert physicians carefully examine the newborn infant and the growing child.

Pathophysiology of uremia. Regardless of cause, the effect of chronic renal failure is similar in all patients. As nephrons are damaged and cease to function, residual nephrons assume increased functional demands, up to the limits of compensatory mechanisms, to maintain body fluid homeostasis.

Reduced renal function is reflected by blood accumulation of end products of protein metabolism, most often measured as urea nitrogen and creatinine, so that a loss of one half of total kidney function is reflected by a doubling of the serum level of both. Further reduction in glomerular filtration rate is represented by a corresponding rise in the blood levels of these waste products. The level of renal function below which untoward effects become manifest is about 30 ml/min/1.73 m^2, or 25% of normal total renal function. When the kidney is no longer able to excrete the hydrogen ion content of the daily diet, acidosis results.

The kidney serves not only as an excretory organ but also has several endocrine functions, one of which is to complete the synthesis of the most biologically active form of vitamin D. The kidney converts 25-hydroxycholecalciferol (25-HCC), synthesized by the liver from vitamin D_3, to 1,25-dihydroxycholecalciferol (1,25-diHCC), which increases the absorption of calcium from the gastrointestinal tract and the kidney and promotes the deposition of calcium in bone. Only a small quantity of the metabolically active 1,25-diHCC is required to effect this latter function, but the diseased kidney requires large quantities of 25-HCC and still greater amounts of vitamin D_3 to synthesize sufficient 1,25-diHCC to reverse the bone disease and hypocalcemia of uremia. Formerly, vitamin D–resistant rickets was the diagnosis given to the patient with renal disease whose rickets responded poorly, if at all, to large doses of vitamin D_3. Persistent hypocalcemia results in adenomatous hyperplasia of the parathyroid glands and secondary hyperparathyroidism. Once uremia is reversed by effective hemodialysis or corrected by renal transplantation, excessive parathyroid hormone produces hypercalcemia, which only subtotal parathyroidectomy corrects. Excess parathyroid hormone has been implicated as directly associated with, if not the actual cause of, many uremic mechanisms.

Another endocrine function of the kidney is to effect the production of erythropoietin, a hormone that stimulates the bone marrow to accelerate the maturation of erythrocytes and to influence stem cells to develop into erythroblasts. As the kidney fails, its production of erythropoietin does also, and a progressive anemia results so that the hemoglobin level expected in a patient with chronic renal failure is less than one half of normal. Because of the insidious onset of uremia, persons are usually well compensated at rest to these reduced levels of hemoglobin and rarely exhibit evidence of cardiac decompensation on the basis of anemia alone; however, exercise tolerance is limited in all patients.

There has been a misunderstanding of long duration in clinical medicine that prompts the automatic restriction of dietary sodium in patients with renal disease. Early in the course of renal failure residual nephrons offset the increase in the filtered sodium load per nephron by increasing their fractional excretion of sodium. The residual nephron excretes less than 1% of filtered sodium under normal circumstances, but in renal failure it may excrete more than 50% so that sodium balance is maintained. To limit sodium intake under these circumstances may become life threatening by producing volume contraction, hypotension, diminished perfusion of the remaining nephrons, and further reduction in renal function. Later in renal failure, however, when there is further reduction in the nephron population, sodium restriction is indicated to minimize volume expansion, which either produces or aggravates hypertension and its control.

On the other hand, the cation most importantly restricted early in renal failure is potassium. The kidney normally excretes most of the dietary potassium; therefore there is little daily variation in the level of serum potassium. An increase in serum potassium of as little as 2 mEq/L above normal can produce changes in the electrocardiogram and altered cardiac rhythm so that potassium metabolism is of paramount importance in an effort to prevent clinical emergencies and possible death.

As renal blood flow is decreased to the failing glomerulus, the response by the kidney is the same as that to any other process compromising blood flow to the kidney. It produces ischemic change, that is, an effort to increase renal blood flow by production of renin, which is converted in plasma to angiotensin I and with one passage through the lung to angiotensin II—the most potent vasoconstrictor agent thus far identified. Secondary hyperaldosteronism results from this pathophysiologic mechanism and further accentuates sodium and fluid retention and hypertension. Therefore at the expense of unwanted alteration in cardiovascular dynamics, the ischemic kidney reacts to increase its own perfusion, and the result is sustained hypertension. Fluid retention and volume expansion further accentuate the hypertension for as long as they are allowed to continue, rendering most conventional forms of antihypertensive therapy ineffective.

Prolonged renal failure is associated with changes in the central and peripheral nervous systems. Uremia may exert a primary effect on the central nervous system and result in psychologic disorders. Peripheral neuropathy in which nerve conduction time is prolonged is manifested by paresthesia, anesthesia, or sometimes pain; is a poorly understood phenomenon; and often is alleviated only by reversal of uremia with intensive dialysis or transplantation.

Clinical findings. The uremic patient may complain of headache, nausea, anorexia, weight loss, malaise, easy fatigability, muscle cramps, and occasional paresthesias. On inspection the patient may display pallor with a characteristic sallow appearance, edema, and malnutrition. The odor of urea or ammonia is detectable often on the child's skin and breath. Hypertension may be absent early in the course of renal failure but eventually becomes a problem in the management of every patient. Clinical evidence of hypocalcemia may be demonstrated. Uremic frost is encountered rarely and only then in the terminal patient in whom progressive renal failure has not been interrupted with some type of dialysis. Because most forms of disease that produce chronic renal failure occur over a period of months and even years, resulting in slowly progressive alterations in body function, patients are often unaware of the dramatic difference in general well-being compared to their previously healthy status.

Management. Chronic renal failure in the child often presents as growth failure when undetected or neglected until a near catastrophe occurs. The devastating toll taken by renal failure on the child who should be actively growing is at best difficult, if not impossible, to reverse. Therefore the goal of therapy for the child with renal failure is directed at early detection of correctable lesions, intervention with gradual dietary restrictions, correction of biochemical abnormalities as they develop, preparation for early hemodialysis, and consideration for renal transplantation earlier in the course of events than is the usual practice for adult-sized persons. Every effort is made to minimize the duration of the uremic process; that is, if acidosis is corrected and hypocalcemia prevented by calcium supplementation or vitamin D therapy, rickets and secondary hyperparathyroidism are less likely to develop.

Diet. The daily caloric intake, essential if growth is to occur in the uremic child, is rarely adequate. When offered food of limited protein content, the taste of which is unenhanced by the virtual elimination of its sodium and potassium content, it becomes an almost impossible task to supply calories sufficient for growth. Dietary protein should be restricted to 1 to 2 g/kg/24 hr and should be of high biologic value, that is, containing mostly essential amino acids, such as eggs, milk, fish, fowl, and veal. Vegetables provide large quantities of nonessential protein, which increase the excretory load of the impaired kidney. The bottle-fed infant can be given a formula with reduced protein and electrolyte content (PM60-40, S-M-A S-26). The balance of caloric intake is offered as carbohydrate and fat within the limits of electrolyte restriction. Any additional calories may be offered as high caloric supplements that are low in volume and contain nearly negligible amounts of sodium and potassium (Cal-Power, Hycal). Products are similarly available for preparation of high caloric desserts and baked goods (Controlyte and resource baking mix).

Fluids and electrolytes. Sodium, both from dietary allowances and alkali therapy, should be restricted on the basis of individual need but not to less than 1 mEq/kg/24 hr. When the serum potassium level nears 6 mEq/L, potassium intake should be limited to 1 mEq/kg/24 hr. The management of hyperkalemia is described on p. 553. Hypokalemia should be prevented in patients with potassium-wasting disease, in those with a history of cardiac decompensation who are now receiving digitalis therapy, and in those receiving diuretics.

For each 100 g protein that is ingested, 70 mEq hydrogen ion must be excreted or buffered. To prevent chronic acidosis and its deleterious effect on growth, alkali (in the form of sodium bicarbonate or combinations of sodium and potassium citrate) is provided in quantities sufficient to maintain clinical acid-base determinations within the normal range.

Daily fluid allowances are calculated on the basis of the insensible water loss (300 to 500 ml/m^2/24 hr), plus any volume of urinary output. Early in the course of renal failure large volumes of urine may not necessitate fluid restriction, but as renal failure progresses, urine output is reduced and daily intake must be decreased proportionally.

Calcium and phosphorus. Hypocalcemia and hyperphosphatemia are common features of untreated chronic renal failure, and the approach to correction is multifaceted. The guiding principle of treatment is for the physician to note that metastatic calcification is more likely to occur when the product of serum concentrations of calcium and phosphorus is greater than 60 mg/dl. Hypocalcemic tetany may not be clinically demonstrable in that acidosis increases the ionized fraction of reduced total serum calcium and is therefore protective to some extent. Correction of the acidosis increases protein binding of calcium, thereby decreasing the ionized fraction of serum calcium; thus tetany may result from aggressive management. Too-rapid restoration of the serum calcium level toward normal will increase the calcium-phosphorus product and may cause calcium deposition in soft tissues. The careful, stepwise correction of this biochemical abnormaility is mandatory and should be directed first toward reducing the serum phosphorus level. This is accomplished best by decreasing the gastrointestinal absorption of phosphate by phosphate binding with an aluminum hydroxide gel, beginning with 100 mg/kg/24 hr in divided doses taken with meals. It is important to remember that some antacid preparations contain magnesium, the accumulation of which can complicate the management of renal failure; therefore only preparations of aluminum hydroxide or trisilicate should be prescribed. Simultaneously with serum phosphate reduction, serum calcium should be increased with supplemental calcium of 10 to 20 mg/kg/24 hr. (Calcium lactate provides 130 mg/g calcium.) One should realize, however, that in the absence of adequate 1,25-dihydroxyvitamin D_3, necessary for intestinal absorption of calcium and phosphate, no amount of calcium supplementation will restore calcium to normal.

Once the serum calcium level is within a clinically safe range, the physician can begin to correct the acidosis with less fear of producing tetany. With serum phosphate reduced within the normal range, vitamin D in increasing doses may be used to enhance the treatment of hypocalcemia by increasing the absorption of calcium through the gastrointestinal tract or to treat renal osteodystrophy. Either 1,25 dihydroxyvitamin-D_3 (14 $\pm$ 10 nanogram/kg/day) or dihydrotachysterol (15 microgram/kg/day) as a single oral dose can be used to control both hypocalcemia and the bone disease of renal failure. Dosage can be increased by 50% at monthly intervals until stable serum concentrations of calcium, phosphorus, parathyroid hormone, and alkaline phosphatase are achieved.

Anemia. Anemia associated with renal failure is related to the decreased production of erythropoietin by the diseased kidney, whereas vitamin and mineral deficiencies are rarely demonstrated. Treatment of the anemia is directed toward improving nutrition, assuring intake of minimal daily vitamin requirements and folic acid, and replacing iron losses resulting from blood loss for laboratory purposes and from hemodialysis. Androgen therapy, given to adult patients, is not considered for the child in whom epiphyseal closure would preclude all hope of continued growth. In some hemodialysis centers the periodic infusion of iron intravenously is advocated as a successful method of maintaining the hematocrit value, even in the patient in whom iron stores appear adequate. The most important aspect of management of anemia associated with chronic renal failure is the minimizing of blood loss, thus reducing the need for blood transfusion; transfusion further suppresses bone marrow activity, risks transmission of hepatitis virus, and sensitizes the patient to common blood antigens, thereby reducing the likelihood of success for a future renal transplant. Blood transfusions should be limited to only those patients whose anemia is symptomatic; for example, one patient may tolerate a hematocrit of 10% to 12% although another becomes symptomatic at 18%. The definitive cure for renal failure–induced anemia is a successful renal transplant because erythropoietin production in the transplanted kidney stimulates the bone marrow to restore the circulating levels of hemoglobin to normal within a few weeks.

Hypertension. The invariable result of chronic renal failure from any etiology is hypertension, and it may be associated with increased renin secretion, secondary hyperaldosteronism, or volume expansion. In either case, volume expansion must be minimized if blood pressure control is to be satisfactory. The physician begins with antihypertensive measures that reduce volume expansion, initially by sodium and fluid restriction and later by diuretic therapy. Hydrochlorothiazide (1 to 2 mg/kg/24 hr) or furosemide (1 to 2 mg/kg/dose at 6 hourly intervals) is frequently used in this regard. When volume expansion has been reduced and hypertension persists, a single antihypertensive agent is introduced and increased to a maximal tolerated safe dose before the addition of another drug. Reserpine, hydralazine, and diazoxide are excellent agents for the inpatient management of acute hypertensive disease, but more consistent control of hypertensive disease is better accomplished with other agents such as alpha-methyldopa (10 mg/kg/24 hr) given in three divided doses, guanethidine (0.2 mg/kg/24 hr) given once daily and increased every 3 to 5 days until the desired effect is achieved or undesirable side effects are realized, or propranolol (1 to 2 mg/kg/24 hr) given in divided doses and increased at 3- to 5-day intervals.

Captopril, a competitive inhibitor of angiotensin-converting enzyme, has been used in a limited number of children with secondary hypertension and varying degrees of renal insufficiency. It should be used only if other measures for controlling blood pressure have not been effective. The usual adult dosage range is 25 to 150 mg three times daily.

Minoxidil, an extremely potent vasodilator, is usually reserved for severe hypertension unresponsive to maximal doses of commonly used antihypertensive agents. The troublesome side effect of increased facial and body hair in children is a major deterrent to its use. The recommended dosage is 0.2 to 2.0 mg/kg/day. It should be administered in conjunction with a diuretic and propanolol.

When medical regimens have failed to control hypertension adequately, bilateral nephrectomy is done, and this is followed by maintenance hemodialysis, after which hypertension becomes a volume-related phenomenon.

Dialysis. Chronic maintenance hemodialysis has been designed for and made available to adult-sized persons (greater than 40 kg body weight). However, at the present time, dialyzers are available to provide the same advantage to infants and children. In a few centers, designed primarily for children, modified equipment and trained personnel provide hemodialysis even to newborn infants. Because the technique of hemodialysis is not within the scope of this book, suffice it to say that this method of treatment is at best an imperfect substitute for the human kidney. Because children receiving maintenance hemodialysis do not grow well, continue to have the problems associated with chronic renal failure, must adhere strictly to dietary regimens, and take increasing quantities of medications, the only indication at the present time for chronic hemodialysis in children is for those considered candidates for renal transplantation.

A recent advance in chronic dialysis therapy in children has been the introduction of chronic peritoneal dialysis. Dialysis is accomplished by the placement of a permanent subcutaneous silastic dialysis catheter. Three chronic peritoneal dialysis regimens have been used. Intermittent peritoneal dialysis (IPD) is performed 3 or 4 nights a week for 14 to 16 hours using an automated dialysis delivery system. Chronic ambulatory peritoneal dialysis (CAPD) is currently the most popular method. CAPD requires four daily fluid exchanges and does not require a machine. A combination of IPD and CAPD is called continuous cycling peritoneal dialysis (CCPD), in which children have 4 to 8 automated cycles at night and a single long exchange during the day. The advantages of peritoneal dialysis over hemodialysis include applicability to small children, less pain, availability of home dialysis, and potentially better rehabilitation to a more normal life-style. Complications of this technique include a very significant incidence of peritonitis and catheter obstruction. When children have had multiple abdominal operations, chronic peritoneal dialysis may not be possible.

Transplantation. Renal allograft survival statistics improve with each year of accumulated experience. Although methods of determining tissue compatibility are inadequately defined and the basis for tissue rejection under seemingly ideal circumstances is poorly understood, satisfactory results have made this procedure routine in most large medical centers. Mortality statistics indicate that transplant-associated deaths are most often the result of infection with unusual organisms, such as fungi and viruses, which causes problems in the immunosuppressed patient and only rarely in the normal population. A 5-year allograft survival of more than 80% for related donor and of 50% in cadaver transplants is reported by several large tansplant centers. The transplant recipient must take prednisone and either azathioprine or cyclophosphamide to prevent rejection of the graft. Long-term steroid therapy, even in small daily quantities, will interfere with the linear growth of the child; therefore alternate-day steroid therapy is advocated by some. When a transplant fails, the patient returns to maintenance hemodialysis and continues to be a candidate for a future transplantation.

ARTERIAL HYPERTENSION

Systemic arterial hypertension is an unusual occurrence during childhood. Although hypertensive cardiovascular disease is reported to affect up to 20% of the adult population, it is estimated to occur in only 1% or 2% of children. However, it may be that hypertension in children has not been seen more often because it is not looked for during infancy or childhood because hypertension is ascribed to adult criteria of blood pressure greater than 140/90 mmHg, rather than compared to the upper limits (+2 SD) above the normal for age.

Moreover, the causes of hypertension follow a different pattern of distribution between the groups in that 90% of adults have essential hypertension, whereas 4 out of 5 children have a demonstrable cause for their hypertension. Again, this may represent a patient population that has been highly selected, since most patients' hypertension was severe; the asymptomatic patients with essential hypertension remained undetected. The categories of disease most commonly associated with hypertension in children are reflux nephropathy with segmental cortical atrophy, renal parenchymal disease, renal vascular disease, renal tumor, coarctation of the aorta, central nervous system tumor, and endocrine disorders including pheochromocytoma, hyperthyroidism, certain forms of congenital adrenal hyperplasia, primary hyperaldosteronism, and Cushing syndrome. Because hypertension is a secondary effect of several specific conditions described elsewhere in this book, only those causes of hypertension that originate with the kidney will be discussed.

Systemic blood pressure is the product of interplay of cardiac output, blood volume, and peripheral vascular resistance; alteration of one or more of these factors will result in a change in blood pressure. Therefore altered neurohumoral stimulation, change in physical dynamics of the cardiovascular system, or both may produce hypertension. As an example, the augmented secretion of catecholamines produces peripheral vasoconstriction and tachycardia, and the result is a rise in blood pressure.

Most long-range studies of hypertension are reported from the adult population, in whom it is widely accepted that 140/90 mmHg is the upper limit of normal systemic arterial pressure and increases above that level indicate hypertension. Normal blood pressure for a newborn infant is 75/40 mmHg, and with age there is a gradual increase in arterial pressure. Levels of pressure within the range of the adult normal are not recorded until some time during adolescence.

The Report of the Task Force on Blood Pressure Control in Children (1977) includes standards for children's blood pressure at various ages, as depicted in Fig. 21-7.

The distribution of blood pressure is displayed by selected percentiles. That is, the position of an individual child's blood pressure is plotted against those of a large group of children. For example, if a 6-year-old boy had a blood pressure of 110 mm Hg systolic and 78 mm Hg diastolic, the chart indicates that his levels are both at the 90th percentile. The boy, compared to his peers, has pressure levels higher than 90% of the population. Because it does not follow that a single high pressure is an abnormal finding, the charts are not intended for use in assessment of an individual child's blood pressure at a single point in time but rather for the plotting of pressures during growth and maturation. Blood pressure values, unlike height and weight in children, will not precisely follow percentile tracks. There is considerable variation in most children's pressures. These charts provide a mechanism for a child's pressure to be recorded so that a pattern over a period of time may be observed.

Blood pressure measurements, like those of weight and height, should be obtained and plotted at least once yearly. Because a single elevated measurement (i.e., greater than the 95th percentile) in an apparently healthy child does not necessarily reflect disease, it is necessary to repeat these measurements over time to obtain a trend.

Physical examination. The method of blood pressure recording in the infant and child is of paramount importance. Before the label of hypertension is attached to any child, the examiner

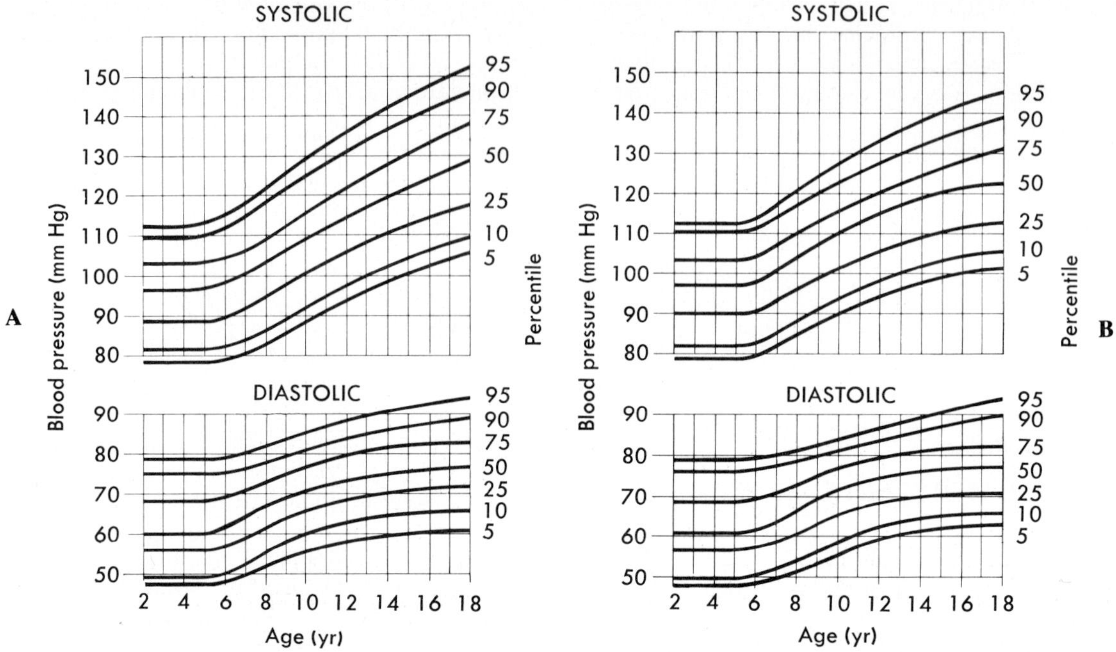

Fig. 21-7 A, Percentiles of blood pressure measurement in boys (right arm, seated). **B,** Percentiles of blood pressure measurement in girls (right arm, seated). (From Report of the Task Force on Blood Pressure Control in Children [prepared by the National Heart, Lung, and Blood Institute], Pediatrics **59**(5), Part 2, May, 1977.)

should ensure that blood pressure has been recorded under optimal conditions, that is, with the patient at rest in both the supine and upright positions and with a pressure cuff that ideally covers two thirds of the arm (measured in length from acromioclavicular junction to elbow), and the bladder of which does not encircle the arm more than once. To complete the examination of a child with suspected hypertension, the physician should compare the blood pressure recorded in the lower extremities to that measured in the upper extremities to detect coarctation of the aorta, should listen over the abdomen and flank for a vascular bruit that may be associated with stenosis or partial occlusion of a renal artery, and should examine the sediment of a freshly voided urine specimen, an abnormality of which would indicate renal parenchymal disease.

The examination of the ocular fundus rarely produces abnormal findings in the hypertensive child, but, when present, the retinal changes are similar to, and are recorded as, those noted in the hypertensive adult. Because the anterior fontanel may remain open throughout infancy and the cranial sutures are easily sprung in the child under the stress of increased intracranial pressure, papilledema is an unlikely finding in hypertensive children.

Laboratory evaluation. A routine urinalysis should be used as a screening test for all hypertensive patients. The finding of hematuria or proteinuria is suggestive of renal parenchymal disease, such as acute glomerulonephritis or any form of chronic glomerular or interstitial nephropathy, whether of primary renal origin or associated with systemic disease—diabetic nephrosclerosis and lupus erythematosus. The serum concentrations of urea nitrogen and of creatinine reflect any serious reduction in renal function, whereas serum electrolytes and carbon dioxide concentration may be abnormal in renal function impairment or in adrenocortical endocrinopathies. A 24-hour urine collection for the quantitative determination of vanillylmandelic acid (VMA) catecholamines aids in establishing the diagnosis of pheochromocytoma.

Plasma levels of aldosterone, corticosterone,

and desoxycorticosterone may be helpful in the diagnosis of an aldosterone-secreting adenoma, bilateral nodular adrenal hyperplasia, glucocorticoid-responsive hyperaldosteronism, or congenital deficiencies of adrenal 11 β or 17 α hydroxylase. A low peripheral venous renin activity may suggest the diagnosis of excessive mineralocorticoid secretion as a cause of hypertension. An increased peripheral venous renin activity may be present in renovascular hypertension or in some renal parenchymal diseases.

Rapid-sequence intravenous pyelogram, voiding cystourethrogram, renal ultrasound, and radionuclide renogram are important noninvasive techniques that may demonstrate or suggest the diagnosis of renovascular hypertension, polycystic renal disease, developmental renal defects, segmental renal atrophy, or obstructive uropathy.

If the investigation up to this point has failed to reveal any abnormality, the diagnostic effort must center on establishing the presence of a vascular lesion that produces relative ischemia to the renal parenchyma and effects the release of renin from juxtaglomerular cells. This pathophysiologic mechanism may result from fibromuscular dysplasia, congenital stenosis, aneurysm, thrombus or extrinsic compression of the renal artery, and intrinsic reduction of blood flow secondary to an atherosclerotic plaque or to an arteriovenous fistula. Assays of plasma renin activity and plasma aldosterone concentration are excellent indicators, when increased, for a renovascular cause of the hypertension, but they do not differentiate between renal ischemia and the rare tumor of the juxtaglomerular cells, and both tests must be interpreted in light of documented sodium intake—best measured in a 24-hour urine collection. The only definitive method of isolating an arterial lesion or excluding renovascular hypertension is selective arteriography and measurement of renin from both renal veins. The affected kidney should evidence an increase in renin activity at least 1½ times over the normal. Renal biopsy is necessary for the definitive diagnosis of renal parenchymal disease and may either precede or be done concomitantly with the arteriographic studies.

Treatment. It is generally accepted from adult studies that morbidity from hypertension (diastolic blood pressure greater than 105 mmHg) can be reduced from 55% to 18% in treated adult patients over a 5-year period of time. Experimental studies in spontaneously hypertensive rats also show that cardiovascular and renal damage can be prevented by treating these animals during gestation and after delivery. The application of these studies to children needs further study. A reduction of blood pressure to a level that is within two standard deviations of the mean for age for young children and below 90 mmHg for adolescents is a reasonable therapeutic goal of antihypertensive therapy in children.

Borderline or mild hypertension may be adequately managed by adherence to a diet restricted in salt and possibly by caloric restriction in obese children. Dietary salt restriction should also be an integral part of the management of all other levels of hypertension in children.

Chronic hypertension is generally managed by a "stepped-care" approach starting with low doses of a particular drug and increasing the dosage until blood pressure is controlled, side effects are unacceptable, or maximal dosages have been achieved. A thiazide diuretic (hydrochlorothiazide) in an oral dose of 1 to 2 mg/kg/day is the initial drug of choice. Volume depletion and hypokalemia are the two major side effects to be prevented. Beta blockers such as propanolol (1 to 10 mg/kg/day) or methyldopa (10 to 40 mg/kg/day) can be added next if adequate blood pressure control is not achieved by diuretics alone. A vasodilator drug such as hydralazine (1 to 5 mg/kg/day) should then be added to the previously established doses of propanolol and hydrochlorothiazide if blood pressure remains elevated. In refractory cases, minoxidil, a potent vasodilator (dosage 0.2 to 2 mg/kg/day), or captopril, a competitive inhibitor of angiotensin-converting enzyme (adult dosage 25 to 150 mg three times daily) that has been used in a limited number of children, may be tried. Infrequently drugs such as guanethidine (0.2 mg/kg/day), a postganglionic sympathetic blocking agent, clonidine (not approved for use in children), or prazosin (pediatric dosage not firmly established) may be tried if previously mentioned drugs are ineffective.

Acute hypertensive emergencies are best managed with either hydralazine intravenously or intramuscularly (0.1 to 0.2 mg/kg every 4 to 6 hr), diazoxide (5 mg/kg intravenous rapidly), or sodium nitroprusside (intravenous drip 0.5 to 8.0 μg—kg—min; concentration of 5 μg/ml). These aggressive measures are usually reserved for diastolic levels of blood pressure of 115 to 130 mmHg or the child who is convulsing or has convulsed secondary to hypertensive encephalopathy. As soon as the patient's condition permits, oral antihypertensive medications should be instituted. In patients who are acutely volume expanded, such as in acute poststreptococcal glomerulonephritis, the addition of a potent diuretic such as furosemide (1 to 2 mg/kg/dose) is recommended.

URINARY TRACT INFECTIONS

(see also p. 914 to 918)

Strictly speaking, bacterial infection of the bladder is termed *cystitis,* whereas infection of the substance of the kidney is termed *pyelonephritis.* It is usually difficult to localize the infection specifically to the bladder or to the kidney. When specific differences in relation to infection of either bladder or kidney need emphasis, these will be pointed out. Otherwise, urinary tract infection (UTI) will be used to identify either or both conditions. UTI should not be diagnosed unless significant numbers of bacteria are demonstrated in a properly collected urine specimen.

Incidence. Studies of healthy newborns indicate that less than 1% have UTI, that males are predominantly affected, and that underlying congenital malformations are rare.

In preschool children UTI occurs more often in girls than boys, affecting as many as 2% of girls and 0.5% of boys. In this age group more than 80% of patients with UTI will have associated congenital malformations that may lead to pyelonephritis, scar formation in the affected kidney, and growth retardation.

Carefully performed screening studies of schoolchildren have demonstrated bacteriuria in 1.2% of girls and 0.03% of boys. Approximately one third of the girls had some symptom referable to the urinary tract when bacteriuria was found.

Etiology. Enteric bacteria are responsible for most urinary tract infections. These include *Escherichia coli, Aerobacter aerogenes, Bacillus proteus, Pseudomonas aeruginosa,* and enterococci. About three fourths of initial infections are caused by *E. coli,* and less than 10% of infections are caused by gram-positive cocci.

Infecting organisms are usually found in pure culture. A mixed bacterial flora from the urinary tract most often results from contamination through improper collection or handling of the urine specimen. Mixed infections may be seen in patients with chronic or complicated infections.

Pathogenesis. The urinary tract is normally sterile above the urethrovesical junction. Bacteria generally reach the urinary tract by ascending from below. Blood-borne infections do occur, as in the neonate with sepsis or in patients with gram-positive infections caused by staphylococci or enterococci.

Bacteria that may enter the bladder are eliminated through normal voiding and the effect of dilution. With bladder outlet obstruction or bladder dysfunction, the normal clearing mechanism of bacteria is inadequate. Bacteria may then multiply and cause UTI. As infection involves the lower ureter, ureteral peristalsis may be affected, and the normally competent ureterovesical junction may become incompetent, allowing reflux of infected bladder urine into the ureters and thus to the renal pelvis. Some patients have congenitally incompetent ureterovesical junctions from abnormal ureteral insertion, abnormal ureteral tunneling into the bladder, or abnormally large ureteral orifices. Other factors that may cause obstruction and contribute to infection are calculi of the urinary tract and abnormal renal vasculature.

Clinical conditions associated with an increased incidence of UTI are hypertension, hypokalemia, diabetes, and cirrhosis of the liver.

Clinical manifestations. Symptoms and signs of acute pyelonephritis vary according to the age of the child. Infants present with fever, anorexia, vomiting, diarrhea, and jaundice. Older children usually present with high temperature, chills, malaise, and abdominal or flank pain.

Signs of progressive renal insufficiency combined with signs of chronic infection define the child who has chronic pyelonephritis. When chronic pyelonephritis is limited to one kidney, symptoms of recurrent unilateral infection without signs of renal insufficiency are evident.

Lower urinary tract infection usually causes few systemic signs except for fever. Urinary frequency, dysuria, enuresis, suprapubic pain, hesitancy, and abnormal urinary odor are also frequently seen.

Poor weight gain or growth retardation in a child should alert the clinician to consider an asymptomatic UTI.

Diagnosis. Diagnosis of UTI may be suspected by the preceding clinical signs and symptoms but requires proof through urine culture and quantitative colony count. Clean-voided, midstream urine specimens obtained from toilet-trained children contain fewer than 10^3 bacteria/ml urine. Colony counts greater than 10^5 are indicative of UTI, especially if only one organism is recovered. Counts between 10^3 and 10^5 are equivocal and must be repeated. In nontoilet-trained children and infants suprapubic aspiration of urine for culture may be necessary. Urine obtained in this manner should be sterile.

Thorough radiographic investigation is recommended in all patients with UTI regardless of their sex. Urologic investigation should be considered in any patient with reflux or obstructive uropathy. The myth of distal urethral stenosis in girls has been demonstrated to be just that—a myth—and should never be the only justification for subjecting a child to the risks of general anesthesia and instrumentation of the urinary tract. Intravenous pyelography may be performed within a week of diagnosis, and the voiding cystogram should be delayed until the urine is sterile.

Treatment. Either oral sulfonamide or ampicillin is generally used in the treatment of acute UTI while awaiting sensitivity studies from the initial urine culture. Subsequent treatment is based on individual patient response and the results of antibiotic sensitivity tests. From 10 to 14 days of treatment are usually sufficient to eradicate the bacteriuria of an initial UTI. The urine will become sterile several days after treatment is started, but clinical improvement may be noted within 24 hours. A repeat urine culture 5 to 7 days after treatment is discontinued is essential to confirm therapeutic success. Subsequently, monthly urine cultures for 3 months, then every 3 months for the balance of a year and twice during the second year after a UTI are necessary to document a cure of the infection and to detect recurrences. Recurrences are more common in the first 2 years after a UTI. Controversy exists in determining the duration of treatment of the child with a recurrent or chronic UTI. Periods of treatment of up to 6 months have been suggested by some investigators. The only drugs proved to be effective in chronic maintenance of a sterile urine are nitrofurantoin (Furadantin) and trimethoprim-sulfamethoxazole.

When definite anatomic abnormalities are demonstrated on intravenous pyelogram or voiding cystourethrogram, urologic consultation may be necessary. The most controversial issue at hand is the management of the patient with vesicoureteral reflux. There is sufficient evidence to support reflux as a pathogenetic mechanism in renal scar formation. These reflux-associated scars may not be manifested radiographically for 5 to 10 years after the time of reflux. Often ureteral reflux will be present during the initial radiographic evaluation, only to disappear subsequent to successful medical therapy of the UTI. It is not known what degree or duration of reflux is required to produce renal scar formation. If scarring does occur, then many, if not all, patients will develop hypertension and after many years without evidence of active infection may present with hypertensive encephalopathy. The child in whom reflux was ever demonstrated should be followed up, therefore, not only with urine cultures but also with serial blood pressure determinations. When the infection does not respond to adequate antibiotic therapy, when the ureter progressively dilates, or when diminishing renal parenchyma is demonstrated, surgical intervention would seem to be appropriate. This approach should in no way delay the surgical correction of obvious obstructive uropathy.

Thus the accepted management of UTI in children begins with the demonstration of significant bacteriuria, follows with appropriate antibiotic treatment and subsequent radiographic investigation of the urinary tract, and includes the correction of obstructive uropathy and adequate long-term follow-up to document cure or to detect a recurrence.

Shane Roy, III
F. Bruder Stapleton

REFERENCES

Poststreptococcal glomerulonephritis

Report of the Task Force on Blood Pressure Control in Children, Pediatrics **59**(supp.):797, 1977.

Roy, S., III, et al.: Prognosis of acute poststreptococcal glomerulonephritis in childhood: prospective study and review of the literature, Adv. Pediatr. **23**:35, 1976.

Roy, S., III, et al.: Second attacks of acute glomerulonephritis, J. Pediatr. **75**:758, 1969.

Idiopathic nephrotic syndrome

Grupe, W.E., et al.: Chlorambucil treatment of frequently relapsing nephrotic syndrome, N. Engl. J. Med. **295:**746, 1976.

Report of the International Study of Kidney Disease in Children: Nephrotic syndrome in children: prediction of histopathology from clinical and laboratory characteristics at time of diagnosis, Kidney Int. **13:**159, 1978.

SELECTED READINGS

Arant, B.S., Jr.: Developmental patterns of renal functional maturation compared in the human neonate, J. Pediatr. **92:**705, 1978.

Nash, M.A., et al.: Renal tubular acidosis in infants and children, J. Pediatr. **80:**738, 1972.

Rodriquez-Soriano, J., et al.: Natural history of primary distal renal tubular acidosis treated since infancy, J. Pediatr. **101:**669, 1982.

Roy, S., III, et al.: Hematuria preceding renal calculus formation in children with hypercalciuria, J. Pediatr. **99:**712, 1981.

Southwest Pediatric Nephrology Study Group: A multicenter study of IgA nephropathy in children, Kidney International **22:**643, 1982.

Stapleton, F.B., et al.: Urinary excretion of calcium following an oral calcium loading test in healthy children, Pediatrics **69:**594, 1982.

Stapleton, F.B., et al.: Hypercalciuria in children with urolithiasis, Amer. J. Dis. Child. **136:**675, 1982.

22 Pediatric Endocrinology

Endocrine disturbances

INTERRELATIONSHIP OF THE HYPOTHALAMUS, ANTERIOR PITUITARY, AND TARGET GLANDS

As a result of their influence on metabolic processes within the cell, hormones control the functions of cells and organs. Endocrine disturbances may therefore be regarded as disturbances in metabolism. Rather than initiating new processes, hormones in increasing or decreasing amounts enhance or diminish the efficiency of metabolic processes.

The glands of internal secretion may be divided into two groups: (1) the anterior pituitary and its target glands, which it controls through tropic hormones (the target glands include the thyroid, adrenal cortex, and gonads); and (2) the posterior pituitary, parathyroid, adrenal medulla, and islet cells of the pancreas.

The anterior pituitary is regarded as the master gland and except for growth hormone and melanocyte-stimulating hormone (MSH) mediates its influence on the target glands by secretion of tropic hormones. Growth hormone and MSH act directly on peripheral body cells. The anterior pituitary is under the regulatory influence of circulating hormones of the target glands and the hypothalamus through neural mechanisms. Indeed, the hypothalamus may be regarded as an organ of internal (hormonal) secretion, which exerts a powerful regulatory influence on anterior pituitary hormones by secreting "tropic-releasing factors" that are transported to the anterior pituitary gland by way of the hypophyseal venous portal system. Evidence indicates that there are releasing factors for the anterior pituitary hormones. In addition, factors have been isolated from the hypothalamus that inhibit the release of anterior pituitary hormones. There are both hypothalamic-stimulating and hypothalamic-inhibiting factors for growth hormone, prolactin, and melanocyte-stimulating hormone. So far, only stimulating factors for adrenocorticotropin, follicle-stimulating hormone (FSH), luteinizing hormone (LH), and thyroid-stimulating hormone (TSH) have been identified.

The secretion of tropic hormones by the pituitary gland is related to the level of circulating hormones of the target glands in a reciprocal manner. Thus thyroxin and hydrocortisone (endogenous or exogenous) suppress TSH and adrenocorticotropic hormone (ACTH), respectively. Conversely, when there is decreased secretion of hormone by the target gland, the pituitary secretes increased amounts of the corresponding tropic hormone. Another but somewhat more complicated example of the reciprocal relationship of two tropic hormones—FSH and LH—of the pituitary gland and its target organ is exemplified in ovarian secretion of estrogen and progesterone. An increase in circulating estrogen levels suppresses the secretion of FSH, with subsequent suppression of estrogen output by the ovary and termination of the proliferative phase of the menstrual cycle. The anterior pituitary gland, however, as a result of decreases in FSH and low progesterone level, elaborates increased amounts of LH; this stimulates corpus luteum formation and production of progesterone in increasing quantities, with the formation of the secretory endometrium, and thus completes a cycle that normally repeats itself every 4 weeks.

The interrelationship of these glands and their secretions is illustrated in Fig. 22-1.

According to Wilkins (1965):

> Alteration in one of the hormones affecting the body may be caused by a disorder arising from any of these centers of control: (1) the brain centers from which impulses pass to the pituitary, (2) the anterior pituitary itself, or (3) the target organs—thyroid, adrenal, or gonad. In diagnosis it

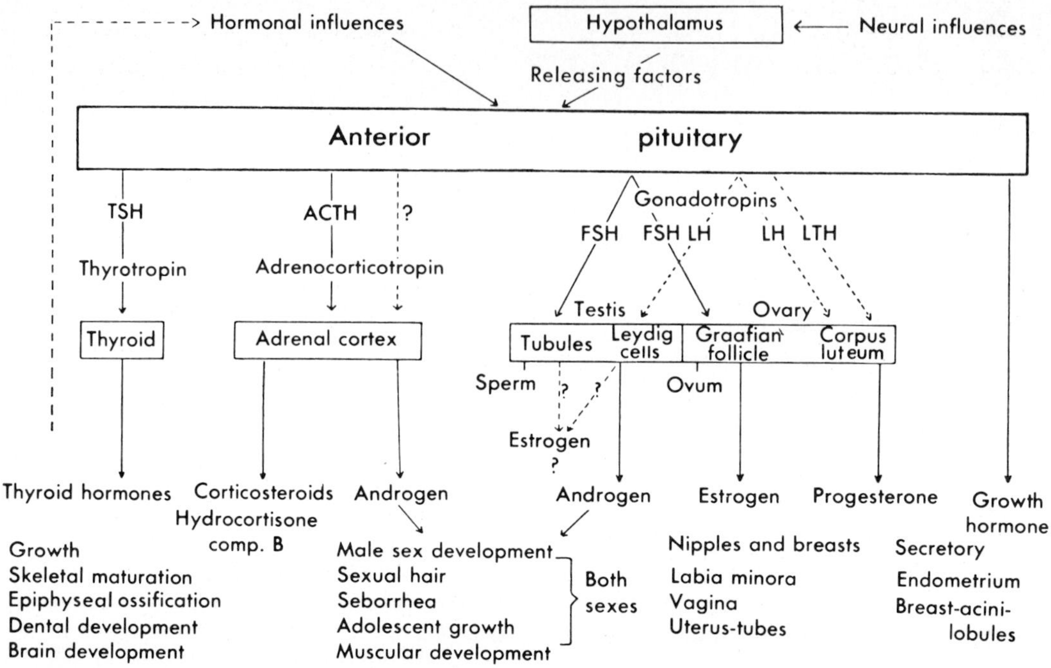

Fig. 22-1. Relations of principal endocrine glands that influence somatic and sexual growth and development. Note that the hormones that exert effects on the body may be increased or decreased by a disorder in (1) the brain, (2) the anterior pituitary, or (3) one of the target glands—thyroid, adrenal, or gonad. (From Wilkins, L., with editorial assistance by Blizzard, R.M., and Migeon, C.: Diagnosis and treatment of endocrine disorders in childhood and adolescence, ed. 3, Springfield, Ill., 1965, Charles C Thomas, Publisher.)

should always be remembered that the primary lesion which gives rise to particular hormonal disturbance may be in any of these levels of control. For example, sexual precocity in a male may be due to a tumor of the testis or adrenal, to premature activity of the pituitary, or to a lesion of the hypothalamus. Sexual infantilism in a female may be due to absence of the ovaries, to pituitary deficiency, or to a hypothalamic lesion.

RELATIONSHIP OF ENDOCRINE GLANDS TO SOMATIC AND SEXUAL GROWTH AND DEVELOPMENT

It is well recognized that endocrine and metabolic disturbances may exert a profound influence on growth and development, but it must be remembered that hormonal and metabolic disorders account for a relatively small proportion of all deviations of sexual and somatic growth and development. The majority of deviations are within the limits of normal variations. To treat an apparent disturbance with potent and expensive agents not only interferes with normal maturation and secretion of glands of internal secretion but also fosters anxiety in the child and parents.

To relate endocrine and metabolic disturbances to aberrations in growth and development, it is essential to become familiar with variations in normal growth and development, to obtain a complete medical and family history, to possess knowledge of the influence of excessive and deficient secretion of the various endocrine and exocrine glands, and to obtain in most instances confirmatory laboratory evidence. Despite a good medical workup, it is not always possible to make a positive diagnosis; limited therapeutic trial and specific hormonal substitution with a subjective evaluation are in order. Needless to say, the age at which aberrations of glandular activity exert their influence is of utmost importance when relating endocrine and metabolic function to growth and development.

Hormones that have direct or indirect influence on growth and development include those secreted by the following glands: (1) anterior pituitary, (2) thyroid, (3) adrenal cortex, (4) gonads, and (5) those glands primarily concerned with metabolism (pancreas, parathyroid, and posterior pituitary). The interrelationships of the endocrine glands that are most involved in somatic and sexual growth and development are illustrated in Fig. 22-1.

Linear or skeletal growth—an interplay of all catabolic and anabolic mechanisms—is related to a host of factors and ceases as a result of fusion of the epiphyses, which normally occurs at adolescence. In the female and the male, closure of the epiphyses usually occurs by age 14 and 16, respectively.

Growth hormone, androgens, and *thyroid hormone* are directly responsible for normal somatic growth and development. Androgens are responsible for the adolescent growth spurt in both boys and girls. Thyroid hormone is essential throughout the entire growing period. *Adrenal glucocorticoids* in pharmacologic amounts (endogenous or exogenous) inhibit growth.

The secretion of gonadotropins and ACTH by the anterior pituitary results in stimulation of the target glands (gonads and adrenals) with resultant development of secondary sexual characteristics (Fig. 22-1).

INTRACRANIAL LESIONS CAUSING ENDOCRINE DISORDERS

A variety of endocrinologic manifestations occur as a result of intracranial lesions caused by direct or indirect involvement of the hypothalamic centers and the anterior and posterior lobes of the pituitary.

Tumors or other lesions of the pituitary gland and infundibulum are infrequent in children, and in most instances symptoms are attributable to lesions in the hypothalamus. As a result of intracranial lesions, there may be (1) stimulation or inhibition of secretion of the anterior pituitary gland, (2) influence on the posterior lobe of the pituitary gland, or (3) direct action on the peripheral organs.

Clinical manifestations of hypothalamic dysfunction include (1) hypothermia, (2) somnolence, (3) adiposogenital syndrome, (4) diabetes insipidus, frequently with hyperthermia, (5) hypothalamic seizures, (6) dwarfism, and (7) sexual precocity or sexual infantilism through regulatory influence of the hypothalamus on the anterior pituitary and its influence in turn on the target glands.

Sexual precocity, along with other possible abnormalities, generally results from a lesion such as a pinealoma. Lesions (inflammations, xanthomas, craniopharyngiomas, gliomas, and teratomas) involving the hypothalamus, optic chiasm, and suprasellar area, as well as infiltrative and destructive lesions of the pituitary, may cause sexual infantilism, sexual precocity, or dwarfism with diabetes insipidus. Eosinophilic adenomas of the pituitary result in gigantism, and on extremely rare occasions basophilic adenoma is associated with Cushing syndrome.

The reader is referred to discussions of the pituitary and target glands for additional information.

PITUITARY GLAND

Embryologically the pituitary gland (hypophysis) may be subdivided into (1) the adenohypophysis (anterior pituitary) and (2) the neurohypophysis (posterior pituitary). The adenohypophysis is derived from somatic ectoderm of the posterior nasopharynx and is further divided into the pars distalis, pars tuberalis, and pars intermedia. The neurohypophysis is derived from neural ectoderm of the diencephalon and comprises the infundibular process, or pars nervosa, and the infundibulum, or neural stalk. The anterior lobe of the pituitary consists of the pars distalis and pars tuberalis of the adenohypophysis. The posterior lobe consists of the infundibular process of the neurohypophysis and pars intermedia of the adenohypophysis.

Circulation of pituitary gland

The pituitary receives its blood from two sources—arterial blood by way of the superior hypophyseal artery, a branch of the internal carotid artery, and venous blood by way of the hypophyseal portal system. This system consists of a capillary bed extending from the median eminence of the tuber cinereum to the lower infundibular stem and empties into a dense network of sinusoidal capillaries of the pars distalis (anterior pituitary). This circulatory arrangement is of major importance in the hypothalamic control of the pituitary and is probably related to the clinical features of certain suprasellar tumors and other lesions in the area that may affect circulation. The central nervous system exerts its controlling influence over the adenohypophysis by humoral factors that are transported by the hypophyseal portal system from the hypothalamus.

The blood supply of the posterior lobe arises from the inferior hypophyseal arteries and is separate from that of the anterior lobe. Venous blood from the anterior and posterior lobes drains into the cavernous sinus.

Hormones of anterior pituitary gland

Growth hormone. Growth hormone (somatotropic hormone [STH]) is under control of growth hormone–releasing hormone (GHRH) from the hypothalamus. It causes nitrogen retention and promotes growth of the body tissues without affecting sexual development. In addition, it has an action on lipid and carbohydrate metabolism. It mobilizes fatty acids from fat stores; patients with a deficiency of growth hormone may have episodes of hypoglycemia, which improves with the administration of growth hormone. A growth hormone–inhibiting hormone is also formed in the hypothalamus, and it has been named *somatostatin*.

The serum concentration of growth hormone increases in response to exercise and to the relative hypoglycemia that occurs after meals. However, the most significant increase occurs 1 to 2 hours after the onset of sleep.

Corticotropin (ACTH). The release of ACTH is dependent on corticotropin-releasing factor (CRF) from the hypothalamus. The plasma levels of ACTH are highest in the morning and lowest at night. It increases the rate of synthesis and secretion of hydrocortisone, and to a lesser extent of androgen, from the adrenal cortex.

Thyrotropic hormone (TSH). The secretion of TSH is regulated by thyrotropin-releasing hormone (TRH) from the hypothalamus; it stimulates the thyroid gland to synthesize and secrete thyroxin and triiodothyronine.

Gonadotropic hormones. The secretion of the gonadotropins—FSH and LH—is controlled by the gonadotropin-releasing hormone (LRH) from the hypothalamus. The release of both FSH and LH probably is stimulated by a single LRH. In the female, FSH acts with LH to bring about synthesis and secretion of estrogen, maturation of the graafian follicle, and ovulation and formation of luteal tissue. In the male they stimulate development of the seminiferous tubules and the production of spermatozoa. LH in the male stimulates the interstitial cells of Leydig to secrete testosterone.

Prolactin (PRL). Prolactin secretion is controlled by prolactin-inhibiting factor (PIF) and prolactin-releasing factor (PRF) from the hypothalamus. It is the principal hormone necessary for growth of the breasts and for lactation. The action of PRL in the male is unknown.

Melanocyte-stimulating hormone (MSH). MSH stimulates pigment formation by skin. There is evidence for the existence of both a melanocyte-releasing hormone (MRH) and a melanocyte-inhibiting hormone (MIH) in the hypothalamus.

Disorders of anterior pituitary gland

Hypopituitarism

Deficiencies of the anterior pituitary hormones may occur singly or in various combinations. The deficiencies are usually partial.

Etiology. The deficiencies may be *idiopathic* or may be the result of a variety of *organic* destructive lesions of the hypothalamus or the adenohypophysis. The commonest organic cause is a craniopharyngioma. Other rare lesions include chromophobe adenomas of the pituitary, hypothalamic tumors, tuberculosis, encephalitis, syphilis, sarcoidosis, tuberous sclerosis, neurofibromatosis, and Hand-Schüller-Christian disease. Deficiencies of the various hormones are most often idiopathic.

Clinical manifestations. *Idiopathic* hypopituitarism is most frequently associated with growth hormone deficiency, either as an isolated event or in combination with other hormone deficiencies. As a result, the presenting complaint is nearly always short stature—hypopituitary dwarfism.

The height and weight of the hypopituitary dwarf are frequently normal for the first 1 to 2 years of life, subsequent to which growth proceeds slowly. The patients appear younger than their chronologic age. Dentition is generally delayed. Manifestations of tropic hormone deficiencies and subsequent target gland deficiencies (hypothyroidism and hypoadrenalism) are usually lacking. Manifestations of hypoglycemia may be present. Sexual development, which is frequently delayed, is absent if a deficiency of gonadotropins exists.

In patients with *organic* lesions the presenting complaint may be solely one of gradual appearance and progression of slow growth in a previously normal child. Unlike idiopathic hypopituitarism, however, severe manifestations of tropic hormone deficiencies (hypothyroidism and hypoadrenalism) and diabetes insipidus are frequently present. The occurrence of diabetes insipidus and anterior pituitary hypofunction should suggest the possibility of an organic lesion. Visual disturbances and/or symptoms of increased intracranial pressure (headache, vomiting, etc.) are frequently present. These may be the presenting complaints and often antedate the manifestations of hormonal deficiency. With lesions involving the hypothalamus, manifestations of hypothalamic dysfunction such as somnolence, temperature disturbances, autonomic epilepsy, and hyperphagia may be present.

Laboratory findings. Small quantities of growth hormone in blood can now be measured by radioimmunoassay (RIA); however, basal levels may be undetectable even in normal children. To demonstrate a deficiency, therefore, the pituitary is stimulated to secrete growth hormone by inducing hypoglycemia with insulin or with the intravenous infusion of L-arginine; a distinct increase (10 to 50 mμg/ml plasma) in the levels of circulating growth hormone occurs in normal persons but not in patients with growth hormone deficiency. Insulin administration must be performed under constant supervision of a physician who is prepared to administer 50% glucose intravenously when signs of hypoglycemia develop. When there is deficiency of TSH, the serum thyroxin and radioactive iodine uptake by the thyroid gland are low; these abnormalities are corrected when a TSH-stimulating test is performed. ACTH deficiency, if present, can be demonstrated by the metyrapone test and a normal response of the adrenal cortex to ACTH administration. The osseous development (bone age) of patients with growth hormone deficiency is usually greatly retarded. Radiologic examination may uncover the cause in cases of organic hypopituitarism, such as sellar or suprasellar calcifications on skull radiographs in patients with craniopharyngiomas, an enlarged sella or destruction of the clinoid processes with pituitary tumors, or the lytic lesions in patients with Hand-Schüller-Christian disease.

Differential diagnosis. The differential diagnosis is essentially one of dwarfism. Organic lesions must be excluded. The more usual causes of short stature include skeletal disorders (chrondrodystrophies, osteogenesis imperfecta, and diseases of the spine), nutritional and metabolic disorders (celiac disease, cystic fibrosis of the pancreas, mucopolysaccharidosis, rickets, hepatic disorders, electrolyte disturbances, nutritional defects, and chronic infections), renal disease (malformations, infections, and acidosis), and circulatory or respiratory disorders (congenital heart disease and pulmonary disease). These conditions are for the most part easily eliminated diagnostically. The conditions with which growth hormone deficiency may be confused are listed in Table 22-1 and are discussed in other sections of this chapter.

Treatment. The ideal form of therapy for somatotropin deficiency is administration of human growth hormone. Its efficacy has been well established, but it is difficult to obtain. Growth hormone of animal origin is ineffective. In patients with TSH and/or ACTH deficiency, replacement therapy with thyroid extract and/or cortisone is indicated. Testosterone is given to males, and estrogens and progestins (cyclic therapy) to females at the age of 15 or 16 years if gonadotropin is deficient, as manifested by the absence of secondary sexual characteristics.

In the presence of organic disease, in addition to replacement therapy, treatment should be directed toward correcting, if possible, the specific underlying disorder.

Specific gonadotropin deficiency (pituitary hypogonadism; pituitary eunuchoidism). Specific gonadotropin deficiency is defined as deficient sexual development resulting from lack of pituitary gonadotropin, without evidence of dwarfism and deficiency of other target gland secretions. The body proportions are eunuchoid, and there are varying degrees of hypogonadism. In males the sexual hair is scanty and feminine in distribution.

These patients must be differentiated from those with primary hypogonadism (such as anorchia and gonadal dysgenesis). It should be remembered that adolescence in rare instances

Table 22-1. Diagnosis of short stature

	Primary hypothyroidism	Constitutional delay	Hypo-pituitarism	Primordial dwarfism	Gonadal dysgenesis
Family history	Occasionally	Often	Rarely	Occasionally	None
Birth weight	Normal	Normal	Usually normal	Often low	Often low
Hypoglycemia	None	None	Not uncommon	None	None
Dental eruption	Delayed	Minimally delayed	Delayed	Normal	Normal
Facial features	Myxedematous	Slightly immature	Immature	Usually normal*	Normal or characteristic†
Dwarfing	Minimal to marked	Minimal to marked	Minimal to marked	Minimal to marked	Usually marked
Sexual development	Infantile‡	Delayed	Infantile	Normal	Infantile except sexual hair
Bone age retardation	Minimal to marked	Minimal to marked	Minimal to marked	None to minimal	None to minimal
Buccal smear	Normal	Normal	Normal	Normal	Usually abnormal (80% chromatin negative)
Water tolerance	Usually normal§	Normal	Often abnormal	Normal	Normal
Insulin sensitivity	Absent	Absent	Usually	Absent	Absent
PBI	Usually low‖	Normal	Often low	Normal	Normal
^{131}I uptake	Usually low‖	Normal	Often low	Normal	Normal
T_4 (RIA)	Low	Normal	Often low	Normal	Normal
TSH (RIA)	Elevated	Normal	Low	Normal	Normal
Growth hormone level	May be decreased	Normal	Decreased	Normal	Normal
Metyrapone	Normal	Normal	Often abnormal	Normal	Normal

*May be progeroid or pinched.
†Hypertelorism, receding mandible, epicanthal folds, low-set ears, low hairline and short neck, broad thick chest, infantile nipples, wide carrying angle, high arched palate, coarctation of the aorta, deeply pigmented nevi, hypoplastic fingernails, genitourinary anomalies, and lymphedema.
‡Rarely, sexual precocity and galactorrhea occur.
§May be abnormal in severe cases.
‖Rare cases of enzymatic defects in thyroid synthesis have normal or elevated protein-bound iodine levels (PBIs) and uptakes.

may occur normally as late as 16 to 18 years of age as a result of delayed release of gonadotropins (delayed adolescence). Such prolonged delayed adolescence is rare in females.

Specific ACTH deficiency. In specific ACTH deficiency the sexual development is adequate except for the absence of sexual hair. There is adequate production of pituitary hormones except for ACTH, as manifested by low levels of urinary 17-ketosteroids and 17-hydroxycorticoids and an abnormal response to the metyrapone test.

It must be remembered that continuous treatment with hydrocortisone or synthetic glucocorticoids for periods longer than 2 to 4 weeks may suppress the pituitary-adrenal axis for significant periods of time after cessation of therapy. Such patients may have circulatory collapse with stress related to surgery, infection, trauma, and so on; therefore during the first year after cessation of therapy, in the event of stressful situations, they should be given 50 to 100 mg/m^2/24 hr of hydrocortisone.

Specific TSH deficiency. Specific TSH deficiency is rare and results in manifestations of hypothyroidism.

Hyperpituitarism

Pituitary gigantism results from excessive production of growth hormone by pituitary tumors. The tumor is usually an eosinophilic adenoma; more rarely, a chromophilic adenoma is present.

Gigantism is usually the presenting complaint, but symptoms of increased intracranial pressure such as headaches may be prominent features. Initially there is symmetric overgrowth of the body, but as the condition progresses acromegalic features are seen: coarsening of the features, broadening of the nose, macroglossia, prognathism, increased spacing of the teeth, and large hands and feet. Manifestations of hyperthyroidism and hyperadrenocorticism are occasionally seen. Hypertrichosis, hyperhidrosis, arthritic complaints, and visceromegaly may be present. In the early stages the patient may have increased libido, but as the disease progresses, pituitary insufficiency develops and is manifested by hypothyroidism, hypogonadism, and hypoadrenocorticism, probably as a result of destruction of the rest of the gland.

The differential diagnosis includes hereditary tall stature, arachnodactyly, hyperthyroidism, and sexual precocity. Radiographs generally reveal enlarged sella turcica and paranasal sinuses and tufting of the phalanges. The bone age is usually normal. Hyperphosphatemia and hyperglycemia with diabetic glucose tolerance curve may be present. The blood growth hormone concentration is increased and is maintained at significant levels with glucose administration.

Various forms of therapy, including external irradiation, heavy particle radiation, local implantation of radioactive yttrium, gold, or strontium, and hypophysectomy are used. Administration of thyroid extract, hydrocortisone, and sex hormones may be indicated.

Cushing syndrome may result from both basophilic and chromophilic adenomas. Visual disturbances, central nervous system symptoms, and hyperpigmentation may be present. Cushing syndrome is discussed on p. 584.

Sexual precocity resulting from hypersecretion of gonadotropins is discussed on pp. 585-586.

POSTERIOR PITUITARY GLAND

The supraoptic and paraventricular nuclei of the hypothalamus, the hypothalamicohypophyseal nerve tracts, and the posterior lobe of the pituitary (neurohypophysis) make up a neurosecretory unit. This unit is the source of the octapeptide hormones *vasopressin* and *oxytocin*. These hormones are produced in the hypothalamic nuclei and are transported along the nerve tracts to the neurohypophysis, where they are stored until liberated into the blood. Contraction of uterine musculature is the predominant effect of oxytocin; it also stimulates milk ejection activity. Vasopressin is the antidiuretic hormone (ADH), which acts on the cellular membranes of the tubular epithelium of the distal convoluted tubules and collecting ducts in the kidney by increasing their permeability to water. An increase in plasma osmolality or a decrease in plasma volume increases secretion of ADH, with resultant retention of water. Painful stimuli, psychic factors, and certain drugs (nicotine, morphine, ether, and barbiturates) may cause antidiuresis.

Diabetes insipidus

Diabetes insipidus results from deficient secretion of ADH or from unresponsiveness of the renal tubule to ADH (nephrogenic diabetes insipidus).

Etiology. Any condition that causes damage to the neurosecretory unit may result in deficient ADH secretion (organic diabetes insipidus). These include operative procedures or trauma to the head, such as basal skull fractures, tumors (particularly craniopharyngiomas), subarachnoid hemorrhages, meningitis, encephalitis, granulomatous lesions of tuberculosis, syphilis, Hand-Schüller-Christian disease, and infiltrative lesions associated with leukemia, Hodgkin disease, and sarcoidosis. It is also associated with the Laurence-Moon-Biedl syndrome. In many instances there is no evidence of disease or injury (idiopathic diabetes insipidus), and the condition may sometimes be hereditary. Nephrogenic diabetes insipidus is a genetically determined renal tubular disorder and occurs nearly always in males. The production of ADH is normal, but the kidneys do not respond.

Clinical manifestations. Polyuria and polydipsia are the principal symptoms of diabetes insipidus. The specific gravity of the urine is below 1.005 or 200 mOsm/kg water. Enuresis may be the first symptom.

If the disorder manifests itself in early life, the infant is irritable and cries excessively from thirst, which is satisfied by giving water but not milk. In contrast to the older child, who compensates for the excessive loss of water by increasing the intake of fluids, the infant exhibits periods of dehydration with hyperelectrolytemia, azotemia, hyperthermia, and circulatory collapse that are relieved by the intake of water. In addition, unexplained fever (caused by dehydration), vomiting, constipation, and failure to gain weight are common manifestations.

When the disorder results from damage to the neurosecretory unit, manifestations of hypothalamic and pituitary tropic hormone dysfunction (obesity, somnolence, disturbance of temperature regulation, emotional disorders, dwarfism, sexual infantilism, or sexual precocity) as well as visual and neurologic disturbances (ocular palsies, papilledema, visual disturbances, and other signs of increased intracranial pressure) may be present.

Diagnosis. The restriction of fluid intake and observations of changes in urine solute concentration (specific gravity and osmolality) are the simplest way of establishing a diagnosis of diabetes insipidus. It should be done under close supervision, with frequent weight checks. It should never be necessary to prolong the period of fluid restriction beyond 24 hours, and if weight loss of 3% to 5% of body weight occurs earlier, it should be terminated to avoid circulatory collapse.

With water restriction the normal subject will increase the urine concentration to 800 mOsm/kg (specific gravity of 1.020). In patients with diabetes insipidus the concentration will not increase above 300 mOsm/kg (specific gravity of 1.008) except with severe dehydration, when it may increase to 800 mOsm/kg (specific gravity of 1.020). If the patient fails to elaborate a concentrated urine, he is rehydrated and a therapeutic test is performed by injecting intramuscularly aqueous pitressin, 0.1 unit/kg body weight, with a maximal dose of 5 units. If the patient is vasopressin responsive, antidiuresis will result and treatment with long-acting vasopressin tannate in oil should alleviate the polyuria and polydipsia. The patient with vasopressin-resistant diabetes insipidus (nephrogenic diabetes insipidus) will not concentrate the urine with vasopressin administration.

Skull radiographs may reveal evidence of organic lesions.

Hypokalemia, hypocalcemia, and chronic renal disease may be associated with polyuria. Patients with thyrotoxicosis may have polyuria. Children with psychogenic ploydipsia may have severe polyuria; however, with fluid restriction they are able to concentrate the urine.

Treatment. Diabetes insipidus resulting from ADH deficiency is satisfactorily treated with intramuscular administration of long-acting (24 to 72 hours) vasopressin tannate in oil, in a dose of 0.5 $ml/m^2/24$ hr. It is important that the active material be thoroughly resuspended in the oil vehicle—hold the ampule under warm running water for 7 minutes, then shake it vigorously. 1-*l*-desamino-8-D-arginine vasopressin (DDAVP), a synthetic vasopressin analogue, is also an effective therapeutic agent. It is administered as an intranasal spray, and its duration of action is 10 to 12 hours. The dose for chilren ranges from 2.5 to 10 μg once or twice daily.

The infant with nephrogenic diabetes insipidus must be given water at frequent intervals to prevent dehydration and a low-solute diet to reduce the osmolar load on the kidney. Chlorothiazide, 1 $g/m^2/24$ hr in three divided doses, has proved beneficial in some cases. Because of frequent side effects, the drug should be used cautiously and only in patients who do poorly with dietary management. The mechanism of action remains uncertain.

THYROID GLAND

The thyroid gland possesses two types of secretory cells, the follicular cells, which secrete thyroid hormones tetraiodothyronine (T_4, or thyroxin) and 3,5,3′-triiodothyronine (T_3), and the parafollicular cells, which secrete calcitonin. The secretion of thyroid hormones is normally in response to TSH from the anterior pituitary. TSH secretion is in response to the effective concentration of thyroid hormones at the pituitary level and the stimulatory effects of the hypothalamic TRH, a tripeptide amide. Factors regulating TRH secretion have not been well established.

By uniting iodine and tyrosine, the thyroid gland synthesizes thyroid hormones and releases them as needed for oxidative metabolism. Dietary intake is the chief source of iodine. Most organic iodines are reduced to iodides during gastrointestinal absorption and then are transported in the blood. Of the iodine absorbed, one third is "trapped" by the thyroid and two thirds is excreted in the urine.

At least five basic enzymatic steps in throxin production by the thyroid gland are present:

1. A trapping enzyme (iodase) removes io-

dides from the blood. The salivary glands, mammary glands, and gastric mucosa also have the ability to trap iodide but are unable to synthesize thyroid hormones.

2. A peroxidase enzyme system influences the oxidation of iodide (I^-) to an active form of iodide (I°), which is instantly attached to tyrosine to form monoiodotyrosine (MIT). The tyrosine molecules are located within the matrix of thyroglobulin. MIT is then iodinated at the 5 position to form 3,5-diiodotyrosine (DIT).

3. One molecule of DIT and one molecule of MIT are enzymatically coupled to form T_3, and two molecules of DIT are coupled to form T_4.

4. Proteolytic enzymes split T_4 and T_3 from the large thyroglobulin molecule, and these are secreted into the bloodstream. Some MIT and DIT are also liberated within the gland.

5. Deiodinating enzymes release iodine from these iodotyrosine (MIT and DIT) molecules for reuse.

Only a small fraction of the circulating thyroxin is free, or unbound. Most of the serum thyroxin is bound to carrier proteins, primarily thyroxin-binding globulin (TBG), and to a lesser degree to thyroxin-binding prealbumin (TBPA) and albumin. Serum T_3 is predominantly bound to TBG and to some small extent to albumin. It is now recognized that the free thyroid hormone is the active hormone and presumably is the feedback regulator of the hypothalamic-pituitary axis.

Several factors influence the levels of TBG and produce secondary alterations in the concentrations of total thyroxin. Increased TBG is found in pregnancy, subjects receiving oral contraceptives, states of estrogen excess, cirrhosis, acute infectious hepatitis, and as an inherited condition. Decreased TBG is found in acromegaly, nephrotic syndrome, hypoproteinemic states, subjects receiving androgens and large doses of glucocorticoids, and as an inherited condition. Furthermore, dilantin and salicylates compete with T_4 for the binding proteins and produce decreased TBG capacity.

Tests of thyroid function

Protein-bound iodine (PBI). In addition to measuring T_4, the PBI measures iodotyrosines, thyroglobulin, and organic and inorganic iodine. For this reason it is not a specific test for evaluating thyroid function and should not be used routinely for this purpose.

Thyroxin. Measurements of serum T_4 by competitive protein binding or by RIA are more specific and accurate methods for determining the levels of circulating T_4 than is the PBI.

T_3 resin uptake. The determination of T_3 resin uptake provides information about the available sites of thyroid-binding proteins and is a good screening test in instances where abnormalities in thyroid-binding proteins are suspected.

Thyroxin-binding proteins. Measurements of thyroid-binding proteins are necessary to interpret the thyroxin levels when abnormalities in thyroid-binding proteins are suspected.

Free thyroxin. The concentration of free T_4 can be estimated by determining the fraction of T_4 that is dialyzable. It is helpful in delineating disorders of abnormal binding proteins.

Serum T_3. Determination of T_3 by RIA is now possible. It is useful in the diagnosis of hyperthyroidism.

Serum TSH. Serum TSH concentrations can be measured by RIA. This is the most sensitive test for the diagnosis of hypothyroidism. Patients with primary hypothyroidism have elevated levels of TSH.

TRH test. TRH administration causes release of TSH from the normal anterior pituitary gland, and peak serum TSH concentrations are reached in 20 to 40 minutes. This test is important in (1) confirming hyperthyroidism, (2) distinguishing hypothalamic from pituitary hypothyroidism, and (3) measuring pituitary TSH reserve.

Iodine 131 uptake. With sensitive scintillation counters, small doses of the isotope ^{131}I should now be used. Adequate amounts range from 1 to 5 μCi. At least two counts should be done—the first count at 4 to 6 hours and the second at 24 hours after the oral dose. In hyperthyroidism the 6-hour uptake may be high and the 24-hour uptake may be as high, normal, or low, depending on the rate of iodine turnover by the gland.

T_3 suppression test. The T_3 suppression test is based on the postulate that if the normal reciprocal relationship exists between thyroxin and TSH, then T_3 will suppress the ^{131}I uptake by 60% or more. After determining the initial ^{131}I uptake, 75 μg of T_3/m^2 is given daily in divided doses for 8 days. A repeat ^{131}I uptake is done on days 7 and 8. The ability to suppress thyroidal uptake is lost in Graves disease and autonomously functioning thyroid nodules.

Hypothyroidism

Hypothyroidism is one of the most common endocrine abnormalities in childhood. The disorder is either congenital (cretinism) or acquired.

Congenital hypothyroidism may be nongoitrous or goitrous. *Congenital nongoitrous hypothyroidism* results from (1) a congenital TSH deficiency, which is a rare and genetically determined condition, and (2) an agenesis or hypoplasia of the thyroid gland, the cause of which is unknown but may be related to defective thyroid primordial cells, abnormal local mesenchymal tissue beneath the primordial cells, or circulating antithyroid substances. Agenesis or hypoplasia is the most frequent cause of congenital hypothyroidism and in some cases it may be associated with maldescent of the thyroid gland.

In *congenital goitrous hypothyroidism* the patients have a deficient synthesis of thyroid hormones. In an attempt to make adequate amounts of hormone, there is an increased TSH secretion, with resultant goiter. It may be caused by (1) enzymatic defects in any of the steps in the synthesis of thyroxin; (2) iodine deficiency (endemic cretinism) during prenatal life secondary to an iodine deficit in the maternal diet (a rare cause); and (3) goitrogens or antithyroid drugs (cobalt, propylthiouracil, *p*-aminosalicylic acid, etc.) ingested by the mother during pregnancy.

Acquired hypothyroidism may be caused by (1) chronic lymphocytic thyroiditis (Hashimoto thyroiditis), the commonest cause; (2) dysgenesis of the thyroid less severe than in cretinism; (3) destructive procedures such as irradiation or surgical thyroidectomy; (4) hypopituitarism or an isolated TSH deficiency; (5) iodine deficiency; or (6) ingestion of goitrogens.

Clinical manifestations. The clinical picture of hypothyroidism depends on the degree and duration of thyroid deficiency regardless of etiology. At birth hypothyroid children may appear normal, and the diagnosis before 6 months of age may be difficult. Nevertheless, suggestive historical and physical findings should prompt investigation. Prolonged physiologic jaundice, mottling of the skin, inactivity, excessive sleeping, slow feeding, minimal crying, and constipation should bring to mind hypothyroidism.

The skin is pale, cool, gray, mottled, scaly, and dry. A yellowish tinge may be noted. The hair may be coarse, dry, brittle, or lusterless with low hairline and hirsutism. The facial features remain infantile and become coarse, with flattened nasal bridge, short upturned nose, and a large thick tongue protruding through an open mouth. Hoarseness and signs of partially obstructed upper airway may be detected. Growth is stunted, with persistent infantile proportions (increased ratio of upper to lower segment). Dental development is delayed. The nervous system is affected in that mental and physical development are delayed. ''Hung up'' deep tendon reflexes (slow relaxation after jerk) are present.

The muscles have poor tone. Protruding abdomen, diastasis recti, and umbilical hernia are present. Cardiovascular manifestations are slow pulse, poor circulation with decreased cardiac output, decreased pulse pressure, and mottled skin. Effects on bones are seen in delayed bone maturation (bone age) and delayed closure of the anterior fontanel.

The most frequent complaint of hypothyroidism during childhood is growth retardation. Other manifestations are cold intolerance, dry skin, excessive sleepiness, muscle aches, and constipation. Less commonly observed is weakness and hypertrophy of muscles. Dry, brittle, and sparse hair is present. Prolonged hypothyroidism in childhood produces lethargy.

Puffy edema of the face and supraclavicular areas and prominent abdomen may suggest obesity. Significant delay in sexual maturation is characteristic of hypothyroidism. However, occasional patients will develop incomplete isosexual precocity, characterized in boys by enlargement of the penis and testes and in girls by enlargement of the breasts and labia minora, as well as menometrorrhagia.

Laboratory findings. The serum T_4 and free T_4 levels are low. The PBI level is usually low but may be normal or elevated in rare cases of enzymatic defects or in thyroiditis. The plasma TSH level is elevated in primary hypothyroidism, while in secondary hypothyroidism the serum TSH level is undetectable. Thyroidal ^{131}I uptake is low or absent in athyrotic hypothyroidism and is increased or normal in patients with enzymatic defects, except in those rare patients who have an enzymatic trapping defect.

Radiographs show delayed bone age. Epiphyseal dysgenesis may also be present. Serum cholesterol, carotene, and creatinine phosphokinase levels may be increased and alkaline phosphatase decreased. However, because of their variability these tests should not be used to diagnose hypothyroidism. Anemia may be present and is corrected only with thyroid therapy.

Treatment. Desiccated thyroid (USP) or synthetic sodium-l-thyroxin (l-T_4) is prescribed. One grain of desiccated thyroid is equal to approximately 100 μg of l-T_4. In neonates and infants a single daily dose of ⅛ to ¼ grain (or its equivalent as l-T_4) is given initially for 4 to 7 days, with subsequent increases of ⅛ to ¼ grain at similar intervals, depending on the patient's response. Under 1 year of age a daily dose of ¾ to 1 grain is usually adequate to maintain euthyroidism. Between the ages of 1 and 6 years, 1 to 2 grains are given daily; between 6 and 12 years, 1½ to 2½ grains; after the age of 12 years 2 to 3 grains are prescribed daily.

Normal growth and development are the aims of therapy. Overdosage with thyroid medications may produce signs and symptoms of hyperthyroidism. It is to be remembered, however, that the previously placid hypothyroid patient becomes more active when the euthyroid state is attained. Adequate thyroid replacement therapy should result in normal values of serum T_4, free T_4, and TSH.

Prognosis. Somatic growth and development can usually be corrected. Ultimate mental attainment, however, depends on the degree of hypothyroidism, age at onset, duration before treatment, and adequacy of therapy. Delayed institution of therapy decreases the chances of normal mental development. As many as 50% of severely hypothyroid infants adequately treated during the first 6 months of life do not achieve an IQ of 90. If the onset of hypothyroidism is more gradual during the first years of life, the prognosis is better. After 2 to 3 years of age, acquired hypothyroidism usually produces no mental retardation if therapy is instituted and continued.

Newborn screening for hypothyroidism

Newborn screening for congenital hypothyroidism has been developed because frequently it takes weeks for infants to manifest signs of the disorder. Most programs employ measurements of T_4 on filter paper blood spots, obtained at the time of discharge from the newborn nursery. If T_4 values are low, the blood should be tested for TSH. The incidence of congenital hypothyroidism is approximately 1 in 4000 newborn infants.

Hyperthyroidism

Hyperthyroidism in childhood is almost always caused by Graves disease. Less common than hypothyroidism, Graves disease occurs in a female-male ratio of 6:1 and shows a significant increased incidence during puberty. The pathogenesis of this disorder is not yet clarified. It is probably caused by a specific genetic defect in immunologic surveillance or control. The defect would permit the specific mutating, self-reactive, forbidden clone of helper T-lymphocytes to survive. These T-lymphocytes would then interact with their complementary antigen, act in or on the thyroid cell membrane, and set up a localized cell-mediated immune response. The clone helper T-lymphocyte will cooperate with the B-lymphocytes to produce thyroid autoantibodies (thyroid-stimulating immunoglobulin, TSI), which appear to be antibodies directed against the TSH receptor, and to stimulate the thyroid follicular cells in a manner indistinguishable from TSH. Some of the TSI are detectable by animal assay, such as the long-acting thyroid stimulator (LATS) assay. The role of stress in the induction of hyperthyroidism may be by reducing immune surveillance in persons with the defect.

Family studies demonstrate familial predisposition to Graves disease. However, neither clinical nor laboratory evidence has substantiated any single mode of inheritance.

Less frequent causes of hyperthyroidism in children include (1) autonomously functioning adenoma of the thyroid, (2) chronic lymphocytic thyroiditis (Hasimoto thyroiditis), (3) McCune-Albright syndrome, (4) thyroid carcinoma, (5) exogenous iodide–induced hyperthyroidism, (6) TSH-producing pituitary tumor, and (7) neonatal Graves disease, in which the mother invariably has active thyrotoxicosis. The toxicosis in the offspring is transient (up to 3 months) and correlates well with the half-life of LATS, a 7S gamma globulin able to traverse the placenta.

Signs and symptoms. The onset of symptoms of hyperthyroidism is usually gradual.

Nervousness, emotional instability, irritability, hyperactivity, tremor, insomnia, and muscle weakness are present. The commonest presenting physical sign is excessive motion. Loss of weight in spite of excessive appetite is often encountered, although some patients gain weight. Vomiting, diarrhea, or increased frequency of stooling may be present. Heat is tolerated poorly. The thyroid gland is diffusely enlarged and smooth, and a bruit may be heard. Exophthalmos, staring expression, increased blinking, inability to converge the eyes, lid lag, and absence of wrinkling of the forehead on upward gaze may be found. Cardiovascular manifestations may include tachycardia, a bounding pulse with a widened pulse pressure primarily caused by increased systolic pressure, systolic murmurs, and cardiomegaly. Sleeping pulse rates are rapid. The hair may be fine and the skin warm, moist, and flushed. Linear growth and bone maturation are generally accelerated.

Fortunately, thyroid crises occur less commonly in children than in adults. These storms are characterized by severe nervousness, vomiting, diarrhea, high temperature, hypertension, and prostration.

Laboratory findings. The T_4 and "free" thyroxin levels are usually elevated. These tests may be normal in the individual with T_3-thyrotoxicosis whose serum T_3 RIA is elevated. Thyroidal uptake of ^{131}I is increased. Thyroid autonomy, one of the characteristics of Graves disease, can be determined by a T_3 suppression test and by the TRH test in questionable cases. Lymphocytosis and leukopenia may exist.

Differential diagnosis includes chorea, psychiatric disturbances, pheochromocytoma, and a nontoxic goiter in a nervous child.

Treatment

Medical treatment. In one program, propylthiouracil (PTU), 200 mg/m^2/24 hr, or methimazole (Tapazole), 20 mg/m^2/24 hr, is given at 8-hour intervals until the patient becomes clinically euthyroid (usually in 6 to 8 weeks), and then the dosage is gradually decreased to half the initial dosage and continued for 2 years. At the end of this period the medication is gradually discontinued.

In another program PTU or methimazole is continued in the full initial dosage, and, when the patient becomes euthyroid, thyroid hormone is introduced in the treatment to prevent induced hypothyroidism and compensatory enlargement of the thyroid. This combined therapy is also continued for 2 years.

Some patients with very large goiters may require larger dosages of PTU or methimazole. Most of the toxic reactions to the medications are mild and do not necessitate discontinuing use. Pruritus, skin rashes, urticaria, nausea, vomiting, vertigo, headache, loss of taste, paresthesias, and arthralgia are among the toxic reactions. Serious complications include neutropenia that cannot be predicted by frequent leukocyte counts, thrombocytopenia, and hepatitis.

After 2 years of medical therapy approximately 40% of patients may relapse and require another course of antithyroid drug or other method of treatment.

Symptomatic treatment is beneficial. A small dosage of phenobarbital produces mild sedation and improves sleep. Reserpine is useful as an antihypertensive and sedative agent. Propranolol (2 to 5 mg/kg/24 hr orally in divided doses every 6 to 8 hours with a maximal daily dose of 120 mg) is useful in the control of tachycardia, restlessness, and tremor.

Surgical treatment. Subtotal thyroidectomy is the treatment of choice in some hospitals. In others it is used when the patient has drug toxicity, recurrent relapses, or when there is lack of compliance. The surgical complications include hypothyroidism, hypoparathyroidism, and damage of the recurrent laryngeal nerve. Hyperthyroidism may recur. It is advisable to control the hyperthyroidism with drug therapy and to administer iodide (Lugol solution, 10 drops t.i.d.) for 10 to 15 days before surgery. Propranolol may also be used.

^{131}I therapy is the method of treatment in some hospitals. We have used this method only in children who cannot be treated medically or surgically.

Goiter

Goiter, or "struma," implies an enlargement of the thyroid gland. The enlargement may be diffuse or nodular. The functional activity of the thyroid gland may be normal (euthyroid goiter), decreased (hypothyroid), or increased (hyperthyroid). Hypothyroid and hyperthyroid goiters have already been mentioned.

The most common conditions producing a euthyroid goiter in children are simple (colloid) goiter and chronic lymphocytic thyroiditis (CLT), or Hashimoto thyroiditis.

Other causes of euthyroid goiters are acute suppurative, acute nonsuppurative, or subacute thyroiditis; adenomatous goiters; carcinoma; and iodide excess.

Simple (colloid) goiter in childhood is more frequent in girls and during puberty. Most patients are asymptomatic, and the thyroid tests are usually normal. Histologically it is characterized by large colloid-filled follicles with flat epithelium. Most adolescent colloid goiters regress spontaneously in 3 years, and hypothyroidism rarely occurs. Full thyroid replacement is indicated for large goiters until the completion of adolescence. Recurrence of the goiter may warrant lifetime replacement therapy.

Thyroiditis implies varying degrees of inflammatory cell infiltration, parenchymal cell destruction, and fibrous replacement. It may be acute, subacute, or chronic.

Acute suppurative thyroiditis may be caused by septicemia or an extension of infection from the neck or upper respiratory tract. Staphylococcal, streptococcal, pneumococcal, *Haemophilus influenzae, Escherichia coli,* and viral infections have been reported as causes of acute thyroiditis. Severe destruction of the thyroid gland rarely occurs during the course of the disease, and thyroid function tests usually remain in the euthyroid range. Specific antibiotic therapy is indicated. If abscess formation occurs, it should be incised, drained, and cultured.

The etiology of subacute thyroiditis is unknown, although a viral cause has been assumed. This is a rare condition in children. The patient frequently has a history of an upper respiratory tract illness. Then the patient develops pain in the thyroid area, extending into the angle of the jaw or behind the ears. Anorexia, malaise, weight loss, and nervousness may be present. The thyroid gland is enlarged and very tender. The patient has leukocytosis, high sedimentation rate, and decreased ^{131}I uptake, which eventually will return to normal. This disease is usually self-limited and of short duration. Aspirin and glucocorticoids are used with variable success.

Chronic lymphocytic (Hashimoto) thyroiditis, an autoimmune condition, is rare before 5 years of age and increases abruptly during puberty. It occurs in a female-male ratio of 9:1. Although lymphocytic thyroiditis may occur in the hypothyroid state, most patients have a diffusely enlarged and firm euthyroid goiter. A few patients complain of mild tenderness in the thyroid gland or of pressure in the neck. Sometimes a history of symptoms suggestive of hyperthyroidism may be elicited. The goiter tends to be firm. A PBI-T_4 iodide difference greater than 2 μg/dl, elevated levels of serum TSH, and positive serum thyroid autoantibodies (antithyroglobulin, antimicrosomal) are frequently found in Hashimoto thyroiditis. Histologic evidence in tissue obtained by needle biopsy may be necessary for the diagnosis.

The treatment of choice for chronic lymphocytic thyroiditis is thyroid hormone replacement to control the hypothyroidism, when present, and to suppress TSH, which is at least partially responsible for the thyroid enlargement. Surgery should be reserved for goiters causing pressure symptoms.

Goiters may be caused by *neoplasms* of the thyroid. *Carcinoma* of the thyroid gland in children is uncommon. The incidence increases with the age of the patient. The female-male ratio is 2:1. In a significant number of cases a history of radiation to the neck or chest is obtained. Histologically the neoplasms are classified as papillary, follicular, medullary, and anaplastic carcinoma. The most frequent complaint is an asymptomatic cervical mass, which may be confined to the thyroid gland or may be lateral to it. Seventy-five percent of patients have cervical lymph node involvement. Thyroid function tests are usually normal. The thyroid scan will indicate the activity of the thyroid mass; in carcinoma it is more frequently inactive. In thyroid cancers a soft tissue x-ray film of the neck is of value to detect calcifications of the psammoma bodies. Surgery is the treatment of choice, followed by replacement therapy.

Benign thyroid neoplasms are contained within a capsule. The pathology of these tumors is varied: embryonal, fetal, follicular, Hürthle cell, and papillary. They usually grow slowly. The treatment is surgical removal.

PARATHYROID GLANDS

Parathyroid hormone, the hormone produced by the parathyroid glands, plays a major role in calcium homeostasis. Its main actions are (1) to increase release of calcium and phosphate from bone by increasing osteoclastic activity, (2) to inhibit renal tubular reabsorption of phosphate, (3) to increase renal tubular absorption of calcium, and (4) to increase the absorption of calcium from the small intestine. It appears that the secretion of parathyroid hormone depends on the calcium ion concentration in extracellular fluid; a fall increases secretion, and a rise decreases secretion.

In addition to parathyroid hormone, *calcitonin,* a hormone secreted by the parafollicular cells of the thyroid gland, plays a role in calcium homeostasis. It is secreted in response to hypercalcemia and decreases serum calcium concentration, apparently by inhibiting bone resorption.

Primary hyperparathyroidism

Primary hyperparathyroidism is a rare disorder in childhood in which there is excessive production of parathyroid hormone with resultant hypercalcemia. It may result from either an adenoma or from idiopathic hyperplasia of a gland(s). Parathyroid adenomas are usually encountered in the older child, whereas the infant is more likely to have hyperplasia.

Hypercalcemia may cause such symptoms as failure to thrive, muscular weakness, anorexia, nausea, vomiting, constipation, abdominal pain, weight loss, bradycardia, and cardiac irregularities. Hypercalcemia may be associated with deposition of calcium in the kidney, resultant nephrocalcinosis, and renal calculi. These may cause polyuria, polydipsia, frequency of urination, nocturia, hematuria, and renal colic. Renal failure may eventually occur. Deposition of calcium may also occur in ligaments, cartilage, conjunctiva, and superficial layers of the cornea where the deposits may be visible by slit-lamp examination. Bone resorption is associated with pain in the back and extremities, deformities, fractures, and radiologic changes. The osseous manifestations (clinical and radiologic) may be absent if the calcium intake is high.

The serum calcium concentration is elevated, and the serum phosphorus level is decreased. The concentration of parathyroid hormone in the plasma is increased. With osseous involvement the serum alkaline phosphatase level may be increased. When renal insufficiency complicates the disorder, the serum phosphorus level increases, the serum calcium may fall to normal levels, and the BUN becomes elevated. Radiographs may show either diffuse demineralization or cystic lesions. A more characteristic sign is subperiosteal erosion of cortical bone, most easily seen in the phalanges. Radiographs of the teeth may show disappearance of the lamina dura. The skull may be either ground-glass or moth-eaten in appearance.

The differential diagnosis includes any disorder that may be associated with hypercalcemia, such as idiopathic hypercalcemia of infancy, vitamin D intoxication, hypophosphatasia, sarcoidosis, thyrotoxicosis, malignant disease with osseous metastases, leukemia, and hypercalcemia as a result of prolonged immobilization.

The treatment of primary hyperparathyroidism is surgical removal of the hyperfunctioning parathyroid tissue.

Secondary hyperparathyroidism

Any disorder that decreases calcium ion concentration in extracellular fluid will result in parathyroid hyperplasia and hyperfunction. Chronic renal insufficiency (hypoplasia of the kidneys, polycystic kidneys, obstructive uropathy, chronic pyelonephritis, chronic glomerulonephritis) is the commonest cause of secondary hyperparathyroidism. Glomerular insufficiency is accompanied by phosphate retention and hyperphosphatemia. This results in decreased extracellular calcium ion concentration and compensatory parathyroid hyperplasia and hyperfunction. As a result, demineralization and cystic lesions of the bone may be produced as well as rachitic changes (renal rickets).

Treatment is directed toward correcting, if possible, the specific disorder, which in many instances may be irreversible. In addition, measures are taken to raise the serum calcium concentration by offering a low-phosphorus diet with administration of calcium lactate and aluminum hydroxide to precipitate phosphate in the intestine and vitamin D (25,000 to 50,000 units daily) to enhance calcium absorption from the intestine. The serum calcium levels should be determined frequently, and, if hypercalcemia results, the dose of vitamin D should be discontinued temporarily until the calcium level returns to normal.

In vitamin D–deficient rickets, severe liver disease, and chronic diarrheal states (malabsorption syndromes), deficient absorption of calcium from the intestines results in secondary hyperparathyroidism. Dwarfism, bone deformities, and joint pain may be present.

Hypoparathyroidism

Hypoparathyroidism may result from removal or damage of the parathyroid glands during thyroidectomy or from aplasia or hypoplasia of the glands. The latter is frequently associated with other developmental defects (thymic aplasia and cardiovascular, optic, and cerebral anomalies). Most often, however, no cause is apparent (idiopathic hypoparathyroidism).

Generalized or focal convulsion is the most frequent presenting symptom. Stiffness, tingling, and numbness of the hands and feet may occur. Tetany (carpopedal spasms) may be evident. Abnormalities of the teeth (premature loss of teeth, delayed dentition, caries, ridging, enamel hypoplasia) and nails (longitudinal ridging, cracking), alopecia, dry scaly skin, cataracts, blepharospasm, keratoconjunctivitis, and photophobia are often present. Infants may manifest laryngospasm. Chronic diarrhea and psychotic symptoms may be present. Nail infections with *Candida albicans* are common. Pernicious anemia, Addison disease, thyroiditis, hypothyroidism, DiGeorge syndrome, diabetes mellitus, and hepatitis are also seen in association with hypoparathyroidism.

In this disorder the serum calcium level is reduced and the serum phosphorus level elevated. The serum phosphatase level is normal or low. Renal function is normal. Bone radiographs are usually normal. Calcification in the basal ganglia may be noted on skull radiographs. The electrocardiogram may show a prolonged Q-T interval.

Conditions that enter into the differential diagnosis are renal insufficiency and other forms of hypocalcemia. Appropriate laboratory determinations should clarify these conditions.

Emergency treatment for tetany or convulsions is the slow intravenous administration of a 10% solution of calcium gluconate (0.5 to 1 ml/min), with careful monitoring of the heart rate. Vitamin D in doses of 25,000 to 200,000 units or 1 to 3 μg of 1,25-hydroxycholecalciferol (1,25[OH]-D) is administered daily for maintenance therapy. The dose is adjusted to maintain the serum calcium level in the low to normal ranges. A low-phosphorus diet is desirable (exclusion of milk, eggs, and cheese). Supplemental calcium (3 to 10 g calcium lactate daily) may be necessary to maintain normocalcemia.

Pseudohypoparathyroidism

In the hereditary condition called pseudohypoparathyroidism the parathyroids are present and are hyperplastic with biochemical changes and clinical manifestations of hypoparathyroidism. When parathyroid extract is administered to these patients, their kidneys do not respond with a phosphate diuresis, nor is there a rise in the serum calcium level or a fall in the serum level of phosphorus. Two clinical types have been described. In type I, there is an insufficient rise in urinary cyclic AMP to the administration of parathyroid hormone. In addition, associated anomalies are present—dwarfism, stocky build, round face, short neck, brachydactylia, and mental retardation. In type II the patients do not manifest the somatic findings present in type I. There is a normal response in urinary cyclic AMP to parathyroid hormone, suggesting that the defect is caused by an inability of the renal cells to respond to an increase in cyclic AMP. As is to be expected, in both types the concentration of serum immunoreactive parathyroid hormone is elevated.

The clinical and chemical findings are similar to those of idiopathic hypoparathyroidism.

Treatment is the same as for idiopathic hypoparathyroidism.

ADRENAL GLANDS

The adrenal gland is composed of two functionally distinct endocrine systems: the *cortex,* which is of mesodermal origin, and the *medulla,* which (like the sympathetic system) is derived from neural ectoderm. The adrenal cortex in the newborn infant consists of a histologically distinct inner zone, known as the "fetal adrenal cortex," and an outer zone of true cortex. Shortly after birth the fetal cortex begins to degenerate and completely disappears by 1 year of age or earlier. The true cortex consists of three zones—the zona glomerulosa, the zona fasciculata, and the zona reticularis.

Hormones of the adrenal cortex—action and control of secretion

Over fifty steroids have been isolated from the adrenal cortex. They differ in their biologic activity, and some of them are physiologically inactive. However, only a few of these are normally secreted into the adrenal vein.

These hormones can be divided into four groups according to their biologic activity: (1) *glucocorticoids,* (2) *mineralocorticoids,* (3) *androgens,* and (4) *estrogens* and *progestins.*

Cortisol (hydrocortisone) is the most important *glucocorticoid* in humans and is secreted at a greater rate (10 to 15 mg/m^2/24 hr) than any of the other adrenal steroids. The principal role of the glucocorticoids is in the control of gluconeogenesis. They promote the deamination of amino acids and their conversion to glucose with a resultant rise in both liver glycogen and blood glucose levels. In addition, they also influence fat, electrolyte, and water metabolism and manifest effects on the cardiovascular, muscular, gastrointestinal, skeletal, hematopoietic, immunologic, and central nervous systems.

The secretion of these compounds is controlled directly by adrenocorticotropin (ACTH) of the anterior pituitary. A rise in free blood cortisol inhibits ACTH secretion and vice versa. In addition to this mechanism, the adrenal cortex is capable of responding to nervous stimuli. Stressful stimuli, for example, surgical stress, act through the nervous system on the hypothalamus to secrete the corticotropin-releasing factor (CRF). This is transported in the hypophyseal portal circulation to the anterior pituitary, where it causes release of ACTH.

The most important *mineralocorticoid* is aldosterone, and it is now generally accepted that it is synthesized in the zona glomerulosa. Its mineralocorticoid activity is 500 times as potent as cortisol and 25 times as potent as deoxycorticosterone (DOC). Like DOC, it promotes sodium retention and potassium loss in the urine. Through its action on the distal convoluted tubule, urine sodium ions are exchanged for hydrogen and potassium ions. When aldosterone is present in excess, there is a rise in serum sodium and a fall in serum potassium levels, with ensuing hypochloremic alkalosis. A lack of aldosterone results in hyperkalemia, sodium loss and hyponatremia, metabolic acidosis, dehydration, and circulatory collapse.

Although the secretion of the glucocorticoids is wholly dependent on ACTH, it affects the secretion of aldosterone to only a comparatively minor degree. Many different factors, which are poorly understood, influence aldosterone secretion. Among these are variations in intravascular volume and changes in the concentration of sodium and potassium in plasma. Evidence has been presented for the existence of an aldosterone-stimulating factor in the kidney—renin.

The main *androgenic steroids* secreted by the adrenal cortex are dehydroepiandrosterone, Δ^4-androstenedione, and 11-beta-hydroxy-Δ^4-androstenedione. They are not produced in appreciable amounts before puberty except for the first few weeks of life. They are responsible for growth of sexual hair, seborrhea, and acne in normal girls at puberty and contribute (together with testosterone from the gonads) to the appearance of these in pubescent boys. They are also protein anabolic and contribute to the growth spurt of puberty.

Feminizing tumors of the adrenal gland, which secrete estrogens and progestins, are extremely rare and will only be mentioned in this discussion.

Hormones of the adrenal medulla—action and control of secretion

The cells of the adrenal medulla respond primarily to splanchnic nerve stimulation to produce epinephrine and norepinephrine. The metabolic effects are well known and include their pressor effect, lipolysis, sweating, hepatic glycogenolysis, hyperglycemia, and central nervous system excitation.

Disorders of the adrenal cortex

Disorders of the adrenal cortex fall in two categories: (1) hypoadrenalism (adrenocortical insufficiency) and (2) hyperadrenocorticism.

Adrenocortical insufficiency

The symptoms of adrenocortical insufficiency may appear abruptly or insidiously, and the deficiency may be temporary or permanent, depending on the etiology.

Acute adrenocortical insufficiency. Although not a frequent occurrence in children, adrenocortical insufficiency may be associated with a variety of conditions.

Etiology. Acute adrenal failure may result from (1) congenital hypoplasia or aplasia of the adrenal glands; (2) hemorrhage into the adrenal gland, which results most frequently from trauma incidental to difficult breech deliveries, asphyxia, violent resuscitative measures, and hemorrhagic diathesis in the newborn infant; (3) fulminating infections causing hemorrhage or necrosis (usually meningococcemia is the underlying disease), but it may occur in the course of other fulminating infections (Waterhouse-Friderichsen syndrome); (4) sudden withdrawal of treatment with cortisone or DOC; (5) salt-losing crisis with congenital adrenal hyperplasia; and (6) failure to administer supportive adrenal steroid therapy during stress, for example, surgery and infections, to patients who are receiving or have recently received steroids.

Clinical manifestations. Usually there is a rapid development of a shocklike picture with hypotension, a weak and rapid pulse, cyanosis, cold and clammy skin, hyperpyrexia, and at times vomiting, diarrhea, rapid respirations, and finally coma. In the newborn infant these manifestations may be indistinguishable from those associated with the more common neonatal conditions of pulmonary infections, sepsis, or intracranial hemorrhage. Since there is no rapid, infallible evidence of adrenocortical insufficiency, treatment must be instituted on suspicion. There is no real danger incurred by unnecessary treatment for a short period, and on recovery diagnostic studies may be undertaken.

Treatment. Therapy must be prompt and vigorous and consists of (1) intravenous administration of isotonic saline containing 5% glucose—the amount administered will depend on the degree of previous depletion and on the size of the patient, but in general it should be given reasonably rapidly at first to replace the fluids and electrolytes that have been lost, at a rate of 2000 to 2500 ml/m^2/24 hr; (2) intravenous hydrocortisone (Solu-Cortef)—an initial dose of 60 mg/m^2 immediately followed by 100 mg/m^2/24 hr by continuous intravenous drip; and (3) norepinephrine (Levophed) intravenously if the circulatory collapse does not respond promptly to the other measures. This form of therapy should be kept up for at least 24 hours or until the patient is out of shock and is able to take adequate fluids and salt by mouth, at which time cortisone can be given orally in divided doses every 6 hours with gradual reduction of the dose to maintenance amounts. In addition, in the presence of infection, specific antibiotic therapy should be added to the preceding regimen.

Chronic adrenocortical insufficiency (Addison disease). Addison disease occurs rarely in childhood.

Etiology. In most instances there is adrenal atrophy of unknown cause (idiopathic). Tuberculosis, once the most frequent cause of Addison disease, is no longer a common etiologic factor. Rare causes include histoplasmosis, coccidioidomycosis, cryptococcosis (torulosis), mycosis fungoides, amyloidosis, and reticuloendotheliosis.

Clinical manifestations. The onset is gradual. Weakness, anorexia, and weight loss are nearly always present. Attacks of vomiting, diarrhea, and abdominal pain commonly occur sometime during the course of the disease and may simulate an acute abdominal condition. There may be episodes of hypoglycemia, and recurrent convulsions are sometimes encountered. There may be an intense craving for salt. Hyperpigmentation of the skin is present in most patients. All the body skin may be dark tan, but the pigmentation is greatest in regions exposed to the sun (face, neck, back of the hands, knuckles) and on the skin of the areolas, genital and perianal regions, elbows, creases of the palms, and operative scars. Nevi are often black. Gray or bluish pigmentation may occur on the lips, gums, tongue, or buccal mucosa. Manifestations of acute adrenocortical insufficiency (acute adrenal crisis) are common and are likely to be precipitated by acute infections and other stressful situations. Hypoparathyroidism and candidiasis (moniliasis) may be associated with Addison disease.

Laboratory findings. It is most important to establish the diagnosis before beginning therapy. Because of the availability of specific ACTH tests, methods formerly employed (sodium deprivation, potassium loading, insulin tolerance test) should not be undertaken because they are somewhat dangerous. The serum sodium and chloride levels may be low and the potassium level elevated. Hypoglycemia may be present. The most definitive test is the measurement of the 24-hour output of urinary 17-hydroxycorticosteroids before and after the administration of ACTH. The urinary 17-hydroxycorticosteroids that may be normal or decreased do not increase when ACTH is given.

Treatment. The treatment of the acute adrenal crisis that develops in the course of Addison disease demands intensive emergency treatment and is the same as has been described for other acute adrenocortical insufficiency states. Patients with chronic adrenal insufficiency require replacement therapy for their deficiencies of mineralocorticoids (aldosterone) and glucocorticoids (cortisol). Some patients with a relatively mild degree of Addison disease do satisfactorily when given substitution therapy with cortisone alone, provided there is a liberal salt intake. Cortisone acetate is administered orally in daily doses of 25 to 50 mg for adults, 25 to 37.5 mg for children, and 15 to 20 mg for infants in three equal doses. This dose should be tripled during stressful situations (severe infections, surgery, or other). Aldosterone is replaced by synthetic salt-retaining steroids given intramuscularly, subcutaneously, or orally. Deoxycorticosterone acetate (DOCA) may be given intramuscularly in single daily injections of 1 to 2 mg, or pellets of free DOC may be implanted subcutaneously every 6 to 12 months. However, oral administration of fludrocortisone, or 9-alpha-fluorohydrocortisone (Florinef), in doses of 0.05 to 0.2 mg once a day is preferred. When the patient is unable to take or retain oral medications, they must be given parenterally.

These dosages should be adjusted to suit the patient. The adequacy of therapy is determined by the maintenance of normal rates of growth and weight gain. Failure to grow may be caused either by the administration of excessive amounts of cortisone or by failure to maintain adequate electrolyte balance. A rapid gain of weight, edema, or hypertension may result from excessive doses of salt-retaining steroid. Excessive cortisone also causes the appearance of cushingoid signs.

Infants have been described with a deficiency of 18-hydroxylase and 18-OH-dehydrogenase enzymes with a resultant inability to synthesize aldosterone. Like "salt losers" with 21-hydroxylase defect (p. 583), manifestations of adrenal insufficiency usually appear during the first days or weeks of life and include anorexia, vomiting, and failure to thrive, with eventual dehydration and circulatory collapse. There is hyponatremia and hyperkalemia; in mild cases the serum sodium and potassium levels may be normal. Urinary 17-ketosteroids and pregnanetriol are normal, and aldosterone secretion rate is decreased. Treatment consists of administration of DOCA and salt.

Adrenocortical hyperfunction

The disorders that are caused by excessive production of adrenocortical hormones may be divided into those in which the predominant manifestations are related to a hypersecretion of (1) adrogenic hormones (adrenogenital syndrome), (2) cortisol (Cushing syndrome), (3) aldosterone (primary hyperaldosteronism), and (4) estrogens.

Adrenogenital syndrome. The adrenogenital syndrome results from excessive secretion of androgenic hormones by the adrenal gland.

Etiology. Overproduction of androgens may be associated either with hyperplasia of the adrenal or with tumors. Hyperplasia may be of unknown etiology, but in most cases it results from inborn deficiency of various enzymes necessary for the biosynthesis of cortisol—congenital adrenal hyperplasia (CAH). This is the commonest form of adrenal disease in infants and children. In an attempt to supply physiologic amounts of cortisol, there is an overproduction of ACTH by the pituitary gland, which in turn results in adrenocortical hyperplasia and overproduction of precursors of cortisol. At the present time five distinct enzymatic defects in the synthesis of cortisol are known—deficiency of 21-hydroxylase (the commonest cause of CAH), 11-hydroxylase, 3-beta-hydroxysteroid dehydrogenase, 17-hydroxylase, and 20,22-desmolase. For discussions on the various precursors of cortisol that are produced in increased amounts and their urinary metabolites, the reader is referred to standard textbooks of endocrinology.

Congenital adrenal hyperplasia is inherited in an autosomal recessive manner.

Clinical manifestations. Virilization results from the overproduction of androgens and incomplete masculinization from deficient production. Salt-losing manifestations are the result of deficient production of mineralocorticoids.

Girls with *congenital adrenal hyperplasia* caused by 21-hydroxylase and 11-hydroxylase defects almost always show evidences of some degree of masculinization at birth (female pseudohermaphroditism), since the disorder of steroidogenesis is present in fetal life. The masculinization is confined to the external genitalia, and the ovary, tubes, and uterus are always normal. The infant is born with an enlarged clitoris and variable degrees of labial fusion. The clitoris may be so enlarged and the labial fusion so complete that the patient is mistaken for a male with undescended testicles. For this reason the disorder should be considered in any infant with abnormalities of the external genitalia. If untreated, such a child develops pubic and axillary hair, acne appears, the voice may deepen, and there is acceleration of linear growth and epiphyseal ossification.

Boys with these defects show no obvious abnormalities at birth. However, they later show signs of excessive somatic development and precocious puberty that may not become evident until 4 or 5 years of age or later. There is enlargement of the penis, scrotum, and prostate, as well as appearance of pubic hair, development of acne, and deepening of the voice. The testes remain small in most cases.

In addition to virilization, other distinctive manifestations may be present in these patients. In about one third of the infants with the 21-hydroxylase defect, manifestations of adrenal insufficiency are seen. The symptoms usually appear during the first days or weeks of life and consist of anorexia, vomiting, diarrhea, failure to thrive or loss of weight with eventual dehydration, and circulatory collapse (salt-losing crisis). These infants are referred to as "salt losers." The aldosterone production in these infants is inadequate and probably accounts for the sodium loss. Patients with the 11-hydroxylase defect have hypertension that returns to normal levels with proper therapy (cortisone administration). The hypertension is believed to result from excessive production of DOC.

In patients with congenital adrenal hyperplasia caused by a deficiency of 17-hydroxylase, there is a deficient synthesis of hydrocortisone and androgens. The external genitalia in boys may show varying degrees of ambiguity. In girls there is no ambiguity of the external genitalia. In addition, there is an increased secretion of mineralocorticoids with resultant hypertension and hypokalemic alkalosis.

Boys with the 3-beta-hydroxysteroid dehydrogenase defect usually show incomplete masculinization (hypospadias, with or without cryptorchidism) of the external genitalia. Girls almost always show evidences of masculinization of the external genitalia. Salt-losing manifestations are frequently present in both sexes.

Male infants with the 20,22-desmolase defect have female external genitalia, since the enzymatic defect prevents synthesis of normal quantities of androgens, whereas girls have no ambiguity of the external genitalia. Also, these infants are incapable of synthesizing adequate amounts of mineralocorticoids, with resulting salt-losing crises.

Androgenic (virilizing) adrenal *tumors* result in masculinization in girls and pseudoprecocious puberty in boys. In boys the manifestations are essentially the same as those occurring with congenital adrenal hyperplasia. In girls they cause masculinization of a previously normal girl.

Laboratory findings. The urinary 17-ketosteroid levels are elevated except in the 17-hydroxylase and 20,22-desmolase defects. The urinary concentration of pregnanetriol is increased in patients with the 21-hydroxylase defect; it may be elevated in the 11-hydroxylase defect but is not elevated in the 3-beta-hydroxysteroid dehydrogenase, 17-hydroxylase, and 20,22-desmolase defects. In patients with the 21-hydroxylase and 11-hydroxylase defect, the plasma concentration of 17-OH-progesterone is increased. The urinary excretion of tetrahydro-S is increased in patients with an 11-hydroxylase defect, as is the plasma compound S concentration. In the 17-hydroxylase defect the urinary excretion of tetrahydro-B and tetrahydro-DOC is increased. In the 20,22-desmolase defect there is failure of synthesis of normal amounts of adrenal steroids. In the salt-losing form of congenital adrenal hyperplasia the serum sodium, chloride, and carbon dioxide content are low and the potassium level is elevated. The bone age is advanced; the degree depends on the age of the patient before diagnosis and treatment. The urinary 17-ketosteroids fall to normal levels in patients with congenital adrenal hyperplasia, *but not* in those with virilizing tumors, with the administration of cortisone. A buccal smear should be done on all newborn infants with ambiguous genitalia. If the results are chromatin positive, the infant should be considered a female pseudohermaphrodite with congenital adrenal hyperplasia until proved otherwise.

Treatment—congenital adrenal hyperplasia. Cortisone is used to treat patients with any of the forms of congenital adrenal hyperplasia. Its administration inhibits the production of corticotropin with a resultant decrease in production of adrenal androgens. It is given intramuscularly for the first 7 to 10 days to bring about a maximum degree of suppression of the urinary

17-ketosteroids. Children under 2 years of age are given 25 mg/24 hr and older patients 50 to 75 mg/24 hr. After attaining maximum suppression a maintenance dose of oral cortisone is administered as follows: 15 to 25 mg/24 hr to children under 2 years of age; 25 to 50 mg/24 hr to children between 2 and 6 years of age; and 50 to 75 mg/24 hr after 6 years of age. During stressful situations such as infections and operative procedures, the dose of cortisone should be tripled. The daily dose of oral cortisone should be administered at approximately 8-hour intervals because it is absorbed rapidly and is effective for only about 6 hours. In addition to cortisone, varying amounts of sodium chloride (2 to 5 g/24 hr) and DOCA (1 to 4 mg/24 hr) are given to infants with the salt-losing disorder. After the maintenance dose of DOCA is established, daily intramuscular injection is replaced by subcutaneous implantation of DOCA pellets. A 125 mg pellet of DOCA is equivalent to daily injections of about 0.5 mg of this drug and will last from 9 to 12 months. During a salt-losing crisis prompt treatment, as outlined for acute adrenal crisis, with administration of intravenous glucose with saline and hydrocortisone is necessary for survival.

Surgical removal is indicated when adrenal tumors are associated with virilization.

Cushing syndrome. Cushing syndrome is rare in childhood.

Etiology. Cushing syndrome is caused by (1) tumors of the adrenal, (2) adrenal hyperplasia, (3) extra-adrenal tumors that produce a corticotropin-like substance, or (4) ACTH-producing pituitary tumors. These pituitary tumors may not become evident until months or years after the onset of the disease.

Clinical manifestations. The predominant manifestations of this syndrome result from the maintenance of abnormally high blood levels of hydrocortisone. In addition, manifestations resulting from the excessive secretion of other adrenal hormones are sometimes present. The signs and symptoms of this syndrome include (1) obesity that characteristically spares the extremities, (2) hypertension, (3) hirsutism, (4) plethora, (5) purple striae, (6) acne, (7) enlarged clitoris, (8) easy bruisability, (9) backache (caused by osteoporosis of the spine), (10) psychoses, and (11) weakness.

Laboratory findings. There may be glycosuria and hyperglycemia with a diabetic glucose tolerance curve and a hypokalemic, hypochloremic alkalosis. The plasma and urinary levels of 17-hydroxycorticosteroids are usually elevated. Administration of dexamethasone, 1.25 mg/45 kg (100 pounds) body weight daily, at 6-hour intervals, causes the output of 17-hydroxycorticosteroids to decrease to less than 2.5 mg daily on the second day of the test in normal subjects but not in patients with Cushing syndrome. This test is valuable in differentiating obese patients with suggestive signs of Cushing syndrome, who not infrequently have slightly elevated levels of urinary 17-hydroxycorticosteroids, from patients with Cushing syndrome. The urinary concentration of 17-ketosteroids may be increased. X-ray examination may show osteoporosis of the vertebrae and enlargement of the sella turcica.

Treatment. It is often difficult to distinguish between adrenal tumor and hyperplasia; surgical exploration is frequently necessary to establish the cause, with extirpation of tumor if one is encountered. When Cushing syndrome is associated with a demonstrable pituitary tumor, hypophysectomy, x-ray therapy or the implantation of radioactive gold or yttrium should be considered. There is a lack of agreement as to the therapy of choice for bilateral hyperplasia; treatment has consisted of pituitary irradiation, subtotal adrenalectomy, and total adrenalectomy.

Hyperaldosteronism. The first case of hypersecretion of aldosterone associated with an adrenal cortical tumor was reported by Conn in 1955. Since this report, a large number of patients with the disorder has been recorded.

Etiology. In most instances excessive secretion of aldosterone is caused by one or more tumors; however, hypersecretion of aldosterone has been reported in association with adrenal hyperplasia.

Clinical manifestations. Hypersecretion of aldosterone results in hypertension, muscular weakness, polyuria, and polydipsia and at times paresthesias, periodic paralysis, tetany, and edema. In patients with bilateral hyperplasia, the hypertension may be malignant.

Laboratory findings. Usually the serum pH, carbon dioxide content, and sodium levels are elevated, and the serum potassium and chloride concentrations are decreased. The urinary excretion and plasma concentration of aldosterone is increased, with normal levels of 17-ketosteroids and 17-hydroxycorticosteroids. The kidneys are unable to concentrate urine normally.

Treatment. Tumors are removed surgically. In instances of hyperplasia, bilateral adrenalectomy is presently recommended.

Disorders of the adrenal medulla

Although no disorder of hyperplasia or hypoplasia of the adrenal medulla has been described, several types of tumors, including neuroblastoma, ganglioneuroma, and pheochromocytoma, arise from this tissue.

Pheochromocytoma. Pheochromocytoma consists of chromaffin tissue and secretes large amounts of epinephrine and/or norepinephrine. Approximately 10% of such tumors are extra-adrenal in location.

Clinical manifestations. Clinical manifestations are caused by hypersecretion of epinephrine and norepinephrine. Hypertension, which may be paroxysmal but is more often sustained, is present. Symptoms and signs associated with hypertensive attacks are anxiety, nervousness, hyperhidrosis, visual disturbances, tachycardia, headache, and peripheral vasomotor episodes. Precordial and abdominal pain, dyspnea, and convulsions may occur. Pulmonary edema and cardiac and hepatic enlargement may develop. Failure to gain weight or weight loss, polydipsia, polyuria, and polyphagia may be present.

Laboratory findings. Screening tests include the phentolamine blocking test and the histamine provocative test. Determinations of VMA (3-methoxy-4-hydroxymandelic acid) concentrations offer the most direct and conclusive tests for overactivity of the adrenal medulla.

Treatment. Treatment consists of surgical removal.

Precocious puberty

In precocious puberty, manifestations of puberty appear earlier than is to be expected. In the United States the average age of onset of puberty is 11 to 12 years in girls and 12 to 13 years in boys. However, it is not unusual for sexual development to occur as early as 8 years in girls and 9 years in boys; sexual development before these ages should be considered precocious and warrants investigation.

At the time of puberty the hypothalamic gonadotropin-releasing hormones (LRH) cause release of the gonadotropic hormones from the anterior pituitary gland, which in turn stimulate the Leydig cells of the testes to secrete testosterone and the ovarian follicles to secrete estradiol. Also, at this time, production of androgens by the adrenal cortex increases. This series of events results in normal sexual development. Precocious puberty therefore may result from a disorder of the gonad, a disorder of the adrenal cortex, or disorders in the brain that cause premature release of pituitary gonadotropins.

In addition to a detailed history and careful examination, the following procedures are undertaken in evaluation of these patients: radiographs of the skull, a skeletal survey to determine bone age and to search for the osseous lesions of polyostotic fibrous dysplasia, a vaginal smear to determine estrogen effect, and urinary 17-ketosteroids. In selected cases additional evaluation includes urinary pregnanediol, pregnanetriol, estrogens, and gonadotropins; computerized axial tomography of the head; pelvic sonography; rectoabdominal examination under anesthesia; and testicular biopsy.

The disorders that cause premature pubertal development may be divided into true precocious puberty and precocious pseudopuberty or incomplete precocious puberty.

True precocious puberty. When there is premature activation of the entire hypothalamic-pituitary-gonadal axis, the pituitary gonadotropins cause development and maturation of the gonads (increase in gonadal size and gametogenesis) and secretion of sex hormones with development of secondary sexual characteristics. True, or complete, precocious puberty results and is always isosexual.

True precocious puberty may be associated with a variety of disorders, or it may be idiopathic. Organic brain lesions include tumors, postencephalitic and postmeningitic lesions, tuberous sclerosis, neurofibromatosis, and hydrocephalus. Craniopharyngioma is an exceedingly rare cause and more often results in sexual infantilism. Hamartoma (hyperplastic group of cells) of the tuber cinereum, unaccompanied by other neurologic manifestations, has been found at autopsy in some cases of sexual precocity. Signs of other hypothalamic dysfunction may be present, such as polydipsia, polyphagia, obesity, sleep disturbances, disturbances in temperature regulation, and emotional instability. Manifestations of increased intracranial pressure or visual disturbances may occur. Since a small and slow-growing tumor may initially produce no signs other than sexual precocity, a prolonged period of thorough observation may be necessary before neurologic manifestations appear. A carefully taken history and physical examination together with radiographs of the skull, electroencephalography, and if indicated, computerized axial tomography of the head should establish the diagnosis of these lesions. Treatment depends on the type of lesion and its location.

McCune-Albright syndrome, consisting of polyostotic fibrous dysplasia of bone and irregular areas of cutaneous pigmentation, is frequently associated with true precocious puberty and occurs almost exclusively in girls. Facial asymmetry may be present. Diffuse or nodular enlargement of the thyroid with or without hyperthyroidism is frequently found. The levels of serum calcium and phosphorus are normal. Radiographs may reveal increased density of the base of the skull or thickening of facial bones, in addition to disseminated areas of osseous rarefaction. The cause of the precocity is not known but is thought to be a congenital defect of the hypothalamus with resultant early release of pituitary gonadotropins.

Hypothyroidism associated with sexual precocity has been encountered. Menstruation has occurred and galactorrhea may be present. Unlike other forms of sexual prococity, there is retardation of linear growth and osseous maturation, as is to be expected with hypothyroidism. Treatment with thyroid hormone results in regression of sexual precocity. It has been postulated that the excessive secretion of thyrotropic hormone that occurs with hypothyroidism is accompanied by an "overlapping" oversecretion of gonadotropins.

Hepatoblastoma is a rare cause of precocious puberty. The tumor is highly malignant, and it has been reported only in males. Gonadotropins have been detected in the urine or blood. It appears that the tumor secretes gonadotropins, which stimulate the Leydig cells to secrete testosterone. Hepatomegaly or a right upper quadrant mass is present. Treatment is surgical, followed by radiation and anticarcinogenic agents.

Choriocarcinomas may secrete excessive amounts of chorionic gonadotropins with resultant precocious puberty. They have occurred in boys in the area of the pineal gland and in girls in the ovary. High levels of urinary chorionic gonadotropins may be present. The tumor is usually highly malignant.

In a large proportion of cases of precocious puberty (approximately 90% of girls with true precocious puberty and 50% of boys with both true and pseudopuberty), no cause can be found. These have been called idiopathic or constitutional precocious puberty. It has been reported as a familial occurrence. Since the diagnosis is made by exclusion, a prolonged period of observation is necessary to exclude an organic cause. As is the case in any type of sexual precocity, there is early acceleration of linear growth and osseous maturation with ultimate early epiphyseal fusion and shortness of stature. Proper psychologic management of the patient and family is the most important aspect of treatment. Medroxyprogesterone acetate, a compound that inhibits gonadotropin production, has been used for treatment of this disorder. This drug needs critical evaluation before its use can be generally recommended as a safe form of therapy. The synthetic antiandrogenic agent cyproterone acetate, which also has progestational properties, has also been used for treatment of this disorder.

Precocious pseudopuberty. Cases of precocious pseudopuberty differ from those of true sexual precocity in that early secretion of gonadotropins does not occur; there is early overproduction of sex hormone by a tumor of the ovary or testis, or by a tumor or hyperplasia of the adrenal. Exogenous androgens or estrogens may also cause this type of precocious sexual development. As is to be expected, the gonads do not develop or mature (no increase in gonadal size or gametogenesis); only secondary sexual characteristics appear. Also, unlike the conditions just discussed in which sexual precocity is always isosexual, the sex hormone that is produced or administered may at times cause heterosexual precocity. For example, androgen-producing tumors in a girl result in precocity inappropriate for a female (clitoral hypertrophy, masculinization, etc.).

Ovarian tumor is a rare cause of sexual precocity. The most commonly encountered neoplasm is the granulosa cell tumor. The tumor is palpable on rectoabdominal examination in most instances. Ascites may be present. Although the isosexual precocity is caused by estrogen production by the tumor, urinary estrogen levels may not be elevated; in most cases normal adult levels are present. There are rare reports of ovarian teratomas, and they resemble the granulosa cell tumor clinically and hormonally. Ovarian thecoma is associated with isosexual precocity, and the levels of urinary pregnanediol may be increased. The neoplasm is seldom palpable. Arrhenoblastomas of the ovary are rare. They cause heterosexual precocity (clitoral enlargement, masculinization) and variable elevations of urinary 17-ketosteroids.

Leydig cell tumor of the testis is a rare cause of sexual precocity. Gynecomastia may be present. The tumor is usually unilateral and palpable, and the contralateral testis is infantile. Excretion of urinary 17-ketosteroids is variable (normal to elevated). The concentration of testosterone in the plasma is increased and does not fall with the administration of hydrocortisone.

Adrenocortical tumors have been associated with overproduction of estrogens or androgens. With the overproduction of estrogens, isosexual precocity in females and heterosexual precocity in males result. The excretion of urinary 17-ketosteroids is usually elevated and is not suppressed by the administration of hydrocortisone. The overproduction of androgen associated with congenital adrenal hyperplasia results in isosexual precocity in males and heterosexual precocity in females.

A careful history must be taken to rule out the possibility of precocity caused by exogenous estrogens, such as the ingestion of birth control pills and the application of estrogen-containing skin creams, or by exogenous androgens. Pigmented nipples are associated with the ingestion of stilbestrol, which is one of the most commonly used estrogens. It must be remembered that none of the anabolic steroids is devoid of androgenic action and would be expected to produce some degree of virilization in both sexes.

Finally, it should be stressed that vaginal bleeding in the absence of secondary sexual development should alert the physician to the possibility of a foreign body in the vagina or of vaginitis, especially if there is a foul discharge. Also, premature thelarche (p. 613) and premature pubarche (p. 613) should not be confused with sexual precocity.

Alvro M. Camacho

Metabolic disturbances

ABNORMALITIES OF CARBOHYDRATE METABOLISM

Insulin-dependent diabetes mellitus

Insulin-dependent diabetes mellitus (also known as juvenile-onset, or type I, diabetes) usually but not always begins before 15 years of age. Although constituting only 8% to 10% of all instances of diabetes, it presents disproportionate problems. Sixty percent of all the cases occur in patients between the ages of 4 and 12 years. Sex distribution between boys and girls is similar.

Insulin-dependent diabetes mellitus is not to be confused with impaired glucose tolerance, characterized by fasting glucose in venous plasma of less than 140 mg/dl and a glucose level of greater than 140 mg/dl at 2 hours following a standard oral glucose tolerance test with 1.75 g glucose/kg up to a maximum of 75 g.

The following characteristics depict the natural history of insulin-dependent diabetes and serve to point out some of the differences from non–insulin-dependent (maturity-onset, or type II) diabetes:

1. Onset is rapid with progression to severe ketoacidosis and possibly coma in a matter of hours or days. The mean duration of symptoms before diagnosis and treatment is 30 days at Le Bonheur Children's Medical Center.
2. Usually within 3 months after initiation of insulin therapy, there tends to be a temporary remission of the diabetic state, commonly referred to as the "honeymoon period." The diabetic state then progresses over a 1- to 5-year period to complete insulin insufficiency. A few patients may continue to produce some insulin for more than 10 years.
3. Insulin replacement is required. Oral hypoglycemic agents are contraindicated.
4. Variations in insulin response are great, with significant swings from hypoglycemia to hyperglycemia influenced by activ-

ity, emotional state, exercise, food, and numerous factors that influence the absorption and/or bioavailability of insulin.
5. Omission of insulin promptly results in extreme hyperglycemia, and within 24 to 48 hours ketoacidosis usually develops.
6. Exercise exerts a definite lowering effect on blood glucose levels particularly if the exercise occurs within a few hours after the subcutaneous injection of regular insulin.
7. Complications occur in a majority of patients with type I diabetes within 20 years after onset, and their rate of progression is rapid. Early manifestations of complications are associated with thickening of glomerular mesangium and capillary basement membranes. This may be reversible if detected early and if good metabolic control is established and maintained.
8. In addition to problems of regulation associated with the lability of type I diabetes, management proves to be difficult in some patients because of poor cooperation associated with immaturity and inadequate insight, as well as a high incidence of infections with anorexia, vomiting, and so on.
9. Psychologic repercussions in the parents and child are frequent.

Etiology

The exact cause of diabetes is not established, but genetic influences play a definite role. It has been established by twin studies that idiopathic diabetes mellitus constitutes a genetically heterogeneous group of disorders. Histocompatibility (HLA) studies have permitted a separation of insulin-dependent from non–insulin-dependent diabetes.

There appears to be heterogeneity within type I diabetes that can be subdivided into at least two subtypes by HLA typing, B8, or Dw3, and B15, or Dw4. Type I diabetes with HLA-B8 is associated with persistent islet-cell antibodies and other autoimmune endocrine diseases, whereas type I diabetes with HLA-B15 is not. If one parent has type I diabetes, less than 10% of the offspring will have type I diabetes. If one child in the family has diabetes, the risk of a sibling developing the disease is 5% to 10%; in monozygotic twins the risk of developing diabetes is about 30% for the nondiabetic twin. The mode of inheritance is not a settled issue.

Other factors that cause hyperglycemia include adrenal hypercorticism (Cushing syndrome), hyperpituitarism, and hyperthyroidism, as well as congenital defects of the pancreas, exhaustion of islet tissue, infections, and toxins such as Vacor rat poison. In recent years, obesity and peripheral resistance to insulin action from alterations in insulin binding to cells or postreceptor defects have been related to the incidence of type II diabetes and glucose intolerance.

An intriguing hypothesis relates to the possible role of viral infections, especially coxsackie virus B, mumps, and rubella, to the onset of type I diabetes. HLA genes are known to be located near immune response genes in mice and are thought to have the same relationship to human response genes on chromosome number 6. Thus it can be hypothesized that there is a genetic predisposition to develop insulin-dependent diabetes mellitus but that some unknown insult must occur that triggers the appropriate and genetically controlled immune response, resulting in islet destruction. The genetic predisposition to diabetes, the immune response, and/or environmental factors are needed to develop insulin-dependent diabetes mellitus. There is some evidence that a virus infection is the unknown insult, whereby new or modified host antigens may be produced and lead to autoimmunization. At the onset of type I diabetes 85% of sera contain antibodies to pancreatic islet cells. However, it is not serum antibodies but cellular immunity, which resides in the lymphocytes and macrophages, that causes the damage. The nature of the islet antigens to which the potential diabetic person becomes autoimmunized have not yet been characterized.

Pathophysiology

The altered metabolic state in diabetes is extensive and not entirely understood. Because of a deficiency of endogenous insulin (failure of synthesis or secretion, abnormal insulins, accelerated degradation, inactive forms, altered tissue binding, or postreceptor defects) glucose use by tissues is impaired and hyperglycemia occurs. Hepatic glycogen synthesis is decreased, and reserves are depleted. Gluconeogenesis is accelerated, and tissue proteins and body fats are catabolized, releasing K^+ and phosphates. Fatty acid synthesis is decreased, and acetyl-CoA production is increased. As a consequence, beta-hydroxybutyric acid and acetoacetic acid are formed at a rate faster than the tissues are capable of using them, and ketonemia with metabolic acidosis occurs. Sodium and potassium are lost in the urine. The hyperglycemia and increase in ketone bodies result in an osmotic diuresis, and large amounts of water as well as electrolytes are lost, with subsequent dehydration, hemoconcentration, and altered renal function.

Clinical manifestations

Clinical manifestations appear suddenly. The early clinical signs and symptoms of diabetes, frequently ushered in by infection, include polyuria, polydipsia, polyphagia, and rapid weight loss. Polyuria and thirst usually appear first. Bed-wetting may be an early symptom in 50% of the patients. Vulvitis is not a frequent early sign in our experience. Ketoacidosis is characterized by dehydration with dry skin, sunken soft eyeballs, sunken fontanel, Kussmaul respiratory pattern, lethargy and somnolence, hypothermia, and tachycardia, which may progress to shock. Abdominal pain, nausea, and vomiting are frequently present.

Laboratory findings

In a patient with untreated diabetes the laboratory findings are as follows: Hyperglycemia with blood sugar frequently greater than 300 mg/dl, glycosuria, and ketosis (ketonemia and ketonuria) are present. Dehydration is found and is usually hypertonic. Uncompensated metabolic acidosis occurs (plasma-base bicarbonate less than 15 mEq/L and pH reduced). Plasma sodium level is variable, with total body deficit. Plasma potassium level is variable (frequently elevated), with a significant body deficit caused by transfer of K^+ out of cells associated with the acidosis, glycogen depletion, and dehydration. This significant loss of potassium must be replaced in therapy of ketoacidosis. Plasma chloride level may be diminished or only slightly elevated, despite a base bicarbonate deficit with an anion gap because of ketonemia and loss of chloride. BUN is elevated. Plasma phosphate levels are normal in the dehydrated state despite body need; the levels decrease during treatment. Plasma glucagon and cortisol levels are elevated before and during the early phase of treatment. Urinalysis shows acid reaction, high specific gravity, glycosuria, and ketonuria. When dehydration and ketoacidosis are present, the hemogram reveals an elevation of hemoglobin and hematocrit levels. Polymorphonuclear leukocytosis is a finding. Serum amylase may be elevated.

Diagnostic tests

Diagnostic tests, including urinalysis and random plasma glucose greater than 200 mg/dl usually suffice in the symptomatic patient. Plasma insulin levels may be of value in the early stages of the disease. The oral glucose tolerance test should be reserved for doubtful cases or patients with asymptomatic hyperglycemia. Fig. 22-2 shows the normal range of plasma glucose levels during oral glucose tolerance tests in the children we have studied. Fasting blood glucose levels are elevated to 140 mg/dl or higher. The glucose tolerance test (frequently unnecessary and to be discouraged) shows a prolonged abnormal elevation, with the 2-hour value and at least one intervening venous plasma glucose value of 200 mg/dl or higher. Postprandial blood glucose levels usually suffice and may be correlated with fasting blood glucose levels.

Differential diagnosis

In differential diagnosis the following conditions must be considered: (1) salicylism; (2) lead intoxication; (3) cerebral injury, infection, or neoplasm; (4) Cushing syndrome; (5) galactosemia and other melliturias; (6) hyperthyroidism with glycosuria; (7) glucosuria in the absence of hyperglycemia, as seen in renal glycosuria and other renal tubular defects; (8) carbohydrate ingestion following periods of decreased caloric intake; (9) conditions associated with K^+ depletion; and (10) non–insulin-dependent type of diabetes in young patients.

Patients may be categorized in stages according to degree of hyperglycemia and disturbance in acid-base balance. The clinical status of the

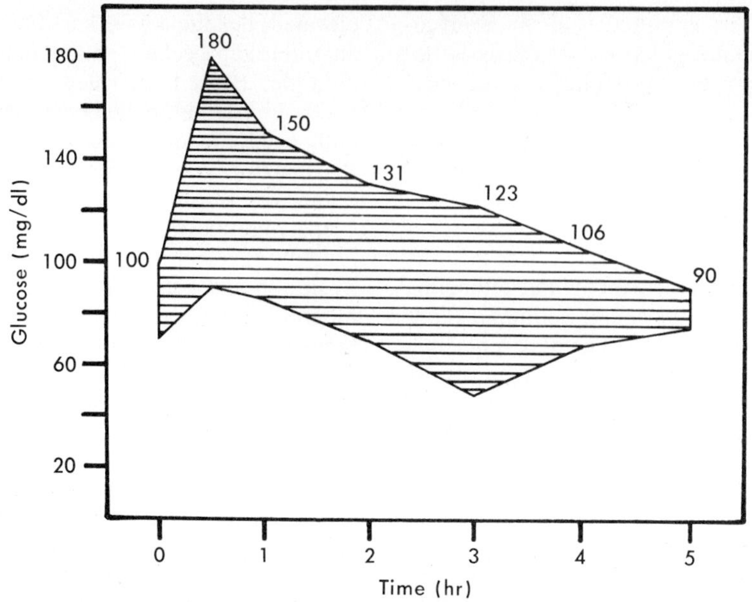

Fig. 22-2. Normal range of plasma glucose (glucose oxidase) during oral glucose tolerance test of forty children, ages 1 year 8 months to 16 years 6 months. To make the diagnosis of impaired glucose tolerance, using the classification of the National Diabetes Data Group, the venous plasma fasting glucose level must be less than 140 mg/dl and the 2-hour OGTT glucose value must be greater than 140 mg/dl. To use this criterion, the patient must have received a high-carbohydrate diet for 3 days before testing, test must be done in the morning, patient must be nonobese, and 1.75 g/kg (maximum, 75 g) of glucose must be used.

patient is equally important in determining treatment.

Stage I
- Glycosuria without ketonuria; minimal dehydration
- Fasting blood glucose >140 mg/dl but <300 mg/dl
- HCO_3^- > 15 mEq/L
- Blood pH—normal range
- Not acidotic clinically

Stage II
- Glycosuria and ketonuria without significant acidosis
- Fasting blood glucose >300 mg/dl
- HCO_3^- > 15 mEq/L
- Blood pH 7.30 to 7.45

Stage III
- Glycosuria, ketonuria, and significant acidosis (Kussmaul respiration, dehydrated skin and subcutaneous tissue, lethargy, etc.)
- Blood glucose usually >300 mg/dl
- HCO_3^- < 15 mEq/L
- Blood pH 7.10 to 7.30

Stage IV
- Glycosuria, ketonuria, with severe acisosis and impending coma or coma
- Blood glucose 500 to 750 mg/dl or higher
- HCO_3^- < 10 mEq/L
- Blood pH <7.10

Management

General considerations for hospital patients. Soon after admission, blood should be obtained for measurements of plasma glucose, ketones, Na^+, K^+, Cl^-, HCO_3^-, BUN, and pH. As stated previously, the oral glucose tolerance test should not be performed unless the diagnosis is questioned. A complete blood cell count and urinalysis are essential. If the patient is in ketoacidosis, vital signs, state of consciousness, intake, output, plasma glucose, Na^+, K^+, HCO_3^-, and blood pH should be monitored at hourly intervals for 4 hours, then every 2 hours until ketoacidosis has cleared. During ketoacidosis it may be necessary to insert an indwelling catheter *aseptically* into the bladder of infants and younger children to obtain urine. Semiquantitative blood glucose levels may be estimated with Dextrostix with a reflectance meter, or with Chemstrip bG with or without a meter. Although potentially of value, plasma electrolyte determinations in stage I and II patients need not be required beyond the time of initial evaluation. Parenteral fluid therapy is not required in the milder cases unless nausea and vomiting occur.

In stages III and IV patients with evidence of circulatory collapse, intravenous administration of 20 ml/kg physiologic saline or plasma should be given rapidly. Dextran must *not* be used because of interference with chemical determinations of glucose levels.

Initial therapy including insulin and fluids in stages III and IV patients should be given intravenously.

During the early phase of treatment, patients should be evaluated by a physician every 2 hours or more often if indicated.

Complete reexamination of the patient is necessary after hydration, and signs of infection should be sought.

The psychologic aspects relative to the parents and child should be considered at the time of hospitalization and throughout management.

Specific measures for hospitalized patients

Stages I and II

Fluids. In stages I and II parenteral fluids are usually unnecessary. However, if the patient is anorectic, maintenance parenteral fluids may be given for the first 6 to 12 hours, calculated in the amount of 1500 to 2400 ml/m^2/24 hr. See Chapter 10 for the principles and specifics of fluid and electrolyte therapy in children. Table 22-2 gives the composition of a replacement and maintenance fluid, or 5% Dextrose in Electrolyte Solution No. 75 can be used with intravenous insulin if plasma electrolytes are normal.

Table 22-2. Composition of replacement and maintenance fluid (omit dextrose when not desired)*

Formula	Concentration
Na^+	77 mEq/L
K^+	35 mEq/L
Cl^-	95 mEq/L
Phosphate	12 mM/L
Glucose	5 g/dl

*This solution may be prepared as follows: One-half strength physiologic NaCl solution—1000 ml, 35 mEq K^+ (½ as KCl; ½ as $K\text{-}PO_4$).

Insulin. In patients with mild alterations, insulin therapy—a mixture of isophane, or NPH (70%), and regular (30%)—may be given to start treatment. Usually an initial dose of 0.2 unit/kg regular insulin is given subcutaneously or intramuscularly, followed by 0.7 to 1 unit/kg/24 hr of the mixture in two divided doses, beginning with two thirds of the daily dose 15 to 30 minutes before breakfast and the remaining third 15 to 30 minutes before supper. This ratio may be altered, if necessary, to meet individual needs. As control is established, normoglycemia is approached, and glucosuria completely disappears, the insulin dose is decreased by decrements of 10%. During the honeymoon period the required dose of insulin may range from 0.1 to 0.4 unit/kg/24 hr. Even with normal 2-hour postprandial blood glucose levels (without insulin), insulin therapy should not be discontinued because in our experience this will shorten the honeymoon period.

As this book goes to press, a NIH-supported multicenter project is underway to determine if intensive insulin therapy using multiple injections of insulin daily or insulin infusion pumps can normalize or improve the metabolic abnormalities seen in type I diabetes. If successful, the next phase of the study will attempt to determine if intensive insulin therapy will prevent or retard the vascular complications. For more details on intensive insulin therapy see the discussion on long-term management.

Diet. As stated previously, parenteral fluids are usually unnecessary in stage I and II patients. The American Diabetes Association (ADA) diet of 1500 kcal/m^2 or 1000 kcal + 100 kcal/year of age should be started promptly, 30%-30%-30% of calories with major meals and 10% as a bedtime snack. For boys over 10 years of age, 200 kcal/year of age may be required for normal growth and to satisfy the appetite. For girls the total caloric intake should not exceed 1800 to 2500 kcal/24 hr unless physical activity is great. (See discussion on long-term management, pp. 593 to 595.)

Stages III and IV. The major aims of early therapy of ketoacidosis, characteristic of these stages, are to replace depleted fluids and electrolytes, to correct the acidosis and hyperglycemia, and to treat shock and/or infection if present.

Fluids. All fluids and insulin are given as continuous intravenous infusions. Two milliliters of a 25% solution (500 mg) of human serum albumin are added to each flask of "hydrating" or "replacement and maintenance" fluids containing insulin to prevent adsorption to glass bottles or plastic containers and tubing. Alternate methods to the use of albumin are (1) infuse the insulin in a more concentrated form (10 units/cc) via pediatric infusion set or syringe pump or (2) allow the first 50 ml of insulin-containing fluid to run through the infusion tubing to saturate the adsorption sites with insulin. Since about one third of the insulin added to a bottle of fluids is adsorbed to the glass if albumin is not present, the dosage of insulin should be doubled to ensure adequate insulin administration when using this method.

INITIAL HYDRATING FLUID (see Table 22-3 for composition). The initial hydrating fluid is given in the amount of 400 ml/m^2 body surface area (SA), infused over a 2-hour period. If the arterial pH is less than 7.0, 1 mEq/kg body weight of additional sodium bicarbonate is infused over a 15-minute period. If necessary, this dose of sodium bicarbonate is repeated in 30 minutes to raise the arterial blood pH to 7.1 or above. Although these small quantities of bicarbonate are not likely to change oxygen transport, overcorrection of pH should be avoided. If the patient initially has vascular collapse, 20 ml/kg body weight of normal saline or plasma are given rapidly intravenously before the hydrating fluid (Table 22-3) is started.

REPLACEMENT AND MAINTENANCE FLUIDS (see Table 22-2 for composition). In the absence of oliguria, the replacement and maintenance fluids are given at a rate of 3600 ml/m^2/24 hr. This fluid contains phosphate, an important ion to be replenished. We have not observed symptomatic or laboratory evidence of hypocalcemia.

Table 22-3. Composition of initial hydrating fluid (omit dextrose when not desired)*

Formula	Concentration
Na^+	123 mEq/L
HCO_3^-	50 mEq/L
Cl^-	73 mEq/L
Glucose	5 g/dl if blood glucose <300 mg/dl No glucose if blood glucose >300 mg/dl

*This solution may be prepared as follows: 7.5% $NaHCO_3$ solution—56 ml; one-half strength physiologic NaCl solution—944 ml alone or in 5% glucose.

However, if severe hypokalemic is being treated K^+ should be given as KCl. When the blood glucose falls below 200 mg/dl, sufficient glucose should be added to the intravenous fluids to raise the glucose content of the fluid to 5 g/dl. The blood glucose should be maintained between 150 and 250 mg/dl. If the blood sugar drops below 100 mg/dl while the 5% glucose and electrolyte solution is being given, the intravenous insulin is stopped until the blood glucose increases above 150 mg/dl.

Insulin. Regular (crystalline) insulin is added to each bottle of initial hydrating fluid and the replacement and maintenance fluids. The amount of insulin is calculated to deliver 0.1 unit/kg/hr. If the intravenous fluids do not contain albumin, 0.2 unit/kg/hr of regular insulin is infused. An initial dose of regular insulin (0.2 unit/kg) is given by intravenous push. If after 1 hour of infusion the blood glucose has not dropped by 10%, then 0.2 unit/kg regular insulin is given as a bolus, followed by the same rate of infusion (0.1 unit/kg/hr). If after 2 hours the blood glucose has not fallen by 10%, insulin resistance should be considered, and larger doses of insulin should be administered (at the rate of 1 unit/kg/hr) by continuous intravenous infusion. When the blood glucose decreases to 200 mg/dl, 5% glucose is added to the intravenous fluids. If the blood glucose falls below 150 mg/dl, the insulin is reduced in the intravenous fluids to 0.05 units/kg/hr.

Other measures and mangement during the acidotic period

1. Monitor blood glucose every 1 to 2 hours until ketoacidosis has cleared.
2. Monitor mental status, temperature, pulse, blood pressure, and rate and depth of respirations.
3. Monitor plasma electrolytes (particularly K^+, Na^+ and HCO_3^-) and arterial blood gases.
4. A complete reevaluation of the patient must be done after hydration to seek signs of infection.

Complications of therapy

1. Cerebral edema. Risk factors include new case of diabetes, hyponatremia, fever of unknown origin and intravenous fluid administration at a rate greater than 4000 ml/m^2/day.
2. Central nervous system acidosis.
3. Hyperchloremic acidosis.
4. Lactic acidosis.
5. Hypernatremia.
6. Hypokalemia.
7. Hypoglycemia.

Treatment following ketoacidosis. Management during the early postacidotic stage consists of establishing appropriate dietary intake while discontinuing intravenous insulin, fluids, and electrolytes and while converting to subcutaneous insulin administration. Because the biologic half-life of insulin is only 4 to 8 minutes, when intravenous insulin is stopped subcutaneous insulin must be started or ketoacidosis will rapidly recur. If doubt exists concerning oral intake of food, the patient may be maintained with parenteral fluid, 1500 ml/m²/24 hr of electrolyte solution number 75, without added insulin during the early phase of feeding. If the serum ketones are present in less than 1:4 dilution, patients usually will accept and retain the ADA diet. From this point, the insulin and diet routine of the patient may be handled in a manner similar to that described for patients in stages I and II (p. 591). However, the insulin requirement at this point may be much higher in patients who have had severe ketoacidosis than in those patients in stages I and II until treatment has been continued for several days.

Long-term management

Adequate control is accomplished when 80% of the preprandial blood glucose values done by Chemstrip bG or Dextrostix with a meter are between 60 and 130 mg/dl and the 2 hour postprandial blood glucose values are less than 180 mg/dl. Glycosolated hemoglobin (Hb A_{1c}), a conjugate of hemoglobin A and glucose, when abnormally high indicates inadequate control for several weeks. Normal values in our laboratory range from 3% to 7.4% of total hemoglobin concentration. We consider a concentration of 8.5% or less in diabetic patients to indicate good control, greater than 8.5% to 11% fair control, and greater than 11%, poor control. Several reports, in addition to our observations, indicate that determinations of Hb A_{1c} levels at 90-day intervals are of great value for following long-term control of diabetes.

Insulin therapy. Insulin requirements are variable but usually do not exceed 0.7 to 1.2 unit/kg/24 hr. As mentioned previously, we recommend mixtures of 30% regular and 70% NPH insulin given twice daily as previously described. Table 22-4 lists characteristics of available types of insulin. The quantity of NPH or regular insulin can be altered depending on the results of self–blood glucose monitoring. To control the blood glucose, more than 2 injections of insulin daily are sometimes required, or portable continuous subcutaneous insulin infusion pumps may be used. It should be kept in mind when using intensive insulin therapy that there is increased risk for potentially dangerous hy-

Table 22-4. Types of insulin and their action

Type of insulin	Time of administration	Onset of action	Peak effect	Duration of action	Probable glycosuria	Probable hypoglycemia	Remarks
Crystalline or regular*	20 minutes before meals subcutaneously, intramuscularly, or intravenously	Within 1 hour	2 hours	6-8 hours	Night	10 AM-12 noon	
Isophane* (NPH)	40-60 minutes before† breakfast subcutaneously	1-2 hours	8-12 hours	18-24 hours	10 AM-12 noon; before breakfast	3-6 PM	
Lente‡	45-60 minutes before† breakfast subcutaneously	2 hours	8-12 hours	20-26 hours	10 AM-12 noon	3-6 PM	Contains no protamine; useful in insulin allergy

*Human insulin of recombinant DNA origin (regular and NPH) when compared to insulin of animal origin has a slightly faster onset of action and is slightly shorter in duration of action.
†When mixed with crystalline insulin, the mixture should be given 15-30 minutes before breakfast or supper.
‡To prevent the loss of the fast acting effect of regular insulin, the insulin mixture should be injected within 5 minutes of loading the syringe unless Mixtard (Nordisk) insulin is used; it is a stable mixture of 70% NPH, 30% regular pork insulin.

poglycemia. When using more than 2 injections of insulin daily approximately one fourth of the total daily dose is given as regular insulin before the three major meals and the remaining one fourth is given as NPH insulin with the injection given at supper or at bedtime. Further adjustments in insulin dosage can be made using self–blood glucose monitoring. Physicians considering the use of intensive insulin therapy should read the article by Skyler et al. Patients using self–blood glucose monitoring have developed ketoacidosis without having marked hyperglycemia. Therefore, to prevent this complication, urine ketones should be checked with Acetest tablets anytime the blood glucose is greater than 240 mg/dl, the patient has an illness, or does not feel well. Doses of insulin greater than 1 unit/kg/24 hr (sometimes less) may result in reactive hyperglycemia (Somogyi effect) and indicate the need for reduced dose of insulin. When doing urine testing, results should be recorded not less than twice daily, particularly before breakfast and supper or more often in the presence of polyuria, polydipsia, or stressful periods.

Insulin requirements are frequently, but not always, increased during infection. Under these conditions 0.1 to 0.2 unit/kg regular insulin is given at mealtimes or at 2 hour intervals if needed, in addition to the usual daily doses of insulin mixture.

As the patient gains tolerance, the insulin dose is decreased by 10% decrements. Similarly, the dose of insulin may be increased when control of diabetes diminishes, as indicated by glycosuria, hyperglycemia, and elevated Hb A_{1c} levels.

Periods of remission early during the course of the disease are variable, with the need for insulin progressively increasing as the child reaches adolescence. Failure to recognize this possibility will lead to the development of hyperglycemia and ketosis. Under these circumstances the daily dose of insulin may exceed 1 unit/kg/24 hr. However, caution must be exercised in preventing reactive hyperglycemia (Somogyi effect).

Dynamic exercise is essential in maintaining control and should be practiced as a daily routine. Intermittent strenuous exercise requires additional calories, rather than a reduction in the dose of insulin. For 2 to 3 hours of such exercise, it is recommended that extra food consisting of 10% of the basic diet be ingested before or during the exercise. Regular strenuous exercise, however, will result in a 10% to 25% reduction of insulin dosage as well as an increase in caloric intake.

Diet. We recommend the use of *Exchange Lists for Meal Planning* by the ADA, which is ideal from a nutritional point of view. We have been using a diet that supplies 20%, 50%, and 30% of the calories as protein, carbohydrate, and fat, respectively. This diet supplies 160 g of available glucose and 50 g of protein per 1000 kcal. Polyunsaturated fats should be selected when available, such as corn oil and liquid margarine. Skimmed milk eliminates a major source of animal fat. The physician, parents, and, if possible, the child should be thoroughly familiar with the exchange system, since it permits a wide range of food selections. This system is available through local chapters of the ADA or from its national headquarters.* For obvious reasons, measured portions of food are preferable to weighed portions.

Caloric allowances. Basic caloric requirements for 24 hours may be determined by using age or surface area, as follows:

1. On the basis of age, allow 1000 kcal for the first year of life, plus 100 kcal for each additional year of age.
2. According to surface area, allow 1500 kcal/m^2.

The maximal daily caloric intake with normal activity usually ranges from 1800 to 2000 kcal for girls and from 1800 to 2400 kcal for boys. When patients are engaging in strenuous work or competitive sports, an additional 200 kcal are allowed every 2 or 3 hours or 10% of 24-hour caloric intake, depending on size of the patient and degree of activity, with a 24-hour intake as high as 3600 to 4000 kcal in older boys. Less optimally, the insulin dosage may be reduced. It is essential to prevent obesity. Ideally, weight should be kept in the normal range proportionate to height. The appropriate diet is one that satisfies the appetite when the patient is under good control and permits ideal growth.

Distribution of calories throughout the day. It is important to consider the normal dietary

*2 park Avenue, New York, NY, 10016.

habits of the child. Ideally, 30% of the calories is allowed at each of the three major meals (7 to 8 AM, 12 to 12:30 PM, 5:30 to 6 PM) and 10% as a snack at 9:00 to 9:30 PM. Frequently, especially in younger children and with activity, midmorning and midafternoon snacks are required. Thus the caloric distribution would be 25% of the calories for each of the major meals, 5% as a midmorning snack, and 10% each as midafternoon and bedtime snacks.

Temporary mild hyperglycemia with glycosuria, in the absence of the Somogyi effect, is tolerated. Complete absence of glycosuria, except during periods of temporary remissions (honeymoon period), is impractical if not impossible to achieve and is unwise if recurrent hypoglycemia, reactive hyperglycemia (Somogyi effect), and psychologic and behavior problems are to be prevented. Repeated episodes of moderate or severe hyperglycemia and ketosis are to be avoided.

Insulin-induced hypoglycemia (insulin reactions), characterized by weakness, headache, pallor, diplopia, sweating, and twitching, is managed by giving sugar, orange juice, milk, or sweetened beverages. If the reaction is severe with loss of consciousness or inability to swallow, glucagon in doses of 1 mg is given subcutaneously, intramuscularly, or intravenously.

Other measures. Measures in addition to insulin therapy and dietary control are recommended. Education of the parents and the child in the problems related to health care and control of diabetes is essential, and will be discussed later with other educational aspects related to total care of the child patient and parents.

The child should be protected against infections insofar as possible, and treatment should be initiated early if they occur. Prophylactic antimicrobial agents are not indicated.

Before surgery and during surgery, maintenance fluids should be administered as outlined on p. 591. Crystalline insulin is usually preferable, and the dosage is adjusted according to the blood glucose results. The urine and blood glucose levels are followed carefully (1) as guides to the adequacy of the insulin dosage and (2) to prevent hypoglycemia with adequate glucose-containing fluid. Postoperatively insulin is given in dosage as governed by glucose content of parenteral fluid therapy, by ability to tolerate the diet, by degree of activity, and so on. Intermediate-acting insulin mixtures used before surgery may be advantageous, depending on the surgical procedure and anticipated caloric intake. The dose may be reduced to as little as 50% of the usual daily dose and complemented by the addition of 0.1 to 0.2 unit/kg regular insulin every 4 to 6 hours. The physician should observe carefully for ketosis and reevaluate insulin dosage and fluid therapy as indicated.

Educational aspects

Because the major responsibility for long-term management of diabetes must lie with the patient and family, teaching the patient about diabetes and how to control it is imperative. The educational program should begin in the hospital as soon as the diagnosis is confirmed and continue during each outpatient visit. The major areas of instruction include general information about diabetes, meal planning, urine testing for glucose and ketones, self–blood glucose monitoring, insulin and adjustment, exercise, general health care, sick day regimen, acute and chronic complications, and community resources. The family and its needs should be evaluated and counseling given as indicated.

Diabetes education should begin as soon as the diagnosis is confirmed. After informing the family and child of the diagnosis and treatment plan, the diabetes education program should be outlined, questions answered, and psychologic support given. An excellent pamphlet entitled *Your Child and Diabetes...What You Should Know* is very helpful to the parents and can be obtained from the ADA.

After the ketoacidosis has been cleared and the emotional tone of the situation has improved, the education program is accelerated. General information about diabetes mellitus and its management is given, such as the prevalence of diabetes, possible causes, and general principles of management. An explanation concerning the differences between non–insulin-dependent and insulin-dependent diabetes mellitus will be helpful in imparting an understanding of why, for instance, insulin injections are necessary rather than an oral hypoglycemic agent.

An important area of discussion is the remission, or honeymoon period, during which insulin dosage needs to be decreased or severe hypoglycemia may occur.

A thorough explanation of meal planning by

a knowledgeable dietitian should include the reasons for meal planning; the exchange system; composition and timing of meals, snacks, and extra food; and how to make adjustments for various situations, for example, growth, appetite, exercise, traveling, parties, restaurants, convenience foods, and school lunches. A demonstration using food models, if available, is helpful. In educating the patient and the family regarding urine testing for glucose and ketones and blood testing for glucose, the reasons for testing methods of collection of specimens, performance of tests, recording of results, and use of results to modify insulin dosage should all be explained.

The role of insulin in the treatment of diabetes should be made clear. In addition, a thorough explanation of the types of insulin to be used, their concentrations, and the dosage and time of injections should be given. The proper use of syringes and the method of rotation of injection sites is demonstrated. The role of physical exercise should be made regarding physical activities. Aspects of general health care should be discussed, including routine medical care, preventive dental care, general hygiene, and care of the skin and feet.

A list of community resources should be made available, with discussion and clarification of their roles. One example is the ADA, which has a number of films, pamphlets, and other resource material on diabetes, insurance, and other topics. Many ADA chapters sponsor summer camps for children with diabetes and have organized parent-youth groups, diabetes education programs, and so on. Another example is vocational rehabilitation programs sponsored by state governments, which are available to help finance college or vocational training and will be helpful to many patients and their parents.

If available, the education and long-term management program can be conducted as a multidisciplinary activity involving the following services: nursing, dietetics, social service, psychology and psychiatry, pharmacy, recreation, and hospital-based teaching.

Complications

Serious complications are relatively rare during childhood. Although some patients are more prone to develop complications than others, good control appears to delay the onset and minimize the progression of complications. Certainly, persistent glycosuria, ketonuria, and hyperlipidemia are to be avoided.

Space permits only a listing of the adverse responses of the host in diabetes. Whether they are a result of hyperglycemia and poor glucose use or a component of the total pathologic picture is uncertain. Capillary basement membrane thickening is the early manifestation of vascular abnormalities. Recent studies by Jackson indicate a reversibility of these lesions through institution of strict control. According to White, the early inception of vascular lesions is evident, but potential reversibility and/or improvement in some vascular lesions were recognized. Poor control of diabetes and infections influence the course of vascular damage. Whether vascular abnormalities precede and are the real cause of diabetes or result from the diabetes remains unanswered. Vascular lesions, however, play a prominent part in the pathogenesis of major complications that increase after puberty and involve the kidneys, eyes, and nervous, musculoskeletal, and reproductive systems. Recently abnormalities in the sorbitol pathway have been implicated in complications related to the nervous system, the lens (cataracts), and atheromas.

Complications may be frequent, multiple, and progressive in type I diabetes. With modern therapy the problems of growth and development have mostly resolved themselves. After 20 years of the disease, complications are more frequent and progress more rapidly in patients with insulin-dependent than in those with non–insulin-dependent diabetes.

- A. Nephropathy
  1. Intercapillary glomerular sclerosis
  2. Nodular glomerular sclerosis
  3. Nephrotic syndrome
  4. Pyelonephritis
- B. Cystitis
- C. Renal and perirenal abscess
- D. Retinopathy
- E. Neuropathy
- F. Thyroiditis
- G. Gangrene
- H. Cutaneous lesions
  1. Infections
     - a. Pyoderma
     - b. Vulvitis and proctitis (candidiasis, or moniliasis)
     - c. Dermatophytoses

2. Xanthoma diabeticorum
3. Necrobiosis lipoidica diabeticorum

I. Brain damage and mental retardation associated with recurrent hypoglycemia (excess insulin) during infancy and early childhood.

J. Psychologic and behavior problems

K. Infertility may occur and the outcome of pregnancy may be affected

L. Crippling complications such as blindness (incidence less than generally thought; healthy second and third generations have been produced)

M. Complications associated with insulin therapy
1. Lipoatrophy and lipoma
2. Infections at sites of injections
3. Allergic sensitivity (switch to pure pork or lente insulin or attempt desensitization with small doses of crystalline insulin)
4. Hypoglycemia
   a. Due to overdosage
   b. Associated with excessive exercise
   c. Due to inadequate caloric intake
5. Paradoxical hyperglycemia (Somogyi effect) associated with excessive insulin administration

N. Decreased mobility of hands and joints

Hypoglycemia

Hypoglycemia is associated with a host of conditions and factors that interfere with the regulation of blood glucose levels, and it may result in symptoms ranging from vague behavior problems to convulsions, coma, and shock, with permanent brain damage or even death.

Of the several methods used for measuring glucose in whole blood, plasma, or serum, only glucose oxidase methods measure "true" glucose. Other methods such as the commonly used ferricyanide AutoAnalyzer method give values 10% to 15% higher than those of glucose oxidase methods. In addition, when interpreting results, consideration should be given to other variables because plasma or serum glucose levels are about 15% higher than those of whole blood, and glucose levels of capillary blood may be as much as 30 mg/dl higher than those of venous blood during the first hour of a glucose tolerance test. The normal overnight fasting true blood glucose level in children ranges between 70 and 100 mg/dl. In contrast to adults, normal children are less able to maintain normal glucose during a prolonged fast. Chaussain (1973) found that a 24-hour fast will cause 1 in 5 children under 9 years of age to have asymptomatic hypoglycemia with a blood glucose level of less than 40 mg/dl. In addition, during the first 3 to 5 days of life, blood glucose levels may be as low as 30 to 60 mg/dl in the absence of symptoms. In older children true blood glucose values below 50 mg/dl are indicative of hypoglycemia. The degree of hypoglycemia may be correlated with true blood glucose values as follows:

Mild, 40 to 50 mg/dl
Moderate, 20 to 40 mg/dl
Severe, below 20 mg/dl

Severity of symptoms is usually, but by no means necessarily, in proportion to the degree of hypoglycemia.

Normal glucose homeostasis. Glucose enters the bloodstream as a result of active absorption from the intestinal tract, conversion of fructose and galactose to glucose by the liver, glycogenolysis in the liver, and glyconeogenesis in the liver, which uses amino acids, glycerol, lactate, and pyruvate. Insulin is secreted by the beta cells of the pancreatic islets in response to several stimuli, including elevated glucose, fructose, amino acids, glucagon, secretin, gastrin, cholecystokinin, and vagus stimulation. The exact mechanism by which insulin lowers blood glucose levels has not been completely defined. It probably acts by increasing cellular permeability to glucose and by induction of liver glucokinase activity. Exogenously supplied glucose either is used as an immediate source of energy or is converted in the liver to glycogen or fat. Since fat carbon is not a ready source of glucose, and since glucose-6-phosphatase is present in the liver and absent in the muscle, liver glycogen is the principal source of endogenous glucose during an overnight fast. During a prolonged fast, the major sources of glucose are lactate and amino acids derived from protein catabolism (glyconeogenesis). Fat breakdown, or lipolysis, releases free fatty acids, which are readily converted in the liver to beta-hydroxybutyric acid and acetoacetic acid. Although many tissues preferentially use lactate, free fatty acids, and ketone bodies as their major sources of energy during fasting, the brain fortunately can also use these substrates. However, some glucose is necessary for normal brain function, which offers an explanation for the central nervous system signs and symptoms that are the result of hypoglycemia. This is an especially important consideration in the prevention of permanent brain damage in the infant under 6 months of age.

Blood glucose homeostasis is dependent on

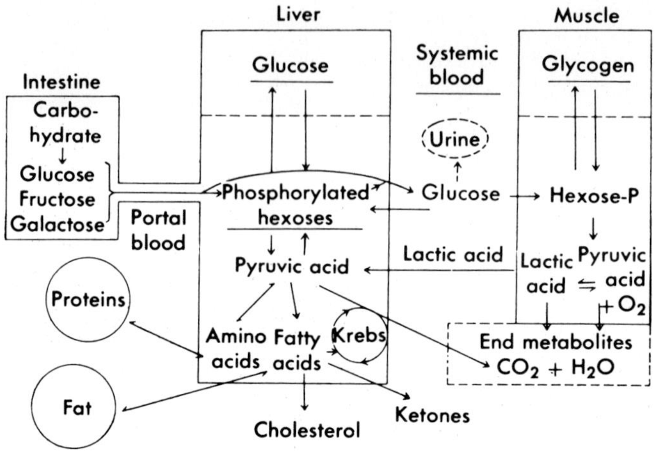

Fig. 22-3. Mechanisms of glucose homeostasis in the body. (From Wilkins, L., with editorial assistance by Blizzard, R.M., and Migeon, C.: Diagnosis and treatment of endocrine disorders in childhood and adolescence, ed. 3, Springfield, Ill., 1965, Charles C Thomas, Publisher.)

Table 22-5. Hormonal control of glucose homeostasis

	Insulin	Catecholamines	Cortisol	Growth hormone	Glucagon	Thyroid hormone
Glucose uptake by muscle	↑	↓	—	↓	—	—
Gluconeogenic amino acids from muscle	↓	↑	↑	↓	—	↑
Activation of lipolysis → free fatty acids and glycerol	↓	↑	↑	↑	—	↑
Insulin secretion	↓	↓	—	—	—	—
Activation of glycogenolytic and gluconeogenic enzymes	↓	↑	↑	—	↑	↑

↑, increase; ↓, decrease; —, no significant effect.

several mechanisms that are summarized in Fig. 22-3 and Table 22-5. Among the factors involved are the following:

1. Insulin secretion and metabolism (Because insulin inhibits lipolysis, glycogenolysis, proteolysis, and glyconeogenesis, a decrease in insulin to basal levels during fasting allows cortisol, epinephrine, glucagon, and growth hormone to maintain normal blood glucose.)
2. Integrity of the liver cells that function in glycogenesis, glucogenolysis, lipogenesis, ketogenesis, glyconeogenesis, and cellular respiration
3. Availability of glycogenic amino acids
4. Presence of cortisol, which stimulates glyconeogenesis and glycogenolysis (Table 22-5)
5. Pituitary growth hormone (Table 22-5), which has an "anti-insulin" action (the mechanism of this action is controversial), stimulates anabolism of protein, and increases the mobilization and use of fat for energy production
6. Glucagon in combination with cortisol (Table 22-5), which stimulates gluconeogenesis
7. Epinephrine (Table 22-5), which stimulates hepatic and muscle glycogenolysis, inhibits peripheral use of glucose, and inhibits insulin release from the pancreatic beta cells

8. Hypothalamus and/or sympathetic nervous system, which apparently control the secretion of epinephrine by the adrenal medulla in response to hypoglycemia
9. Thyroid hormone, which accelerates intestinal absorption of glucose and metabolic processes in general
10. Renal glycosuria with lowered renal threshold for glucose

Most of these factors, which tend to elevate blood glucose levels, are stimulated by hypoglycemia. Since growth hormone, cortisol, thyroid hormone, glucagon, and epinephrine act to elevate blood glucose levels and antagonize the effect of insulin, insufficiency of these hormones may result in hypoglycemia. Current methodology permits determination of the etiology of most cases.

Etiology. Following is an etiologic classification of hypoglycemia.

A. *Ketotic hypoglycemia* (substrate insufficiency)
   Ketotic hypoglycemia is usually seen in short, thin infants and is precipitated by prolonged fast or illness. It is associated with hypoalaninemia and ketosis during hypoglycemia, which usually does not respond to glucagon administration. Catecholamine response to insulin-induced hypoglycemia is poor. Other endocrine functions are normal. It is infrequently seen in the first year of life but is the commonest cause of hypoglycemia in children.
   Patients who have isolated ACTH deficiency, adrenocortical insufficiency, and hypopituitarism may have ketosis and hypoglycemia. In these conditons hypoglycemic episodes are frequently more severe. These patients should be differentiated from those with ketotic hypoglycemia.
B. *Hyperinsulinism (absolute)*
   This is the most common cause of hypoglycemia in infants between 1 week and 1 year of age.
   1. *Islet cell dysmaturation syndrome* is a term proposed by Gabbay to describe a spectrum of islet cell abnormalities, including islet cell adenoma, islet-cell hyperplasia, and nesidioblastosis (the formation of islet cells from pancreatic duct tissue). The syndrome may be seen in infants of diabetic mothers, those with erythroblastosis fetalis, patients with the Beckwith-Wiedemann syndrome, and infants with no apparent predisposing cause. Other terms used to describe infants with this syndrome include *severe persistent or intractable hypoglycemia, leucine-sensitive hypoglycemia,* and *familial hypoglycemia.*
   2. Prolonged excessive (unusual) carbohydrate ingestion, especially with lack of exercise
   3. Delayed but excessive insulin secretion, producing reactive hypoglycemia such as may occur in impaired glucose tolerance.
   4. Neurogenic stimulation of right vagus nerve (frequently functional)
C. *Hyperinsulinism (relative)*
   This is caused by lack of insulin antagonists.
   1. Hypopituitarism (growth hormone, ACTH, and TSH deficiency)
   2. Hypoadrenocorticism (Addison disease) and, rarely, congenital virilizing adrenal hyperplasia
   3. Adrenal medullary insufficiency (hemorrhage, infection, trauma)
   4. Alpha cell (glucagon) deficiency
   5. Failure of secretion of epinephrine in response to hypoglycemia, probably caused by hypothalamic or sympathetic nervous system defect
D. *Dietary insufficiency*
   1. Starvation or stress
      a. Intrauterine (hypoglycemia of the newborn), particularly in term or postmature infants of low birth weight, the smaller of twins, and infants who had fetal distress
   2. Poor intestinal absorption
      a. Deficiency of disaccharide-splitting enzymes
      b. Malabsorption syndromes (celiac disease)
      c. Edema of gastrointestinal tract
      d. Diarrhea
      e. Hypothyroidism
   3. Hyperutilization
      a. Exercise
      b. Fever
      c. Hyperthyroidism
E. *Hepatic disorders*
   1. Inborn errors of metabolism
      a. Glycogen storage diseases (glycogenoses, pp. 662-664)
      b. Galactosemia (deficiency of galactose-1-phosphate uridyl transferase or galactokinase) (p. 656)
      c. Hereditary fructose intolerance (deficiency of fructose-1-phosphate aldolase)
      d. Fructose-1,6-diphosphatase deficiency
      e. Pyruvate carboxylase deficiency (Leigh encephalomyelopathy)
      f. Maple syrup urine disease (block in oxidative decarboxylation of branched-chain keto acids)
   2. Hepatitis, with extensive liver damage (infectious hepatitis and Reye syndrome)
   3. Cirrhosis, advanced
   4. Intoxication (bacterial, organic solvents, heavy metals)
F. *Abnormal losses* (renal glycosuria, either idiopathic or from renal tubular defects)
G. *Iatrogenic*
   1. Excessive insulin in management of diabetes mellitus
   2. Ingestion of drugs (sulfonylurea, salicylates, acetaminophen, etc.)
H. *Tumors*
   Although a few tumors have been shown to produce an insulin-like activity, the mechanism for producing hypoglycemia is unknown.
   1. Hepatoma
   2. Fibrosarcoma
   3. Wilms tumor

Signs and symptoms. Signs and symptoms of hypoglycemia include the following: (1) irritability, fidgetiness, nervousness, and behavior problems; (2) muscle weakness and fatigability; (3) headaches, mental confusion, drowsiness, speech difficulties, and tremors; (4) vertigo and diplopia; (5) paresthesia and hypalgesia; (6) pallor, tachycardia, and shock; (7) coma, with or without convulsions; and (8) in young infants, flushing, sweating, cyanosis, limpness, twitching, and apneic spells.

Permanent brain damage and/or abnormal neurologic signs are especially likely to develop in infants.

Laboratory evaluations. In general, the approach to laboratory evaluation depends on the infant's or child's age and the suspected diagnosis by historical data and physical findings. For the newborn period, see the section on neonatal hypoglycemia (pp. 323-326). Since hyperinsulinemia is the most common cause of hypoglycemia in the first year of life (not including the newborn period), evaluation of insulin and simultaneously measured glucose in the fasting state and postprandially is very helpful in differentiating hyperinsulinism from other causes of hypoglycemia, such as hormonal insufficiency states. At the time the patient has hypoglycemia, measurement of plasma cortisol, growth hormone, glucagon, and amino acids may be very helpful in determining the cause. If the hypoglycemia occurs after 1 year of age and is associated with ketonuria, ketotic hypoglycemia is the most likely diagnosis. Since hypopituitarism and hypoadrenalism can exhibit ketosis and hypoglycemia, a thorough endocrine evaluation is indicated in this group of infants and children.

Glycemic equilibrium should be established by high-carbohydrate feeding for 48 to 72 hours before undertaking diagnostic studies. However, the patient's clinical status may dictate immediate treatment before any testing is done. The reader is referred to standard textbooks on clinical pathology and laboratory methods for detailed descriptions of the tests.

If the patient has an enlarged liver, the differential diagnosis should include glycogen storage disease (GSD), galactosemia, defects in glyconeogenesis, hepatitis, Reye syndrome, and so on. If galactosemia is suspected by finding a reducing substance in the urine that is not glucose, the determination of erythrocyte galactose-1-phosphate uridyl transferase and galactokinase can be made. In fructose-1,6-diphosphatase deficiency, laboratory findings are similar to those found in type I GSD except that glycogenolysis is normal. Patients with fructose-1,6 diphosphatase deficiency have hypoglycemia, hepatomegaly from lipid stores, lactic acidosis, ketoacidosis, hyperlipidemia, and hyperuricemia. Patients with pyruvate carboxylase deficiency have low serum bicarbonate and elevated blood lactate, pyruvate, and alanine. With hepatitis, liver enzymes such as SGOT, SGPT, and alkaline phosphatase are much higher than in GSD. Patients with Reye syndrome have abnormal liver function tests, including hyperammonemia and concomitant encephalopathy.

The following *screening tests* are performed as indicated:

1. Twelve-hour fasting blood glucose test. The period of the fast may be extended to 24 hours or longer. Functional hypoglycemia is said to occur usually within 4 to 6 hours after onset of fast. In patients with ketotic hypoglycemia this test can be terminated with a glucagon tolerance test. In most patients with ketotic hypoglycemia there is little response to glucagon.
2. Prolonged (6-hour) oral glucose tolerance test. A flat oral glucose tolerance curve indicates poor absorption and may be confirmed by a normal intravenous glucose tolerance test. A depressed curve occurs with organic causes of hypoglycemia, such as insulinoma. Progressive fall after 3 hours suggests diminished adrenal or pituitary response to hypoglycemia, alpha cell insufficiency, or, rarely, low threshold renal glycosuria. The determination of insulin and proinsulin may be particularly helpful in cases of reactive hypoglycemia; proinsulin levels are elevated in insulinoma.
3. Urine for glucose and reducing substance. If reducing substance present is not glucose, the differential diagnosis should include galactosemia, aminoacidurias, and hereditary fructose intolerance. Specific sugars, keto acids, and amino acids can be identified with chromatographic and other techniques. Erythrocyte galactose-1-phosphate uridyl transferase can be measured if galactosemia is suspected.
4. Serum thyroxine test.
5. Fasting and postprandial insulin levels un-

related to simultaneous glucose levels.

Other diagnostic tests are performed as indicated:

1. Insulin tolerance test. Increased sensitivity (lack of homeostatic response to induced hypoglycemia) indicates absence of pituitary, adrenal, or pancreatic alpha cell antagonists (relative hyperinsulinism) or hyperresponsiveness and is not to be interpreted to mean a peculiar or allergic response. This test is performed with the patient under close observation and is terminated by the administration of intravenous glucose at the first symptom or sign of severe hypoglycemia. Blood samples are obtained for glucose and growth hormone determinations during the test. Measurement of urinary vanillylmandelic acid and catecholamines before, and in response to, insulin-induced hypoglycemia is used to evaluate adrenal medullary (hypothalamic) response to hypoglycemia.
2. Tolbutamide tolerance test. This test is helpful in patients with suspected insulinoma.
3. Ketogenic diet with frequent blood glucose determinations and observations for onset of ketonuria. This test may have no advantage over observations during a 24-hour fast. The ketogenic diet may have to be continued up to 36 hours, and with any symptoms of hypoglycemia should be terminated readily by glucose administration. The ketogenic diet is continued until the blood glucose level falls below 30 mg/dl or until the patient shows symptoms of hypoglycemia. When the patient becomes ketotic and hypoglycemic, a glucagon tolerance test is performed.
4. Metyrapone and ACTH test for evaluation of pituitary or adrenal insufficiency (see sections on the pituitary gland, pp. 567-572).
5. Leucine tolerance test.
6. Glucagon and/or epinephrine challenge to determine ability of the liver to mobilize glycogen.
7. Fructose tolerance test in selected cases.
8. Exploratory laparotomy is indicated in patients who do not respond to conservative management or who have repeated relapses (insulinoma).

Treatment

General considerations

Neonatal hypoglycemia. Normal blood glucose levels must be maintained by glucose infusions. Adrenal steroids, epinephrine, and glucagon may be needed to prevent severe hypoglycemia and subsequent permanent brain damage. In most cases treatment can be discontinued after a few days, with no further difficulty. In severe cases oral diazoxide may be useful. Successful management eventually depends on accurate diagnosis and application of proper substitution and prophylactic treatment (see discussions on hypopituitarism, adrenal insufficiency, etc.).

Hypoglycemia in older infants and children. The acute attack is treated with the intravenous administration of glucose, and the subcutaneous injection of 0.01 ml/kg of 1:1000 epinephrine or 0.5 to 1 mg glucagon intramuscularly. The intravenous administration of hydrocortisone is indicated in adrenal cortical deficiency states. Dietary measures include frequent feedings of carbohydrate and protein. Attention to the psychologic aspects of the illness in the child and parents is important. Blood glucose can be monitored by the parents using Chemstrip bG or Dextrostix with a reflectance meter.

Specific measures for treatment

Ketotic hypoglycemia. Patients are fed three meals and three snacks daily. The parents should check the urine for ketones with Acetest tablets in the morning and at bedtime daily and more often during illness. When ketonuria develops, high-carbohydrate foods are given until ketonuria clears. If the patient cannot tolerate feedings and/or hypoglycemia develops, intravenous glucose may be required. With patients taking hydrocortisone, the daily dose should be increased to 100 mg/m^2 during a severe infection and 30 mg/m^2 during a mild infection.

Islet cell dysmaturation syndrome. Diazoxide, 8 to 12 mg/kg/24 hr; hydrocortisone, 15 to 30 mg/m^2/24 hr, or a low-leucine formula such as Wyeth S-14 formula may be helpful in specific cases. If the infant has leucine sensitivity, whole milk, which is very high in leucine, should be avoided. Frequent feeds every 2 to 3 hours may control the hypoglycemia. However, partial pancreatectomy with removal of 80% to 95% of the pancreas may be necessary, and is frequently curative. However, diabetes mellitus and/or pancreatic exocrine deficiency may develop later in childhood.

Inborn errors of metabolism. In type I GSD starch and glucose is substituted for lactose in the diet and fat is restricted to 25% of calories.

Portacaval shunt and continuous overnight intragastric feedings of glucose have been successfully employed, as evidenced by reduction in liver size, disappearance of hepatic adenomas, linear growth acceleration, and normalization of biochemical abnormalities. Corn starch taken every 6 hours has also recently been shown to be efficacious. In type III GSD, a high-protein diet with some restriction of carbohydrate is indicated. In galactosemia and hereditary fructose intolerance, the specific causative agents are eliminated from the diet.

Prognosis

Permanent brain damage can be minimized with early diagnosis and treatment directed toward prevention of hypoglycemia. Eventual outcome is dependent on the underlying cause(s) and the adequacy of total therapy.

George A. Burghen
James N. Etteldorf

SEX DETERMINATION, DIFFERENTIATION, AND DEVELOPMENT

Knowledge in the field of abnormalities in sex determination, differentiation, and development has increased greatly in recent years because of advances in methods of investigation of the genetic and biochemical mechanisms involved in sex determination and differentiation, in the hypothalamic-pituitary-gonadal–target tissue axis, in the hypothalamic-pituitary-adrenal axis, and in gonadal function. Evaluation of problems in this field requires competent, properly oriented physicians; many important aspects must be considered in each case. In addition to a carefully taken history and a thorough physical examination, various investigative techniques in the following discussion may be indicated.

Normal sex differentiation and development

The *genetic sex* of an embryo is determined the moment an ovum is fertilized by a sperm. In normal somatic cell division (mitosis) a cell containing 44 *autosomes* and 2 sex chromosomes (XX in the female and XY in the male) gives rise to two daughter cells containing the same 44 + 2 chromosomes. However, by a specialized type of cell division called *meiosis* the cells of the *germ line* undergo a series of two divisions, producing in the female one *ovum* containing 22 autosomes and an X chromosome and in the male four *spermatozoa,* each containing 22 autosomes and either an X or a Y chromosome. In oogenesis one primary oocyte normally gives rise to *one* ovum and two polar bodies, the ovum always containing 22 + X chromosomes; in spermatogenesis one primary spermatocyte produces four mature spermatozoa, two containing 22 + X and two containing 22 + Y. Chance alone determines whether an X-bearing sperm or a Y-bearing sperm fertilizes an ovum. If an X-bearing sperm is contributed by the father, the resulting *zygote* will contain 44 autosomes + XX and is genetically a female. If the sperm contributes a Y chromosome, a genetic male with chromosome constitution 44 + XY results (Fig. 22-4). Abnormalities in the process of meiosis account for some abnormalities in sex determination, whereas abnormalities of an early *mitotic* division of the fertilized egg (zygote) may also produce such abnormalities.

Once the genetic sex of the embryo is determined, the processes of differentiation of the gonads and of the internal and external genitalia begin. Before about 42 days of intrauterine life, the gonads of both XX and XY embryos appear identical. However, even earlier primordial germ cells are identifiable in the allantois and adjacent portions of the yolk sac. As early as 35 to 40 days the migration of primordial germ cells from their point of origin in the hindgut to the gonadal primordia has been observed. The gonadal primordium is derived from mesoblastic and interstitial cells of the midportion of the urogenital ridge. Witschi and others have shown that if the primordial germ cells for any reason fail to migrate to the gonadal primordia, gonadal differentiation does not take place. This suggests that the primordial germ cells in some way serve as inductors of gonadal differentiation.

The genetic mechanisms governing the differentiation of the primitive bipotential gonad into an ovary or a testis are not well understood. The inherent direction of gonadal differentiation is toward an ovary, a direction taken in the absence of a Y chromosome. Evidence gained from the study of the gonads at various stages of differentiation in 45,X fetuses indicates that

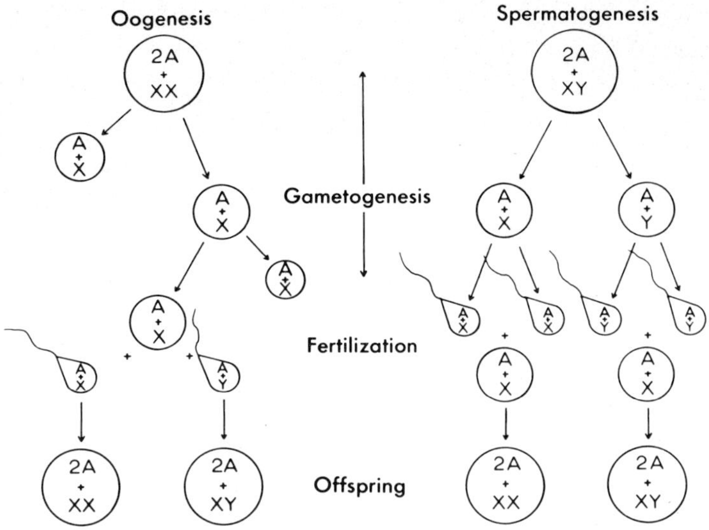

Fig. 22-4. Normal gametogenesis and fertilization: oogenesis on left, spermatogenesis on right. *A* signifies one haploid set of autosomes (22 autosomes); 2*A* signifies two haploid sets of autosomes (44 autosomes). Note that from one primary oocyte only one ovum is formed, whereas from one primary spermatocyte four spermatozoa are formed.

two genetically active X chromosomes in the primordial germ cells are necessary for maintenance of follicle differentiation in the embryonic ovary. In the 45,X fetus primordial germ cells migrate into the gonadal primordium, but follicle formation is defective.

The discovery of the plasma membrane antigen H-Y has shed new light on the process of testicular differentiation. The expression of the H-Y antigen is normally correlated with the presence of a Y chromosome and is assumed to be governed in some manner by a gene located in the Y chromosome. H-Y antigen synthesis is probably also under the control of autosomal or X-linked genes or both. Wachtel and associates, as well as Ohno and other investigators, have presented evidence that this antigen in some manner governs the differentiation of the primitive bipotential gonad to form a testis.

Ohno and colleagues performed an experiment wherein H-Y antigen was stripped from the surfaces of mouse embryonic gonadal cells in rotation culture. When the cells from which H-Y antigen was stripped were allowed to reaggregate, they formed follicle-like structures, while control cells that retained H-Y antigen reaggregated to form seminiferous tubule–like structures. This elegant experiment provides evidence that the presence of H-Y antigen is necessary for testicular differentiation.

In the differentiating testis, primordial germ cells are incorporated into developing testicular cords that appear throughout the gonadal blastema. Connective tissue appears between the testicular cords, and as this occurs, the cords become distinct. Their more peripheral segments become seminiferous tubules, and their central portions become rete cords. The developing seminiferous tubules are lined by two or three layers of Sertoli cells and spermatogonia, the latter derived from primitive germ cells. Leydig cells appear in the testicular interstitium as early as 60 days of embryonic development. Their number increases until in the fourth month of intrauterine life they completely fill the interstitial spaces between the seminiferous tubules. They then gradually decrease in number and disappear completely within the first month of postnatal life. During differentiation of the internal and external genitalia in the male fetus, Leydig cells actively produce androgens.

In the differentiation of the primitive gonad into an ovary, according to Jirásek, the gonadal blastema forms epithelium and interstitial connective tissue. The epithelial elements form irregular groups of cords within the cortical and medullary regions of the differentiating ovary. The cords contain primitive granulosa cells, along with primordial germ cells that have migrated to the gonad. Oogonia derived from the primordial germ cells within the cords divide to form thick zones that consist mostly of oogonia with a few primitive granulosa cells. Thin layers of connective tissue separate the surface epithelium of the embryonic ovary from deeper structures and also separate the cortical cords. Looser connective tissue separates the medullary cords.

Oogonia in the fetal ovary become primary oocytes and enter the prophase of the first meiotic division. The first meiotic division in each primary oocyte is interrupted in late prophase, to be completed only when that specific ovum is ovulated 12 to 50 years later. The stage at which meiosis arrests is called dictyotene.

Within the cords of the fetal ovary primitive granulosa cells surround the primary oocytes in the prophase of first meiosis to form a single layer of flattened follicle cells. This constitutes the primordial follicle. The primordial follicles become completely surrounded by connective tissue to form primary follicles, which contain dictyotene oocytes. The primitive granulosa cells of the ovarian cords either become follicle cells that surround the oocytes in the primordial and primary follicles or fibroblast-like cells in the ovarian stroma. The fetal ovary, even though it contains follicular granulosa cells, has no endocrine function.

In the fetal ovary the oogonia and primary oocytes increase to a maximum of as many as 7 million at 18 to 22 weeks' gestation. Their number then decreases through degeneration to about 2 million at birth. Of these 2 million, only

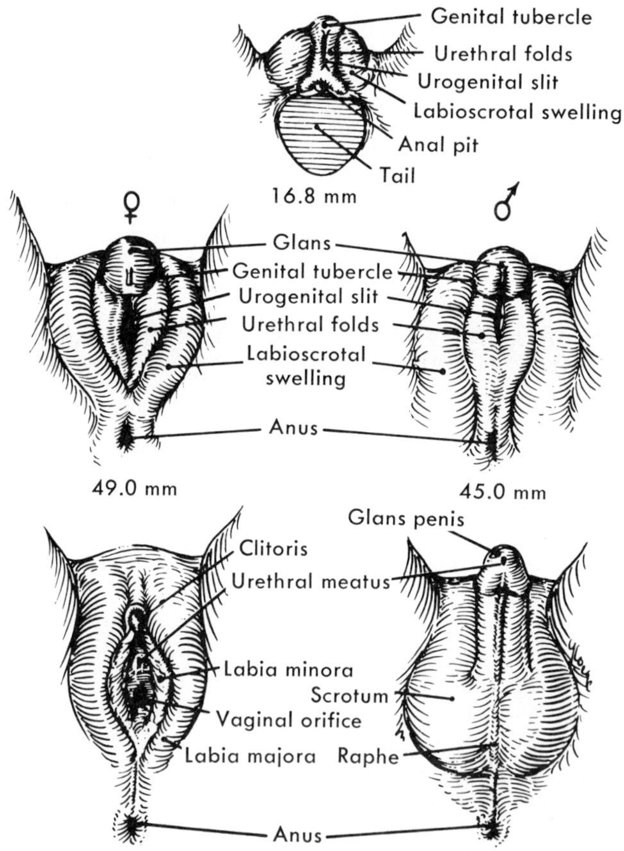

Fig. 22-5. Bipotential primitive external genitalia at top. Changes occuring in female differentiation at left, in male differentiation at right. (From Grumbach, M.M., and Van Wyk, J.J. In Williams, R.H., editor: Textbook of endocrinology, Philadelphia, 1974, W.B. Saunders Co.)

about 400 will be ovulated during the woman's reproductive life. Thus, according to Gillman, most oogonia and oocytes are eliminated before follicle formation, while others degenerate during formation of the primary follicles. Before the end of fetal life the formation of oogonia and oocytes has ceased, and the female is born with all the germ cells she will ever have.

In the presence of an ovary (or in the absence of any differentiated gonad, as will be mentioned later) the internal genital duct system of the embryo will differentiate along female lines. During the third month the müllerian ducts differentiate into fallopian tubes, uterus, and cephalad portion of the vagina, while the wolffian (male) duct system regresses. In both sexes the anlage of the external genitalia are identical until the third month of intrauterine life, consisting (Fig. 22-5) of urogenital sinus, lateral urethral folds and labioscrotal swellings, and anteriorly situated genital tubercle. During the third and fourth months in the female, the urogenital sinus differentiates (Fig. 22-5) into separate vaginal and urethral openings bounded laterally by labia minora and majora, and the genital tubercle forms the definitive clitoris. The caudad portion of the vaginal vault originates from the urogenital sinus, but the cephalad portion is derived from fused müllerian elements. This brief summary of female sex differentiation is schematically represented in Fig. 22-6.

While the fetal ovary has no endocrine secretory function, hormones elaborated by the fetal testis are necessary for male sex differentiation. The fetal testis produces two substances relative to ductal differentiation. One of these is a high molecular weight peptide, the *müllerian suppressive factor,* which actively

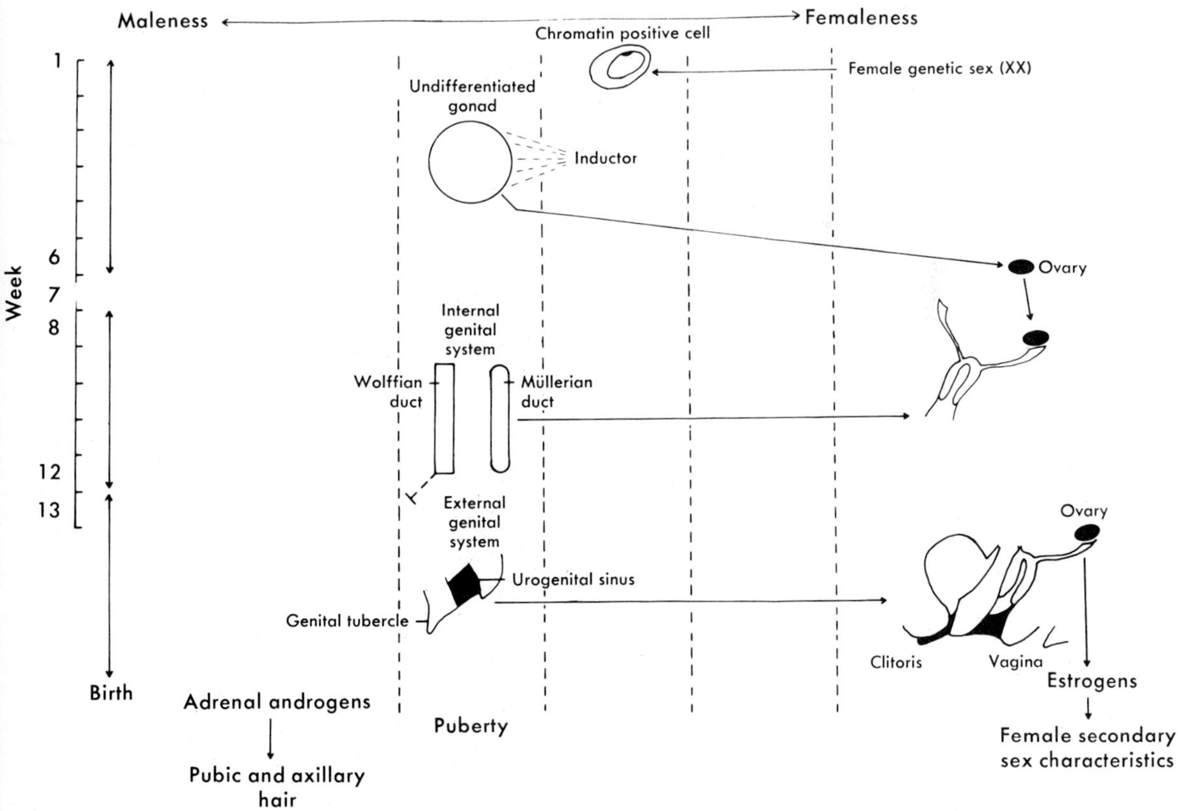

Fig. 22-6. Normal female sex differentiation and development. (Modified from Newman, S., et al.: Postgrad. Med. **27:**488, 1960.)

produces regression of the müllerian duct system in the male fetus. Current evidence indicates that müllerian suppressive factor is secreted by Sertoli cells of the seminiferous tubules. The second substance elaborated by the fetal testis is testosterone. Testosterone, produced by Leydig cells, serves as the inductor of wolffian duct differentiation into epididymis, vas deferens, seminal vesicle, and ejaculatory duct. The actions of both these substances are apparently local and tissue specific; as shown by Jost, in male animals that have been castrated unilaterally during fetal life, the wolffian duct differentiates and the müllerian duct regresses on the side of the remaining testis, whereas on the castrated side the müllerian structures differentiate and the wolffian duct regresses. In addition, implantation of a crystal of testosterone in a castrated fetal animal leads to wolffian duct differentiation on the side containing the crystal, but on that same side müllerian structures also are preserved. This indicates that müllerian suppressive factor is necessary for müllerian regression, and the presence of testosterone alone does not fulfill that function.

Two abnormalities of sex differentiation in humans also bear on this subject. In the male with the complete androgen insensitivity syndrome, in whom testosterone, although present in normal amounts, fails to stimulate wolffian duct differentiation and in whom the external genitalia do not masculinize, müllerian elements are not found. This is apparently because of the normal action of, and normal response to, müllerian suppressive factor even in the presence of androgen insensitivity. On the other hand, in the uterine hernia syndrome, response to androgen is normal so that normal wolffian differentiation and external genital masculinization take place in the affected male, but these patients also have inguinal hernias that are found to contain a uterine horn and adnexa. In this condition the androgenic induction of wolffian duct differentiation occurs normally, whereas müllerian suppressive factor is absent or ineffective. Normally, in the presence of testes the primitive labioscrotal folds fuse to form the scrotum, the urethral folds fuse to form the shaft of the penis, and the genital tubercle becomes the glans penis. The urogenital sinus is enclosed as the posterior urethra. This process occurs under the influence of *circulating androgens* elaborated by Leydig cells of the fetal testes. Male sex differentiation, schematically represented in Fig. 22-7, is complete by the fourteenth week of gestation.

Before the stage of fetal development at which differentiation of the external genitalia takes place, the anlage of the external genitalia acquire the capacity to convert testosterone to dihydrotestosterone through the action of the enzyme 5-alpha-reductase (Fig. 22-8). This plus clinical evidence mentioned later provides proof that while testosterone itself is responsible for wolffian duct differentiation, dihydrotestosterone is the androgen that, in the target cell, mediates masculinization of the external genitalia.

Available evidence indicates that the ability of any cell (except the male germ cell) to respond to androgen depends on the action of a nuclear-cytosol androgen receptor protein, specified by an X-linked gene (Fig. 22-9). Thus masculinization of the bipotential internal and external genitalia is under the control of multiple genetic determinants specific for the following: to govern the differentiation of a testis, to determine the differentiation of Leydig cells within the testis, to control the elaboration of enzymes necessary for the biosynthesis of testosterone and its conversion to dihydrotestosterone, to control the synthesis of müllerian suppressive factor, to mediate the synthesis of nuclear-cytosol androgen receptor protein, and undoubtedly more. As mentioned earlier, in the absence of a testis, internal and external genitalia differentiate along female lines, with the formation of fallopian tubes, uterus, vagina, and female external genitalia. A functional testis is necessary for male sex differentiation; that is, the female sex can be viewed as the *noninduced* sex, the male as the *induced* sex.

Between birth and the onset of puberty, sexual development remains in an essentially stable state. The factors that result in the initiation of puberty are unclear. Current evidence indicates that even in prepubertal life, gonadotropic hormones can be detected in the serum of both males and females. Hypothalamic-pituitary-gonadal interaction is involved in the initiation and progress of puberty. The hypothalamus produces gonadotropin-releasing hormone(s) (LRH), which regulates the activity of the anterior pituitary. Small amounts of estrogens are detectable in the plasma of prepubertal females, as are androgens in prepubertal males. These

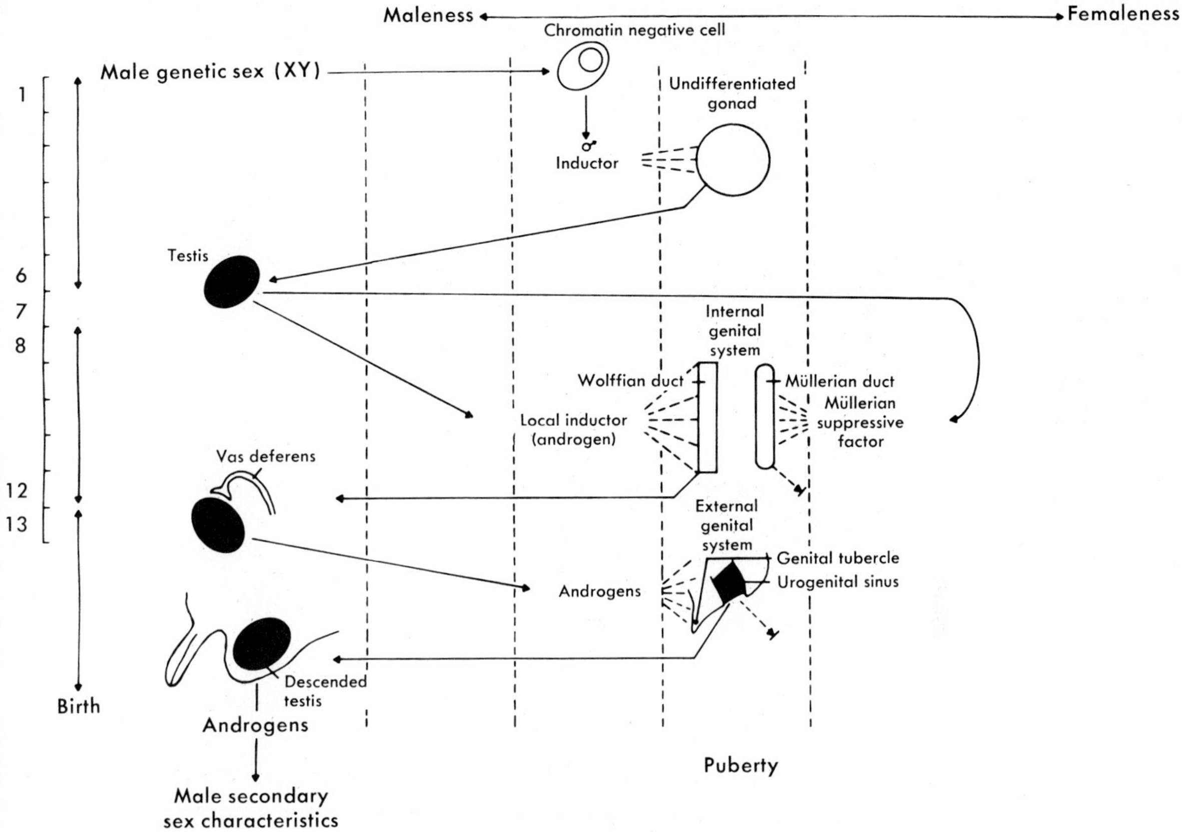

Fig. 22-7. Normal male sex differentiation. (Modified from Newman, S., et al.: Postgrad. Med. **27:**488, 1960.)

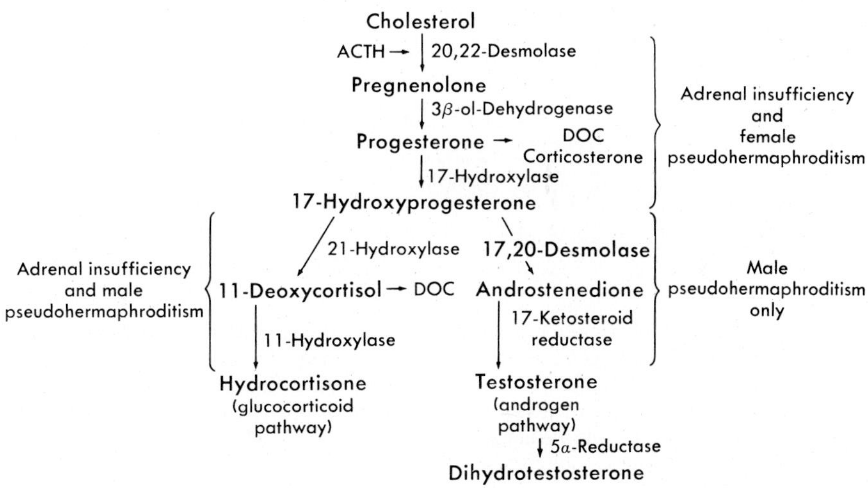

Fig. 22-8. Biosynthesis of cortisol, testosterone, and dihydrotestosterone from cholesterol, showing enzyme systems involved. The first step showing 20-alpha, 22R-desmolase also involves 20-alpha-hydroxylase and 22R-hydroxylase. (Modified from Imperato-McGinley, J., and Peterson, R.E.: Am. J. Med. **61:**251, 1976.)

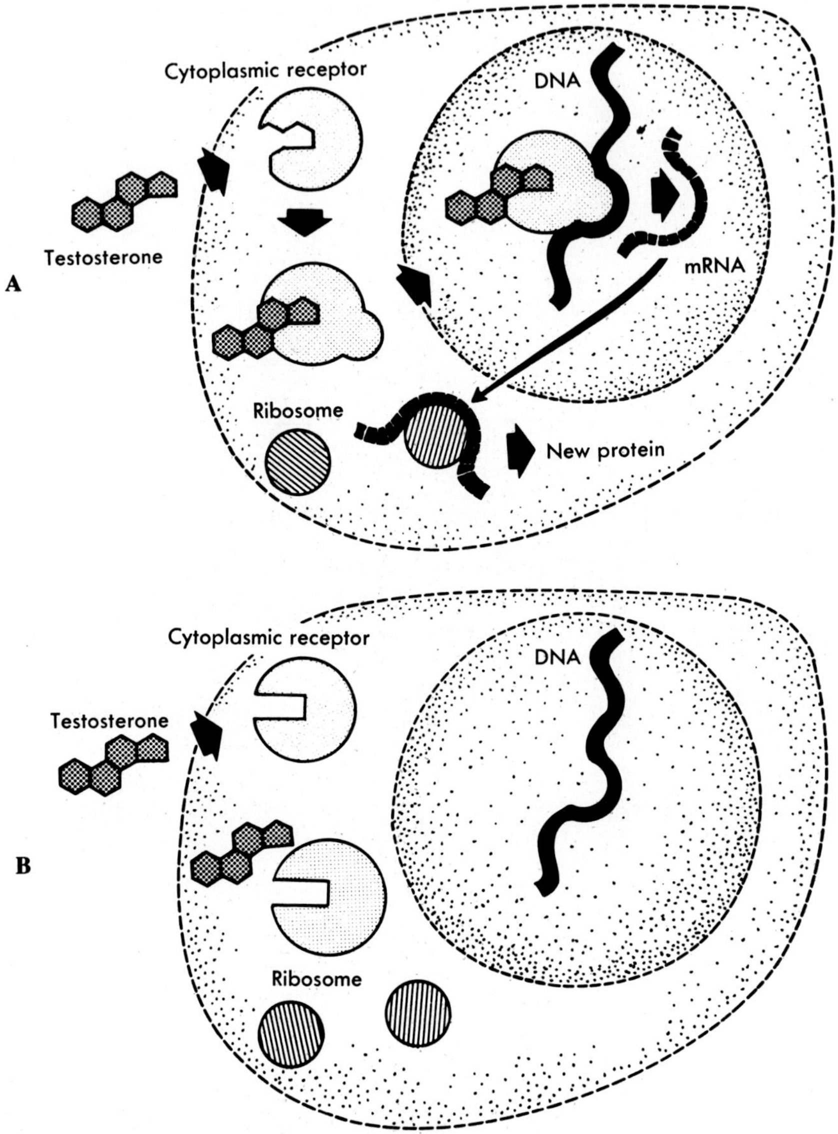

Fig. 22-9. Diagrammatic representation of mechanism of androgen action at cellular site, involving binding of nuclear-cytosol androgen receptor protein and transfer to the nucleus, where androgen-receptor complex binds to genome. **A,** Normal binding. **B,** Situation in androgen insensitivity syndrome. Receptor protein molecule has altered structure, preventing its binding to androgen. (From Imperato-McGinley, J., and Peterson, R.E.: Am. J. Med. **61:**251, 1976.)

small concentrations of sex steroids are sufficient in prepubertal life to suppress the hypothalamic release of LRH, but they are not sufficient to produce the maturation of the sexual apparatus. As the child's age advances, the sensitivity of the hypothalamus to the small amounts of sex steroids decreases. As a result, LRH is produced, resulting in increased pituitary synthesis of the gonadotropins, follicle-stimulating hormone (FSH), and luteinizing hormone (LH). This results ultimately in the increased production of estrogens and androgens to a level sufficient to stimulate maturation of the sexual apparatus. The prepubertal hypothalamic-pituitary-gonadal axis is thus reset at a higher level of secretion of all involved hormones. The age at which puberty begins and the time required for full sexual maturation vary widely, depending at least partly on genetic factors.

In the male interstitial cell-stimulating hormone (ICSH) acts directly on the interstitial cells of the testis, causing them to develop into mature Leydig cells that secrete androgens. Under the influence of androgens, tubules enlarge and mature with the appearance of Sertoli cells and abundant spermatocytes. Under the influence of FSH, complete testicular development occurs, with induction and maintenance of spermatogenesis. Under the influence of testicular and adrenal androgens, the secondary sex characteristics of the mature male appear, growth and skeletal maturation accelerate, and muscle cells increase in size and number. The usual normal sequence of events is shown in Table 22-6.

Sexual maturation in the female begins when FSH stimulation leads to maturation of multiple primary follicles that have been present in the ovary since fetal life. These mature follicles are then able to produce estrogens, and simultaneously the adrenal androgens appear, both factors resulting in the appearance of female secondary sex characteristics. Development of breasts, labia minora, vagina, uterus, and tubes is controlled by estrogen, whereas the appearance of sexual hair and acne and the development of labia majora are governed by androgens. Estrogens and androgens produce accelerated linear growth and skeletal maturation. The cyclic production of estrogens initiates menses, but the first few menstrual cycles are as a rule anovulatory. Ovulation occurs only later under the influence of LH in conjunction with FSH. Not until this occurs is progesterone produced under the influence of LH, resulting in acinar development of the breasts and production of a secretory endometrium.

As can be seen in Table 22-6, puberty in the male normally lags as much as 2 years behind that in the female, resulting in more advanced sexual and somatic maturation in the early teenage girl but ultimately in earlier epiphyseal fusion and shorter stature in the adult female.

Table 22-6. Average approximate age and sequence of sexual characteristics in both sexes

Age (yr)	Boys	Girls
9-10		Growth of bony pelvis Budding of nipples
10-11	First growth of testes and penis	Budding of breasts Pubic hair
11-12	Prostatic activity	Change in vaginal epithelium
12-13	Pubic hair	Pigmentation of nipples Menarche (average, 12.6 to 12.9 yr)
13-14	Rapid growth of testes and penis; subareolar node of breast tissue	Mammae filling in Axillary hair
14-15	Axillary hair; downy hair on upper lip; voice change	Earliest normal pregnancies
15-16	Mature spermatozoa (average, 15 yr; range, 11.25-17 yr)	Acne; deepening of voice
16-17	Facial and body hair; acne	Arrest of skeletal growth
21	Arrest of skeletal growth	

Modified from Wilkins, L.: Diagnosis and treatment of endocrine disorders in childhood and adolescence, ed. 2, Springfield, Ill., 1957, Charles C Thomas, Publisher.

Evaluation of abnormalities of sex determination, differentiation, and development

In addition to a carefully taken history and thorough physical examination, various investigative techniques, summarized in paragraphs that follow, may be used to evaluate abnormalities of sex differentiation and development.

History. Particularly important are (1) family history of aberrations of sex differentiation or development; (2) growth pattern; (3) the mother's pregnancy, with emphasis on the possibility of exposure to progestational drugs; (4) mental development, (5) appearance of the external genitalia at birth, with subsequent change or lack of change; (6) systemic disease or malnutrition; and (7) the exact pattern of the pubertal development of the patient.

Physical examination. A careful, complete physical examination is essential with emphasis on (1) evaluation of growth, with accurate measurements; (2) neurologic examination and mental development; (3) appearance of the genitalia, with impressions gained by rectal and/or pelvic examination; (4) appearance of secondary sex characteristics; and (5) the presence or absence of associated anomalies of systems other than genitalia, with emphasis on minor defects.

Diagnostic studies involving related systems. Studies of the central nervous system and pituitary, thyroid, and adrenal glands are often necessary.

Skeletal maturation. Determination of bone age, and its comparison with height and stage of sexual maturation, is accomplished by radiographic examination of multiple epiphyseal centers.

Hormone levels. Determination of hormone levels in plasma or urine affords valuable information in the evaluation of the infant or child with an abnormality of sex differentiation or development. The following are of value in selected instances: (1) plasma FSH and LH before and after administration of gonadotropin-releasing hormone (LRH); (2) plasma levels of various adrenocortical hormones and their precursors, such as 17-hydroxyprogesterone, 11-deoxycortisol and progesterone; (3) urinary excretion of 17-ketosteroids and 17-hydroxycorticoids; (4) serum and urinary estrogen levels; (5) urinary excretion of pregnanetriol, pregnanediol, and other metabolites; (6) levels of serum and urinary baseline testosterone, its precursors, and its further metabolite dihydrotestosterone, as well as comparison (in prepubertal patients) with levels in response to the administration of human chorionic gonadotropin (HCG); and (7) plasma growth hormone response to various provocative stimuli.

Assay of nuclear-cytosol androgen receptor protein. This technique is available in several laboratories and is a valuable addition to laboratory technology for the investigation of abnormalities of male sex differentiation. Cultured skin fibroblasts, usually of genital origin, are used for this assay.

Testicular incubation studies. The in vitro incubation of fresh testicular slices in the presence of various radioactive-labeled testosterone precursors and measurement of the rate or efficiency of radioactive testosterone synthesis permits the determination, in the testosterone synthetic pathway, of which step is defective. This, by deduction, allows the pinpointing of the enzyme that is deficient.

Buccal smear for sex chromatin. The buccal smear is subjected to two types of evaluation. The first type is the examination by skilled personnel of specially stained cells for the presence of a distinct clump of nuclear chromatin adjacent to the nuclear membrane, which is present when at least two X chromosomes occupy the nuclei of the cells (normal females and abnormal persons with two or more X chromosomes) and absent when only one X chromosome occupies the nuclei (normal males and abnormal persons in whom only one X chromosome is present). In 1949 Barr and Bertram, while studying the neurons of the cat, noted in the nuclei of neurons of some cats a dark-staining mass of chromatin adjacent to the nucleolus. On further investigation they found that this mass of chromatin was present only in the cells of female cats and invariably absent from cells of males. Cells of many tissues of many animals have subsequently been examined, and the same general rule has held: Some of the nuclei of cells of the normal female contain a dark-staining mass of chromatin (Barr body, or *X-chromatin mass,* as shown in Fig. 22-10, *A*), whereas it is not seen in cells of the normal male. In most tissues this mass is adjacent to the nuclear membrane instead of the nucleolus. The most easily obtained source of cells for such examination in the hu-

A 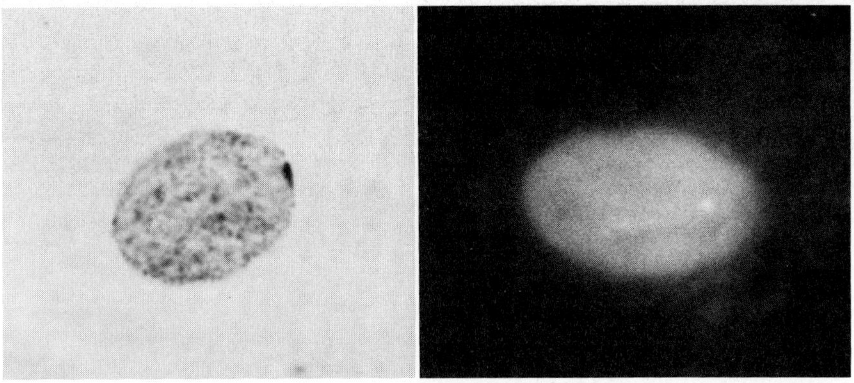 B

Fig. 22-10. A, Cell from buccal mucosa of normal female (could be from any individual whose cells contain two X chromosomes), showing densely staining X-chromatin mass adjacent to nuclear membrane. No such mass is seen in cells from a normal male or from any person whose cells contain only one X chromosome. **B,** Cell from buccal mucosa of a normal male (could be from any individual whose cells contain one Y chromosome) stained with quinacrine mustard and photographed in the fluorescent microscope. This shows a brightly fluorescent point within the nucleus, called a Y-chromatin mass.

man is the buccal mucosa. Thus the buccal smear is the commonly used means of nuclear sexing in the human. If an X-chromatin mass is present, the buccal smear is referred to as *X-chromatin positive;* if no cell in the buccal smear contains an X-chromatin mass, the smear is called *X-chromatin negative*. In our laboratory an X-chromatin mass is seen in the nuclei of 20% to 50% of cells of a buccal smear of a normal female. It is never seen in the normal XY male. If less than 20% of buccal mucosal cells contain an X-chromatin mass, the smear is interpreted as positive, but mosaicism is suspected. The second type of evaluation of the buccal smear is the examination of cells stained with a quinacrine compound in the fluorescent microscope for the presence of a small brightly fluorescent point within the nucleus of the buccal mucosal cell. When metaphase chromosomes of a normal male are stained with quinacrine and examined in the fluorescent microscope, the distal portion of the long arm of the normal Y chromosome is the most brightly fluorescent chromosome segment in the entire karyotype (Fig. 22-11). In interphase cells containing one Y chromosome, that Y appears as the above mentioned brightly fluorescent intranuclear point (Fig. 22-10, *B*). In general, the bright point is seen in only a portion of the buccal mucosal cells. In addition, in cells containing more than one Y chromosome, the maximum number of brightly fluorescent points in interphase cells bears a one-to-one relationship with the number of Y chromosomes. The brightly fluorescent point is referred to as the *Y-chromatin mass*.

Chromosome analysis. Chromosome analysis is performed with cultures of skin fibroblasts, lymphocytes, bone marrow, or other tissues to determine both quantitative and qualitative variations from the normal chromosome complement. In abnormal sex determination and differentiation, abnormalities in the number and/or structure of the sex chromosomes are important, as are sex chromosome complements that, although not truly abnormal, are inconsistent with the genital phenotype. These are described in the discussions of the specific conditions involved.

Vaginal appearance and cytology. These are important for cytologic evaluation and pH determination, which are useful in appraisal of estrogen secretion. In the prepubertal child the pH of the vaginal secretions is alkaline; it changes to acid at puberty. The prepubertal vaginal mucosa consists of a thin layer of epithelial cells; it develops into a stratified squamous epithelium at puberty.

Vaginography. Radiographic contrast studies are helpful in defining the anatomy of the in-

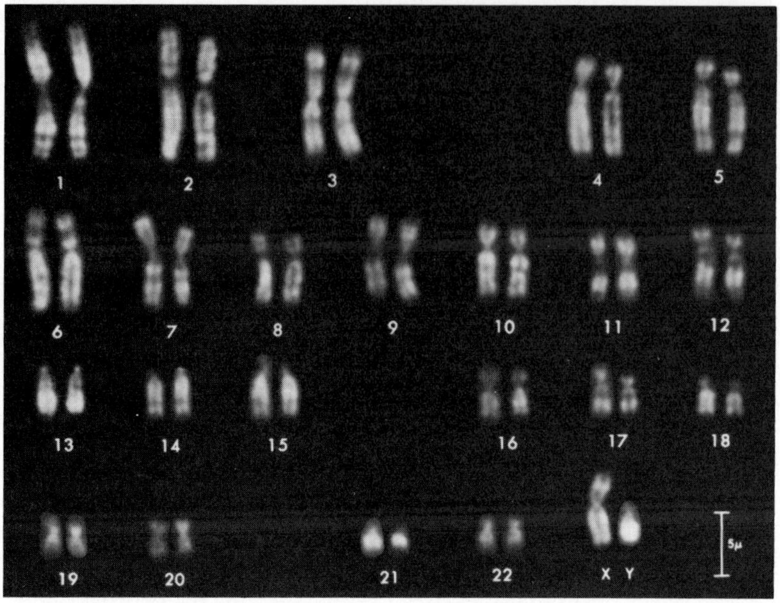

Fig. 22-11. Q-banded (fluorescent) karyotype of a normal male demonstrating intensity of fluorescence of long arm of Y chromosome. (Courtesy A.T. Therapel, Memphis.)

ternal genitalia of phenotypic females and patients with ambiguous genitalia.

Ultrasonography. Pelvic ultrasonography is a nonradiologic, noninvasive technique that, in the hands of an experienced ultrasonographer, permits definition of the pelvic contents of phenotypic females and patients with intersex genitalia.

Laparotomy and gonadal biopsy. Laparotomy and gonadal biopsy are considered in the discussion of the specific conditions involved.

Constitutional variations in normal sexual development

Although the average normal sequence of events in sexual maturation occurs as indicated in Table 22-6, considerable variations in timing and sequence may also occur, the ultimate result being a normal adult male or female. These variations are accounted for (1) by differences in the timing of changes in the hypothalamic-pituitary-gonadal axis, (2) by variations in relative amounts of the sex hormones elaborated by the adolescent gonads and adrenals, and (3) by variations in degree of responsiveness of various end organs. Such normal variations must be differentiated from more serious disorders.

Constitutional variations in normal sexual development to be considered include (1) delayed onset of adolescence, (2) premature thelarche or pubarche, (3) variations such as hirsutism and acne in girls and gynecomastia in boys, (4) menstrual disorders such as amenorrhea and other irregularities, and (5) cryptorchidism.

Delay in onset of adolescence. Delay in onset of adolescence, which results ultimately in a normal adult, may be confused with sexual infantilism.

Clinical features. Important clinical features are (1) failure of adolescent sexual maturation at the expected time; (2) lag in somatic growth and psychic maturation; (3) delay in osseous maturation; (4) frequent family history of similar adolescent pattern; (5) obesity in some cases, particularly in a pectoral and pelvic distribution, producing in the male small-appearing genitalia buried in a pubic fat pad; and (6) eventual normal sexual maturation and function.

Diagnostic aids. Diagnostic aids include (1) evaluation of testicular growth and maturation, such as firmness and size; (2) radiographic examination for bone age; (3) plasma and urinary sex steroid and gonadotropin levels in a range compatible with the developmental level, as well as a normal pituitary-adrenal axis demonstrated by a normal metyrapone test, help to exclude hypopituitarism; (4) in females, normal buccal mucosal X-chromatin pattern, normal chromosome analysis, and normal gonadotropin levels help to differentiate from Turner syndrome; (5) in males, X-chromatin–negative and Y-chromatin–positive buccal smear help to differentiate from Klinefelter syndrome; and (6) observation for a period of 6 to 12 months will usually establish the diagnosis.

Treatment. Usually no treatment is needed. In selected patients emotional problems resulting from delayed development may justify hormonal substitution therapy.

Prognosis. Normal sexual development occurs at later than the average time, resulting in a normal adult.

Premature thelarche. Premature thelarche is the development of breasts in prepubertal females without other signs of pubescence and probably represents either an unusual end organ sensitivity to preadolescent levels of circulating estrogen or intermittent secretion of estrogens by the ovaries.

Clinical features. Clinical features include the following: (1) the condition may occur at any time during infancy or childhood; (2) enlargement is usually bilaterally symmetric; (3) breast enlargement is generally permanent, rarely temporary; (4) the labia, vagina, and uterus remain infantile; (5) pubic hair is absent; and (6) signs of virilization are absent.

Diagnostic aids. The vaginal smear reveals minimal, if any, estrinization. If this is the case in a child with early breast development, a period of observation is warranted before further evaluation is undertaken. Assays for hormone levels (gonadotropins and sex steroids) are all in the prepubertal range and are of little practical value, although estrogen levels have been found elevated in a few cases.

Treatment. Management consists of reassurance that ultimate development will be normal.

Prognosis. Normal adolescence will occur at the usual time.

Premature pubarche. Premature pubarche is the early development of sexual hair without signs of sexual maturation. Its cause is either unusual end organ sensitivity to low levels of androgens or early elaboration of increased amounts of androgens.

Clinical features. Pertinent clinical features are as follows: (1) it is more common in females; (2) lack of other signs of sexual maturation differentiates premature pubarche from true sexual precocity; and (3) absence of rapid virilization and lack of enlargement of clitoris or penis, along with normal urinary sex steroids, differentiates the condition from adrenal tumor or hyperplasia. Root has suggested the term *premature pubarche* for the precocious development of pubic hair with normal-for-age plasma androgen levels and the term *premature adrenarche* for the precocious appearance of sexual hair with elevated plasma androgen levels.

Diagnostic aids. Diagnostic aids are the same as those for premature thelarche.

Treatment. No treatment is indicated other than reassurance that the outcome will be normal.

Prognosis. Normal adolescence will occur at the usual time.

Hirsutism and acne in adolescent girls. Hirsutism and acne are common complaints of pubescent females.

Etiology. The cause is probably a general hypersensitivity of the hair follicles to normal amounts of androgen or possibly an imbalance between the amounts of secreted estrogen and androgen.

Clinical features. The patient may be larger and more muscular than the average child. Adolescence usually progresses normally, and signs of virilization are absent.

Differential diagnosis. In postnatal adrenal hyperplasia or tumor other signs of virilization and elevated plasma and urinary sex steroid levels (and elevated urinary pregnanetriol in adrenal hyperplasia) help to diagnose these conditions. Polycystic ovarian disease can be differentiated with little difficulty on the clinical basis and from the presence of large polycystic ovaries. Drug-induced hirsutism, such as that seen with the administration of androgens, cobalt preparations, and diphenylhydantoin, may rarely be considered, as may hirsutism that sometimes occurs in hypothyroidism.

Treatment. Usually no treatment is justified other than local skin care. Excision and/or wedge resection of polycystic ovaries is performed when indicated in polycystic ovarian disease.

Gynecomastia in adolescent boys. A tiny amount of retroareolar breast tissue occurs temporarily in most pubescent males but occasionally may become prominent enough to create emotional problems.

Etiology. The cause of gynecomastia is unknown. Suggested possibilities have included altered estrogen-androgen ratio, increased estrogen production by the testes, metabolic transformation of androgen to estrogen, hyperthyroidism, and abnormally large amounts of pituitary growth hormone.

Clinical features. Clinical features include the following: (1) breast enlargement is bilateral or unilateral, (2) no other abnormalities of adolescent development are present, and (3) breast enlargement is usually transitory but may be prominent and long lasting.

Differential diagnosis. Klinefelter syndrome can be diagnosed by the presence of small atrophic testes, abnormal buccal sex chromatin pattern, abnormal chromosome analysis, elevated urinary FSH, and testicular biopsy revealing azoospermia and peritubular fibrosis or tubular hyalinization. In a feminizing tumor of the adrenal gland there is a great increase in the excretion of urinary estrogen and elevation of other plasma and urinary sex steroids.

Treatment. Usually no treatment but reassurance is indicated. Mastectomy may be necessary in extreme cases.

Menstrual disorders

Normal delay in onset of menstruation (amenorrhea) and menstrual irregularities may cause concern and merit understanding by the physician.

Delayed menarche. Delayed menarche is ordinarily only of temporary concern.

Etiology. The usual cause of a delay in menstruation is the late onset of adolescence. However, congenital defects of the genital tract, such as imperforate hymen or absence or malformation of the vagina or uterus may be causes.

Clinical features. Generally there is a delay in appearance of other signs of puberty. If a congenital defect is present, careful physical examination will usually elucidate the condition.

Diagnostic aids. Diagnostic aids include the following: (1) lack of an estrogen effect on the vaginal smear, with essentially normal plasma and urinary gonadotropin levels; (2) normal radiographic bone age; (3) normal buccal sex chromatin pattern and chromosome analysis help to differentiate the condition from most forms of gonadal dysgenesis; (4) lack of virilization and normal levels of 17-ketosteroids and pregnanetriol will rule out adrenal causes; (5) vaginography will help to elucidate congenital malformations; and (6) laparotomy may be necessary.

Treatment. Cyclic estrogen therapy is instituted if indicated because of emotional problems.

Menstrual irregularities. Irregularity in timing of menstrual periods and in flow are the two most common conditions.

Etiology. Irregularities in timing of menstrual periods and in flow are common in adolescence. As previously mentioned, the first several menstrual periods after menarche are anovulatory, without the production of a corpus luteum and without elaboration of progesterone. Occasionally thyroid dysfunction may be the cause.

Clinical features. Pertinent clinical features are (1) irregular menstrual cycles, with perhaps months between periods; (2) often, prolonged menstrual periods, with excessive bleeding; and (3) otherwise normal progression of adolescent development.

Diagnosis. Diagnostic aids include the following: (1) family history of similar patterns may be helpful, (2) normal clinical progression of adolescent development, (3) no abnormalities of external or internal genitalia, (4) normal adolescent levels of plasma and urinary gonadotropins and sex steroids, (5) normal estrinization of vaginal mucosa, and (6) normal thyroid function tests unless thyroid dysfunction is present.

Treatment. Usually only reassurance is needed. If irregular menses persist, hormone therapy may be indicated.

Prognosis. Prognosis is generally good. Occasionally irregularities may persist throughout life or until completion of the first pregnancy.

Cryptorchidism. According to Paulsen, failure of testicular descent occurs with a frequency in males at birth of about 10%. By the end of the first year the incidence has decreased to 2% to 3% because of spontaneous descent. Even more descent takes place in childhood so that about 0.4% of adult males have unilateral or bilateral cryptorchidism.

Etiology. Several etiologic factors have been implicated, such as tight inguinal ring, short spermatic artery, and gonadotropin deficiency. However, Sohval and Charny have expressed the view that failure of descent is a result of testicular dysgenesis.

Clinical features. In isolated cryptorchidism the abnormality may be unilateral or bilateral. Spermatogenesis does not occur in the undescended testis.

Diagnosis. The undescended testis is located high within the inguinal canal or is not palpable because of its intra-abdominal position. This is to be differentiated from pseudocryptorchidism, in which the prepubertal testis, although sometimes within the scrotum, often retracts into the inguinal canal. Before a diagnosis of isolated bilateral cryptorchidism is made, the following conditions must be excluded: (1) female pseudohermaphroditism caused by congenital virilizing adrenal hyperplasia (pp. 582 and 584), (2) female pseudohermaphroditism resulting from a nonadrenal cause (p. 633), (3) rare cases of true hermaphroditism, (4) Noonan syndrome (pp. 638-639), (5) Klinefelter syndrome (pp. 627-628), and (6) anorchia (p. 638). The methods of exclusion are mentioned in the appropriate sections.

Treatment. Occasionally the testes apparently have descended, but instead of descending into the scrotum they are located in the perineal, superficial inguinal, or femoral region. When so located, they should be placed surgically in the scrotum as soon as the diagnosis is made. (See pp. 933 to 934.)

The vigor and type of treatment in cryptorchidism center around the question of how long the testis may remain in the abdomen without permanent damage. Recent evidence suggests that irreparable damage may occur if the testis remains in the abdomen past the age of 2 years. Other authors suggest that unless a specific indication for earlier surgical intervention exists, orchiopexy may be delayed until the appearance of the first signs of puberty. A 3-week course of human chorionic gonadotropin (HCG) will result in testicular descent in some cases. If this is not successful, surgery should not be delayed beyond early puberty because (1) spermatogenesis does not occur in undescended testes, (2) irreparable atrophy may eventually ensue, and (3) neoplasia has been shown to be increased as much as fortyfold in a cryptorchid testis in comparison with a scrotal one. On the other hand, evidence is lacking that surgery can be guaranteed to prevent malignancy in the once-cryptorchid testis. One remaining important point is that whenever orchiopexy is performed, testicular biopsy should *always* be obtained.

Prognosis. The spontaneously late-descending testis probably will ultimately function normally. The success of orchiopexy in producing a fully functioning adult testis, regardless of the age at which it is performed, remains controversial. Leydig cell function probably will be normal if testicular dysgenesis is not severe, but some investigators have demonstrated deficient spermatogenesis.

Abnormalities of sex determination/differentiation

Sex differentiation refers to the formation of the gonads, internal ductal system, and external genitalia. Abnormalities of sex differentiation are summarized in Table 22-7 and may be classified as follows: (1) Turner syndrome and variants, (2) XX and XY pure gonadal dysgenesis, (3) Klinefelter syndrome and variants, (4) polysomy Y, (5) incompletely masculinized male (male pseudohermaphrodite), (6) masculinized female (female pseudohermaphrodite), (7) true hermaphroditism, (8) 45, X/46,XY anomaly (gonosomal intersexuality), (9) uterine hernia syndrome, and (10) anorchia. This classification is outlined on pp. 616-621.

Turner syndrome and variants

In 1939 Turner reported seven phenotypic females with sexual infantilism, congenital webbed neck, and cubitus valgus. Much has been learned subsequently about the cause, pathogenesis, and clinical spectrum of this condition. Based on current knowledge, we now prefer to define Turner syndrome as *that spectrum of abnormalities which results from partial or complete monosomy X,* specifically, monosomy for the short arm of the X chromosome. The condition occurs in approximately 1 in 10,000 live female births but is much more common at conception. Recent evidence indicates that the 45,X defect occurs in as many as 1% of human conceptuses.

Etiology. Turner syndrome is caused by an abnormality of the sex chromosomes. In 1954 Polani and associates and Wilkins and associates found that cells from most patients with Turner syndrome lacked the X-chromatin mass and were thus *X-chromatin negative.* In 1959 cells

Text continued on p. 623.

Table 22-7. Types of abnormal sex determination/differentiation

Terminology	Description	Sex chromosome pattern	X-chromatin	Y-chromatin	Etiology
Turner syndrome	Gonadal dysgenesis (wide spectrum of severity) plus somatic anomalies; female phenotype	45,X most common	Negative	Negative	Chromosome aberration: partial or complete monosomy-X
		46,XXp- (deleted X)	Negative or posigive (small)	Negative	
		46,X,ring(X)	Negative or positive	Negative	
		46,X,isochromosome (Xq)	Positive (large)	Negative	
		And various mosaics such as:			
		45,X/46,XX	Negative or positive	Negative	
		45,X/47,XXX	Negative or positive (n − 1)	Negative	
		45,X/46,XXp-	Negative or positive	Negative	
		45,X/46,X,ring(X)	Negative or positive	Negative	
		45,X/46,X,isochromosome (Xq)	Negative or positive	Negative	
		45,X/46,XY	Negative	Negative or positive	
		45,X/47,XYY	Negative	Negative or positive	
		And others			
Pure gonadal dysgenesis	Gonadal dysgenesis, usually without somatic anomalies; female phenotype	46,XX	Positive	Negative	Autosomal mutation in some cases
		46,XY	Negative	Positive	Autosomal or X-linked mutation
Klinefelter syndrome and variants	Testicular dysgenesis; male phenotype with variable anomalies and sometimes mental retardation	47,XXY; 48,XXYY; 48,XXXY; 49,XXXYY; 49,XXXXY; 47,XX(?); Various mosaics	Positive (X − 1)	Positive (1 per Y)	Chromsome aberration
Polysomy Y	Normal male or mental retardation and anomalies; sex differentiation and development usually normal but may be deficient	47,XYY 48,XYYY 46,XY/47,XYY	Negative	Positive (1 per Y)	Chromsome aberration

Gonadal structure						
Form	**Ovarian elements**	**Testicular elements**	**Germ cells**	**External genitalia**	**Genital ducts**	**Secondary sex**
Streak or variably dysgenetic	Stroma only or stroma with a few follicles that may be abnormal	Absent or vestiges, occasionally hilar cells	Absent or scanty (patient almost always sterile)	Female	Female	Usually absent but occasionally present to variable degrees
Tendency to neoplasia	Variable	Variable		Female	Female	Usually absent but may virilize
Streak	Usually stroma only	Absent	Absent (patient sterile)	Female	Female	Absent or minimal feminization
Variable; tendency to neoplasia	Usually stroma only	Absent or vestiges	Absent (patient sterile)	Female or ambiguous	Female	Absent or minimal feminization
Small testes, tubular fibrosis and hyalinization, Leydig cell hyperplasia	Vestiges	Dysgenetic tubules, Leydig cell hyperplasia	Absent (patient sterile)	Male	Male	Male but may be deficient, and associated with gynecomastia
Usually normal testes	Vestiges	Present	Present	Male or rarely ambiguous	Male	Usually normal

Continued.

Table 22-7. Types of abnormal sex determination/differentiation—cont'd

Terminology	Description	Sex chromosome pattern	X-chromatin	Y-chromatin	Etiology
Incompletely masculinized male (male pseudohermaphrodite)	Testicular dysgenesis	46,XY	Negative	Positive	Unknown
	Leydig cell hypoplasia/aplasia	46,XY	Negative	Positive	Unknown
	Defect in testosterone biosynthesis	46,XY	Negative	Positive	
	Conversion of cholesterol to pregnenolone				Autosomal recessive mutation
	3β-Hydroxysteroid dehydrogenase				Autosomal recessive mutation
	17α-Hydroxylase				Autosomal recessive mutation
	17,20-Desmolase				X-linked recessive mutation
	17-Ketosteroid reductase				X-linked or autosomal recessive mutation
	Defect in conversion of testosterone to dihydrotestosterone caused by 5α-reductase deficiency	46,XY	Negative	Positive	Autosomal recessive mutation
	Complete androgen insensitivity syndrome	46,XY	Negative	Positive	X-linked mutation
	Incomplete androgen insensitivity syndrome	46,XY	Negative	Positive	X-linked mutation

Gonadal structure						
Form	**Ovarian elements**	**Testicular elements**	**Germ cells**	**External genitalia**	**Genital ducts**	**Secondary sex**
Dysgenetic testis with varying degrees of differentiation, intra-abdominal	Vestiges	Scattered abnormal seminiferous tubules	Absent or early forms only	Abiguous but variable	Wide variability	Variable but may be absent
Testes in labioscrotal folds, in inguinal canals, or intra-abdominal	Vestiges	Present but Leydig cells few or absent	Early forms only	Female with blind vagina and minimal posterior labial fusion	Male	Absent
Testes in labioscrotal folds, inguinal canals, or intra-abdominal	Vestiges	Present	Present but immature forms only	Female or ambiguous with blind ending vagina	Variable male differentiation but may have prostatic utricle	Variable virilization with breast development in some cases
Testes in labioscrotal folds, inguinal canals, or intra-abdominal	Vestiges	Present	All stages present	Ambiguous minimal virilization but with single urogenital opening	Male	Marked virilization
Testes in labial folds, inguinal canals, or intra-abdominal	Vestiges	Present	Usually absent or early forms only	Female with a blind vagina	Absent	Female (sexual hair minimal or absent)
Testes in labial folds, inguinal canals, or intra-abdominal	Vestiges	Present	Usually absent or early forms only	Ambiguous with a blind vagina	Male or absent	Female

Continued.

Table 22-7. Types of abnormal sex determination/differentiation—cont'd

Terminology	Description	Sex chromosome pattern	X-chromatin	Y-chromatin	Etiology
Masculinized female (female pseudohermaphrodite)	Congenital virilizing adrenal hyperplasia (21-hydroxylase, 11-β-hydroxylase, 3-β-hydroxysteroid dehydrogenase deficiency)	46,XX	Positive	Negative	Autosomal recessive mutation
	Virilizing adrenal tumor	46,XX	Positive	Negative	Unknown
	Exogenous steroids from mother in utero (nonprogressive after birth)	46,XX	Positive	Negative	Progestational or maternal tumor
True hermaphroditism	Ovary and testis, or ovotestis, variable somatic anomalies	46,XX 46,XY 46,XX/46,XY Other mosaics	Positive Negative Variable Variable	Negative Positive Variable Variable	Usually unknown; occasionally autosomal mutation
Gonosomal intersexuality	Varying degrees of gonadal dysgenesis, "mixed" gonadal dysgenesis with varying somatic abnormalities	45,X/46,XY mosaicism	Negative	Variable	Chromosome aberration
Noonan syndrome	Male or female with hypogonadism, multiple anomalies, some similar to Turner syndrome, but others distinct such as mental retardation, pulmonary stenosis	Female 46,XX Male 46,XY	Positive Negative	Negative Positive	Autosomal dominant mutation
Uterine hernia syndrome	Male phenotype with hernia that contains müllerian structures	46,XY	Negative	Positive	Heterogeneous
Anorchia	Male external genitalia with no demonstrable gonadal tissue	46,XY	Negative	Positive	Unknown

	Gonadal structure					
Form	**Ovarian elements**	**Testicular elements**	**Germ cells**	**External genitalia**	**Genital ducts**	**Secondary sex**
Ovaries	Present	Vestiges	Present	Ambiguous or cryptorchid male	Female	Progressive virilization if not treated
Ovaries	Present	Vestiges	Present	Clitoridal enlargement	Female	Progressive virilization if not treated
Ovaries	Present	Vestiges	Present	Ambiguous	Female	Female
Testis and ovary or ovotestis(es)	Present	Present	Present	Usually ambiguous to varying degrees	Variable	Variable
Normal testes; "mixed" gonadal dysgenesis (streak on one side and testis on other, often with neoplasia)	Stroma only in streaks	Present in testes but may be abnormal	Present in testes in some cases	Male, female, or ambiguous	Variable	Variable
Usually normal	Present	Vestiges	Usually present	Female	Female	Usually normal but may be delayed
Normal testis or germinal aplasia or agonadism	Vestiges	Present	May be absent	Male, but often cryptorchid	Male	Variable, often deficient
Testis, in scrotum or cryptorchid	Vestiges	Present	Present	Male, but may be cryptorchid	Male, but with persistent müllerian structures	Male
No gonad demonstrable	Absent	Absent	Absent	Male (small penis)	Male	Absent unless androgen substitution therapy

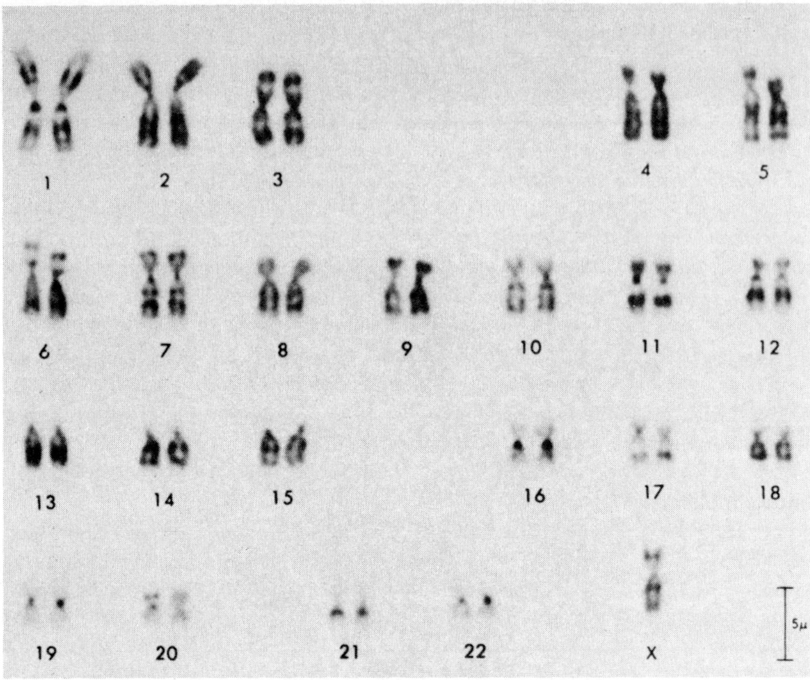

Fig. 22-12. Karyotype of phenotypic female with X-chromatin–negative Turner syndrome, containing only 45 chromosomes with sex chromosome constitution 45,X.

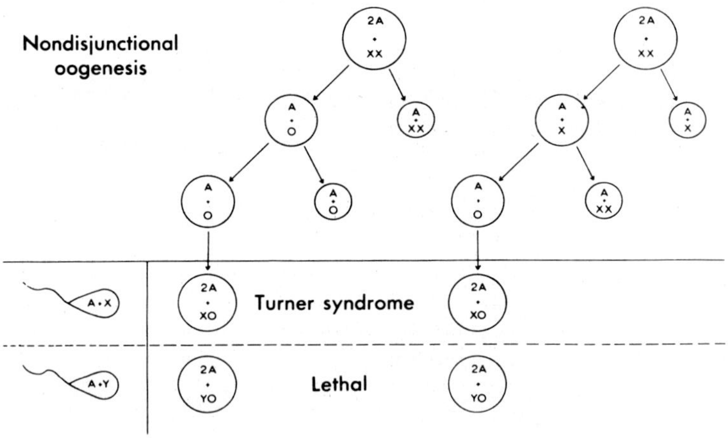

Fig. 22-13. Examples of errors in cell division that may lead to Turner syndrome. *2A* signifies two haploid sets of autosomes (44 autosomes). This depicts meiotic nondisjunction in oogenesis (may also occur in spermatogenesis), leading to ovum containing no sex chromosome: if fertilized by an X-bearing sperm, it leads to 45,X Turner syndrome; if fertilized by a Y-bearing sperm, it leads to a YO zygote that is not viable.

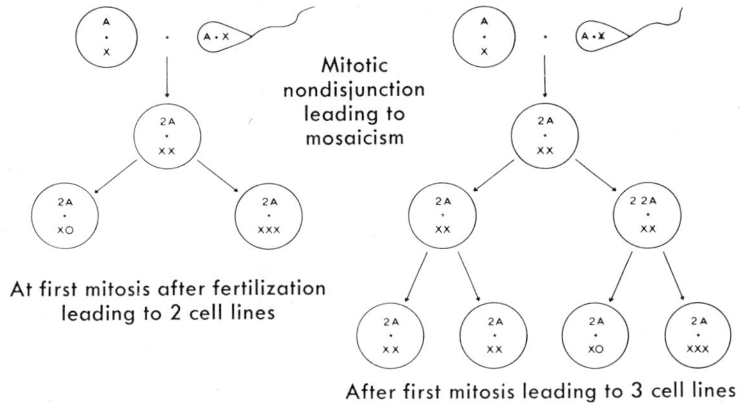

Fig. 22-14. Mitotic nondisjunction in zygote: left, in first cleavage division, mitotic nondisjunction leads to 47,XXX/45,X mosaicism; right, after first cleavage division, mitotic nondisjunction may lead to 47,XXX/46,XX/45,X mosaicism.

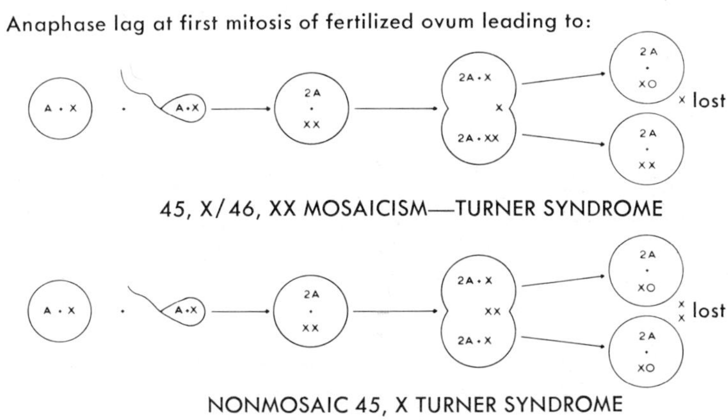

Fig. 22-15. Anaphase lag in cleavage of a 46,XX zygote: above, with loss of X from only one daughter cell, anaphase lag leads to 45,X/46,XX mosaicism; below, with loss of X chromosomes from both daughter cells, anaphase lag leads to nonmosaic 45,X karyotype.

of such patients were found to contain only 45 chromosomes: 44 autosomes and one X chromosome (Fig. 22-12). The second sex chromosome was missing (45,X: *complete monosomy X*). Such a chromosome abnormality may arise through one or more of several mechanisms. *Meiotic nondisjunction* in oogenesis (Fig. 22-13) or spermatogenesis may lead to *complete monosomy X. Nondisjunction* in and early *mitotic* division of the embryo (Fig. 22-14) may lead to *mosaic monosomy X,* the commonest type of which is the presence in the same individual of a 46,XX cell line and a 45,X cell line. Another type is 45,X/46,XY mosaicism (considered in the discussion of gonosomal intersexuality), which in some cases produces Turner syndrome. *Anaphase lag* at the first cleavage division of the zygote may produce mosaic or nonmosaic monosomy X (Fig. 22-15). *Partial monosomy X,* the existence in cells of one normal X chromosome plus a structurally altered second X chromosome, may also produce Turner syndrome. In general, the buccal smear in patients with mosaic monosomy X and partial monosomy X is X-chromatin positive. Less than 20% of nuclei may contain an X-chromatin mass in mosaic monosomy X, whereas the size of the X-chromatin mass may be abnormally large or small in partial monosomy X. Approximately 30% of cases of Turner syndrome are X-chromatin positive. A sex karyotype that includes a normal X chromosome and a tiny centric fragment of either X or Y origin has occasionally been reported in Turner syndrome. Some cases, in which the fragment is presumed to be of Y origin, reveal clitoridal hypertrophy.

Table 22-8 summarizes the chromosome complements found in Turner syndrome. The percentages of the karyotypes in the table are based on data from the Inter-regional Cytogenetic Registry System (ICRS). Of the 651 cases of Turner syndrome on file with the ICRS, the 45,X chromosome complement was found in only 50%.

Pathogenesis. In the presence of a 45,X sex chromosome constitution or a structural abnormality of the second X chromosome, gonadal formation in the embryo is most often defective. Singh and Carr have shown that gonadal differentiation and development are probably normal during the first 3 months of fetal life and that germ cells are abundant. At later fetal stages, however, germ cells are fewer in number and connective tissue is increased. The partially differentiated ovary degenerates to leave a small dysgenetic gonad or fibrous streak. In the presence of such a dysgenetic gonad the internal and external genitalia undergo differentiation exactly as they do in the presence of a normally differentiated ovary. However, in the absence of an ovary the phenotypic female fails to develop at puberty, has no menses, and is sterile (Fig. 22-16). In addition, the sex chromosome abnormality leads to various somatic anomalies.

Table 22-8. Chromosome complements in Turner syndrome

Chromosome complement	Cases (%)
45,X	50
Mosaic: 45,X/46,XX; 45,X/46,XX/47,XXX; 45,X/47,XXX	13
Structural abnormality of X: 46,i(Xq); 45,X/46,X,i(Xq); other mosaics including i(Xq)	28
Cell line including Y chromosome: 45,X/46,XY; 45,X/47,XXYY; etc.	5.5
45,X,mar	3

In reality, the natural history of a normal ovary is progressive degeneration by way of attrition of primordial and primary follicles throughout the life of a female, plus loss through ovulation. This degeneration ordinarily requires four to five decades for completion. In most patients with Turner syndrome, degeneration is complete before the birth of the patient. However, in some cases, follicles may be apparent in infancy; they may remain to allow pubertal development and menses for a limited period in adolescence and young adulthood but rarely permit fertility.

Clinical manifestations. Although few cases present all the possible typical features, these include (Fig. 22-17) (1) significant short stature in virtually all cases; (2) congenital webbed neck and low posterior hairline in 40% to 50% of cases; (3) facies presenting micrognathia, "old" appearance, and low-set and at times malformed ears; (4) so-called shield chest deformity with hypoplastic nipples; (5) congenital heart disease, including coarctation of the aorta, valvular aortic stenosis, and others; (6) anomalies of the urinary tract; (7) increased carrying angle at the elbow (cubitus valgus); (8) numerous pigmented nevi; (9) dysplasia of the fingernails and toenails; (10) mental retardation in a few cases; (11) congenital lymphedema of the limbs; (12) an abnormal pattern of growth characterized by the absence of normally occurring growth spurts; and (13) absence in most cases of sexual development at puberty with primary amenorrhea and sterility. The gonads are replaced by streaks of white fibrous tissue in the mesovarium, which histologically contain cells resembling those of ovarian stroma but no germ cells. The tubes, uterus, and vagina are infantile. Pubic and axillary hair usually appears in adolescence but is sparse.

Diagnosis. Individuals with this condition come to the pediatrician ordinarily for one of three reasons: (1) peripheral lymphedema and webbed neck in a phenotypic newborn female infant; (2) short stature or failure to grow at the normal rate in a phenotypic prepubertal female, with or without associated somatic anomalies; or (3) failure of adolescent development with primary amenorrhea. The patient may occasionally be brought to the physician because of

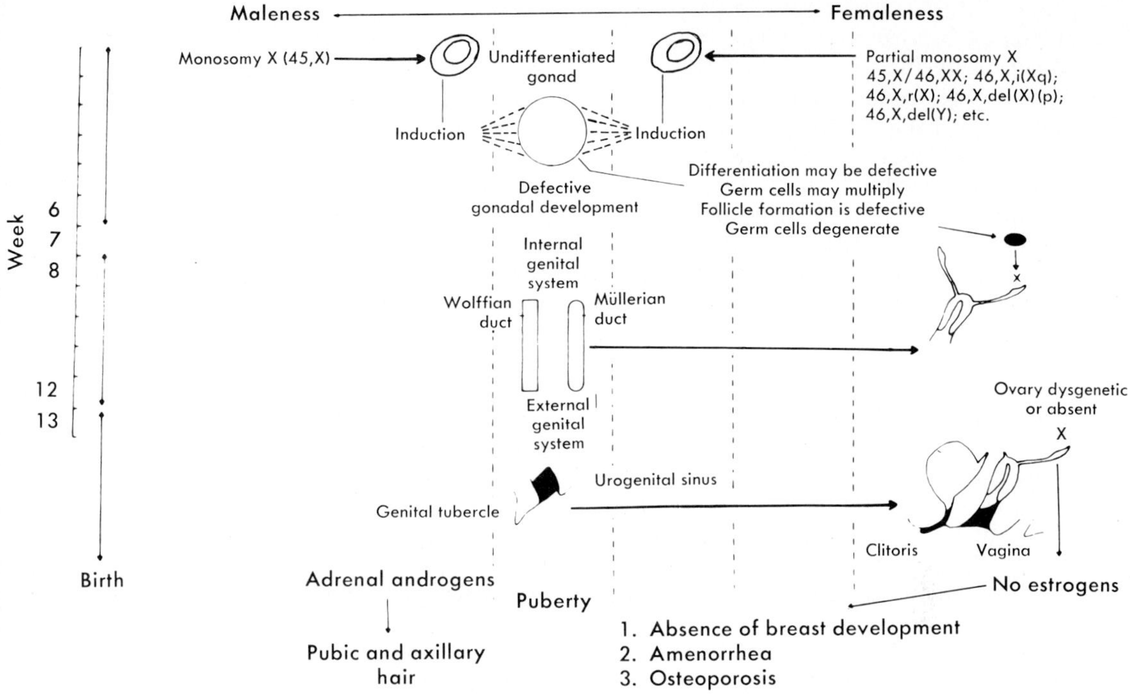

Fig. 22-16. Sex differentiation and development in Turner syndrome. (Modified from Newman, S., et al.: Postgrad. Med. **27:**488, 1960.)

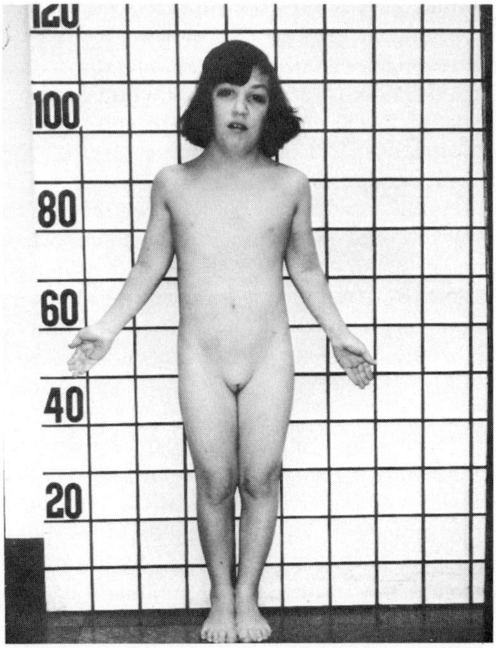

Fig. 22-17. View of typical patient with the 45,X Turner syndrome. Patient is a phenotypic female. External features are described as classic in text.

symptoms of heart disease. When the clinical appearance suggests Turner syndrome or in any phenotypic female with one of the three features—peripheral lymphedema in a neonate, short stature, or failure of sexual development—the following may be of diagnostic aid: (1) a buccal smear that is X-chromatin negative (an X-chromatin positive buccal smear, however, does not preclude the diagnosis), (2) a chromosome analysis that reveals one of the abnormalities noted in Table 22-7, (3) elevated plasma and urinary gonadotropin levels in pubertal or postpubertal patients, and (4) absent or rudimentary ovaries at laparotomy. As indicated previously, an occasional patient may reveal some degree of adolescent development with menses, whereas some may reveal clitoral enlargement and other evidence of virilization. A majority of these are mosaic, the former having a 46,XX as well as a 45,X or structurally abnormal X-bearing cell line, the latter probably being caused by 45,X/46,XY mosaicism and being associated with a predisposition to gonadal neoplasia.

Management. If diagnosis is made before adolescence, the only therapy is practical psychologic support of parents and patient. If webbing of the neck is disfiguring, surgical correction may be undertaken. Cardiac disease requires proper management if present. When the patient fails to develop in adolescence, appropriate hormone therapy will result in breast development, appearance of sexual hair, and maturation of labia and vaginal mucosa; cyclic estrogen administration will produce uterine bleeding simulating menses. Treatment with an anabolic steroid for a period of several years before the institution of estrogen therapy may enhance the height of the patient. No form of therapy will lead to fertility. Excision of gonadal tissue is advocated in all 45,X/46,XY mosaic patients.

XX and XY pure gonadal dysgenesis

In XX and XY "pure" gonadal dysgenesis the patient is a phenotypic female with gonadal dysgenesis but usually without somatic abnormalities of Turner syndrome. The patient may be tall with eunochoid features and may or may not have a variety of other anomalies.

XX pure gonadal dysgenesis. Although most cases are sporadic, gonadal dysgenesis with an XX sex karyotype has been described in multiple siblings. This factor, in addition to parental consanguinity in some families, points to an autosomal recessive genetic mode in this condition. On the other hand, genetic heterogeneity cannot be excluded. Stature is usually normal or tall, and patients present in adolescence because of primary amenorrhea with absent or minimal sex development. Mentality is normal. Pubic hair may be absent or scant. Laparotomy reveals the presence of uterus and fallopian tubes, but instead of ovaries, fibrous streaks are found to contain no follicles.

XY pure gonadal dysgenesis. Both sporadic and familial cases of this condition, also referred to as Swyer syndrome, have been described. The distribution of affected patients in families with multiple affected members suggests a pattern consistent, in some cases, with an autosomal recessive mode of inheritance with genetic male sex limitation and, in other cases, with an X-linked recessive genetic mode. H-Y antigen assays conducted on cells from some affected patients have been negative, suggesting that the etiology of gonadal dysgenesis in those patients is a defect in H-Y antigen synthesis or a qualitative defect in the H-Y antigen molecule, rendering it undetectable. In other cases H-Y antigen is detectable. In the latter category, failure of the testis-inducing influence of H-Y antigen may be explained on the postulate that the function of H-Y antigen requires a cell surface receptor, and that this receptor in H-Y positive cases of XY gonadal dysgenesis is defective.

Genetic heterogeneity in XY gonadal dysgenesis is supported by the occurrence of both H-Y positive and H-Y negative cases. Further genetic heterogeneity is documented by the coexistence in a number of reported cases of various patterns of somatic anomalies. Most patients are of normal or tall stature. Symptoms include primary amenorrhea and absent or minimal sex development. Body proportions may be eunuchoid. A few patients exhibit evidence of virilization. Laparotomy reveals uterus and fallopian tubes, but only fibrous streaks or neoplastic tissue are present instead of normally differentiated testes. In one series, gonadal tumors were found in 26% of 76 cases. These were, for the most part, gonadoblastomas and dysgerminomas.

Diagnosis. The diagnosis should be suspected in a phenotypic female otherwise normal except possibly a eunuchoid habitus, who has primary amenorrhea and absent or deficient feminization. The buccal smear is X-chromatin positive if the sex chromosome constitution is XX, X-chromatin negative if it is XY. The diagnosis is occasionally made incidentally in a prepubertal patient at the time of appendectomy or laparotomy for another reason when ovaries are found to be replaced by fibrous streaks. Even in an adolescent female with the clinical features of this condition, laparotomy is necessary for the diagnosis.

Management. Estrogen substitution therapy is indicated just as it is in Turner syndrome. The patient should be told that she is normal except that her ovaries failed to develop normally, resulting in the need for estrogen therapy, and that she should adopt any desired children. The excision of any rudimentary gonadal tissue is advocated in cases of XY gonadal dysgenesis because of the predisposition to neoplasia.

Klinefelter syndrome and variants

In 1942 Klinefelter and associates described a group of phenotypic males with azoospermia, small testes, intact Leydig cells, increased FSH excretion in urine, gynecomastia, normal or decreased urinary 17-ketosteroid excretion, defective development of secondary sex characteristics, and hyalinization of seminiferous tubules. Subsequently, many variations of the classic syndrome have been reported. Mental retardation and skeletal defects are common, although many victims of Klinefelter syndrome are of normal intelligence and have only problems of sterility.

Etiology. In 1956 Plunkett and Barr reported that about 80% of their patients had X-chromatin–positive buccal smears. In 1959 Jacobs and Strong reported a sex chromosome abnormality in the X-chromatin–positive Klinefelter syndrome. The karyotype included 47 chromosomes with sex chromosome constitution XXY (Fig. 22-18). The probable mechanism responsible for this karyotype is nondisjunction

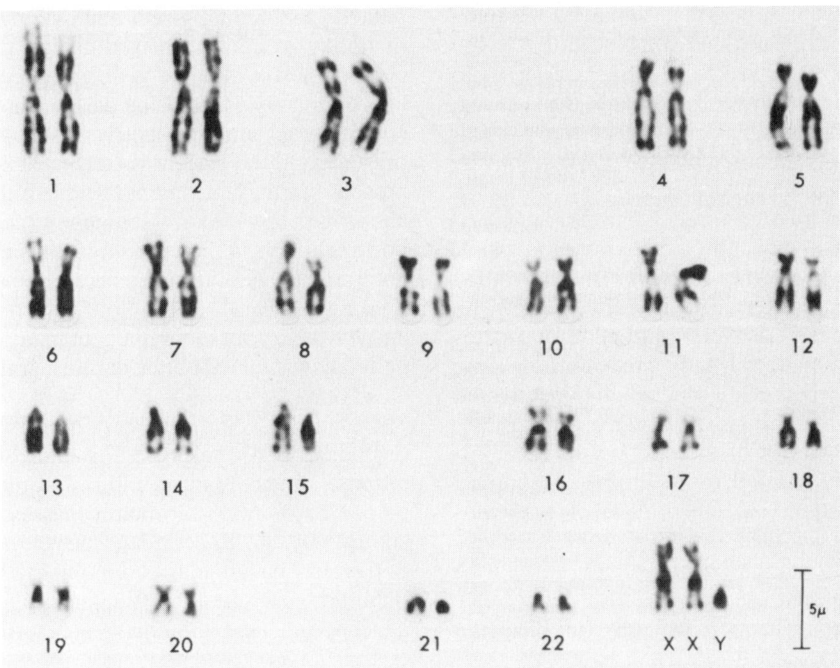

Fig. 22-18. 47,XXY Karyotype of Klinefelter syndrome. (Courtesy A.T. Therapel, Memphis.)

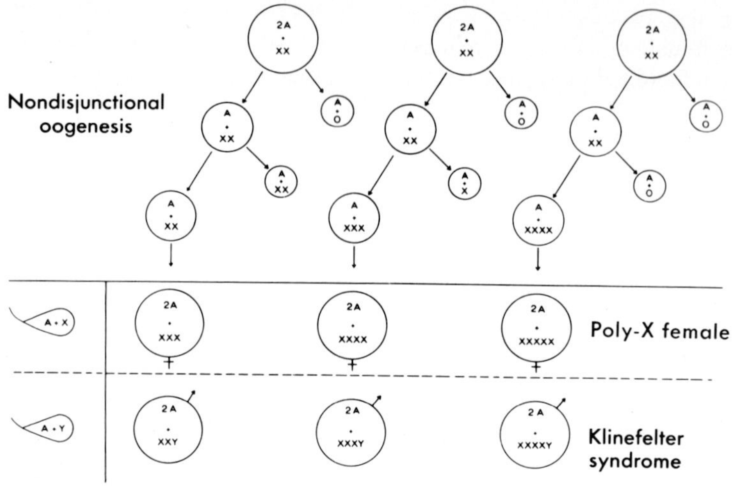

Fig. 22-19. Examples of nondisjunction in oogenesis that may result in Klinefelter syndrome if fertilized by a Y-bearing sperm or in the poly-X female if fertilized by an X-bearing sperm. Nondisjunction in spermatogenesis may also lead to either condition. *2A* signifies two haploid sets of autosomes (44 autosomes).

at meiosis (Fig. 22-19). Since the presence of two X chromosomes is necessary for an X-chromatin–positive buccal smear, the basis for an X-chromatin–positive buccal smear in Klinefelter syndrome became apparent. Subsequently, sex chromosome constitutions XXXY, XXXXY, XXYY, XXXYY (Fig. 22-19), and many mosaics have been found. In these cases, because of the single X origin of the X-chromatin mass, as specified by the *Lyon hypothesis,* nuclei of buccal mucosal cells may contain a maximum of two or three X-chromatin masses—one less than the total number of X chromosomes in the nucleus (the so-called "X − 1" rule referred to in Table 22-7). The Lyon hypothesis (in oversimplified terms) states that in any somatic cell only one X chromosome is genetically active, all others being inactivated through formation of an X-chromatin mass. Current knowledge of the etiology of Klinefelter syndrome has led us to limit its definition to *the phenotypic male with clinical and laboratory abnormalities resulting from the presence of two or more X chromosomes, along with one or more Y chromosomes*. XXY Klinefelter syndrome occurs in approximately 1 in 1000 live male births.

Clinical manifestations. Patients are phenotypic males. The patient is seldom seen before puberty, and the diagnosis in prepubertal cases is made usually in X-chromatin surveys of consecutive newborn infants and of mentally defective children. A small proportion of affected patients are mentally retarded. Varying degrees of failure of adolescent virilization may occur. Gynecomastia of some visible degree occurs in approximately 20% of the cases. The testes are small, firm, and insensitive. Azoospermia is present, and the patient is sterile. Sexual hair is present but may be sparse. The habitus is often abnormal; lower body segment exceeds upper body segment, although arm span is not usually greater than height. In general, those patients with more complex aneuploidy, such as XXXY and XXXXY, are more likely to manifest mental deficiency, skeletal abnormalities, and shortness of stature.

Diagnosis. When the condition is suspected on the basis of the preceding clinical manifestations, a buccal smear will reveal the presence of one or more X-chromatin masses. Chromosome analysis will define the karyotype. Urinary gonadotropins are elevated in pubertal and postpubertal cases, and testicular biopsy reveals azoospermia and the changes described previously.

Management. Patients are sterile and should be so advised, with proper guidance and counseling to help avoid psychologic problems. Mastectomy may be indicated if gynecomastia is a problem. Androgen substitution therapy is often helpful in stimulating virilization and seems to be useful in avoiding psychologic problems. Mental retardation may be a limiting factor.

Polysomy Y

The first reported patient with an XYY sex chromosome constitution was the normal father of a child with Down syndrome. A few patients have exhibited hypogonadism and/or cryptorchidism. Most affected patients have been found in surveys of tall inmates of criminal institutions. The majority of reported patients have been tall and aggressive with antisocial tendencies. This biased sampling may have led to an extremely limited view of the total phenotypic spectrum of Y-polysomy.

Incompletely masculinized male (male pseudohermaphroditism)

Male pseudohermaphroditism is present in a genetic male (XY) who has two testes but in whom the external genitalia may resemble those of the normal female or may be ambiguous. The term *pseudohermaphroditism* indicates agreement between genetic sex and basic gonadal sex, with abnormal gonadal, or target cell, function resulting in abnormal genital anatomy. The following outline of abnormalities of sex differentiation leading to abnormal genitalia includes a comprehensive classification of male pseudohermaphroditism:

- I. Incompletely masculinized male (male pseudohermaphroditism)
  - A. Type with female external genital phenotype
    - 1. Leydig cell aplasia (testicular unresponsiveness to LH and HCG)
    - 2. Complete or very severe biochemical defect in androgen biosynthesis
      - a. Defect in conversion of cholesterol to Δ^5-pregnenolone caused by a defect in enzyme system that includes 20-alpha-hydroxylase, 22R-hydroxylase, and 20,22-desmolase
      - b. 17-alpha-hydroxylase deficiency
      - c. 17,20-desmolase (lyase) deficiency
    - 3. Complete androgen insensitivity syndrome
      - a. Cytosol-binding protein defect demonstrable
      - b. Cytosol-binding protein defect not demonstrable
  - B. Type with intersex genitalia
    - 1. Testicular dysgenesis (dysgenetic male pseudohermaphroditism)
    - 2. Defects in androgen biosynthesis
      - a. Defect in conversion of cholesterol to Δ^5-pregnenolone caused by a defect in enzyme system that includes 20-alpha-hydroxylase, 22R-hydroxylase, and 20,22-desmolase
      - b. 3-beta-hydroxysteroid dehydrogenase deficiency
      - c. 17-alpha-hydroxylase deficiency
      - d. 17,20-desmolase (lyase) deficiency
      - e. 17-ketosteroid reductase (17-beta-hydroxysteroid oxidoreductase) deficiency
    - 3. Defect in conversion of testosterone to 5-alpha-dihydrotestosterone caused by deficient 5-alpha-reductase activity in androgen-responsive target tissues
    - 4. Incomplete androgen insensitivity syndrome
      - a. Cytosol-binding protein defect demonstrable
      - b. Cytosol-binding protein defect not demonstrable
    - 5. Others, usually with associated nongenital anomalies
- II. Masculinized female (female pseudohermaphroditism)
  - A. Congenital virilizing adrenal hyperplasia
    - 1. 21-hydroxylase deficiency
    - 2. 11-beta-hydroxylase deficiency
    - 3. 3-beta-hydroxysteroid dehydrogenase deficiency
    - 4. 17-alpha-hydroxylase deficiency
  - B. Virilizing adrenal tumor
  - C. Masculinization of the fetus by maternally derived hormonal effect
    - 1. Maternal virilizing ovarian tumor during pregnancy
    - 2. Maternal consumption of progestational agents, testosterone and related steroids, or ? stilbestrol during pregnancy
  - D. Others, usually with associated nongenital anomalies
- III. True hermaphroditism
  - A. With identifiable sex chromosome abnormality
  - B. Without identifiable sex chromosome abnormality
- IV. Gonosomal intersexuality (mixed or asymmetric gonadal dysgenesis)
- V. Uterine hernia syndrome (defect in synthesis of, secretion of, or response to müllerian duct–inhibiting factor)
- VI. XY female with dysgenetic gonads (XY pure gonadal dysgenesis)
- VII. Anorchia

Type with female external genital phenotype. Male pseudohermaphroditism with female external genitalia represents essentially a complete failure of masculinization of the external genitalia of the male fetus. The definition of male pseudohermaphroditism dictates that testes be present. Such a clinical picture has been described as the result of Leydig cell hypoplasia or aplasia, of severe defects in the conversion of cholesterol to testosterone (Fig. 22-8) and its further metabolism to dihydrotestosterone, and of insensitivity of target cells to normally synthesized androgen. Cases have been described in which a phenotypic female had testes that contained few or no histologically identifiable Leydig cells. In the absence of Leydig cells in the fetal testis, androgens are not elaborated and male differentiation of the external genitalia does not occur. The reported patients with this variety of male pseudohermaphroditism were sexually infantile. They had identifiable vasa deferentia and epididymides. While the authors of one report suggest that testosterone of *Sertoli cell* origin may have been responsible for wolffian duct differentiation, it was more likely the result of Leydig cell–produced testosterone in early embryogenesis. Leydig cells, then, could have no longer been present at the time of external genital differentiation.

A number of enzymes are necessary for the conversion of cholesterol to testosterone. Defects in every enzymatic step involved have been reported. At least three such defects have been described in severe enough form that no masculinization of the male fetus occurred, resulting in a male pseudohermaphrodite with a female external genital phenotype (Fig. 22-8). These include a defect in the conversion of cholesterol to pregnenolone—a step that involves the three enzymes 20-alpha-hydroxylase, 22R-hydroxylase, and 20-alpha,22R-desmolase—and a defect in 17 alpha-hydroxylase. This has also been called lipoid hyperplasia of the adrenal gland because of the accumulation of lipid material in cells of the adrenal cortex. Both these defects produce adrenal insufficiency as well as male pseudohermaphroditism, since the same defective metabolic step is necessary for cortisol biosynthesis. The majority of patients with a defect in the conversion of cholesterol to pregnenolone have died in infancy of adrenal failure, but several have survived to later childhood. These two defects are inherited in an autosomal recessive manner. A third defect in testosterone biosynthesis, involving the enzyme 17,20-desmolase, has been described in male pseudohermaphrodites with female phenotypes. 17,20-Desmolase deficiency is inherited apparently in an X-linked recessive manner. Since this enzyme is not involved in cortisol biosynthesis, this type of male pseudohermaphroditism is not accompanied by adrenal failure. In each of these forms of male pseudohermaphroditism caused by defective testosterone biosynthesis and in that caused by Leydig cell aplasia, müllerian suppressive factor is normally produced. As a result, affected patients have neither wolffian nor müllerian duct structures.

A distinct type of male pseudohermaphroditism occurs even in the presence of normal Leydig cells and normal synthesis of testosterone. It is the result of the insensitivity of target cells in the anlage of the male internal and external genitalia to biologically active androgens, and on the basis of current knowledge it is termed the *androgen insensitivity syndrome*. In this condition, historically termed the "complete testicular feminization syndrome," the patient appears to be a normal female who may have inguinal hernias containing masses that on examination or biopsy are found to be testes. The patients feminize at puberty with normal breast development (Fig. 22-20). Pubic and axillary hair is scanty. Although they feminize at puberty, patients with the androgen insensitivity syndrome have no uterus or other müllerian or wolffian derivatives, and thus have primary amenorrhea. The external genitalia appear normal. The vagina ordinarily is only a few millimeters in depth and invariably ends as a blind pouch. The diagnosis should be suspected in any phenotypic female child with inguinal hernias containing masses. The buccal smear is always X-chromatin negative and Y-chromatin positive, and the sex chromosomes are XY. A history of similarly affected siblings or "aunts" may be elicited. The condition is inherited in an X-linked manner.

Much progress has been made in elucidating the pathogenesis of the androgen insensitivity syndrome. The testes of affected patients produce normal male amounts of testosterone and dihydrotestosterone, but target tissues do not respond to these androgens. The administration of testosterone or dihydrotestosterone to such patients produces none of the effects usually attributable to androgens. Defective binding of testosterone and dihydrotestosterone to cultured genital skin fibroblasts has been demonstrated in some humans with the *complete* androgen insensitivity syndrome. This appears to be the result of an inability of testosterone and dihy-

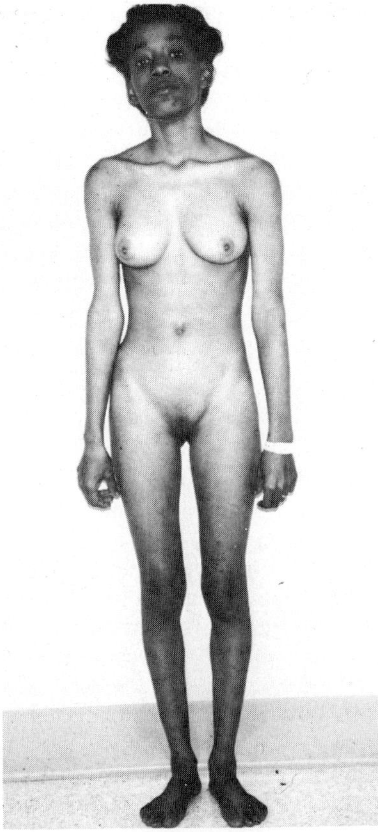

Fig. 22-20. Sixteen-year-old patient with the complete form of the androgen insensitivity syndrome. Note normal breast development and scant pubic hair.

drotestosterone to bind to the previously mentioned nuclear-cytosol androgen receptor protein, a process necessary for androgen action. In the normal situation the nuclear-cytosol receptor protein binds to androgen within the cytoplasm of the target cell (Fig. 22-9). This complex then enters the nucleus where it binds to the genome, thereby activating genes necessary for male sex differentiation. In the androgen insensitivity syndrome the nuclear-cytosol receptor protein is either deficient (Fig. 22-9) or, because of altered structure, its binding to androgen is quantitatively or qualitatively defective. In some cases of the androgen insensitivity syndrome, however, androgen binding appears to be normal. The abnormality here could possibly involve a structural alteration of the portion of the receptor molecule that recognizes and binds to appropriate portions of the genome. The facts that plasma LH is elevated in the androgen insensitivity syndrome and that LH can be suppressed in affected patients by administered estrogen but not by androgen are evidence that cytosol binding of androgens is also defective in the hypothalamus, thus interrupting the normal hypothalamic-pituitary-gonadal axis. Other possibilities in androgen-insensitive patients include a partial deficiency of cytosol receptor protein or a mutation in a gene determining another protein necessary for androgen action.

At any rate, androgen insensitivity results in the lack of differentiation of the wolffian duct system and lack of masculinization of the external genitalia. At the same time, the mechanism that produces müllerian duct regression is fully functional. The end result is absence in the pelvis of both male and female ductal structures, with female differentiation of the external genitalia. Pubertal feminization is produced by testicular-derived estrogen. Estrogen is produced normally by the testis, and the absence of breast development in the normal male is attributable to a balance between androgen and estrogen influence. In the androgen insensitivity syndrome that balance is interrupted and estrogen influence is unopposed.

Patients with the complete androgen insensitivity syndrome *must* be reared as females. The terms *male, testes, intersex,* or any word which suggests that the patient is anything other than a female should be avoided in discussing the condition with the family or the patient. The question arises as to what should be done with the testes. Some authors advocate the removal of the testes *only after* pubertal development is complete. Others recommend removal of gonads before puberty, as soon as the diagnosis is made. After the gonads are removed, estrogen replacement therapy is necessary. Menses cannot be induced, and the patient is sterile. However, she can function normally in sexual intercourse if her vagina is adequate. If not, surgical enlargement of the vaginal vault is indicated.

Type with intersex genitalia. Several etiologic bases exist for the type of male pseudohermaphroditism with ambiguous external genitalia.

1. In a few patients with ambiguous external genitalia and an XY sex chromosome complement, gonads have been found that, while con-

taining testicular elements, are not normal testes. It has been suggested that these structurally dysgenetic testes are also functionally abnormal and lead to defective masculinization.

2. Defects in three enzyme systems mediating the conversion of cholesterol to testosterone have been discussed as causes of male pseudohermaphroditism with female external genitalia. Defects, perhaps less severe, in the same enzymes have been described in male pseudohermaphrodites with ambiguous genitalia. It is not difficult to visualize different, perhaps allelic, mutations involving genes that code for the same enzymes, one of which produces a more severe functional defect than the other.

In addition, recent advances in the technology of steroid biochemistry have demonstrated deficiencies of 3-beta-hydroxysteroid dehydrogenase and 17-ketosteroid reductase in cases of male pseudohermaphroditism. Thus a defect in every enzyme operating in the conversion of cholesterol to testosterone (Fig. 22-8) has been found in male pseudohermaphroditism. In contrast to the androgen insensitivity syndrome, patients with defects in testosterone biosynthesis, as a rule, masculinize at puberty, with further phallic enlargement and appearance of body hair. Some, at the same time, experience breast development, while others do not. All these defects except 17,20-desmolase deficiency are inherited in an autosomal recessive manner. 17,20-Desmolase deficiency appears to be the result of a mutation in an X-linked gene. Because 20-alpha-hydroxylase, 22R-hydroxylase, 20,22 desmolase, 3-beta-hydroxysteroid dehydrogenase, and 17-alpha-hydroxylase are necessary for both cortisol and testosterone synthesis (Fig. 22-6), a defect in any of these enzymes produces adrenal failure as well as male pseudohermaphroditism.

3. A form of male pseudohermaphroditism has been described wherein patients are born with minimal signs of masculinization of the external genitalia. However, at puberty the patients virilize with phallic enlargement, deepening of the voice, appearance of body hair, and increase in muscle mass. The extent of the phallic enlargement is such that a functional penis results. This condition was described in a large inbred isolate by Imperato-McGinley and Peterson and was shown to be caused by a defect in the conversion of testosterone to dihydrotestosterone, resulting from a deficiency (Fig. 22-8) of the enzyme 5-alpha-reductase. 5-Alpha-reductase deficiency has been documented in a number of other cases of male pseudohermaphroditism and may be the most common type with ambiguous genitalia. It is inherited as an autosomal recessive trait.

In patients with this form of male pseudohermaphroditism, the internal genital duct system is masculinized, with epididymis, vas deferens, seminal vesicle, and ejaculatory duct. At the time of wolffian duct differentiation of the male fetus, the capacity to convert testosterone to dihydrotestosterone in the normal state has not developed. These two facts indicate that wolffian duct differentiation is testosterone dependent. However, the capacity to convert testosterone to dihydrotestosterone *is* present in the tissues of the urogenital sinus and external genitalia *before* the onset of male external sex differentiation. Thus in the genetically determined absence of 5-alpha-reductase one would expect normal wolffian duct differentiation but defective masculinization of the external genitalia.

4. Some patients present the picture of androgen insensitivity syndrome except that they have clitoridal enlargement and are not devoid of body hair. They feminize at puberty, just as do patients with the complete form of the syndrome, and the genetic mode appears to be identical to that in the complete form. A defect in nuclear-cytosol androgen receptor protein has been described in several patients with this *incomplete androgen insensitivity syndrome*. Perhaps this involves a less severe defect in nuclear-cytosol receptor protein than that in the complete form of the syndrome.

5. Reifenstein syndrome, pseudovaginal perineoscrotal hypospadias, Lubs syndrome, and Gilbert-Dreyfus syndrome are all terms used historically to describe various types of male pseudohermaphroditism. They are all based on phenotype alone and were coined before the advent of contemporary techniques for the investigation of the causes of male pseudohermaphroditism. For example, reinvestigation of the families originally described by Reifenstein has shown that affected patients have the incomplete androgen insensitivity syndrome. Pseudovaginal perineoscrotal hypospadias has been shown in some instances to be the result of a defect in testosterone biosynthesis and in others a deficiency of 5-alpha-reductase. As a result of the advances in recent years, all these descriptive

terms should be discarded in favor of more specific terms that specify the exact mechanism involved, as listed in Table 22-7 and in the outline on p. 629.

In the isolated prepubertal patient with male pseudohermaphroditism, the specific diagnosis is not readily apparent. Even in the pubertal or adult patient—in whom feminization suggests the incomplete androgen insensitivity syndrome, while masculinization points more to a defect in testosterone biosynthesis or 5-alpha-reductase deficiency—the diagnosis may be in question. Efforts should be made in every case to ascertain the diagnosis, since prognosis and genetic mechanisms differ in the various types. In the pubertal patient, measurements of plasma levels of testosterone and its precursors should identify any defect in testosterone biosynthesis; in the prepubertal patient such measurements must be preceded by several days of HCG stimulation of the testes. Activity of 5-alpha-reductase and of nuclear-cytosol androgen receptor protein should be measured in cultured genital skin fibroblasts.

Masculinized female (female pseudohermaphroditism)

Female pseudohermaphroditism is defined by the presence of two ovaries in a genetic female (XX) with ambiguous or "cryptorchid male" external genitalia. The condition is most often produced by masculinization of the female fetus by extragonadal androgen (see Table 22-7 and the outline on p. 629). The commonest cause is congenital virilizing adrenal hyperplasia, which is discussed in detail elsewhere (p. 582). Several cases of clitoridal enlargement and labial fusion have been caused by the administration of progestational agents to the mother of the patient during pregnancy. The type caused by congenital adrenal hyperplasia is progressive after birth, whereas that caused by progestational agents given to the pregnant mother is not progressive after birth. Female pseudohermaphroditism may rarely be caused by a virilizing disorder in the pregnant mother of the patient. Isolated cases with no demonstrable cause, some with accompanying somatic anomalies, have been described.

True hermaphroditism

True hermaphroditism is characterized by the presence of both ovarian and testicular gonadal tissue in the same individual—that is, either bilateral ovotestes, an ovary on one side and a testis on the other (in which case the genital duct systems on each side will correspond to the gonad on that side), or an ovotestis on one side and a testis or ovary on the other side.

Etiology. The cause is unknown in many cases. Some patients have chromosome abnormalities. Several 46,XX/46,XY true hermaphrodites have been reported. This abnormality is attributable to a phenomenon known as chimerism, the presence in a single individual of cells derived from different (usually two) zygotes, in this case an XX and an XY zygote. This could occur, for example, through the fusion of an XX and an XY zygote or very early embryo. Both XX and XY true hermaphrodites have also been described. Etiologic possibilities in the XY true hermaphrodite include (1) undetected mosaicism or chimerism in which an XX cell line, although not detectable, is present and (2) a mutant gene. Similar possibilities exist for XX true hermaphroditism, that is, undetected mosaicism or chimerism in which an XX cell line, although not detectable, is present and (2) a mutant gene. Similar possibilities exist for XX true hermaphroditism, that is, undetected mosaicism and a single gene mutation. However, another possibility is a Y-to-X translocation or a Y-autosome translocation in which male determinants ordinarily present in the Y chromosome have been transferred (but the transferred segment is not visible) to an X chromosome or an autosome. Translocation or undetected mosaicism seem most plausible in view of the observation that H-Y antigen is detectable in most XX true hermaphrodites.

Clinical manifestations. Innumerable variations in the formation of internal and external genitalia are possible, as shown in Fig. 22-21. Pubertal development may be predominantly male or female.

Diagnosis. This condition, although rare, should be suspected in any patient with ambiguous external genitalia. The buccal smear may be either X-chromatin positive (karyotype XX or any mosaic that includes an XX or poly-X cell line) or X-chromatin negative. Chromosome analysis may reveal the underlying cause in cases resulting from a chromosome abnormality. Family history may be important. Actual diagnosis depends on the demonstration of both ovarian and testicular tissue at laparotomy.

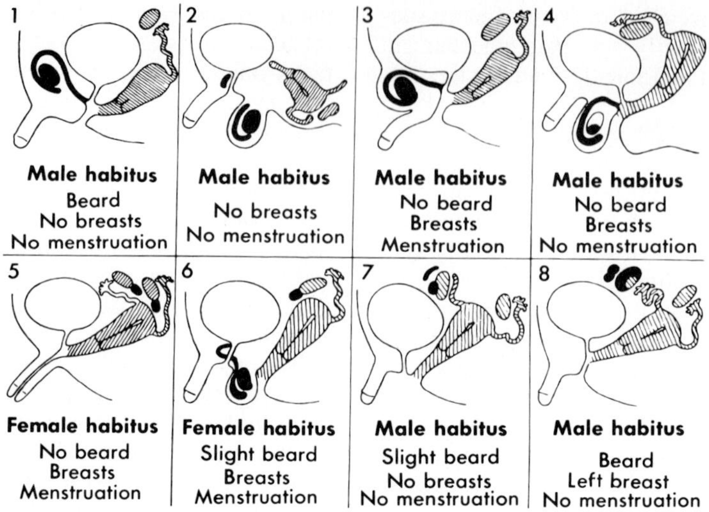

Fig. 22-21. True hermaphrodites. Diagrams in the upper row show a testis on one side and an ovary on the other. In each case the differentiation of the genital duct corresponds to the sex of the gonad on the same side. In the lower row there is an ovotestis on one or both sides, and considerable variation is shown in the development of the genital ducts and external genitalia. True hermaphrodites show much variation in the habitus and in the development of secondary sex characteristics. (Diagrams correspond to various cases collected by Hugh H. Young.) (From Wilkins, L., et al.: Pediatrics **16:**287, 1955.)

45,X/46,XY abnormality (gonosomal intersexuality)

Gonosomal intersexuality is considered separately because its clinical spectrum may vary from that of the phenotypic female with Turner syndrome on one extreme, through the entire gamut of intersex phenotypes, to a normal fertile male phenotype on the other extreme. The most commonly encountered phenotype is the presence of intersex genitalia, and the most common gonadal abnormality is "mixed" gonadal dysgenesis.

Gonosomal intersexuality should be suspected in *any* X-chromatin–negative intersex individual who is found to have a uterus. In gonosomal intersexuality a streak gonad may be found on one side and a dysgenetic testis on the other side. Alternatively, both gonads may be streaks or both may be dysgenetic testicles. The dysgenetic gonads in *all* such cases are predisposed to neoplastic transformation and should be excised.

Uterine hernia syndrome. Uterine hernia syndrome is a rare condition in externally normal males who have, in addition, müllerian duct derivatives. Its etiology remains in question but it has been reported in multiple siblings and in monozygotic twins. Its occurrence in maternal half-siblings suggests X-linked recessive inheritance. The pathogenetic mechanism probably is deficient action of or response to müllerian suppressive factor elaborated by the fetal testis. All reported patients have a 46,XY karyotype. Cryptorchidism is common, and abdominal exploration reveals the presence of testes (which may occupy the position of ovaries) and wolffian duct structures, along with uterus, fallopian tubes, and a vagina that opens into the posterior urethra. Fertility has been reported, although in one case each testicle contained a gonadoblastoma. Müllerian duct derivatives should be removed. The finding of gonadal neoplasia raises the question of the advisability of gonadectomy as well.

Diagnosis and management of patients with ambiguous external genitalia

Complete investigation is indicated in patients with (1) ambiguous external genitalia, (2) masses in the inguinal region or labia of phenotypic females, (3) absence of palpable testes in phenotypic males or individuals with hypospadias, (4) history of the mother having received a progestational agent during the pregnancy of an infant with ambiguous external genitalia, and (5) history of siblings or other relatives with a similar abnormality.

The management of the complete androgen insensitivity syndrome is discussed on p. 631.

Proper sex assignment as early as possible is extremely important in patients with ambiguous external genitalia.

1. The presence of an X-chromatin–positive buccal smear, an XX sex karyotype, the finding of a uterus on rectal examination, electrolyte imbalance in some cases, the presence of elevated urinary 17-ketosteroids and pregnanetriol, and the presence of elevated plasma 17-hydroxyprogesterone and progesterone are indicative of female pseudohermaphroditism caused by congenital adrenal hyperplasia. This condition is discussed in more detail in the section on the adrenal gland. These patients should *always* be reared as females. The diagnosis of this condition is most important, since with proper medical and surgical treatment these patients are potentially *fertile*.

2. A history of the administration of progestational agents during pregnancy to the mother of an infant with ambiguous genitalia, an X-chromatin–positive buccal smear, an XX sex karyotype, absence of elevated urinary 17-ketosteroids and pregnanetriol or of plasma 17-hydroxyprogesterone, a palpable uterus by rectal examination, and lack of progressive virilization after birth indicate virilization caused by the progestational agent. No treatment is indicated, but if clitoridal enlargement is a problem, clitoridectomy or clitoridal recession may be advisable. Separation of labial fusion is routinely necessary. These patients should *always* be reared as females and are potentially fertile.

3. The management of male pseudohermaphroditism encompasses the problem of sex assignment in the affected infant, the question of gonadectomy, the prognosis relative to sexual function, and the use of hormone substitution therapy. Historically, if a diagnosis of male pseudohermaphroditism has been made for an infant with ambiguous genitalia, the assignment of a female sex has been most prudent. The choice of sex assignment in male pseudohermaphroditism has been based on the question of whether the available external genitalia, specifically the phallus, is large enough that with surgery to repair the hypospadias, it could be ultimately a functioning penis. The answer most often has been negative. A female sex assignment still is probably the best choice unless the phallus is well developed. However, a small phallus in the infant with 5-alpha-reductase deficiency or 17-ketosteroid-reductase deficiency may enlarge to the size of a functional penis at puberty. Thus exact diagnosis is important as a basis for sex assignment.

If a female sex assignment is made, removal of the testes is in order. In the incomplete androgen insensitivity syndrome, the same approach may be taken as in the complete syndrome. In all other forms, some degree of masculinization at puberty is the rule, and so the testes should be removed before that age, preferably as soon as the diagnosis is established. It should be emphasized that the testes should *not* be removed *before* a specific diagnosis is established because the presence of a testis is necessary for some diagnostic procedures.

All male pseudohermaphrodites are sterile, with the possible exception of some who have 5-alpha-reductase deficiency. Complete spermatogenesis has been seen in testicular biopsies from affected patients, and patients do have erections and ejaculations. However, the severe hypospadias may preclude natural insemination, and no case of fertility has been reported in a 5-alpha-reductase deficient male. If a female sex assignment is made, plastic surgery is necessary to remove the enlarged clitoris and to form a vagina. If a shallow separate vaginal vault is already present, it may have to be deepened surgically.

If a male sex assignment is made, for example, in an older child with the incomplete androgen insensitivity syndrome, testosterone therapy may be necessary to raise plasma testosterone levels high enough to induce masculinization. If a female sex assignment is made and the testes removed, estrogen substitution therapy must be used beginning in early adolescent years and continuing until or after the usual age of menopause. With proper surgical and hormone therapy the possibility of normal sexual function is maximized. Needless to say, continued intensive psychologic support is mandatory.

4. The general rules applicable to the management of male pseudohermaphroditism also apply to true hermaphrodites, except that if the

patient is to be reared as a female and an ovary and a testis are present, the testicular tissue should be removed and the ovary left. If the phallus is adequate for the formation of a penis or if a male gender has previously been established in an older child, any vagina, uterine structures, or ovarian tissue should be removed. Male pseudohermaphrodites and true hermaphrodites are almost invariably sterile. The parents of infants with ambiguous external genitalia, and the patients themselves when they are older, need intelligent long-term guidance.

Abnormal sexual development—failure of sexual development (sexual infantilism)

Failure of sexual development is to be differentiated from simple delayed adolescence by its persistence and by the frequency of accompanying abnormalities. Causes of sexual infantilism are considered in the following discussions and summarized in the following outline and in Table 22-9.

- I. Central nervous system
  - A. Hypothalamus
    - 1. Congenital anomalies
      - a. Isolated bihormonal gonadotropin deficiency
      - b. Craniopharyngioma
      - c. Tuberous sclerosis or neurofibromatosis
      - d. Absence of gonadotropin-releasing hormone(s)
        - (1) Familial
        - (2) Sporadic
    - 2. Other central nervous system sites
  - B. Inflammatory processes
    - 1. Encephalitis
    - 2. Granuloma (e.g., sarcoid)
  - C. Tumors
    - 1. Hypothalamic
    - 2. Pineal
    - 3. Optic chiasm
  - D. Trauma
  - E. Miscellaneous syndromes
    - 1. Kallman syndrome
    - 2. Laurence-Moon-Bardet-Biedl syndrome
    - 3. Ataxia-hypogonadism syndrome
    - 4. Nevoid basal cell carcinoma syndrome
    - 5. Biemond syndrome
    - 6. Carpenter syndrome
    - 7. Crandall syndrome
    - 8. Ichthyosis-hypogonadism syndrome
    - 9. Kraus-Ruppert syndrome
- II. Pituitary
  - A. Congenital anomalies
    - 1. Aplasia
    - 2. Hypoplasia
    - 3. Absence of gonadotropins
      - a. Panhypopituitarism
      - b. Isolated bihormonal gonadotropin deficiency
      - c. Isolated luteinizing hormone deficiency
      - d. Isolated follicle-stimulating hormone deficiency
  - B. Inflammatory processes—granuloma
  - C. Tumors
  - D. Trauma
- III. Gonads
  - A. Congenital anomalies
    - 1. Syndromes of gonadal dysgenesis
      - a. Turner syndrome
      - b. Pure gonadal dysgenesis
      - c. Ovarian failure caused by X-autosome translocation
    - 2. Testicular defects
      - a. Klinefelter syndrome
      - b. Anorchia
      - c. Noonan syndrome
      - d. Prader-Willi syndrome
  - B. Inflammatory process, testicular—orchitis
  - C. Trauma
    - 1. Ovarian—bilateral torsion of ovarian pedicle
    - 2. Testicular
      - a. Bilateral testicular torsion
      - b. Atrophy following bilateral orchiopexy
  - D. Tumors, bilateral, requiring gonadectomy
- IV. Systemic disease
  - A. Cardiorespiratory disease
  - B. Gastrointestinal disease
  - C. Urinary tract disease
  - D. Endocrine disease
  - E. Malnutrition

Three systems are directly involved in sex development: (1) the central nervous system, which stimulates; (2) the pituitary gland, which secretes the gonadotropins; and (3) the gonads themselves, which must be responsive to these stimuli. Abnormalities involving any of the three principal systems may result in aberrations in pubertal development, for example, failure of maturation or precocious puberty.

Central nervous system defects

Any lesion that prevents the synthesis of gonadotropin-releasing hormones (LRH) will result in sexual infantilism.

Clinical manifestations. Symptoms in addition to sexual infantilism depend on the location of the abnormality. Other signs of hypothalamic dysfunction, such as irregularities of temperature, somnolence, or diabetes insipidus, may occur. Papilledema, visual field defects, or motor disturbance may result from an expanding lesion at the base of the brain. Accompanying

Table 22-9. Gonadotropin deficiency with associated anomalies

Condition	Somatic features	Gonadal features	Mode of inheritance
Ataxia-hypogonadism syndrome	Cerebellar ataxia	Bihormonal gonadotropin deficiency	Autosomal recessive X-linked recessive
	Chorioretinal degeneration in one type		
Nevoid basal cell carcinoma syndrome	Basal cell nevi, jaw cysts, broad facies	Bihormonal gonadotropin deficiency Cryptorchidism	Autosomal dominant
	Anosmia in one family	Unilateral absence of testis	
Biemond syndrome (? relationship to Laurence-Moon-Biedl syndrome)	Obesity, iris coloboma, mental retardation, polydactyly	Bihormonal gonadotropin deficiency	Autosomal recessive
Carpenter syndrome	Acrocephalosyndactyly, preaxial polydactyly, telecanthus, epicanthal folds, downward slanting eyes, flat nasal bridge, broad cheeks, micrognathia, coxa valga, obesity, mental retardation, abdominal hernias	Bihormonal gonadotropin deficiency	Autosomal recessive or (?) autosomal dominant
Crandall syndrome	Growth hormone deficiency alopecia, neurosensory deafness	Bihormonal gonadotropin deficiency	Autosomal recessive (?)
Ichthyosis-hypogonadism syndrome	Congenital ichthyosis	Bihormonal gonadotropin deficiency	X-linked (?)
Kallman syndrome	Anosmia or hyposmia, hypoplasia of olfactory tract, cleft lip and palate, deafness, unilateral renal aplasia	Bihormonal gonadotropin deficiency Small testes Infantile genitalia Failure of secondary sex development Primary amenorrhea Cryptorchidism	Probably autosomal dominant
Kraus-Ruppert syndrome	Severe mental retardation, microcephaly, syndactyly of second to fourth toes	Bihormonal gonadotropin deficiency	Autosomal recessive
Laurence-Moon-Bardet-Biedl syndrome	Retinitis pigmentosa, mental retardation, polysyndactyly, obesity, progressive renal disease	Bihormonal gonadotropin deficiency	Autosomal recessive

Modified from Simpson, J.L.: Disorders of sexual differentiation, New York, 1977, Academic Press, Inc.

growth hormone deficiency may produce shortness of stature.

Pituitary defects

Congenital aplasia, or destruction by space-occupying lesions, of the pituitary gland produces a deficiency of multiple tropic hormones. Panhypopituitarism (multitropic pituitary hormone deficiency) encompasses a deficiency of two or more pituitary tropic hormones, growth hormone deficiency being a constant feature. It appears also that gonadotropic hormones are virtually always deficient and, in addition, TSH and/or ACTH may be deficient. Whereas gonadotropin deficiency results in sexual infantilism, the most obvious feature of multitropic pituitary hormone deficiency is growth failure caused by growth hormone deficiency. This type of dwarfism is proportionate and is characterized by increased subcutaneous tissue, a high-pitched voice, and wrinkled skin. Gonadotropin deficiency produces lack of facial and body hair, small testes, and small penis. If TSH and/or ACTH is deficient, symptoms of hypothyroidism and/or hypoadrenalism will be apparent. The etiology of multitropic pituitary hormone deficiency is heterogeneous, the majority of cases being sporadic with undetermined specific etiology. Pedigree analysis indicates that the condition may be inherited in some instances. Some of those pedigrees indicate an autosomal recessive mode of inheritance, while others point to X-linked recessive inheritance.

In isolated bihormonal gonadotropin deficiency both FSH and LH are deficient. Clinical manifestations in the male include failure of appearance of secondary sex characteristics, lack of facial hair, small penis, scant body hair, small prostate, and small testes. Testicular biopsy reveals immature seminiferous tubules and absent Leydig cells. Affected females have primary amenorrhea, underdevelopment of breasts, and may have a eunuchoid habitus. Clinical features vary widely, and symptoms may be much less pronounced than those presented here. Plasma LH and FSH are very low to undetectable, and response to LRH is variable. In some cases no response occurs, suggesting a pituitary origin as the problem, while other patients do respond, pointing to the hypothalamus as the site of the abnormality. Gonadotropins may be administered in an effort to treat bihormonal gonadotropin deficiency, and at least one patient so treated has become pregnant.

Instances of isolated LH deficiency and of isolated FSH deficiency have been described. In isolated LH deficiency the testes of the affected male contain normal numbers of germ cells but practically no Leydig cells. Secondary sex development does not occur and affected males have high-pitched voices, poor muscle mass, and scant facial hair. It has been suggested that isolated LH deficiency is in reality one end of a widely varying spectrum of bihormonal gonadotropin deficiency.

Isolated FSH deficiency has produced primary amenorrhea in an affected female. As in isolated LH deficiency, isolated FSH deficiency may be another variant of bihormonal gonadotropin deficiency.

A number of conditions have been described in which hypogonadotropism is accompanied by other anomalies. These are summarized in Table 22-9. It may be that most, if not all, cases of isolated bihormonal or isolated single gonadotropin deficiency represent variants of Kallman syndrome.

Gonadal defects. Gonadal defects include gonadal dysgenesis (Turner syndrome), testicular disorders, and prepubertal castration. In these conditions normal pituitary mechanisms for elaboration of gonadotropins are present, but defective gonads are unable to respond to stimuli. The term *gonadal dysgenesis* refers to a group of conditions wherein there is complete or almost complete failure of differentiation of the embryonic anlage of the gonads into either definitive testes or ovaries and to other abnormalities of gonadal differentiation to be discussed later.

Gonadal dysgenesis. The group of conditions comprising gonadal dysgenesis is discussed on pp. 615-627.

Testicular disorders

Testicular disorders include Klinefelter syndrome, anorchia, Noonan syndrome, and Prader-Willi syndrome.

Klinefelter syndrome. Klinefelter syndrome is discussed on pp. 627-629.

Anorchia. Anorchia is significant only if it is bilateral.

Etiology. The etiology of anorchia is unknown. Genetic factors have been postulated in some cases, but, in all likelihood, anorchia is etiologically heterogeneous. Pathogenesis apparently involves some destructive process involving a testis that was functionally active during the embryonic period of sex organ differentiation.

Clinical manifestations. Both testes are absent. The penis may be small but is unambiguously well differentiated. The postpubertal habitus is eunuchoid, and secondary sex characteristics fail to appear. Sexual hair is present but diminished. There may be associated genitourinary anomalies.

Noonan syndrome. Reports of the so-called male Turner syndrome have appeared in the past and dealt with phenotypic males who have varying degrees of hypogonadism and of somatic abnormalities similar to some of those in Turner syndrome in phenotypic females.

Etiology. After it was recognized that affected

males have normal male karyotypes, several females, labeled mistakenly as examples of Turner syndrome but with no chromosomal abnormality, were recognized as manifesting the same somatic phenotype as affected males. The condition was noted in full and half siblings, in mother and son, in mother and daughter, and in father and son. Noonan syndrome is a common condition, perhaps as common as 1 in 1000 live births. Its genetic mode has not been well worked out, but it may be inherited as an autosomal dominant with widely variable expressivity. Genetic heterogeneity cannot be excluded. It is *not* caused by a chromosome abnormality.

Clinical manifestations. The following features are found in varying percentages of documented cases: (1) short stature, 72%; (2) mental retardation of mild to severe degree, 61%; (3) low-set or malformed ears, 85%; (4) epicanthal folds, 51%, with or without ptosis of one or both eyelids; (5) hypertelorism, 84%; (6) downward slanting palpebral fissures, 83%; (7) high or narrow palatal arch, 65%; (8) dental malocclusion, 52%; (9) micrognathia, 70%; (10) low posterior scalp hairline, 80%; (11) webbed neck, 78%; (12) shield-shaped chest with a proximal pectus carinatum–distal pectus excavatum, 75%; (13) congenital heart disease, 55%—the most commonly encountered lesion being pulmonary valvular or infundibular stenosis; other cardiac lesions include peripheral pulmonary artery stenosis, patent ductus arteriosus, atrial septal defect, and tetralogy of Fallot; (14) cubitus valgus, approximately 85%; (15) renal anomalies, 27%; and (16) peripheral lymphedema at some time, about 35%. The typical facial and somatic phenotype is shown in Fig. 22-22. Hypogonadism is variable, being reported more commonly in males than in females. Unilateral or bilateral cryptorchidism occurs in 70% of affected males, and gonadal function has varied in reported cases from complete agonadism to normal function with fertility. In affected females puberty may be delayed, but eventual normal ovarian function is the rule.

Prader-Willi syndrome. The etiology of Prader-Willi syndrome is discussed on p. 146. The condition is a rare cause of sexual infantilism, especially in males.

Clinical features. Affected children are obese and mentally retarded. Hypotonia, decreased activity, and poor feeding in early infancy give way to a voracious and uncritical appetite. Cryptorchidism and small genitalia are features in childhood.

Prepubertal castration

Prenatal causes of prepubertal castration are not included.

Etiology. In females prepubertal castration may be caused by pelvic infections or oophorectomy performed because of neoplasia or cysts. In males it may be caused by trauma, bilateral testicular torsion, and circulatory failure after orchidopexy, resulting in complete fail-

A 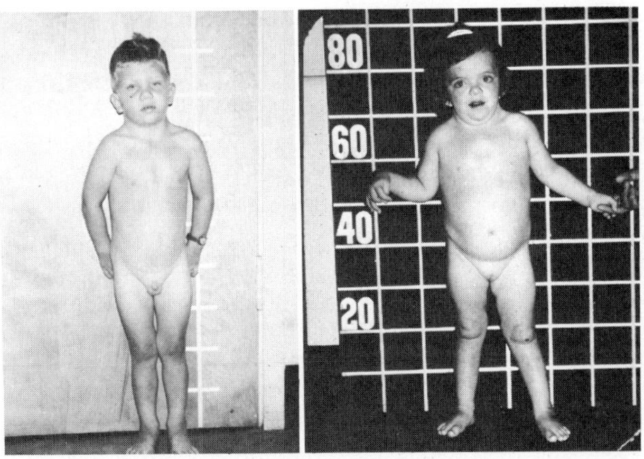 B

Fig. 22-22. Typical Noonan syndrome. **A,** Male. **B,** Female.

ure of pubertal development. (In contrast, orchitis and cryptorchidism may result in sterility, but masculinization is normal.)

Clinical features. There is a failure of pubertal development in males and females, accompanied by a tall eunuchoid habitus, presence of sexual hair, and sterility.

Systemic diseases

Diseases involving systems other than the hypothalamic-pituitary-gonadal axis may produce a delay in, or failure of, sexual maturation. Severe cardiac or respiratory disease may result in general growth delay, as can nutritional disturbances, including those caused by gastrointestinal lesions. Urinary tract disease with compromised renal function may likewise impair growth and development. Hypothyroidism can produce severe impairment of growth, which unless treated will prevent adolescent development. Adrenal insufficiency and poorly controlled diabetes mellitus can produce delayed adolescence. Early enzymatic blocks in sex steroid biosynthesis, such as 17-hydroxylase deficiency, preclude normal production of testosterone and estrogens and result in failure of sexual development.

Diagnosis of sexual infantilism

In the evaluation of patients with failure of sexual development, the first question to be answered is whether the patient represents simply a delay in adolescence that will ultimately proceed normally with a normal but late result, or whether the patient has a permanent failure of sexual development.

History. Important points include history of the sequence of events to date relative to growth and sexual maturation. Significant short stature suggests Turner syndrome or panhypopituitarism. Any significant deviation from an established pattern suggests a systemic condition such as acquired hypothyroidism. History designed to reveal abnormalities of other systems is most important. Visual difficulties and diabetes insipidus suggest a central nervous system lesion. History of pregnancy, labor, delivery, and neonatal course is important. Family history of similar patterns of sexual development in ultimately normal relatives would favor delayed adolescence rather than permanent failure. Family history of permanent failure in a female might suggest pure gonadal dysgenesis.

Physical examination. As an extension of the preceding, particular attention is paid to measurement of height, upper and lower segments, and arm span and to the exact status regarding sexual maturation. General assessment of other body systems provides useful information as to the possibility of systemic disease. Neurologic assessment, including visual field measurement, can provide information regarding the presence of an intracranial lesion. Somatic anomalies such as short stature, typical facies, webbing of the neck, cubitus valgus, and other features mentioned previously suggests Turner or Noonan syndrome. In males similar findings with or without mental retardation make Noonan syndrome a prime possibility. Gynecomastia in the presence of sexual developmental failure suggests Klinefelter syndrome.

Diagnostic tests. Preliminary evaluation designed to differentiate permanent sexual infantilism from delayed adolescence includes radiographic evaluation of bone age and—in all girls, as well as those boys in whom Klinefelter syndrome is suggested—a buccal smear for X- and Y-chromatin determination. Depending on the results of the latter, chromosomel analysis may be indicated. Unless these preliminary studies point to a specific abnormality, a period of observation may be in order. If the preliminary studies indicate further evaluation or if after a period of observation sexual development does not proceed, further evaluation may include the following:

1. Evaluation of other systems, such as skull and chest radiographs, computerized tomography of the head, blood count, determination of renal function, serum electrolytes and blood glucose, and evaluation of pituitary-thyroid and pituitary-adrenal axes.
2. Determination of specific plasma gonadotropin (FSH and LH) concentrations; if a pituitary or central nervous system lesion is at fault, low levels of gonadotropins would be expected, whereas elevated concentrations would point to a gonadal lesion.
3. Response of plasma FSH and LH to the administration of luteotropin-releasing hormone (LRH). In bihormonal gonadotropin deficiency,

a response would suggest a hypothalamic abnormality, producing LRH deficiency, while a lack of response would point to an abnormality in the pituitary gland, resulting in its inability to respond to LRH.

4. Plasma and urinary concentrations of sex steroids, with specific measurements of testosterone and its precursors in males before and after the administration of human chorionic gonadotropin; in gonadal lesions, testosterone response would be abnormally low.

5. Visualization of the internal genitalia of affected females by laparoscopy or laparotomy, which may reveal dysgenetic gonads or ovarian lesions. The diagnosis of anorchia is ordinarily made at the time of surgery for suspected bilateral cryptorchidism. Testicular biopsy of affected males may demonstrate tubular hyalinization in Klinefelter syndrome.

Management of sexual infantilism. Management depends, of course, on the basic abnormality and may involve treatment of such systemic diseases as diabetes mellitus, hypothyroidism, or cardiac defect. In general, once simple delayed adolescence has been excluded and a specific diagnosis made, substitution therapy should be undertaken. Naturally the timing of such therapy is important to avoid compromising ultimate height. Thyroid hormone should be used if hypothyroidism is a factor. Estrogen-progesterone substitution therapy in females and testosterone in males should be employed. Psychologic support is also an important part of successful management.

Robert L. Summitt

GENERAL REFERENCES

Insulin-dependent diabetes mellitus

Brodoff, B.N., and Bleicher, S.J., editors: Diabetes mellitus and obesity, Baltimore, 1982, The Williams & Wilkins Co.

Ellenberg, M., and Rifkin, H., editors: Diabetes mellitus—theory and practice, ed. 3, Garden City, N.Y., 1982, Medical Examination Publishing Co., Inc.

SELECTED READINGS

Parathyroid glands

Breslau, N.A., and Pak, C.Y.C.: Hypothyroidism, Metabolism **28:**1261, 1979.

DeLuca, H.F.: Vitamin D: revisited 1980, J. Clin. Endocrinol. Metab. **9:**3, 1980.

Root, A.W., and Harrison, H.E.: Recent advances in calcium metabolism. I. Mechanisms of calcium homeostasis, J. Ped. **88:**1, 1976. II. Disorders of calcium homeostasis, J. Ped. **88:**177, 1976.

Tsang, R.C., et al.: Pediatric parathyroid disorders, Ped. Clin. North. Am. **26:**223, 1979.

Adrenal glands

Dixon, R.B., and Christy, N.P.: On the various forms of corticosteroid withdrawal syndrome, Am. J. Med. **68:** 224, 1980.

Finkelstein, M., and Shaefer, J.M.: Inborn errors of steroid biosynthesis, Physiol. Rev. **59:**353, 1979.

Juan, D.: Pheochromocytoma: clinical manifestations and diagnostic tests, Virology **17:**1, 1981.

Interrelationship of the hypothalamus, anterior pituitary, and target glands

Daughaday, W.H.: The adenohypophysis. In Williams, R.H., editor: Textbook of endocrinology, ed. 5, Philadelphia, 1974, W.B. Saunders Co.

Korsgaard, O., et al.: Endocrine function in patients with suprasellar and hypothalamic tumors, Acta Endocrinol. **83:**1, 1976.

Plotkin, L.P., et al.: Comparison of physiological and pharmacological tests of growth hormone function in children with short stature, J. Clin. Endocrinol. Metab. **48:**811, 1979.

Thyroid gland

Barnes, H.V., and Blizzard, R.M.: Antithyroid drug therapy for toxic diffuse goiter (Graves disease): Thirty years experience in children and adolescents, J. Ped. **91:**313, 1977.

Committee on Drugs: Treatment of congenital hypothyroidism, Pediatrics **62:**413, 1978.

Fisher, D.A., and Klein, A.H.: Thyroid development and disorders of thyroid function in the newborn, N. Engl. J. Med. **304:**702, 1981.

Fisher, D.A., et al.: Screening for congenital hypothyroidism: results of screening 1 million North American infants, J. Ped. **94:**700, 1979.

Hung, W., et al.: Clinical, laboratory, and histologic observations in euthyroid children with goiters, J. Ped. **82:**10, 1973.

Klein, R.Z.: Neonatal screening for hypothyroidism, Adv. Ped. **26:**417, 1979.

Insulin-dependent diabetes mellitus

Alberti, K.G.M.M., et al.: Home blood glucose monitoring: does it improve diabetic control per se? In Peterson, C.M., editor: Diabetes management in the '80's—the role of home blood glucose monitoring and new insulin delivery systems, New York, 1982, Praeger Publishers.

American Diabetes Association, Inc.: Exchange Lists for Meal Planning, 2 Park Avenue, New York, New York, 10016.

Andersen, O., et al.: Immunological aspects of diabetes mellitus, Acta Endocrinol. **83:**15, 1976.

Berger, M., et al.: Absorption kinetics and biologic effects of subcutaneously injected insulin preparations, Diabetes Care **5:**77-91, 1982.

Bodansky, H.J., et al.: Risk factors associated with severe proliferative retinopathy in insulin-dependent diabetes mellitus, Diabetes Care **5**:97-100, 1982.

Bruck, E., and MacGillivray, M.H.: Posthypoglycemic hyperglycemia in diabetic children, J. Pediatr. **84**:672, 1974.

Bunn, F.H., et al.: The glycosylation of hemoglobin: relevance to diabetes mellitus, Science **200**:21, 1978.

Burghen, G.A., et al.: Comparison of high-dose and low-dose insulin by continuous intravenous infusion in the treatment of diabetic ketoacidosis in children, Diabetes Care **3**:15-20, 1980.

Burghen, G.A., et al.: Insulin and proinsulin in normal and chemical diabetic children, J. Pediatr. **89**:48, 1976.

Creutzfeldt, W., et al.: The genetics of diabetes mellitus, New York, 1976, Springer-Verlag New York, Inc.

Ensinck, J.W., and Williams, R.H.: The endocrine pancreas & diabetes mellitus. In Williams, R.H., editor: Textbook of endocrinology, ed. 6, Philadelphia, 1981, W.B. Saunders Co.

Goldstein, D.E., et al.: Hemoglobin A_{1c} levels in children and adolescents with diabetes mellitus, Diabetes Care **3**:503-507, 1980.

Hare, J.W., and Rossini, A.A.: Diabetic comas: the overlap concept, Hosp. Pract. **14**:95-108, 1979.

Kaye, R.: Diabetic ketoacidosis—the bicarbonate controversy, J. Pediatr. **87**:156, 1973.

Kitabchi, A.E., and Burghen, G.A.: Treatment of acidosis in diabetic children and adults. In Brodoff, B.N., and Bleicher, S.J., editors: Diabetes mellitus and obesity, Baltimore, 1982, The Williams & Wilkins Co.

Kitabchi, A.E., et al.: Problems associated with continuous subcutaneous insulin infusion (CSII), Horm. Metab. Res. **12**(suppl):271-276, 1982.

Kitabchi, A.E., et al.: Evaluation of a portable insulin infusion pump for outpatient management of brittle diabetes, Diabetes Care **2**:421-424, 1979.

Malone, J.I., et al.: Diabetic vascular changes in children, Diabetes **26**:673-679, 1977.

National Diabetes Data Group: Classification and diagnosis of diabetes mellitus and other categories of glucose intolerance, Diabetes **28**:1039-1057, 1979.

Paulsen, E.P.: Hemglobin A_c in childhood diabetes, Metabolism **22**:269, 1973.

Rosenbloom, A.L., et al.: Cerebral edema complicating diabetic ketoacidosis in childhood, J. Pediatr. **96**:357-361, 1980.

Rosenbloom, A.L., et al.: Chemical diabetes, Metabolism **22**:209, 1973.

Rosenbloom, A.L., and Giordano, B.P.: Chronic over treatment with insulin in children and adolescents, Am. J. Dis. Child **131**:881, 1977.

Rudolf, M.C.J., et al.: Effect of intensive insulin treatment in linear growth in the young diabetic patient, J. Pediatr. **101**:333-339, 1982.

Schmidt, M.I., et al.: The dawn phenomenon, an early morning glucose rise: implications for diabetic intraday blood glucose variation, Diabetes Care **4**:579-585, 1981.

Skyler, J.S., et al.: Algorithms for the adjustment of insulin dosage by patients who monitor blood glucose, Diabetes Care **4**:311-318, 1981.

Symposium on blood glucose self-monitoring, Diabetes Care **4**:392-426, 1981.

Tamborlane, W.V., et al.: Outpatient treatment of juvenile-onset diabetes with a preprogrammed portable subcutaneous insulin infusion system, Am. J. Med. **68**:190-196, 1980.

Winter, R.J., et al.: Diabetic ketoacidosis: induction of hypocalemia and hypomagnesemia by phosphate therapy, Am. J. Med. **67**:897-900, 1979.

Wishner, W.J., and Young, R.M.: Psychosocial issues in diabetes, Diabetes Care **1**:45-48, 1978.

Hypoglycemia

Chaussain, J.L.: Glycemic response to 24 hour fast in normal children and children with ketotic hypoglycemia, J. Pediatr. **82**:438, 1973.

Cornblath, M., and Schwartz, R.: Major problems in clinical pediatrics: disorders of carbohydrate metabolism in infancy, ed. 2, Philadelphia, 1976, W.B. Saunders Co.

Ensinck, J.W., and Williams, R.H.: Disorders causing hypoglycemia. In Williams, R.H., editor: Textbook of endocrinology, ed. 6, Philadelphia, 1981, W.B. Saunders Co.

Pagliara, A.S., et al.: Hypoglycemia in infancy and childhood. Part I. J. Pediatr. **82**:365, 1973.

Pagliara, A.S., et al.: Hypoglycemia in infancy and childhood. Part II. J. Pediatr. **82**:558, 1973.

Scully, R.E., et al.: Case records of the Massachusetts General Hospital, N. Engl. J. Med. **299**:241, 1978.

Stanley, C.A., and Baker, L.: Hyperinsulinism in infants and children: diagnosis and therapy, Adv. Pediatr. **23**:315, 1976.

Sex determination, differentiation, and development

Barr, M.L., and Bertram, E.G.: A morphological distinction between neurones of the male and female and the behavior of the nucleolar satellites during accelerated nucleoprotein synthesis, Nature **163**:676-677, 1949.

Charny, C.W., and Wolgen, W.: Cryptorchidism, New York, 1957, Paul B. Hoeber.

Charny, C.W.: The spermatogenic potential of the undescended testis before and after treatment, J. Urol. **83**:697-705, 1960.

Imperato-McGinley, J., et al.: An unusual form of male pseudohermaphroditism. A model of 5α-reductase deficiency in man, J. Clin. Invest. **53**:35a, 1974.

Imperato-McGinley, J., et al.: Steroid 5α-reductase deficiency in man. An inherited form of male pseudohermaphroditism, Science **186**:1213-1215, 1974.

Jirasek, J.E.: Morphogenesis of the genital system in the human. In Blandau, R.J., et al., editors: Morphogenesis and malformation of the genital system, White Plains, N.Y., 1977, The National Foundation—March of Dimes.

Jirasek, J.E.: Principles of reproductive embryology. In Simpson, J.L., editor: Disorders of sexual differentiation, New York, 1977, Academic Press, Inc.

Jost, A.: Hormonal factors in the sex differentiation of the mammalian foetus, Philos. Trans. R. Soc. London, Ser. B. **259**:119-131, 1970.

Jost, A.: Problems in fetal endocrinology: the gonadal and hypophysical hormones, Recent Prog. Hormone Res. **8**:379-418, 1953.

Ohno, S.: The role of H-Y antigen in primary sex determination, J.A.M.A. **239**:217-220, 1978.

Ohno, S., et al.: Testicular cells lysostripped of H-Y antigen organize ovarian follicle-like aggregates, Cytogenet. Cell Genet. **20:**351-364, 1978.

Paulsen, C.A.: The testes. In Williams, R.H., editor: Textbook of Endocrinology, ed. 5, Philadelphia, 1974, W.B. Saunders Co.

Root, A.W.: Endocrinology at puberty. II. Aberrations of sexual maturation, J. Pediatr. **83:**187-200, 1973.

Singh, R.P., and Carr, D.H.: The anatomy and histology of XO human embryos and fetuses, Anat. Rec. **155:**369-384, 1966.

Sohval, A.R.: Histopathology of cryptorchidism: A study based upon the comparative histology of retained and scrotal testes from birth to maturity, Am. J. Med. **16:**346-362, 1954.

Summitt, R.L.: Genetic forms of hypogonadism in the male, Prog. Med. Genet. **3:**1-72, 1979.

Summitt, R.L.: Turner syndrome. In Bergsma, D., editor: Birth defects atlas and compendium, White Plains, N.Y. 1979, The National Foundation—March of Dimes, pp. 1056-1058.

Wachtel, S.S., and Koo, G.C.: H-Y antigen in gonadal differentiation. In Austin, C.R., and Edwards, R.G., editors: Mechanisms of sex differentiation in animals and man, London, 1981, Academic Press, Inc.

Wachtel, S.S., and Ohno, S.: The immunogenetics of sexual development, Prog. Med. Genet. **3:**109-142, 1979.

Witschi, E., et al.: Genetic, developmental and hormonal aspects of gonadal dysgenesis and pseudohermaphroditism, J. Clin. Endocr. Metabol. **16:**922-923, 1956.

23 Inborn Errors of Metabolism

Inborn errors of metabolism (IEM) are inherited disorders of intermediary metabolism, all defects ultimately based in an alteration of the DNA structure. Most are inherited as autosomal recessive disorders, some as X-linked disorders, and a few (acute intermittent porphyria) are autosomal dominant disorders. These conditions are usually the result of an altered rate (absent, reduced, enhanced) of an enzyme reaction (phenylalanine hydroxylase) or altered structure of a nonenzyme protein (hemoglobin). The effects of these altered proteins are found in aberrant metabolic pathways (phenylketonuria), disordered feedback regulation (acute intermittent porphyria), abnormal membrane function (hypercholesterolemia), altered intracellular compartmentation (alpha-1-antitrypsin deficiency), and distorted cell or tissue architecture (sickle cell anemia). Currently, over 125 areas of metabolism are represented, and, with the defects and their types and subtypes, over 200 inherited metabolic diseases have been described. Not all are clinically evident in the pediatric age group, but the majority can be biochemically detected then. The ultimate diagnosis and confirmation of these disorders generally depends on assessment of accumulated or missing metabolites in body fluids (urine, plasma, cerebrospinal fluid); enzyme analyses of a body fluid, tissue, or cultured tissue; description of structural protein variation; or, as is rapidly evolving, by analysis of the genes themselves by restriction endonucleases. Although definite "cures" for genetic diseases are not currently available, dietary treatment, prevention of new cases (recurrence-risk counseling, carrier screening, prenatal diagnosis) and palliative procedures constitute treatment. Replacement or modification of deficient products or proteins, restrictive diets to limit substrate accumulation, inhibitors, enzyme amplification, and organ transplantation are currently in use as treatment. Genetic engineering techniques involving replacement of a deleterious mutant gene with a normal one may eventually provide a cure for inborn errors of metabolism. Truly, this is an exciting time for the development of novel treatment modalites for genetic diseases.

For the student, resident, or private practitioner of pediatrics, the most common problem with the categorization of these disorders is to know when to suspect them, as each may be so rare as to be seen only a few times during one's practice. However, becase of the high recurrence risk to the families of affected persons, it is of the utmost importance to recognize symptoms of inborn errors, to include them in a wider differential diagnostic evaluation, and to obtain appropriate screening studies for them. This chapter outlines those symptoms that should alert one to an inborn error of metabolism and guide one to an appropriate differential diagnosis. For a general reference, M. Ampola's *Metabolic Diseases in Pediatric Practice* is an inexpensive and primarily clinical reference for these diseases. The book also provides information on genetic centers in the United States from which one can obtain further information.

ACUTE INBORN ERRORS OF METABOLISM (IEM)

Those inborn errors included here are conditions that present clinically either in the newborn period (common) or anytime thereafter with symptoms of a life-threatening nature. The box on p. 645 lists the symptoms common to many. These symptoms, each taken alone or with others, are also found in more commonly occurring neonatal diseases, such as sepsis, intraventricular bleeding, primary cardiorespiratory abnormalities, gastrointestinal obstruction, and acute liver diseases.

However, if the clinician has thought of an

ACUTE PRESENTATION OF SELECTED IEM

Emesis and diarrhea	Metabolic acidosis
Lethargy	Jaundice
Respiratory distress	Hypoglycemia
Seizures	Electrolyte disturbance
Coma	Unusual odor (body tissue or fluid)

IEM as a possibility in differential diagnosis, then screening studies may be pursued concurrent with other standard evaluation. The box on p. 646 is a brief list of symptoms and the more commonly associated inborn errors manifesting them. Initial treatment for acute IEM disorders may include vigorous alkali and fluid therapy for metabolic ketoacidosis; high glucose intake ($D_{10}W$ with or without Intralipid) to prevent catabolism of body proteins; restriction of dietary protein (e.g., Mead-Johnson 80056 formula); exchange transfusion in hyperbilirubinemic disorders; peritoneal or hemodialysis in cases of hyperammonemia or intractable metabolic acidosis; and cofactor supplementation if known or suspected to be needed.

Symptoms that are not necessarily life-threatening but which should alert the clinician to an inborn error of metabolism are many, but usually include:

1. Liver or splenic enlargement (lysosomal storage, carbohydrate, amino acid, and organic acid disorders)
2. Coarse facies (mucopolysaccharidoses, mucolipidoses, GM_1-gangliosidoses, mannosidoses, fucosidoses)
3. Neutropenia, thrombocytopenia (organic acidurias)
4. Developmental delay (phenylketonuria, aminoacidurias, organic acidurias, urea cycle disorders, homocystinuria, galactosemia, congenital lactic acidosis, storage disorders, Lesch-Nyhan syndrome)
5. Failure to thrive (aminoacidurias, organic acidurias, cystinuria, congenital lactic acidosis, storage disorders)

LABORATORY DIAGNOSIS

Metabolic screen is the standard term for a screen of various metabolites (amino acids, organic acids, carbohydrates, mucopolysaccharides) in urine. However, the term differs for each laboratory and the clinician should know exactly what is needed and what is provided in a particular laboratory. The qualitative tests listed in the box on p. 647 are those performed in most IEM laboratories associated with genetics, endocrine, or developmental disciplines. The quantitative tests require specialized equipment and techniques and qualified interpretation. With these tests, one can usually determine which patients need further evaluation by enzyme analysis of plasma, leukocytes, or skin fibroblasts. Remember, these are only screening tests; if clinically suspicious, one should pursue further testing in the face of negative screening. For example, patients with Sanfilippo syndrome, MPS-III, may have a negative MPS spot test but a positive urine uronic acid test or ^{35}S-sulfate incorporation into fibroblasts.

AMINOACIDURIAS

Phenylketonuria and the hyperphenylalaninemias

Phenylketonuria (PKU) is the most common disorder of the hyperphenylalaninemias, which are autosomal recessively inherited. It is panethnic and occurs in the United States with a frequency of about 1:11,000 births. Untreated patients usually present after 6 months with developmental delay, "musty" odor, fairer skin than their family, eczema, and eventually seizures and psychotic behavior. A metabolic screen of urine will reveal phenylketone elevation and plasma quantitative phenylalanine usually greater than 20 mg/dl. Phenylalanine hydroxylase, catalyzing the conversion of the essential amino acid phenylalanine to tyrosine, is virtually absent in the liver of affected patients. Quantitative phenylalanine and tyrosine determinations in response to a phenylalanine load usually suffices to distinguish phenylketonuria from milder forms of hyperphenylalaninemias. A plasma phenylalanine value greater than 20 mg/dl and presence of urinary phenylketones on a regular protein diet, or when presented with a challenge of L-phenylalanine, is usually sufficient to make the presumptive diagnosis of PKU and immediately begin treatment.

Persistent and transient hyperphenylalaninemia may present initially as classical PKU, but because of relative ease of treatment, may be challenged at 6 months and found to have lower plasma phenylalanine than previously. Dietary treatment may then be reevaluated for discontinuation. Hyperphenylalaninemia may also be

SYMPTOMS OF ACUTE INBORN ERRORS OF METABOLISM

Vomiting

Congenital adrenal hyperplasia (electrolyte disturbance)
Urea cycle disorders (hyperammonemia)
Organic acidurias (toxicity secondary to elevated organic acid)
Branched-chain amino acid disorders (maple syrup urine disease [MSUD], toxicity of elevated substrate)
Miscellaneous and less common disorders (phenylketonuria, galactosemia, hereditary fructose intolerance, Wolman disease, female carrier for urea cycle disease [ornithine carbamyl transferase deficiency])

Diarrhea

Congenital lactose deficiency
Glucose-galactose malabsorption
Chloridorrhea, familial
Wolman disease

Jaundice

Galactosemia (elevated galactitol toxic to liver)
Hereditary fructose intolerance
Tyrosinemia
Alpha-1-antitrypsin deficiency
Carnitine deficiency
Miscellaneous and less common disorders (hereditary spherocytosis, glycolytic red blood cell defects, Crigler-Najjar syndrome, hypothyroidism, Wolman disease)

Lethargy and coma

Urea cycle disorders
Organic acidurias
Branched chain aminoacidurias
Hyperglycinemia, nonketotic
Carnitine deficiency

Seizures

Hyperglycinemia, nonketotic
Maple syrup urine disease (MSUD)
Organic acidurias
Congenital adrenal hyperplasia
Glycogen storage diseases I and III (hypoglycemia)
Congenital lactic acidosis

Unusual odor (body or body fluids)

Maple syrup urine disease (sweet)
Isovaleric acidemia (sweaty feet, fruity)
Phenylketonuria, tyrosinemia (musty)
Methionine malabsorption (Oasthouse, dried malt or hops)
Hypermethionemia (rancid butter)
Beta-methyl-crotonyl-CoA-carboxylase deficiency (cat urine)

detected with deficiency of the cofactor, tetrahydrobiopterin, caused by deficiency of dihydropteridine reductase, and by enzyme deficiencies in biopterin synthesis. These patients, usually 1% to 2% of all hyperphenylalaninemic patients, may have abnormal biopterin metabolites in urine, and the enzyme deficiencies are usually detectable in skin fibroblasts. Transient neonatal and hereditary tyrosinemia may result in elevations of plasma phenylalanine, necessitating measurement of tyrosine simultaneously with phenylalanine quantitation in initial evaluation of hyperphenylalaninemia.

The pathophysiology of neurologic effects in untreated cases is based on the presumed toxic effect of phenylalanine and phenylketones on myelin formation. Lipids and proteolipids are decreased.

LABORATORY EVALUATION OF IEM

Qualitative Tests (urine metabolic screen)

Characterization of urine sample (Bili-Lab Stix, specific gravity, creatinine)
Wet-tube methods
- Ferric chloride (wet tube/dip sticks) (PKU, tyrosinemia, MSUD, histidinemia, Oasthouse, alkaptonuria, etc.)
- Cyanide-nitroprusside (cystine and homocystine metabolites)
- Nitrosonaphthol (tyrosine metabolites)
- Dinitrophenylhydrazine (keto acids)
- Clinitest (reducing substances)

Mucopolysaccharide screening (Berry spot test, acid albumin turbidity, CTAB precipitation)
Paper chromatography
- Carbohydrates
- Organic acids
- Glycoproteins

Amino acids (high-voltage paper electrophoresis, with or without subsequent paper chromatography; thin layer chromatography, less desirable)

Quantitative tests

Amino acids (plasma, urine, cerebrospinal fluid, amniotic fluid; ion-exchange chromatography or gas chromatography [GC])
Organic acids (urine, plasma; GC or GC–mass spectrometry [GC-MS])
Mucopolysaccharides (urinary uronic acid)
Orotic acid (urine, elevated in some urea cycle disorders)
Enzymatic determinations in plasma, leukocytes, skin fibroblasts, affected tissue (brain, liver, and amniocytes)

The detection of these autosomal recessively inherited conditions is primarily now achieved in most states by mandatory screening of newborn blood, usually within 48 to 72 hours after birth. The Guthrie test, a bacterial inhibition assay, detects elevations of phenylalanine from a filter paper spot filled with the infant's blood. If an elevation is detected, usually greater than 4 mg/dl, the referrer is notified to send a follow-up sample to the referral laboratory for quantitation of phenylalanine and tyrosine. If the elevation persists, especially if greater than 12 mg/dl, and the tyrosine is normal, the child and family are referred to the nearest facility specializing in such treatment for further documentation of the type of PKU, counseling, and initiation of treatment.

If classical PKU is diagnosed, a diet low in phenylalanine (Lofenalac plus supplemental protein) is instituted to maintain plasma phenylalanine between 4 and 10 mg/dl. Because Lofenalac alone is not sufficient for phenylalanine requirements, the amount and type of protein supplement should be determined by a metabolic nutritionist in conjunction with monitoring the plasma phenylalanine. Phenylalanine can be monitored weekly during the first few months, and then every few months in ensuing years. Discontinuation of the diet may occur by age 6 to 8 years in some patients. Others may show learning problems or behavioral changes and are aided by continuation of the diet. Persons with either transient or persistent hyperphenylalaninemia may initially have values that require dietary intervention. However, when challenged and found not to have classical PKU, the diet may be discontinued if the plasma phenylalanine remains below 15 mg/dl and no ketonuria is observed. Many hyperphenylalaninemias have elevations only up to 12 to 15 mg/dl, never spill phenylketones, do not have any clinical sequelae themselves, and are therefore detected only on newborn screening surveys. The cofactor deficiencies do not respond to low-phenylalanine diet alone, and 5-OH-tryptophan, dopa, and carbidopa are being used as additional treatment, although with variable success. European studies in which the missing cofactor is provided are promising.

An increasingly important aspect of PKU is the occurrence of microcephaly, mental retardation, and congenital heart disease in children born of women with untreated PKU or undetected hyperphenylalaninemia. Among offspring of women whose elevation of phenylalanine is greater than 20 mg/dl during pregnancy, mental retardation and microcephaly are seen in 90% and 70%, respectively. Although the proportion of offspring affected decreases with decreasing phenylalanine level, even when the maternal phenylalanine level is between 3 and 10 mg/dl (a goal of dietary treatment during pregnancy) there is still an increase in these birth defects. Therefore it is not clear that even strict phenylalanine restriction will completely abolish the teratogenic effect. It is currently recommended that all women with hyperphenylalaninemia be counseled regarding their risks and if desired begin a diet, when appropriate, before conception.

Prenatal diagnosis of PKU has not been available because of the virtual lack of measurable activity of phenylalanine hydroxylase in readily accessible tissues. However, new advances in recombinant DNA research have allowed isolation of a cDNA probe to a portion of the gene by restriction endonuclease analysis, allowing characterization of clinical types and family studies in leukocytes, skin fibroblasts, and amniotic fluid cells. Likewise, these analyses may eventually be used to characterize suspected carriers.

Maple syrup urine disease

Maple syrup urine disease (MSUD) is an autosomal recessively inherited deficiency of branched-chain ketoacid decarboxylase, an enzyme in the catabolism of the branched-chain amino acids—leucine, isoleucine, and valine. Classically, symptoms are of acute onset in the first week of life, with lethargy, anorexia, vomiting, seizures, coma, and death. A sweet odor appears in body sweat and urine. Hypoglycemia and a profound metabolic ketoacidosis are found, and elevation of the amino acids and their keto acids—isocaproic, 2-methylvaleric, and isovaleric acids—occurs. A dinitrophenylhydrazine (keto acid) spot test and a ferric chloride test will be abnormal, but quantitative amino acid and organic acid analyses are required for presumptive diagnosis and eventual treatment monitoring. Elevation of leucine and its organic acid appear to be responsible for the central nervous system symptoms. Acute treatment consists of vigorous fluid and alkali therapy, accompanied by institution of high-calorie, nonprotein formula (Mead-Johnson 80056) if vomiting has ceased. However, elevated leucine levels may necessitate peritoneal dialysis or hemodialysis for removal of the toxic compounds. Definitive diagnosis depends on demonstration of enzyme deficiency in leukocytes or fibroblasts. The amount of residual activity may help to predict the extent of dietary restriction. This is accomplished by restricting the branched-chain amino acids to an amount that maintains growth with the least ketoacidosis (e.g., Mead-Johnson MSUD Diet Powder). Intercurrent infections and high-protein intake may precipitate ketoacidotic episodes. Cofactor therapy with thiamine has been successful in some patients. Prenatal diagnosis is available. *Intermittent* and *intermediate* forms occur, with either intermittent episodes of ketoacidosis triggered by infection or cases with constant but intermediate elevations of the branched-chain amino acids, resulting in retardation.

Hypervalinemia (failure to thrive, vomiting, and hyperactivity) and *hyperleucineisoleucinemia*, (seizures, failure to thrive, and mental retardation) may be isolated branched-chain amino acid transaminase defects. Other abnormalities of branched-chain amino acids are found in the section on organic acidurias.

Urea cycle enzymopathies

The urea cycle disorders result from deficiencies of enzymes in the urea cycle pathway. All except arginase deficiency may present in both neonatal and chronic forms. Acute episodes present with lethargy, vomiting, seizures, coma, and death. Ammonia is usually 10 to 20 times elevated, and peritoneal dialysis, hemodialysis, or exchange transfusion may be required to remove ammonia and urea precursors. Hyperammonemia caused by a primary urea cycle enzymopathy must be differentiated from transient hyperammonemia of prematurity, parenteral alimentation of amino acid solutions, Reye syndrome, and organic acidurias.

Carbamyl phosphate synthetase deficiency. Carbamyl phosphate synthetase (CPS) deficiency is an autosomal recessively inherited urea cycle disorder with onset usually in the neonatal period and characterized by vomiting, lethargy, hypothermia, hypotonia, irritability, and opisthotonus. Profound hyperammonemia plus nonspecific hyperaminoacidemia, elevated serum transaminases, normal to low BUN, and normal orotic acid are found. Symptoms of *partial CPS deficiency* include episodic hyperammonemia, particularly after increase in protein content of formula or food; interim hyperammonemia is mild, and citrulline is low or absent. Developmental delay is seen and a CT scan may reveal cortical atrophy or ventricular dilation. Although the deficiency is measurable in liver biopsies, rectal and duodenal biopsies also possess the enzyme and are useful diagnostically. Most have less than 10% of control activity, although up to 50% activity has been noted in partial forms. Treatment currently consists of a low-protein diet (1 to 1.5 gm/kg), sodium benzoate (excrete NH_3 as hippuric acid), and arginine supplementation. However, survival past infancy for patients with the complete form has been rare; death normally occurs during acute hyperammonemic episodes refractory to peritoneal dialysis and sodium benzoate.

Ornithine carbamyl transferase deficiency. Ornithine carbamyl transferase (OCT) deficiency is X-linked in inheritance and is the most common urea cycle abnormality. Hemizygous males are affected in the majority of cases, presenting within days of life as in CPS deficiency. In addition to marked hyperammonemia, hyperaminoaciduria, hypocitrullinemia, and orotic aciduria distinguish OCT deficiency from CPS deficiency. Liver biopsy for specific enzyme determination is usually not necessary because these findings apparently are unique. Duodenal and rectal tissue analysis may be helpful for diagnosis. Heterozygous females may present in the newborn period or may be totally asymptomatic, depending on the proportion of body cells with the active X chromosome containing the altered OCT gene. Many heterozygous females have episodes of vomiting, headache, lethargy, and slurred speech, sometimes associated with protein intake or infections, and therefore appear to have migraine. Some males have shown later onset in infancy and childhood, with variable residual activity of OCT. Liver, duodenal, or rectal biopsy during well periods may be required to distinguish OCT deficiency from recurrent Reye syndrome. Asymptomatic female carriers may be detected by observing hyperammonemia and orotic aciduria levels after protein or alanine loading. Although prenatal diagnosis is not yet available other than by sex detection, recombinant DNA methods may soon yield a cDNA probe for the OCT gene, thus making initial diagnosis, carrier determination, and prenatal diagnosis available on easily obtainable tissues. Treatment currently is similar to that for CPS deficiency, and a few males are surviving infancy with variable neurologic outcome.

Citrullinemia. Citrullinemia is an autosomal recessively inherited disorder with deficiency of arigininosuccinic acid synthetase. Neonatal, subacute, and late onset forms exist. Citrulline elevation of 4 to 200 times normal, hyperammonemia, orotic aciduria, and metabolic acidosis are usually present. Enzyme activity is measurable in fibroblasts and amniotic fluid cells. Neonatal forms are now surviving (with variable mental status) on protein restriction, sodium benzoate, and increased arginine supplementation to increase excretion of NH_3 as citrulline.

Argininosuccinic aciduria. Argininosuccinic aciduria (argininosuccinate lyase deficiency) is an autosomal recessive disorder with some neonatal and predominantly subacute and late onset clinical forms. The latter present with psychomotor retardation, seizures, and intermittent ataxia in the first 1 to 2 years of life. Dry, brittle hair (trichorrhexis nodosa) is seen. Argininosuccinic acid and its metabolites are excreted in large amounts in urine along with increased amounts of citrulline. Plasma arginine and ornithine may be reduced. Diagnosis may be ascertained by assay of the enzyme in erythrocytes or fibroblasts, but tissue variation exists. Prenatal diagnosis is possible in those with fibroblast enzyme deficiencies. Treatment consists of protein restriction, arginine supplementation, and variable additions of sodium benzoate.

Argininemia. Argininemia (arginase deficiency), an autosomal recessive disorder, is the rarest of the urea cycle enzymopathies. Motor difficulties present from infancy to 2 years, lower extremity spasticity (scissoring or 'tip-toe' gait) ensues and progresses to spastic diplegia, and irritability, vomiting, tremors, and choreoathetosis progress to seizures, psychosis, and severe mental retardation. Argininemia is a consistent finding, and serum transaminases are elevated. Hyperammonemia and orotic aciduria are variably present. Erythrocytes and leukocytes are assayed for activity. Prenatal diagnosis by fetoscopy is available. Therapy is aimed at restricting arginine by restricting protein, supplementing other essential amino acids, and adding sodium benzoate.

Lysinuric protein intolerance. Lysinuric protein intolerance (hyperdibasic aminoaciduria) may also present with intermittent episodes of hyperammonemia and requires a low-protein diet and arginine supplementation.

Transient neonatal hyperammonemia. Transient neonatal hyperammonemia results from immature argininosuccinate synthetase and is usually self-limited, after requiring vigorous attention initially.

Nonketotic hyperglycinemia

Nonketotic hyperglycinemia (NKH) is an autosomal recessively inherited disorder that characteristically presents in the neonatal period with hypotonia and lethargy, usually requiring respirator assistance. Less frequently, mental retardation and seizures may be the chief complaint. Myoclonic or tonic-clonic seizures are seen and hiccuping may be frequent. An electroencephalogram may show hypsarrhythmia or a burst suppression pattern. Neutropenia may be seen. Plasma glycine is usually elevated 4 to 5 times and the cerebrospinal fluid:plasma glycine ratio is elevated (normally less than 0.02) up to 0.17 ± 0.09. Loading with glycine results in a rise in plasma glycine without a rise in serine, thus supporting a defect in the glycine cleavage system. Exchange transfusion may lower the glycine level in severe neonatal cases, and sodium benzoate may lower the glycine level in less severe cases. Neither appear to appreciably alter the clinical course. Glycine acts as a postsynaptic neurotransmitter inhibitor; block of this inhibition with strychnine has met with variable clinical results. Recent successes with diazepam treatment have been noted.

Tyrosinemia

Hereditary tyrosinemia, tyrosinosis, and other terms have been proposed for an autosomal recessive condition that usually presents in the neonatal period with failure to thrive, vomiting, diarrhea, hepatomegaly, and "cabbage-like" odor. A chronic form with chronic liver disease, renal tubular dysfunction, and rickets presents by age 1 year. If either is untreated, death occurs. Bilirubin, liver enzymes, cholesterol, alpha-fetoprotein, and prothrombin time are increased. Spot tests for tyrosine and its metabolites (*p*-hydroxyphenyl-pyruvic and *p*-hydroxyphenyl-lactic acids) are positive, plasma tyrosine is increased to 6 to 12 mg/dl, and methionine may be elevated to 1 to 5 mg/dl. Glycosuria, phosphaturia, and a generalized aminoaciduria may also be present. Succinylacetoacetate and succinylacetone are elevated in urine. Because of the difficulty in distinguishing this condition from neonatal hepatitis, the latter two compounds should be determined, as it is thought their elevation only occurs in patients with hereditary tyrosinemia. Fumarylacetoacetate hydrolase is deficient in liver biopsies in affected patients. Treatment currently consists of restricting phenylalanine and tyrosine in the diet (e.g., Mead-Johnson 3200AB), with additional restriction of methionine as needed. Prenatal diagnosis is not yet available because the enzyme is not routinely found in appreciable amounts in skin or leukocytes.

Another tyrosine abnormality is *tyrosine aminotransferase deficiency,* (Rickner-Hanhart syndrome), with corneal erosions, hyperkeratoses, and mental retardation, treatable by restricting dietary tyrosine and phenylalanine. *Neonatal tyrosinemia* usually occurs in premature infants, is asymptomatic, usually detected incidentally, and may be treated with dietary restriction, with tyrosine values returning to normal within weeks to months.

Homocystinuria

Homocystinuria is a term used for one of the more common defects in transsulfuration, cystathionine beta-synthase deficiency. This autosomal recessively inherited condition is probably underdiagnosed because of the seemingly unrelated symptoms in the ocular, skeletal, central nervous, vascular, and other systems. Mental retardation and, less frequently, seizures develop within the first 1 to 2 years. Thromboembolic episodes in the carotid, coronary, renal, or pulmonary vessels occur during childhood or thereafter. Malar flushing, livedo reticularis, skeletal findings of osteoporosis and "fish" vertebrae, and the classical ocular findings of ectopia lentis and iridodonesis occur between 2 and 10 years of age. Urine screening reveals an increase in homocystine by cyanide-nitroprusside spot test and amino acid electrophoresis. False-negative results may be encountered in the milder, pyridoxine-responsive forms if the patient is taking vitamins. Plasma amino acids reveal an increase in methionine in addition to homocystine. The enzyme deficiency is confirmed in skin fibroblasts and is prenatally diagnosable. Methionine determinations on filter-paper blood spots have been performed in several newborn screening surveys, resulting in estimates of 1 in 60,000 to 1 in 200,000 in frequency. Treatment has consisted of a low-methionine diet and cofactor therapy in pyridoxine-responsive patients.

Cystathioninuria (alpha-cystathionase deficiency) and hepatic *methionine adenosyltransferase deficiency* result in apparently no consistent phenotype and are autosomal recessively inherited.

Other inborn errors of amino acid metabolism

Histidinemia. Histidinemia is an autosomal recessively inherited condition resulting from deficiency of histidase. Although initial cases were described with mental retardation and speech defects, this condition appears to have no consistently abnormal phenotype when ascertained through newborn screening surveys in the United States and Canada, although Japanese cases appear more involved.

5-Oxoprolinuria. 5-Oxoprolinuria (pyroglutamic acidemia) is an autosomal recessively inherited condition presenting with severe central nervous system effects (quadraparesis, cerebellar disturbances, incoordination, speech dysarthrias) and severe metabolic acidosis. 5-Oxyprolinuria results and increased hemolysis is seen. Glutathione synthetase is deficient and results in alteration of the gamma-glutamyl cycle. Other errors in this cycle include an erythrocyte-limited glutathione synthetase deficiency, and deficiencies in gamma-glutamylcysteine synthetase, gamma-glutamyl transpeptidase, and 5-oxoprolinase.

Iminoacidopathies. The iminoacidopathies (proline and hydroxyproline), including *hyperprolinemia type I* (proline oxidase deficiency), *type II* (delta-pyroline-5-carboxylate dehydrogenase deficiency) and *hydroxyprolinemia* (hydroxy proline oxidase deficiency), all occur without apparent clinical sequelae. However, *prolidase deficiency* may result in chronic dermatitis, leg ulcers, splenomegaly, abnormal facies, and mental retardation. Urinary imino acid–containing peptides increase.

Disturbances of ornithine metabolism. Two distinct genetic disorders occur in ornithine metabolism. The *hyperornithinemia-hyperammonemia-homocitrullinuria* (H-H-H) syndrome is an autosomal recessively inherited condition with symptoms related to hyperammonemia. Transport of ornithine into the mitochondria may be defective and treatment with a low-protein diet may be useful. *Gyrate atrophy* of the choroid and retina results in progressive degeneration beginning in the first decade and is caused by a deficiency of ornithine-delta-aminotransferase. Arginine-restricted diets and pyridoxine have shown promising results in halting progression of chorioretinal degeneration.

Two types of hyperlysinemia exist. *Periodic hyperlysinemia* results from an increased protein load, in turn competing with the last enzyme, arginase, in the urea cycle, causing hyperammonemia. Low-protein diets appear to be useful. *Persistent hyperlysinemia* appears to have no characteristic clinical symptoms.

Disturbances in folate metabolism. Several defects occur in folate acid metabolism. *Methylene tetrahydrofolate reductase deficiency* is the most common of the folate disorders, resulting in central nervous system defects that present from infancy to childhood as seizures, apneic episodes, developmental delay, and hyperactivity. No effective treatment is available. *Congenital folate malabsorption* from the small intestine may result in failure to thrive, megaloblastic anemia, and occasionally severe central nervous system dysfunction. High oral doses or parenteral therapy of folic acid are required. *Dihydrofolate reductase deficiency* may result in stillbirths and abortions or, in living cases, failure to thrive and megaloblastic anemia. Treatment with folinic acid has been used in therapy. *Formiminotransferase deficiency* syndromes may result in central nervous system problems or milder problems, and treatment with folic acid may be used in some.

Other disorders. No specific consistent clinical features have yet been assigned to the *hypersarcosinemias*. Although cases are reported with mental deficiency, it is not clear whether the deficiency in sarcosine dehydrogenase in these patients is a bias of ascertainment, as many patients with the same deficiency are clinically normal.

Hypercarnosinemia, (carnosinase deficiency) is an autosomal recessive disorder resulting from inability to split carnosine to beta-alanine and histidine. Myoclonic seizures and psychomotor retardation are usually apparent in the first year of life, although some enzymatically proved cases show no symptoms. *Hyper-beta-alaninemia* is another disorder of beta-alanine metabolism, resulting in severe neurologic symptoms in the neonatal period. No successful treatment exists for either of these conditions.

Two types of *hyperlysinemia,* with and without hyperammonemia, occur as a result of degradative defects in the catabolism of lysine. Symptoms in the former are those of hyperammonemia. The latter form has no consistent clinical presentation. *Hyperpipecolic acidemia* occurs further in the catabolic pathway, is sometimes found in Zellweger syndrome, and is an autosomal recessively inherited condition with psychomotor retardation and hepatomegaly. No enzyme defect has been ascertained. A low-protein or low-lysine diet may be useful.

Transport defects of amino acids

Cystinuria. Cystinuria is the most common amino acid transport defect and probably one of the most common inborn errors of metabolism, with an overall prevalence of about 1 in 7000 detected in newborn screening. Clinical symptoms of this autosomal recessive disorder are related to defects in renal transport, with cystine stone formation and resulting obstructive symptoms. Although cystinuria occurs in both sexes, males are more severely affected. Onset may occur anytime during childhood or as late as age 90, but usually presents during the second to third decade. Recurrent urinary tract infection, hypertension, and renal failure may occasionally be the presenting complaints. Cystine crystals may be seen in a concentrated urine sediment. The cyanide-nitroprusside spot test has been used as a screen, although it is not specific (see p. 647). High-voltage paper electrophoresis distinguishes the elevation of cystine, along with arginine, ornithine, and lysine. All suspected cases should have quantitative amino acid tests performed on a 24-hour urine specimen and documentation of normal plasma amino acids. Analysis of stones may reveal cystine, but the lack of cystine does not rule out cystinuria, as calcium stones may form in cystinuric patients secondary to infection from cystine stones. Heterozygotes may also show many positive tests but rarely have symptoms and do not have characteristic elevations of quantitated urinary amino acids. Although classically cystine and the dibasic amino acids are elevated in urine, conditions have been described in which each cystine elevation occurs alone and vice versa, resulting in current proposals for three possible reabsorptive sites. Genetic classification into three types is based on excretion profiles in heterozygotes and intestinal transport studies in homozygotes, the latter of which have no symptoms. The excretion of greater than 250 mg cystine/mg creatinine is abnormal, and values of greater than 300 mg are associated with stone formation. Treatment currently consists of conservative medical therapy, including diluting the cystine (about 4 liters of fluid per day evenly distributed), alkalinizing urinary pH, and restricting excessive methionine in the diet. Failing that, D-penicillamine is used, which combines with cystine to form the more soluble cystine-penicillamine compound. Renal failure from repeated obstruction and infection may require renal transplantion.

Familial iminoglycinuria. Familial iminoglycinuria is an autosomal recessive, benign inborn error of renal tubular transport of proline, hydroxyproline, and glycine, and should be distinguished from the iminoacidemias. Intestinal transport defects may also be involved. Elevations of iminoaminoacids occur in urine but not plasma.

Hartnup disease. Hartnup disease is an inborn error of renal tubular and jejunal transport of the following amino acids; alanine, serine, threonine, asparagine, glutamine, valine, leucine, isoleucine, phenylalanine, tyrosine, tryptophan, histidine, and citrulline. Clinically this probable autosomal recessively inherited condition presents with an intermittent red, scaly, pellagra-like rash after sunlight exposure; cerebellar ataxia; behavioral changes; and frequently mental retardation. Diagnosis is based on the symptoms and the massive aminoaciduria. Excretion of indican from intestinal decomposition of tryptophan may be observed. The pathophysiologic relationships appear to be related to central nervous system toxicity from decomposition products, decrease in kynurenine nicotinamide from tryptophan resulting in dermatologic problems, and variable malnutrition from loss of essential amino acids. Treatment with oral nicotinamide is successful.

ORGANIC ACIDURIAS

The organic acidurias are inherited metabolic disorders of the nonamino organic acids and cause a variety of symptoms. These conditions should be considered in (1) acute or chronic sustained metabolic acidosis; (2) unusual body fluid odor; (3) recurrent vomiting; (4) neurologic dysfunction, such as seizures, ataxia, and unusual movements; (5) acute disease in infancy, especially with hyperammonemia or acidosis; (6) familial, atypical, or recurrent Reye syndrome; and (7) any inherited disease of obscure cause. Because of advancement in techniques capable of detecting these compounds—gas chromatography (GC) and mass spectrometry (MS)—the clinical description and etiology of many are available. Screening for excesses of urinary organic acid metabolites may be achieved by GC alone or GC-MS.

Below is a list of the organic acidurias according to their area of metabolic dysfunction; the more common disorders are discussed further. Most have had an enzymatic deficiency defined, thus making specific diagnosis, prognosis, and rational therapies available. Because many present with acute metabolic ketoacidosis, intensive fluid, alkali, and calorie intake are initially required. Peritoneal dialysis, hemodialysis, or exchange transfusion may be necessary. Chronic treatment usually consists of a low-protein diet (1-1.5 gm/kg/day), as many acidurias occur in degradative pathways of essential amino acids. Some are vitamin or cofactor responsive. Others, such as the lactic acidoses, present challenges for chronic, long-term treatment. Prenatal diagnosis is available for those with specific enzyme deficiencies detectable in amniotic fluid cells or in whom the amniotic fluid contains a diagnostic metabolite.

Methylmalonic acidemia. Methylmalonic acidemia is the most common such disorder detected thus far and therefore the most investigated. Symptoms may appear within the first few days of life in an otherwise healthy infant as feeding difficulties, vomiting, lethargy, seizures, and life-threatening metabolic acidosis. Later onset may include recurrent vomiting, failure to thrive, and developmental delay which, with an intercurrent infection or protein loading, may present with an acute episode.

ORGANIC ACIDURIAS

Leucine metabolism

Isovaleric acidemia
3-Methylcrotonylglycinemia
3-OH-3-methylglutaric acidemia

Isoleucine and valine metabolism

2-Methyl-3-hydroxybutyric acidemia
Propionic acidemia
Methylmalonic acidemia

Lysine and tryptophan metabolism

2-ketoadipic acidemia
Glutaric acidemia, I and II
Jamacian vomiting sickness

Miscellaneous

D-Glyceric acidemia
Pryoglutamic acidemia
Tyrosinemias
Hyperglycerolemia
Lactic acidemias
Ketosis
Dicarboxylic acidurias
Acetoacetyl-CoA thiolase deficiency
Multiple carboxylase deficiency
Succinyl-CoA: 3-keto-acid CoA transferase deficiency

Laboratory studies in the acute episodes reveal metabolic ketoacidosis, frequently neutropenia or thrombocytopenia, hypoglycemia, and mild to moderate hyperammonemia. A metabolic screen will reveal positive keto acids, hyperglycinuria, and presence of methylmalonic acid on the paper chromatography pattern. Plasma amino acids usually reveal a marked hyperglycinemia. Urinary organic acids, both in acute and interim specimens by GC-MS reveal marked elevation of methylmalonic acids. During periods of ketoacidosis, other organic acids and their glycine conjugates may be present. Autopsy findings are nondiagnostic and may reveal fatty infiltration.

There are currently at least six separate enzymatic defects that result in the clinical condition, resulting from autosomal recessively inherited enzymatic deficiencies in conversion of methylmalonyl CoA to succinyl-CoA (mutase), and metabolism of adenosylcobalamin (B_{12}), the cofactor required for mutase activity. Acquired, severe B_{12} deficiency will result in a similar clinical presentation. Enzymatic deficiencies are measurable in leukocytes and skin fibroblasts. Methylmalonyl CoA is a metabolite in the degradative propionate pathway of the essential amino acids isoleucine, valine, threonine, and methionine; the odd-chain fatty acids; and cholesterol side chains. Acute therapy for methylmalonic acidemia includes intravenous alkali therapy, administration of 10% dextrose solution, and concurrent therapy for underlying infections. High-calorie intake should be instituted as quickly as possible without accompanying protein intake until cessation of ketosis. Exchange transfusions or peritoneal dialysis may be used in cases with significant hyperammonemia or for removal of organic acid metabolites. Base formulas without protein are available (Mead-Johnson 80056) and are useful in both acute and chronic therapy. Prenatal diagnosis is available by enzyme detection in amniotic fluid cells. Methylmalonic acid is increased in amniotic fluid. In utero effects on the developing fetus have not been proved, but some fetal effects are thought to be present in some cases. This has precipitated treatment in utero of one B_{12} responsive fetus. Chronic treatment presently consists of limiting the diet in protein (1 to 1.5 gm/kg/day high-quality protein) and in excess intake of certain lipids in those forms with the mutase abnormality. The other forms are, in general, B_{12} responsive. This usually decreases the frequency of acute episodes, although intercurrent infections resulting in endogenous protein catabolism may still require acute therapy. Careful metabolic and dietary monitoring are required.

Propionic acidemia. Another autosomal recessive organic aciduria in the pathway of isoleucine and valine metabolism is propionic acidemia, with similar clinical onset as methylmalonic acidemia. Similar laboratory findings are seen, including hyperglycinemia, and organic acids in urine include primarily tiglylglycine, propionylglycine, and methylcitric acids. Propionyl CoA carboxylase deficiency is measured in leukocytes and skin fibroblasts. Treatment consists of a low-protein diet (see previous section), although a few have been responsive to biotin, a cofactor in the enzymatic reaction. Prenatal diagnosis is available by measurement of the enzyme deficiency in amniotic cells and by measuring methylcitrate in the fluid.

Disorders of pyruvate and lactate metabolism. Two autosomal recessive inborn errors of metabolism in pyruvate metabolism have been reported—pyruvate dehydrogenase complex (PDHC) and pyruvate carboxylase (PC) deficiencies. Secondary disorders altering pyruvate metabolism may be distinguished clinically from these two inborn errors, including inherited abnormalities in oxidative (mitochrondrial) pathways subsequent to PDHC, usually presenting with progressive muscular disease. Enzyme deficiencies in the gluconeogenic pathways subsequent to pyruvate carboxylase (i.e. fructose and glycogen storage abnormalities), also result in changes in the pyruvate metabolism. Inborn errors of biotin metabolism may also alter pyruvate carboxylase activity. Acquired secondary effects affecting pyruvate metabolism include anoxia, dietary thiamine deficiency, diabetes, and Reye syndrome.

Pyruvate carboxylase deficiency has been reported to occur in patients with congenital lactic acidosis and severe developmental delay. Few patients are reported with adequate documentation of biochemical abnormalities in multiple tissues, including fibroblasts. Parents have intermediate enzyme deficiency. Clinically, seizures develop within 3 months, accompanied by hypotonia, posturing, and severe, progressive retardation. Histopathologic changes have been noted in brain, kidney, muscle, and liver. Other reports of pyruvate carboxylase deficiency are primarily based on liver enzyme determinations. The association with the condition of Leigh encephalopathy is not clear, but may be a secondary deficiency.

Deficiency of the pyruvate dehydrogenase complex has been reported in over 50 patients. This intricate and complex series of reactions converts pyruvate oxidatively to CO_2 and acetyl CoA. Three enzymes are involved: pyruvate dehydrogenase, dihydrolipoyltransacetylase, and dihydrolipoyldehydrogenase. Patients exhibit psychomotor retardation, hypotonia, microcephaly, abnormal reflexes, and apparent lactic acidosis within the first year or two of life. Death from progressive changes may occur within the first decade. Milder pyruvate dehydrogenase deficiencies have been reported in ataxic patients without apparent severe developmental delay.

Diagnoses of these disorders depend on careful analysis of these enzymes. Pyruvate, lactate, and alanine are usually elevated in patients with primary pyruvate abnormalities, resulting in pyruvate to lactate ratios in the normal range. Secondary disorders usually have an altered pyruvate/lactate ratio. Patients with pyruvate dehydrogenase complex deficiency usually develop excessive pyruvate after a glucose load. Patients with pyruvate carboxylase deficiency or other gluconeogenic defects do not increase their blood glucose after an alanine challenge. Treatment, aside from acute and chronic alkali therapy, has been aimed at cofactor supplementation and dietary alteration, depending on the deficient step, and has been variably successful. Prenatal diagnosis is available in some families.

Glutaric aciduria, type I. Type I is an autosomal recessively inherited disorder that may present subsequent to normal development by age 3 to 20 months. Macrocephaly from birth is frequent. Acute episodes of emesis and encephalopathy associated with minor infections may be presenting complaints, accompanied by hypoglycemia, metabolic acidosis, and hepatomegaly. Neurologically, hypotonia, lack of head control, athetoid movements, and dystonia and chorea are usually present. Milder cases have been reported and are usually associated with a higher residual enzyme activity. Glutaryl-CoA dehydrogenase, an enzyme in the catabolic pathway of lysine and tryptophan, is deficient in leukocytes and skin fibroblasts. Glutaric acid is the organic acid consistently elevated, with 3-hydroxyglutaric and glutaconic acids variably present. Glutaric acid elevations may affect neurotransmitter function. Attempts at treatment have included a low-lysine diet, cofactor supplementation (riboflavin) and the GABA analogue baclofen (Lioresal). Prenatal diagnosis is available.

Glutaric aciduria, type II. Type II is distinguished from type I by its clinical symptoms and organic acid pattern. Acute onset of profound hypoglycemia, metabolic acidosis, and unusual odor (sweaty feet) have occurred in the neonatal period, but older cases with additional encephalopathy and hyperammonemia are also reported. Lactic, glutaric, 2-hydroxyglutaric, ethylmalonic, adipic, suberic, and sebacic acids appear in the urine. An enzyme defect in the mitochondrial electron transport system of acyl-CoA and sarcosine dehydrogenase is proposed. Treatment has generally been unsuccessful, with several patients having acidosis resistant to alkali therapy.

Jamaican vomiting sickness. Jamaican vomiting sickness may be confused with the glutaric acidurias by clinical symptoms and organic acid pattern, but is distinguishable by eliciting a history of ingestion of the unripe ackee fruit. It is usually limited geographically to areas in which that fruit is in plentiful supply. The toxins, alpha-aminopropionic acid (hypoglycine A) and its gamma glutamyl conjugate (hypoglycin B) appear to inhibit fatty acid oxidation enzymes and glutaryl-CoA dehydrogenase, and indirectly gluconeogenesis. Profound hypoglycemia, acidosis, and pathologically fatty degeneration of the liver and kidneys is seen. Urine excretion reveals metabolites increased, resulting from inhibition of several acyl-CoA-dehydrogenases, and from the action of methylenecyclopropylacetic acid. Treatment is with acute carbohydrate and alkali therapy and avoidance of the fruit.

MELITURIA

Melituria is the condition involving increased urinary excretion of any one of several simple sugars. A Benedict test (usually Clinitest) will detect the ability of certain 5-carbon and 6-carbon sugars to reduce copper heating. A glucose-oxidase test (usually Clinistix) is specific for glucose alone. Thus these two tests help to determine the need for further identification of urinary sugars. Sugars resulting in a positive test for urinary reducing substances are glucose, galactose, fructose, lactose, mannose, xylose, xylulose, ribose, maltose, and arabinose. Sucrose does not give a positive reaction. False-positive reactions may occur when other compounds are present, such as homogentesic acid, sialic acid, Renografin, and large antibiotic dosages (Keflin, ampicillin, penicillin, and streptomycin). False-negative reactions are known to occur, especially if the diet does not contain a particular sugar at the time of urine testing. Normally, no sugar should be present in the urine. However, patients on intravenous dextrose and premature infants may excrete glucose. Small amounts of galactose may be present in the urine of neonates. Small amounts of lactose are seen in infants and lactating women. Increased consumption of sugars not needed or those sugars not metabolized (xylose) may lead to increased excretion.

Several inborn errors of sugar metabolism occur (Table 23-1). Classically, if the urinary glucose-oxidase test is negative and the Benedict test positive, further screening by paper or thin-layer chromatography is required to tentatively identify the excessive sugar. However, because many affected patients may also be receiving additional intravenous dextrose and therefore give a positive glucose-oxidase, it is best to reevaluate any positive Benedict test by repeating the test when the patient is on oral intake alone, or identifying the sugar by paper chromatography. Thereafter, specific enzyme analysis may be performed to confirm an enzyme deficiency and dietary sources altered to prevent further metabolite accumulation.

Galactosemia

At least two different enzymatic defects, both of which are inherited in an autosomal recessive manner, may produce galactosemia.

Transferase deficiency. The more common and severe defect is a deficiency of galactose-1-phosphate uridyl transferase. In this deficiency, galactose can be converted to uridine diphosphogalactose and glucose-1-phosphate, a necessary step for metabolism of galactose. Galactosemia and galactosuria result and accumulation of galactitol is thought to be toxic to the lens. Origin of liver and brain toxicity is not clear. Manifestations appear shortly after birth and include vomiting, listlessness, weight loss, jaundice, hepatomegaly, cataracts, and neonatal E. coli sepsis. If treatment is not instituted early, cataracts and mental retardation are likely to occur. It is suggested that all jaundiced neonates be tested for reducing substances while on a lactose-containing formula. Hepatic failure and death are late complications. Early dietary restriction of galactose by use of nonlactose-containing formulas and continued restriction of lactose-containing foods provides effective treatment. Diagnosis is established by demonstrating absence or severe deficiency of the enzyme in erythrocytes or fibroblasts. Prenatal diagnosis is available. Intermediate values may be found in erythrocytes from unaffected heterozygotes.

Table 23-1. Disorders of carbohydrate metabolism

Sugar	Reducing property	Disorder(s)
Glucose	+	Diabetes Renal transport defects (Fanconi syndrome) Glucose-galactose malabsorption
Galactose	+	Galactosemia: galactose-1-P uridyl transferase deficiency Galactokinase deficiency Liver disease
Fructose	+	Essential fructosuria Fructose intolerance Tyrosinemia
Lactose	+	Lactose intolerance Lactase deficiency
Xylulose	+	Pentosuria
Sucrose	−	Disaccharide intolerance

Galactokinase deficiency. A deficiency of galactokinase results in the inability to convert galactose to galactose-1-phosphate, resulting in galactosemia and galactosuria. Cataracts may be the first and only abnormality, and all children with cataracts should be screened for galactosuria. Additionally, any infant with a positive urinary galactose screen without other symptoms should be screened for galactokinase deficiency, as dietary alteration prevents cataract formation. Erythrocyte and fibroblasts reveal the deficient activity.

Hereditary fructose intolerance

This autosomal recessively inherited disorder of fructose metabolism may be detected in an acutely ill neonate, a chronically ill child or young adult, or an asymptomatic adult. This variation results because the array of symptoms depend on the amount and consistency of sucrose or fructose ingestion. Infants who are switched to nonlactose-containing formulas may have poor feeding, vomiting, and failure to thrive. Gastrointestinal discomfort, liver disease, hypoglycemia, and shock occur less frequently. Laboratory findings are those of liver failure, proximal renal tubular dysfunction, aminoaciduria, and reducing substances in urine. The formula may be switched to one containing lactose and many families begin to avoid the sweet foods that result in such symptoms as abdominal distention, hepatomegaly, failure to grow, irritability, tremor, drowsiness, jaundice, hemorrhages, and diarrhea. Thus many persons remain undiagnosed because they have treated themselves unknowingly.

If fructose is identified in the urine of such a patient, an intravenous fructose tolerance test is performed (200 mg/kg, 20% solution). Affected persons first show a rapid fall in serum phosphate (accumulation of fructose-1-P), then serum glucose, and then a rise in urate and magnesium. Measurement of the deficient enzyme fructose-1-P aldolase B is possible in biopsy of liver or small intestine, but not erthyrocytes or fibroblasts. Treatment consists of elimination from the diet of all sucrose, fructose, or sorbital.

Essential (benign) fructosuria

Essential fructosuria results from a deficiency of fructokinase, which normally converts fructose to fructose-1-phosphate. There are no clinical symptoms; it is an autosomal recessively inherited disorder.

Essential (benign) pentosuria (L-xylulosuria)

Excretion of L-xylulose in urine occurs in persons who lack the enzyme L-xylulose reductase. This pathway serves no essential function in humans and the condition is benign and symptomless, inherited in an autosomal recessive manner, and occurs almost exclusively among Jews.

LYSOSOMAL STORAGE DISORDERS

The lysosomal storage diseases make up the major group of the inborn errors of metabolism that result in storage. The lysosome is the compartment of the cell functioning in the breakdown of large molecular weight molecules. The enzymes contained therein are acid hydrolases and there are about 40 such enzymes known. When a primary lysosome with enzymes converges with a pinocytotic vesicle containing extracellular, macromolecular material, acid hydrolysis occurs. When an acid hydrolase is either absent or deficient, material accumulates within the lysosome, resulting in enlargement, malfunction, and death to the cell involved. Tissues and organs affected are those in which the macromolecular compound normally is synthesized and catabolized, thus resulting in a wide variety of clinical symptoms. Table 23-2 lists both the lysosomal and glycogen storage disorders by age of onset and whether the central nervous system or the visceral organs, or both, are predominantly involved.

Mucopolysaccharidoses

These storage disorders have emerged in the past 10 years as distinct genetic entities from the prototype Hurler syndrome. Each of these conditions is characterized clinically by disturbances in the connective tissue caused by accumulation of mucopolysaccharides (glycosaminoglycans) and thus have a wide range of expression, depending on the particular mucopolysaccharide stored and the tissue in which it normally occurs. Tissues most involved include eye, brain, liver, skin, and musculoskeletal system. Qualitative screening tests detect excessively excreted urinary mucopolysaccharides (see p. 647). There are seven types, catego-

Table 23-2. Clinical presentations of selected storage disorders

	Predominant tissue system involved		
	Central nervous	**Visceral**	**Central nervous/visceral**
Onset: Early infancy to 6 months	Tay-Sachs Sandhoff Globoid cell leukodystrophy	Wolman Glycogen storage disease type I Glycogen storage disease, type II Glycogen storage disease, type IV	Gaucher, type 2 Niemann-Pick, type A GM_1-Gangliosidosis, Mucolipidosis II Farber Mannosidosis type I Sialidosis, type II (infantile and congenital forms)
Onset: 6 months to 2 years	Metachromatic leukodystrophy (infantile) GM_1-gangliosidosis (juvenile)	MPS-VI (Maroteaux-Lamy) MPS-IV (Morquio) Glycogen storage disease, type III Glycogen storage disease, type VI	MPS-IH (Hurler) MPS-II (Hurler) MPS-VII (beta-glucuronidase, mild) Fucosidosis Mannosidosis type II
Onset: 2 years to adolescence	Metachromatic leukodystrophy (juvenile) MPS-III (Sanfilippo) Sialidosis, type I	Gaucher, type I Niemann-Pick, type B Fabry MPS-IS (Scheie) ML-III Cholesterol-ester storage disease Glycogen storage disease, types V and VII	Gaucher, type III Niemann-Pick, type C MPS-I Hurler-Scheie MPS-VII (beta-glucuronidase, milder) Sialidosis, II (juvenile) Aspartylglycosaminuria

rized by their phenotype and specific lysosomal enzyme deficiency. Further clinical variability occurs in three types, and one type has multiple enzyme deficiencies. Many reveal inclusions in circulating lymphocytes and therefore peripheral blood smears should be evaluated when considering these disorders. Radiographically, varying degrees of *dysostosis multiplex* are seen, comprised of an elongated sella turcica, anterior spatulate ribs, anterior vertebral wedging, diaphyseal flaring of long bones, and proximal narrowing on the diaphyses of shortened metacarpal bones. All but one type are autosomal recessively inherited (type II Hunter syndrome is X-linked). All are prenatally diagnosable in cultured amniotic fluid cells.

Hurler syndrome (MPS I-H). This condition is detected between 6 months and 1 year, manifesting developmental delay, hirsutism, stiff joints, lumbar lordosis, hepatosplenomegaly, and nasal breathing. Progression of these features as well as coarsening of facies, scaphocephaly, communicating hydrocephalus, corneal clouding, short stature, claw-hand deformity, deafness, and cardiac involvement occur over the next few years. Features of dysostosis multiplex usually seen are medial flaring of the clavicle, shallow orbits, vertebral "wedging" at the thoracolumbar level, and flaring of iliac wings. Patients with the Hurler syndrome usually die before 10 years of age of either respiratory or heart failure. The lysosomal hydrolase, alpha-L-iduronidase, is deficient (less than 5%) in body tissues, resulting in cellular accumulation and urinary excretion of heparan sulfate and dermatan sulfate, the natural substrates of this enzyme. Prenatal diagnosis is available. There is no successful treatment to date, although skin grafts and bone marrow transplants have been attempted to provide a source of enzyme.

Scheie syndrome (MPS I-S). This autosomal recessive condition is characterized by normal intelligence, milder features of visceral storage, and is rarer than Hurler syndrome. Corneal clouding, retinal degeneration, and glaucoma occur. Stiff joints, especially of the hands and feet, are present. Coarse facies are present but not as severe as in MPS-IH. Aortic valve changes are known to occur. Height is normal.

The enzyme alpha-L-iduronidase is also decreased, using several substrates. Biochemical differences presumed to exist between the Hurler and Scheie types await further molecular characterization.

Hurler-Scheie compound (type I H-S). This is a disorder that is thought to be a genetic compound of type I-H and type I-S, with intermediate clinical phenotype but similar deficiency of alpha-L-iduronidase. Moderate mental retardation may be present. Severe and limiting dysostosis multiplex, arachnoid cysts around the sella turcica, and characteristic receding chin are clinical manifestations that occur with progression, in addition to other storage characteristics. Death occurs in the late teens or twenties.

Hunter syndrome (MPS-II). There are two forms of this X-linked recessive condition, one severe and one mild, both revealing deficiency in iduronate sulfatase. The most distinctive clinical difference between this and other forms of MPS is the lack of corneal clouding, although older patients may develop lesions detectable only on slit-lamp examination. Additionally, pebbly ("peu de orange") areas of skin are found in the infrascapular region. Laryngotracheal abnormalities are manifested by a hoarse voice and airway obstruction. Pachymeningitis cervicalis may result in hydrocephalus or cervical cord impingement. Chronic pseudopapilledema probably occurs secondary to optic nerve sheath involvement. Cardiac, skeletal, and other somatic changes are as in MPS-IH. Management is symptomatic. Mortality occurs in the early teens in the severe form; survival into the eighth decade is known for the milder forms. Although intermediate values of iduronate sulfatase may occur in obligate carrier females, generally it is difficult to classify a woman at risk for being a carrier because of overlap into the normal range. All women at risk for carrying the gene for MPS-II are offered amniocentesis as the only reliable method to detect an affected fetus.

Sanfilippo syndrome (MPS-III). This form of mucopolysaccharide storage disorder is characterized by four subtypes that are clinically indistinguishable but biochemically separate. Severe and progressive mental retardation is the key clinical presentation, beginning with behavior changes within the first 2 to 3 years of age. Although patients may begin regular school, most are institutionalized before the second decade. Somatic evidence of storage disease is mild, but coarse facies, hirsutism, and mitral valve involvement progress with age. Because of the mild somatic complaints, less severe radiologic changes, and the fact that usual qualitative screening tests may be negative, Sanfilippo syndrome is the most frequently underdiagnosed mucopolysaccharide storage disorder. Most patients die in their early twenties. Of four lysosomal enzymes involved in the degradation of heparan sulfate—heparan N-sulfatase (type A), N-acetyl glucosaminidase (type B), glucosamine N-acetyl transferase (type C), and N-acetyl-glucosamine-6-sulfatase (type D)—one is deficient in tissues in each type. These are all measurable in skin fibroblasts and amniotic fluid cells. This autosomal recessive MPS form is estimated to have an occurrence rate of 1 in 25,000 in the Netherlands, four times as common as Hurler syndrome.

Morquio syndrome (MPS-IV). Morquio syndrome is an autosomal recessively inherited condition characterized primarily by skeletal storage and severe radiologic dysostosis multiplex. Symptoms become evident between 1 and 2 years of life, with prominence of the rib cage and slightly coarse facies. Over the next few years, genu valgum, short trunk, prominent sternum, platyspondyly, short neck, and broad mouth develop. Growth may cease in severe cases after 7 years. Nonskeletal somatic storage is mild. Progressive deafness occurs. Intelligence is usually normal, and corneas are minimally cloudy. Severe neurologic sequelae may develop from complications secondary to hypoplasia of the odontoid process of C_2, resulting in atlantoaxial instability and cord injury with neck hyperextension. Acute or chronic cervical myelopathy develops in most patients. Patients should be cautioned regarding sudden neck movements or hyperextension with surgical anesthesia, and should be evaluated frequently for possible vertebral fusion. Although patients may live into their sixties, patients with severe forms may not live past the second decade because of their compromised cardiorespiratory status with severe pectus deformities. The severe type A is deficient in galactosamine-6-sulfate sulfatase, and the milder type B is deficient in keratan sulfate–specific beta-galactosidase, both lysosomal enzymes involved in the degradation of this predominantly skeletal mucopolysaccharide. These deficiencies are measurable in skin fibroblasts and amniotic fluid cells.

Maroteaux-Lamy syndrome (MPS-VI). Three clinical forms of varying severity are seen in this autosomal recessive disorder. Severe forms may resemble Hurler syndrome (MPS-I) in skeletal, ocular, cardiac, and facial characteristics, but are distinguisable by their normal intelligence. Atlantoaxial subluxation may occur and changes in the femoral heads may be severe. Survival is into the second decade, although mild cases may survive longer. Because of the deficiency of N-acetyl-galactosamine 4-sulfate sulfatase, dermatan sulfate accumulates and is excreted. Diagnosis is made by enzymatic determination on skin fibroblasts and can be made on amniotic fluid cells.

Sly syndrome (MPS-VII). Sly syndrome may have variable and milder manifestations of classical MPS symptoms, some with normal intelligence. Only a dozen cases have been reported and a clinically uniform picture has not emerged. Deficiency of beta-glucuronidase, apparently specific for degradation of the heparan and dermatan sulfates that accumulate, is found in all, although some are reported with residual activity. Any patient with an MPS disorder not clinically or enzymatically categorized into the other forms should have tissue examined for this enzyme.

Mucolipidoses

Originally classified as disorders with features of mucopolysaccharidoses and the lipidoses, further study now permits the original type I to be classified into the sialidoses (see Glycoproteinoses pp. 660-662). Mucolipidosis (ML) types II and III share common biochemical causes but have different phenotypes. Both are autosomal recessively inherited diseases.

ML type II or pseudo-Hurler polydystrophy clinically presents as Hurler syndrome, although even earlier and more severely. Joint restriction with tight and puffy skin are problems. Gingival hyperplasia and less corneal clouding also help to distinguish it from Hurler syndrome. Death occurs within 5 years from cardiac and respiratory problems.

Alternatively, patients with *ML-III* present much like those with intermediate Maroteaux-Lamy syndrome at 4 to 5 years of age, with stiffness of fingers, elbows, hips, and knees. Carpal tunnel compression may be a complication. These patients have been confused with patients suffering from juvenile rheumatoid arthritis. Growth impairment and mild mental retardation may be present. Mildly coarse facies may be seen, and radiographically unique features distinguish it from other MPS disorders.

Biochemically, urine screening in both disorders is negative for excessive mucopolysacchariduria. The basic defect involves the lack of a normal posttranslational modification of lysosomal acid hydrolases, the addition of a phosphate group to a mannose chain. Normally the resulting mannose-6-phosphate is involved in transport recognition to the lysosome. With transport altered, there is a decrease of intracellular and increase of extracellular lysosomal acid hydrolases. Therefore plasma may be used to screen for elevations of acid hydrolases. Beta-hexosaminidase A and arylsulfatase A are commonly tested, revealing ten- to twenty-fold elevations. Skin fibroblast cell extracts are deficient in many hydrolases. Distinguishing between ML-II and ML-III is currently by clinical phenotype. Treatment other than palliative is currently unavailable. Prenatal diagnosis by amniocentesis is possible by detection of increased acid hydrolases in the fluid and decreased acid hydrolases in amniotic fluid cells, and by direct measurement of the deficient enzyme.

Glycoproteinoses

Glycoproteins are formed by addition of oligosaccharides to serine, threonine, or asparagine amino acid residues of proteins. Degradation of these groups are by specific lysosomal acid hydrolases, and deficiencies in these enzymes result in glycoprotein storage disorders that clinically and radiologically resemble mild mucopolysaccharidoses. All have vacuolated lymphocytes on peripheral smear. All are autosomal recessively inherited and prenatally diagnosable.

Mannosidosis presents either as an *infantile (type I)* or a milder *juvenile onset (type II)* form. Coarse facies, psychomotor retardation, some degree of dysostosis multiplex, and other mild MPS-like features occur. Distinctive ocular findings include superficial opacities of the cornea and posterior lenticular opacities in a spoke-like pattern. Survival of type I mannosidosis may be as late as 10 years, although patients with type II survive into adulthood. Characteristic "high mannose" glycoproteins may be seen in the urine, but definitive diagnosis rests on determining deficiency of alpha-mannosidase in skin fibroblasts. Prenatal diagnosis is available.

Fucosidosis is similar clinically to mannosidosis in its MPS-like features and in early and later onset forms. Coarsening of the facies is milder. Increased sodium chloride in sweat occurs in type I and angiokeratoma occurs in type II. Characteristic fucoside-containing residues are found in urine. Fucosidase is the enzyme deficient in skin fibroblasts.

The *sialidoses* are also divided into two types: *type I,* without somatic involvement (cherry-red spot, myoclonus); and *type II,* with somatic storage (coarse facies, dysostosis, multiplex). These are further subdivided into age of onset categories. Onset of type I is usually in the second decade, with decreasing visual acuity, gait disturbances, myoclonus, and ophthalmologic abnormalities. Type II may be divided into congenital infantile and juvenile forms, the former presenting with hydrops fetalis and ascites and in the latter, the development of a combination of MPS-like features with macular cherry-red spot and myoclonus. The enzyme, alpha-neuraminidase, is deficient in fibroblasts from all these types.

Aspartylglycosaminuria clinically presents with mild MPS-like features with progressive mental deterioration. Aspartylglycosamine is elevated in urine and aspartylglycosaminidase is deficient in skin fibroblasts.

Sphingolipidoses

The sphingolipidoses comprise a group of inherited metabolic disorders characterized by the accumulation of certain glycolipids and phospholipids known collectively as the sphingolipids. These compounds are stored predominantly in the cells of the reticuloendothelial and nervous systems. In the reticuloendothelial system the accumulated sphingolipids apparently originate from the membranes of senescent erythrocytes and leukocytes. In the nervous system, neuronal gangliosides are probably the sources of the accumulated sphingolipids. The possibility of a sphingolipidosis should be considered in any infant with progressive mental or motor deterioration or both. Each of the sphingolipidoses results from the deficiency of a lysosomal enzyme necessary for the degradation of a particular sphingolipid that accumulates in excess. The determination of the specific enzyme deficiencies in leukocytes or skin fibroblasts now permits accurate and specific diagnosis of affected patients. Detection of heterozygotes is possible for the mutant allele responsible in selected diseases. Prenatal diagnosis of the affected fetus is available through enzyme analysis of the amniotic fluid cells. Treatment of the sphingolipidoses has been mostly supportive. Current efforts concern enzyme replacement therapy in several of the sphingolipidoses, such as Gaucher disease.

Farber lipogranulomatosis is an autosomal recessive disorder characterized by painful and progressively deformed joints, subcutaneous nodules, and progressive laryngeal involvement secondary to lipid storage. Ceramide and ganglioside storage may result in nervous system dysfunction. Death usually occurs within a few years. Deficiency of lysosomal acid ceramidase is detected in skin fibroblasts, leukocytes, and amniocytes, resulting in storage of ceramide. No therapy is currently available.

Niemann-Pick disease *types A, C,* and *D* are covered in Chapter 29. In *type B* (chronic, nonneuronopathic form), visceral storage of sphingomyelin is extensive. Clinically, patients have protuberant abdomen, respiratory difficulties, and short stature. Hepatosplenomegaly, pulmonary infiltrates, and foam cells in bone marrow are seen. Intellect is normal and the central nervous system is not involved. Retinal changes may occur. Affected persons usually survive into adulthood. Sphingomyelinase is deficient as measurable in skin fibroblasts, leukocytes, or tissue extracts. Prenatal diagnosis is available.

Gaucher disease is the most commonly occurring of the lipidoses, resulting in storage of glucocerebroside. Three clinical types have been described. *Type 1,* the "adult," chronic, nonneuronopathic form, may present anytime from birth to older age. Splenomegaly, hepatomegaly, and hematologic problems related to hypersplenism are the usual presenting complaints. In patients whose onset is early in childhood, respiratory problems secondary to infiltrative pulmonary storage may develop. Recurrent bone pain is seen and differentiation from osteomyelitis must be made. Neurologic involvement is not seen. Bone marrow aspirates reveal typical Gaucher cells ("crumpled silk" or "wrinkled tissue paper" cystoplasm). Deficiency of glucocerebrosidase in skin fibroblasts confirms the diagnosis. Enzyme replacement is being attempted, particularly in the younger patients with Type 1. *Types 2* and *3* are covered in Chapter 29 and have major neurologic involvement in addition to visceral storage.

Fabry disease is an X-linked storage disorder in hemizygous males characterized by pain and paresthesias in the extremities, angiokeratoma of skin, corneal and lenticular opacities, and renal impairment. Symptoms result from storage of glycosphingolipid in the endothelium and smooth muscle of blood vessels, ganglion cells, heart, kidneys, eyes, and other tissues. Heterozygous females are usually asymtomatic. Rarely, they may be as affected as males. Corneal epithelial dystrophy is usually seen on slit-lamp examination of heterozygotes and is used to detect carrier females. Deficiency of alpha-galactosidase in skin fibroblasts confirms the diagnosis. Phenytoin may relieve the pain and paresthesias. Major sequelae result from the renal impairment and if severe enough may require renal transplant. Enzyme therapy is being attempted. Prenatal diagnosis is available in amniocytes.

The *gangliosidoses* are covered in Chapter 29, and include the GM_2-gangliosidoses, Tay-Sachs and Sandhoff diseases, and the GM_1-gangliosidoses.

Wolman disease and *cholesteryl ester storage disease (CESD)* are both autosomal recessive disorders resulting from massive accumulation of cholesteryl esters and triglycerides in most body tissues. *Wolman disease,* which is more severe than CESD, has its onset during infancy with hepatosplenomegaly, steatorrhea, abdominal distension, adrenal calcifications, and failure to thrive. Death usually occurs in the first year of life. CESD may not be detected until adulthood, with hepatomegaly being the only complaint. Deposits of lipid occur throughout the body. Hyperbetalipoproteinemia is common, and premature atherosclerosis is present. Deficiency of acid lipase is confirmed in skin fibroblasts from both diseases, with CESD having the greater residual activity. No specific therapy is available.

OTHER STORAGE DISORDERS

Carnitine deficiency

Systemic carnitine deficiency is an apparently autosomal recessively inherited lipid storage disorder. Clinically, recurrent episodes of nausea, vomiting, confusion, or coma, as seen in Reye syndrome, present in early childhood. Slow, progressive muscle weakness occurs, the only clinical manifestation of a distinct myopathic form. During acute episodes, hypoglycemia, ketoacidosis, lactic acidosis, elevated plasma glutamic transaminase activities, and increased urinary decarboxylic acids occur. Muscle biopsy reveals lipid storage, as in the myopathic form. However, serum carnitine is deficient in the systemic form both during and between acute episodes, which distinguishes it from Reye syndrome. Carnitine is important in the transport of long-chain fatty acids into the mitochondria, where they are oxidized. Hepatic synthesis is the primary source of human carnitine, and a defect in this transport system is postulated. Treatment with supplemental carnitine has met with variable results.

Glycogenoses

Defects in the enzymatic synthesis or degradation of glycogen, the principal storage form of carbohydrates in animals, result in a group of disorders called the glycogenoses. The clinical manifestations of these disorders result from excessive storage of glycogen of normal or abnormal structure in affected tissues, primarily the liver, muscle, heart, or kidney. Most are inherited in an autosomal recessive manner, and each enzyme alteration may affect selected tissues. Many are diagnosable by leukocyte or skin fibroblast enzyme assay and are therefore available for prenatal diagnosis or early neonatal screening in at-risk siblings. Other glycogenoses require tissue biopsy for enzyme assay.

Type I: hepatorenal (von Gierke disease). Clinical features of hepatorenal gycogenosis include prominent abdomen, hepatomegaly (often from birth), and proportionate short stature. Xanthomas of fundus and extremities, bleeding diatheses (platelet abnormalities), flabby musculature, and diarrhea commonly occur frequently. Seizures secondary to hypoglycemia may occur early. Patients may live into adulthood, with the abdomen becoming less prominent. If uric acid is elevated, symptoms of gout may develop. Autosomal recessive inheritance is established. Laboratory findings usually include fasting hypoglycemia, unresponsiveness to epinephrine and glucagon challenges, elevations in lactate, pyruvate, triglycerides, phospholipids, cholesterol, and uric acid, without ketosis. Radiographic enlargement of the kidney is seen, and hepatomas depress isotope uptake in liver. Aminoaciduria, glycosuria, and phosphaturia may be seen.

Diagnosis rests on liver biopsy, which reveals elevations of normal structure glycogen and absence of *glucose-6-phosphatase*. Treatment by continuous intragastric feeding plus frequent high-carbohydrate meals has been successful, resulting in growth, correction of circulating abnormal metabolites, and regression of hepatomas. Portacaval shunting improves the condition of many patients, but hypoglycemia persists.

Type II: generalized (Pompe disease). Generalized glycogenosis is an autosomal recessively inherited condition that usually is ascertained in the first 6 months of life. The condition manifests profound hypotonia, muscle weakness, and congestive heart failure and massive cardiomegaly. Most patients die by 1 year of age. Electrocardiography (ECG) reveals giant QRS complexes and shortened P-R interval. There is no hypoglycemia nor other circulating abnormal metabolites as in type I. Electromyography (EMG) reveals pseudomyotonic and high-frequency discharges and fibrillations. Tissues of primary storage are the heart, muscle, liver, and central nervous system. Two other forms present in infancy, early childhood, or adulthood. Muscle weakness, cardiac involvement, similar EMG abnormalities, and slow progression occur. These patients appear to have the same enzyme defect as in classical type II glycogenosis but the storage is not marked. The lysosomal enzyme, alpha-1,4-glucosidase (acid maltase) is absent in muscle, leukocytes (if renal isozyme removed) and skin fibroblasts, making this condition prenatally diagnosable. There is no replacement treatment yet available.

Type III: limit dextrinosis (Cori disease). Patients with dextrinosis or Cori disease are clinically like type I but may have muscle involvement (wasting and weakness), splenomegaly, cardiomyopathy, and no renal enlargement. An adult form with progressive muscle weakness and cardiac hypertrophy occurs. Progression of the disease is milder and the liver may return to normal size by puberty. Laboratory findings include consistently elevated serum transaminases and fasting hypoglycemia, but variability in plasma lipids and responses to epinephrine and glucagon. Liver biopsy reveals abnormal glycogen accumulation (limit dextrin-like) and absence of amylo-1,6-glucosidase (debrancher enzyme). Enzyme deficiencies are also seen in leukocytes, muscle, and skin fibroblasts but may vary with clinical subtype and method of assay. Diagnostic studies should include enzyme analysis on all these tissues for appropriate genetic counseling, prenatal diagnosis, and ascertainment of sibling cases before development of clinical symptomatology. Treatment may include frequent feedings and high-protein diet in some cases and continuous intragastric feeding for those with hypoglycemia.

Type IV: amylopectinosis (Anderson disease). Clinically, evidence of hepatosplenomegaly, failure to thrive, developmental delay, and hypotonia are found within the first few months of life in patients with amylopectinosis. Electrocardiographic abnormalities are variable. Laboratory values include elevated serum transaminases and variable responses to glucagon and epinephrine challenges, both likely secondary to the severe early cirrhosis that develops. Infants with this apparently autosomal recessive condition usually die by age 2 years. The glycogen concentration in the liver and other tissues is usually not increased but instead is abnormal in structure and less soluble. Liver extracts, leukocytes, and skin fibroblasts reveal decreased alpha-1,4-glucan:alpha-1,4-glucan 6-glucosyltransferase (brancher) activity. Muscle glycogen appears normal. Prenatal diagnosis is possible.

Type V: muscle phosphorylase deficiency (McArdle disease). These patients present primarily with increased fatigability during childhood and adolescence. Painful muscle cramps develop after strenuous exercise in the second to fourth decades, and muscle wasting and weakness predominate thereafter. Myoglobinuria develops with severe cramps. The defect in conversion of glycogen to lactate blunts the rise of venous lactate from a limb performing ischemic exercise. Muscle tissue exhibits increased glycogen content. Less than 1% of the enzyme muscle phosphorylase is found. Liver phosphorylase is normal. Patients tolerate moderate exercise, and hypoglycemia does not occur. The condition appears to be autosomal recessively inherited. Treatment consists of prevention of renal failure caused by myoglobinuria. Isoproterenol, which increases free fatty acids and blood flow to muscle, has been tried with some success.

Type VI: hepatic phosphorylase deficiency (Hers disease). Patients with type VI glycogenosis may no longer be a distinct group. Clinical symptoms were milder than type I, and the liver showed an increased glycogen level and only 25% of normal hepatic phosphorylase. Some patients showed deficient leukocyte phosphorylase activity. It is important to measure the phosphorylase-activating system to distinguish this condition from phosphorylase *b* kinase deficiency. These are not distinguishable by tolerance tests. It is likely that such cases have been misclassified enzymatically and inheritance remains uncertain.

Type VII: muscle phosphofructokinase deficiency (Tarui disease). Patients with type VII glycogenosis resemble those with type V (McArdle disease), and findings in family studies so far are consistent with autosomal recessive inheritance. A severe infantile form associated with respiratory complications and resulting in death at 6 months has been reported. Hyperuricemia and gout have been found in one patient. Muscle and erythrocyte phosphofructokinase activity is less than 5% of normal. Glycogen accumulation may result from activation of glycogen synthetase by the accumulated glucose-6-phosphate reported.

Type VIII: hepatic phosphorylase b kinase deficiency. Patients that have been classified enzymatically appropriately usually present with hepatomegaly alone. Liver and leukocyte phosphorylase *b* kinase is less than 10%, resulting in slow activation of phosphorylase. Pedigree analysis with preponderance of affected males and in vitro tissue studies in the few affected females support X-linked recessive inheritance, although two other families have shown an autosomal recessive type.

Other abnormalities in glycogen metabolism. One female has been reported with asymptomatic hepatomegaly and was normoglycemic but had an abnormal glucagon response. Liver and muscle show glycogen accumulation, and a cyclic AMP-dependent kinase deficiency was postulated. Another case with cirrhosis resulting in death at 14 months of age showed accumulation in all organs of a low molecular weight glycogen. Patients with partial deficiency of phosphoglucomutase in liver and muscle and muscle alone have been reported. Cases with profound hypoglycemia after prolonged fasting have revealed absent glycogen synthase. However, because this enzyme is regulated by insulin and may be labile during tissue extraction, these cases are not always distinct from those with ketotic hypoglycemia. Up to 13 types of glycogen storage diseases have been reported.

DISORDERS OF PLASMA LIPIDS

Plasma lipids comprise phospholipids, cholesterol and cholesterol esters, triglycerides, and free fatty acids. All except the free fatty acids are transported in the blood associated with proteins known as lipoproteins. The lipoproteins may be separated by electrophoretic or ultracentrifugation techniques into four classes: alpha (high density, or HDL), beta (low density, or LDL), pre-beta (very low density, or VLDL), and chylomicrons. Most disorders of the plasma lipids result from an excess or deficiency of one or more of the lipoprotein classes, with resultant alterations in plasma cholesterol or triglyceride concentration (Table 23-3).

Hyperlipoproteinemia. Hyperlipoproteinemia should be considered when a patient presents with any of the following: xanthomas, hepatosplenomegaly, hypertriglyceridemia, hypercholesterolemia, recurrent attacks of abdominal pain, or a family history of premature vascular disease. The *primary* hyperlipoproteinemias (p. 666) are all familial and must be distinguished from *secondary* causes of hyperlipoproteinemia. Following is an outline of the causes of secondary hyperlipidemia and hyperlipoproteinemia:

- Exogenous
  - Alcohol
  - Contraceptives
  - Steroid therapy
- Endocrine and metabolic
  - Diabetes mellitus
  - Hypothyroidism
  - Hypopituitarism

- Steroid therapy
- Lipodystrophy
- Acute intermittent porphyria
- Pregnancy

Storage diseases
- Glycogen storage disease
- Cystine storage disease
- Gaucher disease
- Juvenile Tay-Sachs disease
- Tay-Sachs disease
- Niemann-Pick disease

Hepatic
- Congenital biliary atresia
- Benign recurrent intrahepatic cholestasis
- Hepatitis
- Biliary cirrhosis

Renal
- Nephrotic syndrome
- Chronic renal failure
- Hemolytic-uremic syndrome

Miscellaneous
- Burns
- Anorexia nervosa
- Systemic lupus erythematosus
- Klinefelter syndrome
- Idiopathic hypercalcemia
- Werner syndrome
- Progeria (Hutchinson-Gilford syndrome)

Currently the primary hyperlipoproteinemias are classified into five phenotypes by a combination of the plasma cholesterol and triglyceride concentrations, appearance of plasma after sitting in the refrigerator for 24 hours, and a definitive pattern after lipoprotein electrophoresis.

Type II, familial hypercholesterolemia (FH), is the most common disorder in adults and children. Affected heterozygote frequencies vary between 1 in 200 to 500, making this autosomal dominant condition the most common inborn error of metabolism. Mass neonatal screening programs and their subsequent follow-up studies have successfully identified the heterozygous state. The homozygous state is usually evident clinically at birth or shortly thereafter. Radioisotopic studies in fibroblasts suggest a defect in removal of LDL from the circulation, resulting in three proposed genetic defects: LDL–receptor negative, LDL–receptor defective, and defective LDL internalization. Prenatal diagnosis of homozygous FH has been made.

The familial hypertriglyceride disorders are all far less frequent, especially in children. *Type IV (familial hypertriglyceridemia)* presents very rarely under age 20 years. *Familial combined hyperlipidemia (FCH)* is a syndrome comprised of three lipoprotein patterns (IIa, IIb, and IV) in equivalent proportions of affected adult relatives (there is no category in the Fredrickson scheme). Premature vascular disease is the predominant symptom. Autosomal dominant inheritance is proposed. *Familial type I hyperlipoproteinemia* results from an apparently autosomal recessively inherited defect in postheparin lipolytic activity of lipoprotein lipase (LPL), resulting in a fivefold increase in the half-life of chylomicrons. This disorder usually presents before age 10 years. At-risk heterozygotes cannot yet be reliably detected. Absence of the cofactor of LPL, apolipoprotein C-II, has been recently described, resulting clinically in hypertriglyceridemia and hypercholesterolemia. This is a rare, autosomal recessive disorder, currently limited to a Caribbean inbred kindred.

Type V hypertriglyceridemia is compatible with either a defect in increased synthesis or decreased clearance of VLDL. A defect in LPL structure has been proposed. The plasma VLDL in *type III hyperlipoproteinemia* is composed of two species: normal VLDL, and a "beta" VLDL (more cholesterol, less triglyceride, and an increased minor apolipoprotein, apoE). It is extremely rare in persons less than 20 years of age.

Screening for hyperlipidemia has included detection of at-risk relatives and mass neonatal programs. The latter are complex because of changing normal lipid values with increasing age. Currently, children over 1 year of age who have relatives with clinical or biochemical symptoms of hyperlipidemias should have cholesterol and triglyceride levels determined. Follow-up specimens should be obtained every 2 to 3 years or more frequently if the child is obese. The mean and ranges for normal plasma lipid concentrations are listed in Table 23-4.

Hypolipoproteinemia. *Abetalipoproteinemia* (acanthocytosis, Bassen-Kornzweig syndrome) results from an absence of beta-lipoproteins. The plasma contains no chylomicrons, VLDL, or LDL. Cholesterol, phospholipid, and triglyceride concentrations are reduced. Steatorrhea and bizarrely shaped erythrocytes (acanthocytes) may be seen in early childhood; weak-

Table 23-3. Primary hyperlipidemia and hyperlipoproteinemia in childhood*

Type	Lipid	Lipoprotein	Plasma supranate/infranate	Clinical symptoms	Therapy	Genetics/ prevalence
I Familial hyperlipoproteinemia	↑↑↑TG ↑CHO	↑↑↑CHY N-↓HDL, LDL	Cream/clear	Abdominal pain, xanthomas, hepatosplenomegaly, lipemia retinales	↓Fat diet, 10-15 g/day ↑MCT	?AR/Rare
IIa Familial hypercholesterolemia	↑↑↑CHO	↑↑↑LDL	Clear/clear	Homozygote: Planar xanthomas (buttocks, extensor surfaces, between fingers, popliteal fossa), premature vascular disease Heterozygote: Tendon xanthomas (Achilles tendonitis)	Dietary: ↓CHO ↑polyunsaturates Drug: Cholestyramine	AD/Common
IIb	↑↑CHO,TG	↑LDL,VLDL	Clear/turbid	See familial combined	Hyperlipoproteinemia	(FCH)
III	N-↑CHO,TG	↑'beta'VLDL	Creamy/turbid	Premature vascular disease, xanthomas, (striata palmaris, tendons)	Dietary: Calorie and CHO reduced Drug: Clofibrate (±nicotinic acid)	Polygenic/Rare
IV	↑TG	↑VLDL	Turbid/turbid	Adults: Premature vascular disease, xanthomas, glucose intolerance, uric acid	Dietary: ↓TG	AD/Rare
V	↑↑↑TG, ↑CHO	↑↑CHY,VLDL	Creamy/turbid	Pancreatitis, eruptive xanthomas, lipemia retinalis, glucose intolerance	Dietary: ↓TG	AD/Rare

*Fredrickson classification. *AD,* Autosomal dominant; *AR,* autosomal recessive; *CHO,* cholesterol; *TG,* triglyceride; *LDL,* low-density lipoprotein; *VLDL,* very low density lipoprotein; *HDL,* high-density lipoprotein; *CHY,* chylomicrons.

Table 23-4. Suggested "normal limits" for plasma lipid concentrations (mg/dl)

Age (yr)	Cholesterol, mean and 90% limits	Triglycerides, mean and 90% limits
0-19	175 (120-230)	65 (10-140)
20-29	180 (120-240)	70 (10-140)
30-39	205 (140-270)	75 (10-150)
40-49	225 (150-310)	85 (10-160)
50-59	245 (160-330)	95 (10-190)

ness, nystagmus, ataxia, and retinitis pigmentosa develop later. This disorder appears to be inherited in an autosomal recessive manner. A defect of a major apolipoprotein, apoB. Vitamin supplementation, especially A, D, E, and K, may result in clinical improvement.

Patients with *hypobetalipoproteinemia* may have acanthositosis, but usually no neurologic or cardiac findings, and generally have less risk for vascular disease. Low LDL, cholesterol, and triglycerides are found. A neurologic picture similar to Friedreich ataxia is seen in some persons.

Familial high–density lipoprotein (HDL) deficiency (Tangier disease) results from defective synthesis of alpha-lipoprotein. The plasma contains no HDL. Plasma cholesterol concentrations are low, whereas triglyceride concentrations are normal. Clinical manifestations result from excess deposition of cholesterol esters and include hepatosplenomegaly, lymphadenopathy, enlarged tonsils having a characteristic gray yellow or orange color, characteristic foam cells in bone marrow and rectal mucosa, and peripheral neuropathies. This disorder is inherited in an autosomal recessive manner.

Familial lecithin-cholesterol acyltransferase deficiency results in greatly reduced levels of plasma cholesterol esters. Plasma triglycerides are often increased, and pre-beta lipoproteins cannot be distinguished on electrophoresis. Clinical manifestations include corneal opacities, anemia, accelerated atherosclerosis, and proteinuria.

ABNORMALITIES OF PURINE AND PYRIMIDINE METABOLISM

The purines (adenine, guanine, inosine) and pyrimidines (cystosine, thymine, uracil) are components of such molecules as DNA and RNA; adenosine monophosphate, diphosphate, triphosphate, and other nucleic acid phosphate sources of energy and cofactors; and nicotinamide adenine dinucleotide. Purines may be synthesized by the body from precursor molecules (glutamine, glycine, and ribose), may be ingested, or may be "recycled" from catabolized purines. The excreted catabolic end product is uric acid. Some of the abnormalities of purine metabolism are the result of a defect in the recycling pathway, producing an excess of uric acid. A defect in pyrimidine metabolism, called orotic aciduria, is the result of a defect in pyrimidine synthesis whereby an intermediate precursor, orotic acid, cannot be converted to later precursors.

Gout. Gout is a disorder or group of disorders characterized by elevated serum levels and excessive urinary excretion of uric acid, recurrent episodes of acute arthritis, and in some cases tissue deposits (tophi) of uric acid salts. Acute gout is predominantly a disease of the adult male. Children with gout show neither male predominance nor predilection for involvement of the feet to the degree seen in adults. The arthritis may be chronic and disabling, but acute attacks characteristically respond to the drug colchicine. Urate deposits in the parenchyma of the kidney may lead to renal complications, and nephrolithiasis may occur. Most patients have the idiopathic primary form of gout. Some patients, however, have been shown to exhibit a partial deficiency of the enzyme hypoxanthine-guanine phosphoribosyltransferase (HPRT), a defect in the purine recycling pathway. This defect is inherited as an X-linked recessive trait.

Gout may occur in other genetically determined conditions, such as glycogen storage disease type I, some forms of glucose-6-phosphate dehydrogenase deficiency, and partial adenine-phosphoribosyltransferase deficiency. Secondary gout occurs in certain conditions involving decreased renal clearance of urates or increased nucleic acid turnover; the latter may be seen in leukemia or hemolytic anemia. Among persons with hyperuricemia, manifestations of gout develop earlier and more frequently in males than in females. The serum level (and, by inference, the tissue level) of uric acid may be reduced by the use of agents that enhance uric acid excretion, such as probenecid and sulfinpyrazone, or by agents that inhibit uric acid synthesis. This latter category includes allopurinol, which seems to inhibit uric acid synthesis primarily by its action as an inhibitor of the enzyme xanthine oxidase, which catalyzes the conversion of xanthine to uric acid.

Lesch-Nyhan syndrome. The Lesch-Nyhan syndrome is a rare X-linked recessive condition in which the absence of the enzyme HPRT occurs. In affected hemizygous males, this results in an excessive production of uric acid. Clinical manifestations include severe mental retardation, choreoathetosis, spasticity, and a peculiar behavioral reaction characterized by self-mutilation and aggression toward others. Affected infants appear normal at birth, but developmental retardation becomes apparent by age 3 to 5 months, and the full-blown picture appears by age 2 years. The neurologic manifestations are not the result of hyperuricemia and the cause is not clearly understood. Later complications of hyperuricemia may include the formation of uric acid stones in the urinary tract and gouty arthritis. Some patients with less complete deficiency of HPRT may have only gout, but some may also have central nervous system manifestations. Hyperuricemia with its noncentral nervous system manifestations may be treated successfully with allopurinol, but the central nervous system problems are not affected by such therapy. Diazepam, haloperidol, and phenobarbital are helpful in controlling movement.

Xanthinuria. Xanthine is an intermediate catabolite of purines and the immediate precursor of uric acid. Xanthinuria is a rare disease resulting from significant deficiency of the enzyme xanthine oxidase, and it is inherited in an autosomal recessive manner. Xanthine oxidase deficiency results in low blood and urine levels of uric acid, and its replacement as the primary end product of purine catabolism by xanthine and hypoxanthine. Clinical manifestations include the appearance of xanthine calculi in the urinary tract and a myopathy associated with xanthine and hypoxanthine deposits in skeletal muscle. Therapy, except for dilution of urine by high fluid intake, remains experimental.

Hereditary orotic aciduria. Orotic acid is an intermediate in the synthetic pathway of pyrimidines from aspartic acid. Orotic aciduria results from a metabolic block in pyrimidine synthesis distal to the orotic acid step. It is inherited in an autosomal recessive manner and is of special interest because evidence indicates a deficiency of *two* enzymes, orotate phosphoribosyltransferase and orotidine-5′-phosphate decarboxylase. This apparent exception to the "one gene–one enzyme" principle has been explained tentatively as a mutation in a gene coding for the enzyme orotidine-5-phosphate decarboxylase, which leads to a defect in its combination with orotate phosphoribosyltransferase necessary for the activity of both enzymes.

Affected infants (only a few reported) appear normal at birth, but during the first year of life a megaloblastic anemia appears, which is resistant to conventional therapy. Infants become pale and reveal growth and developmental retardation. The urine of affected infants contains large amounts of orotic acid. This relatively insoluble compound precipitates out as needle-shaped crystals when the urine is cooled. The orotic aciduria and the anemia respond promptly to the administration of large amounts of uridine. The developmental and growth problems also improve.

Jewell C. Ward

REFERENCES

Ampola, M.: Metabolic diseases in pediatric practice, Boston, 1982, Little, Brown & Co.

Genetic disorders and birth defects. In Rudolph, A.M., and Hoffman, J.J.E., Epstein, C.J., editors: Pediatrics, New York, 1982, Appleton-Century-Crofts.

Stanbury, J.B., et al.: The metabolic basis of inherited disease, ed. 5, New York, 1983, McGraw-Hill Book Co.

Acute inborn errors of metabolism

Aleck, K.A., and Shapiro, L.J.: Genetic-metabolic considerations in the sick neonate, Pediatr. Clin. North Am. **25:**431-451, 1978.

Burton, B.K., and Nadler, H.L.: Clinical diagnosis of the inborn errors of metabolism in the neonatal period, Pediatrics **61:**398-405, 1978.

Laboratory diagnosis of IEM

Kelly, S.: Biochemical methods in medical genetics, Springfield, Ill., 1977, Charles C Thomas, Publisher.

Aminoacidurias

Goldsmith, L.A.: Tyrosinemia and related disorders. In Stanbury, J.B., et al.: The metabolic basis of inherited diseases, ed. 5, New York, 1983, McGraw-Hill Book Co.

Mudd, S.H., and Levy, H.L.: Disorders of transsulfuration. In Stanbury, J.B., et al.: The metabolic basis of inherited diseases, ed. 5, New York, 1983, McGraw-Hill Book Co.

Nyhan, W.L.: Non-ketotic hyperglycinemia.In Stanbury, J.B., et al.: The metabolic basis of inherited diseases, ed. 5, New York, 1983, McGraw-Hill Book Co.

Scriver, C.R., and Clow, C.L., Phenylketonuria: epitome of human biochemical genetics, New Eng. J. Med. **303:**1336-1342, 1394-1400, 1980.

Tanaka, K., and Rosenberg, L.E.: Disorders of branched chain amino acid and organic acid metabolism. In Stanbury, J.B., et al.: The metabolic basis of inherited diseases, ed. 5, New York, 1983, McGraw-Hill Book Co.

Tourian, A., and Sialbury, J.B.: Phenylketonuira and hyperphenylalaninemia. In Stanbury, J.B., et al.: The metabolic basis of inherited diseases, ed. 5, New York, 1983, McGraw-Hill Book Co.

Walser, M.: Urea cycle disorders and other hereditary hyperammonemic syndromes. In Stanbury, J.B., et al.: The metabolic basis of inherited diseases, ed. 5, New York, 1983, McGraw-Hill Book Co.

Organic acids

Adams, R.D., and Lyon, G.: Neurology of hereditary metabolic diseases of children, New York, 1982, McGraw-Hill Book Co.

Chalmers, R.A., and Lawson, A.M.: Organic acids in man: the analytical chemistry, biochemistry and diagnosis of the organic acidurias, New York, 1982, Chapman & Hall.

Goodman, S.I., and Markey, S.P.: Diagnosis of organic acidemias by gas chromatography-mass spectrometry, New York, 1981, Alan R. Liss, Inc.

Meliturias

Gitzelmann, R., et al.: Essential fructosuria: hereditary fructose intolerance, and fructose -1,6.-diphosphatase deficiency. In Stanbury, J.B., et al.: The metabolic basis of inherited disease, ed. 5, New York, 1983, McGraw-Hill Book Co.

Segal, S. Disorders of galactose metabolism. In Stanbury, J.B., et al.: The metabolic basis of inherited disease, ed. 5, New York, 1983, McGraw-Hill Book Co.

Lysosomal and other storage diseases

Beudet, A.L.: Disorders of glycoprotein degradation: mannosidosis, fucosidosis, sialidosis, and aspartylglycosaminuria. In Stanbury, J.B., et al.: The metabolic basis of inherited disease, ed. 5, New York, 1983, McGraw-Hill Book Co.

Brady, R.O., and Barranger, J.A.: Glucosylaramide lipidosis: Gaucher's disease. In Stanbury, J.B., et al.: The metabolic basis of inherited disease, ed. 5, New York, 1983, McGraw-Hill Book Co.

Desnik, R.J., and Sweeley, C.C.: Fabry's disease: α-galactosidase A deficiency. In Stanbury, J.B., et al.: The metabolic basis of inherited disease, ed. 5, New York, 1983, McGraw-Hill Book Co.

Grossman, H., and Dorst, J.P.: The mucopolysaccharidoses. In Kaufman, H., editor: Progress in pediatric radiology, vol. 4, Chicago, 1973, Year Book Medical Publishers, Inc.

McKusick, V.A., and Neufeld, E.F.: The mucopolysaccharide storage diseases. In Stanbury, J.B., et al.: The metabolic basis of inherited disease, ed. 5, New York, 1983, McGraw-Hill Book Co.

Neufeld, E.F., and McKusick, V.A.: Disorders of lysosomal enzyme synthesis and localization: I-cell disease and pseudohurler polydystrophy. In Stanbury, J.B., et al.: The metabolic basis of inherited disease, ed. 5, New York, 1983, McGraw-Hill Book Co.

Abnormalities of plasma lipids

Goldstein, J.L., and Brown, M.S.: Familial hypercholesterolemia. In Stanbury, J.B., et al.: The metabolic basis of inherited disease, ed. 5, New York, 1983, McGraw-Hill Book Co.

Kwiterovick, P.O.: Disorders of lipid and lipoprotein metabolism. In Rudolph, A.M., and Hoffman, J.J.E., editors: Pediatrics, New York, 1982, Appleton-Century-Crofts.

Purine and pyramidines

Kelley, W.M., and Wyngaarden, J.B.: Clinical syndromes associated with hypoxanthine-guanine phosphoribosyltransferase dificiency. In Stanbury, J.B., et al.: The metabolic basis of inherited disease, ed. 5, New York, 1983, McGraw-Hill Book Co.

Kelley, W.M.: Hereditary orotic aciduria. In Stanbury, J.B., et al.: The metabolic basis of inherited disease, ed. 5, New York, 1983, McGraw-Hill Book Co.

24 Cystic Fibrosis

Cystic fibrosis (CF) is the most common lethal genetic disease in white populations. Although the complex of signs and symptoms that make up this syndrome has been recognized since 1938, the basic biochemical defect remains unknown. CF affects virtually every organ system, most importantly the lungs, pancreas, intestinal mucous glands, and sweat glands. A common pathogenetic mechanism underlying the involvement of the major target systems seems to be the blockage of ducts and air passages with abnormally viscous secretions.

GENETICS AND PREVALENCE

CF is inherited as an autosomal recessive disorder. It occurs in approximately 1 in 2000 live births in white populations, and about 1 in 17,000 births in American blacks; it is virtually unheard of in oriental populations. More than 5% of the white population are presumed to be heterozygous for CF. Currently, there is no test that can identify heterozygotes or detect CF in utero. It is estimated that there are now between 15,000 and 30,000 patients with CF in the United States.

CLINICAL MANIFESTATIONS

Gastrointestinal tract

Exocrine pancreatic insufficiency is present at birth in approximately 90% of patients and is manifest by maldigestion of fats and protein with consequent malabsorption, steatorrhea, and failure to thrive. Patients may come to the physician with evidence of deficiencies of fat-soluble vitamins. Bowel obstruction, a result of thickened intestinal mucus and pancreatic insufficiency, may be present at birth (meconium ileus) in 10% of patients, or later in life (meconium ileus equivalent) in 20% to 25%. Rectal prolapse, caused by the same factors, is seen in 20% of CF patients in the first years of life. Intussusception is much less common, but CF patients account for a significant portion of the patients with intussusception after 1 year of age. Liver pathology, including nonspecific steatosis and the specific lesion, focal biliary fibrosis, is common histologically, but cirrhosis with clinically important manifestations such as hepatic failure or portal hypertension with hypersplenism and/or bleeding esophageal varices is, fortunately, rare. Adolescents or adults with clinically intact pancreatic function may have acute pancreatitis.

The absence of gastrointestinal manifestations often delays the diagnosis of CF.

Sweat glands

CF patients have a defect in sodium reabsorption from the ducts of their sweat glands. This leads to the characteristic high salt content of CF sweat and provides the basis for the sweat test (discussed later). CF patients lose more salt during exercise in the heat than normal persons and may experience heat prostration. Infants may be brought for medical care with hyponatremia and hypochloremia.

Respiratory tract

The upper respiratory tract is involved in most patients, with radiographic evidence of pansinusitis. This is seldom clinically bothersome to the patient, but occasionally is helpful diagnostically. Nasal polyps may be found in 10% to 15% of patients.

The lower respiratory involvement in CF accounts for well over 90% of the morbidity and mortality. Although the lungs are histologically normal at birth, obstructive pulmonary disease, beginning in the small airways, eventually is present in almost all patients. Recurrent cough and/or wheeze, which may be diagnosed as recurrent bronchiolitis, bronchitis, or pneumonia, are often the first indications of pulmonary involvement. As the disease progresses, hyperinflation, crackles, and rhonchi become apparent.

The older child (6 to 7 years and older) who is able to cooperate in the pulmonary function laboratory produces tests with a pattern of obstructive airways disease: decreased vital capacity, decreased forced expiratory volume in 1 second, decreased peak expiratory flow, and increased residual volume, indicative of air trapping. These obstructive changes show varying responses to bronchodilator inhalation, with which some patients apparently improve while others actually worsen. Exercise testing typically shows reduced exercise tolerance and fitness, with a comparatively large minute volume for the oxygen consumed, presumably because of greater than normal dead space ventilation. Typically a higher than normal proportion of the ventilatory capacity is required at peak work loads. The pulmonary function and exercise tests are relatively sensitive tools for following progression of disease in the older, cooperative child.

Chronic pulmonary infection, with acute exacerbations, is characteristic of CF patients. *Staphylococcus aureus, Hemophilus influenzae,* and a variety of gram-negative organisms may be involved in the early stages, but eventually the vast majority of patients become colonized with *Pseudomonas aeruginosa*. Many patients have *Pseudomonas* at diagnosis. There seems to be a unique relationship between CF patients and *Pseudomonas*; at least half of all patients are colonized with a peculiar mucoid strain of this organism that is seldom seen in other human disease states. A similarly mucoid strain of *Escherichia coli* has been isolated from a group of CF patients. Recently, other organisms, such as *Aspergillus fumigatus* and *Pseudomonas cepacia* have become increasingly important as pulmonary pathogens. Despite the universal finding of chronic pulmonary colonization and infection, extrapulmonary infection is unusual, indicating that any defect in defense mechanisms is limited to the lungs. Pulmonary defenses are almost certainly inhibited by viscid mucus. Mucociliary transport rates are dramatically reduced in CF patients. There may be circulating factors that inhibit the phagocytosis of *Pseudomonas* by pulmonary alveolar macrophages.

The chain of events caused by chronic infection with acute exacerbations begins with bronchiolitis and leads through bronchitis to bronchiectasis, peribronchial fibrosis, and progressive loss of pulmonary function.

Pulmonary complications include hemoptysis, segmental and lobar atelectasis, and pulmonary hypertension leading to cor pulmonale.

Other organ systems

The reproductive tract is involved in most male patients, with atresia of the vas deferens and consequent obstructive azoospermia and sterility. In female patients, thick cervical mucus often results in decreased fertility. Delayed puberty may be seen in either sex as a consequence of chronic illness. Some adolescents and adults display a unique pattern of hyperglycemia and abnormal glucose tolerance tests, but almost never have ketoacidosis or diabetic nephropathy or retinopathy. Long bones and adjacent joints may be involved with pulmonary hypertrophic osteoarthropathy. Digital clubbing is a nearly universal finding in patients with even mildly abnormal lung function.

DIAGNOSIS

Because the basic biochemical defect of CF has not yet been identified, diagnosis must rest on the clinical features of the disease. Currently the accepted criteria for diagnosis are: (1) a positive sweat test (a sweat chloride concentration greater than 60 mEq/L on a sample of at least 100 mg, obtained after maximal stimulation by pilocarpine iontophoresis), (2) chronic obstructive pulmonary disease, (3) exocrine pancreatic insufficiency, and (4) family history of the disease. Most experts require at least two of these criteria for establishing a diagnosis, and the diagnosis is almost never made without a positive sweat test. Recently a new system of diagnostic criteria has been proposed (Stern et al., 1982). The sweat test is theoretically simple, but false positives and false negatives are very common in tests performed outside established CF centers.

It must be stressed that the key to making the diagnosis is a high index of suspicion in the presence of any of the manifestations. Table 24-1 lists the indications for a sweat test. Most physicians are sufficiently aware of the disease that few children with the triad of growth failure, steatorrhea, and chronic pulmonary disease escape diagnosis. However, atypical patients, especially those who have no clinically apparent pancreatic involvement (as many as 15% of all

Table 24-1. Indications for sweat testing

Pulmonary	Gastrointestinal	Other
Chronic cough	Meconium ileus, steatorrhea, malabsorption	Family history of cystic fibrosis
Recurrent or chronic pneumonia		
Staphylococcal pneumonia	Rectal prolapse	Failure to thrive
Recurrent bronchiolitis	Childhood cirrhosis (portal hypertension or bleeding esophageal varices)	Salty sweat, salty taste when kissed, salt frosting of skin
Atelectasis		
Hemoptysis		
Mucoid *Pseudomonas* infection	Hypoprothrombinemia beyond newborn period	Nasal polyps
		Hyponatremia, hypochloremia, and heat prostration, especially in infants
		Pansinusitis
		Aspermia

From Wood, R.E., et al.: Cystic fibrosis, Am. Rev. Respir. Dis. **113:**833-878, 1976.

CF patients) or who have normal growth, may escape diagnosis for years. There is no such thing as a child who "looks too good" to have CF.

It must finally be emphasized that this is a disease in which early diagnosis and institution of an aggressive treatment program make a difference in quality and length of life. Efforts at pursuing this diagnosis will be rewarded by the family's peace of mind in the case of a negative result and the knowledge of improved outlook for the child in the event of a positive result.

TREATMENT

Cystic fibrosis is a complex disease, and patients require a comprehensive care program. This is usually best carried out in, or at least coordinated from, a specialized center where many different specialists are available. Therapy is aimed primarily in three directions: pulmonary, gastrointestinal, and psychologic.

Pulmonary therapy

The goal of pulmonary therapy is to prevent or delay progression of the pulmonary lesion. These goals are accomplished through the relief of airway obstruction and the control of infection.

Therapy of obstruction. Chest physical therapy with percussion and postural drainage is the mainstay of most treatment programs, despite the lack of definitive studies to indicate ideal time for instituting this treatment or benefits of various techniques. Most patients undergo therapy to all pulmonary segments at least once and up to 4 times daily, with increases at the time of clinical exacerbation. Many patients have found that mechanical percussors ease this arduous task.

Exercise. Various investigators have shown aerobic exercise (jogging and swimming) to be beneficial for CF patients in terms of increased fitness and work capacity, and there is some suggestion that it may be as effective as traditional chest physical therapy in relief of pulmonary obstruction. However, until a definitive study is available most experts advise the use of exercise *and* chest physical therapy.

Aerosol therapy. Continuous aerosol therapy came into and out of vogue in the past 20 years with no adequate evaluation. Intermittent aerosols are much more widely used but are also somewhat controversial. Intermittent aerosols have been used to deliver various types of medications. Bronchodilators clearly increase airflow in some patients, but make no difference in many, and in a few actually reduce airflow (perhaps because of a reduction in bronchomotor tone in airways kept patent only by abnormally high tone). Mucolytic agents (e.g., acetylcysteine) are favored by many, and are effective in the test tube, but may cause irritation, bronchoconstriction, and bronchorrhea in vivo. Vasoconstrictors (e.g., phenylephrine) are commonly used to reduce mucosal edema, although their efficacy has yet to be established. Finally, antibiotics (especially aminoglycosides and the anti-*Pseudomonas* penicillin derivatives) have been delivered by aerosol, apparently with favorable results.

Therapy of infection. There is general agreement that antibiotic treatment has probably been the single most important factor in the greatly improved prognosis in CF. Colonization and infection with *Staphylococcus* and later *Pseudomonas* are nearly universal, and clinical exacerbations of pulmonary disease have been convincingly linked to worsening infection. *Staphylococcus* and *Hemophilus* may occasionally be eliminated from the bronchial tree in CF, but once *Pseudomonas* colonization is established it is almost never eradicated. It may, however, be controlled.

Antibiotic strategies. Some centers advocate continuous "prophylactic" antibiotic treatment. There is some concern that this approach might lead to the early emergence of drug-resistant flora. Another approach is to restrict the use of antibiotics to times of exacerbation of pulmonary disease, as evidenced by increased symptoms or signs (such as cough or sputum production), or worsening chest radiograph or pulmonary function test results. Since some patients, especially those with advanced disease, will suffer exacerbation whenever they are not being treated with antibiotics, virtually continuous treatment is occasionally indicated. Still a third approach is to treat patients with full-dose drugs, based on culture results, for 2 to 3 weeks every 1 or 2 months if there is any evidence of pulmonary disease. It is not clear at present which strategy is most successful. A cornerstone of most successful treatment programs is frequent physician evaluation of patients, including bacteriologic evaluation of respiratory tract flora. Oral antibiotics (dicloxacillin, cephalosporins, amoxicillin, trimethoprim with sulfamethoxazole, tetracyclines, and chloramphenicol) are often adequate when the offending organism is *Staphylococcus* or *Hemophilus,* and even on occasion when *Pseudomonas* is the only organism isolated in culture.

Intravenous antibiotics are indicated when the patient does not respond promptly to outpatient oral administration of antibiotics. The important consideration in the decision to hospitalize a patient and begin parenteral therapy is whether the child is sicker than his own baseline, and not whether the child seems dreadfully ill. It is clear that a tremendous amount of lung can be lost irreversibly while a child still looks reasonably well. Because *Pseudomonas aeruginosa* is usually the offending organism, intravenous therapy is commonly carried out with an aminoglycoside and an anti-*Pseudomonas* penicillin. Intravenous antibiotics are usually administered during hospitalization, but in carefully selected cases may successfully be administered at home.

Aerosolized antibiotics may be effective in many patients colonized with *Pseudomonas*. In those who have severe airways obstruction, aerosol penetration into the lung may be limited and render this form of treatment less valuable. Patients who cannot tolerate certain drugs (e.g., colistin) intravenously may do well with the same drugs delivered by aerosol.

Pulmonary complications

Pneumothorax. Many pneumothoraces will eventually resolve with simple chest tube drainage but may recur at a rate of between 50% and 100%. Therefore it is advisable to enlist some form of prevention. The instillation of chemical sclerosing agents has been used with some success. In our patients, the most sucessful treatment for early resolution of the pneumothorax, prevention of subsequent episodes, and least morbidity has been open thoracotomy through a small subaxillary incision and identification and exision of any apical blebs, stripping of the apical pleura, and manual abrasion of the remainder of the accessible pleura.

Hemoptysis. Hemoptysis is a common complication and, although terrifying to patient and family, rarely is severe enough to require transfusion. Deaths have been reported but are exceedingly rare. Hemoptysis is thought to be the result of local infection eroding a small vessel. As such, the appropriate treatment for all but the most overwhelmingly brisk bleeding is reassuring the patient and family and initiating or continuing aggressive treatment of pulmonary infection, including chest physical therapy and antibiotics. In some patients, hemoptysis may be associated with vitamin K deficiency, because of malabsorption of fat-soluble vitamins, or with the platelet aggregation defect seen with carbenicillin or ticarcillin therapy.

Gastrointestinal therapy

The main goal of gastrointestinal therapy is to establish good nutrition. Since replacement pancreatic enzyme preparations and especially enteric coated preparations (Pancrease, Cotazym-S) became available, this once insurmountable problem has become quite manageable.

The correct dosage of enzymes is decided by trial and error, titrating against the symptoms and signs of maldigestion and malabsorption (steatorrhea, abdominal discomfort, excessive hunger, and poor weight gain). Supplemental vitamins, especially fat-soluble A, D, E, and K, are recommended in twice the usual daily doses. Diet need not be specially tailored for the CF patient as long as adequate balanced calories are supplied. Especially with good enzyme replacement, more psychologic harm than nutritional good may be done with painstaking attention to a special "CF diet," which would contribute to the patient's feeling different from family and peers.

Gastrointestinal complications. Meconium ileus and meconium ileus equivalent can usually be treated with careful administration of diatrizoate methylglucamine (Gastrografin) enemas. Rectal prolapse is treated by gentle manual pressure on the protruding rectum and is prevented by adjustment of diet and enzymes to reduce bulky stools. There is no treatment yet for the uncommon cirrhosis, but endoscopic sclerotherapy may be lifesaving and may obviate the need for portocaval shunting in the rare cases of symptomatic esophageal varices.

Psychologic considerations

The emotional burdens of a genetic, incurable, progressive, life-shortening, financially draining, and activity-limiting disease on patient and family are great. It is remarkable how well the large majority of patients and families adjust. Issues that patients must face include education and vocation, marriage, reproduction, medical expenses, independent living, and anticipation of disability and death. Establishing and maintaining a positive, optimistic yet realistic attitude are extremely important. These goals are attainable especially if the primary physician shares these attitudes and maintains a close supportive relationship with the patient and family. Knowledge of the tremendously improved prognosis over the past 2 decades facilitates such an attitude.

Miscellaneous treatment considerations

Hyperglycemia occurs in a small but important group of patients with CF and may require insulin therapy. Salt loss may be excessive, especially during exertion in warm weather. Infants may require small amounts of supplemental salt, but older children and adolescents will regulate their salt intake quite adequately if given free access to the salt shaker. Salt tablets are not necessary and may be harmful.

PROGNOSIS

Almost all children with cystic fibrosis died before school age when the disease was first recognized in the late 1930s. Institution of specialized CF centers and comprehensive, aggressive treatment programs beginning in the 1950s has improved prognosis tremendously. National median survival age was 10.6 years in 1966, and 20.0 years in 1981. There are currently many patients in their late teens and early twenties with excellent lung function, and, at the end of 1981, 16.2% of patients in the United States were 21 years or older. Survival probably depends on several factors, including inherent severity of the disease, aggressiveness of the treatment program as prescribed by the physician and carried out by the patient and family, and some degree of chance, especially concerning contact with various bacterial and viral pathogens. In general, the survival of male patients is better than that of female. Perhaps most importantly, long-term prognosis may depend on the timing of diagnosis and institution of treatment. Several studies indicate that those CF patients who are diagnosed and who begin an aggressive treatment program before the onset of irreversible pulmonary damage have significantly better pulmonary function and survival than those only discovered and treated after considerable pulmonary tissue has been lost.

David M. Orenstein

The author gratefully acknowledges the contributions of Robert E. Wood, Ph.D., M.D., to this chapter.

REFERENCES

Stern, R.C., et al.: Obstructive azoospermia as a diagnostic criterion for the cystic fibrosis syndrome, Lancet **19:**1401-1404, 1982.

SELECTED READINGS

Orenstein, D.M., et al. The effect of early diagnosis and treatment in cystic fibrosis: a 7-year study of 16 sibling pairs, Am. J. Dis. Child. **131:**973-975, 1977.

Wood, R.E.: Cystic fibrosis: diagnosis, treatment, and prognosis, South. Med. J. **72:**189-202, 1979.

Wood, R.E., et al.: State of the art: cystic fibrosis, Am. Rev. Respir. Dis. **113:**833-878, 1976.

25 The Host Defense System

From the time of birth the human organism is bombarded with foreign substances, many of which are potentially harmful. Examples of these include infectious agents, pollutants of all types, and pollens. Despite this barrage of antigenic material, most humans manage to cope with their environment very well. This chapter outlines the defense mechanisms that the host employs to protect itself and briefly discusses some of the disorders of this defense system.

NONSPECIFIC DEFENSE MECHANISMS

Nonspecific defense mechanisms are primitive in a phylogenetic sense but remain highly effective in protecting man from his environment. The nonspecific defense system can be thought of as consisting of three components: physical, cellular, and humoral (Table 25-1).

Generally, the first line of host defense is the mechanical barrier represented by the skin and mucous membranes lining the respiratory and gastrointestinal tracts. In addition to the physical barrier itself, nonspecific factors such as the unsaturated fatty acids in the skin, gastric secretions in the stomach, and cilia lining the respiratory tree may contribute to the overall barrier effect.

Table 25-1. Nonspecific host defense mechanisms

Physical	Cellular	Humoral
Skin	Phagocytic cells	Lysosomes
Mucous membranes	Neutrophils	Interferon
	Macrophages	Complement
Mucociliary system	Monocytes	Lactoferrin
	Eosinophils	Lymphokines
	Reticuloendothelial system	

If the mechanical barriers are penetrated, both nonspecific cellular and humoral factors contribute to protection of the host. Of particular importance are the phagocytic cells and humoral factors such as complement (C′), interferon, and lymphokines.

Nonspecific defense mechanisms are not nearly so well studied as are the specific immune mechanisms of defense. Yet when considered together, these nonspecific factors play an extremely important role in preserving the well-being of the host.

SPECIFIC IMMUNE MECHANISMS

The last 15 to 20 years have brought an enormous increase in our understanding of the immune system. A comprehension of immune mechanisms has become necessary in order to appreciate new developments in areas as diverse as rheumatology, oncology, dermatology, organ transplantation, allergy, infectious disease, and nephrology. Many of the basic concepts in these areas have been derived from studying patients with various aberrations in their immune system.

It is now evident that the lymphocyte is the cell line responsible for most immune reactions. Two main types of immunity are now recognized: (1) cell-mediated immunity (CMI) and (2) humoral immunity.

Cell-mediated immunity. Precursors of lymphocytes that are responsible for CMI come under the influence of the thymus gland and are known as T cells. Embryologically the thymus is derived from the third and fourth pharyngeal pouches. After migrating through the thymus, T cells distribute peripherally to the paracortex of the lymph nodes and the white pulp of the spleen. The majority of circulating lymphocytes in the blood are also T cells.

T cells are thought to be important in host defense against certain viral, fungal, and protozoal infections, and in recognizing mutant or malignant cells.

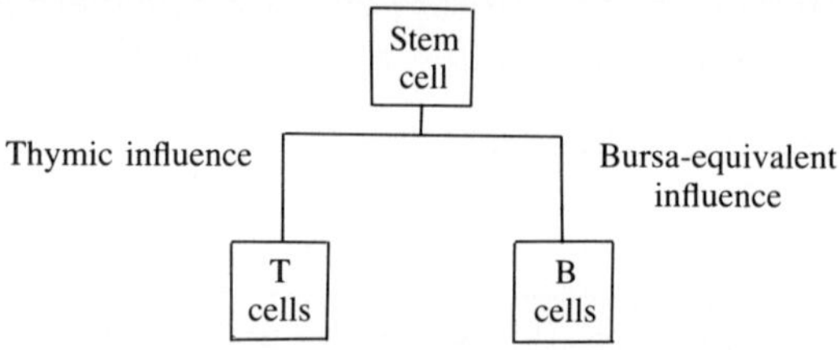

T cells	B cells
1. Direct cytolysis	1. Immunoglobulin synthesis and specific antibody production
2. Delayed hypersensitivity	2. Protection against bacterial and some viral infections
3. Protection against some viral, protozoal, and fungal infections	
4. Graft vs host reactions	
5. Lymphokine production	
6. ? Immune surveillance	
7. T helper cells	
8. T suppressor cells	

In the human fetus, T cell activity has been identified as early as 10 to 14 weeks. By the time of birth the newborn has a full complement of cells bearing the cell surface characteristics of T helper-inducer cells and T cytotoxic-suppressor cells.

T helper cells are necessary for some humoral responses to occur. This T cell subpopulation also is necessary for the induction of the differentiation of other T cell subpopulation functions. T suppressor cells may dampen certain humoral and cellular immune functions. Cytotoxic T cells share some membrane antigen markers with the T suppressor cell population. Monoclonal antibodies that recognize these T cell subpopulations are currently being used to dissect the role of these T cells in immune responses. Some of the more commonly used monoclonal antibodies are listed in Table 25-2.

Humoral immunity. Lymphoid cells that eventually differentiate into antibody-secreting plasma cells are classified as B cells. In the chicken these cells come under the influence of a hindgut organ known as the bursa of Fabricius. Removal of this organ in ovo ablates the capacity of the bird to produce immunoglobulins.

In man a bursal equivalent has not been identified. It is clear that the differentiation of B cells does not follow the same pathway of differentiation as does that of T cells. In contrast to T cells, they tend to accumulate in the lymphoid follicles and germinal centers of the lymph nodes and in the red pulp of the spleen. They constitute only 5% to 15% of the peripheral blood lymphocytes. Some of the characteristics useful in differentiating T cells and B cells are listed in Table 25-2.

In the fetus, B lymphocytes are detectable by 10 to 14 weeks. Although the major immunoglobulin found in cord blood is maternal IgG, the fetus is capable of responding to antigenic stimulation, as evidenced by specific IgM antibodies in neonates infected in utero with agents such as cytomegalovirus and *Toxoplasma*.

The final product of B cell differentiation is the plasma cell, which produces immunoglobulin. Five classes of immunoglobulin have been identified in man.

IgG. IgG is the major immunoglobulin class found in serum. It has a half-life of 21 days and is the principal type of antibody appearing in a secondary immune response. There are four

Table 25-2. Characteristics of T cells and B cells

T cells	B cells
Surface markers	***Surface markers***
T cell receptor for sheep erythrocytes; reacts with monoclonal antibodies OKT3, OKT11, Leu 4	Usually IgM or IgD
T helper-inducer cells react with monoclonal antibodies OKT4, Leu 2	Receptor for C3b
T cytotoxic-suppressor cells react with monoclonal antibodies OKT8, Leu 3	Receptor for Epstein-Barr virus
Functional properties (in vitro)	***Functional properties (in vitro)***
Undergo blastogenic transformation to certain plant lectins such as phytohemagglutinin and concanavalin A	Can synthesize immunoglobulin under appropriate conditions
Acts as the responding cell in mixed leukocyte cultures	Acts as a stimulator cell in mixed leukocyte cultures
Acts as a direct cytotoxic cell	

subclasses of IgG: IgG1, IgG2, IgG3, and IgG4. IgG is the only immunoglobulin transported across the placenta from the maternal to the fetal circulation. It is evenly distributed between the intravascular and extravascular space.

IgM. IgM is the principal immunoglobulin class found in a primary antibody response. It has a half-life of 4 to 5 days. IgM is found on the surface of B cells, where it can bind to specific antigens. An elevated IgM in cord blood suggests an immune response by the fetus to foreign antigens, including infectious agents.

IgA. The IgA immunoglobulin occurs in two forms. In the circulation it exists as a monomeric molecule. In external secretions, IgA plays a role in protecting the mucous membranes. In the secretions it exists as a dimer and is bound to a unique polypeptide known as the secretory component.

IgD. The IgD immunoglobulin exists in minute quantities in the circulation. Along with IgM, it is the immunoglobulin found most frequently on B lymphocytes. Its exact function is not well understood at the present time.

IgE. The IgE immunoglobulin class is associated with immediate hypersensitivity reactions. It exists in small quantities in the circulation. Through its Fc fragment (crystallizable) it binds to tissue mast cells and circulating basophils. When two IgE molecules bound to these cells are bridged by an antigen such as ragweed pollen, the cells then can release mediators of the allergic response, such as histamine and slow reactive substance of anaphylaxis (SRS-A or leukotriene).

Other lymphocyte subpopulations. A third population of lymphocytes is now recognized in man. These cells are not clearly T cell or B cells by standard criteria. They are called null cells. Within this population are cells responsible for natural killer cell activity and antibody-dependent cell-mediated cytotoxicity.

CONDITIONS OF IMPAIRED HOST DEFENSE

Nonspecific mechanisms. Defects in any of the nonspecific mechanisms of defense can potentially lead to increased problems with infectious agents. For example, patients with severe burns or acute eczema display increased susceptibility to skin infections. The best-studied abnormalities of the nonspecific defense mechanisms are those involving deficiencies or dysfunctions of the complement systems and those involving defects in phagocytosis.

Complement. The complement system consists of a series of separate serum proteins that act in an interrelated fashion. In addition, there are other serum proteins necessary for modulation of the complement system. Complement has a number of biologic functions, including facilitating opsonization, immune adherence, and acting as a chemotactic factor. There are two pathways of complement activation–the classic and the alternative pathways. Deficiencies in the functioning of either pathway of activation can result in impaired host defense.

Phagocytic disorders. Impaired phagocytosis can result from either inadequate numbers of phagocytic cells or from functionally abnormal cells.

Quantitative abnormalities–neutropenia. There are both hereditary and nonhereditary forms of neutropenia. Kostmann syndrome is an autosomal recessive form of neutropenia in which there appears to be adequate precursor cells in the marrow. Cyclic neutropenia is characterized by a cyclic decrease of neutrophils occurring approximately every 21 days. Schwachman-Diamond syndrome consists of neutropenia, pancreatic insufficiency, and malabsorption. Neutropenia can be associated with a number of immunodeficiency states. Acquired neutropenias can be the result of drugs, radiation, neoplasms, and numerous other causes.

Qualitative abnormalities. Qualitative defects in phagocytosis exist when there are adequate numbers of phagocytic cells but defective function of these cells. The whole process of phagocytosis is complex, and there are a number of areas in which functional defects can exist. For example, in order for phagocytes to ingest foreign material, they must first be attracted to the area of inflammation. Deficiencies in chemotactic factors such as C3a and C5a can result in failure of the phagocytes to enter an area of inflammation. A few patients have been described who have factors in their serum that inactivate chemotactic factors. The best-recognized defects in phagocytic function include the following.

Chédiak-Higashi syndrome. Patients with Chédiak-Higashi syndrome have oculocutaneous albinism, photophobia, and increased frequency of infections. Their polymorphonuclear cells have giant intracytoplasmic granules. Leukocytes of these patients ingest organisms normally but fail to kill them. These patients also are thought to have poor natural killer cell activity.

Lazy leukocyte syndrome. Patients with lazy leukocyte syndrome have recurrent infections, particularly of the skin, gingivae, and middle ear. This entity probably results from a decreased response to chemotactic factors caused by an intrinsic leukocyte defect. These patients are generally neutropenic as well.

Chronic granulomatous disease. Children with chronic granulomatous disease are plagued with severe, recurrent infections of the skin, lungs, and reticuloendothelial system. The underlying defect is an inability of the patient's leukocytes to kill ingested organisms. The exact enzymatic defect that leads to this is not known, but it results in an inability of the leukocyte to generate a respiratory burst. Catalase-positive bacteria such as staphylococci and Enterobacteriaceae are particularly bothersome to these patients. The most common form of transmission of this disease is as an X-linked recessive trait. The other mode of inheritance is autosomal recessive. This condition can be diagnosed in the laboratory by the failure of the patient's phagocytes to reduce nitro blue tetrazolium (NBT test).

Defects of specific immunity. It is now recognized that very few, if any, of the immunodeficiency states represent a pure isolated defect of a single cell type. Despite this, it is still useful to think of immunodeficiencies as being functional defects of either antibody production, abnormal T cell function, or a combination of the two.

Antibody deficiencies

Transient hypogammaglobulinemia of infancy. Patients with transient hypogammaglobulinemia have a delay in their ability to synthesize IgG until well after their maternal IgG has been catabolized. Recent studies suggest that this disorder may be secondary to inadequate T helper cell activity.

Infantile X-linked agammaglobulinemia (Bruton type). Patients with Bruton agammaglobulinemia have low or absent immunoglobulins of all classes. They do not make antibody to specific antigens. They are particularly susceptible to infections with encapsulated pyogenic organisms such as *Haemophilus influenzae*, *S. pneumoniae*, and *Streptococcus* organisms. They may have difficulty handling certain viruses such as hepatitis, poliovirus, and echovirus. These patients lack B cells in their peripheral blood or in their lymph nodes.

Common variable agammaglobulinemia (B type or acquired). Patients with common variable agammaglobulinemia differ from those with the X-linked form in that most of the former have at least some detectable B cells in their circulation. These patients are as a rule diagnosed at a later age than those with X-linked agammaglobulinemia. This implies either that the disease is acquired or that these patients have fewer problems with infections at earlier ages. They can have prominent lymphoid tissue and can have malabsorption problems secondary to persistent infection with *Giardia lamblia*. Current evidence suggests that in at least some of these patients excessive T suppressor cell activity or inadequate T helper cell activity contributes to the immunodeficiency.

Selective IgA deficiency. Selective IgA deficiency is by far the most common immunodeficiency, the incidence ranging from 1 in 500 to 1 in 700 persons. Many persons with this entity are asymptomatic. Others have difficulty with respiratory tract infections. A high proportion of these patients are also deficient in IgG_2 or IgG_4. Patients with complete absence of IgA may develop anti-IgA antibodies. In some of these patients anaphylactic reactions have been reported following infusion of blood products.

X-linked immunodeficiency with hyper-IgM. Patients with an X-linked deficiency may have absent IgG and IgA but markedly elevated levels of IgM. Specific IgM antibodies may exist to some antigens but not to others. Infection is common and is frequently caused by the same type of organisms seen in patients with agammaglobulinemia.

T cell defects

DiGeorge syndrome. DiGeorge syndrome is the result of maldevelopment of the third and fourth pharyngeal pouches. These patients have hypoplastic or absent parathyroid and thymus glands. Other congenital anomalies, including peculiar facies and cardiac lesions, may also be present. Hypocalcemic tetany is a common mode of presentation. These patients are very susceptible to infections with viral, protozoal, fungal, and gram-negative organisms.

Nezeloff syndrome. Patients with Nezeloff syndrome have a hypoplastic thymus gland with absent Hassell corpuscles. They do not have the endocrine abnormality of those with DiGeorge syndrome. Immunoglobulin levels may be normal or elevated. Some of these patients have been found to be deficient in the enzyme nucleoside phosphorylase.

Combined dysfunction of T cells and B cells

Severe combined immunodeficiency (SCID). A marked deficiency in T cell function and low or absent immunoglobulin levels characterize patients with SCID. The mode of inheritance in these patients may be X-linked recessive, autosomal recessive, or sporadic. Some with the autosomal recessive form of this disease have been found to be deficient in the enzyme adenosine deaminase. Despite functional abnormalities, some patients with SCID have cells that bear markers for either T cells or B cells.

Wiskott-Aldrich syndrome. Patients with Wiskott-Aldrich syndrome have problems with recurrent infection and with thrombocytopenia and eczema. They may have variable immunoglobulin abnormalities, with a decreased IgM and increased IgA and IgE being the most common pattern. An increased incidence of malignancy has been observed in patients with this disorder.

Ataxia-telangiectasia. Clinically, patients with ataxia-telangiectasia have progressive cerebellar ataxia, recurrent sinorespiratory infections, and oculocutaneous telangiectasia. Many have a selective deficiency of IgA. They also show an increased incidence of malignancy.

OTHER DEFECTS OF THE IMMUNE SYSTEM

Hyper-IgE syndrome. The hyper-IgE syndrome manifests itself by severe skin and respiratory tract infections, with staphylococcal organisms being particularly bothersome. Serum levels of IgE are markedly elevated. The other common features of this disorder include atopic dermatitis and defective neutrophil chemotaxis.

X-linked lymphoproliferative syndrome. X-linked proliferative syndrome is characterized by marked lymphoid hyperplasia. Several families with this disorder have been described. Patients affected with this disorder may develop fatal mononucleosis, lymphomas, or hypogammaglobulinemia after an infection with Epstein-Barr virus. The condition appears to be caused by an inability to mount a normal immune response to Epstein-Barr virus.

Acquired immunodeficiency syndrome (AIDS). AIDS, a new condition originally reported in adult male homosexuals and intravenous drug users, has also occurred in a few children. In this condition there is a marked T cell deficiency and patients develop infections with viruses, *Pneumocystis carinii* and other opportunistic infections.

Many other aberrations of the immune system may exist. Most of these are not well-defined at present and include chronic mucocutaneous candidiasis, immune deficiency with short-limb dwarfism and cartilage-hair dysplasia, immunodeficiency with thymoma, and reticular dysgenesis.

EVALUATION OF THE PATIENT FOR IMMUNE DEFICIENCY

Most patients with a deficiency in host defense will present with a history of either recurrent infections or unusual or severe infections. It is important when evaluating such patients to consider whether their problem is caused by abnormalities of the specific defense system or nonspecific defense mechanisms. Examples of the latter might include individuals with anatomic abnormalities such as tracheoesophageal fistulas, sequestered lobes of the lung, or bronchogenic cysts. Aside from anatomic considerations, certain disorders such as cystic fibrosis should be considered.

The most important element in determining the appropriate approach to evaluating a patient with recurrent infections is to take a detailed history. In obtaining the history, it is important to inquire about the frequency, site, and type of infections. The family history should be looked into, particular questions being asked about infectious problems and childhood deaths.

The physical examination should include height and weight, careful palpation for lymphoid tissue, and examination of the skin for signs of scarring secondary to infection.

Laboratory studies are necessary to make a specific diagnosis of abnormal host defense. An outline of evaluation of the patient for immune deficiency follows:

I. History
II. Physical examination
III. Laboratory
  A. Cell-mediated immunity (CMI)
    1. Total lymphocyte count (normal, greater than 1000 to 1500/mm^3)
    2. Delayed hypersensitivity skin tests to antigens such as *Candida albicans,* streptokinase-streptodornase (SKSD), and dinitrochlorobenzene (DNCB)
    3. X-ray film for thymic shadow
    4. Percent lymphocytes forming rosettes with sheep erythrocytes
    5. Monoclonal antibody studies
    6. In vitro responses to mitogens, antigens, and allogeneic cells
  B. Humoral immunity
    1. Quantitative immunoglobulins—IgG, IgA, IgM, IgD, and IgE
    2. Specific antibody—isoagglutinins, other antibody assays to specific antigens such as diphtheria, tetanus, *H. influenzae,* pneumococcal polysaccharide, rubella, and salmonella O and H antigens
    3. Quantitation of circulating B cells by detection of surface immunoglobulin
  C. Complement deficiency
    1. Total hemolytic complement (CH50)
    2. Individual complement components
  D. Phagocytosis
    1. Quantitate the absolute number of granulocytes
    2. NBT test
    3. Bacterial phagocytosis
    4. Chemotactic assays

In general, it is useful to think of impaired host defense as resulting from defects in one of the following four areas: (1) antibody production, (2) T cell function, (3) phagocytosis, or (4) complement.

The initial evaluation of a patient with suspected impaired host defense should include a complete blood count, including determination of hemoglobin, absolute neutrophil count, absolute lymphocyte count, and platelet count. A low hemoglobin may be a tipoff to the presence of chronic infection or of a hemoglobinopathy such as sickle cell disease, in which case infection is a serious problem. A platelet count is useful when Wiskott-Aldrich syndrome is under consideration.

In pediatrics, quantitative immunoglobulins are of more use than protein electrophoresis. Tests for specific antibody such as isohemagglutinins can be very helpful. Routine evaluation of CMI should include intradermal skin tests with ubiquitous antigens such as *Candida albicans* and streptokinase-streptodornase.

More specialized laboratory studies might include immunofluorescence of peripheral blood mononuclear cells to determine the percentage of B cells. T-lymphocyte subpopulations can be enumerated with the use of monoclonal antibodies. In vitro lymphocyte stimulation tests are of use in detecting T cell function.

The most readily available complement studies are a total hemolytic complement and a C3 and C4 level. The most useful tests of phagocytic function are the NBT test and studies evaluating bacterial phagocytosis.

THERAPY

Antibody deficiency. The important consideration in patients with humoral disorders is to supply them with a source of specific antibody. Currently, three alternative modes of therapy exist. Gamma globulin (which is more than 95% IgG) can be administered intramuscularly. Empirically it has been found that an initial dose of 1.2 ml/kg can be given, followed by 0.6 ml/kg every 3 or 4 weeks.

The second form of therapy is administration of intravenous gamma globulin (Gammimune). With this form of therapy, higher levels of IgG can be obtained. The standard dose of intravenous gamma globulin is 100 to 150 mg/kg every 4 weeks.

The third form of therapy is intravenous infusion of plasma. This has several advantages. It provides all five classes of immunoglobulin, it is less painful, and higher levels of immunoglobulin can be attained. In addition, the potential donor can be immunized with vaccines, and specific antibody can thus be transfused into the immunodeficient recipient. This form of therapy also has disadvantages. The risk of serum hepatitis is greater, the infusion itself is more time consuming than intramuscular injection, and it can be performed only in areas that have adequate blood bank facilities.

T cell dysfunction. Therapy for T cell disorders is far less satisfactory than that for humoral deficiencies. A few patients with DiGeorge syndrome have been successfully reconstituted immunologically with fetal thymus transplants.

A number of agents have been touted as helping patients with defects in their CMI. Among these are transfer factor, thymosin, and levamisole. At present there have been few controlled studies proving the efficacy of any of these.

Combined T cell and B cell dysfunction. Immunologic reconstitution with HLA-identical bone marrow or fetal tissues has been reported to be successful in patients with a number of different immunodeficiencies. The most widely accepted indication for this form of therapy is in severe combined immunodeficiency in which bone marrow reconstitution can be a definitive form of therapy.

Other therapy. A mainstay in the therapy of every immunodeficient patient is the appropriate treatment of any infectious process with antibiotics. Some patients, for example, those with chronic granulomatous disease, appear to benefit from continuous antistaphylococcal or sulfonamide agents. However, many patients with immunodeficiency need antibiotic therapy only with acute infections.

Henry G. Herrod

SELECTED READINGS

General reviews

Ammann, A., and Wara, D.: Evaluation of infants and children with recurrent infection, Curr. Probl. Pediatr. **5:**11, 1975.

Buckley, R.H.: Immunodeficiency, J. Allergy Clin. Immunol. **72:**627, 1983.

Miller, M., editor: The child with recurrent infections, Pediatr. Clin. North Am. **24:**1, 1977.

Stiehm, E.R., and Fulginiti, V.A.: Immunologic disorders in infants and children, ed. 2, Philadelphia, 1980, W.B. Saunders Co.

Specific reviews

Babior, B.: Oxygen-dependent microbial killing by phagocytes, N. Engl. J. Med. **298:**659, 721, 1978.

Diamond, B.A., et al.: Monoclonal antibodies, N. Engl. J. Med. **304:**1344, 1981.

Johnston, R.B., and Stroud, R.M.: Complement and host defense against infection, J. Pediatr. **90:**169, 1977.

Stiehm, E.R.: Fetal defense mechanisms, Am. J. Dis. Child. **129:**438, 1975.

26 Allergic Diseases

The term *allergy* denotes a state of altered reactivity from repeated contact with antigenic substances. *Allergy* is also defined as "an acquired, qualitatively altered capacity of living tissue to react, induced by a specific allergen."

An antigen (allergen) is any substance capable of stimulating the production of antibodies and reacting with them, thereby producing the manifestations of allergy. Their number is countless. The strongest antigenic substances are usually proteins, and their antigenic specificity depends on their chemical structure. Some carbohydrate and lipid substances may also become antigens. Simple chemicals usually combine with a serum protein to produce a haptene, which may be antigenic.

Development of the allergic state depends on the nature of the antigen as well as degree and duration of exposure. Inherited predisposition may set the stage for the development of allergy. All persons are potentially allergic, varying only in degree. Although atopic persons are more likely to develop hypersensitivity, nonatopic persons may do so under proper circumstances.

An antigen may stimulate the production of several classes of antibodies (immunoglobulins) with different functions. The antibodies produced may result in responses that are neutral, beneficial, or harmful. At present, five classes of immunoglobulins have been identified.

The identification and characterization of various immunoglobulin classes, including IgE, the allergic antibody, and newer knowledge of the function of sensitized lymphocytes have enabled Gell and Coombs (1968) to classify hypersensitivity diseases. They have divided hypersensitivity reactions into four types, depending on the mechanism by which they produce cellular and tissue injury. This chapter will concentrate on features of the type I anaphylactic reaction. Examples of type I reactions are immediate skin tests, passive transfer tests, bronchial inhalation testing, in vitro radioallergosorbent testing (RAST), and atopic diseases. The common atopic diseases are allergic eczema, urticaria, gastrointestinal allergy, allergic conjunctivitis, allergic rhinitis, asthma, and anaphylaxis.

Additional knowledge acquired since the original Gell and Coombs classification has necessitated modification of the classification. The modified classification is shown in Table 26-1. An additional miscellaneous group (type V) has been added to include more recently described mechanisms of tissue injury such as antireceptor antibody–induced disease, antibody-dependent cell-mediated cytotoxicity, and cutaneous basophil hypersensitivity.

In type I reactions, allergens enter the body through inhalation, ingestion, transepidermal penetration, or parenteral injection. Allergens come into contact with immunocompetent B preplasma cells that produce the IgE antibodies that have affinities for the specific allergen that stimulated their production. Although IgE is the antibody responsible for the vast majority of allergies, a subclass of IgG has been incriminated in the production of symptoms in some patients. Specific IgE antibodies passively sensitize target cells—mast cells in tissue or basophils in blood—at distant sites. The IgE antibodies interact through the Fc fragment of their heavy chain with a receptor site on the mast cell and the basophil cellular membrane. Allergic patients appear to differ from nonallergic persons in antigen specificity of cell-bound IgE antibodies and in the greater amount of histamine released from mast cells when challenged by allergens. A more detailed discussion on the historical background, structure, biologic and immunologic properties, functions, quantitation, synthesis, and serum level of IgE may be found in a reference text (Ishizaka and Ishizaka, 1978).

Specific IgE antibodies do not cross the pla-

Table 26-1. Classification of immunologically induced disease

Type	Name	Antibody	Mediators and/or cells	Examples
I	Immediate hypersensitivity or anaphylactic hypersensitivity	IgE, IgG (?)	Mast cell and basophil contents	Allergic rhinitis, allergic asthma, anaphylaxis
II	Cytotoxic	IgG, IgM	Complement; polymorphonuclear lysosomal contents	Immune hemolytic anemias and Goodpasture disease
III	Immune complex	IgG, IgM	Complement; polymorphonuclear lysosomal contents	Serum sickness, systemic lupus erythematosus
IV	Cell-mediated immunity; delayed hypersensitivity	None	Lymphocytes; lymphokines	Contact dermatitis
V (miscellaneous)	Antireceptor or antieffector antibody disease	IgG	Antibody interference with normal receptor or effector activity	Graves disease and insulin-resistant diabetes mellitus
	Antibody-dependent cell-mediated cytotoxicity (ADCC)	IgG	Numerous cells, including mononuclear cells, eosinophils, polymorphonuclear cells	Role in production of disease not clearly established
	Cutaneous basophil hypersensitivity (CBH)	IgG (?)	Basophils, lymphocytes	Contact dermatitis?

From Lieberman, P.L., and Crawford, L.V.: Management of the allergic patient, New York, 1982, Appleton-Century-Crofts.

centa, are inactivated by heating and sulfhydryl-reducing agents, are elevated in allergic disease, and will passively sensitize human and monkey skin. Skin-sensitizing antibody cannot be demonstrated by routine serologic methods such as precipitation or complement fixation. Although this antibody does not cross the placenta, it is present in trace amounts in cord blood, and the average adult level is 100 units/ml. Shortly after birth, neonatal synthesis increases rapidly. Levels of IgE continue to rise to peak values between the ages of 10 and 13. There is a wide variation of IgE serum level in normal subjects, but elevation above 325 units/ml is abnormal. Patients with allergic diseases, parasitic infection, and some cell-mediated immune (CMI) defects have elevated serum levels of IgE. On reexposure, the allergen bridges two adjacent cell-fixed IgE molecules, which induces a release of chemical mediators: histamine, slow reactive substance of anaphylaxis (SRS-A), eosinophilic chemotactic factor (ECF-A), bradykinin, and prostaglandins, as well as many other newly identifiable substances (Fig. 26-1). The activation of enzymes by the allergen-antibody bridge is responsible for the release of chemical mediators. The release of chemical mediators also involves glycolysis and is calcium dependent.

These released chemical mediators are responsible for the clinical reaction that occurs in the patient. Histamine results in (1) dilation of small venules, (2) increased capillary permeability, (3) contraction of smooth muscle of large blood vessels and bronchioles, and (4) stimulation of irritant receptors. The principal action of SRS-A in humans is bronchoconstriction. SRS-A is inhibited by arylsulfatase found in eosinophils. Bradykinin release results in bronchoconstriction, vasodilation, and increased capillary permeability. ECF-A is responsible for the chemotaxis of eosinophils to the site of the allergic shock organ. In allergic rhinitis, histamine and ECF-A are probably the most important mediators, and histamine, SRS-A, and ECF-A are the important mediators of asthma. Table 26-2 lists the mediators, chemotactic factors, and cytotoxic substances and enzyme constituents of the mast cell granules and notes their structure, inactivators, functions, and activities.

In cytotoxic or cytolytic reactions (Gell and Coombs type II) there is injury or death to the cell. The antigens are cellular antigens or noncellular antigens absorbed on the cell membrane. The reaction is mediated by two classes of immunoglobulin, IgG and IgM. In the majority of reactions of this type complement sys-

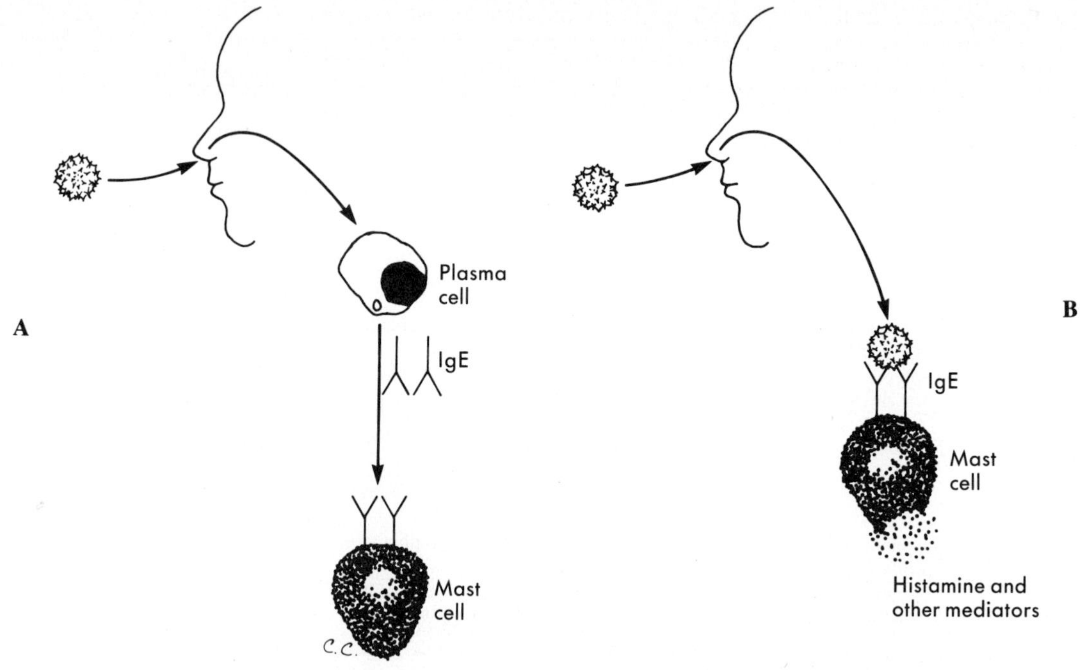

Fig. 26-1. IgE synthesis is induced by mucosal exposure to antigen. **A,** IgE produced rapidly fixes to mast cells and basophils. **B,** On re-exposure to antigen, cell-bound IgE and antigen union produces mast cell (basophil) degranulation and mediator release. (From Lieberman, P.L., and Crawford, L.V.: Management of the allergic patient, New York, 1982, Appleton-Century-Crofts.)

tem is activated. Injury is produced by the irritant effect of this antigen-antibody combination and by cytolysis caused by the complement activation.

Examples of this type reaction are transfusion reaction, hemolytic anemia of the newborn, drug-induced hemolytic anemia, and Goodpasture syndrome. In transfusion reaction the incompatible blood cells from the donor react with the recipient's isohemagglutinins. The complement system is activated, resulting in lysis of cells. In drug-induced hemolytic anemia the drug is absorbed to the cell protein and may act as a hapten. The red blood cell is destroyed when the drug antibody binds the drug antigen on the cell. In hemolytic anemia of the newborn, Rh antibody produced by a previous sensitization in the mother crosses the placenta and binds with the Rh antigen of an Rh positive fetus and destroys the red cells. In the glomerulonephritis of Goodpasture syndrome, antiglomerular basement membrane antibodies react with glomerular membrane antigen and, with the help of complement, cause tissue damage.

In toxic complex or arthus reactions (Gell and Coombs type III), antigen reacts with precipitating antibodies IgG or IgM to form precipitating complexes in blood vessels, resulting in vascular damage and thrombosis. Toxic complexes are more readily formed in the zone of moderate antigen excess. These precipitating complexes fix complement and result in an inflammatory response. The activation of C5, C6, and C7 results in chemotaxis of polymorphonuclear leukocytes that liberate enzymes that damage blood vessels. Examples of type III reactions are Arthus reactions, serum sickness, drug hypersensitivity, poststreptococcal and lupus nephritis, and hypersensitivity pneumonitis caused by inhalation of organic dusts and fungi.

Important examples of the delayed type of reaction are contact dermatitis, homograft reactions, and tuberculin and histoplasmin skin reactions. These reactions are type IV (Gell and Coombs, 1968) and are mediated by cellular sensitivity. Type IV reactions can be transferred to a normal subject by lymphoid cells or leukocyte extract but not by serum. The reaction

Table 26-2. Mast cell (basophil) granular contents

Mediator	Structure	Inactivator(s)	Comment
Mediators exerting effect on smooth muscle and vasculature			
Histamine	β-Imidazolyethyl-amine	Histamine methyl-transferase and histaminase	Increased vascular permeability, smooth muscle contraction via direct effect and irritation of vagal nerves (acetylcholine release)
Slow-reacting substance of analphylaxis (SRS-A)	leukotriene	Arylsulfatase	Prolonged and vigorous smooth muscle contraction, increased capillary permeability
Prostaglandins	20-carbon, aliphatic fatty acids	—	Various effects, including increased venular permeability, smooth muscle contractions, platelet aggregation—effects dependent on type and organ (see text)
Thromboxane	20-carbon, aliphatic fatty acids	—	Smooth muscle contraction
Platelet aggregating factor (PAF)	Lipid	Phospholipase (contained in eosinophil)	Role in human immediate hypersensitivity unproven; postulated indirect effect by release of serotonin from platelets
Basophil kallikrein	Polypeptide	—	Indirect effect via production of kinin
Chemotactic factors			
Selective eosinophil chemotactic factors (ECF-A, ECF)	Polypeptides and oligopeptides	Aminopeptidase and carboxy-peptidase A	Chemotaxis, mainly of eosinophils
Neutrophil chemotactic factors (NCF)	Protein	—	Chemotaxis, mainly of neutrophils
Hydroxyeicosatetraenoic acid (HETE) and hydroxyheptadecatrienoic acid (HHT)	Similar to prostaglandins	—	Derived from arachidonic acid (lipoxygenase pathway); chemotactic for polymorphonuclear leukocytes and eosinophils
Cytotoxic substances and enzymes			
Superoxide radical and hydrogen peroxide	H_2O_2	Peroxidase	Potentially toxic to many cells
Arylsulfatase	Protein	—	Destroys SRS-A
Trypsin and chymase	Protein	Proteolysis	Role unknown
Exoglycosidases	Protein	Unknown	Role unknown; may be important in tissue repair
Miscellaneous			
Heparin	Proteoglycan	—	Anticoagulation; anticomplement activity

From Lieberman, P.L., and Crawford, L.V.: Management of the allergic patient, New York, 1982, Appleton-Century-Crofts.

is delayed from 12 to 24 hours after exposure to the antigen and is usually local. Contact dermatitis is most often caused by chemically active compounds of low molecular weight. Many of the antigens are haptenes—simple chemicals that have combined with tissue proteins. In this type of reaction, antigen contact of sensitized thymus-dependent (T) lymphocytes is followed by blast formation and release from the lymphocytes of a number of biologically active factors called lymphokines (Fig. 26-2). Lymphokines are responsible for a variety of activities, such as inhibition of macrophage migration, macrophage chemotaxis, neutrophil chemotaxis, killing of target cells, blast transformation of nonsensitive lymphocytes, inhibition of virus replication, and transfer of activity to uncommitted lymphocytes.

Pathogenesis of allergic diseases. *Heredity* is generally considered to be the single most important factor in the development of hypersensitivity. Various studies have revealed that 40% to 80% of allergic persons have a family history of allergy. It is further estimated that a

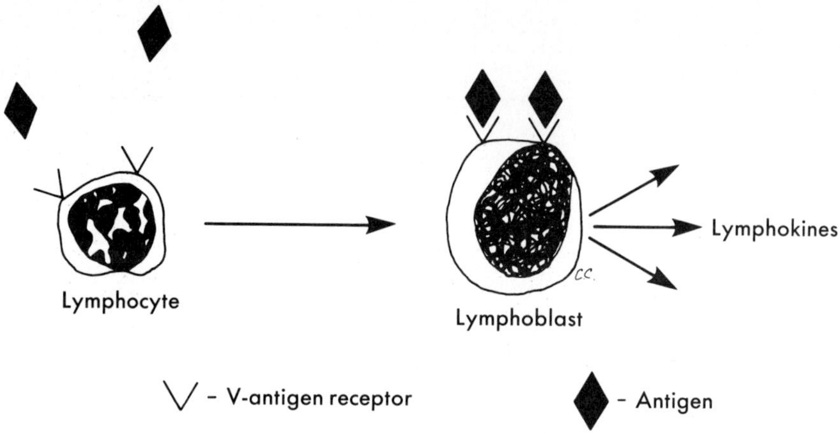

Fig. 26-2. Type IV tissue injury. (From Lieberman, P.L., and Crawford, L.V.: Management of the allergic patient, New York, 1982, Appleton-Century-Crofts.)

bilateral family history of allergy is present in about 35% of allergic patients. Of the allergic syndromes, asthma seems more influenced by heredity than allergic rhinitis, atopic eczema, or gastrointestinal allergy. However, there are many allergic children whose family histories are free of major allergic disease. In children with a bilateral family history, allergic disease is often more severe and appears at an earlier age. Heredity appears to have no relationship to the type of allergic disease or to the specific sensitizers.

Age is of utmost importance in the allergic diathesis. In the first year eczema is frequent, and asthma is infrequent. Eczema is less common after the third year. It tends to be more persistent when it develops in later childhood. Hay fever becomes more frequent in later childhood. However, the degree of exposure influences the incidence of hay fever, and this varies in different parts of the country. Urticaria is a commonly recurring syndrome in early infancy as well as throughout childhood. Chronic urticaria is rare in childhood. Allergic diseases in infants and children show a predominance of eczema in the first year, followed later by a decreasing incidence of eczema and a rising incidence of asthma and hay fever.

The nature and degree of exposure to allergens is a generally underestimated factor in the pathogenesis of the allergic state. Recent evidence tends to support this statement (Matthew et al., 1977). Exposure to allergens may start even before birth. Congenital transmission of sensitization in utero is thought to explain the explosive allergic response that occurs in certain infants partaking of a food for the first time. Positive skin reactions obtained to foods before actual ingestion by the infant suggest that the allergic reaction is caused by either active or passive sensitization in utero. In the first few months the young infant may be exposed to many new food antigens. Because of the immaturity of the intestinal tract at this age, the infant more readily absorbs native antigens into the bloodstream. As the child gets older, he is exposed to a greater variety and volume of environmental inhalants, such as house dust, feathers, animal hairs and danders, cotton lint, wool, and jute. Although the factor of heredity is most important, development of hypersensitivity also depends on intensity of exposure and on specific sensitizing qualities of the allergen. As the child's world also begins to include the outdoors, exposure to pollens and atmospheric molds occurs.

Prophylaxis of allergy in potentially allergic children. Physicians have an excellent opportunity for prophylaxis of allergy in their routine care of potentially allergic children.

Foods are the most important allergens in the first 6 months of life. Cow's milk is the most abundant foreign protein infants are exposed to in the first few months. For the potentially allergic child, breast-feeding will eliminate exposure to this important food allergen and is to be recommended. Some authorities have recommended the use of soybean formulas rather than cow's milk for infants who are unable to be breast fed.

Foods should be introduced singly. Mixed foods are to be avoided. Foods other than milk should be introduced slowly and not before 2½ to 3 months of age. Allergenic foods such as eggs should be avoided for 6 to 9 months. Most food antigens are made less allergenic by cooking. Thus it is best to serve well-cooked foods. Because of transplacental transfer of potent food allergens, such as milk and eggs, diets of mothers with a strong family history of allergy should not contain excessive amounts of these foods. There is a greater tendency to absorb unsplit native proteins from the intestinal tract after episodes of diarrhea. Therefore after a bout of diarrhea in the potentially allergic child, foods should be returned to the diet slowly and in a well-cooked state.

In potentially allergic young infants, environmental inhalants become important even in the first year. Severely allergic infants under 1 year of age are often sensitive to foods, but also in most cases they develop sensitivity to environmental inhalants. Such allergens become important in the first year and remain so throughout life. Preparation of the infant's nursery to minimize contact with house dust, animal hairs and danders, wool, and so on is most important in the prophylaxis of allergic disease.

Diagnostic methods. It is a mistaken and often costly belief that infants and young children are not suitable subjects for comprehensive allergic testing. Because of this erroneous opinion, many children are denied the workup they need and deserve. Although infants and young children may spontaneously outgrow hypersensitivity or may develop immunologic tolerance by continual natural contact, their allergies may persist into adult life. Therefore comprehensive evaluation of severely allergic infants and early action to control their hypersensitivity are strongly indicated to diminish the frequency and severity of their disease later on.

Simple methods of management should be tried before more complicated tests and procedures. The younger the infant or child, the less complicated the allergic state, and the more likely that simple procedures will prove effective. Psychic trauma of allergic skin testing has been overemphasized. Most allergic children tolerate the mechanics of skin testing with no emotional crisis. The important diagnostic procedures are (1) history; (2) special laboratory studies; (3) elimination procedures, primarily foods and environmental inhalants; and (4) allergic skin testing. Additional diagnostic techniques that are often helpful are serum IgE levels, RAST, bronchial inhalation testing, and pulmonary function tests.

History. A detailed allergic history is the single most important procedure in the diagnosis and management of allergic conditions. It is the key to establishing the diagnosis of allergy, suggests the most likely allergenic offenders, serves as a guide in determining the kind and strength of antigens to use in testing, and is necessary for proper interpretation of skin testing. The history is of particular importance in the differential diagnosis of allergic disorders, especially in children under 2 years of age in whom many nonallergic causes of eczema and wheezing exist.

In taking the allergic history, which may require as much as an hour's time, it is often best to have a relative or friend accompany the mother to manage the child. The history is best taken in two stages. The mother is asked to relate the suggestive symptoms of allergy from the first month on, in chronologic order year by year, with emphasis on seasonal variation or other cause and effect. At this point the historian may also suggest possible allergic symptoms that may be related to disorders of the skin or the gastrointestinal and respiratory tracts. During this stage significant points in the history are best recorded on a blank sheet of paper.

After a broad allergic picture has been established, one proceeds to the second stage. Here, a printed allergic history form is of great help in obtaining additional valuable information. Generally, about half the useful information is obtained from the mother's detailed history and the other half from the answers to questions in the routine allergy history sheets. Examples of allergic history sheets may be found in standard textbooks on allergy. Physicians primarily interested in children may find some modification necessary. An adequate allergy history sheet should include specific questions about family history, past personal history of allergic syndromes, physical environment, dietary history, immunization history, and detailed questions regarding the present allergic complaint.

Special studies. Certain laboratory procedures aid greatly in the management of allergic children. Sometimes they also help establish that an allergic state exists. They may also aid in the detection of complicating infections that frequently occur.

Blood count. Peripheral eosinophilia exceeding 7% is often present in the allergic state. Counts over 25% are seldom found in allergic disorders; they suggest other disease states such as parasitosis (especially visceral larva migrans), collagen diseases, eosinophilic leukemia, Loeffler syndrome, and familial eosinphilia. Adrenocortical hormone therapy depresses the tendency to eosinophilia.

Leukocytosis with a shift to the left is often present when allergic rhinitis or asthma is complicated by bacterial infection.

Cytology of mucus (nasal, conjunctival, bronchial, and gastrointestinal). Eosinophils respond specifically to hypersensitivity reactions and are attracted to the shock organ. Eosinophilia of 10% or more in nasal, bronchial, or conjunctival secretions suggests an allergic reaction. Because cytology of nasal secretions closely parallels that of bronchial secretions, studies of nasal secretions are particularly important in young children who cannot cough up mucus. In many cases of atopic eczema, eosinophilia in nasal mucus precedes clinical manifestations of allergic rhinitis. Such eosinophilia in infants with eczematoid dermatitis strongly suggests that the eczema is allergic and that allergic rhinitis or asthma may develop later.

Nasal smears also help detect superimposed bacterial infections, in which neutrophils predominate and there are many bacteria.

It is important to remember that eosinophils are present in the nasal mucus of 25% to 30% of infants less than 3 months of age.

In cytologic studies for eosinophilia the Hansel* stain is superior to Wright stain.

In older children nasal secretions are collected by having the patient blow his nose on wax paper. In young infants mucus is obtained by use of a soft rubber bulb syringe. In older children bronchial secretions may be coughed into a bottle after the mouth has been washed several times. The mucus material from conjunctival smears should be collected from inner canthus.

Eosinophilia in gastrointestinal mucus is of some aid in diagnosing gastrointestinal allergy. However, the cells are difficult to demonstrate and may be absent when such allergy is present. At other times they can be found in the stools of infants with parasitic infestations and can thus be misleading.

Radiographs. Chest radiographs should be obtained whenever a child has the first attack of asthma, in patients refractive to sympathomimetic drugs, and in those with complications such as infections, atelectasis, and middle lobe syndromes. Radiographs of paranasal sinuses help establish the diagnosis of purulent sinusitis complicating allergic rhinitis, particularly in older children.

Pulmonary function tests. Pulmonary function tests are impractical in infants and preschool children. However, in children older than 6 years they are valuable in differential diagnosis, in estimating progress of antiasthmatic therapy, and in evaluation of bronchodilator drugs. Timed vital capacity and the expiratory flow rates are the most useful measurements for large airway obstruction. The maximal mid-expiratory flow rate is more sensitive for detecting airway obstruction, particularly in the small airways. The maximal expiratory rate can be measured simply in the office by the Wright peak flowmeter or Puffmeter and correlates well with the degree of obstructive impairment in asthma.

Miscellaneous laboratory tests. Various laboratory procedures—histoplasmin and tuberculin skin tests, determination of sweat electrolytes, serum immunoglobulins, serum electrophoretic studies, bacteriologic cultures, and Gram stains of mucus from the nose, eyes, and bronchi—are often indicated as an aid in differential diagnosis of syndromes such as tuberculosis, histoplasmosis, and fibrocystic disease. Diagnostic techniques helpful in diseases of CMI are total lymphocyte count, a battery of skin tests for delayed hypersensitivity, x-ray film for thymic shadow, lymph node biopsy, transformation of lymphocytes by antigen and mitogen, and T cell and B cell counts.

Elimination procedures. Elimination of foods or environmental allergens is often of great help in establishing the cause of an allergic

*Lide Laboratories, Inc., St. Louis, Mo.

disorder. The younger the child, the more restricted is contact to allergens. The less severe allergic state is more likely to be controlled by a simple elimination procedure. As stated previously, for children under 2 years of age the commonest allergens are foods and environmental inhalants. Therefore for allergic disease, whether gastrointestinal, dermal, or respiratory, an elimination diet may be tried. In this age group, however, with a seasonal pattern of allergic disease the elimination diet is unlikely to be effective. The child with respiratory allergy who may have symptoms the first winter, improves greatly in the summer, and then flares up again the second winter is probably allergic to environmental inhalants.

If indicated by age and allergic history, young infants can be offered the following hypoallergic diet: (1) milk substitute, (2) rice cereal, and (3) two fruits, two vegetables, lamb, and aqueous multiple vitamins. If in 7 to 10 days the allergic syndrome disappears or greatly improves, various food groups can be added one at a time at weekly intervals. The most important foods—milk and wheat—are added first. If this causes exacerbation of the allergy, the offending foods should be eliminated for 6 months before another trial. After milk and wheat have been introduced successfully, foods can be added according to biologic groups because members of these groups are antigenically related. If the allergic disease is not improved appreciably in the 10-day trial period, a regular diet for a child of that age is reinstituted, except that eggs and egg products are not permitted. In this case it can be assumed that foods are not the major offender. If the response to a hypoallergic diet does not suggest a food etiology, trial of environmental control is then undertaken. Specific instructions for maintenance of a dust-free room are included in most standard texts on allergy or can be obtained by writing to any of the major allergy supply laboratories.

Environmental inhalants are important etiologic factors. Asthma or eczema caused by these allergens tends to be worse in the winter because the child stays indoors much of the time and because the house is kept closed. This increases concentration of house dust also containing other environmental allergens, such as feathers, wool, animal hairs and danders, jute, and kapok. In addition, if the detailed allergic history reveals that sneezing, coughing, and wheezing occur on contact with house dust, fuzzy toys, or feathers, the importance of environmental inhalants is more conclusive. Parents of these young allergic children should be taught that it is important to continue these routine environmental control procedures throughout the childhood years.

Specific tests. Skin testing is of great importance in diagnosis and management of the severely allergic child. Such tests are performed only after failure to identify offending allergens by history and elimination procedures. Elimination procedures are more likely to be successful in the allergic child under 2 years of age. Later, the allergic state becomes complicated by sensitivities to a wider range of allergens, and in most cases skin testing is indicated. Allergens strongly suspected by the history, such as wheezing or coughing on contact with grass or angioedema after ingestion of peanuts, can be substantiated by appropriate skin tests. However, the most important objective is to detect allergens that are unsuspected, even after a detailed allergic history. Skin tests also suggest to some extent the degree of sensitivity; therefore they help determine the starting point for hyposensitization treatment.

A tremendous amount of specific information can be obtained from early comprehensive skin testing of young children with major allergic syndromes such as asthma. There are few chronic diseases in which so much improvement can be achieved. The combination of a detailed allergic history and intelligent skin testing aids greatly in the rehabilitation of the young allergic cripple and helps forestall or lessen the inroads of allergy in later years.

Selection of allergens. Different allergic skin tests are indicated for individual patients; the choice depends on the patient's age and clinical history. In infancy, foods and environmental inhalants or a combination of both are the most important allergens. Pollen sensitivity is rarely noted in the first year. It usually requires one season of exposure to a pollen to become sensitized. However, during the second year some children begin to show sensitivity to pollen. Therefore in the infant under 2 years of age, if the history correlates with pollen hypersensitivity, pollen testing is indicated.

When allergic symptoms occur chiefly during

midwinter months, environmental inhalants should be highly suspected, as discussed previously. When exacerbation of allergic symptoms corresponds with a specific pollen season, pollen testing is indicated. However, when the child has allergic manifestations throughout the year, comprehensive testing of foods, environmental inhalants, pollens, and molds is indicated. Most children with perennial symptoms are sensitive to a number of allergens.

Scratch tests. Scratch tests are best performed on the flexor surface of the forearm or on the back. Areas of dermatitis, skin infection, or other disorders are to be avoided. Test sites are wiped with benzalkonium chloride (Zephiran), 1:5000. Scratches should be about 3 to 6 mm (⅛ to ¼ inch) in length and sufficiently superficial not to draw blood. Liquid or powdered antigens may be used. Powdered antigens are placed on a drop of 0.1N sodium hydroxide at the scratch site. The extracts are then gently rubbed into the scratch with the flat end of a toothpick. Scratch tests are read within 15 to 20 minutes.

Intracutaneous tests. Intracutaneous tests are stronger than scratch tests. In general, a scratch test is roughly equal to a 1:10,000 intradermal test. Intradermal tests for environmental inhalants, pollens, and molds are performed only after a negative or slightly positive scratch test. Antigens giving a strongly positive scratch test should never be injected intradermally. Food antigens may be irritating when injected intradermally. Therefore tests for food sensitivity are best done by the scratch technique.

The most commonly used dilution for intracutaneous skin testing is 1:1000, and the volume injected is 0.01 to 0.02 ml. Occasionally, when 1:1000 dilutions are negative, it may be necessary to progress to 1:500 or 1:200 tests. The best intradermal testing sites are the outer aspect of the upper arm and the flexor surface of the forearm. About eight intradermal tests on one arm is maximal for children. Intracutaneous tests are read in 10 to 15 minutes.

Passive transfer tests. The skin-sensitizing antibody can be tested for by the passive transfer (Prausnitz-Küstner) test. Such tests may be used when eczema is so extensive that there is no suitable body area for testing the patient and in vitro RAST are not available. However, steroid treatment may improve eczema to a point at which direct skin testing is possible. Risk of transmitting serum hepatitis limits the use of this test.

Nonallergic recipients are injected intradermally with 0.05 to 0.1 ml of the patient's serum on the volar surface of the forearm. After 24 hours the sites are tested with the indicated extracts in a 1:1000 dilution. The volume injected is 0.02 ml, and the sites are read in 15 minutes on the same scale as for direct intradermal tests. Serum to be tested is first passed through a Seitz filter and tested for syphilis. Sera from infants or children with a past history of jaundice should not be used.

Mucous membrane tests. The conjunctival test is best suited for testing of inhalant allergens, particularly pollens. It is also employed to test for sensitivity to serum to be administered. Often a pollen suspected by the history fails to produce a reaction by the scratch and intradermal tests. The chief disadvantage of the conjunctival test is the limitation of testing to only one antigen. A drop of aqueous pollen extract or a 1:10 dilution of serum is dropped into the conjunctival sac on the inner lower lid. A control test with the diluting fluid is performed in the other eye. The test is read in 2 to 5 minutes. Conjunctival or scleral redness, pruitus, and congestion indicate a positive reaction.

Other mucous membrane tests, such as bronchial inhalation tests, are accurate but cumbersome and may cause severe constitutional reactions. Bronchial inhalation challenge procedures in clinical practice have been used more extensively in Europe than in the United States. They have been employed in this country primarily as an investigative tool and secondarily as a clinical diagnostic tool. Methacholine inhalation tests are being used with increasing frequency as a diagnostic technique in asthma (Townley et al., 1965). Over 70% of asthmatic children have significant bronchospasm following exercise. A positive exercise-induced bronchospasm (EIB) test in a child is additional confirmatory evidence that the child is asthmatic. For more information the reader is referred to a recent symposium on exercise and asthma (Pediatrics, 1975).

Immunologic tests. Increased interest in immunology in the past 15 years has resulted in many attempts to develop both in vivo and in vitro diagnostic techniques for the study of clinical allergy. The RAST is an in vitro analogue of the cutaneous skin test and will detect allergen-specific IgE. It uses the principles of the Coombs antiglobulin test and is slightly less sensitive than cutaneous allergy tests. More information may be obtained from a recent symposium (Evans, 1975). Of increasing research interest are in vitro tests that measure histamine release from leukocytes of allergic patients after incubation with specific antigens. The basophil degranulation test has been used in an attempt to identify both anaphylactic and skin-sensitizing antibodies in the sera of allergic patients. The test is positive when 25% of the cells over and above the degranulation noted in the saline control show evidence of degranulation. The sera of allergic patients can passively sensitize the skin of primates.

Another immunoassay, the enzyme-linked immunosorbent assay (ELISA), has been employed to detect specific IgE antibody. The ELISA depends on linkage of an enzyme to an antibody. When the antibody combines with antigen, the enzyme is activated and exerts its effect on its substrate. The substrate, when acted on by the enzyme, undergoes a color change that can be quantified. The ELISA has certain advantages over the RAST test; it is less expensive and does not require radioactive maerial. However, its applicability in clinical allergy testing has not been studied extensively, and at present it is primarily used as a research tool (Ward, 1979). At the present time the determination of specific allergens depends primarily on clinical history and cutaneous tests for confirmation.

Patch tests. Patch tests are indicated only in cases of contact dermatitis. They are more difficult to perform and evaluate in young children than in adults. Liquid or powdered material to be tested is applied to a piece of gauze or filter paper, covered with a larger square of cellophane, and then covered by adhesive tape. The test is read at 48 hours. However, if itching occurs before 48 hours, the patch should be removed immediately. Positive reactions are localized areas of dermatitis, primarily erythema and vesicles.

Interpretation of tests. The major objective is to demonstrate that an allergen suspected from the history gives a positive reaction, thus confirming its etiologic role. However, testing may also reveal sensitivity to unsuspected allergens, thereby helping to clarify the cause. It should be emphasized that adequate diagnosis demands correlation of the history and the tests.

Tests for inhalants, pollens, molds, and environmental allergens are usually more accurate than food tests. Because skin test reactions depend on skin reactivity of the particular patient, a control test is necessary for proper interpretation. The younger the child, the less likely are scratch tests to be positive. Negative scratch tests do not preclude sensitivity. If the suspected inhalants give negative results on scratch testing, intradermal tests should be performed.

In interpretation it should be remembered that antihistamines and sympathomimetic medication may reduce skin reactivity. Also, the skin of infants is more likely to react to test material with erythema and to a lesser degree with whealing. The older child reacts with less erythema but more whealing.

In the interpretation of scratch tests the general reactivity of the skin should be noted. If all the tests react, the patient probably has dermographic skin. Only definitely positive reactions should be recorded. More mistakes are made by overreading tests than by underreading them. Interpretation of skin tests should be individualized to the patient. General rules are as follows: 1+ = a mild erythema, 2+ = moderate erythema with definite whealing, 3+ = severe erythema with wheals and pseudopods, and 4+ = severe erythema with large wheals and pseudopods.

One must be particularly careful in interpreting food tests. Young infants often outgrow hypersensitivity to food. Skin tests may still be positive when the child is no longer allergic to the food. Thus a positive test to a food may indicate past or present sensitivity. However, the tests help narrow suspected foods to a small group. Then by elimination-provocative diets, only foods that currently produce symptoms need be eliminated. No food should be eliminated from the diet solely on the basis of a positive skin test.

When the primary shock organ is the gastrointestinal tract, and when there is no associated dermal or respiratory sensitivity, skin tests are most often negative. In this instance the testing approach is by elimination-provocative diets.

SPECIFIC TREATMENT

Specific treatment of the allergic state includes removal of allergens and immunotherapy to allergens that cannot be removed. The less complicated the allergic state, the more likely the simpler procedure—removal of allergens—will be successful. However, in more complicated allergic diseases such as perennial allergic rhinitis or perennial asthma, multiple allergic factors are usually involved. Therefore a comprehensive antiallergic program combining removal of allergens and immunotherapy is often necessary.

Removal of offending allergens. Sensitivity to food antigens is more common in young infants, particularly those with atopic eczema and nonseasonal asthma. However, such children often develop immunologic tolerance to many of these foods as they grow older. If unquestionable evidence of food hypersensitivity exists, the food should be eliminated for a period of 6 months. Then the allergenic food may be reinstituted into the diet at 6-month intervals to determine whether tolerance has developed. Sensitivity to fish and nuts is less likely to be outgrown than sensitivity to milk, eggs, wheat, vegetables, and fruits.

The clinical importance of foods positive by skin tests but negative by history must be substantiated by elimination-provocative diets. Essentials are (1) testing suspected foods one at a time, (2) testing at a time when the child is asymptomatic, (3) eliminating test foods for a period of 3 days before trial, and (4) serving more of test foods than the average portion. Because a positive skin test to foods may mean present or past sensitivity, elimination of the food is indicated only if symptoms are reproducible by its ingestion.

Environmental inhalants are frequent causes of atopic eczema, allergic rhinitis, and asthma. House dust is the commonest of these allergens. However, sensitivity to feathers, jute, animal hairs and danders, cotton lint, kapok, and wool occurs frequently. If sensitivity to a specific environmental inhalant is established by history, skin test, or a combination of both, elimination of the antigen should be accomplished insofar as possible for the whole house.

When the child is sensitive to house dust, the most important room is the bedroom. Infants or young children often spend up to 75% of their time in the bedroom. Mattresses and box springs should be encased with dustproof material. All upholstered furniture should be removed from the bedroom. Synthetic pillows should replace the feather ones. Hair pads and carpets should be removed, and washable cotton throw rugs should be installed. Stuffed toys should be removed from the bedroom. It is best to give written instructions for control of house dust.

For the pollen-sensitive child an air-conditioned bedroom is a great aid. Attic or window fans may cause greater exposure to pollens and should be eliminated. The patient may be sent to a pollen-free locality if the allergy is severe and cannot be controlled by avoidance of exposure and by hyposensitization.

Molds are present in the air to some extent all year. Therefore mold-sensitive patients are exposed to a certain degree at all times. Mold counts are much higher in older furniture, barns, and damp, musty areas. When the child is mold sensitive, the mattress should be encased in plastic material, and the child should not play in barns or musty, damp areas.

Immunotherapy against a specific antigen. Immunotherapy is indicated when avoidance of the allergen is impossible.

Amounts of antigens injected should be small enough not to induce a reaction but large enough to produce some increase in tolerance. Beginning with an initial injection chosen with regard to the patient's degree of hypersensitivity, as revealed by history and confirmed by testing, doses are gradually increased until an amount is reached that protects but gives no side effects. Injections are usually given once or twice a week.

The three principal types of immunotherapy programs are (1) coseasonal, (2) preseasonal, and (3) perennial.

Coseasonal treatment. Coseasonal treatment is the least satisfactory of the three treatment plans but is occasionally indicated when a severely pollen-sensitive patient arrives for treatment during the season and has had no previous injection therapy.

Preseasonal immunotherapy. Preseasonal immunotherapy treatment is indicated when pollens alone are the main cause of asthma or hay fever. In this type, pollen injections are started 2 to 3 months before the season to allow for the maximal tolerated dosage before the onset of the pollen season.

Perennial immunotherapy. Perennial immunotherapy is indicated in the most severely allergic children because those with perennial asthma or allergic rhinitis are usually sensitive to several antigens that cannot be removed, particularly pollens, molds, and house dust. Injections are given at weekly intervals. Sometimes the maximal dose must be reduced during the pollen season because of increased incidence of constitutional reactions.

Immunotherapy is best instituted by physicians having experience with this type of therapy. Uncomfortable and occasionally severe constitutional reactions may follow such injections. Epinephrine, 1:1000, and a tourniquet should always be on hand. Before an injection is given, the patient is always questioned as to any previous local or constitutional reaction. The skin is cleaned with benzalkonium (Zephiran) chloride or alcohol, and the injection is given on the outer surface of the upper arm. After receiving the injection, the patient should wait 20 minutes in the physician's office.

ATOPIC DISEASES

Serum sickness. The greater the amount of serum administered, the higher the incidence of serum sickness. Serum from different species varies in its ability to provoke serum sickness. Horse serum is more antigenic, avian serum less antigenic, and beef serum is midway between horse and avian sera.

The clinical syndrome of serum sickness results not only from serum injections but may also occur after injection of penicillin or other antibiotics.

Serum sickness usually occurs in persons who have never had any experience with the foreign serum protein. The incubation period is from 6 to 14 days. Accelerated serum reactions occur immediately after the injection in patients previously sensitized to serum proteins. Such reactions are likely to be more severe than delayed reactions and may be fatal.

Clinical manifestations. The most striking manifestations are skin lesions, usually urticarial but at times scarlatiniform, morbilliform, erythema multiforme, or purpuric. The dermatitis may spread over the entire body and form edematous areas. Pruritus is intense and usually lasts from 3 to 7 days. The fever may be low grade or high. Lymphadenopathy is commonly present, the most prominent nodes being those draining the injected area. Enlargement of lymph glands may precede fever and the exanthema by several days. Polyarthritis is present in about 20% of patients. It varies from mild stiffening of joints to joints that are hot, red, swollen, painful, and tender. Joints commonly involved are the knees, ankles, elbows, wrists, and the small joints of the hands and feet. Neurologic complications are often present. At times there is leukocytosis and at other times leukopenia. The sedimentation rate is often increased.

Prognosis. Severity and duration of the disease are related to the amount of serum administered. In general, serum sickness is a self-limited disease. Occasionally death occurs from pericardial effusion or edema of the glottis.

Prophylaxis. When the history indicates previous reaction to horse serum, therapeutic serums from other animals, such as bovine serum, should be used. Even if there is no history of sensitivity to horse serum, it may be present. Therefore, before any foreign serum is injected, the patient should be skin tested. Intradermal injection of 0.02 ml of a 1:1000 dilution of the serum is preferred. Physiologic saline solution (0.02 ml) is injected in the other arm as a control.

Treatment. For more severe serum sickness, steroid therapy is indicated. In most cases troublesome symptoms may be controlled within 48 to 72 hours. Doses of steroids are gradually decreased, and treatment is discontinued within 7 to 8 days. In less severe cases, steroids are not indicated. Antipruritics such as calamine lotion and colloid baths are indicated for itching. Antihistamines, ephedrine (10 to 25 mg by mouth), or epinephrine (1:1000, 0.2 ml subcutaneously) may give symptomatic relief. Analgesics may be indicated for joint pains and sedatives for restlessness.

Anaphylaxis in children. Anaphylaxis includes that type of hypersensitivity which results from parenteral injection of antigens.

Etiology. Anaphylaxis is an immediate type of allergic reaction, different from the atopic immediate type of reaction in that heredity does not seem to be an important factor. Anaphylactic reactions in children are most often precipitated by injected antigens, such as heterologous antisera, antibiotics, and insect venoms. When the specific antigen is injected, there is a prompt antigen-antibody reaction, with the release of certain chemical mediators such as histamine. The reaction is generalized and characterized by dilation and increased permeability of the small blood vessels, smooth muscle spasm, hypotension, and shock.

Clinical manifestations. The more severe the anaphylactic reaction, the quicker will be the onset of symptoms after injection of the specific antigen. Clinical manifestations are often present in the skin and respiratory and circulatory systems. In less severe reactions, onset of symptoms may be slightly delayed, and itching and flushing of the skin, which is associated with urticaria, may appear first. This may be followed by respiratory complaints of tightness in the chest, cough, wheezing, dyspnea, and cyanosis. In the more severe episodes the reaction may appear almost immediately, causing severe hypotension, circulatory failure, absent pulse, pallor, and coma.

Treatment. Before any potential antigenic substance is injected, a careful history of possible previous reactions must be obtained. Antigens giving allergic reactions previously will in most cases give a more severe reaction if injected again. Children should always be skin tested with a heterologous serum before it is injected.

If the injection or insect bite causing anaphylaxis is on the extremity, a tourniquet should immediately be placed proximal to the injection or bite. Epinephrine, 1:1000, from 0.3 to 0.5 ml, should be injected intramuscularly at the site of the injection. The same dose is injected in the opposite extremity. Steroids, even given intravenously, are slower in action and are not as beneficial as epinephrine in a rapidly progressing anaphylactic reaction. However, steroids given for a longer period may be of benefit in urticaria and angioedema. If circulatory collapse occurs, 1 ml nikethamide (Coramine) may be injected. Dyspnea should be treated by oxygen. In persons with severe laryngeal edema, tracheostomy is indicated.

Although serum and other injectables causing previous allergic reactions can be avoided, the child who is severely allergic to insect venom presents a difficult problem. The most severe reactions are to stings of bees and wasps. Treatment is by immunotherapy, which is usually successful in increasing tolerance.

Gastrointestinal allergy. Many nonallergic causes of diarrhea, vomiting, and colic are erroneously labeled gastrointestinal allergy. However, sensitivity in the gastrointestinal tract does occur, generally to foods but sometimes to drugs and inhalants. Gastrointestinal allergy to food occurs more frequently in the first year and decreases in incidence in older children.

The allergic reaction may occur throughout the intestinal tract. A food allergen may produce swelling of the lip and tongue or intestinal spasm if instilled in the rectum. Also, the antigen may be absorbed into the circulation from the upper gastrointestinal tract and transferred to the shock organ in the lower intestinal tract. Thus diarrhea and anal itching may occur within minutes after ingestion of an allergic food.

Clinical manifestations. Symptoms may be related to any portion of the gastrointestinal tract. There may be edema of the lips and tongue, associated with itching of the pharynx and difficulty in swallowing. Epigastric distress and colicky-type pains are frequent. Recurrent diarrhea with abundant mucus, often blood streaked, is commonly associated with these symptoms.

Diagnosis. A carefully taken history is the most important aid in diagnosis of gastrointestinal allergy. A family or personal history of allergy may be suggestive. A food diary, recording daily intake of all foods in relationship to time and type of gastrointestinal symptoms, is often most helpful. Foods suspected from the history or food diary should be given a clinical trial by the elimination-provocative diet. Finding eosinophils in rectal smears is suggestive, but other conditions such as parasitic infestations may also cause eosinophilia in the rectal mucus. Allergic skin tests, so helpful in other types of atopic disease, are of limited value in gastrointestinal allergy.

Treatment. The most effective treatment is complete elimination of the causative food. If sensitivity exists to several foods or if the food cannot be avoided, a hypoallergic heat-denatured diet may be of value. Most foods processed by heat or dehydration are rendered less allergenic. Thus evaporated milk, hard-boiled eggs, precooked cereals, and boiled vegetables are preferable to foods cooked less well. Hyposensitization has not been successful in food allergy. Attempted hyposensitization to food extracts is dangerous and unsuccessful. Epinephrine parenterally or ephedrine orally may relieve symptoms of allergic abdominal pain. Antihistamines and belladonna are also useful agents in controlling intestinal spasm.

Eczema. Eczema is the most common and important dermatologic disease of infants and young children. Several types with diverse and complex etiology are encountered in pediatric practice: (1) allergic infantile eczema (atopic eczema), (2) seborrheic eczema, (3) infectious eczematoid dermatitis, (4) contact dermatitis, (5) neurodermatitis, and rarely (6) nummular eczema. The most common types are allergic infantile eczema and seborrheic infantile eczema. Proper management necessitates that the specific type be ascertained because treatment of the various types differs considerably. Eczema is not a disease; it is only the dermal manifestation of a variety of etiologic conditions and results from a series of histologic changes. The characteristic polymorphous lesions include erythema, papules, vesicles, scaling, and lichenification.

Allergic infantile eczema (atopic eczema) results from a specific antigen-antibody mechanism. In this type there is (1) high family incidence of allergic disease; (2) often association of, or progression to, respiratory allergy; (3) positive dermal reactions; (4) presence of circulating Prausnitz-Küstner antibodies; and (5) tendency to blood eosinophilia. However, final proof of allergic eczema is clearing of the skin when the specific allergen is removed and reappearance of the eczema on reexposure.

The most common factors in allergic eczema are foods, environmental inhalants, pollens, or some combination of these allergens. In children under 2 years of age, the most common allergens are foods and environmental inhalants. By the third year, pollen eczema becomes much more frequent. It is uncommon for a child with severe eczema or asthma to be sensitive to only one type of allergen. As the allergic child grows older, there is decreasing sensitivity to food and increasing sensitivity to pollens. Environmental inhalants are frequent factors in eczema at all ages, even in the first year of life.

Infants and young children may outgrow their hypersensitivities spontaneously or may develop immunologic tolerance through continued natural contact. On the other hand, allergic eczema that appears in the very young child may persist into adult life.

The incidence of allergic infantile eczema is greater in families that contain a higher than normal percentage of persons with allergic rhinitis, asthma, urticaria, angioedema, or eczema. In about 50% of the patients, allergic eczema begins before the age of 6 months and in about 95% before the age of 2 years.

Clinical manifestations. Allergic eczema usually starts as an erythematous eruption on the cheeks and spreads peripherally to involve the remainder of the face. It may then become generalized or may involve the outer aspects of the forearms and legs. In older infants or children bilateral involvement of the antecubital and popliteal areas is common. Lesions vary from redness of the skin in the erythematous acute stage to thickened lichenification in the chronic stage. Vesiculation, papules, weeping, and crusting often occur. Pruritus is severe, and the child is most irritable and may sleep poorly.

Eosinophilia is usual. If nasal symptoms are present, eosinophilia may be noted in smears of nasal mucus. Skin tests to various allergens may be positive. Passive transfer antibodies can sometimes be demonstrated.

Approximately one half of the infants with allergic eczema progress to allergic rhinitis or asthma later on.

Differential diagnosis. The most common types of eczema to be differentiated are seborrheic eczema (seborrheic dermatitis), contact dermatitis, and, to a lesser extent, infectious eczemoid dermatitis. Table 26-3 lists the relative importance of diagnostic techniques in the differential diagnosis of the common types of eczema in children.

Seborrheic eczema. Seborrheic eczema is thought to be caused by an abnormality of the sebaceous glands. The predominant viewpoint is that there is a defect in the quantity or composition of the sebum.

Seborrheic eczema is not ordinarily associated with a strong family history of eczema. Approximately 50% of all infants have at some time a mild seborrheic dermatitis of the scalp, the so-called cradle cap, during the first several months of life.

Seborrheic eczema is likely to start as greasy crusts of the scalp, especially over the frontal and parietal regions, with extension to the postauricular areas as a pink, scaly eruption. As seborrhea becomes generalized, it is more likely to involve areas that contain more abundant se-

Table 26-3. Relative importance of diagnostic techniques in common types of eczema in children

Diagnostic technique	Atopic	Contact	Seborrheic	Infectious
History	+ + + +	+ + + +	+ + +	+ +
Physical examination	+ + + +	+ + + +	+ + + +	+ + + +
Eosinophilia	+ +	0	0	0
Nasal cytology	+	0	0	0
Elimination procedures	+ +	+ +	0	0
Scratch intradermal test	+ +	0	0	0
Patch test	0	+ + + +	0	0
IgE serum	+ +	0	0	0
RAST	+ +	0	0	0

From Crawford, L.V.: Differential diagnosis of pediatric allergic diseases. In Crawford, L.V., editor: Pediatric allergic diseases—focus on clinical diagnosis, Garden City, N.Y., 1977, Medical Examination Publishing Co., Inc.
+ + + + = Very important; + + + = important; + + = helpful; + = occasionally helpful; and 0 = negative.

baceous glands and flexural regions, such as the axillary, inguinal, antecubital, and popliteal areas.

Lesions of seborrheic dermatitis are of two principal types: (1) a scaly erythematous eruption that involves the scalp, postauricular region, and trunk and (2) a moist flexural type that is characterized by erythema, exudation, and maceration in the umbilical, inguinal, axillary, antecubital, and popliteal flexures. Both major types of lesions may exist in the same patient. Other seborrheic lesions seen at times are waxy yellow plaques with larger scales than those usually seen in allergic eczema. Lichenification does not occur.

A child with extensive seborrheic eczema is often happy and has little or no pruritus. There is no tendency for children with seborrheic eczema to develop asthma.

Infectious eczematoid dermatitis. Infectious eczematoid dermatitis must also be differentiated from atopic eczema. It is usually secondary to some pruritic skin condition. Purulent discharge from the ears and nasal discharge are also frequent causes. Treatment of the primary disorder is needed to improve infectious eczematoid dermatitis.

Symptomatic treatment. It must be appreciated that no combination of symptomatic agents, such as antihistamines, local medication, ultraviolet light, x-ray therapy, or steroids, will completely control a case of allergic eczema unless the excitant (ingestants, contactants, inhalants) are eliminated.

Hospitalization often dramatically improves the condition of a child with severe allergic eczema because environmental inhalants are more adequately controlled. However, because of danger of contracting complicating pyogenic as well as herpes simplex infections, hospitalization is not indicated unless the eczema is severe.

In the management of allergic eczema it is important to *eliminate responsible foods*. However, it is equally essential to avoid unnecessary and prolonged dietary restrictions. If a child does not improve during a 10-day trial period on a hypoallergic diet, he is unlikely to improve during a prolonged trial period. Aqueous multiple vitamin preparations, which are in most cases hypoallergic, are often restricted unnecessarily, and because of this, there is a higher incidence of scurvy in children with eczema. A trial of unsaturated fatty acids may be warranted; for this purpose, soybean oil in a dose of 2 to 4 teaspoons for each feeding may be used.

Itching and irritability warrant *sedation*. Barbiturates and chloral hydrate are the drugs of choice. A good plan is to give the longer-acting phenobarbital (Luminal) before bedtime and to use the shorter-acting pentobarbital sodium (Nembutal) as needed as the child awakens during the night.

In allergic eczema the use of *antihistamines* in divided doses has not appeared to be worthwhile. However, on occasion, the practice of prescribing the total daily dose of diphenhydramine (Benadryl), 4 mg/kg (2 mg/lb), before bedtime may aid in controlling the extreme nocturnal itching because of its combined sedative and antipruritic action.

The use of *elbow splints* is important in protecting the skin in cases of severe eczema. In hospitalized children the wrists and ankles may be tied to the sides of the crib, but the mother may not accept such restraints at home. The local procedure of greatest help is *bandaging of the extremities*. The ointment of choice is applied to the arms and legs and is covered with one layer of high-grade cotton cloth; an outside layer of 2-inch Ace bandage is employed. This dressing is changed only once every 24 hours.

Soap acts as an irritant in most forms of eczematoid dermatitis. On the other hand, some cleansing agent must be used to prevent pyogenic infection. The detergent sodium lauryl sulfate is a useful soap substitute.

Colloid baths relieve the itching for short periods of time and are most useful before bedtime. Two cups of cornstarch are added to a tub of warm water, and the child is soaked for 10 to 15 minutes. There are good commercial oatmeal preparations available.

Because of extreme pruritus, allergic eczema is much more likely than other types of eczema to become secondarily infected. If infected areas are moist or oozing, a wet dressing should be used until drying occurs. Potassium permanganate solution (1:5000 to 1:10,000), gentian violet (2%), and benzalkonium chloride (1:5000) represent *antiseptic soaks* of great value. Wet dressings containing antibiotics with little tendency to cause skin sensitization are highly effective against secondary infections. These are prepared to contain 1 to 2 mg of the drug for each milliliter of physiologic saline solution.

In the absence of secondary pyogenic infection, choice of *local preparations* depends on the stage of the dermatitis. In the acute exudative stages, wet dressings or soaks of Burow solution (1:20) or potassium permanganate (1:5000) are useful. Ointments should not be applied to oozing areas. After the weeping stage has been corrected, the ointment prescribed should be tested on a small area of skin three or four times every 24 hours to detect any previous skin sensitization.

For chronic eczema with papulation and lichenification, *tar preparations* are usually helpful therapeutic agents. Coal tars should not be used during the summer months because of their photosensitizing effect. Because of possible toxic effects on the kidneys, routine urine examinations are indicated in patients treated with tars. The two most common tars used are coal tar and wood tar, and on occasion a patient may respond much better to one type of tar than to the other. Tar preparations stronger than 3% are seldom used for children.

Steroid ointments and *creams* in strengths of 0.01% to 1% are among the most effective local agents available in the treatment of infantile eczema.

Because of its dangers, long-continued systemic steroid therapy should not be prescribed lightly. Short-term courses of dexamethasone to depress the eczematoid reaction are sometimes indicated to clear the skin enough for skin testing or to aid in control of severe eczema when other measures have been unsuccessful. Steroid hormones relieve only temporarily the symptoms of allergic eczema, and when they are discontinued, the eczema often reappears in more severe form than before.

Specific treatment. Along with the other measures mentioned, a *hypoallergic diet* is prescribed as follows: (1) milk substitute; (2) rice cereal; (3) two fruits, apples and apricots; (4) two vegetables, carrots and string beans; (5) beef, and (6) aqueous multiple vitamin preparation (egg products are not permitted).

After 10 days the infant returns for follow-up observations. If the eczema has disappeared or improved greatly, various food groups are added one at a time at weekly intervals. The most important foods, milk and wheat, are added first. If this causes an exacerbation of the eczema, the offending food should be eliminated for a period of 6 months before another trial is attempted. After milk and wheat are tried, foods can be added according to biologic groups, since these groups are antigenically related. If the eczema is not improved appreciably in the 10-day trial period, a regular diet for a child of that age is prescribed, with the exception that eggs and egg products are not permitted.

If the response to the hypoallergic diet does not suggest a food etiology, an attempt at *environmental control* is then undertaken, as described previously.

Pollen eczema is more prevalent in older children and has a seasonal pattern that corresponds to the local pollen season. Specific *immuno-*

therapy treatment by injection of pollen extracts proves effective at times. Immunotherapy for pollen eczema is not as successful as for pollen asthma and is controversial. In addition, it is easier to cause a flare-up of eczema than of asthma with immunotherapeutic injections. In more severe allergic eczema, allergic skin testing is indicated to facilitate a more precise environmental control program and possible immunotherapy.

Urticaria and angioneurotic edema. Acute urticaria and angioneurotic edema occur more commonly in children, whereas chronic urticaria is more common in adults. Many stimuli, both allergic and nonallergic, may cause these conditions.

Etiology. The incidence of urticaria in the general population is estimated to be from 15% to 40%. This is much higher than the 10% incidence of atopic diseases, such as hay fever and asthma.

Foods are the most common allergens causing urticaria in children, especially shellfish, nuts, berries, and eggs. Drugs, both as ingestants and injectants, are the next most frequent cause in children. The injectable drug antigens such as penicillin may cause acute or delayed urticaria and angioedema. Infectious agents, bacterial and parasitic, may also be causative.

In some persons, heat and cold cause histamine release and urticaria. This phenomenon has been called physical allergy.

Emotional or psychic stimuli may also result in release of acetylcholine, which in turn results in the liberation of histamine with the production of urticaria.

Despite these facts, the cause of acute urticaria remains obscure in approximately one third of affected children. Fortunately, urticaria is usually a self-limited disease in pediatrics.

Clinical manifestations. The disease is so well known that the parent generally makes the diagnosis. Lesions vary from erythema with little edema to elevated, intensely itching, massive wheals with giant pseudopods. These usually appear in crops in successively different sites.

Episodes of urticaria may or may not be associated with angioneurotic edema. Common sites for this localized edema are the lips, eyelids, ears, face, hands, and knees. Occasionally angioneurotic edema may result in severe respiratory distress. Angioedema is characteristically nonpitting and nonpruritic.

Treatment. Although generally a self-limited condition, an etiologic diagnosis should be made, if possible. A detailed allergic history is most important, but skin testing is usually unnecessary. The use of food diaries and elimination diet is often of help in pinpointing specific food allergens. Any food or drug that can be implicated as a cause of urticaria and angioedema should be avoided. If urticaria is associated with bacterial infections or parasitic infestations, these should be treated with the appropriate antibiotics or anthelminthic drugs. Persons sensitive to heat and cold should avoid such exposure as much as possible.

Depending on the severity of the attack, different drugs are useful in the palliative treatment of urticaria and angioedema. Antihistamines help prevent formation of new wheals but have no effect on those already present. The dose necessary to obtain symptomatic relief in urticaria is usually twice that which gives relief in allergic rhinitis. Epinephrine is still the drug of choice for massive urticaria and angioedema and for severe pruritus. Epinephrine in oil affords more prolonged relief. After the initial response to epinephrine, ephedrine may be given orally. In patients not responding to antihistamines and sympathomimetic drugs, steroids may be used. Prednisolone may be given in a dose of 20 mg in the first 24 hours, and then the dose is decreased daily until the maintenance dose is determined. Antipruritics such as calamine lotion or soothing colloid baths help relieve pruritus.

Allergic rhinitis. Allergic rhinitis is characterized by mucosal edema and hypersecretion of mucus. It is the commonest allergic disease, afflicting 5% to 10% of the population. It usually begins in childhood. The two forms are hay fever (seasonal rhinitis) and nonseasonal (perennial) allergic rhinitis.

Etiology. The most important causes of seasonal allergic rhinitis are pollens. In such instances, symptoms correspond to the period of pollination of the causative plant. However, other allergic factors may be responsible for seasonal occurrence of nasal symptoms. Some airborne fungi have seasonal atmospheric peaks. Also, the patient may have more contact in certain seasons with other inhalant allergens such as animal hairs. Perennial allergic rhinitis is usually caused by other inhalant allergens rather than pollens. However, there are many such patients also sensitive to pollens.

The term *vasomotor rhinitis* is reserved for a syndrome identical to perennial allergic rhinitis. However, in this condition no allergic etiology can be incriminated. It is thought to be caused by neurogenic, infectious, or psychosomatic factors.

Clinical manifestations. If contact with the allergen is strong, explosive and uncontrolled attacks of sneezing occur, associated with rhinorrhea and tearing. In seasonal hay fever the conjunctiva is often involved, causing lacrimation and redness. More acute cases have associated itching of the nose, palate, and pharynx, and sneezing often occurs in paroxysms. Nasal congestion and stuffiness may be the most prominent symptoms in the chronic type. In such cases, itching is not as severe but is more prolonged and leads to the habit of rubbing the nose, called the allergic salute. In chronic cases the nasal mucosa is grossly edematous and purple-gray in appearance, and there is a copious watery discharge. However, in young children the appearance of the nasal mucosa is sometimes not distinctive.

Approximately 30% to 50% of the children with untreated allergic rhinitis develop asthma. Also, bacterial infections are frequent complications. When this occurs, the nasal mucus changes from a clear to purulent discharge, cells change from eosinophils to neutrophils, and fever and general malaise may be present. Important ear complications may occur, such as gross hearing loss, purulent otitis media, and serous otitis. Older children with chronic allergic rhinitis may develop nasal polyps, either in the antra or nasal cavity. Nasal polyps may cause obstruction.

Diagnosis. The history usually suggests the cause of pollen or seasonal hay fever, the patient's symptoms corresponding to a locally occurring pollen season. The cause of nonseasonal allergic rhinitis may be suggested by a history of sneezing on contact with some environmental inhalants such as house dust or feathers.

Recurrent nasal symptoms associated with peripheral eosinophilia of more than 5% suggests allergic rhinitis; with nasal mucus eosinophilia of more than 10%, it is pathognomonic. When bacterial infections occur, a shift from eosinophils to neutrophils takes place, and bacteria are often seen. Diagnosis of allergic rhinitis may be further substantiated by selective allergic skin tests. The number and types of tests are indicated by the history and by knowledge of the most common local pollens and their pollinating seasons. Table 26-4 lists the relative importance of diagnostic techniques in the differential diagnosis of the most common causes of chronic nasal obstructions in children.

Treatment. The most satisfactory treatment is elimination of causative allergens, such as foods and environmental inhalants. Although contact with pollens and molds cannot be eliminated, methods previously outlined may prove helpful.

If allergens cannot be removed or controlled by symptomatic medication, immunotherapy is indicated. This is particularly true if there have been major complications such as recurrent sinobronchial infections, hearing loss secondary to serous or infectious otitis media, or nasal polyps.

For symptomatic relief of hay fever, antihistamines are most useful. Antihistamines can be

Table 26-4. Relative importance of diagnostic techniques in the most common causes of nasal obstruction in children

Diagnostic technique	Allergic rhinitis	Vasomotor rhinitis	Adenoid hypertrophy
History	+ + + +	+ +	+ +
Physical examination	+ + + +	+ + +	+ + + +
Eosinophilia	+ +	0	0
Cytology	+ + + +	0	0
X-ray film	0	0	+ + +
Skin test	+ + + +	0	0
RAST	+ +	0	0
Mucous membrane	+	0	0

From Crawford, L.V.: Differential diagnosis of pediatric allergic diseases. In Crawford, L.V., editor: Pediatric allergic diseases—focus on clinical diagnosis, Garden City, N.Y., 1977, Medical Examination Publishing Co., Inc.
+ + + + = Very important; + + + = important; + + = helpful; + = occasionally helpful; and 0 = negative.

Table 26-5. Features of the four antihistamine groups

Group	Prototype	Structure	Comment
Ethylenediamines	Tripelennamine (pyribenzamine)	Ethylamine side chain connected to nitrogen	Effective for nasal symptoms, main side effects probably gastric irritation and drowsiness, usually not used for skin problem.
Ethanolamines	Diphenhydramine (Benadryl), carbinoxamine (Clisten, Rondec)	Ethylamine connected to oxygen	Potent antihistamine; used for cutaneous and respiratory symptoms, major side effect is related to production of drowsiness.
Alkylamines	Chlorpheniramine (Chlor-Trimeton, Teldrin), brompheniramine (Dimetane), triprolidine (Actifed)	Ethylamine connected to carbon	Most commonly employed class, probably least apt to cause drowsiness.
Miscellaneous	Cyproheptadine (Periactin), hydroxyzine (Atarax, Vistaril)	Ethylamine contained in heterocyclic ring	Potent antipruritic; perhaps most tranquilizing of the antihistamine groups; employed to treat allergic disease; mainly used for cutaneous disorders but recently applied effectively for rhinitis.

classified into four groups. The groups, prototype drugs, and structural features, are noted in Table 26-5. However, they are not as effective in perennial allergic rhinitis as in seasonal hay fever. The antihistamine may be used in conjunction with ephedrine or some other sympathomimetic medication for relief of nasal blocking. The dose for children is ⅛ to ¼ grain. Phenylephrine hydrochloride (Neo-Synephrine) is an effective vasoconstrictor for short periods of time—about an hour. Because of their tendency to cause rebound effects on the nasal mucosa, nose drops are best used sparingly. They are often more helpful if restricted to use before bedtime. If antihistamines and ephedrine fail to give symptomatic relief of rhinitis, atropine sulfate in a dosage depending on the weight of the child may lessen the rhinitis. For swelling and itching of eyelids the following prescription may be helpful: epinephrine, 1:1000, 8 ml; tetracaine (Pontocaine), 65 mg; boric acid, sufficient to make 30 ml. Steroids suppress the allergic inflammation of seasonal hay fever and perennial allergic rhinitis. However, in most cases symptomatic treatment combined with specific immunotherapy procedures will control the symptoms, and steroids are not indicated.

Bronchial asthma. Allergic bronchial asthma is by far the most serious allergic disease in the pediatric age group. It is an atopic disease in which the shock organs are the mucosa, smooth muscles, and vessels of the bronchioles. It is characterized by a wheezing type of dyspnea resulting from generalized obstructive emphysema caused by spasm of the bronchi and bronchioles, with outpouring of thick tenacious secretions in the bronchial lumen.

In bronchial asthma, in addition to the importance of the immunologic reaction, defects in the autonomic nervous system may be significant. The parasympathetic system mediated by cholinergic activity incites bronchoconstriction, whereas sympathetic adrenergic activity produces bronchodilation. Stimulation of beta-adrenergic receptors generally results in bronchodilation, but mechanisms that block beta-adrenergic activity may result in increased bronchospasm in asthma.

Onset may be at any age, although it is somewhat less frequent in infancy. Asthma is usually the result of sensitivity to foods, environmental inhalants, pollens, mold spores, or some combination of these allergens. Occasionally bacterial allergens are incriminated as causative agents. In the young child allergic asthma is frequently complicated by episodes of respiratory infections.

Pathology. Although asthma is a disease of

low mortality in children, it is characterized by high morbidity. Pathologic changes are generalized throughout the bronchial tree but are pronounced in the smaller bronchioles.

Essential features are spasm of the bronchiolar musculature, mucosal edema, and hypersecretion of thick, tenacious material from the bronchial glands. Mucosal edema is responsible for the thickened bronchi. Secretions from the mucous glands add to obstruction caused by bronchial spasm and bronchial edema. A state of generalized emphysema results from the obstruction. Asthma is frequently complicated by intercurrent pulmonary infections. Patchy areas of atelectasis are frequently present, and occasionally a thick mucous plug is responsible for more massive atelectasis.

The typical acute attack is usually caused by a combination of bronchial spasm, bronchial edema, and presence of mucoid secretions in the bronchial lumen. Normally the bronchi dilate and elongate on inspiration and contract and shorten on expiration. Therefore obstructive changes embarrass respiration more on expiration, causing the expiratory wheezes and tracheal rales often heard.

In chronic bronchial asthma there is generalized vascularization, mucosal thickening, and hypertrophy of mucous glands and fibers of the bronchial musculature. Emphysema may finally result and is the most important cause of pulmonary disability in adults. As emphysema develops, the thoracic cage becomes fixed in a position of expiration, the diaphragm is depressed, and accessory muscles of respiration are called into play.

Symptoms. The onset may be gradual or fairly abrupt. However, in most patients there are varying degrees of sneezing, recurrent rhinorrhea, or nasal stuffiness for a period of time before progression to the asthmatic state. Many children who develop asthma have a past history of allergic eczema.

In the early stages, attacks are generally paroxysmal. Allergic asthma seldom starts with a wheezing attack of long duration. In fact, if the first attack of asthma is prolonged, other causes of bronchial obstruction should be ruled out. As the allergic state progresses, however, continuous wheezing may be present.

The attack is usually preceded by several days of increased nasal symptoms. Often these are followed by a dry, hacking, intractable cough caused by an increase in allergic response or a superimposed bacterial infection. As bronchial edema and bronchospasm increase in severity, there is tightness of the chest, and the child develops an audible wheeze. Accessory respiratory muscles are used to a greater extent. As the attack progresses, sweating becomes prominent, and the child appears anxious and may become cyanotic.

In a typical attack there are generally sibilant or sonorous rales throughout the lung fields. In addition, there is usually a prolongation of the expiratory phase, accompanied by bilateral expiratory wheezes. Percussion reveals generalized hyperresonance. The older child has a tendency to sit upright with the shoulders forward to use the accessory muscles of respiration. This is usually in contrast to infants who appear to be comfortable in the supine position. In infancy the prolonged expiratory phase is frequently not apparent. Young infants with allergic asthma often develop inspiratory and expiratory wheezes, with tracheal rales.

At first the attacks are generally periodic, with a nocturnal tendency. If the first attack of wheezing is prolonged, it suggests some nonallergic cause such as a foreign body. Although at first the condition usually clears completely, the frequency and duration of the attacks may increase as the degree of sensitivity increases.

Status asthmaticus is a state in which persistent asthma is present, lasting days or weeks. In this stage there is usually poor response to epinephrine or other symptomatic drugs.

Diagnosis. The diagnosis is a clinical one and depends on the history, physical examination, and laboratory findings. Any process leading to narrowing or constriction of the bronchial pathway may result in the asthmatic type of wheezing, more so in infancy than later on. A positive family history of allergic diseases is often found. Typical atopic eczema may coexist, or there may be a history of previous eczema. In most cases bronchial sensitivity has been preceded by nasal sensitization. Therefore most asthmatic children will give a history of sneezing, nasal stuffiness, rhinorrhea, and allergic salute. Bilateral obstructive emphysema, dyspnea, and expiratory wheezing dramatically relieved by epinephrine administration point to asthma. The cytology of mucus coughed up from the bronchial tract or of nasal mucus will reveal a predominance of eosinophils. If 10% or more of the cells in the nasal mucus are eosinophils, it is suggestive of allergic respiratory tract disease. The blood may show eosinophilia. Chest radiographs reveal emphysema and sometimes evidence of superimposed infection or atelectasis.

In children the most common condition to be differentiated from bronchial asthma is acute infectious bronchitis. Acute infectious bronchitis generally responds poorly to epinephrine. Fever is present and often leukocytosis without eosinophilia. The nasal cytology is characterized by a predominance of neutrophils. There is usually a negative family history of allergic disease.

A foreign body in the bronchus may simulate an asthmatic attack. If there is any doubt, radiologic examination is mandatory. A metallic foreign body may be identified by a simple chest radiograph. On the other hand, a nonopaque foreign body may be somewhat more difficult to detect. Substances such as peanuts that release irritative products are accompanied by inflammation. Often fluoroscopy is of more value than plain films in diagnosis of a foreign body. If history, examination, and x-ray studies are inconclusive, bronchoscopic examination of the child should be performed.

In infancy the syndrome of bronchiolitis may also simulate an attack of asthma.

Children with cystic fibrosis develop recurrent cough, wheezing, and bronchial infection.

Congenital laryngeal stridor is a frequent cause of dyspnea in children under 1 year of age. This is the most common syndrome that is mistaken for asthma in the first few months of life.

Pertussis may be confused with asthma. The history of exposure to persons with pertussis may suggest the diagnosis. Leukocyte counts are not dependable, but an increase in the total count, as well as a high percentage of lymphocytes, is suggestive.

Congenital lobar emphysema may be confused with allergic asthma. The chest radiographs show a large area of localized translucence, with the heart shifted away from the affected area.

Congenital vascular rings may compress the trachea or bronchi and produce expiratory wheezing, which must be differentiated from bronchial asthma. The most common such anomaly is a double aortic arch. Symptoms usually begin in the first few months of life. An esophagram and angiocardiograms may be necessary for diagnosis.

Many types of masses in the chest may cause obstruction by pressure on bronchial walls. The most common causes of extrinsic obstruction are enlarged lymph nodes, especially tuberculous nodes and those of Hodgkin disease.

An enlarged thymus gland is occasionally incriminated as the cause of asthma. This is rarely if ever true.

Table 26-6 lists the relative importance of

Table 26-6. Relative importance of diagnostic procedures in common causes of wheezing in children

Diagnostic technique	Allergic asthma	Infectious asthma	Bronchiolitis	Foreign bodies	Cystic fibrosis	Vascular rings
History	+ + + +	+ +	+ +	+ + + +	+ + + +	+ +
Physical examination	+ + + +	+ + + +	+ + + +	+ + + +	+ +	+ +
Eosinophilia	+ +	0	0	0	0	0
Cytology	+ + +	0	0	0	0	0
Other laboratory findings	0	WBC, culture	0	0	Sweat test	0
X-ray film	+ +	+ +	+ +	+ + + +	+ +	+ + + +
Skin test	+ + + +	0	0	0	0	0
IgE serum	+ +	0	0	0	0	0
RAST	+ +	0	0	0	0	0
Mucous membrane	+ +	0	0	0	0	0
Pulmonary function	+ +	0	0	0	+ +	0

From Crawford, L.V.: Differential diagnosis of pediatric allergic diseases. In Crawford, L.V., editor: Pediatric allergic diseases—focus on clinical diagnosis, Garden City, N.Y., 1977, Medical Examination Publishing Co., Inc.
+ + + + = Very important; + + + = important; + + = helpful; + = occasionally helpful; and 0 = negative.

diagnostic procedures in the differential diagnosis of some of the more common causes of wheezing in children.

Complications. The most common complications are pulmonary infections, especially in asthmatic children less than 5 years old.

Bronchiectasis is an extremely rare complication of severe chronic asthma, but early tubular dilation of the bronchi is usually reversible if the asthma can be brought under control.

Atelectasis is not an uncommon complication. It may be small and patchy or massive because of collapse of an entire lobe.

Mediastinal or subcutaneous emphysema, with or without associated pneumothorax, is a relatively rare complication of childhood asthma.

The most frequent complication of longstanding asthma is emphysema. Acute emphysema is always present during an attack of asthma and generally disappears when the asthma is quiescent. Recurrent attacks foster development of persistent emphysema.

Deaths from bronchial asthma in childhood are uncommon. Several studies on the status of patients with asthma 20 years after onset during childhood would indicate that the mortality from asthma is 1% to 2%. However, with improvements in fluid therapy and use of antibiotics and steroids, death from an acute asthmatic attack may now be less common.

Symptomatic treatment. In the acute asthmatic attack, the immediate need is symptomatic relief. After this is achieved, a careful allergic study to help the patient avoid further attacks is indicated. The elimination of exposure to the offending allergen is the most effective form of treatment. In many cases, pollens and atmospheric mold spores cannot be avoided, and a trial of immunotherapy is warranted.

The four most important points in treating acute asthmatic attacks in children are (1) institution of symptomatic treatment early in the attack, (2) appropriate oral use of bronchodilators, (3) maintenance of hydration, and (4) treatment of any coexisting bacterial infection.

In the acute severe attack, *epinephrine hydrochloride,* 1:1000, should be administered subcutaneously in a dose of 0.01 ml/kg, not to exceed 0.3 ml subcutaneously. If the expiratory peak flow does not improve at least 16%, the older child is usually unresponsive to the second injection. However, if some improvement results from the first injection of epinephrine, a second injection may be repeated in 20 minutes. Because of the short duration of action of aqueous epinephrine after the demonstration of responsiveness, an injection of epinephrine suspension, 1:200 in a dose of 0.005 ml/kg, may be indicated because of the longer duration of action. Failure to respond to three doses of 1:1000 aqueous epinephrine or to one dose of aqueous epinephrine and one inhalation treatment of a nebulized bronchodilator indicates a state of status asthmaticus, which requires hospitalization.

Xanthines such as aminophylline (intravenously) or theophylline (orally) are considered first-line bronchodilators. The dose recommended is 6 mg/kg every 6 hours around the clock for children up to the age of 9 years, 5 mg/kg in children age 9 to 15, and 4 mg/kg in adolescents over 15. Because of the wide range in the bioavailability of theophylline, therapy is best monitored by theophylline blood levels. Side effects of nausea and vomiting and central nervous system stimulation may be troublesome. Because of the unpredictability of absorption of aminophylline suppositories, these are not recommended.

Ephedrine sulfate has for many years been a useful bronchodilator. Its major drawbacks are side effects such as palpitation, nervousness, and tremors. It is more useful in preventing a mild episode of bronchospasm from progressing to a severe attack. The dose is 0.5 to 1 mg/kg every 4 to 6 hours.

Isoproterenol hydrochloride may be used by inhalation or sublingually. By inhalation the dose is 0.25 to 0.5 ml in 1.5 to 8.5 ml saline every 4 to 8 hours. Side effects are palpitation, tachycardia, headache, tremor, and insomnia. Overuse of inhalations of isoproterenol may result in an increase in the irritability of the bronchi and aggravation of the asthma.

A change in the position of one of the phenolic hydroxyl groups of isoproterenol produces a decrease in the inactivation of this compound in the gastrointestinal tract, resulting in a much longer duration of action. *Metaproterenol* may be given orally or by inhalation. The oral dose is 0.5 mg/kg every 6 to 8 hours, not to exceed 20 mg four times a day. The side effects of metaproterenol as compared to isoproterenol are the same but of lesser degree.

Terbutaline is somewhat similar structurally to metaproterenol but has been changed by the addition of a methyl group to the *N*-alkyl position. This change results in a longer duration of action and a greater selectivity for the beta$_2$-adrenergic receptors, resulting in decreased tachycardia. Terbutaline may be given orally, by inhalation, or by subcutaneous injection. In older children the oral dose is 0.075 mg/kg, or 1.5 mg three times a day. The subcutaneous injection dose is 0.01 mg/kg to a maximum of 0.25 mg/kg. Side effects include tremors, tachycardia, nausea, and headaches.

Albuterol (salbutamol) has recently become available for use in the United States. It is marketed as Proventil and Ventolin. At present it is available for use in a metered dose cartridge nebulizer and 2 mg and 4 mg tablets. It is a selective beta$_2$-agonist with prolonged duration of action and reduced cardiac side effects. A pediatric suspension is scheduled to be marketed in this country in the near future and will probably be the oral bronchodilator of choice.

In the acute attack, maintenance of adequate *fluid balance* is important. Dehydration fosters inspissation of mucus, the most frequent predisposing factor in the development of status asthmaticus. If adequate fluids cannot be retained orally, parenteral fluid therapy is mandatory to compensate for losses from inadequate intake, vomiting, hyperventilation, and sweating. In the mild asthmatic attack, the child should be encouraged to increase his oral intake of fluid to maintain hydration. If the child becomes dehydrated, 5% glucose in normal saline, 12 ml/kg or 360 ml/m^2 for the first hour, is indicated. Maintenance requirement is 50 to 60 ml/kg/24 hr or 1500 ml/m^2/24 hr.

Iodide may help reduce the viscosity of the mucus. Saturated solution of potassium iodide (1 grain/drop) may be used routinely for asthmatic children. The dose is 1 grain per year of age, up to 15 grains three times a day. Sodium iodide may be added to intravenous fluids. The side effects include gastric irritation, rhinorrhea, parotitis, and acnelike skin reaction. Occasionally prolonged administration of iodides leads to hypothyroidism, which usually disappears after the drug is discontinued.

Antihistamines are of little value in the acute asthmatic attack in children. Because of their drying effect on bronchial mucus, they may even aid in production of mucous plugs.

Sedation is contraindicated in treating a severe asthma attack because of the respiratory depression produced by drugs such as phenobarbital. In mild episodes, chloral hydrate, 15 mg/kg rectally, may be given for extreme restlessness.

Cromolyn sodium has no antihistaminic, bronchodilating, or antiinflammatory effects. It prevents mast cell degranulation and release of chemical mediators induced by antigen-antibody reactions. If the asthma is uncontrolled by bronchodilators, a trial of 20 mg four times a day by inhalation is indicated. Approximately 60% of children will be responsive to this type of therapy. A 2- to 4-week trial is indicated. If the patient is unresponsive, treatment with cromolyn sodium may be discontinued.

Steroids are important in the treatment of severe status asthmaticus or intractable asthma. In status asthmaticus the recommended dose is hydrocortisone, 7 mg/kg, immediately followed by 7 mg/kg/24 hr, or dexamethasone, 0.3 mg/kg, immediately followed by 0.3 mg/kg/24 hr intravenously. In uncontrolled intractable asthma, the chronic use of corticosteroids may be occasionally indicated. If this is required, an attempt to manage the patient by alternate-day prednisone therapy should be made. Chronic intractable asthmatics may often be managed by beclomethasone dipropionate topical aerosol in a dose of 400 to 800 μg/24 hr, making oral steroid therapy unnecessary.

Oxygen therapy is indicated for the hospitalized asthmatic patient. Therapy is always done with humidified oxygen delivered by mask. Results of arterial blood gas studies may indicate that oxygen therapy may be discontinued.

Antibiotics or *chemotherapeutic agents* are of great value when bacterial infections complicate asthmatic attacks. If infection is present, there is fever, leukocytosis, specific physical findings, and poor response to sympathomimetic drugs. If antibiotics are indicated by clinical or x-ray evidence of infection, ampicillin, 150 mg/kg/24 hr, is recommended in status asthmaticus. Adjustment of therapy may be needed if a specific bacterial pathogen is isolated.

In status asthmaticus, if the pH is below 7.3 and the base deficit is greater than 5 mEq/L, intravenous *sodium bicarbonate* is indicated in the dose of 2 mEq/kg body weight. Arterial blood gases should be monitored and additional bicarbonate may be indicated.

Children in status asthmaticus must be closely monitored for signs of impending respiratory failure. Low level of consciousness, cyanosis, $Paco_2$ above 65 torr and Pao_2 of less than 50 torr when receiving 100% oxygen are indications for intravenous isoproterenol or assisted ventilation. These children should be treated in an intensive care unit with controlled mechanical ventilation by a team of trained nurses, anesthetists, and pediatric allergists.

In chronic asthma in older children, particularly in those prone to secondary bronchial infections, attempts to improve bronchial drainage and ventilatory functions should be used. These include (1) use of small-particle nebulization for aerosol administration, in addition to oral bronchodilators; (2) postural drainage after nebulization; and (3) pursed-lip expiration and pulmonary diaphragmatic exercises.

Ophthalmologic allergy. Conditions of the eye of interest to physicians dealing with allergic children are atopic conjunctivitis, vernal conjunctivitis, and dermatoconjunctivitis (Gell and Coombs, 1968).

Atopic allergic conjunctivitis. Atopic allergic conjunctivitis is often associated with hay fever. The seasonal eye symptoms may appear with or without minimal nasal symptoms. Pollens are by far the most common etiologic allergens, but environmental inhalants and molds may be implicated occasionally.

In atopic conjunctivitis, redness and edema of the conjunctiva with intense itching and tearing are the cardinal symptoms. Conjunctival smears reveal a predominance of eosinophils. Symptomatic relief may be obtained by irrigating with equal parts of 1:1000 epinephrine and 0.5% tetracaine (Pontocaine). Antihistamines may also be of benefit. Cortisone eyedrops are less rapid in action.

If allergic conjunctivitis cannot be controlled by symptomatic medication, immunotherapy with appropriate pollens or molds may be indicated.

Vernal conjunctivitis. Vernal conjunctivitis is recurrent, at times clearly allergic but in other instances of unknown cause. Eye symptoms may persist throughout the year but are often more intense in the spring and fall. There is usually lacrimation, extreme pruritus, and photophobia. The diagnosis is suggested by the appearance of hard, flattened papillae on the upper palpebral conjunctivae that have been described as having a cobblestone appearance. There is generally associated edema of the limbal conjunctivae, with a thick, milklike exudate over the palpebral conjunctivae. Eosinophils are often found in the discharge. Symptomatic treatment is essentially the same as that for atopic conjunctivitis.

Dermatoconjunctivitis. Dermatoconjunctivitis is a contact dermatitis involving the eyelids, with an associated conjunctival reaction. The allergens are usually local medications applied to the eye. Sulfonamide drugs, penicillin, and local antiseptics are the most potent sensitizers. Treatment depends on recognition of the reaction and avoidance of medication. Symptomatic treatment of choice is local application of cortisone eyedrops.

Drug allergy. As newer and more complex drugs are added to the armamentarium, drug sensitivities increase. Such reactions must be differentiated from those resulting from other mechanisms, such as drug idiosyncrasy, drug toxicity, or side effects (secondary effects) of the drug. Major factors that influence development of drug hypersensitivity are hereditary predisposition and route of administration. Such reactions are much more common after local application of the drug to the skin or mucous membranes. The second most frequent route is parenteral administration; the least common route is oral administration. Also, certain drugs are innately more likely to produce hypersensitivity reactions.

Clinical manifestations. Clinical manifestations may be varied and are immediate or delayed. It usually takes about 7 days for a patient to become sensitive to a drug that has never been administered to him previously. If there has been previous sensitization, allergic symptoms may occur almost immediately. They vary from an anaphylactoid reaction to sneezing, wheezing, itching, redness of the eyes, or asthma. A delayed type of serum sickness reaction generally occurs in 3 days to 4 weeks and is more commonly seen between 7 and 10 days. This syndrome is characterized by urticaria, angioedema, lymphadenopathy, fever, arthralgia, and occasionally central nervous system symptoms. Skin eruptions are probably the most common manifestations of drug sensitivity. Beside an urticarial reaction, drugs may cause morbilliform, scarlatiniform, vascular, pustular, or bullous lesions. Among the less common but more severe effects of drug allergy are vascular manifestations such as polyarthritis, erythema nodosum, and lupus erythematosus. Sulfonamide drugs have been more frequently implicated. The most common hematologic manifestation is allergic purpura—a reaction involving capillary endothelium as well as platelets.

Treatment. The most important aspect of drug allergy is prevention. The physician should avoid needless use of drugs, especially those with a high index of sensitization. Before a heterologous serum is given, testing by intracutaneous or conjunctival method is recommended. However, a carefully taken history is more important than skin testing in avoiding severe reactions to drugs. In general, positive skin tests usually indicate drug sensitivity, but a false test may be misleading. Skin tests also do not detect those children who develop serum sickness–like reactions. Furthermore, there is danger of serious reaction in skin testing drug-sensitive children.

For symptomatic relief of acute drug reactions the following are indicated: (1) application of a tourniquet proximal to the site of an injected drug; (2) injection of 0.2 ml epinephrine, 1:1000, near the area of drug injection; (3) injection of 0.5 ml epinephrine, 1:1000, intramuscularly in the opposite extremity; (4) administration of an antihistamine after the epinephrine; (5) intravenous administration of fluids and vasopressor agents; (6) combating circulatory collapse by administration of oxygen for dyspnea and cyanosis; and (7) tracheostomy in rare instances of severe laryngeal edema.

Children with anaphylactoid purpura from drug sensitivity must be observed closely for renal involvement, a common occurrence.

Lloyd V. Crawford

REFERENCES

Crawford, L.V.: Differential diagnosis of pediatric allergic diseases. In Crawford, L.V., editor: Pediatric allergic diseases—focus on clinical diagnosis, Flushing, N.Y., 1977, Medical Examination Publishing Co., Inc.

Evans, R., editor: Advances in diagnosis of allergy: RAST, Miami, 1975, Symposia Specialists, Publishers.

Coombs, R.R.A., and Gell, P.G.H., editors: Clinical aspects of immunology, ed. 2, Philadelphia, 1968, F.A. Davis Co.

Ishizaka, K., and Ishizaka, T.: Immunology of IgE-mediated hypersensitivity. In Middleton, E., Jr., et al.: Allergy principles and practice, ed. 2, vol. 1, St Louis, 1983, The C.V. Mosby Co.

Lieberman, P.L., and Crawford, L.V.: Management of the allergic patient, New York, 1982, Appleton-Century-Crofts.

Matthew, D.J., et al.: Prevention of eczema, Lancet **1:**321, 1977.

Symposium on Exercise and Asthma, Pediatrics **56:**5 (supp. 2), 1975.

Townley, R.G., et al.: Comparative action of acetyl-beta-methylcholine, histamine, and pollen antigens in subjects with hay fever and patients with bronchial asthma, J. Allergy **36:**121, 1965.

Ward, H.A.: Immunoassays, Pathology **11:**341, 1979.

27 Infectious Diseases

Bacterial diseases

BACTEREMIA

The term *bacteremia* refers to the presence of bacteria in the blood. The term *septicemia* (sepsis) refers to bacteria in the blood causing serious illness.

Etiology

Considering the large number of bacterial species present in the environment, relatively few species are commonly responsible for bacteremia in the immunocompetent host. Neonates may become bacteremic with gram-negative enteric bacilli, group B streptococci, *Haemophilus influenzae,* or *Listeria monocytogenes*. Meningitis, pneumonia, or septic arthritis frequently accompanies bacteremia in this age group. *Streptococcus pneumoniae* bacteremia occurs at all ages in association with focal infection, and children under the age of 2 years may become bacteremic with this organism in the absence of focal infection. *Haemophilus influenzae* type b bacteremia occurs commonly in children under the age of 5 years and uncommonly in older children, usually in association with focal infections such as meningitis, epiglottitis, pneumonia, or cellulitis. *Neisseria meningitidis* bacteremia occurs at all ages. This organism frequently infects in the absence of focal infection, although meningitis, pneumonia, or septic arthritis may be present. Other bacterial species occasionally responsible for sepsis in the immunocompetent host include *Salmonella* species, *Staphylococcus aureus,* and group A streptococci. Sepsis may also occur in a high percentage of immunocompetent hosts who are exposed to highly virulent species of bacteria such as *Brucella, Francisella tularensis, Salmonella typhi,* and *Yersinia pestis*.

The immunocompromised host may become bacteremic with any of a wide variety of bacterial species including those that commonly infect the immunocompetent host and *Staphylococcus epidermidis,* non-group A streptococci, many species of gram-negative enteric bacilli, *Pseudomonas* species, *Listeria monocytogenes, Corynebacterium* species, and anaerobes.

Epidemiology and pathogenesis

Factors that predispose to bacteremia and septicemia include age less than 2 months, presence of foreign bodies or indwelling prosthetic devices, traumatized tissues, cancer, immunosuppressive agents such as chemotherapy and corticosteroid therapy, recent antimicrobial therapy, congenital malformations, congenital or acquired disorders of the immune system including absence or hypofunction of the spleen, and certain genetic disorders such as diabetes mellitus, cystic fibrosis, and galactosemia.

Transient bacteremia occurs in healthy individuals during activities such as routine dental care. In addition, bacteria may occasionally enter the blood spontaneously through the nasopharynx, lungs, skin, or gastrointestinal tract. These bacteria are usually rapidly cleared by circulating polymorphonuclear leukocytes and by macrophages in the liver, spleen, and lungs. Bacteremia may also occur secondary to a focal infection. Conversely, bacteremia may be primary, and focal infections may result from hematogenous seeding of the tissue.

Septicemia results when bacteria enter the bloodstream or multiply within the bloodstream in greater numbers than are cleared from the circulation and eventually reach a level causing serious illness. Considering that the concentration of bacteria in a favorable liquid medium may double every 30 minutes, it is theoretically possible for one bacterium to result in 10^6 colony forming units in 10 hours. This potential for extremely rapid growth of bacteria justifies the efforts to diagnose and treat bacterial infections on an emergent basis.

Clinical manifestations

In the young infant even serious infections may produce minimal clinical manifestations. The temperature may be increased, decreased, or normal. Poor feeding, lethargy, vomiting, apnea, pallor, irritability, jaundice, petechiae, and hypotension may be present. In the older child the level of activity, the respiratory pattern, and appetite may be helpful in assessing the degree of illness. The skin should be inspected for presence of petechiae, purpura, and ecthyma gangrenosum. An elevated white blood cell count with a left shift is cause for concern, but an unexplained decreased white blood cell count should create even greater concern.

Diagnosis

If septicemia is suspected on clinical grounds, cultures of the blood, spinal fluid, and urine should be obtained while antimicrobial therapy is being prepared for intravenous administration. Accessible sites of focal infection should also be cultured. Culture of the pharynx, rectum, and skin can be helpful in some circumstances. Radiographic examination of the chest should be considered in the initial evaluation.

Microscopic examination of a gram-stained preparation of the cerebrospinal fluid, urine, or material from a localized site of infection may reveal the infecting organism. Rarely, a gram-stained buffy coat or whole blood smear may reveal bacteria. Gram-stained preparations of petechial scrapings may reveal meningococci. Countercurrent immunoelectrophoresis and latex agglutination tests for bacterial antigens are most helpful in the child who has received antibiotics before cultures are obtained.

A history of contact with *H. influenzae* type b or meningococcal infection during the preceding month may be critical to the early diagnosis of bacteremia.

Treatment

The infant younger than 3 to 4 weeks of age with suspected sepsis is usually treated with ampicillin and an aminoglycoside. Alternate antimicrobial combinations may be indicated if infection with *S. aureus* or resistant gram-negative bacilli is suspected.

The older infant or child with suspected sepsis requires individualization of antimicrobial therapy based on clinical manifestations and local epidemiologic considerations. For example, in the presence of pyuria, an aminoglycoside should be administered. For suspected sepsis in children over 1 month of age with no indication as to the etiology, broad-spectrum coverage of likely etiologic organisms is recommended. One reasonable approach to therapy would be to administer the combination of ampicillin, chloramphenicol, and a penicillinase-resistant penicillin, thus providing adequate therapy for *N. meningitidis*, streptococci, *H. influenzae, S. aureus, Salmonella* species, *Listeria monocytogenes, Rickettsia* species, and many gram-negative bacilli. The length of antimicrobial therapy varies depending on the organism, underlying illness, site of infection, and response to therapy.

A high index of suspicion for infection must be maintained in the management of the immunocompromised host. Principles of treatment include early diagnosis and prompt therapy with broad-spectrum antimicrobial agents. In the absence of a likely etiologic organism, treatment may consist of an aminoglycoside, a penicillinase-resistant penicillin, and carbenicillin.

Supportive care should include oxygen and fluid and electrolyte management. Fresh frozen plasma, blood, vasopressors, and advanced life support are administered as required.

Prevention

Prophylaxis following exposure to systemic *Haemophilus influenzae* type b or *Neisseria meningitidis* infections is discussed with bacterial meningitis.

BACTERIAL MENINGITIS

Meningitis is an acute infectious disease characterized by fever, inflammation of the meninges with accompanying stiffness of the neck, and subsequent dysfunction of the central nervous system.

Etiology and epidemiology

The etiology of meningitis includes many species of bacteria and viruses as well as a few species of fungi and parasites. However, the vast majority of life-threatening cases are of bacterial etiology. Each year in the United States over 20,000 children develop bacterial meningitis.

Bacterial meningitis in the first 3 weeks of

life is most commonly caused by group B *Streptococcus, E. coli,* or other gram-negative enteric bacilli. Neonatal meningitis is discussed in greater detail in Chapter 15. Bacterial meningitis in infants over 3 weeks of age and in older children most frequently is caused by *H. influenzae* type b, *S. pneumoniae,* or *N. meningitidis*. Other bacterial species are occasionally isolated from children with meningitis including group A *Streptococcus,* gram-negative enteric organisms, *S. aureus,* and *Mycobacterium tuberculosis*.

Pathogenesis

Bacterial meningitis usually occurs following bacteremia resulting from spontaneous entry of organisms colonizing the upper respiratory tract. Invasion by direct extension is less common, but may occur from purulent infection of the paranasal sinuses, mastoids, or rarely from an abscess contiguous to the meninges. Bacteria may also gain entry to the central nervous system through penetrating wounds, lumbar puncture, neurosurgical procedures, and midline dermal sinus tracts.

Pathologic findings

The brain is hyperemic, edematous, and contains exudate in the subarachnoid space. The exudate is composed of fibrin, white cells, red cells, and the organisms. Purulent meningitis may block the foramina of Luschka and Magendie, the sylvian aqueduct, or the foramen of Monro. Thromboses may occur in the meningeal veins or venous sinuses. Destructive changes may be present in the cerebral cortex. Infection and exudate about the cranial nerves may cause deafness, blindness, or facial weakness.

Meningococcal infection may cause lesions in other areas, such as petechiae from septic thrombi localizing in vessels of the skin and hemorrhages in serosal surfaces and mucous membranes. Purulent lesions may develop in the peritoneum, pericardium, or pleura. Acute adrenocortical insufficiency, characterized pathologically by the presence of hemorrhages in the adrenal glands, may occur. Ecchymotic areas may be so extensive that they subsequently slough.

Clinical manifestations

Clinical manifestations observed at initial examination are influenced by age of the patient, nature of the infecting organism, duration of the disease, degree of effectiveness of the antecedent therapy, and the presence of an underlying disease.

Older children react like adults in that the onset of meningitis is likely to be abrupt with fever, chills, headache, and vomiting being the characteristic symptoms associated with or quickly followed by changes in sensorium. The patient is extremely irritable and restless and often becomes delirious. Later, stupor and coma may occur. Seizures may occur at any stage of the illness. Examination reveals stiff neck and positive Kernig and Brudzinski signs.

During the newborn period and for the first 6 months of life the infant may not show classical symptoms and signs of meningitis. Early symptoms of meningitis in the newborn include unexplained apnea, respiratory distress, and seizures. Older infants often exhibit irritability alternating with drowsiness, poor feeding, and high-pitched cry. Fullness or distention of the anterior fontanel may occur. By the time the older infant develops a stiff neck and positive Kernig and Brudzinski signs, permanent neurologic damage may have occurred. Nonspecific manifestations include fever, anorexia, and failure to gain weight. Meningococcal meningitis may be associated with petechiae, purpura, or profound hypotension.

Diagnosis

In the absence of contraindications, a lumbar puncture should be performed if there is the slightest suspicion of meningitis. Contraindications most commonly encountered include presence or suspicion of a mass lesion with greatly increased intracranial pressure, presence of large areas of infected skin overlying the lumbar spine as may occur in burns, and respiratory or circulatory instability in the critically ill patient. If meningitis is suspected on clinical grounds and a lumbar puncture is contraindicated, antimicrobial therapy should be administered without the benefit of cerebrospinal fluid examination and culture. Antimicrobial therapy should not be delayed for the amount of time required to schedule, perform, and interpret such diagnostic tests as computerized tomography of the head.

If there are no contraindications to lumbar puncture, the procedure should be performed immediately. As the subarachnoid space is entered, the pressure of the fluid should be recorded. If greatly increased intracranial pressure is encountered unexpectedly, only a few drops of cerebrospinal fluid should be removed. If the pressure is not excessively elevated, the fluid may be collected in three tubes—one for the determination of glucose and protein content, one for cell count and examination of the centrifuged sediment, and one for culture and sensitivity. Special media will be required for tubercle bacilli and fungi. Blood cultures should also be obtained.

In acute bacterial meningitis the cerebrospinal fluid pressure may be elevated, but this is sometimes difficult to interpret when the child is crying. The appearance of the fluid may be clear in the earliest phase of the infection, but generally has the appearance of ground glass to a definite cloudiness. The cell count is usually greatly elevated, but may be only slightly increased in the early stage of infection. Bacterial meningitis produces a polymorphonuclear leukocytic response in over 90% of the cases. Gram stain of the centrifuged sediment frequently reveals the causative organism.

The cerebrospinal fluid glucose level is typically reduced in bacterial meningitis, generally in proportion to the severity and duration of the disease. However, it may be normal initially. The cerebrospinal fluid glucose level should be compared with a blood glucose level obtained just before lumbar puncture. Normally the cerebrospinal fluid glucose level is two thirds or more of the blood sugar level. The protein content of the cerebrospinal fluid is usually increased.

In approximately 15% of pediatric patients with meningitis the causative organism cannot be demonstrated by smear or culture because of prior therapy. Countercurrent immunoelectrophoresis and latex particle agglutination tests are useful in establishing the diagnosis in patients with negative cultures. These tests detect bacterial antigen in body fluids (blood, cerebrospinal fluid, and urine).

Differential diagnosis. Acute bacterial meningitis must be differentiated from other entities that cause meningeal irritation. Viral (aseptic) meningitis is the most common of these conditions. Viral meningitis usually produces predominantly lymphocytic pleocytosis of moderate degree, but in the initial stages the cellular response may be polymorphonuclear. The glucose content of the fluid is usually normal, the smear negative for bacteria, and the bacterial culture sterile.

Tuberculous meningitis is suggested by the presence of pleocytosis that is predominantly lymphocytic, a reduction in glucose content, a moderate rise in protein level, and the fact that organisms are not grown from the fluid on the usual media. Acid-fast bacilli may be seen in a smear of the centrifuged sediment of the fluid but are best found in the pellicle that forms when the tube of fluid is kept overnight. The tuberculin test is almost invariably positive, and the chest radiograph generally reveals evidence of tuberculosis.

In cases with atypical features, consideration should be given to unusual etiologies of meningitis including *Herpes simplex, Histoplasma capsulatum, Coccidioides immitis, Toxoplasma gondii,* and free-living amoebae.

Treatment

The principles of treatment are: (1) appropriate antimicrobial drug therapy in a dosage and by a route that results in adequate levels at the site of infection, (2) rapid identification of the causative organism and determination of its antibiotic susceptibility, (3) adjustment of antimicrobial therapy on the basis of bacteriologic findings, (4) continuation of antimicrobial therapy until clinical signs have disappeared and the cerebrospinal fluid has been sterilized, (5) supportive care and symptomatic management, (6) observation for and treatment of complications, and (7) long-term rehabilitation when required.

Although the etiologic organism can frequently be seen and identified on gram-stained centrifuged cerebrospinal fluid sediment, even experienced observers occasionally incorrectly identify the causative agent. Thus, initial selection of antimicrobial therapy should not be based solely on examination of the gram-stained sediment. Broad-spectrum coverage is preferred until the etiology of the infection is confirmed by culture and sensitivity results. Antimicrobial therapy for neonatal meningitis is discussed in Chapter 15. For infants over 3 weeks of age and for children, initial coverage should include ampicillin (300 mg/kg/24 hr in six divided doses) and chloramphenical (75 to 100 mg/kg/24 hr in four divided doses) administered intravenously. In patients with meningitis associated with trauma, dermal sinus tracts, central nervous system shunts, or parameningeal infections, antistaphylococcal antibiotic therapy should be included. Once the etiologic agent and sensitivity are established, single drug therapy is usually preferable. Patients should receive therapy at least 7 days for *N. meningitidis* and 10 days for *H. influenzae* or *S. pneumoniae*. In general, patients should be afebrile at least 3 days before therapy is discontinued.

Patients with meningitis require close monitoring. Neurologic status and serum electrolytes should be evaluated frequently until the patient has stabilized. Patients should initially receive nothing by mouth, and intravenous fluid administration should be restricted as required to maintain a normal serum sodium concentration. Once the patient has stabilized, daily measurement of head circumference and transillumination are recommended.

The patient should be evaluated neurologically during convalescence and at intervals of 3 to 4 months during the succeeding year. Early detection of residual brain damage permits intelligent counseling of parents and planning for long-term management of the child.

Treatment of complications (see also pp. 785-787)

Although almost half the infants with acute bacterial meningitis develop some degree of subdural effusion, in only about 10% is it clinically significant. Effusions are more common in *H. influenzae* and *S. pneumoniae* meningitis. The subdural effusion may be unilateral or bilateral. Subdural effusions usually do not require tapping. However, it may be beneficial in the presence of increased intracranial pressure or focal neurologic deficits. One may also consider subdural taps in the presence of prolonged fever to differentiate subdural effusion from subdural empyema, a rare complication that may require neurosurgical intervention.

Waterhouse-Friderichsen syndrome is a catastrophic complication usually associated with meningococcal meningitis, but it may occur in other types of infection. This syndrome is caused by bilateral adrenal hemorrhage. The patient may develop profound hypotension. Petechial and ecchymotic lesions may spread rapidly. Vomiting and prostration are often present. Shock is treated by the intravenous administration of electrolyte solutions and blood. Pharmacologic doses of corticosteroids may be useful in combating the hemodynamic and metabolic alterations associated with this condition.

Inappropriate secretion of antidiuretic hormone is a rather frequent complication of bacterial meningitis. This is caused by increased secretion of antidiuretic hormone (ADH) and is manifested by hyponatremia, inappropriately concentrated urine relative to serum hypotonicity, and increased urinary excretion of sodium in the absence of dehydration and with normal renal and adrenal function. This condition may result in cerebral edema. Treatment consists of fluid restriction.

Prevention

Young children who are in household contact with patients with systemic *H. influenzae* type b infections have recently been shown to be at greatly increased risk of *H. influenzae* infection. Evidence is accumulating that there is a similar risk for exposure in a day-care setting. The American Academy of Pediatrics has recently recommended rifampin prophylaxis for all persons in household contact with *H. influenzae* type b disease in households where there are children less than 4 years old. Rifampin prophylaxis may also be considered for day-care center children and personnel who are in contact with a person infected with *H. influenzae* type b. Also, patients with infection should receive rifampin prophylaxis before discharge because standard therapy does not eradicate the nasopharyngeal carriage. The recommended dose of oral rifampin is 20 mg/kg/day (maximum 600 mg/day) given once daily for 4 days. Rifampin is not recommended during pregnancy.

All persons in household and day-care contact with patients with *N. meningitidis* infection should receive antimicrobial prophylaxis. These persons may be given oral rifampin, 5 mg/kg every 12 hours for 4 doses for infants less than 1 month of age, and 10 mg/kg every 12 hours for 4 doses (maximum: 600 mg/dose) for infants and children over 1 month. A vaccine is available that reduces susceptibility to meningococcal serogroups A, C, Y, and W135.

BRUCELLOSIS

Brucellosis is an infectious disease characterized chiefly by prolonged fever. *Brucella* organisms are gram-negative aerobic bacilli. The organisms are intracellular parasites with a predilection for cells of the reticuloendothelial system. Four species of *Brucella,* named for their major reservoir, are pathogenic in man: *B. abortus* (cattle), *B. melitensis* (sheep and goats), *B. suis* (swine), and *B. canis* (dogs). Brucellosis is usually acquired by contact with infected animals or by consumption of unpasteurized milk or other dairy products. The incubation period is typically 5 to 35 days but may be longer. Pathologic changes are hyperplasia of the reticuloendothelial tissue, formation of granulomas, and areas of focal necrosis in the liver, spleen, and lymph nodes.

Clinical manifestations

Although severe clinical manifestations sometimes appear suddenly, gradual onset with a subacute or chronic course is more characteristic. The disease usually begins with low-grade fever, which increases and at times is high. The fever may last for a few weeks, several weeks, or many months. With a prolonged clinical course there is a tendency to have periods of fever for 1 to 2 weeks separated by fever-free intervals of variable length. Other systemic manifestations include headache, malaise, chills or chilly sensations, muscle aches and pains, anorexia, irritability, fatigability, progressive weakness, weight loss, and anemia. Less common are cough, diarrhea, and joint pains, with or without manifestations of arthritis. Enlargement of the liver and spleen occurs rather frequently, especially in more prolonged illness. A variety of other manifestations may appear, including hepatitis, nephritis, endocarditis, pericarditis, pleuritis, peritonitis, meningitis, encephalitis, osteomyelitis, and subcutaneous abscesses.

In acute cases there may be moderate leukocytosis, but leukopenia with relative lymphocytosis is more common.

Diagnosis

The diagnosis of brucellosis should be considered in patients with a prolonged febrile illness, especially if there is a history of exposure to animals or unpasteurized dairy products. The organism may be recovered from blood, bone marrow, urine, or local lesions. Bacteremia, if present, is usually of a low level. Thus several blood cultures are recommended. The laboratory should be advised if brucellosis is suspected so that special media may be used and cultures will be held for at least 3 weeks. Agglutination titers greater than or equal to 1:160 are suggestive of acute or chronic disease, but of greater significance is the demonstration of a rising titer in serial samples. The intradermal skin test is not of value in the individual patient.

Differential diagnosis includes many conditions capable of causing prolonged fever with systemic manifestations. These include typhoid or paratyphoid fever, malaria, tuberculosis, tularemia, bacterial endocarditis, infectious mononucleosis, lymphoma, rheumatic fever, and rheumatoid arthritis. Brucellosis should also be considered in diagnostically difficult cases of meningitis, pleurisy, pericarditis, and peritonitis.

Treatment

Early treatment is important in preventing prolonged morbidity. In cases of mild to moderate severity tetracycline should be given orally in a dosage of 40 mg/kg/24 hr (maximum 2 g/day), divided into four doses and continued for 3 weeks. In cases of greater severity, streptomycin should be added in a dosage of 20 mg/kg/24 hr (maximum 1 g/day), divided into two doses intramuscularly for 2 weeks. In children under the age of 9 years, chloramphenicol 75 to 100 mg/kg/24 hr (maximum 4 g/day), divided into four doses orally or intravenously may be substituted for tetracycline to avoid staining developing teeth. Adrenocorticosteroid therapy may prove useful in the extremely ill child with severe toxemia but is not indicated in the average case. The course of steroid therapy should be brief. Convalescence may be prolonged and characterized by weakness and fatigability.

DIPHTHERIA

Diphtheria is an acute infectious disease characterized by presence of a local membranous lesion containing bacteria that elaborate a potent exotoxin. Absorption of this exotoxin, an inhibitor of protein synthesis, may produce severe systemic illness.

Etiology and epidemiology

The causative organism, *Corynebacterium diphtheriae,* is a pleomorphic gram-positive bacillus. Only toxigenic strains cause diphtheria. Rarely, *C. ulcerans* may be associated with an illness indistinguishable from diphtheria.

The disease is contracted via direct contact with an infected individual or carrier. Inanimate objects rarely serve as sources of infection. The portal of entry is usually the upper respiratory tract, with the formation of the membrane in the oropharynx, nasopharynx, or laryngotracheal tree. Rarely, the portal of entry is the conjunctiva, skin, external genitalia, or the external ear. The incubation period is usually 2 to 6 days.

Infants born of mothers immune to the disease are passively protected for 3 to 6 months, but infants of nonimmune mothers are susceptible. Active immunization is achieved and maintained by injections of diphtheria toxoid at periodic intervals. Details of immunization against diphtheria are discussed in Chapter 11.

Pathologic findings

The potent exotoxin elaborated by *C. diphtheriae* produces local epithelial degeneration and an outpouring of serous and fibrinous material that coagulates to form a pseudomembrane containing the bacilli, dead and dying cells, fibrin, and white and red blood cells. Tissues contiguous to the membrane are acutely inflamed, congested, edematous, and sometimes hemorrhagic. The membrane may be whitish gray, dirty gray, or darker and is adherent to the mucous membrane. Bleeding occurs when it is dislodged. Laryngotracheal diphtheritic membranes are less firmly adherent.

The absorbed exotoxin affects all cells, but, clinically, damage to the heart, kidneys, and peripheral nerves are most prominent. Myocardial degeneration, edema, and mononuclear cell infiltrate are seen in fatal myocarditis. The heart is dilated, and the myocardium is flabby and pale. Tubules and interstitial tissue bear the brunt of the renal damage. Tubular cells undergo degeneration and necrosis, and the interstitial tissue is acutely inflamed. Sensory as well as motor nerve fibers may be involved pathologically, despite the fact that motor symptoms predominate. Degeneration of myelin and axonal swelling are seen microscopically.

Clinical manifestations

General symptoms. The usual manifestations of an acute illness are present, including malaise, headache, anorexia, and fever. Prostration varies: some children show little systemic effect and others are overwhelmed by the toxemia (Fig. 27-1).

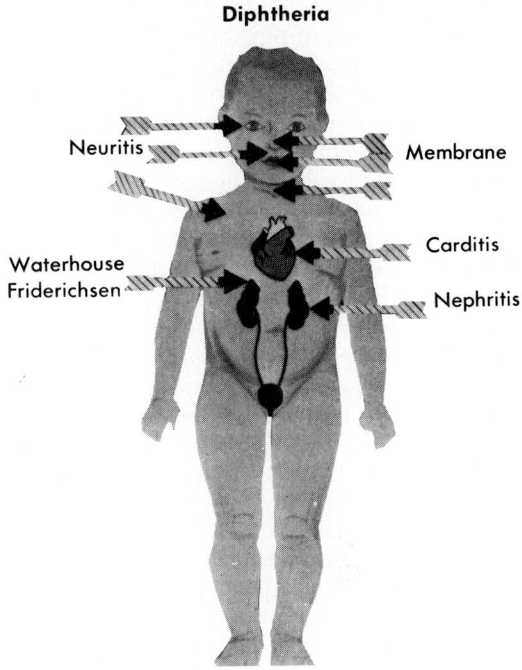

Fig. 27-1. Diphtheria and its complications.

Local manifestations. *Nasal diphtheria* may exist as an isolated entity or in combination with pharyngeal diphtheria. The child may not appear to be seriously ill. Unilateral or bilateral nasal discharge that becomes serosanguineous and is associated with excoriation of the upper lip is characteristic. Careful inspection reveals the presence of a pseudomembrane, and a positive culture confirms the clinical impression of diphtheria.

In *pharyngeal diphtheria,* inflammation of the tonsils and pharynx progresses from simple redness and swelling to the formation of a follicular tonsillar exudate that rapidly coalesces to form a pseudomembrane. The adherent membrane often extends to involve the soft palate, uvula, and anterior tonsillar pillars. It may spread to the nasopharynx, the pharynx, the larynx, and even the trachea. The cervical nodes may become swollen and tender. The throat is painful, swallowing is difficult, and the voice may become muffled.

Laryngotracheal diphtheria is usually the most serious form of diphtheria because of the potential for airway obstruction and the frequency with which bronchopneumonia supervenes. In approximately 75% of cases of laryngotracheal diphtheria, a membrane is also present in the pharynx or nose.

The child with the laryngotracheal form of the disease develops a brassy cough, is hoarse, gradually loses his voice, and suffers progressive interference with respiration. The membrane may become detached a few days after onset of the disease, causing complete obstruction of the airway and asphyxiation. Pieces of membrane may break off and be coughed up or inhaled deeply into the bronchial passages, causing atelectasis, emphysema, or pneumonia.

Other diphtheric syndromes have been described. Infrequently, the diphtheritic membrane may be on the skin at the site of pyoderma or a wound, on the conjunctiva, in the external auditory canal, in the vulvovaginal area, or even on the unhealed umbilicus of the newborn infant or at the site of circumcision. When such lesions are small, there is relatively less absorption of toxin, and systemic manifestations may be mild.

Specific toxic effects. Toxic degenerative damage to myocardial fibers and the conduction system usually occurs during the first 2 weeks of illness, but may occur as late as 6 weeks. The incidence of myocarditis may be as high as 10% with a mortality of 50% to 75%. This complication is recognized by combinations of the following manifestations: hepatomegaly, vomiting, dyspnea, rales in lung bases, venous congestion and stasis, tachycardia out of proportion to fever, weak pulse, muffled first heart sound, blowing systolic murmur replacing the first heart sound, arrhythmias, cardiac enlargement, hypotension, and electrocardiographic changes. Electrocardiographic changes frequently consist of some element of heart block.

Neuritis occurs in up to 10% of cases, and except for palatal paralysis it occurs later in the course than myocarditis (3 weeks or more). Diphtheritic neuritis is characterized by bilateral distribution, involvement of motor instead of sensory nerves, and complete recovery in most instances.

Palatal and/or pharyngeal paralysis is the most common manifestation and tends to appear during the first 3 weeks of the disease. It results in a nasal quality to the voice and regurgitation of fluids through the nose. Paralysis of ocular muscles occurs during the third week, manifested by loss of accommodation, dilation of the pupils, strabismus, or ptosis. A progressive generalized paralysis may appear after the fourth week. Phrenic nerve paralysis may develop as late as 4 to 8 weeks into the course of illness.

Toxic renal damage may result in decreased urine volume, proteinuria, pyuria, casts, and at times mild generalized edema.

Diagnosis

The initial diagnosis of diphtheria is usually made on clinical grounds.

A history of primary immunization against diphtheria, followed by appropriate booster injections of diphtheria toxoid, makes the diagnosis very unlikely. However, immunization does not provide absolute protection. Obviously, knowledge of contact with a known case of diphtheria strengthens the clinical impression.

Definitive diagnosis depends on isolation of *C. diphtheriae* from the site of invasion and subsequent demonstration of toxigenicity by guinea pig inoculation or an in vitro assay. Swab culture should be obtained from beneath the membrane if possible and plated on blood agar, Loeffler blood serum agar, and a selective tellurite-containing medium. A fluorescent antibody technique is available that permits rapid identification of *C. diphtheriae* in a large percentage of cases. Examination of stained smears from diphtheritic lesions is unreliable.

A negative culture does not exclude the possibility of diphtheria, especially if the patient has received prior antibiotic therapy. Group A streptococci are often isolated from diphtheritic lesions. Their presence does not disprove diphtheria but does merit penicillin therapy.

Differential diagnosis. The differential diagnosis of diphtheria varies according to location of the lesion. Nasal diphtheria must be distinguished from ethmoiditis, self-induced ulcerations, and foreign body in the nose. Presence of a diphtheritic membrane and the associated serosanguineous discharge facilitates these distinctions.

Pharyngeal diphtheria must be differentiated from other entities that produce pseudomembranous lesions on the tonsils and pharynx. The diphtheritic membrane is generally darker, tougher, and more adherent than lesions caused by other conditions, such as streptococcal pharyngitis, viral pharyngitis, infectious mononucleosis, and herpetic infection.

Laryngotracheal diphtheria may present greater difficulty in diagnosis, especially when there is no visible pharyngeal or nasal membrane. Conditions to be considered include croup, epiglottitis, acute laryngitis, laryngotracheobronchitis, foreign body, retropharyngeal abscess, and peritonsillar abscess. A carefully taken history and a thorough physical examination usually suffice to differentiate most of these conditions. The most difficult to distinguish is acute laryngotracheobronchitis. If there is any doubt, laryngoscopy, sometimes in conjunction with bronchoscopy, may be necessary. Visualization of the larynx also permits obtaining cultures if a diphtheritic lesion is present. In addition, it furnishes evidence of the degree of subglottic edema, which is often present and may necessitate tracheostomy.

Diagnosis of diphtheria of the skin, vulvovaginal area, umbilicus, and other areas requires knowledge of the appearance of diphtheritic lesions and a sufficiently high index of suspicion to consider that any pseudomembranous lesion, especially if associated with a serosanguineous discharge, may be diphtheritic.

Treatment

Antitoxin. The most important aspect of treatment is early administration of diphtheria antitoxin in amounts sufficient to neutralize circulating exotoxin. Once the exotoxin penetrates the target cell, the antitoxin is no longer effective. Antitoxin dosage is purely empiric. The suggested range for pharyngeal or laryngeal disease of 48 hours duration is 20,000 to 40,000 units; for nasopharyngeal lesions, 40,000 to 60,000 units; for extensive disease of 3 or more days duration or in any patient with brawny swelling of the neck, 80,000 to 120,000 units. After testing for sensitivity (eye, 1:10 dilution or skin, 1:100 dilution) the antitoxin should be given intravenously to neutralize toxin as rapidly as possible. If the patient is sensitive to antitoxin, he should be desensitized.

Antitoxin is probably of no value for cutaneous lesions, but vigorous cleansing with soap and water and topical antimicrobials are recommended. If the condition is severe with punched-out lesions, penicillin or erythromycin should be given systemically.

Hypersensitivity reactions to antitoxin occur in up to 10% of patients (less frequently in children). Accordingly, the physician should have available epinephrine and other agents to counteract severe reactions when antitoxin is administered.

Antibiotics. Antibiotics are not a substitute for antitoxin, but *C. diphtheriae* can be eliminated in up to 95% cases when antibiotics are given for 14 days. Erythromycin may be administered for 14 days in a dosage of 40 mg/kg/24 hr, or procaine penicillin G may be given intramuscularly (300,000 units daily for those less than 9 kg and 600,000 units for those more than 9 kg) for 14 days.

Supportive care. The child should be hospitalized and observed carefully for a minimum of 2 weeks; this period should be extended if there are complications. Daily physical examinations should be performed, especially with reference to the status of the heart. An electrocardiogram should be obtained at the onset of illness and should be repeated at frequent intervals until it has been established that damage to the myocardium is not continuing.

A liquid or soft diet should be offered. Patients who are unable to swallow may be fed by nasogastric tube. In severe cases intravenous fluid administration is indicated. If airway obstruction exists, special caution should be exercised in the use of sedatives that may lessen the child's respiratory efforts.

Immunization. Only about half of those recovering from diphtheria acquire immunity. Therefore immunization with toxoid should be provided.

Complications

Myocarditis. Although congestive heart failure in diphtheritic myocarditis is relatively refractory to treatment, the usual anticongestive measures should be employed. Fluid and salt intake should be restricted, diuretics should be administered and oxygen and sedatives may be required.

Neuritis. Management of neuritis is symptomatic. Palatal paralysis may necessitate use of nasogastric tube feedings. Respiratory paralysis is managed by mechanical ventilation.

Laryngotracheal diphtheria. Because asphyxiation may occur from interference with respiration in laryngotracheal diphtheria, the quality of respiration should be evaluated initially and frequently thereafter. Mild cases, diagnosed and treated early, may need no special therapy other than humidified oxygen. Tracheostomy is indicated, however, when the child becomes increasingly restless and anxious and shows an increasing degree of respiratory distress.

Prevention

Isolation. The patient should be isolated until three negative cultures of involved areas have been obtained at 24- to 48-hour intervals after completion of antibiotic therapy.

Management of persons in contact with patients. Persons in household and similar contact should be examined daily for 7 days for symptoms and signs of early diphtheria. A booster injection should be given to persons who have completed a primary series. Previously immunized persons with positive cultures for *C. diphtheriae* should be treated with penicillin or erythromycin for 7 days and recultured after completion of therapy; they should be retreated if cultures remain positive. Persons who have not received primary immunization with diphtheria toxoid should be treated with antibiotics immediately and immunized; the series should be completed in those individuals who received only a partial series.

Management of carriers. Carriers are healthy individuals who harbor *C. diphtheriae* in the nasopharynx and/or throat. Although *C. diphtheriae* strains isolated from carriers are often nontoxigenic, most authorities agree that all carriers should be treated. A single course of treatment with penicillin or erythromycin eradicates the carrier state in up to 90% of patients. If the organism is not eradicated by the first course of antibiotic, a second course may be administered.

PERTUSSIS (WHOOPING COUGH)

Pertussis, an acute infectious disease of the respiratory tract, is characterized by paroxysms of coughing terminating in an inspiratory whoop.

Etiology and epidemiology

The causative organism is *Bordetella pertussis* (rarely *B. parapertussis*). It is transmitted by direct contact (droplet spread) from a patient with the disease, or indirectly by freshly contaminated articles. The period of infectivity is considered to begin about 1 week after exposure, when the patient is in the catarrhal stage of the disease, and to extend through the first 3 weeks of the paroxysmal stage and sometimes longer. The incubation period is 7 to 14 days.

The newborn infant receives no transplacental passive protection from the mother and is thus vulnerable in the first months of life. Approximately 40% of deaths from the disease occur within the first 5 months of life. The disease is worldwide in distribution and occurs endemically and epidemically. No age is exempt.

Pathologic findings

Pertussis produces an acute catarrhal inflammation of the respiratory tract. The causative bacilli grow among the cilia of the trachea and bronchi and cause necrosis of the midzonal and basilar areas with infiltration of polymorphonuclear cells. Peribronchial infiltration and interstitial pneumonitis occur. Obstruction to smaller air passages is caused by thick, tenacious mucus. This material and inflammatory swelling of the mucosa produce obstruction that leads to patchy areas of emphysema or atelectasis. These obstructive phenomena, along with inflammatory changes and the pulmonary distention incidental to severe paroxysms, may lead to bronchiectasis. Bronchopneumonia may be caused by *B. pertussis* itself or may result from secondary bacterial invasion by common pathogens of the respiratory tract.

In severe cases there may be small focal hemorrhages in the brain, and permanent damage to the brain may result from hypoxia. Subconjunctival hemorrhages can occur because of elevated venous pressure during paroxysms.

Clinical manifestations

The clinical picture of pertussis is divided into three phases: catarrhal, paroxysmal, and convalescent.

Catarrhal stage. The catarrhal stage lasts for 7 to 14 days. Initially symptoms and signs are indistinguishable from those of an ordinary acute upper respiratory tract infection or bronchitis. The child has coryza, sneezing, lacrimation, cough, and slight elevation of temperature. The cough gradually becomes more frequent and paroxysmal.

Paroxysmal stage. A typical paroxysm is

characterized by a rapid succession of explosive coughs during which the child cannot take a breath, followed by a long drawn-out inspiration through the narrowed glottis that produces a high-pitched crowing sound, or whoop. Such paroxysms may occur several times within a few minutes until the child coughs up thick, tenacious mucus. Vomiting often follows the paroxysm. Paroxysms may be of such intensity that at their height the child's face becomes livid or cyanotic, the eyes bulge and are deeply congested, and the tongue protrudes. Immediately after a paroxysm the child may be confused and exhausted. As many as 50 such paroxysms can occur in a 24-hour period. Because of elevated venous pressure during paroxysms, puffiness may develop about the eyes, and conjunctival hemorrhages are not uncommon. Convulsions can occur during paroxysms, apparently caused by hypoxia. Infants may require artificial respiration when the attacks are unusually severe.

Paroxysms often occur spontaneously or may be precipitated by cold air, cold liquids, pressure on the trachea, tobacco smoke, or dust.

This stage of the disease lasts for a variable period. Usually the paroxysms increase in severity for 2 weeks or so, maintain their peak intensity for another week, and then gradually diminish in severity over a period of 1 to 2 weeks.

Convalescent stage. Convalescence is characterized by gradual diminution of cough, cessation of vomiting, return of appetite, gain in weight, and improvement in strength. Intercurrent infections of the respiratory tract may cause a return of paroxysmal coughing during the next weeks or months.

Diagnosis

Differentiation from an acute infection of the upper respiratory tract, or bronchitis, is not difficult in the typical case but may prove puzzling in the catarrhal stage. Since the asymptomatic carrier state occurs rarely, if ever, isolation of the causative organism from a nasopharyngeal culture on Bordet-Gengou medium is diagnostic. The immunofluorescent antibody technique is frequently useful for rapid diagnosis. The white blood cell count and differential count may aid in diagnosis: pertussis characteristically causes leukocytosis with lymphocytosis. Leukocytosis of 20,000 to 30,000 cells/mm^3, with more than 60% lymphocytes, occurs commonly toward the end of the catarrhal stage. Extremely high counts up to 100,000/mm^3 or more may occur.

Because of the pronounced leukocytosis, differentiation from leukemia, infectious lymphocytosis, and various conditions that cause a leukemoid reaction may be required when clinical manifestations of pertussis are atypical or when the paroxysmal stage has not yet begun.

Occasionally in an infant in which vomiting is a prominent feature of pertussis, differentiation from gastroesophageal reflux may be difficult.

Pertussis is not the only entity that may produce paroxysmal coughing. In some instances the physician must consider foreign body in the air passages, enlarged tracheobronchial lymph nodes (usually of tuberculous origin), acute bronchiolitis, bronchopneumonia, and the severe cough sometimes present in patients with cystic fibrosis. Adenoviruses have been associated with a pertussis-like syndrome.

Treatment

Specific therapy. There is no dramatically effective specific therapy for pertussis, but erythromycin administered in a dosage of 50 mg/kg/day for 10 days does shorten the period of communicability. When administered early in the course of pertussis, erythromycin may modify or prevent severe disease. Ampicillin is not effective.

There is no evidence that pertussis immune globulin (human) is efficacious in treating or preventing the disease.

General care. The child should be placed in respiratory isolation from susceptible individuals only until a course of erythromycin therapy has been completed. Patients mildly to moderately affected may be managed at home. Those more severely infected, particularly infants, deserve hospital care. Factors previously mentioned that precipitate paroxysms should be avoided. A well-ventilated room of normal temperature is advisable. Small frequent feedings are preferable to larger amounts taken less often. Nutrition may be better maintained if the child is fed immediately after a severe paroxysm. Maintenance of fluid and electrolyte balance may require parenteral administration, especially when vomiting occurs frequently.

Humidification of inspired air may diminish the viscosity of tenacious secretions and thus facilitate their expectoration. This may be achieved by nebulization with a bedside machine, if the patient does not require oxygen, or in a plastic tent if he does need oxygen. Mechanical suction should be available. During a paroxysm some relief may be obtained by gentle aspiration of obstructive secretions. Excessive sedation may dangerously depress the cough reflex and depth of respiration, thus fostering accumulation of secretions and increasing the risk of occlusion of smaller air passages.

Prevention

Active immunization. Active immunization is discussed in Chapter 11.

Persons exposed to pertussis. Persons exposed to pertussis should receive chemoprophylaxis with erythromycin for a period of 10 days after exposure is ended. Persons under 7 years of age who are exposed to but previously immunized against pertussis should also receive a booster dose of vaccine unless a booster dose was given within the past 6 months.

Jerry Shenep

SALMONELLOSIS (INCLUDING TYPHOID FEVER)

The genus *Salmonella* is divided into three species on the basis of biochemical reactions: *S. typhi* (one serotype), *S. choleraesuis* (one serotype), and *S. enteritidis* (over 1700 serotypes). *Salmonella typhi* seems to be strictly adapted to humans, whereas the other species show no preference between man and a wide variety of animals. *S. enteritidis, S. typhimurium,* and *S. heidelberg* are the most common causes of human salmonellosis. The clinical syndromes of salmonellosis are: gastroenteritis (enterocolitis), enteric fever (typhoid and nontyphoid fever), bacteremia, local infections, and chronic carriage.

Typhoid fever

Typhoid fever is a systemic infection caused by *S. typhi* and characterized by fever, gastrointestinal and systemic manifestations, and at times localized inflammatory lesions.

Etiology and epidemiology

The organism is transmitted by the fecal-oral route. It is acquired most commonly in the United States by direct and indirect contact with chronic carriers. Food handlers who are carriers are particularly dangerous sources of infection. Poor sanitation with inadequate disposal of human feces can result in contamination of food or water. Water-borne typhoid fever is uncommon in the United States but is a major epidemiologic source in underdeveloped countries. The incubation period is 7 to 21 days, usually about 2 weeks. The period of communicability exists as long as the organism is excreted in the stool.

Pathologic findings

Invasion occurs in the upper small bowel where the organism penetrates the mucosa and enters the lymphatics and bloodstream. Phagocytosis takes place, but the organism is not killed and continues to proliferate intracellularly in the reticuloendothelial cells (liver, spleen, bone marrow, and lymph nodes). Secondary invasion of the bloodstream occurs from these sites and probably coincides with the onset of clinical manifestations. Large numbers of organisms are excreted in the bile, causing reinfection of the bowel. Aggregates of lymphoid tissue in the intestinal mucosa (Peyer's patches) become swollen mainly in the lower ileum. Necrosis and ulceration may occur at these sites, producing hemorrhage and perforation. The mesenteric lymph nodes are acutely inflamed. The spleen is deeply congested and often enlarged. Localized infection (often abscesses) can occur, resulting in arthritis, periostitis, osteomyelitis, endocarditis, pneumonitis, meningitis, or pyelonephritis. The myocardium may be damaged by endotoxin liberated by destruction of the organisms. Leukopenia is usually present.

Clinical manifestations

In general, the older the child the more severe and prolonged the manifestations. In the young child the disease is often so mild that it is confused with simple gastroenteritis. Onset of infection is gradual. The disease begins with fever, headache, malaise, anorexia, vomiting, and at times chilly sensations. A nonproductive cough is often present in the early stages. There may be only a few loose stools daily, or diarrhea may be severe enough to cause dehydration and acid-base imbalance. Mild abdominal distention may be noted. Severe abdominal distention with a silent bowel is a manifestation of hypokalemia. The spleen is often enlarged. Rose spots, erythematous maculopapular lesions on the trunk and extremities, are uncommon in children. The average patient is mentally alert, but there may be a variable degree of clouding of the sensorium, which can progress to stupor or coma. Toxic myocarditis, meningitis, arthritis, pneumonitis, osteomyelitis, or urinary tract infection may develop. The usual clinical course lasts 1 to 3 weeks, but relapses sometimes occur. Although infrequent in children, gastrointestinal hemorrhage and intestinal perforation are the most severe life-threatening complications of *S. typhi*.

Diagnosis

Definitive diagnosis rests on isolation of the organism or on serologic tests. Cultures should be obtained from the blood, stool, and urine. The blood culture is positive in approximately 90% of patients in the first week of the disease, 75% in the second week, and 60% in the third week. Stool cultures are positive in about 50% to 60% of cases during the first and second week; they are more frequently positive in the third week.

The serologic agglutination test (Widal) detects the presence of agglutinins against antigens of the causative organism. Of the three antigens—O, H, and Vi—antibodies against the O antigen are the most indicative of present active infection. A titer of 1:160 or higher is considered diagnostic, but demonstration of a rising antibody level in subsequent tests is more conclusive.

In the differential diagnosis one must consider other types of *Salmonella* infection, brucellosis, bacillary dysentery, influenza, malaria, subacute bacterial endocarditis, miliary tuberculosis, infectious mononucleosis, pneumonia, meningitis, and sepsis.

Treatment

Antibacterial therapy. Initial therapy should be intravenous chloramphenicol, 50 to 100 mg/kg/day (maximum 2 g/day), or ampicillin 100 to 200 mg/kg/day. Once the oral intake is adequate, oral antibiotic therapy may be instituted. Amoxicillin, 100 mg/kg/day may be substituted for ampicillin. There is an increasing rate of antibiotic-resistant *Salmonella,* particularly those strains from outside the United States. Antibiotic sensitivities should be performed on all *Salmonella* isolates to ensure appropriate therapy. Antibiotic therapy should be for 14 days. Trimethoprim-sulfamethoxazole (TMP-SMZ) (10 to 12 mg/kg/day TMP, 50 to 60 mg/kg/day SMZ) has been found to be effective therapy for salmonellosis, including *S. typhi*. Cephalosporins, although having in vitro activity against *Salmonella,* have not shown clinical usefulness.

The temperature usually returns to normal about the third day, symptoms abate, and general improvement occurs. About 10% to 20% of patients relapse and can be treated with the same course of therapy.

For the neonate, the dosage of chloramphenicol should not exceed 25 mg/kg/day.

Supportive care. Supportive care is of great importance. Maintenance of adequate fluid and electrolyte balance ranks first in this respect. Liquids and a soft diet are usually tolerated well in the acute stage. The diet should be supplemented as the patient improves. Antipyretic therapy such as with acetaminophen or salicylates should be avoided, as it can produce hypothermia. Tepid sponge baths can be used for fever control. Prednisone, 2 mg/kg/day for 3 to 4 days, may be of benefit in the severely toxic and delirious patient. The routine use of steroids for fever and symptom control is not indicated.

Complications such as gastrointestinal hemorrhage and perforation, or the localized inflammatory manifestations of the disease, are managed along standard lines applicable to the particular circumstance. Local public health regulations must be followed concerning management of convalescent chronic carriers. Chronic carriage is defined as fecal excretion of *Salmonella* for at least 1 year. Children do not become carriers as frequently as adults. Ampicillin (or amoxicillin) or TMP-SMZ (8 mg/kg/day TMP, 40 mg/kg/day SMZ) for 3 to 4 weeks have been used successfully to treat *S. typhi* carriers. Failures are not uncommon.

Nontyphoidal salmonellosis

Nontyphoidal *Salmonella* infections in humans are much more common than typhoid fever and have become a significant public health problem. Many infections are asymptomatic. The most common clinical manifestation is gastroenteritis, although enteric fever, bacteremia, and localized infection can occur.

Epidemiology

Humans usually acquire the infection through contact with infected domestic animals or pets and foods such as poultry, meat, eggs, and milk products. A relatively large inoculum of *Salmonella* organisms (in comparison with *Shigella*) is required to produce clinical manifestations.

Pathologic findings

Pathologic findings are similar to those produced by *S. typhi* except that a polymorphonuclear inflammatory response occurs in the bowel in contrast to the mononuclear response seen in tyhpoid fever.

Clinical manifestations

It should be emphasized again that inapparent infection is common and contributes to difficulties in controlling the spread of this organism.

Gastroenteritis. Gastroenteritis is the most common clinical syndrome of nontyphoidal *Salmonella* infection. The incubation period ranges from several hours to about 3 days. The course may be that of simple, mild diarrhea with low-grade fever, minor systemic manifestations, and no appreciable disturbance of fluid and electrolyte balance. In cases of moderate severity the temperature is higher, and anorexia, nausea, vomiting, abdominal pain, and diarrhea are more intense. The stools may contain pus and blood. Dehydration, acidosis, and other disturbances of electrolyte balance are more likely to occur. In more severe cases all the findings mentioned are present to an increased degree, and the infection may be life threatening. The onset can be explosively abrupt and characterized by severe nausea, vomiting, cramping abdominal pain, fever, and profuse diarrhea. Extreme toxicity, prostration, and shock are possible. The usual picture is mild to moderate gastroenteritis lasting only a few days, often followed by persistently positive stool cultures.

Enteric fever (paratyphoid fever). The paratyphoid syndrome is like typhoid fever but milder, and the course is somewhat shorter. Any of the findings seen in typhoid fever may occur, including rose spots and splenomegaly. The incubation period varies from 1 to 12 days.

Localized infection. A variety of localized infections may occur, accompanying the enteric fever or gastroenteritis, or following a relatively benign bacteremia (with or without fever). These include meningitis, endocarditis, purulent arthritis, osteomyelitis, soft tissue abscesses, pneumonia, and pyelonephritis. Patients with sickle cell disease are particularly likely to develop salmonella osteomyelitis. Chronic carriage of nontyphoidal *Salmonella* is rare in children.

Diagnosis

Definitive diagnosis depends on isolation of the organism. Serologic studies are not particularly valuable in the diagnosis of nontyphoidal salmonellosis. The organisms may be recovered from cultures of the blood, fresh stool, rectal swab, urine, or pus aspirated from local lesions. The differential diagnosis is virtually the same as for typhoid fever.

Treatment

Gastrointestinal *Salmonella* infections usually require only supportive care. Although several antibiotics have been shown to have in vitro activity against *Salmonella* organisms, there is little proof that they shorten the course of the illness, and there is substantial evidence that they prolong the convalescent carrier state. However, when salmonellosis is severe, especially when there is bacteremia and localized infection, and when the patient has chronic gastrointestinal disease, a hemoglobinopathy, or is immunosuppressed, chloramphenicol or ampicillin should be administered. During the first year of life, antibiotic therapy for salmonellosis is often indicated. All *Salmonella* isolates should have antibiotic sensitivities performed because of the increasing rate of resistance. TMP-SMZ is an alternative antibiotic.

Sandor Feldman

SHIGELLOSIS (BACILLARY DYSENTERY)

Shigellosis is an acute infectious disease characterized by fever, abdominal pain, tenesmus, and diarrheal stools. Shigellosis in which diarrheal stools contain mucus, pus, and blood is sometimes referred to as bacillary dysentery.

Etiology and epidemiology

The disease is caused by organisms in the genus *Shigella,* which is divided into four serogroups: *S. dysenteriae, S. flexneri, S. boydii,* and *S. sonnei*. Infections caused by *S. dysenteriae* and *S. boydii* are rare in the United States. The bulk of cases are caused by *S. flexneri* and *S. sonnei*.

The incubation period is 1 to 7 days (usually 3 to 4 days). The mode of transmission is by the fecal-oral route, directly from patients with active disease or asymptomatic carriers or indirectly via contaminated fomites, water, or food. Flies may be vectors. Poor hygiene and crowded living conditions are the most important factors in spread of the disease. Custodial institutions and day-care centers are high-risk settings. All ages may be infected, but the highest attack rate is in the age group 1 through 4 years. There is no immunization available at present.

Pathology and pathogenesis

Shigellosis is essentially a local infection of the colon and the lower ileum. Bacteremia and extraintestinal infections have been reported but are rare. There is an acute inflammation of the mucosa characterized by engorgement of vessels, pinpoint hemorrhages, edema, and outpouring of excessive quantities of mucus. A fibrinopurulent yellow membrane forms on the mucosa, sloughs in a patchy manner, and leaves shallow ulcerations that usually do not affect the submucosa and rarely perforate. They heal by granulation and epithelialization. Inflammatory cellular infiltration of the bowel wall causes it to be thickened. The mesenteric lymph nodes are swollen.

Clinical manifestations

Intensity of clinical manifestations varies, ranging from patients who are virtually asymptomatic to those who are critically ill. *S. dysenteriae* in particular may have a fulminating onset. In general, mild forms of shigellosis outnumber those of moderate or severe degree.

Patients with the mild form are ill only a few days. They have few if any constitutional symptoms; pass only a few stools daily, which may not contain blood, pus, or mucus; and suffer little fluid and electrolyte imbalance.

Shigellosis of moderate severity usually has an abrupt onset with temperature in the range of 39° to 40° C (102° to 104° F), anorexia, vomiting, and abdominal pain. Diarrhea may not appear until 12 to 24 hours or longer after onset of illness. Early in the course the stools are loose to watery in consistency, contain undigested food particles, and are yellow or green. Later the stools become more frequent, 10 or more daily, and contain blood, pus, and mucus. Because of anorexia and vomiting they may contain little food residue. Mucus appears in the stool in abundance—clear, flecked, or streaked with blood. Tenesmus is common and, combined with rapid weight loss and poor muscle tone, may lead to prolapse of the rectum. The untreated child rapidly becomes dehydrated and acidotic, and shock may ensue. Dehydration is manifested by weight loss, poor tissue turgor, dry mucous membranes, sunken eyes, and depressed anterior fontanel. Acidosis may be indicated by Kussmaul respiration. If water is lost out of proportion to electrolytes, hypernatremia will develop. The untreated child or one whose parenteral fluid therapy did not include replacement of large losses of potassium in the diarrheal stools may develop abdominal distention and ileus. In severe cases acute renal failure can occur. Seizures may occur associated with electrolyte disorders or high fever, but seizures may also occur in patients with shigellosis in the absence of fever and electrolyte disturbances. Some strains of *Shigella* produce a toxin capable of inducing seizures, delirium, and nuchal rigidity.

With early diagnosis and treatment, rapid improvement occurs. In untreated disease the acute manifestations ordinarily last 1 to 2 weeks. One or more additional weeks may be required for the stools to return to normal.

The severe form of dysentery is generally caused by *S. dysenteriae,* which is uncommon in the United States. Typically the onset is fulminating. The child has sudden high temperature, may have seizures, and may become delirious, stuporous, or comatose. A stiff neck and positive Kernig and Brudzinski signs may develop, simulating meningitis. The first stool may not appear until many hours or a day or so later, thus multiplying diagnostic difficulties. Abdominal cramping and tenesmus are severe, and the diarrheal stools are explosive.

Shigellosis occasionally progresses to a

chronic form that may last weeks or months. Periods of diarrhea alternate with intervals when the stools are relatively normal. Low-grade fever is common. The child fails to regain weight or may continue to lose weight. Muscle tone is poor. Edema may develop as a result of hypoalbuminemia. Anemia caused by nutritional impairment and infection is common, and vitamin deficiencies may ensue.

Diagnosis

The diagnosis is established by isolation of shigellae from stool or rectal swab cultures or cultures taken from local lesions in the colon via the sigmoidoscope. A methylene blue or Wright-stained smear of the stool may reveal neutrophils and red blood cells; their presence suggests that diarrhea is caused by *Shigella* or other pathogenic bacteria.

Mild cases without blood in the stool and without appreciable cramping or tenesmus must be differentiated by culture. A presumptive diagnosis on clinical grounds is easier in cases of moderate severity. The differential diagnosis includes infection with *Salmonella,* enterotoxigenic *E. coli, Campylobacter, Yersinia,* viruses, and diarrhea of noninfectious etiologies.

Abdominal pain simulating that of appendicitis may occur before the onset of diarrhea. Shigellosis can produce neurologic abnormalities simulating meningitis and necessitating examination of the cerebrospinal fluid. Rare complications of shigellosis include conjunctivitis, nonsuppurative arthritis, vaginitis, intussusception, and bacteremia with metastatic foci of infection.

Treatment

The chief causes of morbidity and mortality in the early stages of shigellosis are dehydration and acidosis. Accordingly, parenteral fluid and electrolyte therapy are the most important aspects of treatment (see Chapter 10).

Drugs that inhibit intestinal peristalsis should not be used, since they do not reduce fluid and electrolyte losses and they may prolong or aggravate clinical illness. Isolation should be continued until stool cultures are negative.

Antimicrobial therapy of shigellosis has been complicated in recent years by an increasing resistance of this organism to previously effective and relatively nontoxic antibiotics. This multiple drug resistance is mediated by resistance-transfer factors. Most shigellae are now resistant to sulfonamides, and many are resistant to ampicillin and tetracycline. Nonabsorbable oral antibiotics have not been proved effective clinically, despite susceptibility by in vitro testing. Resistance to chloramphenicol and TMP-SMZ is not yet a significant problem. Several studies indicate that TMP-SMZ is just as effective clinically and bacteriologically as ampicillin in the treatment of infections caused by susceptible shigellae. Accordingly, TMP-SMZ would seem to be the current drugs of choice for the treatment of shigellosis pending results of in vitro susceptibility tests, especially in areas experiencing a high incidence of ampicillin resistance among shigellae. Asymptomatic individuals who are unlikely to transmit the organism to others need not be treated.

Jerry Shenep

SCARLET FEVER

Scarlet fever is an acute infectious disease caused by group A streptococci that produce erythrogenic toxin. It is characterized by fever, headache, vomiting, sore throat, and rash. A schematic diagram of the clinical course of a typical case is shown in Fig. 27-2. Some of the clinical manifestations and complications are indicated in Fig. 27-3.

Etiology and epidemiology

Strains of group A streptococci that produce erythrogenic toxin are capable of causing scarlet fever. The pathogenesis of the rash caused by the erythrogenic toxin is not completely understood. However, hypersensitivity to the toxin in a previously sensitized individual appears to play a role. Scarlet fever should be viewed as a syndrome of streptococcal pharyngitis with a rash.

Group A streptococci are acquired from infected individuals by direct contact or indirectly by contaminated fomites. The individual transmitting the organism may have a streptococcal infection, usually pharyngitis, or may be an asymptomatic carrier. The incubation period of scarlet fever is generally 2 to 5 days. The period of infectivity lasts until the organism is fully eradicated.

The disease is more common in winter and

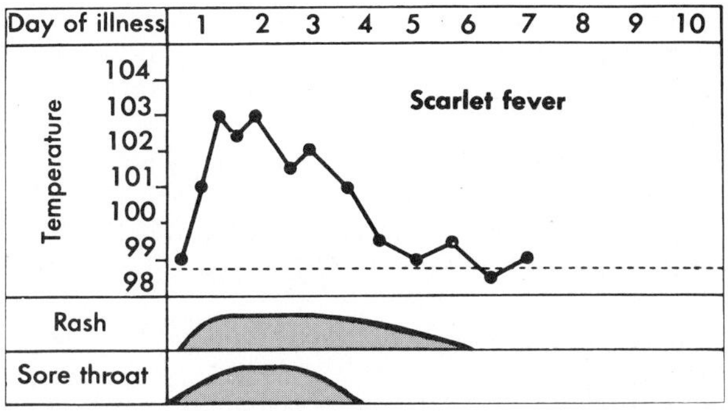

Fig. 27-2. Schematic diagram of a typical case of untreated uncomplicated scarlet fever. Rash usually appears within 24 hours of onset of fever and sore throat. (From Krugman, S., and Katz, S.L.: Infectious diseases of children, ed. 7, St. Louis, 1981, The C.V. Mosby Co.)

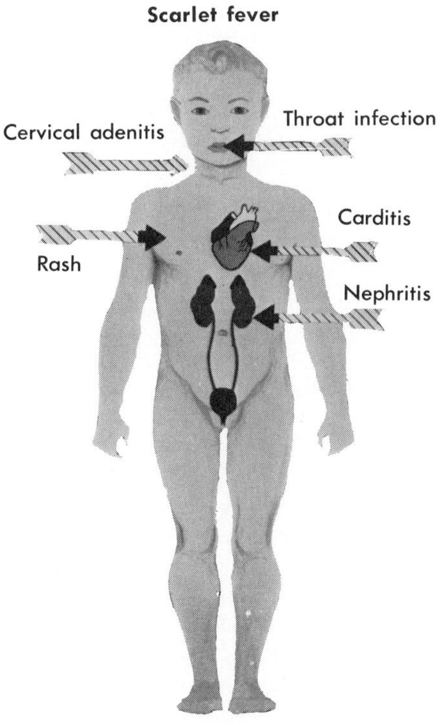

Fig. 27-3. Clinical manifestations and complications of scarlet fever.

spring. It occurs endemically and epidemically. More than 50% of cases appear in children 3 to 8 years of age. Passive immunity, as of yet not completely understood, appears to exist for the first 6 months of life, and the infection is rare in infancy.

Scarlet fever may result from streptococcal wound infection; it is then known as surgical scarlet fever.

Pathologic findings

With the exception of the acute inflammatory changes of the skin, pathologic changes in scarlet fever are like those of any other group A streptococcal infection. Since the portal of entry is usually the pharynx, acute pharyngitis and tonsillitis are common. Although streptococcal pharyngitis may be deceptively mild, in typical cases the pharynx is beefy red and edematous, and the tonsils are acutely inflamed. A follicular tonsillar exudate develops rapidly, spreads, and may coalesce to form a pseudomembrane. The soft palate and uvula are often erythematous and edematous. Punctate petechiae may develop on the soft palate. Regional lymph nodes become enlarged, painful, and tender. Otitis media frequently develops, and the paranasal sinuses are often infected. The infection may extend to involve the larynx and lower respiratory tract. Bacteremia is a rare complication. Postinfectious complications such as rheumatic fever or glomerulonephritis may develop after a latent period of 1 to 3 weeks. Today, when compared to several decades ago, scarlet fever is of a milder nature.

Clinical manifestations

Scarlet fever may be a relatively mild disease, but in the typical case the onset is abrupt with high temperature, headache, vomiting, malaise, sore throat, and abdominal pain from mesenteric lymphadenitis.

The pharyngeal, tonsillar, and palatal lesions have been described previously, and the regional complications of streptococcal pharyngitis (otitis media, cervical lymphadenitis, and paranasal sinusitis) have also been mentioned. The dorsum of the tongue becomes coated and the papillae become red and swollen, giving the appearance of "white strawberry tongue." Within a few days the coating disappears, leaving a shiny red tongue with prominent papillae—"red strawberry tongue."

The rash appears on the first to the third day, reaches full development in 2 days, and lasts approximately 5 days. The eruption consists of diffuse redness that blanches on pressure and superimposed tiny papules. Punctate petechiae may occur in severe cases. The rash begins at the base of the neck and on the chest and axillae. It then spreads to involve most of the body, tends to be less severe on the face, and spares the area around the mouth (circumoral pallor). The antecubital fossa may have a dark red streak, perhaps with pinpoint petechiae (Pasta's sign). As the rash disappears, it fades and eventuates in brawny desquamation. The skin of the palms and soles may peel in large pieces, and in severe cases skin casts of the tips of the fingers may be shed.

Diagnosis

Scarlet fever must be differentiated from other eruptive fevers, especially measles, rubella, exanthem subitum, Kawasaki disease (mucocutaneous lymph node syndrome), allergic reactions, and infectious mononucleosis with a rash. Such distinctions are generally not difficult when one takes into consideration presence of the disease in the community, history of exposure, possible presence of streptococcal infection within the family, details of the clinical picture, positive culture for group A streptococci, and a peripheral leucocytosis with neutrophilia. Demonstration of a rising antistreptolysin (ASO) titer, or titers of other antibodies to streptococci, during convalescence gives retrospective support to the diagnosis.

Treatment

The general care and symptomatic management of a child with scarlet fever is the same as for any child with a group A streptococcal infection. (see pp. 380-381.)

Specific therapy consists of administration of penicillin in sufficient dosage to control the infectious manifestations and maintenance of penicillin levels for a period long enough to eradicate the organism (usually 10 days). In the penicillin-allergic child, erythromycin is the alternate drug of choice.

Sandor Feldman

STAPHYLOCOCCAL INFECTIONS

Staphylococci are gram-positive cocci that occur in clusters. Coagulase-positive strains are classified as *S. aureus* and coagulase-negative strains are classified as *S. epidermidis*. Staphylococci produce several potent exotoxins. Strain differences in exotoxin production are partially responsible for the variety of clinical syndromes produced by staphylococcal infections.

Epidemiology

Colonization with *S. epidermidis* is universal and colonization with *S. aureus* is common (more than 10% of the population). The organism is most commonly spread by direct contact. Several factors predispose to staphylococcal infections: antimicrobial therapy to which the colonizing strain is resistant, foreign bodies including intravenous catheters, wounds, and infections with other bacteria and viruses.

Clinical manifestations

S. aureus produces several distinct clinical syndromes including pyogenic infections, food poisoning, staphylococcal scalded skin syndrome, and toxic shock syndrome. *S. epidermidis* is responsible for bacteremia and meningitis in the immunocompromised host.

Pyogenic infection. *S. aureus* is responsible for a variety of pyogenic infections including impetigo, carbuncles, furuncles, cellulitis, osteomyelitis, septic arthritis, endocarditis, pericarditis, meningitis, lymphadenitis, deep tissue abscesses, and pneumonia. Abscess formation is typical. Fever and local inflammation may be severe. Bacteremia usually occurs secondary to a focal infection, although the focal infection may be minor. This fact emphasizes the importance of proper management of focal infections.

Food poisoning. Ingestion of improperly refrigerated food contaminated with enterotoxin-producing staphylococci may result in food poisoning. The illness usually occurs within 7 hours of ingestion. Vomiting and diarrhea with low-grade or absent fever is characteristic.

Staphylococcal scalded skin syndrome (SSSS). Several forms of SSSS have been described. The most severe form is characterized by generalized bullous desquamation of large areas of the skin. The term *Ritter disease* has been used to refer to this syndrome in infants. SSSS is difficult to distinguish clinically from toxic epidermal necrolysis (TEN), a disease that usually occurs in adults. TEN is not associated with staphylococcal infection, is usually drug-induced, and is pathologically distinct from SSSS. In TEN, the entire epidermis is damaged, in contrast to localization of damage to the superficial layers of the epidermis in SSSS.

Localized forms of SSSS also occur. Bullous impetigo usually is localized to the periumbilical or perineal areas, or other moist areas of young children. Bullous impetigo also occurs in conjunction with varicella (bullous varicella). In this form bullous lesions may occur wherever varicella lesions are located.

Staphylococci may occasionally produce a rash indistinguishable from that of scarlet fever.

Toxic shock syndrome (TSS). TSS is a newly recognized syndrome characterized by fever, erythematous macular rash (sunburn-like) with subsequent desquamation (especially of the finger tips and toes), hypotension, and variable occurrence of mucous membrane inflammation, diarrhea, renal dysfunction, liver dysfunction, cardiopulmonary dysfunction, leukocytosis with left shift and central nervous system dysfunction (delirium or hallucinations). The syndrome appears to be caused by the absorption of an exotoxin elaborated by some strains of *S. aureus*. Blood cultures are negative, but *S. aureus* is usually isolated from the nares, throat, vagina, rectum, or from a focal infection such as a cutaneous abscess or pleural effusion. Most cases have occurred in conjunction with the use of tampons, but TSS also occurs in males and in children.

Diagnosis

The diagnosis of the various staphylococcal syndromes is suspected on clinical grounds and is confirmed by Gram-stain and culture of purulent tissue, blood, cerebrospinal fluid or, in the case of SSSS and TSS, by surface culture. The diagnosis of staphylococcal food poisoning depends on demonstration of the organism in contaminated food.

Treatment

Staphylococcal pyogenic infections should receive prompt attention. Since relatively few strains of *S. aureus* are sensitive to penicillin, a penicillinase-resistant penicillin such as methicillin or oxacillin is usually employed in the initial therapy. In certain medical centers, infections with methicillin-resistant *S. aureus* have become common enough to warrant use of vancomycin for patients with suspected nosocomial infection. The dose, route, and duration of therapy depends on the clinical setting. As a general rule, an abscess must be drained for resolution of the infection.

Staphylococcal food poisoning is managed by supportive care.

SSSS should be managed with supportive care and systemic antimicrobial therapy. Since only the superficial layers of the epidermis are affected, complete resolution generally occurs.

TSS requires intensive supportive care. Systemic antibiotic therapy should be employed. Prompt removal of foreign bodies and drainage of abscesses with extensive saline irrigation of the involved area may prevent further absorption of exotoxin.

The therapy of *S. epidermidis* infections must be guided by the antibiotic sensitivities of the isolate. Vancomycin has proved to be among the most effective of antibiotics.

All patients with draining lesions containing *S. aureus* should be placed on wound isolation. Also patients with SSSS and TSS should be placed on wound isolation to prevent spread of the responsible exotoxin-producing staphylococcal strains.

Jerry Shenep

TETANUS

Tetanus is a preventable disease caused by *Clostridium tetani,* an anaerobic spore-bearing organism. It is characterized by muscular rigidity, paroxysmal spasms, and respiratory difficulties.

Etiology and epidemiology

Four factors are involved in the development of tetanus: (1) presence of tetanus spores, (2) injury to tissues, (3) conditions in the wound suitable for multiplication of anaerobic organisms, and (4) susceptibility of the patient. Tetanus spores are widespread in nature. They are passed in the feces of herbivorous animals and commonly exist in the soil of barnyards and farms. However, they also contaminate the soil of cities. Human feces may contain the organism. So ubiquitous is *C. tetani* that one must assume that most wounds, however trivial, may have been contaminated by *C. tetani* spores.

Tetanus spores enter the body through wounds and, if conditions are favorable, elaborate two exotoxins: (1) tetanospasmin, responsible for clinical manifestations, and (2) tetanolysin. Puncture wounds and penetrating injuries, especially those causing devitalization of tissue, afford ideal anaerobic conditions, particularly when foreign bodies are present. Tetanus spores may enter the body through a wound small enough to attract little or no attention.

Clinical manifestations

The incubation period averages 8 days but may vary from 3 days to 3 weeks. Extensive and massively contaminated injuries favor a short incubation period. As a general rule, the shorter the incubation period, the more severe the clinical manifestations.

The manner of onset varies. The first manifestations are usually tightness and tenseness of jaw muscles. In other instances muscles of the neck, back, abdominal wall, or extremities are first affected. Headache, backache, restlessness, apprehensiveness, and difficulty in opening the mouth constitute a fairly typical picture at onset. The slightest noise or the gentlest touch may elicit muscular spasms lasting several seconds. Contractions of facial muscles produce the called sardonic smile (risus sardonicus). The neck becomes extremely stiff, the back arches into opisthotonos, the abdominal wall is boardlike, the extremities are tensely extended, and the fists are clenched. There is sweating, rapid pulse rate, anxious expression, and complete mental clarity. Eventually the muscles maintain a more or less constant state of rigidity.

The severe spasms may involve muscles of respiration and the larynx, sometimes proving fatal. Muscular contractions may be so intense as to cause compression fractures of the thoracic vertebrae.

Pulmonary complications (atelectasis and pneumonia) are rather frequent in tetanus.

As the patient recovers, paroxysmal seizures occur less and less frequently, muscular rigidity subsides gradually, and the need for sedation is correspondingly reduced. Full disappearance of muscular rigidity may require weeks.

Diagnosis

The manifestations of tetanus are so distinctive that there is usually little difficulty in diagnosis. Local conditions impairing ability to open the mouth may simulate the trismus of tetanus: peritonsillar abscess, severe dental infections, mumps, and arthritis of the temporomandibular joint. In early stages differentiation from meningitis may require examination of cerebrospinal fluid. Neonatal manifestations of brain injury or developmental defect may cause stiffening spasms like those of tetanus, but circumstances of labor and delivery and many other features aid in differentiation. Phenothiazine toxicity may cause tetanic-like spasms with opisthotonos, but concomitant presence of oculogyric crises, relaxation of muscles between spasms, and the dulled sensorium from overtranquilization aid in differentiation. Hypocalcemic tetany of the newborn infant or of an older infant is easily distinguished by chemical findings and the presence of carpopedal spasm.

Treatment

Therapy may be considered from the standpoint of prevention and active management.

Prevention. All individuals should be actively immunized against tetanus by toxoid injections. Reinforcing booster injections should be given at periodic intervals (see p. 191). When an individual sustains a tetanus-prone injury, it is essential to cleanse the wound thoroughly, remove any foreign material that might be present, and débride the wound carefully to remove necrotic tissue that might favor an anaerobic environment.

Despite the well-known need for universal immunization against tetanus, many individuals have never been immunized or have lapsed immunity through failure to receive booster injections. It is not always a simple matter to know what action to take at the time of injury. Guidelines are presented in Table 27-1 for tetanus prophylaxis in wound management.

When tetanus immune globulin (human) (TIG) is employed for wound prophylaxis, the recommended dosage is 250 to 500 units intra-

Table 27-1. Guide for tetanus prophylaxis in wound management

History of tetanus immunization (doses)	Clean, minor wounds		All other wounds	
	Td*	TIG†	Td	TIG
Uncertain	Yes	No	Yes	Yes
0-1	Yes	No	Yes	Yes
2	Yes	No	Yes	No‡
3 or more	No§	No	No‖	No

From Report of the Committee on Infectious Diseases, Evanston, Ill., 1982, American Academy of Pediatrics.
*Tetanus and diphtheria toxoids.
†Tetanus immune globulin.
‡Unless wound is more than 24 hours old.
§Unless more than 10 years since the last dose.
‖Unless more than 5 years since the last dose.

muscularly. If TIG is not available, tetanus antitoxin (equine or bovine) (TAT) should be employed at a dosage of 3000 to 5000 units intramuscularly, after testing for sensitivity.

Active treatment

Specific. TIG should be employed, if available, at a dosage of 500 to 7000 units intramuscularly. The optimum weight-adjusted dosage for infants and young children has not been established. It has been recommended that a portion of the dose be infiltrated around the wound. If TIG is not available, TAT is recommended in a dosage of 50,000 to 100,000 units (with a portion of the dose administered intravenously). Dosages as low as 10,000 units have been found to be effective in children. Sensitivity testing should be performed before administration of TAT. However, the results of such testing are not entirely reliable, and the possibility of a serious reaction should always be anticipated when TAT is administered.

If the wound source is apparent, it should be opened and débrided. Penicillin G kills the vegetative forms of *C. tetani* and should be administered in therapeutic dosages for 7 to 10 days to terminate further exotoxin production.

Nonspecific. The patient should be placed in a quiet, darkened room, and sensory stimuli should be reduced to a minimum. Constant nursing care is mandatory. Treatment of tonic spasms and seizures requires agents that (1) reduce sensory input and central nervous system excitability, (2) lower reflex activity and decrease motor output, and (3) inhibit transmission of excess motor-nerve activity to effector muscles. Short-acting barbiturates, phenothiazine drugs, and diazepam are commonly used for these purposes. When the disease is severe and when adequate facilities for artificial respiration are available, neuromuscular blocking agents are often employed. In the management of severe cases of tetanus it is advisable, when possible, to have an anesthesiologist skilled in maintenance of respiration on the treatment team.

TUBERCULOSIS

Tuberculosis is a chronic infectious disease characterized by an extremely variable clinical course. Both *Mycobacterium tuberculosis* and *M. bovis* are pathogenic for humans. However, *M. bovis* infection is uncommon in the United States. Both the incidence of tuberculosis and the death rate because of the disease have decreased dramatically in developed countries since 1900. The decline was apparent before the introduction of chemotherapy and was largely the result of improved living conditions. However, the decline accelerated with the introduction of antimicrobial therapy, and by 1970 the death rate for children in the United States was 0.3 per 100,000 population. Unfortunately, the number of new active cases has not decreased as rapidly as the death rate. In 1974 there were more than 30,000 new active cases reported in the United States; approximately 1200 cases occurred in children under 5 years of age.

Epidemiology

Most children who contract tuberculosis first become infected in their lungs. The disease is usually contracted by droplet infection, the source generally being some person in close contact with the child. The source is usually a tuberculous adult. The younger the child, the more likely he is to have contracted his infection from someone in frequent close contact.

Predisposing factors. Evidence suggests that differences in tuberculosis attack rates result from differences in socioeconomic status and living conditions rather than racial factors. Age has a strong influence on the disease. Infants more commonly develop progressive extension of the initial lesion in the lung, miliary tuberculosis, and tuberculous meningitis. During puberty and adolescence there is an increased tendency to develop chronic pulmonary tuberculosis caused by endogenous reinfection. During adolescence girls more commonly develop chronic pulmonary tuberculosis than do boys. Immunosuppressive drugs and corticosteroids may facilitate the development of reinfection (chronic) tuberculosis.

Terminology

The current terminology for pulmonary tuberculosis refers to initial (primary) infection and reinfection (chronic) tuberculosis. Children who have acquired initial infection early in life may develop chronic tuberculosis long before the adult years, and to an increasing degree individuals are reaching young adulthood before developing initial infection. When progression of the disease develops after an initial tuberculous infection is considered under control, one speaks of exogenous reinfection if new organisms have gained entry and of endogenous reinfection if protective barriers are broken down and the original lesion spreads.

Pathogenesis

In the initial infection, tubercle bacilli enter the lungs and establish a site of infection called the initial focus. Although host defenses in the lung respond to the initial infection, some organisms reach regional (hilar) lymph nodes through the lymphatics, and others reach distant organs (liver, spleen, kidneys, bones, central nervous system, etc.) by the hematogenous route. The pulmonary parenchymal lesion (initial focus), the subsequent lymphangitis, and the resultant hilar adenopathy together compose the primary complex. The sequence is the same when initial infection occurs in any other body site. The initial focus usually heals. The regional adenopathy also heals steadily in the usual case.

Infants have much less capacity to contain the initial tuberculous infection (Fig. 27-4), and a progressive initial focus may develop. The infection may spread via blood vessels or lymphatics, causing massive hematogenous dissemination (miliary tuberculosis), or it may erode into a bronchial lumen and by bronchogenic dissemination produce extensive tuberculous bronchopneumonia.

Clinically silent tuberculous foci in various organs that resulted from initial hematogenous dissemination may not always remain silent. If the immune status of the host is compromised, these lesions may progress and cause clinical manifestations. An example is the development of tuberculous meningitis from rupture of the contents of a small focus into the ventricular system or into the subarachnoid space.

The child's subsequent response to the organism is governed to some degree by hypersensitivity to the protein fraction of the tubercle bacillus that develops as a consequence of initial infection. The hypersensitivity response is ac-

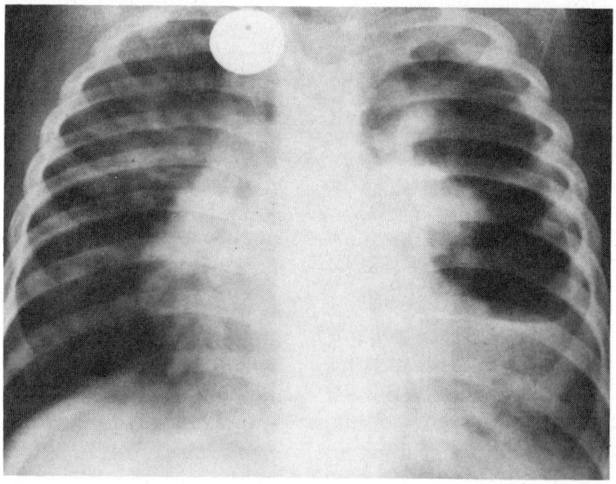

Fig. 27-4. Infant with advanced pulmonary tuberculosis. Note widespread nodular infiltrate, left hilar adenopathy, and left pleural effusion. (Courtesy Dr. W. Webster Riggs, Le Bonheur Children's Medical Center, Memphis.)

celerated when reinfection occurs and tends to localize the organisms at the site of entry and prevent lymphatic progression. Accordingly, reinfection (chronic) pulmonary tuberculosis usually remains a pulmonary disease.

Clinical manifestations

Tuberculosis may exist without clinical manifestations, or it may cause signs and symptoms ranging over a broad spectrum of intensity. These findings may be of a general nature—fever, malaise, anorexia, and weight loss—or they may be related to the site of infection—the lungs, brain, kidneys, bones, and so on.

Initial (primary) tuberculosis. In the initial pulmonary infection host defenses are usually able to limit the infection after it has caused a small parenchymal lesion, lymphangitis, hilar adenopathy, and subsequent minimal hematogenous dissemination. In the 2 to 10 weeks required for the development of tuberculin hypersensitivity, the child may not appear ill. With the development of tuberculin hypersensitivity there may be fever, and, rarely, erythema nodosum or phlyctenular conjunctivitis. Investigation reveals a positive tuberculin test. In an infant the chest radiographs might reveal an infiltrative lesion and enlargement of the hilar glands (without cough or abnormal physical findings). In an older child the radiograph is often normal. Initial tuberculosis is usually insidious in onset and clinically occult.

The child, usually an infant, who is unable to limit the spread of the parenchymal lesion develops a progressive initial focus. He exhibits persistent fever, malaise, anorexia, pallor, anemia, weakness, and weight loss. However, extensive tuberculous lesions often produce minimal abnormal physical findings. Cough may or may not be present.

In initial tuberculosis, hilar glandular involvement is constant and tends to be excessive in relation to the usual small size of the parenchymal lesion. With the passage of time the glands generally decrease in size, residual calcification being the only permanent evidence of involvement. Occasionally the tuberculous hilar glands cause clinical difficulty by pressure on or extension of infection into contiguous structures (Fig. 27-5). Infants and young children are more disposed to these complications than are older children.

Clinical manifestations of bronchial involvement depend on the degree to which air exchange is embarrassed. Expiratory wheezing may be the first and only sign, although a paroxysmal brassy cough may be present. Later, emphysema may occur distal to luminal narrowing. When the obstruction becomes more complete, atelectasis occurs. Finally, bronchiectasis tends to develop in the atelectatic area.

Reinfection (chronic) pulmonary tubercu-

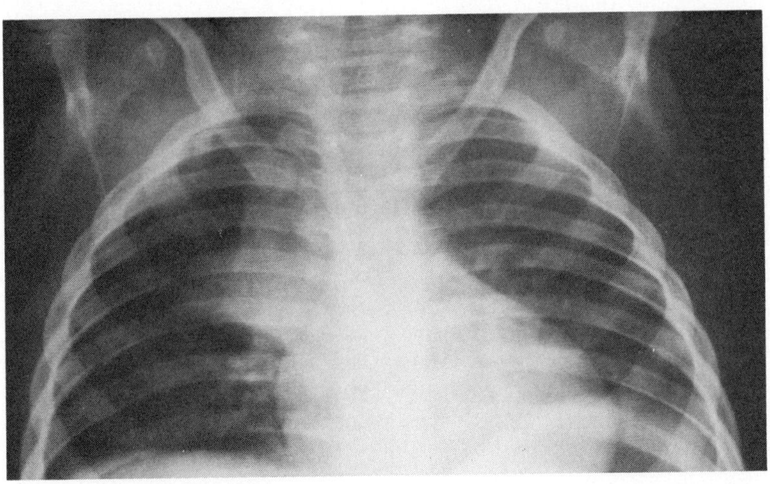

Fig. 27-5. Tuberculosis. Note large right hilar lymph node and atelectasis of right upper lobe. (Courtesy Dr. W. Webster Riggs, Le Bonheur Children's Medical Center, Memphis.)

losis. Chronic tuberculosis may be of exogenous origin, but it is usually endogenous (extension of a previous initial lesion). Clinical manifestations of these two types of reinfection are identical, but there is obvious need to search for a new tuberculous contact in case the reinfection is exogenous in origin.

The pathologic pattern of reinfection tuberculosis differs from that of the initial form. The pathologic changes have a predilection for the apex, greater tendency to cavitation, and little or no hilar glandular enlargement.

Clinical manifestations vary. The child may have only minimal symptoms such as low-grade unexplained fever and malaise. With more extensive progression temperature increases, malaise becomes more intense, anorexia and weight loss ensue, anemia develops, and cough and chest pain may occur. Hemoptysis does not occur as commonly in children as in adults.

If the parenchymal lesion is small, there may be no abnormal physical findings. If it is somewhat larger, chest findings have more tendency to be abnormal.

Tuberculous pleurisy. A pleural effusion must be considered tuberculous until proved otherwise. In view of the fact that cultures of the pleural fluid are often negative for tubercle bacilli, the physician must depend on a positive tuberculin test and a distinctive radiograph or one highly suggestive of tuberculosis to establish the diagnosis.

Clinical manifestations vary according to extent of the effusion and nature of the underlying pulmonary lesion. The effusion often develops about a year or so after the primary infection.

Miliary tuberculosis. Massive hematogenous dissemination produces miliary tuberculosis. Miliary tuberculosis occurs chiefly in infants and young children. It usually appears 6 to 12 months after primary infection. It often develops without antecedent evidence of tuberculous disease; less commonly it follows known infection. Tuberculous meningitis may accompany miliary tuberculosis and early signs of concomitant meningitis may be masked by those of miliary tuberculosis.

Early clinical manifestations may be limited to irritability, anorexia, fever, and malaise. Fever may be sustained but more often is intermittent. Polymorphonuclear leukocytosis may be present. The course is steadily downhill, with increasing toxemia, fever, prostration, and weight loss. The spleen frequently enlarges, as may the liver and peripheral lymph nodes. Respiratory manifestations are lacking in the first week or two, but then the child may develop tachypnea and fine crepitant rales.

Diagnosis may be difficult in the initial stages: clinical findings resemble those of many other

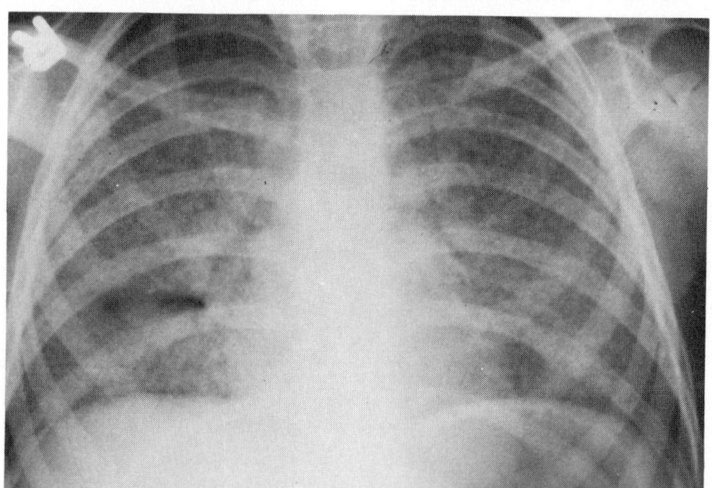

Fig. 27-6. Miliary tuberculosis. Note homogeneous distribution of multiple small nodules. (Courtesy Dr. W. Webster Riggs, Le Bonheur Children's Medical Center, Memphis.)

diseases. If the physician knows that the infant or young child formerly had primary tuberculosis, suspicion of the presence of miliary tuberculosis is increased. If a tuberculin test is applied and found to be positive, it would also strongly suggest the diagnosis. After the disease has been present 2 to 3 weeks, fine granular densities occur in a generalized pattern throughout both lung fields. These lesions begin to enlarge, and the radiograph reveals the so-called snowstorm appearance (Fig. 27-6). Death occurs in 4 to 8 weeks, unless specific therapy is applied early and vigorously.

Tuberculous meningitis. Tuberculous meningitis is one of the most serious complications of tuberculosis. It usually originates within a year after the initial infection but may have its onset much later. Meningitis may occur as a complication of miliary tuberculosis.

Clinical manifestations. Although there may be imperceptible transition from one stage to another as the disease progresses, it is traditional to speak of three phases: (1) the prodromal stage of invasion with nonspecific symptoms, (2) the stage of clear-cut meningeal manifestations, and (3) the terminal stage of paralysis, coma, and death.

First (prodromal) stage. The onset may be so insidious that diagnosis remains in doubt for 1 to 2 weeks. Nonspecific symptoms include irritable disposition, drowsiness, restless sleep, loss of appetite, constipation, abdominal pain, low-grade fever, headache, and perhaps vomiting.

Second (meningeal) stage. As the disease progresses, classic signs of meningeal irritation develop, including stiff neck and back, positive Kernig, Brudzinski, and Babinski signs, bulging of the anterior fontanel, and exaggeration of deep tendon reflexes. The sensorium is clouded, temperature increases, and vomiting becomes more frequent. Examination of eyegrounds reveals papilledema and in some instances peripherally located pathognomonic choroidal tubercles. Cranial nerve palsies may appear, always suggestive of tuberculosis in the clinical setting of meningitis. Muscle twitching, tremors, and paralysis of one or more extremities may occur. If untreated, the second stage lasts about 7 to 10 days.

Third (terminal) stage. Stupor progresses to coma. The pupils become dilated and fixed, the corneal reflex is absent, deep tendon reflexes disappear, emaciation and scaphoid abdomen are notable, and irregular respiration develops.

Tuberculous adenitis. Although tuberculosis involves regional glands wherever primary infection begins, the term *tuberculous adenitis* is usually reserved for disease of the superficial glands. Cervical glandular involvement is the most common form, but is now rare in the United States. Cervical nodes may be infected by hematogenous dissemination or as a result of primary invasion of the tonsil or other area of the pharynx. Several glands are generally involved, preference being exhibited for the deeper chains. As a rule the glands enlarge to a moderate degree and remain enlarged for a long while without producing other symptoms. Caseation necrosis with subsequent calcification is common. The glands may enlarge, adhere to each other, and form irregular nodular masses. The infection approaches the skin, which becomes dusky red and thin. Finally, rupture occurs, and there is a thick discharge and a chronic draining sinus with subsequent disfiguring scarring.

Diagnosis involves differentiation from disorders such as atypical mycobacterial adenitis, pyogenic adenitis, lymphoma, leukemia, tularemia, and actinomycosis. Presence of a positive tuberculin test points toward, but does not prove, a diagnosis of tuberculous adenitis. If calcification is revealed in a radiograph of the neck, the diagnosis of tuberculosis is greatly strengthened. At times the physician must resort to biopsy and culture.

Diagnostic tests and procedures

Tuberculin test. Initial infection initiates development of hypersensitivity to the protein fraction of the tubercle bacillus, first detectable 2 to 10 weeks later by a positive reaction to tuberculin.

The tuberculin test is the single most important test to determine whether a child or adult has been infected with the tubercle bacillus. Unless there is a probability of earlier exposure to tuberculosis, it should be performed first at 6 to 12 months of age, before routine immunization against measles. Although the Committee on Infectious Diseases of the American Academy of Pediatrics (1982) recommends *routine* tuberculin testing when an infant is 12 months old and every one to two years thereafter, frequency of testing also depends on risk of exposure and prevalence of tuberculosis in the population. Knowledge that the child's test has converted from negative to positive permits the early institution of isoniazid therapy and hopefully prevents extension of the initial infection. Any child or adolescent who at any time is shown to have a positive tuberculin test should be treated with isoniazid for a period of 1 year, whether or not the test is known to have recently converted from negative to positive.

Purified protein derivative tuberculin (PPD) has virtually replaced old tuberculin (OT) in the United States. The U.S. Reference Standard PPD (PPD-S) was prepared by Seibert in 1939 and adopted as the international standard tuberculin by the World Health Organization in 1952. The standard dose of PPD tuberculin is 5 tuberculin units (TU) in 0.1 ml of Tween stabilized solution. There are a number of techniques for administration of PPD, but the Mantoux is the most accurate test. Multiple puncture tests (tine, Heaf, Applitest, Mono-vacc, etc.) should be considered as screening procedures rather than diagnostic tests.

The volar surface of the forearm is the preferred site for testing. The Mantoux test is read as follows at 48 to 72 hours:

1. Erythema without induration—negative
2. Induration less than 5 mm—negative
3. Induration greater than 5 mm but less than 10 mm—doubtful (repeat at a different site)
4. Induration greater than 10 mm—positive

A negative reaction to tuberculin testing usually means that the individual has never been infected with the tubercle bacillus. However, reactions may be falsely negative, and it is important to recognize the circumstances under which this may occur:

1. Intercurrent diseases (rubeola, varicella, etc., may suppress the tuberculin reaction for as long as 4 weeks)
2. Viral vaccines (vaccines for rubeola, etc., may also suppress the reaction for about 4 weeks)
3. Corticosteroids and immunosuppressive agents
4. Cellular immune deficiency diseases
5. Severe malnutrition
6. Overwhelming tuberculous infection
7. Testing too early
8. Impotent testing material
9. Faulty technique

Studies indicated when the tuberculin test is positive. When the tuberculin test is first found to be positive, a search should be made for the source and the child should be evaluated as to the status of the disease. If a pulmonary infiltrative lesion is detected by radiography, gastric washings should be performed in an attempt to culture the tubercle bacillus. Other studies may be indicated when it is thought that the tuberculous lesion may be elsewhere (kidneys, bone, etc.).

Members of the family, and other close contacts should have a carefully taken physical history, a physical examination, a chest radiograph, and/or a tuberculin test.

Identification of the tubercle bacillus by smear or culture. It is best to rely on cultures to make a firm diagnosis of tuberculosis. If the child with pulmonary infection is producing sputum, this may be cultured. If not, an aerosol-induced sputum may prove useful in the child old enough to cooperate. In a child of any age gastric washings can be obtained for examination. Early in the morning before breakfast a tube is passed into the stomach, and the contents are aspirated and placed in a sterile container. The stomach is then lavaged with sterile water, these washings are aspirated and added to the material in the container, and cultures are then performed. When tuberculous meningitis is suspected, the centrifuged sediment of the cerebrospinal fluid should be examined for tubercle bacilli, with the Ziehl-Neelsen or Kinyoun stain, or specimens of sediment should be stained with auramine-rhodamine and examined with ultraviolet light for fluorescence. The cerebrospinal fluid should also be cultured, of course, but treatment should be instituted immediately on clinical grounds and should not be postponed until the results of the culture are reported.

Radiographic studies. Radiographic studies may support the opinion that the child has pulmonary or osseous tuberculosis. However, similar radiographic findings are present in other diseases. Therefore caution should be exercised in interpretation of x-ray studies, and the diagnosis should not be made on this evidence alone, especially when the tuberculin test is negative.

Biopsy. Biopsy is infrequently required for diagnosis of tuberculosis. However, when the tuberculin test is positive, when there is no discharge to be cultured, and when the diagnosis of tuberculosis is still doubtful, biopsy of accessible lesions may establish a definite diagnosis. This would apply to a primary ulcerated skin lesion, other skin manifestations of tuberculosis, and sometimes to a cervical lymph gland.

Treatment

General care. Patients with asymptomatic initial infection can be managed as outpatients and require no restrictions of activity except avoidance of competitive sports during the active stage of disease. They should receive all immunizations, including rubeola vaccine (with isoniazid prophylaxis for 6 weeks).

Febrile children with more severe disease should be kept at bed rest and gradually allowed to walk following defervescence. Those with complications should be hospitalized until afebrile and until their condition has stabilized to the point where home care is possible. Isolation is necessary only for the duration of contagion, which in the usual case is relatively brief. Children with initial infection are seldom, if ever, contagious. The patient with chronic tuberculosis is contagious only so long as the sputum is positive for *M. tuberculosis* and significant coughing is present.

Chemotherapy. Asymptomatic initial tuberculosis (including tuberculin conversions) should be treated with isoniazid daily for a period of at least a year. The recommended dosage of isoniazid for this purpose is 10 to 20 mg/kg/24 hr (maximum 300 mg), administered as a single dose. Isoniazid is also used alone when chemoprophylaxis is required in a patient known to have had previous tuberculosis (measles, measles vaccine, corticosteroid therapy, etc.). Toxic effects of this drug include hepatotoxicity, peripheral neuritis, and toxic encephalopathy. Hepatotoxicity is rare in children. Peripheral neuritis in children has been reported only in association with accidental poisoning. Toxic encephalopathy is rare and is rapidly reversible with withdrawal of the drug.

Combined drug therapy is recommended, at least initially, for all symptomatic and/or complicated tuberculosis. Combined therapy is used for two reasons—to hasten bacteriologic conversion and to delay or prevent development of drug resistance. Triple drug therapy is seldom if ever necessary. Combined therapy with isoniazid and rifampin is recommended for initial therapy of all forms of tuberculosis except asymptomatic initial infection (treated with isoniazid alone). Rifampin has practically replaced streptomycin in the therapy of tuberculosis in children. In mild disease rifampin is sometimes discontinued and isoniazid administered alone, when acute illness has subsided and cultures have converted to negative. When prolonged therapy is required for severe or complicated disease, another drug may be substituted for rifampin after a variable period of initial therapy. Chemotherapeutic agents in this category, which are used to delay development of resistance, include para-aminosalicylic acid (PAS), ethambutol, and ethionamide.

Rifampin toxicity is rare in children. Transient abnormalities of liver function, as well as nausea and vomiting, have been reported. An orange-red color may be noted in the stool, urine, and other secretions of patients receiving the drug. Rifampin is administered in a single daily dose of 10 to 20 mg/kg (maximum 600 mg).

Para-aminosalicylic acid is generally poorly tolerated by children because of its gastrointestinal side effects. It is used solely to delay emergence of drug resistance. The recommended dosage is 200 to 300 mg/kg/24 hr in 2 to 4 doses.

Ethambutol is gradually replacing PAS in the treatment of older children and adults. The major toxic side effect of this drug is retrobulbar neuritis. Accordingly, it should not be used in children (under the age of 6 years) who cannot be tested reliably for visual acuity and color blindness. Ethambutol is administered in a dosage of 25 mg/kg/24 hr for 2 months and then 15 mg/kg for the duration of therapy. Monthly ophthalmologic examination should be performed.

Ethionamide is relatively well tolerated by children, although gastrointestinal side effects and hepatotoxicity have been reported. The recommended dosage is 20 to 30 mg/kg/24 hr (maximum 500 to 1000 mg) in three doses.

Other drugs available for the treatment of drug-resistant tuberculosis include kanamycin, viomycin, pyrazinamide, and cycloserine. The only generally accepted indications for corticosteroid therapy in tuberculosis are actual or impending block in tuberculous meningitis and respiratory distress in tuberculous endobronchitis. Surgical procedures are seldom necessary in the treatment of tuberculosis in children.

Immunization. BCG immunization is indicated only when contact with active tuberculosis cannot be avoided in the family or community. Accordingly, this procedure is rarely necessary in the United States. BCG should not be given to individuals with comprised immune status caused by underlying disease or immunosuppressive drug therapy.

INFECTIONS WITH UNCLASSIFIED MYCOBACTERIA (ATYPICAL MYCOBACTERIA)

Unclassified mycobacteria are organisms morphologically similar to *Mycobacterium tuberculosis* but distinguishable by laboratory methods. In humans these organisms may produce infection that simulates tuberculosis. Furthermore, such infection may result in cross-reaction to tuberculin solution derived from *M. tuberculosis,* generally causing a tuberculin reaction from 5 to 9 mm in diameter. Thus, when an individual has a tuberculin reaction of less than 10 mm induration, infection with unclassified mycobacteria should be suspected. If a repeat tuberculin test is also equivocal, the individual should be tested with tuberculin solution prepared from these organisms.

Unclassified mycobacteria causing disease in humans are usually grouped according to the Runyon classification:

Group I	Photochromogens (*M. Kansasii, M. marinum*)
Group II	Scotochromogens (*M. scrofulaceum*)
Group III	Nonphotochromogens (Battey bacillus, (*M. avium*—intracellulare)
Group IV	Rapid growers (*M. fortuitum*)

Infection with unclassified mycobacteria has been reported from many areas of the world. In the United States such infections occur more frequently in the southeastern states, particularly those bordering the Gulf of Mexico. They have also been reported from the central and southwestern states. Transmission from one person to another has not been demonstrated.

Pathologic changes in tissues are almost identical with those caused by *M. tuberculosis.*

Clinical manifestations greatly resemble those of tuberculosis. In children the principal lesion is lymphadenitis, particularly of the cervical nodes. In most areas of the United States granulomatous lymphadenitis is more often caused by unclassified mycobacteria than by the tubercle bacillus. Cervical lymphadenitis is generally submandibular and unilateral. General manifestations of illness are usually absent. There is no history of tuberculous contact in associates or family, the chest radiograph is negative, and the tuberculin skin test results in an area of induration generally 5 to 9 mm in diameter. Skin testing with tuberculin of the specific mycobacterium causing the disease results in a much stronger reaction than with tuberculin test material prepared from *M. tuberculosis.* Conclusive diagnosis is best established by culture and identification of the causative mycobacterium. Treatment is early excision of affected nodes.

Another lesion of clinical importance is swimming pool granuloma, caused by *M. marinum.* This organism has been recovered from water, especially swimming pools. Infection of the skin is considered to result from abrasions of the skin acquired while entering or leaving the pool. Chronic ulcerative granulomatous skin lesions develop at the site of inoculation about 2 to 3 weeks after infection, persist for weeks or months, and leave a scar on healing.

Unclassified mycobacterial disease of the lungs occurs uncommonly in children, *M. kansasii* usually being the etiologic organism. A few cases of widely disseminated mycobacterial infection have been reported in children. Although the unclassified mycobacteria tend to be resistant to most of the older chemotherapeutic agents, many are susceptible to rifampin by in vitro testing, and limited clinical studies suggest that this drug may be effective in vivo.

Revised by Fred F. Barrett

TULAREMIA

Tularemia is a febrile infectious disease that has several clinical presentations depending on the portal of entry and the size of the inoculum.

Etiology and epidemiology

The causative organism, *Francisella tularensis,* was first isolated in Tulare County, California, in 1912. The organism is a pleomorphic gram-negative coccobacillus. Humans are highly susceptible and usually become infected by contact with infected animals or by bites of insects, most commonly ticks and flies. Major animal sources include rabbits, squirrels, deer, cats, mice, and rats. Other animals, including birds, fish, and amphibians, may rarely be sources of infection. The disease has also occasionally been transmitted via ingestion of contaminated water, inhalation of aerosols, and by the bites of mosquitoes or mites. Tularemia occurs year round. The incubation period is usually about 3 days, but may vary from a few hours to 3 weeks.

Pathogenesis

A local lesion may occur at the portal of entry, usually the skin, conjunctiva, oropharynx, respiratory tract, or gastrointestinal tract. The disease spreads via the lymphatics and bloodstream. The organism survives as an intracellular parasite. Secondary lesions may occur in a variety of organs. Lesions are characterized by focal necrosis early in the course and by granuloma formation later. Occasionally patients develop fulminant disease with subsequent death.

Clinical manifestations

Manifestations of tularemia vary with the inoculum and portal of entry. All forms of the disease include fever. Hepatomegaly and splenomegaly occur frequently. A variety of rashes have been reported.

In *ulceroglandular tularemia,* the primary site of infection is the skin. A papule may appear initially that develops into a painful ulcer. Regional lymphadenitis occurs frequently. When lymphadenitis occurs in the absence of an identifiable skin lesion, the disease is referred to as *glandular tularemia*. When the portal of entry is the conjunctival sac, the disease is referred to as *oculoglandular tularemia*. In this form there may be multiple ulcers present in the conjunctiva along with inflammation of the surrounding tissues. *Oropharyngeal tularemia* usually occurs as a result of eating improperly cooked infected meat. In this form of the disease, pharyngitis may be associated with cervical adenitis. When the disease is acquired as a result of aerosolization of organisms, diffuse or localized pulmonary disease results. This form of the disease, *pneumonic tularemia,* may occur as a result of exposure in a bacteriology laboratory. Occasionally, the disease may present a clinical picture similar to typhoid fever. In this form, *typhoidal tularemia,* fever, sore throat, cough, and diarrhea with subsequent septic shock may occur. The portal of entry in typhoidal tularemia is usually ingestion or aerosolization. In the presence of septicemia, multiple systems may be infected, including the central nervous system and skeletal system.

Diagnosis

A careful history and physical examination are essential to increase the index of suspicion of tularemia. The organism can be cultured on special media, but culturing the organism is dangerous for laboratory personnel and should be attempted only in designated laboratories. In most cases the diagnosis is confirmed by serologic tests. A bacterial agglutination test is most commonly employed. Agglutination titers of 1:160 or greater are suggestive of past or recent infection, but demonstration of a fourfold or greater rise in titer or rapidly falling titer are more supportive of the diagnosis. Agglutination titers usually become detectable 1 to 4 weeks after onset of illness and peak from 4 to 8 weeks. Cross-reactive antibody has been reported with brucellosis, proteus OX19, and infectious mononucleosis.

The differential diagnosis varies with the clinical presentation of the illness. Ulceroglandular, glandular, and oculoglandular tularemia must be differentiated from infections with common bacterial pathogens, sporotrichosis, cat-scratch disease, and mycobacterial infections. Pneumonic tularemia requires differentiation from other bacterial and fungal etiologies of pneumonia. Typhoidal tularemia must be differentiated from typhoid fever and other bacterial septicemias.

Treatment

Suspected cases of tularemia should be treated with streptomycin, 30 mg/kg/24 hr in two divided doses administered intramuscularly for at least 7 days. Gentamicin is an effective substitute. Tetracycline and chloramphenicol are also effective, but these antibiotics are not recommended as they are associated with a greater risk of relapse. Administration of corticosteroids may be considered if septic shock is present.

Prevention

Exposure to ticks should be minimized. Wild animal meat should be cooked thoroughly. Rubber gloves may provide protection when handling wild animals. Laboratories with inexperienced personnel should not attempt to culture the organism.

Spirochetal diseases

SYPHILIS

Syphilis is a diverse disease caused by *Treponema pallidum,* a spiral motile organism. After the introduction of penicillin the incidence of syphilis decreased dramatically, and there was hope that the disease might be eliminated in the United States. However, in recent years the total number of reported cases has increased, as has the number of cases of congenital syphilis.

Epidemiology

Acquired syphilis is transmitted by sexual contact. Congenital syphilis results from transplacental acquisition of the organism. The mother of the congenitally syphilitic child is herself invariably infected. *T. pallidum* apparently does not cause disease in the fetus in the first months of gestation. Therefore serologic testing and treatment can be carried out in sufficient time to avert fetal infection. However, the fetus can be infected by syphilis contracted later in the pregnancy after an earlier serologic test has been reported to be negative. Therefore it is advisable to perform a serologic test late in pregnancy as well as early. The mother often shows no clinical evidence of the disease.

Pathologic findings

Acquired syphilis in the older child or adolescent results in similar pathologic changes to those that occur in the adult.

Pathologic findings in congenital syphilis depend on the intensity and time of transplacental spirochetemia. When the infection is intense, death may occur in utero. When it is less severe, the infant may be born prematurely, heavily infected. A milder result is the birth of a full-term obviously infected infant. Finally, the infant might show no clinical evidence of the disease at birth, but signs and symptoms may appear weeks or months later.

In contrast to acquired syphilis, in which the spirochetes invade the body more slowly and in smaller numbers, congenital syphilis is a bacteremic illness from its inception. Thus the organisms enter almost all the tissues of the body, particularly the central nervous system, liver, lungs, bones, skin, spleen, kidneys, and pancreas. Low-grade inflammatory reaction and subsequent fibrosis are the principal pathologic changes. Parenchymal destruction and fibrosis alter structure and function of many organs.

Clinical manifestations

Clinical manifestations in children and adolescents with acquired syphilis are similar to those of adults with acquired syphilis, except in the younger child the chancre of primary syphilis is not common. Thus, syphilis may not be evident until the secondary stage manifestations of early condyloma and mucous patches appear.

Clinical manifestations of congenital syphilis may appear early, within the first 2 years, or may not appear until later, sometimes many years afterward. Although clinically evident manifestations may be present at birth, the syphilitic newborn usually appears normal. About three fourths of such infants show signs and symptoms of syphilis within the first few months of life. The pattern of involvement varies greatly. There may be only general manifestations of syphilis, such as anemia and failure to thrive. More commonly, distinctive syphilitic lesions of the skin, mucous membranes, and bones appear. Generalized glandular enlargement, splenomegaly, and hepatomegaly are present in one third to one half of infected infants. The most characteristic lesions of early syphilis are rhinitis, skin rash, and involvement of the bones. Interstitial keratitis, deafness, deformities of the teeth, periostitis, arthritis, and syphilitic gummas are more characteristic of late congenital syphilis. Not uncommonly, the late lesions appear as the first evidence of infection.

Syphilitic rhinitis (snuffles). Syphilitic rhinitis occurs within the first weeks or months of life in one third to two thirds of infected infants. Invasion of the nasal mucous membrane by spirochetes produces swelling, obstruction to breathing, and the outpouring of a profuse, infectious, and at times blood-tinged discharge. It frequently excoriates the upper lip. Its persistence and association with other signs of syphilis distinguish it from the common cold. Group A streptococcal infection may be superimposed on syphilitic rhinitis.

Skin lesions. Skin lesions of early congenital

syphilis are characterized by great variability. The commonest type consists of round or oval, slightly raised, red-to-copper–colored maculopapular lesions about the size of a dime, present anywhere on the body. They are nonpruritic, fade slowly, assume a brownish color, and finally leave a temporary pigmented appearance. Shallow ulcerated lesions, reddened at the margins, may occur and may be mistaken for impetigo. Black infants are particularly likely to develop annular or circinate lesions that are raised, curved, or tortuous. They are often present on the face near the mouth and are followed by temporary depigmentation. The palms and soles may present a dry red scaling appearance, or large vesicles may develop, rupture, and leave raw oozing surfaces. Bullous lesions (syphilitic pemphigus) may appear distal to the elbows and knees and represent more intense involvement of the skin. Painless syphilitic paronychiae may be present on several fingers. Subsequent scarring of the matrix may result in a clawlike nail.

In late congenital syphilis, syphilitic gummas may develop in the subcutaneous tissues, break down, drain, and produce punched-out ulcers.

Mucocutaneous lesions. Early congenital syphilis frequently produces lesions about the nares, mouth, vagina, and rectum. Circumoral syphilitic inflammation causes moist oozing areas that crack, become secondarily infected, and result in puckering scars radiating from the mouth, called *rhagades*. Toward the end of the first year or somewhat later, condylomas may develop about the vaginal or anal orifices. These are raised and flat and have moist surfaces.

Osseous involvement. Characteristic radiographic changes of the bones are present in more than 90% of patients within the first months of life, and symptoms referable to the bones are common (Fig. 27-7). Syphilitic osteochondritis affects the epiphyseal lines, resulting in a disturbance of orderly formation of bone and weakness that may lead to painful epiphyseal separation. Such pathologic fractures occur most commonly at the wrists and to a lesser extent at the upper end of the humerus. The epiphyseal area is swollen, painful, and tender, and the infant avoids pain by not using the part (syphilitic pseudoparalysis). Bone lesions of such severity occur only in the first months of life. The presence of wrist-drop or the observation that an infant's arm hangs limply by the side should always call to mind the possibility of syphilis. The pseudoparalysis of scurvy does not occur so early. Syphilitic dactylitis may occur in the first months of life. Generally, more than one finger is affected, proximal phalanges are principally involved, there are fusiform swellings, and the fingers are slightly tender. The dactylitis of sickle cell disease can be distinguished by hematologic findings. Syphilitic periostitis is also common, as are moth-eaten areas of diminished density seen in skeletal radiographs.

Late luetic periostitis also commonly occurs. Periostitis chiefly affects long bones, causing thickening and new bone formation. Forward bowing of the tibia (saber shin) is a characteristic example. Periosteal lesions develop slowly, are often painful, and are frequently tender to palpation. Syphilitic gummas may develop in bones, especially those of the skull, causing painful tender swellings that break down and discharge. Destructive lesions of the nasal septum may cause collapse of the nasal bridge, producing a saddle nose.

Joints. Syphilitic arthritis rarely occurs in early congenital syphilis but is a relatively common late manifestation. Although almost any joint may become involved, the knee joints are more frequently affected, usually bilaterally (Clutton joints). The arthritis may be acute and painful, or may develop insidiously without pain or fever. The knees become moderately stiff, fluid accumulates in the joint capsule, and fluctuation is demonstrable.

Teeth. Deformities of the permanent teeth may result from early syphilitic infection. Although caused at an early age, their appearance occurs at the time of eruption of the permanent teeth. Hutchinson teeth are deformities of the permanent upper central incisors characterized by crescentic notching of biting edges, a tapering toward the biting edge (screwdriver teeth), small size, abnormal spacing, and deviations from normal alignment. Moon molars (mulberry molars) are knobby deformities of occlusal surfaces of the first permanent molars. The simultaneous presence of interstitial keratitis, deafness, and Hutchinson teeth is known as the Hutchinson triad, but this combination is rare.

Lymph nodes, liver, and spleen. Generalized enlargement of lymph nodes, splenomeg-

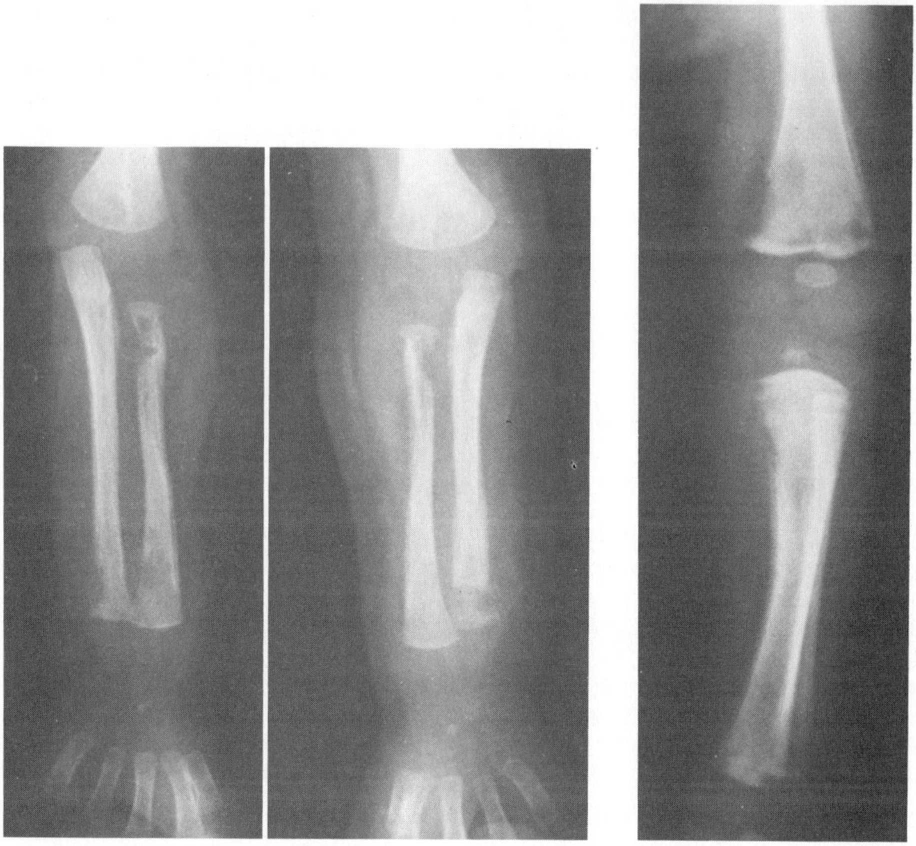

Fig. 27-7. Infantile syphilis in a 2-month-old infant showing periosteal reaction and focal destruction in metaphyses. (Courtesy Dr. W. Webster Riggs, Le Bonheur Children's Medical Center, Memphis.)

aly, and hepatomegaly are common findings in early congenital syphilis. Syphilis may produce persistent jaundice in the newborn.

Ocular lesions. Syphilitic choroiditis may occur in the first months of life. Iritis may occur later. Interstitial keratitis is the most frequent late lesion. It usually appears between 6 and 14 years of age, is ordinarily bilateral, and is characterized by opacity of the cornea associated with pain, photophobia, lacrimation, and impaired vision. Early diagnosis and prompt treatment result in rapid recovery without residual defect. Choroiditis, retinitis, and optic atrophy are less commonly seen in late congenital syphilis.

Nervous system. Infection of the nervous system occurs commonly in early congenital syphilis. The spinal fluid is frequently abnormal; there is an increase in cells, chiefly lymphocytes, a rise in protein, and positive tests for syphilis. Rarely, syphilitic meningitis occurs, and hydrocephalus may develop. Syphilitic involvement of the brain may lead to seizures and mental retardation. One of the most important reasons for early diagnosis and treatment is to avoid the danger of residual defects of the brain.

In late congenital syphilis, Argyll-Robertson pupils may develop, and other cranial nerve palsies can occur. Sudden onset of permanent deafness may occur in childhood from involvement of the eighth cranial nerve. Emotional instability and progressive mental deterioration may accompany meningovascular syphilis. Severe episodes of restlessness, headache, vomiting, and dizziness may occur. Paresis and tabes rarely occur in children.

Other lesions. Nephrotic syndrome and other glomerulopathies have been reported in early congenital syphilis. The liver can become cirrhotic or the seat of syphilitic gummas, sometimes with accompanying ascites. Paroxysmal hemoglobinuria, precipitated by exposure to cold, is seen in late syphilis.

Diagnosis

When florid infantile syphilis is present, or characteristic lesions of late or acquired syphilis occur, the diagnosis can be strongly suspected on clinical grounds alone.

Radiographs of the long bones are especially helpful in the diagnosis of congenital syphilis in the early months of life (Fig. 27-7). They may also be of diagnostic aid in late syphilis.

The diagnosis is established by appropriate laboratory tests. Darkfield examination of lesions, especially in severe congenital syphilis, may reveal the presence of spirochetes. Serologic tests for syphilis (STS) are essential, particularly when clinical manifestations are vague or even lacking. Two general categories of STS are available—nontreponemal and treponemal. The best known of the nontreponemal tests are the Venereal Disease Research Laboratories (VDRL) and the rapid plasma reagin (RPR) tests. The VDRL is inexpensive, well controlled, easily quantitated, and continues to be the most reliable screening test for syphilis. The fluorescent treponemal antibody-absorption test (FTA-ABS) is the most frequently used treponemal test. This test should be used only to confirm the results of the sensitive but less specific VDRL. The FTA-ABS specific for IgM is not reliable. Tests for syphilis can be quantitated to express the degree of seropositivity, and serial tests can be employed to demonstrate a rising titer (active infection) or a falling titer (absence of syphilis or cured syphilis). False positive tests may result from a wide variety of conditions.

A false positive STS may occur in a noninfected infant from passive transfer of maternal antibodies. Serial tests in such instances show a gradually diminishing titer, a negative reaction almost invariably occurring by the age of 3 months. Thus a seropositive asymptomatic infant in the first weeks of life should not be treated for syphilis unless he is born of an untreated syphilitic mother, or unless the STS demonstrates a rising titer (active syphilitic infection). In such circumstances radiographs of the long bones are helpful in diagnosis.

Tests of the cerebrospinal fluid, such as the VDRL, are valuable in the diagnosis of neurosyphilis.

Treatment

Treatment of the infant with congenital syphilis should be started at birth if the mother's treatment was inadequate, if antibiotics other than penicillin were used, or if her treatment status is unknown. A lumbar puncture should be performed before instituting therapy for congenital syphilis, and treatment should be based on the following cerebrospinal fluid findings:

Abnormal cerebrospinal fluid findings	Aqueous crystalline penicillin G, 50,000 units/kg/24 hr in two intramuscular or intravenous doses should be administered for 10 days. Aqueous procaine penicillin G, 50,000 units/kg/24 hr intramuscularly daily for 10 days is an acceptable alternative therapy.
Normal cerebrospinal fluid findings	A single injection of benzathine penicillin G, 50,000 units/kg, should be administered. If neurosyphilis cannot be excluded, the treatment regimens outlined under abnormal findings should be employed.

Older children with congenital syphilis need not receive more penicillin than recommended for adults with acquired syphilis of more than 1 year's duration. Erythromycin and tetracycline can be used in older children who are allergic to penicillin (tetracycline should not be used in children less than 8 years of age).

Secretion isolation should be carried out until the patient has been treated a minimum of 24 hours.

A febrile reaction of unknown etiology, Herxheimer's reaction, may occur during the first 24 hours of treatment. This reaction is particularly likely in infants with severe forms of congenital syphilis. However, the reaction is generally mild.

Repeat quantitative nontreponemal tests should be performed 3, 6, and 12 months after treatment. When treatment is initiated early during the course of the disease, about 80% of patients will be seronegative within 6 months, 90% in 12 months, and almost all are seronegative after 2 years. Patients with neurosyphilis should be reevaluated every 6 months for at least 3 years. Repeat cerebrospinal fluid examinations should be performed in patients with neurosyphilis.

Treatment and followup guidelines for adults apply to older children and adolescents with acquired syphilis.

LEPTOSPIROSIS

Leptospirosis is a diverse illness of humans and animals that can be caused by any one of the over 100 recognized serotypes of the spirochete *Leptospira interrogans*. The serotypes most frequently associated with human disease are *icterohaemorrhagiae* and *canicola*. The animal reservoirs of leptospires include rodents, dogs, cats, hogs, horses, and cattle. Animals excrete the spirochete in their urine, and humans usually become infected through contact with infected urine or contaminated water. Direct contact with infected animals, usually dogs or cats, may also result in infection. Infection may occur by way of the conjunctivae or nasopharynx. Leptospirosis is diagnosed far less frequently than infection actually occurs.

Clinical manifestations

Leptospirosis may present a variety of clinical manifestations ranging from minor to severe. The severity of illness does not seem to be serotype specific. After an incubation period of 2 to 20 days, clinical manifestations begin with fever (sometimes chills), malaise, headache, and myalgia. Gastrointestinal symptoms may be present. An important early diagnostic finding is conjunctival inflammation. Since the leptospire has a predilection for liver, kidneys, muscles, and blood vessels, the physician may note jaundice, proteinuria, azotemia, or hematuria, as well as hemorrhages in the skin, gastrointestinal tract, or central nervous system. Anemia and thrombocytopenia may develop. A variety of rashes also may occur. The clinical syndrome of aseptic meningitis is a common manifestation. The clinical course may be biphasic.

Diagnosis

Early in the course of the illness, the causative organism may be cultured from blood or cerebrospinal fluid with special media. Later in the illness, the organism may be cultured from the urine. The diagnosis may also be established by means of serologic studies.

Differential diagnosis includes other forms of aseptic meningitis, brucellosis, infectious hepatitis, serum hepatitis, infectious mononucleosis, acute nephritis, mucocutaneous lymph node syndrome, and toxic shock syndrome. Treatment with penicillin early in the course of the illness may shorten duration of symptoms.

Prevention implies avoidance of contact with water that might possibly have been infected by animals and avoidance of close contact with the animals themselves.

Jerry Shenep

Viral diseases

CAT-SCRATCH DISEASE

Cat-scratch disease is a syndrome characterized by subacute regional lymphadenitis that is usually preceded by an injury to the skin distal to the affected node. Although the syndrome is frequently associated with the scratch of a cat, a variety of traumatizing objects have been reported (splinters, pins, fishhooks, thorns, etc.). A variety of viral and bacterial agents (psittacosis-lymphogranuloma venereum groups, herpes simplex, atypical mycobacteria) have been proposed as the etiologic organism of cat-scratch disease, but none has been confirmed. The disease has worldwide distribution and is apparently not transmissible from one human being to another. The incubation period varies from 10 to 30 days.

There is a local lesion at the site of inoculation in approximately one half the cases. The area becomes red and swollen and may become ulcerated and crusted. The lesion is indolent and slow to heal. About 1 to 3 weeks later there is painful inflammatory enlargement of the regional lymph nodes. The glands may become massively enlarged and tender to palpation, and the overlying skin is reddened. In about one half the cases the gland suppurates. Affected nodes may remain enlarged for a variable period of time, often weeks or months, and in some cases more than a year elapses before they return to normal size. Since the wound of entry is generally on the hands, the epitrochlear and axillary nodes are usually affected. Involvement of the inguinal and cervical nodes occurs less commonly. In the oculoglandular form conjunctivitis is associated with enlargement of the preauricular and cervical nodes.

Clinical manifestations

At onset of glandular swelling systemic manifestations of acute illness may occur. These include fever, malaise, headache, anorexia, nausea, vomiting, abdominal pain, chills or chilly sensations, and generalized aching. The fever is usually short in duration and moderate in degree, but the temperature can be high and in some cases persists for weeks or months.

Atypical manifestations include maculopapular rash, erythema nodosum, purpura, pneumonia, pharyngitis, mesenteric adenitis, osteolytic lesions, and encephalomyelitis. Encephalitis usually appears in the second week of glandular swelling and is characterized by abrupt onset, high temperature, convulsions, and coma. Neurologic abnormalities may last for weeks or months, but full recovery almost invariably ensues. The cerebrospinal fluid generally has a moderate increase in lymphocytes and protein content.

Diagnosis

The diagnosis is based on clinical findings and a positive intracutaneous test with antigen prepared from pus aspirated from a bubo of the patient. Differential diagnosis requires consideration of pyogenic adenitis, tularemia, tuberculous adenitis, infectious mononucleosis, ratbite fever, lymphogranuloma venereum, lymphoma, and Hodgkin disease. The encephalitic form is not difficult to diagnose if the physician keeps in mind the peculiar combination of encephalitis associated with regional adenitis.

Treatment

Treatment of cat-scratch disease is purely symptomatic, with the exception of aspiration drainage of fluctuant nodes if they become progressively enlarged. This is preferable to incision and drainage, which may produce a sinus tract with prolonged discharge.

James G. Hughes

CHICKENPOX (VARICELLA)

Chickenpox (varicella) is an extremely common, highly contagious infection caused by a virus and characterized by constitutional symptoms and the appearance of a specific rash.

Etiology

Chickenpox and herpes zoster are caused by the same virus, varicella-zoster (V-Z), a member of the herpes virus group. Varicella is the primary infection whereas herpes zoster is most often reactivation of a latent V-Z virus. The role of host defenses and inciting events that cause reactivation of the latent virus are not clearly understood.

Epidemiology

Chickenpox occurs most commonly in children 2 to 8 years of age. It occasionally affects the newborn infant. It is one of the most common contagious childhood infections and is transmitted by contact with an affected person (droplet infection). Vesicle fluid contains numerous contagious viral particles. In the hospital the virus may be carried from one person to another by a third individual. Transmission through air in the hospital may also occur. Incubation period is usually 14 to 16 days but ranges from 10 to 21 days.

The disease is usually contagious 24 hours before appearance of the rash and for about 5 to 6 days thereafter. Once crusts have begun to form the patient is no longer contagious. Virus particles decrease in quantity as the vesicular fluid becomes thick and cloudy. Chickenpox may be transmitted from a mother with the disease to the newborn infant, giving rise to so-called congenital chickenpox. The newborn infant is usually passively protected for 3 to 6 months if the mother is immune to varicella.

Pathologic changes

Skin lesions begin as macules, progress to papules, and then form vesicles. Initially these vesicles are filled with clear fluid, but they are rapidly invaded by polymorphonuclear cells and become cloudy. Soon afterwards they rupture and produce crusts that adhere to the skin for approximately 1 week. Secondary infection may occur, leading to cellulitis, bacteremia, and perhaps distant pyogenic complications.

Mucus membrane lesions also occur, usually in the mouth, pharynx, and vagina. Conjunctival lesions are rare. Patients with compromised host defenses and otherwise normal adults are at significant risk to develop V-Z dissemination to the lungs, liver, and brain.

Clinical manifestations

Initial manifestations are malaise, fever, headache, and anorexia. The rash appears within about 24 hours. It usually begins on the face and neck and spreads to the trunk and extremities. Scattered small red macules and papules within 24 hours develop into vesicles. The skin lesions do not erupt in one crop, but in successive crops, so that various combinations of macules, papules, vesicles, and crusts are seen. Ulcerations within the mouth may cause pain and may interfere with eating and swallowing. Similar lesions of the vagina may cause burning pain on urination.

The skin lesions are intensely pruritic. Scratching frequently results in secondary infection and scarring. Staphylococci or streptococci may be the secondary invaders. Cellulitis, furunculosis, or erysipelas may occur. Invasion of the bloodstream may lead to various pyogenic complications such as pyarthrosis or osteomyelitis. Nephritogenic streptococci can infect the lesions of varicella and cause acute nephritis.

Fever is in proportion to severity of the eruption. In some patients only a few skin lesions occur with little or no temperature elevation. Patients whose condition is characterized by extensive eruption generally have a high temperature.

Adults are more likely to have severe disease, with dissemination to deep organs, that is, lungs, liver, and brain. Visceral dissemination occurs in 25% to 30% of children receiving steroids and other immunosuppressive drugs for cancer, nephrotic syndrome, and other conditions. Children with congenitally impaired cell-mediated immunity are also at high risk for disseminated varicella. Significant mortality occurs in those patients with lung and brain involvement. Rarely, hemorrhagic varicella, in which there is bleeding into vesicles secondary to thrombocytopenia and/or deficient clotting factors, occurs. Varicella in the neonate may disseminate to deep organs. Encephalitis, including cerebellar ataxia, has been reported following varicella. Varicella is one of the most common antecedent infections associated with Reye syndrome. Also the use of salicylates has been associated with Reye syndrome. Fever control with compounds other than salicylates should be considered for children with varicella (and any influenza-like illness).

In the usual case, the child has fever for approximately 7 days, a rash for about 5 days, and crusting and eventual separation of the crust over a period of 4 to 5 days, making the total duration of skin manifestations approximately 9 to 10 days.

Diagnosis

Chickenpox requires differentiation from several other conditions characterized by skin manifestations.

Smallpox. It is traditional to discuss the differential diagnosis between chickenpox and smallpox; however, the two infections are not likely to be confused. Smallpox has been eradicated worldwide. Chickenpox has a short prodromal period of about a day, whereas smallpox has a period of about 3 days, during which there are severe constitutional symptoms before the rash appears. Chickenpox produces crops of macules, papules, vesicles, and crusts in various stages of development, distributed mainly on the trunk, with the extremities affected to a lesser degree. On the contrary, smallpox produces one single crop of lesions, and they are generally most numerous on the extremities and face instead of on the trunk. The skin lesions of chickenpox are more superficial than those of smallpox. Smallpox lesions are much firmer to palpation than those of chickenpox. They are umbilicated, whereas those of chickenpox are not.

Herpes zoster. Herpes zoster is produced by reactivation of the latent V-Z virus. The vesicular eruption of herpes zoster is usually localized to a dermatone distribution corresponding to a peripheral nerve and is generally unilateral. Zoster is uncommon in childhood. However, children with cancer receiving immunosuppressive therapy have an occurrence rate of approximately 10%. Visceral dissemination following zoster in this latter group of children is unusual.

Impetigo. Lesions of impetigo may look like those of chickenpox, but they do not appear in crops. Mucous membranes are not involved, and constitutional symptoms are unusual.

Rickettsialpox. Rickettsialpox produces vesicles similar to those of chickenpox, but the vesicles are smaller and are superimposed on papules. Crusts usually do not develop. There is a primary eschar on the part of the body where the causative organisms gained entry, and systemic manifestations of fever, chills, general malaise, and backache are common.

Treatment

A live, attenuated vaccine is being evaluated in children at high risk for disseminated varicella, that is, those receiving immunosuppressive therapy. Information on efficacy and duration of immunity is not yet available. Passive immunization with V-Z immune globulin is available for those patients susceptible to varicella who are at high risk for disseminated disease following a close exposure to an active case of the infection. High-risk factors are underlying malignancy, congenital or acquired immunopathy, immunosuppressive therapy, or a newborn of a mother with varicella. Passive immunization must be given within 96 hours of exposure at a dosage of 1 vial per 10 kg body weight. Varicella is prevented in 60% of patients receiving this passive immunization; in the remaining 40% the infection usually is mild.

Since chickenpox is mild and without serious morbidity and mortality in the otherwise healthy child, antiviral therapy is not indicated. However, in the child at high risk for disseminated infection with serious morbidity and mortality, antiviral therapy with either vidarabine or acyclovir should be considered.

The child with chickenpox should be confined until free of fever. Pruritus can be allayed by sedation, antihistamines, local applications such as calamine lotion, or starch baths. The skin should be kept as clean as possible to minimize the risk of secondary bacterial infection. Fingernails should be manicured short and kept clean. If secondary skin infection occurs, appropriate antibiotics are employed. If encephalitis develops, supportive care should be afforded.

INFECTIOUS MONONUCLEOSIS

Infectious mononucleosis is characterized by fever, pharyngitis, lymphadenopathy, splenomegaly, atypical lymphocytes in the peripheral blood, and presence of heterophil antibodies. This infection is caused by a herpes virus (Epstein-Barr), which was originally detected in cultures of Burkitt lymphoma cells.

Etiology and epidemiology

Infectious mononucleosis is an infection of children and adolescents. The young child may have a subclinical infection or a nonspecific upper respiratory tract infection. The adolescent and young adult usually develop the typical clinical picture of infectious mononucleosis. Most cases are sporadic but may occur in epidemic form in college dormitories and military camps. The incubation period ranges from 10 to 60 days. The mode of transmission is by direct intimate contact ("kissing disease") or by droplet infection from the secretions of the upper respiratory tract. The period of communicability is unknown, but virus can be isolated from throat secretions several months after recovery from infection.

Pathologic findings

Infectious mononucleosis is a generalized disease causing enlargement of lymphoid tissue throughout the body, particularly in the lymph nodes, spleen, and tonsils. The liver usually has mild lymphocytic and monocytic portal infiltration. Chronic liver damage is very rare. Mononuclear infiltrates may be found in almost any organ.

Clinical manifestations *(Fig. 27-8)*

Epstein-Barr virus induces a broad spectrum of illness in children. It may range from the mild upper respiratory tract infection of infants to the classical picture of infectious mononucleosis in the young adult. There is usually a prodrome of less than 1 week. The acute phase of the illness lasts for 1 to 2 weeks. The convalescent phase may be 4 to 6 weeks. The findings of fever, pharyngitis, cervical lymphadenopathy, splenomegaly, and lymphocytosis in the peripheral blood are very suggestive of infectious mononucleosis. Fever is variable in degree and duration. It is present in over 90% of patients and usually resolves over a 10 to 14 day period. Temperature range is 38° to 39° C (100° to 104° F) but may reach 40° to 41° C (104° to 105° F). Anorexia and malaise are characteristic of the infection and may persist into

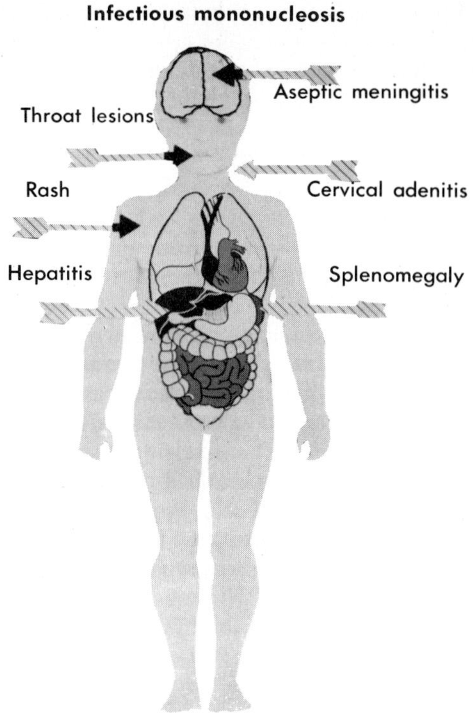

Fig. 27-8. Chief clinical manifestations in infectious mononucleosis.

the convalescent phase. Sore throat is the most common complaint, occurring in over 75% of symptomatic patients. Pharyngitis is present in over 85% of the patients, but less than half of these will have exudate covering the tonsils.

Lymphadenopathy occurs in over 95% of the patients and is the most common sign of infection. Cervical lymph nodes are usually enlarged and tender. Lymph nodes anywhere in the body may be enlarged.

Splenomegaly of varying degree is present in about one half of the cases. Rupture of the spleen, although rare, may occur spontaneously or from minor trauma.

Hepatitis, as evidenced by elevated serum transaminases, occurs in 80% to 90% of patients. An enlarged liver is found by palpation of the abdomen in less than 20% of the patients. Hyperbilirubinemia is uncommon.

Skin rashes of various types may occur in the first week of disease. The eruption is usually an erythematous macular or maculopapular rash but may be morbiliform, scarlatiniform, vesicular, urticarial, or petechial. Over 90% of patients with mononucleosis who receive ampicillin will develop a maculopapular rash.

Central nervous system involvement occurs in less than 10% of patients, but accounts for one half of the deaths caused by Epstein-Barr virus. The major manifestation is that of meningoencephalitis. Infectious polyneuritis (Guillian-Barré syndrome) and transverse myelitis are serious consequences of the infection and account for a significant proportion of the deaths.

Pneumonitis occurs occasionally with cough and radiographic findings similar to those of atypical pneumonia. Pericarditis may occur but is rare. Thrombocytopenia purpura is sometimes a complication.

Diagnosis

Definitive diagnosis is based on laboratory findings in the presence of a compatible clinical picture. Peripheral blood characteristically reveals the presence of atypical lymphocytes (Downey cells) that constitute at least 10% of all lymphocytes. The atypical lymphocytes are not pathognomonic of infectious mononucleosis, as they occur in many viral infections. The leukocyte count is usually elevated, with monocytes and lymphocytes accounting for 50% to 70% of the total white cell count.

The heterophil antibody test, based on development of agglutinins to sheep red blood cells, is useful in diagnosis. It usually becomes positive within the first week of the disease, but it may not become positive for several weeks and in some cases the test is never positive. When the serum of the patient with infectious mononucleosis is exposed to guinea pig kidney, it will subsequently agglutinate sheep red blood cells; after exposure to beef red blood cells it will not. These absorption tests are used to differentiate the naturally occurring antibody (Forssman antibody) to sheep red blood cells and the antibody of serum sickness from the antibody of infectious mononucleosis. A rapid 2-minute slide test (monospot) has replaced the more cumbersome Paul-Bunnell heterophil agglutination tests. Within 1 to 2 years heterophil antibodies can no longer be detected.

A recent development has been the specific Epstein-Barr virus serology. An immunofluorescent IgG antibody to viral capsid antigen (VCA) is readily available. This antibody can be detected at clinical presentation of infectious mononucleosis and persists lifelong. Also available in many laboratories is a test for antibody against Epstein-Barr nuclear antigen (EBNA), which usually can be detected 3 to 4 weeks after onset of illness and persists lifelong. Thus the patient who has antibody to VCA but not to EBNA has recent-onset infectious mononucleosis. Presence of both antibodies and a negative monospot test suggests the illness is not infectious mononucleosis.

Differential diagnosis. Differential diagnosis depends on the clinical picture presented by the particular patient. The pharyngeal manifestations may simulate those of diptheria, streptococcal pharyngitis, adenovirus pharyngitis, or agranulocytic infection. Generalized lymphadenopathy, fever, and malaise require consideration of Hodgkin disease, leukemia, brucellosis, typhoid fever, other *Salmonella* infections, hepatitis, and tularemia. Nervous system manifestations necessitate differentiation from the entities that produce aseptic meningitis, encephalitis, and infectious polyneuritis (Guillian-Barré syndrome). Because the skin eruption is so variable, scarlet fever, drug rash, and allergic skin eruptions must also be considered. Enlargement of the mesenteric lymph nodes may cause pain similar to that of appendicitis.

Treatment

Treatment consists of symptomatic management and observation for unusual manifestations of the disease. Recovery of full strength is often slow, and the patient may require supervision of activity for several weeks.

INFLUENZA

Influenza is an acute, highly communicable viral infection affecting principally the respiratory tract and occurring periodically in epidemics and occasionally in pandemics.

Etiology and epidemiology

There are three major types of influenza virus: A, B, and C. Type C is an infrequent cause of infection in man.

Types A and B are responsible for most of the significant outbreaks of influenza. Type A tends to undergo antigenic drift and shift, producing epidemics of varying intensity. Antigenic drifts are relatively minor changes within an influenza A subtype, whereas antigenic shifts are the production of new subtypes in which the population has little or no immunity. Antigenic drifts occur every 1 to 3 years, producing epidemics. Antigenic shifts occur infrequently and produce world-wide pandemic influenza. Strain variations of type B occur much less frequently than do type A.

Influenza is communicable through droplet infection. Infected individuals excrete virus from their upper respiratory tract 1 day before and through the fifth day of illness. Antibodies appear rapidly and can be demonstrated by serologic techniques. Incubation period is 1 to 3 days. Children provide a major pool of susceptible hosts for influenza epidemics.

Pathologic findings

Influenza produces severe inflammation of the upper respiratory tract, as well as the larynx, trachea, bronchi, and bronchioles. Ciliated columnar epithelium is destroyed. In severe cases there is edema of the upper and lower respiratory tracts, and a serosanguineous exudate may appear. Submucosal hemorrhages may occur. In fatal cases without complicating bacterial infection the lungs may present an edematous, hemorrhagic appearance. The alveolar ducts may be lined with a hyaline membrane. Myocardial edema with interstitial mononuclear cell infiltration may be present. Extensive damage to the respiratory tract epithelium caused by the influenza virus paves the way for secondary bacterial invasion. Common organisms encountered in this circumstance are *Staphylococcus,* group A *Streptococcus, Streptococcus pneumoniae,* and *Haemophilus influenzae*. Secondary infection increases morbidity and mortality.

Clinical manifestations

Influenza generally begins abruptly, often with chills and fever, 38° to 41° C (100° to 105° F). The throat feels dry and is painful. Hoarseness may be present. Initially, there may be a bothersome dry hacking cough that later may become productive. The face is flushed and there is pharyngeal hyperemia, conjunctival congestion, and clear watery nasal discharge. Often in the younger child there is abdominal pain, nausea, and vomiting. Croup-like symptoms may also occur in the younger child and infant.

Severe prostration out of proportion to degree of fever is a common manifestation. Frontal headache and pain in the eyes are made worse by ocular movements. Myalgias are characteristic.

Uncomplicated influenza usually lasts for 5 to 7 days. The patient recovers rapidly, although there may be weakness, fatigability, and cough for weeks afterwards.

Secondary bacterial infections are usually heralded by the return of fever and symptoms associated with the infected organ, that is, productive cough, ear pain, or headache. Pneumonia, otitis media, and sinusitis are the most common secondary bacterial infections. After appropriate cultures, antibiotic therapy should be instituted and based on the most likely etiologic agents, as discussed in the previous section.

In uncomplicated influenza the leukocyte count may be slightly elevated at onset, followed by leukopenia with decreased numbers of granulocytes. Secondary bacterial infection should be suspected when leukocytosis persists or appears after onset.

Diagnosis

Public health laboratories maintain surveillance for influenza viruses. Epidemics are usually known shortly after their appearance, making diagnosis relatively easy. In sporadic cases, or before epidemics appear, the diagnosis can be established only by isolation of virus in the upper respiratory tract or the demonstration of a four fold rise in antibody titer.

Treatment

Treatment of uncomplicated influenza is symptomatic and follows the supportive lines of therapy indicated for other acute infections of the respiratory tract. Chemoprophylaxis with rimantadine or amantadine, instituted early in an outbreak of influenza A or B, can result in markedly decreased rates of infection. Side effects from both drugs, although less with rimantadine, involve the gastrointestinal system with nausea, vomiting, and abdominal pain, and the central nervous system with insomnia, ''jitteriness,'' and difficulty in concentration. These side effects subside with discontinuing the drug. Prophylactic antibiotic therapy is ineffective.

Active immunization. Vaccination for the otherwise normal healthy child is not recommended. Vaccination is recommended for children at high risk for complications, such as those with heart disease, pulmonary disease, diabetes, renal disease, and blood dyscrasia and those receiving immunosuppressive therapy for a variety of disorders. It should be noted that the antibody response in this latter group is only 50% as compared to 85% in the nonimmunosuppressed child. The inactivated (formalin-treated) influenza vaccines are licensed for use in the United States. In children, split-virus vaccine requiring two doses 4 weeks apart are used because of less side effects than with whole virus vaccine. The Guillain-Barré syndrome has only been associated with the swine influenza vaccine of 1976. A new, live, attenuated, cold-adapted intranasal influenza vaccine is under investigation and may replace the killed vaccine.

Reye syndrome)

Reye syndrome is an increasingly recognized hepatic and central nervous system complication of influenza (also of chickenpox and less often of other viruses) infections. It appears more commonly following influenza B than influenza A virus infection. This syndrome occurs almost exclusively in children between the ages of 2 and 6 years and has a mortality of 10% to 40%. There also has been an association between Reye syndrome and aspirin administration in children with influenza (and chickenpox). Alternatives to salicylates should be considered for fever control in children with influenza-like illnesses (and chickenpox).

MUMPS

Mumps is a common contagious infection caused by mumps virus. It is characterized by painful, tender swelling of the parotid or other salivary glands and by a predilection to affect the testicles, ovaries, pancreas, and central nervous system. The principal findings are shown in Fig. 27-9.

Etiology and epidemiology

The disease is caused by a myxovirus that is transmitted by direct contact with a patient (droplet spread). The period of infectivity is considered to be from a few days before the first symptoms until about 9 days following the onset of parotid swelling. The patient is usually isolated until the swelling has subsided or until other manifestations have cleared. The incubation period is 14 to 21 days.

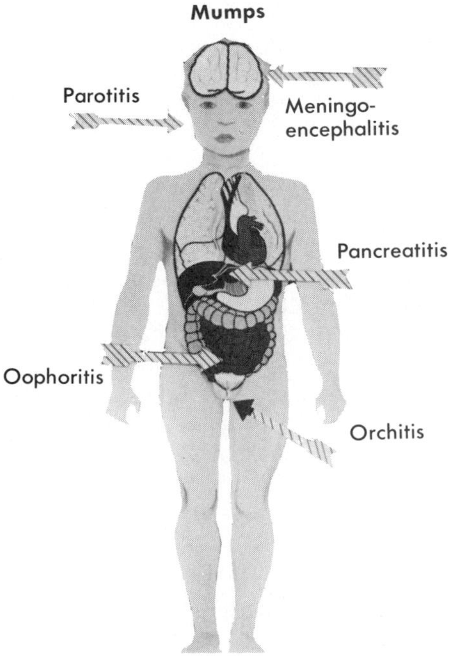

Fig. 27-9. Mumps and its complications.

Mumps occurs endemically and epidemically. Of infected individuals, only about two thirds have apparent disease; the other one third are subclinically infected. This high rate of subclinical mumps explains why many persons after repeated close exposure to mumps fail to contract the infection.

Transplacental passage of antibody probably accounts for the low incidence of infection during the first 6 months of life. It occurs most commonly in the age group 5 to 10 years. A single attack affords permanent immunity.

Pathologic findings

Mumps is a generalized infection but with a predilection for certain tissues. The salivary glands, especially the parotid glands, are usually involved and become swollen and edematous. The interstitial tissue is congested and infiltrated with lymphocytes. Cells lining the ducts degenerate and become necrotic. The ducts become plugged with debris and inflammatory cells. The testicles may show congestion, edema, perivascular lymphocytic accumulations, focal hemorrhage and degeneration, and necrosis of the germinal epithelium. Similar changes may occur in the ovaries or pancreas. Meningoencephalitis, encephalitis, myelitis, or neuritis may occur.

Clinical manifestations

Individuals infected with the mumps virus usually exhibit typical clinical evidence of the disease, but others have clinical mumps without salivary gland swelling or show no signs at all. The infection often begins with fever, headache, vomiting, anorexia, and malaise, followed in 1 or 2 days by swelling of the parotid gland.

Involvement of salivary glands. The parotid glands are usually affected, sometimes unilaterally but much more often bilaterally. One parotid gland may be swollen a few days before the other. The first distinctive symptom is pain immediately below the ear and at the angle of the jaw that increases with palpation or with chewing. Swelling soon follows and may become extensive. The ear is pushed upward and outward, and pain and tenderness become progressively severe. Peak enlargement is reached by about the third day. The gland returns to normal size in another 3 to 7 days. Submaxillary glandular swelling produces a mass anterior to the angle of the jaw and below the anterior border of the masseter muscle. Sublinguinal glandular involvement produces a swelling beneath the chin, a little to one side and in the floor of the mouth. Pouting and redness of the orifice of the parotid duct may be present.

Orchitis. Orchitis rarely occurs before puberty, but 20% to 30% of postpubertal males will develop unilateral testicular involvement. Approximately 2% to 15% have bilateral involvement, but even then permanent sterility is unusual. Orchitis, often accompanied by epididymitis, tends to occur toward the end of the first week or in the early part of the second week. The testicle swells rapidly and is extremely tender. Concomitantly, systemic manifestations become accentuated. Fever, chills, headache, nausea, vomiting, and abdominal pain often accompany the testicular swelling. Acute manifestations of orchitis last about 4 to 7 days. As the local symptoms regress and temperature falls, the testicles become softer in consistency and in about one half of cases undergo subsequent atrophy.

Oophoritis. Oophoritis occurs rarely in prepubertal girls, but in adult females it has an incidence of about 5%. Symptoms are fever, abdominal pain, nausea, and vomiting. Sterility has not been reported.

Pancreatitis. Pancreatitis is a rare complication of mumps in childhood. It produces abdominal pain, nausea, vomiting, and is associated with prostration, fever, and chills. Full recovery ordinarily follows.

Central nervous system. Mumps is a neurotropic virus. Central nervous system involvement is the most common extrasalivary gland manifestation of the infection. Cerebrospinal fluid pleocytosis occurs in 50% of patients with mumps; however, only 10% will have clinical meningitis. Onset is usually 4 days after the parotid swelling but may occur as early as 1 week before or as late as 2 weeks after parotitis. Laboratory findings are like those of any aseptic meningitis. Males are affected more commonly than are females. Symptoms usually resolve within 1 week. Sequelae are very rare. Encephalitis, transverse myelitis, and neuritis are rare complications (less than 1%).

Diagnosis

The usual case of mumps can be diagnosed readily on clinical grounds alone. However, when meningoencephalitis or one of the less common complications occurs as the sole clinical manifestation laboratory tests may be of assistance. A fourfold or greater increase to antibody titer between acute- and convalescent-phase specimens is considered diagnostic. The mumps skin test is not reliable and should not be used. Serum amylase from salivary gland involvement is usually elevated during the first week of the infection.

Differential diagnosis. Differentiation from acute cervical lymphadenitis is ordinarily not difficult. Careful attention to the location, contour, and consistency of the swelling should suffice for this distinction. Suppurative parotitis is a pyogenic inflammation of the gland and produces the usual signs of inflammation. The gland is swollen, painful, and tender, and the overlying skin is generally red and hot. Pressure on the gland forces pus from Stensen's duct. The peripheral white count is usually elevated with a neutrophilia. Recurrent parotitis is a condition in which the child has repeated episodes of parotid swelling. History of previous attacks should be sufficient to differentiate this condition from mumps. Calculus in Stensen's duct is rare in childhood. Tumors of the parotid gland usually offer little trouble in diagnosis because of the lack of general symptoms of mumps and the nature of the local findings.

Treatment

The acutely ill child prefers to remain in bed, but those with mild forms of the disease suffer no harm from being up and about the house. The danger of orchitis does not appear to be increased by limited activity. However, postpubertal males should not indulge in strenuous exercise. Fever is controlled by the usual means. The pain of salivary gland swelling may be relieved by aspirin or codeine. Treatment of pancreatitis and oophoritis is symptomatic. Parenteral fluid therapy may be required for the persistent vomiting associated with pancreatitis. Treatment of central nervous system complications is also symptomatic.

Persons in contact with cases of mumps

There is no reliable procedure for preventing susceptible persons in contact with mumps from contracting the disease. However, the communicability of mumps is rather low in comparison with other contagious diseases. Furthermore, as mentioned previously, many individuals who cannot recall having had mumps have been subclinically infected in the past and are immune. Mumps-immune globulin is commercially available but is of unproven efficacy. A highly efficacious live mumps vaccine is available and is usually given along with the live measles and rubella vaccine at 15 months of age. The mumps vaccine is discussed in more detail on p. 194.

GERMAN MEASLES (RUBELLA)

German measles (rubella) was a very common contagious infection of viral etiology. The availability of a live, attenuated rubella vaccine since the late 1960s, combined with aggressive vaccination programs, has seen a marked decline in the number of cases of rubella in children in this country. The infection is characterized by mild constitutional symptoms; mild fever; swelling and tenderness of posterior cervical, occipital, and retroauricular lymph nodes; and the eruption of a maculopapular or morbilliform rash. A schematic diagram of the clinical cause of a typical case is shown in Fig. 27-10.

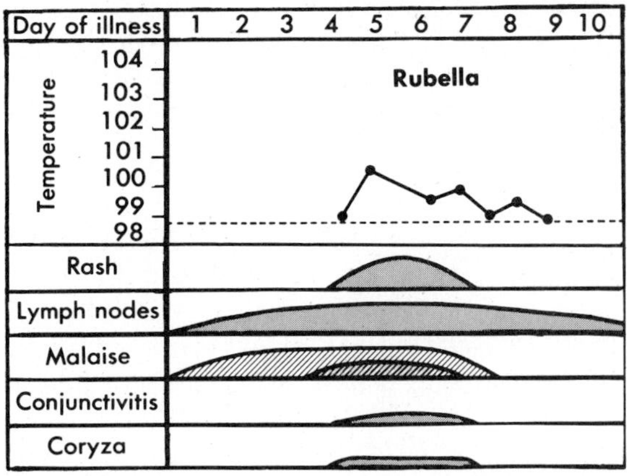

Fig. 27-10. Schematic diagram illustrating typical course of rubella in children and adults. Lymph nodes begin to enlarge 3 to 4 days before rash. Prodromal symptoms (malaise) are minimal in children (shaded area). In adults there may be a 3- to 4-day prodrome (hatched areas). Conjunctivitis and coryza, if present, are usually minimal and accompany the rash. (From Krugman, S., and Katz, S.L.: Infectious diseases of children, ed. 7, St. Louis, 1981, The C.V. Mosby Co.)

Etiology and epidemiology

Rubella is transmitted by droplet spread. The period of infectivity is considered to extend from 7 days before to approximately 5 days after appearance of the rash. The incubation period ranges from 14 to 21 days. Transplacental transmission to the fetus may occur, producing malformations and/or widely disseminated disease, as discussed on pp. 319 and 321. With rare exceptions, permanent immunity follows a single attack. An effective vaccine is available for active immunization (p. 194).

Rubella occurs endemically throughout the world and periodically appears in epidemic form. Infants are usually protected against the disease for the first 5 to 6 months of life because of transplacental immunity from a mother who has had rubella. The disease occurs more frequently in young children and adults. Congenital rubella, caused by transplacental transmission of the virus, is discussed on pp. 319-321.

Clinical manifestations

In a young child appearance of the rash is usually the first sign of illness. In adolescents and adults there is often a prodromal period lasting 1 to 5 days.

Prodromal manifestations. Prodromal manifestations consist of fever, usually low grade, generalized malaise, loss of appetite, headache, rhinorrhea, mild sore throat, cough, and swelling of lymph nodes in areas previously mentioned.

Enanthem. Occasionally in the later prodromal stages, or coincident with the appearance of the rash, an enanthem (Forcheimer spots) consisting of red spots or petechiae appears on the soft pallet or uvula. These lesions may be pinpoint or blotchy. They are not pathognomonic of rubella, as they are similar in appearance to lesions associated with scarlet fever and other viral infections.

Exanthem. Rubella causes a rash that lasts about 3 days. It begins on the face, spreads downward, and disappears later in the same sequence. The lesions are pale, rose-colored maculopapules, usually round or oval, generally discrete, but sometimes blotchy and confluent.

Lymph nodes. Rubella causes generalized lymphadenopathy, but tender swelling of the posterior cervical, occipital, and retroauricular nodes are characteristic of the disease. Tenderness decreases shortly after appearance of the rash, but the nodes may remain enlarged for several weeks.

Complications

Complications are uncommon. It is estimated that encephalitis occurs approximately once in every 6000 cases. Arthritis and arthralgia are common complications of the infection. This occurs in 25% of prepubertal children and occurs even more commonly in adolescents and adults. Females are more likely to be affected than males. Onset of joint symptoms usually follows the rash by several days. Duration of joint symptoms is variable, lasting from several days to several weeks. Sequela are unusual. Fingers, knees, and wrists are the joints commonly involved.

Diagnosis

Typical rubella does not usually pose a diagnostic problem. Rubella may resemble several other conditions that produce a rash. The distribution of the lymphadenopathy, combined with the other features of the infection, helps in differential diagnosis.

Rubeola is differentiated by a much more severe prodromal period, pronounced coryza, cough, conjunctivitis, and presence of Koplik spots. Exanthem subitum (roseola infantum) is distinguished by sudden onset of high temperature in a small child with almost no other manifestations and the appearance of the rash on the third or fourth day as the temperature falls abruptly. Scarlet fever is associated with sore throat, tonsillar exudate, and leukocytosis instead of leukopenia. The throat culture is positive for group A streptococci, and the rash is generally more diffuse, blanches on pressure, and avoids the circumoral area.

Infectious mononucleosis with rash may simulate rubella, but the blood count, blood smear and mono spot test help make the distinction. Drug rashes and eruptions of serum sickness may be confused with rubella. Skin rashes associated with enteroviruses and respiratory viruses may pose problems in diagnosis. Enterovirus infections tend to occur in the summer and fall and are associated with gastrointestinal symptoms. Respiratory viruses, although also occurring in winter and spring, usually have more prominent coryza, cough, and pharyngitis.

Rubella in pregnancy

The main purpose of the campaign to eradicate rubella by active immunization is to prevent acquisition of rubella during pregnancy and subsequent fetal infection. The susceptible pregnant woman who had an exposure to rubella within the preceding 72 hours can receive 20 ml of immune serum globulin. The congenital rubella syndrome is not necessarily prevented if the mother had a subclinical infection. Although large numbers are not available, inadvertent vaccination of pregnant women has not lead to the congenital rubella syndrome.

MEASLES (RUBEOLA)

Rubeola is a highly contagious viral infection, characterized by fever, coryza, conjunctivitis, cough, Koplik spots, and a distinctive generalized maculopapular rash. A schematic diagram of the clinical course of a typical case is shown in Fig. 27-11. The principal findings are shown in Fig. 27-12.

Etiology and epidemiology

The measles virus is transmitted by droplet spread. The incubation period is about 10 days. There is a prodrome of 3 to 4 days and the rash typically appears on the fourteenth day. Patients are highly infectious during the late prodromal phase and for about 48 hours after the onset of the rash.

The infection is worldwide, and, before widespread use of the measles vaccine, epidemics and endemics occurred every 2 to 5 years, lasting for 3 to 4 months. Typically, measles occurs in the winter and spring. Worldwide immunization programs have drastically reduced the incidence of measles. The United States hopes to be measles-free by the end of the 1980s.

Pathologic findings

Acute inflammatory changes occur in the conjunctiva, the nasopharynx, the oral mucosa, and the epithelium of the respiratory tract. Bronchopneumonia may occur from secondary infection. There is generalized lymphoid hyperplasia with presence of giant cells in the tonsils, adenoids, lymph nodes, spleen, and appendix. Perivascular lymphocytic cuffing of small blood vessels, with associated congestion and edema, is observed. Pathognomonic Koplik spots in the buccal mucosa are produced by inflammation of the submucous glands. Encephalitic lesions consist of edema, congestion of small blood vessels, perivascular collections of lymphocytes, and petechial hemorrhages, followed by demyelination.

Clinical manifestations

The prodromal stage occurs 10 to 11 days after exposure and is characterized by marked

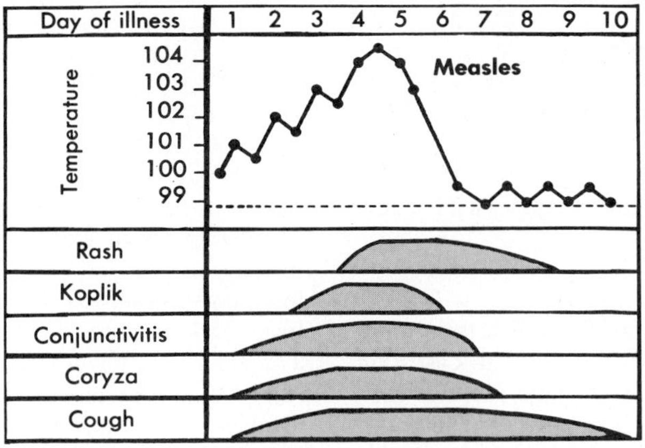

Fig. 27-11. Schematic diagram of clinical course of a typical case of measles. Rash appears 3 to 4 days after onset of fever, conjunctivitis, coryza, and cough. Koplik spots usually develop 2 days before rash. (From Krugman, S., and Katz, S.L.: Infectious diseases of children, ed. 7, St. Louis, 1981, The C.V. Mosby Co.)

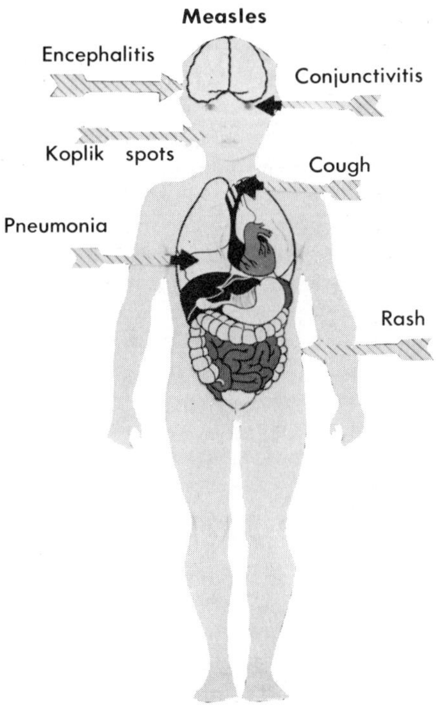

Fig. 27-12. Major manifestations of measles.

malaise, progressive fever, conjunctivitis, coryza, and cough. These symptoms are progressive. Temperatures ranging from 39.5° to 41° C (103° to 105° F) are not unusual. One to two days before the rash erupts, Koplik spots appear. They are tiny gray-white papules (''grains of sand'') on a dull, red base on the buccal mucosa opposite the molars. Soon after appearance of the rash, Koplik spots are no longer visible. Koplik spots have also been noted on the mucous membranes of the lower lip and near the gum, on the caruncle of the eye, and on the vaginal mucosa. These spots are pathognomonic of rubeola.

Conjunctivitis. Severe conjunctival infection and edema are characteristic of measles. First evidence of conjunctivitis is a transverse line of hyperemia on the conjunctiva of the lower lid near the margin. Conjunctival infection then becomes intense and generalized, the caruncle is inflamed, the lids become swollen, lacrimination is present, and photophobia occurs. Conjunctivitis clears as the temperature falls.

Rash. The rash usually appears 3 to 4 days after onset of illness. It begins as a maculopapular, erythematous eruption at the hairline, on the forehead, on the back of the neck, and behind the ears. It spreads downward to reach the feet in about 3 days. The rash is most common on the face, neck, and upper trunk and arms. It begins to fade about 3 to 4 days after its appearance in the same sequence as it occurred.

The initial red lesions blanch on pressure, but the subsequent brownish-stained ones do not. Brawny desquamation finally occurs, and the skin returns to normal. One to two days after appearance of the rash, fever and other clinical manifestations begin to resolve. The only exception is the cough, which may persist for several weeks.

Diagnosis

A typical case of measles, as just described, is easily diagnosed. However, not all cases are typical. In the pre-eruptive stage measles may be confused with an ordinary upper respiratory tract infection, but the presence of conjunctivitis should alert the physician to the possibility of measles. Observation for Koplik spots should rapidly establish the diagnosis.

Rubella is not so severe an infection, causes noticeable enlargement of the posterior cervical and occipital lymph nodes, and does not cause severe conjunctivitis, photophobia, cough, or Koplik spots. Exanthema subitum (roseola infantum) causes sudden high temperature in small children, but the rash appears after the temperature falls. Furthermore, roseola does not produce conjunctivitis, cough, and Koplik spots. Scarlet fever characteristically causes sore throat, tonsillar exudate, and cervical lymphadenitis. The blanchable rash is more diffusely red and avoids the area around the mouth (circumoral pallor). With scarlet fever there is a leukocytosis, whereas with measles there is a leukopenia. A rash similar to that of measles may occur as a result of drug sensitivity or with serum sickness. Other entities such as adenovirus exanthema may be confused with measles. Serologic studies are rarely needed for retrospective diagnosis.

Complications

Measles may produce a variety of complications, the most common of which are those of the respiratory tract. The complications of measles may be caused by the virus alone, by superimposed bacterial infection, or by a combination of the two.

Respiratory tract. The intense inflammation of the respiratory tract favors development of otitis media, cervical lymphadenitis, laryngitis, laryngotracheitis, and bronchopneumonia. Superinfection usually accounts for the otitis media. Moderate cervical glandular swelling may result from measles, but complicating pyogenic adenitis may also occur. Inflammatory changes in the larynx and trachea can be so severe as to cause obstruction to the airway, at times necessitating tracheostomy. Bronchopneumonia, the most common serious complication of measles, is said to occur in about 10% of cases, especially in the younger age group. Secondary bacterial infections should be suspected if high spiking fever persists longer than expected, or there is a recurrence of fever. Often there is leukocytosis rather than the leukopenia of uncomplicated measles. After appropriate cultures, antibiotic therapy should be instituted. *Pneumococcus, Streptococcus pyogenes,* and *Haemophilus influenzae* are the most common etiologic agents. *Staphylococcus aureus* may produce a severe pneumonia and empyema.

Encephalitis. Approximately 1 in every 1000 children who contract measles develops encephalitis. This complication may prove fatal or permanently damaging. It usually appears within the first 6 days of the rash but may occur before or after the rash.

Other complications. In rare instances measles causes extensive confluent hemorrhages into the skin (black measles) and bleeding from the nose, mouth, and intestinal tract. Fever appears abruptly and increases to high levels. The child becomes delirious, may have convulsions, and becomes stuporous or comatose. Measles may cause purpura of the thrombocytopenic or nonthrombocytopenic type. Occlusion of the lumen of the appendix by intense lymphoid hyperplasia may cause appendicitis. Measles may cause temporary reversal of the tuberculin test from positive to negative and favors extension of pulmonary tuberculosis.

Compromised hosts. Children with cancer and other disorders for which they are receiving immunosuppressive chemotherapy or radiation therapy are at high risk for severe and fatal measles. Often there is an extensive giant-cell pneumonia caused by direct invasion of lung parenchyma by the virus. Superinfection of the lungs with enteric gram-negative bacilli, *Staphylococcus aureus,* or enterococci also can occur in these compromised hosts. Children with low or absent immunoglobulins usually have an uncomplicated course. However, children with impaired cell-mediated immunity or marked malnutrition can have a severe and fatal course.

Pregnancy. Measles during the first trimester of pregnancy is associated with a high risk of spontaneous abortion. There is about a 10% risk for fetal wastage if measles occurs during the first trimester. Congenital anomalies associated with rubella are not found with rubeola.

Subacute sclerosing panencephalitis (SSPE). Panencephalitis is a chronic demyelinating cerebral degenerative disease. There is a strong association between SSPE and measles as evidenced by high antibody titers to measles virus in both the peripheral blood and cerebrospinal fluid. The exact pathogenesis and relationship to measles is unknown. The risk following natural infection is about 1 per 100,000 infections. It tends to occur in children who have had measles in the first few years of life. The onset of symptoms can be from 4 to 17 years following measles. Widespread vaccination programs have seen a decline in SSPE. It is estimated that the risk of SSPE is about 1 per 1,000,000 vaccinations. This entity is discussed in more detail on p. 788.

Atypical measles. Atypical measles has been reported to occur in children who received the killed measles vaccine, or killed vaccine followed by live vaccine, and several years later were exposed to wild virus. It is believed to be caused by hypersensitivity to the virus. The incubation period is similar to that of typical measles. The prodrome of 1 to 2 days is characterized by high fever of 39.5° to 41° C (103° to 105° F), headaches, abdominal pain, and myalgias. Unlike classical measles, the rash begins peripherally and may be urticarial, maculopapular, hemorrhagic, or even vesicular. Pulmonary symptoms are usually present, and a chest radiograph reveals marked infiltrates usually out of proportion to the clinical findings. Koplik spots are not seen. The infection tends to be quite severe and somewhat more prolonged than regular measles. Fatalities have not been reported.

Prevention and modifications

Measles vaccine is discussed on pp. 193-194. The child should be isolated from the onset of illness until 4 or 5 days after the rash appears. Therapy is essentially symptomatic, consisting of fever control, bed rest, and fluid management. The severe photophobia usually necessitates placing the patient in a dimly lit room. The cough should be treated symptomatically in a manner similar to that of other respiratory tract infections. Prophylactic antibiotics are of little benefit. Antibiotics should be used for the treatment of secondary bacterial infections. Measles encephalitis is managed symptomatically by aspirin or codeine for headache, sedation for irritability, and drugs for control of convulsions if they occur.

Sandor Feldman

ENTEROVIRAL INFECTIONS (POLIOMYELITIS, COXSACKIEVIRUS, AND ECHOVIRUS)

Enteroviruses have the common qualities of being small, being resistant to adverse factors, serving as transient inhabitants of the intestinal tract of humans, causing similar changes in tissue cultures, being worldwide in distribution, causing epidemics of illness chiefly in warm seasons, and having a predilection to infect the nervous system.

Poliomyelitis

Poliomyelitis is an acute viral disease occurring endemically and epidemically throughout the world and characterized by a tendency to produce variable degrees of paralysis. In areas where widespread active immunization has been achieved, its incidence has been dramatically reduced. In some areas of the world it has been virtually eliminated.

Etiology and epidemiology

The disease is caused by any one of three polioviruses—type 1, type 2, or type 3. Type 1 is the most frequent cause of paralytic poliomyelitis, type 3 is next in frequency, and type 2 is the least frequent.

When an individual becomes infected, the virus can be recovered from the oropharynx for about 1 week, but multiplication in the intestinal tract results in large quantities of virus being passed in the stools for a variable period, sometimes for weeks. Transmission by droplet infection may occur, but the principal mode of spread appears to be the fecal-oral route.

Although poliomyelitis may affect adults, even the elderly, it is predominantly a disease of the young.

The usual incubation period is 7 to 14 days. The period of communicability is more difficult to define, since it is impossible to predict how long the virus will be passed in the stools. The virus is generally present in the stool during the first week and may be excreted for 4 to 6 weeks or longer. Immunization against poliomyelitis is discussed elsewhere (p. 193).

Pathologic findings

Poliomyelitis selectively damages special areas in the central nervous system, and the neurologic manifestations vary with the particular sites involved. Neuronal injury may be mild and reversible (in which case full recovery ensues), sufficiently severe to destroy the cells and cause permanent loss of function, or so extensive and so intense as to cause death of the patient.

The anterior horn cells are affected in paralytic disease. Among the more serious but less frequent lesions are those that involve the respiratory and vasomotor centers in the medulla. Medullary nuclei of cranial nerves may also be damaged.

Clinical manifestations

There are four possible consequences of infection with poliovirus: (1) clinically inapparent asymptomatic infection, (2) abortive poliomyelitis, a minor illness with nonspecific manifestations, (3) nonparalytic poliomyelitis with the aseptic meningitis syndrome, and (4) paralytic poliomyelitis.

Inapparent infection. Most individuals who become infected with poliovirus exhibit no clinical manifestations.

Abortive poliomyelitis. The next most common type of infection is a minor illness with no manifestations pathognomonic of poliomyelitis. Clinical findings include fever, headache, sore throat, nausea, vomiting, anorexia, malaise, and vaguely localized abdominal pain.

Nonparalytic poliomyelitis. This clinical form is essentially a nonparalytic aseptic meningitis syndrome. It may occur as the initial evidence of illness or may appear after an afebrile period following the abortive form. In addition to the symptoms just described with reference to abortive poliomyelitis, there are now findings referable to the nervous system, such as pain and stiffness of the posterior muscles of the neck, back, and legs.

Examination of the cerebrospinal fluid reveals an increase in cells and a moderate increase in protein.

Paralytic poliomyelitis. Paralytic poliomyelitis may appear a few days after the patient has seemed to recover from the abortive type of the disease, or it may begin with all the manifestations of the nonparalytic aseptic meningitis syndrome discussed previously. Depending on sites of neuronal involvement there are four forms—spinal, bulbar, bulbospinal, and encephalitic.

Spinal form. The spinal form consists of manifestations referable to involvement of nerves arising from the spinal cord. Paralysis is associated with symptoms and signs of the nonparalytic form of the disease. It appears within a day or two after these manifestations occur. Impending paralysis may be indicated by muscle pain, hyperesthesia, tremors in the extremities, or changes in deep tendon reflexes.

Paralysis occurs usually within 2 to 5 days after the onset of illness. It is not likely to develop or to become more extensive after the temperature has returned to normal.

Muscle pain and spasm are present in the early stages and sometimes last for weeks. The child tends to avoid using the affected muscles, giving a false impression that paralysis has developed in these areas. Respiratory difficulty can arise because of phrenic nerve paralysis. This may be associated with paralysis of muscles of the chest wall. The urinary bladder may become paralyzed and retain urine, and there may be atony and distention of the bowel, causing constipation.

The subsequent fate of affected muscles is unpredictable. In muscles destined to recover completely or partially there is gradual recovery of muscle strength and a return to normal of the deep tendon reflexes. Although most improvement occurs within the first months after onset, gradual improvement may be noted for 12 to 18 months. Muscles that have continued to be paralyzed for a period of several weeks undergo atrophy.

Bulbar and bulbospinal form. Bulbar poliomyelitis may occur without associated manifestations of the spinal form, but combinations of these two types are more common. The bulbar type is life threatening but fortunately occurs in only about 10% of patients with the paralytic disease. Involvement of the tenth cranial nerve is particularly important. When this nerve is affected, there is weakness or paralysis that interferes with swallowing and respiration. The soft palate, pharynx, and larynx are affected. The voice assumes a nasal quality as palatal paralysis develops or becomes hoarse when the vocal cords are paralyzed.

When the respiratory center is affected, respirations are shallow, irregular, and interspersed by periods of apnea. Consequently the patient suffers from insufficient ventilation and decreased ability to clear secretions. In the bulbospinal form of the disease these difficulties may be combined with weakness or paralysis of the diaphragm and/or the respiratory muscles of the chest wall.

Encephalitic form. Clinical manifestations of this form are those of encephalitis in general. Disturbances in personality and sensorium occur. The patient may become irritable, disoriented, delirious, stuporous, or comatose. Gross tremors or convulsions may develop.

Diagnosis

Definitive diagnosis is based on laboratory studies. Recovery of poliovirus from the feces and throat establishes the fact that the patient harbors the virus. If clear-cut clinical disease is also present, the diagnosis of poliomyelitis is virtually certain. Demonstration of a rise in antibody titer to poliovirus in paired serum samples taken 2 to 3 weeks apart constitutes proof of the disease. Suspect cases should be reported to the Centers for Disease Control.

The cerebrospinal fluid is generally abnormal, and the cell count is usually elevated in the range of 10 to 500 cells. Initially the cells may be predominantly polymorphonuclear, but subsequently lymphocytes predominate. At first the protein content is generally slightly elevated and may increase up to 300 mg/dl within 2 to 3 weeks. No organisms are demonstrable by smear, and cultures are negative. The glucose content is normal.

Paralytic poliomyelitis must be differentiated from conditions that cause the aseptic meningitis syndrome and from conditions that cause pseudoparalysis or actual paralysis. Pseudoparalysis occurs when there is pain in an extremity and the patient prefers not to move it. In former years, when scurvy and congenital syphilis were more prevalent, pseudoparalysis caused by syphilitic osteochondritis or scurvy often led to the presumptive diagnosis of poliomyelitis. Today unrecognized trauma, sometimes inflicted in the home, and toxic synovitis, especially of the hip joint, may pose diagnostic problems. The joint pain of septic arthritis or rheumatic fever and the bone pain of acute osteomyelitis may also result in reluctance to use an extremity.

Muscular weakness or actual paralysis may occur in many conditions, in some instances simulating paralysis of poliomyelitis. Paralysis may result from infection with certain strains of coxsackie virus or echovirus. A more frequent cause of diagnostic difficulty is the Guillain-Barré syndrome (acute polyneuritis). Tick paralysis is a rare possibility.

Treatment

Treatment of the abortive form of poliomyelitis is entirely symptomatic. The child is confined to bed until he is afebrile and seems well. Strenuous activity should be avoided because of the possible effect of overexertion encouraging onset of the paralytic form. Treatment of the nonparalytic or aseptic meningitis form is also symptomatic. However, because of pain and stiffness of muscles of the neck, back, and extremities, analgesics alone may prove insufficient to control discomfort, and heat may be required. As in the abortive form, strenuous exertion should be avoided during the acute illness.

All children with the paralytic form should be hospitalized, regardless of how minor the paralysis may seem at the moment. Hospitalization affords much closer observation for indications that the disease is advancing, thus permitting early action to be taken when necessary.

Since improper positions in bed favor development of contractures that make rehabilitation more difficult, boards are placed beneath the mattress, the knees are supported in a slightly flexed position, the feet are maintained at right angles to the legs by means of a footboard or otherwise, and the hips and spine are kept in straight alignment. (All physiotherapeutic measures should be under the guidance of the orthopedist or physiatrist.)

Inability to swallow, present in the bulbar or bulbospinal form, necessitates special management such as gravity drainage and suction or tracheostomy. Unless there are other reasons why tracheostomy must be performed, gravity drainage and suction may be tried first. Parenteral fluid therapy is employed for the first few days, after which it may be possible to give a liquid diet by an indwelling nasogastric tube.

Respiratory difficulties present the most complicated problem in therapy. When there is weakness or paralysis of the respiratory muscles of the chest wall and/or the diaphragm, mechanical assistance for respiration is required, with or without tracheostomy. It is essential that the physician and personnel using these machines have complete familiarity with them. The patient must be observed frequently and carefully, and management must be individualized to the patient's needs. Laboratory facilities must be available for the various tests required for skilled care (blood gas determinations, pH, etc.).

The blood pressure should be followed carefully, because hypertension and hypotension frequently occur and require therapeutic action. The heart should be examined frequently in the acute phase of the disease to detect evidence of arrhythmia or decompensation necessitating digitalization. The possibility of intercurrent pneumonia should be kept constantly in mind. The urine should be examined periodically to detect unsuspected infection of the urinary tract, especially in patients requiring catheterization. Hyperpyrexia, sometimes of dangerous degree, may occur in the bulbar form. The biochemical dangers of prolonged immobilization should also be considered.

Coxsackievirus infections

Coxsackieviruses are divided into two major groups—A and B.

Etiology and epidemiology

Coxsackieviruses may be recovered from the pharyngeal secretions and feces of humans as well as from raw sewage. The human being appears to be the only host. Transmission from one individual to another takes place mainly in warm seasons of the year by the fecal-oral route. Although coxsackieviruses are definitely related to certain disease states, recovery of the organism from the stools does not always imply an etiologic relationship to current symptoms.

Pathologic findings

Although much is known concerning the pathologic lesions produced by these organisms in suckling mice and monkeys, less is known about the lesions they produce in humans. Myositis, hepatitis, carditis, and encephalomyelitis have been noted in infections produced by one or another strain of these viruses.

Clinical manifestations

Only a few of the many clinical syndromes ascribed to the coxsackieviruses will be described.

Herpangina. Herpangina is an acute, febrile self-limited disease occurring in the summer with a predilection for young children. Discrete vesicular lesions are found on the anterior tonsillar pillars and sometimes the soft palate, uvula, tonsils, pharynx, and posterior buccal mucosa. The vesicles are small and grayish and have a red areola around them. They rupture to leave small ulcers. There is headache, general malaise, vomiting, and temperature of 39° C (103° F) or more, as a rule. Treatment is symptomatic. This syndrome is caused by several strains of coxsackievirus group A.

Acute lymphonodular pharyngitis. Acute lymphonodular pharyngitis resembles herpangina and is caused by the coxsackievirus A-10. Symptoms are fever, headache, and sore throat. Small white or yellowish nodular lesions are seen on the uvula, anterior tonsillar pillars, and posterior pharynx. They subside without vesiculation or ulceration. Treatment is symptomatic.

Hand, foot, and mouth disease. This acute self-limited entity is caused by coxsackievirus group A. It is characterized by fever, malaise, presence of vesicular and ulcerative lesions in the mouth, and maculopapular rash and vesicles on the hands and feet. Sometimes a transient erythematous rash is seen on the extremities and buttocks.

Epidemic myalgia (pleurodynia; devil's grip; Bornholm disease). Epidemic myalgia is characterized by recurrent knifelike, excruciating pain in the muscles of the chest wall and perhaps upper abdomen. Occasionally, tenderness and swelling are found at sites of myositis. The child has a moderate to high temperature, general malaise, anorexia, and headache. The disease is self-limited, and the treatment is symptomatic. This illness is caused by strains of coxsackievirus group B.

Aseptic meningitis. One of the more common manifestations of infection with certain strains of coxsackievirus groups A and B is the development of aseptic meningitis. Fever, headache, vomiting, stiff neck and back, positive Kernig and Brudzinski signs, and abnormal cerebrospinal fluid are all signs of this disease. The number of white blood cells is elevated to several hundred per cubic millimeter or perhaps more, and there is usually a lymphocytic preponderance (initially polymorphonuclear leukocytes may predominate). The disease is self-limited, and treatment is symptomatic.

Encephalomyocarditis of the newborn. Small outbreaks of encephalomyocarditis caused by coxsackievirus group B, types 1 to 5, have occurred in newborn infants. These infants have fever and perhaps diarrhea and then develop symptoms and signs of cardiac decompensation, which is often fatal. Tachycardia, cardiomegaly, hepatomegaly, electrocardiographic signs of myocarditis, and finally circulatory collapse are the typical clinical manifestations.

Echovirus infections

The echoviruses are enteroviruses that have many similarities to polioviruses and coxsackieviruses. They cause a variety of clinical syndromes.

The term ECHO refers to *enteric cytopathogenic human orphan* viruses. They are found in the feces of humans and damaged cells in cell culture and were originally said to be orphans because they could not be related to any disease. Subsequent investigations proved their etiologic roles in several disease syndromes.

Aseptic meningitis is one of the most common expressions of infection with these organisms, and it has the clinical findings previously mentioned in the discussion of coxsackieviruses. In addition, certain types of echoviruses produce muscular weakness and paralysis like those of poliomyelitis. Some strains produce maculopapular eruptions associated with general symptoms of febrile illness. Diarrhea and undifferentiated febrile illness may be produced by echoviruses.

Mycotic diseases

NORTH AMERICAN BLASTOMYCOSIS

Etiology and epidemiology

Blastomyces dermatitidis is the etiologic agent of North American blastomycosis. The majority of cases in the United States occur in the southeast, although sporadic cases are found in other states. Several cases have been reported in Canada. The highest incidence is in men between the ages of 30 and 40 years; the disease is rare in children. The natural habitat is unknown, and human-to-human transmission does not occur.

Pathogenesis

The respiratory tract is usually the portal of entry. From pulmonary lymph nodes and parenchymal lesions the infection may disseminate by hematogenous, lymphogenous, or local extension. Any organ may be involved except the intestine.

The lesion is one of suppuration and granulomatous reaction with giant cells, and the organism is seen as a double-contoured budding yeast cell.

Clinical manifestations

There are three clinical forms of the disease—pulmonary, cutaneous, and disseminated. The pulmonary type resembles tuberculosis. The course of the cutaneous lesions is that of a papule or pustule, which ulcerates and progresses to a large, chronic granulomatous lesion. In the disseminated form the signs and symptoms are related to the organs involved, which may include the central nervous system, abdominal viscera, muscle, and bone.

Diagnosis

Skin tests and serologic studies are of little use in diagnosis. On examination of exudate or biopsy of the lesions the parasitic yeast phase is found in active lesions. Isolation of *B. dermatitidis* in culture is necessary for diagnosis. Specimens can be cultured on Sabouraud dextrose agar.

Treatment

Amphotericin B is the drug of choice (p. 760), although hydroxystilbamidine has been used successfully.

CANDIDIASIS

Etiology and epidemiology

Candida albicans is the usual cause of candidiasis, although other *Candida* species occasionally cause disease. *C. albicans* may exist as a saprophyte or may cause disease in humans and several of the lower animals. It is a normal inhabitant of the throat, intestinal tract, and vagina.

Pathogenesis

Candidiasis is encountered in newborn infants and in older children who may have underlying disease (such as malignant neoplasms or endocrinopathies) or immune deficiency disorders or who have been subjected to broad-spectrum antibiotics or immunosuppressive drugs. Oral candidiasis of the neonate is usually acquired from the maternal vagina or breast.

Clinical manifestations

Candidiasis may be manifested in one or more of the following forms.

Infection of the mucous membranes. Thrush is the most frequently encountered form of candidiasis and is easily recognized as white, plaquelike lesions on the oral mucosa, tongue, or soft palate. The underlying mucous membrane is slightly inflamed. Similar lesions may occur in the vagina. Enteric infection is frequently associated with oral thrush.

Paronychia and onychia. Inflammations of the nail fold and nail matrix are possible manifestations.

Pulmonary infection. Pulmonary infection may be acute or chronic, occurring either as pneumonitis or bronchitis.

Cutaneous candidiasis. Cutaneous candidiasis occurs in four forms: (1) intertriginous—erythematous, papulovesicular, and confluent lesions of the gluteal folds, groin, axillae, or neck; (2) generalized—may be chronic and usually is associated with underlying endocrinopathy or defect of the immune mechanism; (3) congenital—generalized dermatitis acquired in utero, which is extremely rare; and (4) granuloma, a rare form with horny crusts on granulomatous lesions.

Systemic candidiasis. Hematogenous dissemination of *C. albicans* may result in generalized infection involving lungs, kidney, central nervous system, liver, spleen, and other organs. This form of candidiasis is always secondary to an underlying disease that compromises the host's response to infection.

Diagnosis

Careful correlation of clinical manifestations with repeated isolation of *C. albicans,* as well as demonstration of the organism in inflamed tissue, is required to establish a diagnosis of visceral or systemic candidiasis. Serum antibody titers are of no diagnostic help. Infections localized to the skin and mucous membranes are usually characteristic enough to establish a diagnosis by inspection.

Treatment

Nystatin is the drug of choice for oral, enteric, and cutaneous candidiasis. Intravenous amphotericin B is required for the systemic disease (p. 760). Flucytosine is useful in some types of systemic candidiasis along with amphotericin B. Miconazole and ketoconazole are new drugs with some effect against certain types of candidiasis.

COCCIDIOIDOMYCOSIS

Etiology and epidemiology

Coccidioidomycosis is a frequent infection in children of the dusty and dry areas of southern California, Arizona, New Mexico, and southwestern Texas. The etiologic agent, *Coccidioides immitis,* is found in the soil. Human-to-human transmission does not occur.

Pathogenesis

A focal pneumonitis occurs after inhalation of *C. immitis*. Most of the pulmonary lesions heal spontaneously. Less frequently, hematogenous dissemination may result in lesions of nearly all viscera and tissues. The histologic response resembles that of tuberculosis.

Clinical manifestations

More than half the patients with the pulmonary form have no symptoms; the remainder have fever, cough, and chest pain. Some of the children have a maculopapular rash. The symptoms usually abate in 1 to 2 weeks. Chronic pulmonary fibrosis and cavitation rarely occur in children.

With disseminated coccidioidomycosis, symptoms and signs may appear abruptly or insidiously, and clinical findings depend on the organs involved. Visceral organs, lungs, lymph nodes, bones, joints, and the central nervous system are most frequently involved.

Diagnosis

A reaction to the coccidioidin skin test indicates recent or past infection. Complement-fixation and precipitin tests are reliable. Examination of exudates and tissue, employing Grocott stain, demonstrates the large thick-walled spherules filled with endospores, which are diagnostic. *C. immitis* may be cultured on Sabouraud dextrose agar.

Treatment

Amphotericin B is the drug of choice for the treatment of disseminated coccidioidomycosis (p. 760). The pulmonary form does not require therapy, except in rare cases of chronic progressive pulmonary disease. Two new drugs, miconazole and ketaconazole, are being evaluated in the treatment of this condition.

CRYPTOCOCCOSIS (TORULOSIS)

Etiology and epidemiology

The monomorphic yeast *Cryptococcus neoformans* is the causative agent of cryptococcosis. Infection is more likely to occur in patients with debilitating disorders such as cancer, diabetes mellitus, and Hodgkin disease. The organism is most frequently found in pigeon excreta, although pigeons are not hosts to *C. neoformans*.

Pathogenesis

Tubercle-like lesions develop after inhalation of *C. neoformans*. Hematogenous dissemination may occur, with the central nervous system being the most frequent site for secondary infection.

Clinical manifestations

Pulmonary symptoms resemble those of tuberculosis. There is sudden or insidious onset of central nervous system signs and symptoms of increased intracranial pressure and meningeal irritation. Osteolytic bone lesions, endocarditis, lymphadenopathy, and cutaneous lesions are rare forms of cryptococcosis.

Diagnosis

The diagnosis is made by isolation of *C. neoformans* in culture from tissue specimens or by demonstrating the large halolike capsule of budding yeast cells with an india ink preparation of cerebrospinal fluid. Studies to detect cryptococcal antigen in body fluids, especially the cerebrospinal fluid, may be of help in making a rapid diagnosis.

Treatment

Amphotericin B is the drug of choice (p. 760). The drug flucytosine has synergistic activity and should be given with amphotericin B.

HISTOPLASMOSIS

Etiology and epidemiology

The etiologic agent of histoplasmosis is *Histoplasma capsulatum*. Its habitat is the soil, and infection occurs by inhalation of airborne spores. Human-to-human transmission does not occur. Approximately 30 million people in the United States have been infected with *H. capsulatum*. Although the disease occurs in temperate and tropical climates around the world, the majority of cases in the United States are found in the eastern central states.

Pathogenesis

Inhaled spores enter macrophages and are carried as yeast forms to the peribronchial and hilar lymph nodes, where a granulomatous reaction occurs. This primary complex, similar to that of tuberculosis, remains localized in most patients and eventually heals by calcification. Hematogenous dissemination may occur, producing lesions within the spleen, liver, bone marrow, and other organs.

Clinical manifestations

The spectrum of clinical manifestations is broad, varying from an asymptomatic infection to a fulminating and fatal disease. In general, five clinical forms can be delineated as follows: (1) inapparent infection, (2) acute pulmonary form, (3) chronic pulmonary form, (4) acute disseminated form, and (5) chronic histoplasmosis. Inapparent infection is manifested only by conversion of the histoplasmin skin test from negative to positive.

The acute pulmonary form is an influenza-like illness with cough, fever, chest pain, and malaise. Radiographs reveal hilar adenopathy and pulmonary infiltration.

The chronic pulmonary form occurs infrequently in children and is characterized by exacerbations and remissions of pulmonary disease leading to cavitation.

The acute disseminated form is uncommon and occurs most frequently in children less than 2 years of age. The onset may be insidious or acute with cough, fever, hepatosplenomegaly, purpura, and mucocutaneous lesions. Pancytopenia may occur. The radiograph usually reveals pneumonitis, which may be miliary, with diffuse mottled infiltrates.

Chronic histoplasmosis is rare in children; it resembles chronic cavitary tuberculosis of adults, or it may progress to a prolonged disseminated form.

Diagnosis

A reaction of 5 mm or greater of induration to the histoplasmin skin test indicates past or present infection with *H. capsulatum*. Accordingly the skin test is not helpful in diagnosis.

Agar gel precipitin and agglutination tests demonstrate antibodies early in the course of disease. Complement-fixation tests measure antibodies, appearing 2 to 4 weeks after onset of infection. A titer of 1:8 to the yeast or mycelia antigen suggests infection. Skin tests may influence antibody titer, especially to the mycelia (histoplasmin) antigen and should not be used if histoplasmosis is suspected.

The yeast form of *H. capsulatum* in large mononuclear cells may be specifically identified by Giemsa stain in bone marrow or biopsy specimens.

Isolation of *H. capsulatum* in culture of sputum, bone marrow, urine, or other specimens establishes the diagnosis. Brain heart infusion agar is a suitable medium.

Treatment

Primary pulmonary histoplasmosis almost invariably subsides spontaneously and requires only supportive therapy. The mortality in acute disseminated histoplasmosis is 80% if untreated. Specific therapy with amphotericin B is indicated.

Amphotericin B must be administered intravenously with daily infusions. The initial dosage is 0.25 mg/kg/24 hr. The amount is increased daily until the dosage of 1mg/kg/24 hr is attained, and therapy is continued for approximately 4 to 6 weeks. Amphotericin B is nephrotoxic, and renal function must be carefully monitored. Anemia, hypokalemia, and hypocalcemia are also frequent side effects. Sulfonamides have also been used in therapy but are not considered the drugs of choice in serious cases. Early studies with ketoconazole suggest this drug has promise for the treatment of histoplasmosis.

OTHER MYCOSES AND MYCOTIC-LIKE INFECTIONS

The actinomycetes, *Nocardia* and *Actinomyces* species, are considered to be higher bacteria with some features of the lower fungi.

Actinomycosis is a chronic granulomatous disease that may be arbitrarily divided into three clinical types—cervicofacial, thoracic, and abdominal. Abscess formation with draining sinuses characterizes the disease. *Actinomyces israelii* is the species most frequently responsible for the infection. Penicillin is the drug of choice and should be administered for a long period of time.

Nocardiosis is usually caused by *Nocardia asteroides*. The lung, brain, and liver are the most frequent sites for infection. Sulfadiazine should be given over an extended period.

Phycomycosis

Patients with diabetes mellitus or cancer or those receiving immunosuppressive therapy are susceptible to infection from Phycomycetes organisms, especially *Mucor* and *Rhizopus* species. Sites of predilection are the lung, gastrointestinal tract, head and neck structures, and brain. These large aseptate organisms initiate suppurative necrosis and may penetrate arterial walls to cause thrombi and infarcts. Amphotericin B should be used in therapy, and surgery should be considered for localized lesions.

Aspergillosis

Species of *Aspergillus* are usually saprophytic but may cause disease in the susceptible host. Pulmonary lesions may be similar to those of tuberculosis. Allergic bronchopulmonary aspergillosis is an asthmalike illness in which the clinical manifestations indicate a hypersensitivity to organisms in the respiratory tract. Systemic aspergillosis is always secondary to an underlying chronic disease. Chronic conjunctivitis, mucopurulent nasal discharge, and cutaneous abscesses suggest systemic aspergillosis. Generalized disease requires therapy with intravenous amphotericin B (p. 760).

Walter T. Hughes

Rickettsial diseases

The rickettsial diseases comprise a group of acute, often life-threatening, infections caused by rickettsiae—small, gram-negative, pleomorphic, coccobacilli that are intermediate between bacteria and viruses. They inhabit the alimentary tract of arthropod vectors and infect animals and humans. Rickettsial diseases are worldwide in distribution, and individual types of rickettsiae exhibit a predilection for particular geographic regions. Only three of these conditions will be discussed: Rocky Mountain spotted fever (tick-borne typhus), murine typhus (endemic typhus), and rickettsialpox.

ROCKY MOUNTAIN SPOTTED FEVER (TICK-BORNE TYPHUS)

Rocky Mountain spotted fever is an acute febrile illness caused by *Rickettsia rickettsii*. It is transmitted to humans by ticks and is characterized by abrupt onset, headache, fever, and a characteristic skin rash.

Etiology

Ticks become infected by feeding on a variety of wild animals that constitute the natural reservoir of the organism. After ingestion the rickettsiae penetrate the tick's intestinal wall and eventually reach the salivary glands, through which the tick is capable of transmitting the disease to a new host. The rickettsiae are passed transovarially from generation to generation. Humans become infected by the bite of the tick or by contamination when removing the tick from the body of another person or a dog. The disease has now been reported from 44 states. Two thirds of cases occur in Appalachian states, especially Maryland, Virginia, North Carolina, and Georgia.

Tick vectors vary from one geographic area to another. In the Rocky Mountain states the wood tick *(Dermacentor andersoni)* is the principal vector. In the Appalachian states the dog tick *(D. variabilis)* is the usual vector. In the Gulf Coast states the Lone Star tick *(Amblyomma americanum)* is usually the transmitting arthropod.

Exposure to ticks is most likely to occur in persons whose occupations require them to frequent the woods, or in the increasing number of Americans who seek wooded areas for recreation. It is important to note that humans may not be infected by the tick's bite until the tick has been attached to the skin for several hours.

Pathologic findings

The rickettsiae invade primarily small blood vessels, especially in the skin, subcutaneous tissue, myocardium, and central nervous system. Endothelial cells swell, proliferate, and degenerate, leading to formation of thrombi that may partially or completely block the vascular lumen. Smooth muscle cells of arterioles and small blood vessels may be invaded, causing degenerative changes, focal necrosis, rupture, and consequent petechiae or ecchymoses. Capillaries undergo mononuclear inflammation, fibrous thrombosis, increased permeability, and transudation of fluid high in protein, the latter accounting for generalized edema. Disseminated intravascular coagulopathy may occur.

Clinical manifestations

After an incubation period of 3 to 12 days the disease begins abruptly with fever, severe headache, severe malaise, anorexia, generalized muscular aching, sometimes vomiting, and occasionally chills. Usually within 4 to 5 days after onset, but sometimes earlier, the characteristic rash appears. It generally begins on the wrists, ankles, and lower legs and spreads rapidly to involve the entire body, including the palms, soles, and scalp. The fact that palms and soles are involved is of importance in differential diagnosis. The typical lesion begins as an erythematous macule but soon becomes purplish, maculopapular, and petechial. As the fever falls, the lesion begins to fade, leaving a pigmented area. Gangrene of the skin may occur in severe cases.

Because of increased capillary permeability edema may appear 3 to 4 days after onset, generally first seen in the face but soon noted in the extremities.

At onset patients are usually irritable or apathetic and may progress to stupor or coma. Signs of meningeal irritation may appear early in the course of the disease, with or without mild abnormalities of the cerebrospinal fluid. More severe neurologic manifestations may occur.

The electrocardiogram may show minor changes, reflecting myocardial vascular damage. Frank cardiac failure can occur in severe cases.

The liver may be slightly enlarged, but jaundice is uncommon. The spleen may be enlarged.

With early diagnosis and proper treatment the course of the disease is mild and greatly abbreviated. Untreated patients are ill for 2 to 3 weeks, and severely ill patients recover in 3 to 4 weeks. Before the advent of treatment with chloramphenicol or tetracyclines the overall mortality was high, but with modern therapy few patients now die from this disease.

Diagnosis

Differential diagnosis includes other types of rickettsial diseases (especially murine typhus and rickettsialpox), meningococcemia, infectious mononucleosis, rubella, measles, and ECHO viral infections.

Leukopenia occurs during the first week, and leukocytosis appears during the second week. Anemia is not characteristic but may occur when the disease is unusually severe. Traces of albumin are often present in the urine. Mild azotemia is often present, and oliguria or anuria may occur in severe disease. A highly characteristic finding in Rocky Mountain spotted fever is the presence of a low serum sodium concentration, usually below 130 mEq/L. Minor electrocardiographic abnormalities may be noted. Liver function studies may be abnormal. In the second week of the disease serum protein values may be reduced.

The Weil-Felix reaction is helpful in establishing a presumptive diagnosis of a rickettsial disease, but it is not specific for Rocky Mountain spotted fever. Aggulutinins against three types of *Proteus vulgaris* may appear (OX-19, OX-2, OX-K) from the fifth to twelfth day of illness. Highest titers are generally obtained against the OX-19 strain but sometimes against the OX-2 strain. A single convalescent serum titer of 1:320 is considered diagnostic of a rickettsial disease, but demonstration of rising titer in paired serum specimens is stronger evidence. The complement-fixation antibody test for *R. rickettsii* constitutes positive evidence of infection with this particular organism.

Treatment

Because serologic proof of a rickettsial disease is not available until the second week of the illness and because of the rapidity with which the disease may progress, the physician should initiate treatment based on clinical suspicion. Tetracycline or chloramphenicol should be administered until 4 to 6 days after the patient has become afebrile.

Prevention

Since ticks may not infect an individual for several hours after attaching themselves to the skin, persons frequenting wooded areas should examine themselves after possible exposure. Children should be examined by parents when they return from areas of possible exposure. Ticks should never be removed by detaching them with bare fingers; juices of the crushed ticks may cause infection.

A vaccine is available for protection against Rocky Mountain spotted fever.

MURINE TYPHUS (ENDEMIC TYPHUS)

Etiology

Murine typhus is an acute febrile rickettsial disease caused by *R. mooseri*. It is similar to, but milder than, epidemic typhus. Geographic distribution in the United States includes the southeastern states, particularly those bordering the Gulf of Mexico.

Rats constitute the natural reservoir for the rickettsiae causing this disease. After the flea has ingested the blood of an infected rat, the organisms multiply in the flea's intestinal tract. When the flea bites a human being, infected feces are deposited at the site of the bite. Irritation from being bitten leads to scratching, which inoculates the organisms into the skin, causing infection. Inhalation of infected, dry flea feces may also cause the disease.

Pathologic findings

Pathologic changes follow the general pattern of rickettsial diseases as described in the discussion of the pathologic course of Rocky Mountain spotted fever.

Clinical manifestations

Clinical manifestations begin after an incubation period that ranges from 6 to 14 days. Onset is abrupt, with headache, backache, muscular pains, arthralgia, sometimes gastrointestinal disturbances, and fever that lasts about 9 to 14 days. An erythematous macular rash appears, usually on the fourth or fifth day. It starts on the trunk, spreads to the extremities, and usually does not involve the palms, soles, or face. Some affected children have no rash.

Mild edema may occur from vascular damage. Mild pharyngeal hyperemia and complaint of sore throat may be present. Central nervous system symptoms rarely occur. The death rate is extremely low.

Laboratory findings include leukopenia during the first week and leukocytosis afterward.

There may be slight lowering of the serum proteins when edema is present.

Diagnosis

Serologic surveys have shown that the disease occurs far more commonly than is reported. The Weil-Felix reaction may become positive but is nonspecific. The complement-fixation antibody test should be employed to establish a precise diagnosis of murine typhus.

Treatment and prevention

Treatment consists of supportive care and administration of either tetracycline or chloramphenicol. Prevention is difficult to achieve but obviously involves control measures for reduction of the rat population.

RICKETTSIALPOX

Etiology

Rickettsialpox is caused by *R. akari*. It is transmitted to humans by the bite of the mouse mite and is characterized by a local lesion at the site of the bite, subsequent fever, systemic manifestations, and a diagnostically distinctive rash.

Clinical manifestations

After an incubation period of 7 to 10 days, a local lesion develops at the site of the bite in almost all cases. The lesion is a firm, red papule 0.5 to 2 cm in diameter that develops a vesicle in its center, which ruptures, crusts, and leaves an eschar for 2 to 3 weeks or longer. Regional nodes may enlarge and become tender but do not suppurate.

About a week later general manifestations of illness develop, with fever, chills or chilly sensations, generalized aching, and sometimes eye pain and photophobia. In about 1 to 3 days after onset of fever the characteristic rash appears. It is scattered indiscriminately, showing no predilection for trunk or extremities. Lesions begin as erythematous maculopapules that enlarge and are soon surmounted by vesicles. The regress in 4 to 7 days, leaving no scar. The presence of the local eschar at the site of infection and the peculiar maculopapular lesions topped by vesicles is sufficient to alert the physician to the proper diagnosis. In about one third of cases there is an enanthem similar to the exanthem. After onset of systemic manifestations the duration of the disease is usually 7 to 10 days. Complications are extremely rare, and no deaths have been reported in the United States.

Diagnosis

Diagnosis should be relatively simple in the typical case. Chickenpox is about the only disease with which rickettsialpox could be confused. In chickenpox the lesions erupt in crops and vary in stages of development, and the vesicles are not superimposed on the tops of papules.

Precise diagnosis rests on the complement-fixation antibody test that distinguishes rickettsialpox from other rickettsial infections. It is to be noted that rickettsialpox does not produce a positive Weil-Felix reaction to *Proteus* organisms. There is usually leukopenia with relative lymphocytosis during the first week of the disease.

Treatment

Treatment consists in administration of tetracycline or chloramphenicol.

James G. Hughes

PNEUMOCYSTIS CARINII PNEUMONIA

This infection occurs almost entirely in immunocompromised patients, but has been recognized in debilitated as well as otherwise healthy infants.

Etiology

P. carinii is a protozoan-like agent with global distribution.

Pathology

The infantile form of *P. carinii* pneumonia is characterized by a generalized interstitial plasma cell pneumonitis. The pneumonitis in older children and adults who are immunocompromised is a diffuse bilateral alveolar disease.

Clinical manifestation

The infantile form has a subtle onset with marked tachypnea, rales, and little or no fever. The child-adult form has an acute onset with fever, tachypnea, and no rales. In both types the disease remains localized to the lungs. Untreated, the mortality rate for the infantile form is about 50%, whereas in children and adults the mortality rate is almost 100%.

Diagnosis

The chest radiograph reveals a diffuse interstitial pneumonitis with no unique characteristics. A definitive diagnosis requires the demonstration of *P. carinii* organisms in lung parenchyma obtained by biopsy or in fluid obtained by needle aspiration of the lung.

Treatment

Trimethoprim-sulfamethoxazole is the drug of choice. Pentamidine isethionate is equally effective but has severe adverse effects.

Isolation. Active cases should be isolated from immunocompromised individuals through respiratory precautions.

CHLAMYDIA INFECTIONS

Two species of chlamydiae, *C. trachomatis* and *C. psittaci,* cause disease in man as well as in lower animals.

Chlamydia trachomatis

Etiology and epidemiology

C. trachomatis is an obligate intracellular parasite transmitted from infected mothers to newborn infants. Approximately 2% to 13% of pregnant women harbor the organism. Sexual transmission occurs, and direct transmission from infected material is possible.

Pathology

In trachoma the organism infects the conjunctival epithelial cells, causing subepithelial infiltration of lymphocytes and proceeding to the development of follicles. Infected epithelial cells contain cytoplasmic inclusion bodies. Fibroblasts and neovascularization invade the affected area and a pannus forms. With *C. trachmatis* pneumonitis of infancy an intense interstitial lymphoid infiltration is seen around the bronchioles and blood vessels and in the alveoli. The airway is often filled with mixed inflammatory cells.

Clinical manifestations

Several clinical types of infections occur. Inclusion conjunctivitis is usually noted 1 to 2 weeks after birth with congestion, edema, and minimal discharge.

Trachoma is a chronic follicular conjunctivitis associated with repeated infections that may result in blindness.

Lymphogranuloma venerum is a local lesion of the urogenital tract with regional (inguinal) lymphadenitis.

C. trachomitis urethritis will cause pain on urination.

Pneumonitis is seen usually in infants 1 to 4 months of age, manifested by staccato cough, tachypnea, wheezing, and rales. The course is subtle onset with little or no fever. Chest radiograph reveals hyperinflation and diffuse interstitial and patchy alveolar infiltration.

Diagnosis

The organism can be cultured in McCoy, HeLa, or L-cells. Scrapings of conjunctiva or tracheal aspirates stained with Giemsa stain reveals intracytoplasmic inclusions. A microimmunofluorescent antibody titer of 1:32 is strongly suggestive in infants with pneumonitis but is not of much diagnostic help in other types of the infection. The infantile pneumonitis is often accompanied by eosinophila and elevation of immunoglobulin G levels.

Treatment

Erythromycin, tetracycline, or sulfonamides are used in the treatment of *C. trachomatis* infections.

Isolation precautions. Respiratory isolation of infants with pneumonitis and secretion precautions for eye infections are recommended.

Chlamydia psittaci

C. psittaci is an uncommon cause of acute pneumonitis in adults and even less common in children. The major source for transmission is birds. Tetracycline is the drug of choice for treatment.

Walter T. Hughes

GENERAL REFERENCES

American Academy of Pediatrics: Report of the Committee on Infectious Diseases, ed. 19, Evanston, Ill., 1982, The Academy.

Krugman, S., et al., editors: Infectious diseases of children, St. Louis, 1977, The C.V. Mosby Co.

Remington, J.S., and Klein, J.O.: Infectious diseases of the fetus and newborn infant, ed. 2, Philadelphia, 1983, W.B. Saunders Co.

Feigin, R.D., and Cherry, J.D., editors: Textbook of pediatric infectious diseases, Philadelphia, 1981, W.B. Saunders Co.

Wedgewood, R.J., et al.: Infectious diseases of children, New York, 1982, Harper and Row, Publishers, Inc.

SELECTED READINGS

Bacteremia

Feigin, R.D.: Bacteremia and septicemia. In Vaughan, V.C., III, et al., editors: Textbook of pediatrics, Philadelphia, 1979, W.B. Saunders Co.

McCarthy, P.L., et al.: Bacteremia in children: an outpatient clinical review, Pediatrics **57:**861, 1976.

Myers, M.G., et al.: Complications of occult pneumococcal bacteremia in children, J. Pediatr. **84:**656, 1974.

Teele, D.W., et al.: Bacteremia in febrile children under 2 years of age: results of cultures of blood of 600 consecutive febrile children seen in a "walk-in" clinic, J. Pediatr. **87:**227, 1975.

Bacterial meningitis

Balagtas, R.C., et al.: Secondary and prolonged fevers in bacterial meningitis, J. Pediatr. **77:**957, 1970.

Davis, S.D., et al.: Partial antibiotic therapy in *Haemophilus influenzae* meningitis: its effect on cerebrospinal fluid abnormalities, Am. J. Dis. Child. **129:**802, 1975.

Dodge, P.R., and Swartz, M.N.: Bacterial meningitis: a review of selected aspects. II. Special neurologic problems, postmeningitic complications and clinicopathological correlations, N. Engl. J. Med. **272:**954, 1965.

Feigin, R.D.: Bacterial meningitis beyond the neonatal period. In Feigin, R.D., and Cherry, J.D., editors: Textbook of pediatric infectious disease, Philadelphia, 1981, W.B. Saunders Co.

Feigin, R.D., et al.: Countercurrent immunoelectrophoresis of urine as well as of CSF and blood for diagnosis of bacterial meningitis, J. Pediatr. **89:**773, 1976.

Kaplan, S.L., and Feigin, R.D.: The syndrome of inappropriate secretion of antidiuretic hormone in children with bacterial meningitis, J. Pediatr. **92:**758, 1978.

Leinonen, M., and Herva, E.: The latex agglutination test for the diagnosis of meningococcal and *Haemophilus influenzae* meningitis, Scand. J. Infect. Dis. **9:**187, 1977.

Report of The Committee on Infectious Diseases: *Hemophilus influenzae* infections; meningococcal infections, ed. 19, Evanston, Ill., 1982, American Academy of Pediatrics.

Brucellosis

Buchanan, T.M., et al.: Brucellosis in the United States, 1960-1972, Medicine **53:**403, 1974.

Fox, M.D., and Kaufmann, A.F.: Brucellosis in the United States, 1965-1974, J. Infect. Dis. **136:**312, 1977.

Street, L., Jr., et al.: Brucellosis in childhood, Pediatrics **55:**416, 1975.

Yow, M.D.: Brucellosis. In Feigin, R.D., and Cherry, J.D., editors: Textbook of pediatric infectious diseases, Philadelphia, 1981, W.B. Saunders Co.

Diphtheria

Brooks, G.F., et al.: Diphtheria in the United States, 1959-1970, J. Infect. Dis. **129:**172, 1974.

Hodes, H.L.: Diphtheria, Pediatr. Clin. North Am. **26:**445, 1979.

McCloskey, R.V., et al.: The 1970 epidemic of diphtheria in San Antonio, Ann. Intern. Med. **75:**495, 1971.

Morgan, B.C.: Cardiac complications of diphtheria, Pediatrics **32:**549, 1963.

Pertussis (whooping cough)

Balagtas, R.C., et al.: Treatment of pertussis with pertussis immune globulin, J. Pediatr. **79:**203, 1971.

Linneman, C.C., and Perry, E.B.: Bordetella parapertussis: recent experience and a review of the literature, Am. J. Dis. Child. **131:**560, 1977.

Nelson, J.D.: The changing epidemiology of pertussis in young infants: the role of adults as reservoirs of infection, Am. J. Dis. Child. **132:**371, 1978.

Olson, L.C.: Pertussis, Medicine **54:**427, 1975.

Pittman, M.: Pertussis toxin: the cause of the harmful effects and prolonged immunity of whooping cough—a hypothesis, Rev. Infect. Dis. **1:**401, 1979.

Report of the Committee on Infectious Diseases: Pertussis (whooping cough), ed. 19, Evanston, Ill., 1982, American Academy of Pediatrics.

Salmonellosis

Black, P.H., et al.: Salmonellosis—a review of some unusual aspects, N. Eng. J. Med. **262:**811, 1960.

Cherubin, C.E., et al.: Septicemia with non-typhoid salmonella, Medicine **53:**365, 1974.

Dixon, J.M.S.: Effect of antibiotic treatment on duration of excretion of Salmonella typhimurium by children, Br. Med. J. **2:**1343, 1965.

Hornick, R.B.: Non-typhoidal salmonellosis. In Hoeprich, P.D., editor: Infectious diseases: a modern treatise of infectious processes, ed. 3, New York, 1983, Harper & Row, Publishers, Inc.

Hornick, R.B.: Typhoid fever. In Hoeprich, P.D., editor: Infectious diseases: a modern treatise of infectious processes, ed. 3, New York, 1983, Harper & Row, Publishers, Inc.

Nelson, J.D.: Salmonella infections. In Wedgewood, R.J., et al., editors: Infections in children, New York, 1982, Harper & Row, Publishers, Inc.

Nelson, J.D., et al.: Treatment of Salmonella gastroenteritis with Ampicillin, Amoxicillin, or placebo, Pediatrics **65:**1125, 1980.

Shigellosis (bacillary dysentery)

Duncan, B., et al.: *Shigella* sepsis, Am. J. Dis. Child. **135:**151, 1981.

DuPont, H.L., and Hornick, R.B.: Adverse effect of lomotil therapy in shigellosis, J.A.M.A. **226:**1525, 1973.

Hornick, R.B.: Shigella infections. In Feigin, R.D., and Cherry, J.D., editors: Textbook of pediatric infectious diseases, Philadelphia, 1981, W.B. Saunders Co.

Keusch, G.T., and Jacewicz, M.: The pathogenesis of shigella diarrhea. V. Relationship of shiga enterotoxin, neurotoxin, and cytotoxin, J. Infect. Dis. **131**(suppl.):33, 1975.

Nelson, J.D., et al.: Endemic shigellosis: a study of fifty households, Am. J. Epidemiol. **86:**683, 1967.

Nelson, J.D., et al.: Trimethoprim-sulfamethoxazole therapy for shigellosis, J.A.M.A. **235:**1239, 1976.

Rosenberg, M.L., et al.: Shigellosis in the United States: ten-year review of nationwide surveillance, 1964-1973, Am. J. Epidemiol. **104:**543, 1976.

Scarlet fever

Breese, D.R., and Hall, C.B.: Beta hemolytic streptococcal diseases, Boston, 1978, Houghton Mifflin Co.

Krugman, S., and Katz, J.: Infectious diseases of children, ed. 7, St. Louis, 1981, The C.V. Mosby Co.

Mandel, G.L., et al.: Principles and practices of infectious diseases, New York, 1979, John Wiley & Sons, Publishers, Inc.

Staphylococcal infections

Aranow, H., Jr., and Wood, W.B., Jr.: Staphylococcic infection simulating scarlet fever, J.A.M.A. **119:**1491, 1942.

Christensen, G.D., et al.: Nosocomial septicemia due to multiple antibiotic-resistant *Staphylococcus epidermidis,* Ann. Intern. Med. **96:**1, 1982.

Davis, J.P., et al.: Toxic-shock syndrome: epidemiologic features, recurrence, risk factors, and prevention, N. Engl. J. Med. **303:**1429, 1980.

Manzella, J.P., et al.: Toxic epidermal necrolysis in childhood: differentiation from staphylococcal scalded skin syndrome, Pediatrics **66:**291, 1980.

Melish, M.E.: Staphylococcal infections. In Feigin, R.D., and Cherry, J.D., editors: Textbook of pediatric infectious diseases, Philadelphia, 1981, W.B. Saunders Co.

Peacock, J.E., Jr., et al.: Methicillin-resistant *Staphylococcus aureus:* introduction and spread within a hospital, Ann. Intern. Med. **93:**526, 1980.

Shulman, S.T., and Ayoub, E.M.: Severe staphylococcal sepsis in adolescents, Pediatrics **58:**59, 1976.

Tetanus

LaForce, F.M., et al.: Tetanus in the United States (1965-1966), epidemiologic and clinical features, N. Engl. J. Med. **280:**569-574, 1969.

Weinstein, L.: Current concepts—Tetanus, N. Engl. J. Med. **289:**1293-1296, 1973.

Adams, J.M., et al.: Modern management of tetanus neonatorum, Pediatr. **64:**472-477, 1979.

Tuberculosis

Krugman, S., and Katz, S.L.: Infectious diseases of children, ed. 7, St. Louis, 1980, The C.V. Mosby Co.

Report of the Committee on Infectious Diseases: Tuberculosis, ed. 19, Evanston, Ill., 1982, American Academy of Pediatrics.

Smith, M.H.D., and Marguis, J.R.: Tuberculosis and other mycobacterini infections. In Feigin, R.D., and Cherry, J.D., editors: Textbook of pediatric infectious diseases, 1981, W.B. Saunders Co.

Atypical mycobacteria

Schaad, U.B., et al.: Management of atypical mycobacterial lymphadenitis in childhood: a review based on 380 cases, J. Pediatr. **95:**356-360, 1979.

Schuit, K.E., and Powell, D.A.: Mycobacterial lymphadenitis in childhood, Am. J. Dis. Child. **132:**675-677, 1978.

Tularemia

Boyce, J.M.: Recent trends in the epidemiology of tularemia in the United States, J. Infect. Dis. **131:**197, 1975.

Hughes, W.T.: Tularemia in children, J. Pediatr. **62:**495, 1963.

Hughes, W.T.: Oculoglandular tularemia: transmission from rabbit, through dog and tick, to man, Pediatrics **36:**270, 1965.

Miller, R.P., and Bates, J.H.: Pleuropulmonary tularemia: a review of 29 patients, Am. Rev. Respir. Dis. **99:**31, 1969.

Tyson, H.K.: Tularemia, an unappreciated cause of exudative pharyngitis, Pediatrics **58:**864, 1976.

Yow, M.D.: Tularemia. In Feigin, R.D., and Cherry, J.D., editors: Textbook of pediatric infectious diseases, Philadelphia, 1981, W.B. Saunders Co.

Syphilis

Centers for Disease Control: Sexually transmitted diseases treatment guidelines, 1982, Morbidity and Mortality Weekly Report **31:**50S, 1982.

Hill, L.L., et al.: The nephrotic syndrome in congenital syphilis: an immunopathy, Pediatrics **49:**260, 1972.

McCracken, G.H., and Kaplan, J.M.: Penicillin treatment for congenital syphilis: a critical reappraisal, J.A.M.A. **228:**855, 1974.

Wilfert, C., and Gutman, L.: Syphilis. In Feign, R.D., and Cherry, J.D., editors: Textbook of pediatric infectious diseases, Philadelphia, 1981, W.B. Saunders Co.

Wilkinson, R.H., and Heller, R.M.: Congenital syphilis: resurgence of an old problem, Pediatrics **47:**27, 1971.

Leptospirosis

Feigin, R.D., and Anderson, D.C.: Leptospirosis. In Feigin, R.D., and Cherry, J.D., editors: Textbook of pediatric infectious diseases, Philadelphia, 1981, W.B. Saunders Co.

Wong, M.L., et al.: Leptospirosis: a childhood disease, J. Pediatr. **90:**532, 1977.

Cat-scratch disease

Carithers, H.A.: Oculoglandular disease of Parinaud. A manifestation of cat scratch disease, Am. J. Dis. Child **132:**1195, 1978.

Margileth, A.M.: Cat-scratch disease in 65 patients: evaluation of cat scratch skin test antigen in 109 subjects, Clin. Proc. Child Hosp. DC **27:**213, 1971.

Torres, J.R., et al: Cat-scratch disease causing reversible encephalopathy, J.A.M.A. **240:**1628, 1978.

Chickenpox (varicella) and herpes zoster

Arbeter, A.N., et al.: Live attenuated varicella vaccine: immunization of healthy children with the OKA strain, J. Pediatr. **100**(6):886-893, 1982.

Feldman, S., et al.: Herpes zoster in children with cancer, Am. J. Dis. Child **126:**178, 1973.

Feldman, S., et al.: Varicella in children with cancer: 77 cases, Pediatrics **56:**388, 1975.

Weller, T.H.: Varicella and herpes zoster, N. Engl. J. Med. **309:**1362, 1434, 1983.

Infectious mononeucleosis

Evans, A.S., et al.: Seroepidemiologic studies of infectious mononucleosis with EB virus, N. Engl. J. Med. **279:**1121, 1968.

Henle, G., et al.: The Epstein-Barr virus, Berlin, 1979, Springer-Verlag.

Henle, G., and Henle, W.: Observations on childhood infections with the Epstein-Barr virus. J. Infec. Dis. **121:**303, 1970.

Niederman, J.C., et al.: Infectious mononeucleosis: clinical manifestations in relation to EB virus antibodies, J.A.M.A. **203:**205, 1968.

Rapp, C.E., and Hewetson, J.F.: Infectious mononeucleosis and the Epstein-Barr virus, Am. J. Dis. Child **132:**78, 1978.

Sumaya, C.V.: Primary Epstein-Barr virus infections in children, Pediatrics **59:**16, 1977.

Influenza

Boyer, K.M., and Cherry, J.D.: Influenza viruses. In Feigin, R.D., and Cherry, J.D., editors: Textbook of pediatric infectious diseases, Philadelphia, 1981, W.B. Saunders Co.

Cory, L., et al.: A nationwide outbreak of Reye's syndrome. AM. J. Med. **61:**615, 1976.

Dolin, R., et al.: A controlled trial of amantadine and rimantadine in the prophylaxis of influenza A infection, N. Engl. J. Med. **307:**580, 1982.

Wright, P.F., et al.: Influenza A infections in young children, N. Engl. J. Med. **296:**829, 1977.

Mumps

Krugman, S., and Katz, S.L.: Infectious diseases of children, ed. 7, St. Louis, 1981, The C.V. Mosby Co.

Marcy, S.M., and Kibrick, S.: Mumps. In Hoeprich, P.D., editor: Infectious diseases: a modern treatise of infectious processes, ed. 3, Philadelphia, 1983, Harper & Row, Publishers, Inc.

German measles (rubella)

Krugman, S., and Katz, S.L.: Infectious diseases of children, ed. 7, St. Louis, 1981, The C.V. Mosby Co.

Cherry, J.D.: Rubella. In Feigin, R.D., and Cherry, J.D., editors: Textbook of pediatric infectious diseases, Philadelphia, 1981, W.B. Saunders Co.

Measles (rubeola)

Cherry, J.D.: Rubeola. In Feigin, R.D., and Cherry, J.D., editors: Textbook of pediatric infectious diseases, Philadelphia, 1981, W.B. Saunders Co.

Krugman, S., Katz, S.L.: Infectious diseases of children, ed. 7, St. Louis, 1981, The C.V. Mosby Co.

Enteroviruses and Coxsackievirus

Baron, S., editor: Medical microbiology, Menlo Park, Calif., 1982, Addison-Wesley Publishing Co.

North American blastomycosis

Steele, R.W., and Abernathy, R.S.: Systemic blastomycosis in children, Ped. Infect. Dis. **2:**304-307, 1983.

Mycoses

Galgiani, J.H.: The deep mycoses. In Wedgewood, R.J., et al., editors: Infections in children, New York, 1982, Harper & Row, Publishers, Inc.

Hughes, W.T.: Systemic candidiasis: a study of 109 fetal cases, Pediatr. Infect. Dis. **1:**11, 1982.

Coccidioidomycosis

Drutz, D.J., and Catanzaro, A.: Coccidioidomycosis: state of the art [in 2 parts]. Ann. Rev. Resp. Dis. **117:**559-585, 1978.

Histoplasmosis

Wheat, J., et al.: The diagnostic laboratory tests for histoplasmosis, Ann. Intern. Med. **97:**680-685, 1982.

Rickettsial diseases

Hattwick, M.A.W., et al.: Rocky Mountain spotted fever: epidemiology of an increasing problem, Ann. Intern. Med. **84:**732, 1976.

Haynes, R.E., et al.: Rocky Mountain spotted fever in children, J. Pediatr. **76:**685, 1970.

Kelsey, D.S.: Rocky Mountain spotted fever, Pediatr. Clin. North Am. **26:**367, 1979.

Older, J.J.: The epidemiology of murine typhus in Texas, 1969, J.A.M.A. **214:**2011, 1970.

Pneumocystis carinii

Ruskin, J., and Hughes, W.T.: *Pneumocystis carinii*. In Remington, J., and Klein, J.D., editors: Infectious diseases of the fetus and newborn infant, Philadelphia, 1983, W.B. Saunders Co.

Chlamydia

Beem, M.O., and Saxon, F.M.: Respiratory tract colonization and a distinctive pneumonia syndrome in infants infected with *Chlamydia trachomatis*, N. Engl. J. Med. **296:**306, 1977.

28 Parasitic Infestations

HELMINTH INFECTIONS

Effectively coping with human roundworm infestation necessitates an understanding of the life cycle of these parasites and their pathogenicity. Diagnostic methods, therapeutic specificity, and dosage tolerance must be familiar facts. Of equal importance is a basic knowledge of the in vivo and in vitro methods of propagation of roundworms. These facts are essential in programming preventive measures for initial infection or reinfection.

Ascaris lumbricoides (large roundworm of intestine)

Ascaris lumbricoides infection is most prevalent in children living in warm climates. A mature female worm is about 20 to 35 mm in length; the male averages 15 to 30 mm.

Although a female may produce up to 200,000 eggs daily, they are infertile unless males are present. Outside the body the fertilized egg is resistant to most types of chemicals. However, direct sunlight and moist heat of 80° C (176° F) or above are lethal factors. When the developed infective egg is ingested in food, drink, or other contaminated sources, it passes through the stomach and is hatched in the duodenum or upper jejunum. The larva penetrates the intestinal wall and enters the portal or lymphatic system to be carried to the lungs. The larva burrows into the alveolus and, after a short growth period, is carried up the respiratory tree, over the epiglottis to the esophagus and stomach, and eventually into the small bowel. In the small intestine it develops to the adult form. In humans the total incubation period is about 2 to 3 months.

Clinical manifestations. The spectrum of clinical symptoms depends on the extent and severity of the infection. Characteristic symptoms of intestinal ascariasis in children are loss of appetite, fretfulness, nervousness, and a protuberant abdomen. Nutritional disturbances are proportional to the degree of infestation. Severe symptoms include colicky abdominal pain, nausea, vomiting, and hematemesis. When heavy infestation exists, a large number of worms may lead to intestinal obstruction. Infrequently they may perforate the bowel wall and cause acute peritonitis. Rare cases of laryngeal and tracheal obstruction caused by ascarids and their eggs have been reported.

Hepatic involvement may be a consequence of larval migration. Focal eosinophilia and granulomas develop in and around the tracts of the larval migration, causing fibrosis of the periportal and interlobular spaces.

In the lungs intense local infiltrations of eosinophils, epithelioid cells, and macrophages develop in the alveoli, producing a specific type of pulmonary pathology referred to as "Ascaris pneumonitis." The radiographic picture of scattered mottling of the lung fields may suggest tuberculosis or viral pneumonia. Pulmonary symptoms are those of dyspnea, cough (either dry or productive), musical and wheezing rales (rarely crepitant), and high temperature, often reaching 38.3° C (101° F). High, transient eosinophilia is often found. Ascaris pneumonitis, which rarely persists for more than 1 week, is one form of Löffler pneumonia.

Diagnosis. The diagnosis of ascariasis is often made when the patient or parent brings to the office a worm that has been passed or reports that such a worm has been passed. Diagnosis may, of necessity, be based on finding the eggs in direct fecal films. If these smears are negative, centrifugation of a small specimen and reexamination should be performed. The zinc sulfate centrifugal-flotation technique, which has been devised for the concentration of helminth eggs and protozoal cysts, provides a much higher concentration and is recommended as a routine procedure. It should be noted that infertile eggs are too heavy to float in this solution.

Treatment. Several drugs are available that provide excellent cure rates. Pyrantel pamoate (Antiminth) has the advantage of being effective in a single dose of 10 mg/kg administered as a suspension not to exceed 1 g. The drug is nonstaining and may be given with food at any time of the day. The main adverse reactions are gastrointestinal (nausea, vomiting, cramping). Minor transient elevations of SGOT have occurred in a small percentage of patients. Piperazine hexahydrate (Antepar) in the form of syrup, wafer, or tablet is effective in a single dose of 75mg/kg/24 hr for 2 consecutive days, with a maximum daily dose of 3.5 g. In severe infections the treatment course may be repeated with either drug after a 1-week interval. Mebendazole (Vermox) is considered by some to be the drug of choice in the treatment of all intestinal nematodes except Strongyloides. Side effects with this drug are rare and the dose schedule is the same for all patients. The effective dose is 100 mg given twice daily for 3 days. It is generally recommended that treatment be repeated in 2 weeks.

Because the parasite egg requires development outside of the human host, children and adults should be educated in the use of sanitary latrines or toilets. This problem is most common in communities with low economic and social standards and therefore is a very real public health problem based largely on poverty and poor living conditions. If a treated child is returned to the environment in which he contracted an intestinal nematode, the chances are high that infection will recur.

Enterobius vermicularis (oxyuris, the pinworm, or seatworm)

Infection by *Enterobius vermicularis* has no seasonal variation. It differs from infection by *Ascaris* in that there is no developmental stage outside the body. The mature female worm measures 8 to 13 mm in length, the male averages 2 to 5 mm.

The adult worms live with their heads attached to the mucosa of the distal small bowel, cecum, appendix, and colon. The gravid female, as her uterus becomes more and more distended with eggs, releases herself from the intestinal wall and wanders from level to level in the bowel lumen. She commonly migrates out of the anus, especially at night, and deposits her embryonated eggs on the perianal skin.

The pinworm requires neither an intermediate host nor a period of development outside the body. Ingested eggs hatch in the duodenum or upper jejunum. The larva then passes down the bowel, where it grows, attaching directly to the bowel wall. The time from ingestion to maturity is about 2 to 3 weeks.

The most common methods of infection and reinfection are (1) directly from anus to mouth by way of the fingers from scratching the perianal area; (2) by way of contaminated clothes, bed sheets, or any household objects; and (3) the air of bedrooms, which may be contaminated and then breathed in. Rarely, persons may maintain an infection even though their personal hygiene is satisfactory. This occurs when the eggs hatch on the perianal area and migrate back into the lower bowel.

Clinical manifestations. The primary symptom of oxyuriasis is related to the migration of the female worm out of the bowel onto the perianal area, causing an intense and aggravating anal pruritus. Children, as a result of the pruritus, become fretful, sleep poorly, develop anorexia, and in general have a poor disposition. On occasion the worms migrate into the vagina, where their presence may initiate inflammation with leukorrhea. Of importance also is the reported association between enterobiasis and cystitis in young girls. There is also recent evidence that pinworms may cause enuresis in children. Severe abdominal complaints are unusual with this infection.

Diagnosis. Diagnosis of oxyuriasis is based on recovery of the eggs from the feces, from swabbings of the perianal area, or from recognizing the female on the perianal skin. Use of clear cellophane tape is recommended for recovering the eggs from the perianal area. The search for these eggs should continue daily for at least a week before one excludes the possibility of pinworm infection.

Treatment. As in the therapy of ascariasis, pyrantel pamoate (Antiminth) has the advantage of being effective in a single dose. The same dose of 10 mg/kg is administered orally not to exceed 1 g. Pyrvinium pamoate (Povan) is also effective as a single dose of 5 mg/kg. As with pyrantel, gastrointestinal symptoms may occur with the use of this drug. Pyrvinium has the disadvantage of staining the stool bright red; should vomiting occur, the sight of bright red vomitus may be frightening if the patient and parents are not forewarned. Mebendazole (Vermox) is a newer but equally effective single-dose anthelminthic drug administered in a dose of 100 mg. It is recommended that treatment with any of these, if well tolerated, be repeated in 2 weeks.

The policy of treating whole families without proved infection in some members is open to question. If infections recur in various family members, all members of the family should be treated and all the hygienic measures stressed.

Giardiasis

Giardia lamblia is a protozoan parasite associated with diarrheal illness occurring in both endemic and epidemic forms. Reproduction of the organism is by binary fission, with motile trophozoites living primarily in the lumen of the duodenum and proximal jejunum. These trophozoites, under certain conditions, transform into cystic forms that have walls providing resistance to a variety of adverse environmental conditions. The organisms in the cystic form are excreted in the feces. Except for trichomoniasis, giardiasis may be the most common protozoal infection in this country.

Infection is acquired by the ingestion of *Giardia* cysts from food or water contaminated with infected feces. Contaminated drinking water is thought to be the most common source of outbreaks of this infection. Cysts remain viable in water for 3 months, resisting chlorination sufficient to kill bacterial pathogens. Transmission by close contact under conditions of poor sanitation probably is significant in families, crowded institutions, and in some endemic areas.

There are several host factors that affect susceptibility to infection and severity of symptoms, including achlorhydria and hypochlorhydria and immunologic deficiencies. Symptomatic giardiasis has also been reported in infantile X-linked agamaglobulinemia.

Epidemiologic studies show an incubation period varying from 2 to 35 days, with 15 days as an average. Travelers returning from endemic areas have shown maximum incubation periods of up to 8 weeks. Parasites first appeared in the stool of volunteers on the average of 9 days after ingestion of *Giardia* cysts.

It is important to note that the prevalence of endemic infection is greatest in the age group of 1 to 6 years. Although infection has been documented in a 3-week-old baby, the incidence is low in the first year of life.

Patients with giardiasis need not be isolated, but precautions should be taken such as increased attention to personal hygiene, appropriate disposition of soiled linen or underclothing, and proper disposal of fecal material.

Clinical manifestations. Diarrhea, acute or chronic, intermittent or continuous, is the cardinal manifestation of giardial infection. Although many persons with giardiasis are asymptomatic, diarrheal disease of varying severity and duration is common. The occurrence of loose, frequent, foul-smelling stools that may appear watery or greasy is the most common complaint. Malaise, anorexia, nausea, abdominal discomfort, cramping or distention often associated with weight loss may occur. Low-grade fever has been reported in acute giardiasis, but is rare. Uncommon complaints include vomiting and urticaria. The progress of giardiasis is variable. In the acute, self-limiting form, symptoms disappear within a few weeks after the onset of illness, but chronic, persisting, or intermittent symptoms may occur. In the immunodeficient patient, persistence of infection for years has been documented.

The chronic form of giardiasis may mimic celiac disease, and tests of gastrointestinal absorption may be abnormal. Secondary intestinal disaccharidase deficiency with milk intolerance has been reported. Growth failure associated with chronic diarrhea may be the initial finding.

Laboratory findings include anemia, which is probably related to the degree of malabsorption, and normal white blood cell counts. Radiologic studies of the intestine may be normal or may show evidence of thickening of the mucosal folds of the duodenum and jejunum. Segmentation of the barium column, dilation of bowel loops, hypersecretion, and hypermobility may also be seen.

Changes in other systems, although reported, have not been confirmed. These include involvement of the eyes, joints, and urinary tract as well as behavioral disorders.

Diagnosis. Giardiasis should be considered in the differential diagnosis of children who have diarrheal disease, malabsorption, and abdominal pain. Diagnostic tests currently of value are fecal examinations by direct, wet films and by concentration techniques and the examination of duodenal contents or duodenal mucosa biopsies.

Trophozoites can be seen in diarrheal feces if a wet preparation is made from a fresh specimen and stained with Lugol iodine. Solid stools are more likely to contain cysts than trophozoites. Formol-ether concentration increases the value of the study, but this procedure, which destroys the trophozoites, should not be the only method of examination employed if giardiasis is suspected. Cyst excretion is inconsistent and unpredictable; several specimens obtained on different dates should be examined before accepting a negative result. A minimum of three specimens should be examined and those should be collected with intervals of at least 1 or 2 days between specimens. The use of oily laxatives, antidiarrheal compounds containing bismuth or kaolin, and nonabsorbable antacids should be avoided until the collection of fecal specimens is complete.

Examination of duodenal contents or duodenal biopsy is valuable but should be used as an adjunct to a series of fecal examinations. The Entero-Test, a device that allows for collection of duodenal contents by means of a length of nylon yarn, is another means of collecting material for examination. This method requires the patient to swallow a gelatin capsule that, when digested, releases a weighted length of nylon yarn. When retrieved from the small bowel, mucous adherent to the yarn is removed, stained, and examined. Generally, fecal examination in combination with examination of duodenal contents has a high success rate in diagnosis.

At present there are no diagnostically useful serologic tests for giardiasis, although circulating antibody has been detected in some patients.

Treatment. There is considerable debate concerning the relative efficacy of the drugs currently used for the treatment of giardiasis. Results of clinical investigations are confusing because of variations in doses, duration of treatment, and because of the use of differing criteria for cure. Quinacrine hydrochloride (Atabrine) and furazolidone (Furoxone) are approved for use in the United States for *Giardia* infections. Although metronidazole (Flagyl) is considered the drug of choice by some clinicians, it is not approved in this country for the treatment of giardiasis although it is available for treatment of amebiasis and trichomoniasis.

Quinacrine hydrochloride is considered by many authorities to be the drug of choice, with cure rates of up to 100% being reported after a single course. The dosage is 7 mg/kg of body weight (maximum 300 mg) divided into three daily doses for 7 days. For young children it is useful to have the medication made up in a flavored syrup to mask the bitter taste. The most common side effects of nausea, vomiting, and abdominal pain often may be avoided by administering quinacrine with meals. Yellow discoloration of the skin and gingiva have been reported with prolonged administration. It should not be used by pregnant women or by patients with cirrhosis. Furazolidone appears to have less efficacy than quinacrine, with a cure rate of 70% to 80%. The dosage is 5 mg/kg (maximum 400 mg) divided into four doses daily for 5 days. Nausea, vomiting, headache, and malaise are common side effects. Hypersensitivity has been reported, with various manifestations of urticaria, morbilliform rash, fever, arthralgia, and hypertension. It should not be used in infants under 1 month of age.

Metronidazole appears to be nearly as effective as quinacrine. There is suggestion that it may be less effective in recently acquired infections. The dosage is 10 to 20 mg/kg divided into three doses daily for 10 days. It has also been used successfully in single doses of 2 gm daily for 3 days in adults and in proportional doses for children. Side effects are infrequent when the drug is used in the smaller doses, although nausea and other gastrointestinal symptoms may occur. It should be avoided in the first trimester of pregnancy and during lactation.

In summary, based on current information, quinacrine is the drug of choice for treatment of giardiasis in this country. Treatment failures usually respond to a second course of therapy with the same or alternate drug.

Asymptomatic persons with giardiasis should be treated to avoid spread of the infection to others and to prevent the development of symptoms at some future date. Attempts at chemoprophylaxis with any of the available drugs is not recommended. Travelers to countries in which the water supply may be contaminated may consider chemical treatment of that water with iodine. Tincture of iodine (2% iodine) may be added, 1 or 2 drops per glass of water or 5 drops to a quart or liter, and should be allowed to stand for 30 minutes. Water may be made safe by boiling, but often this is not convenient for the traveler.

Hookworm

Hookworm infection in humans on the North American continent is caused primarily by *Necator americanus* and, to a lesser extent, *Ancylostoma braziliense* and *Ancylostoma caninum*. *Ancylostoma duodenale* ("Old World hookworm") is more common in Europe, North Africa, and the Middle and Far East.

A. braziliense and *A. caninum* are parasites that are present along the southeastern Atlantic coast and the Gulf Coast. They have never been reported as an intestinal infection of humans; they produce a skin disease known as "creeping eruption" or cutaneous larva migrans. Intestinal infection with these species appears to be limited almost exclusively to canine and feline hosts.

N. americanus lives attached to the mucosa of the midportion of the small intestine. Females measure approximately 9 to 11 mm in length; males average 7 to 9 mm. The eggs of this worm require development outside the body. They are deposited on soil (moist, sandy humus in a warm locality), and some hatch. The larva that emerges is infective for human beings. After making contact with human skin, especially the interdigital skin of the feet, it penetrates through the tissues until it reaches the venous circulation. The larva is carried to the lungs, where it penetrates into the alveoli and progresses up the respiratory tree over the epiglottis. The larva is then swallowed and passes through the stomach to the small intestines. As it travels through these organs, the larva continues to develop; after it reaches the intestine it achieves maturity. The time interval from penetration of the skin until the eggs appear in the stool is about 5 weeks.

Clinical manifestations. The early symptoms are caused by penetration of the infective larvae through the skin. This "ground itch" consists of itching, edema, and erythema, which, if irritated by scratching, may become secondarily infected with skin bacteria.

The intestinal symptoms depend on the degree and duration of the infection and the age of the patient. Children are more severely affected than adults. Hookworm causes more extensive damage to the bowel than do the other worm infections. Anemia is usually present because of chronic blood loss caused by the attached worms. Bacterial invasion of the traumatized intestinal wall is common. In heavy worm infestation, nutritional deficiencies develop, manifested by the typical "potbelly" appearance caused by anasarca and hypoproteinemia.

Diagnosis. Diagnosis of intestinal hookworm infection is contingent upon finding typical hookworm eggs in the feces. If eggs are not recovered in three unconcentrated films of feces, the number of hookworms present is usually not sufficient to produce clinical disease.

Treatment. Therapy in severe infestation may necessitate whole blood transfusions to replace losses of blood and protein. Iron replacement may also be indicated. Effective drugs in treating intestinal hookworm include pyrantel pamoate given in a single dose of 10 mg/kg or mebendazole in a dose of 100 mg twice daily for 3 days.

In "creeping eruption" or "ground itch" the lesions are treated topically for pyogenic infection and then frozen locally with ethyl chloride spray to kill the larvae in situ. Thiabendazole in a 10% aqueous suspension applied locally may also be used. When local therapy fails, thiabendazole may be given orally (5 mg/kg/dose twice daily for 2 successive days).

Humans initiate the extrinsic phase of the life cycle of the hookworm by discharging eggs on the soil and in turn picking up the infection by direct contact with the soil. Prophylaxis therefore consists of proper sanitary disposal of human excreta, treatment of infected cases with proper follow-up examination, and wearing of shoes to protect the feet from infected soil.

Visceral larva migrans

Visceral larva migrans is a syndrome typically diagnosed in children 1 to 4 years of age with a history of pica. It is characterized by chronic extreme eosinophilia, hepatomegaly, pulmonary infiltration, fever, weight loss, cough, and hyperglobulinemia. It results from penetration of internal organs by nematode larvae of *Toxocara canis* and, less commonly, *Toxocara cati,* which have similar life cycles in the dog and cat, respectively.

There are several ways the child may come into contact with the eggs and ingest them: (1)

by direct contamination of the hands and especially the fingers from contact with a nursing dog or cat or its immediate environment; (2) indirectly by contact with objects contaminated with infective eggs; or (3) by ingestion of soil containing larvae or infective eggs. Periodic deworming of household dogs and cats should be stressed as a preventive measure.

After an egg is swallowed and hatched in the upper alimentary tract, the larvae migrate through the viscera. Unlike the larval migration of *Ascaris lumbricoides,* these larvae are prevented from carrying out their complete migration by the intense eosinophilic infiltration and development of granulomatous reactions along their path in the liver and lungs, and ectopically in the eye, brain, and myocardium.

Clinical manifestations. The clinical course varies from a benign, relatively asymptomatic illness to a severe life-threatening one. The intensity of clinical manifestations depends on the number of eggs ingested, the number of larvae present in the body, the frequency and pattern of larval migration, the organ(s) involved, and the immune or allergic responses evoked in the patient. Leukocyte counts between 30,000 and 100,000/mm^3, with 50% to 90% eosinophils, are not unusual. This eosinophilia may persist for months. Concentration of serum albumin is usually normal, whereas the gamma globulins (IgG, IgM, and IgE) are usually elevated. Elevated anti-A and anti-B titers are frequently noted in children because *toxocara* larvae contain surface antigens that stimulate isohemagglutinin. Mild pulmonary involvement is common, but severe respiratory distress is rare. Neurologic manifestations include focal and generalized seizures. Ocular involvement, typically unilateral, is not uncommon, and the complaints include visual loss, strabismus, and, more rarely, eye pain.

Diagnosis. The infection may be identified only after the incidental finding of hypereosinophilia and usually in children with a history of pica. A definitive diagnosis depends on the demonstration of larvae in the tissue from biopsy material, enucleated eyes, or autopsy specimens. The presence of *toxocara* species is not detected by stool analysis because the larvae rarely become mature in humans. Until recently, immunodiagnostic tests have lacked sufficient sensitivity and specificity, mainly because they used antigens prepared from adult *toxocara* or *ascaris* worms. Testing with larval antigens or their metabolic products has been shown to be more sensitive, and such antigens have been adapted to the enzyme-linked immunosorbent assay.

Treatment. Specific treatment for visceral larva migrans consists of the oral administration of thiabendazole (25 mg/kg twice daily for 5 to 10 days). The total daily dose should not exceed 3 g. In severe disease this course of treatment may be repeated in 4 weeks. Hepatosplenomegaly, when present, gradually subsides with therapy, as does the elevated peripheral leukocyte count. The percentage of eosinophils and the isoagglutinin (anti-A and anti-B) titers may remain elevated for several years. Adrenal corticosteroids may be beneficial in severe cases, particularly in those with extensive pneumonitis and myocarditis, where their anti-inflammatory effect may be lifesaving. They are also indicated in active disease of the eye.

Amebiasis

Amebiasis is an intestinal infection caused by *Entamoeba histolytica*. The infection may occur in the absence of definite clinical symptoms or it may be characterized by attacks of dysentery or diarrhea. Symptoms associated with the nervous and gastrointestinal systems are not uncommon. The symptom complex known as "amebic dysentery" is only one phase of amebiasis, dysentery occurring in only a small proportion of infections with *E. histolytica*. *E. coli* and all other species of amebae except *E. histolytica* are harmless commensals living in the human intestine.

When cysts of *E. histolytica* are ingested in contaminated food or water, they traverse the upper gastrointestinal tract, excysting in the lowest portion of the ileum. A single, four-nucleated ameba is liberated from each of these cysts. The motile trophozoites burrow into the intestinal wall by aid of a cytolytic substance and by means of pseudopodic movement. The extent of this intestinal invasion determines the symptomatology associated with the various types. In temperate regions the majority of these infections are followed by prompt healing of the lesions, with little or no symptomatology.

Infection with *E. histolytica* probably does not occur without associated intestinal damage.

It appears in tissues as a motile trophozoite. Such forms are not uncommon in the lumen of the bowel. When conditions arise that prevent the penetration of the tissues, such as diarrhea, the trophozoites round up in the lumen, and cysts are formed that may be found in the feces. These cysts, which are the infective agents, do not occur in the tissues. Motile trophozoites are not usually found in stools except when diarrhea occurs.

Pathologic findings. The pathology of amebiasis varies from microscopic necrosis of the mucous membrane to extensive ulceration involving any or all layers of the large intestine. In carriers the lesions most frequently detected are microscopic areas of necrosis of the mucous membrane. In cases in which exacerbations of acute dysentery have occurred, the intestinal wall is usually greatly thickened and the normal tissue is replaced by dense fibrous scar tissue. The typical microscopic pathology of amebiasis is characterized by the absence of significant cellular infiltration, as is usually found in bacterial invasion of the intestine. The amebae are found both within and between the glands of the intestine, in the submucosa and muscular coats, and in blood vessels and lymphatics.

Clinical manifestations. Symptoms vary from slight disturbances of the intestinal tract to severe "amebic dysentery." In children, symptoms are frequently absent or mimic other gastrointestinal disorders. Dysentery is rare except in the tropics and subtropics.

Children and adults who are symptomatic carriers of *E. histolytica* manifest minor attacks of diarrhea that may last a few hours to a few days. Frequently, alternating periods of constipation and gaseous distention of the lower abdomen are noted. Not infrequently, nausea and vomiting and headaches may alternate with a ravenous appetite. Myalgia and malaise are common. Children who are carriers may fail to gain weight properly and may be mildly anemic. Eosinophilia is typically absent.

In amebic enteritis the same symptoms are manifested, but to a more severe degree. Colic associated with foul, watery stools containing blood and mucus frequently occurs. Amebic dysentery is a progression of the basic illness and is much more severe in character and effect than simple enteritis. The number of bloody, mucoid stools varies from 15 to 30 during 24 hours. In uncomplicated attacks of dysentery the temperature may be normal. However, the patient may rapidly become dehydrated and exhibit concomitant problems in electrolyte balance.

The most serious complication of amebiasis is amebic abscess of the liver, which may occur in "carriers" who have never exhibited severe diarrhea or dysentery. Abscesses in other organs, such as brain and lung, are extremely rare. Strictures of the intestine, as a result of adhesions and cicatrices of healed ulcers, may be sequelae of amebiasis.

Diagnosis. The diagnosis of amebiasis in any of its various stages rests on the demonstration of *E. histolytica*. Examination of the feces demands experience because of the necessity of differentiating this parasite from the other intestinal amebae. *Entamoeba coli* and *E. nana,* which may be found in the stool, should not be considered pathogens. In examining the feces for *E. histolytica,* it should be remembered that the motile or trophozoite stage will be found only in fluid or semifluid stools, whereas the cysts are found only in semiformed or formed stools.

Specimens should be examined within 1 hour of passage. If delays are anticipated, the specimen should be held in the refrigerator (4° C) or preserved in formalin and polyvinyl alcohol fixative. Antimicrobial agents cause amebae to disappear from the stool.

Serologic examination is a useful adjunt to the diagnosis of amebiasis. The various tests employed, including indirect hemagglutination, indirect immunofluorescence, countercurrent immunoelectrophoresis, and agar gel diffusion, are not all useful for extraintestinal amebiasis. They are somewhat less helpful for active intestinal infection and of least assistance for the asymptomatic patient who is passing cysts.

Treatment and prevention. Prophylaxis includes the prevention of contamination of food and drink with the cysts of *E. histolytica*. The most common mode of transmission appears to be person to person; therefore it is important to examine contacts of recently diagnosed patients.

Because of the potential significant side effects (subacute myelo-opticoneuropathy) of diodohydroxyquin, as well as its relative ineffectiveness, it is no longer recommended as a major form of therapy for intestinal amebiasis. Diloxanide furoate (Furamide) has been recommended by some as the drug of choice for patients passing cysts. The recommended dose is 20 mg/kg/24 hours in three doses for 10 days. There has been minimal toxicity observed; primarily nausea, vomiting, diarrhea, and urticaria. Metronidazole treatment of patients with extraintestinal or symptomatic intestinal amebiasis has generally been successful. This current recommendation has been made despite concern about carcinogenicity in rats, and its action as a mutagen in bacteria. The known cardiac and neurologic toxicity of emetine is great enough to outweigh the potential toxicity of metronidazole in man. The recommended dose of metronidazole is 50 mg/kg/24 hours in three divided doses by mouth (not to exceed 2.4 g/day) for 10 days. Some authorities would combine this therapy, in mild to severe intestinal disease, with diodohydroxyquin in a dose of 30 to 40 mg/kg/24 hours in three doses for 20 days (not to exceed 2 g/day).

The permanent disappearance of the cysts of *E. histolytica* from the feces should be used as the index of cure. Weekly examination of the stools should be performed for at least 3 months after cessation of treatment.

Hershel P. Wall

SELECTED READINGS

Blumenthal, D.S.: Intestinal nematodes in the United States, N. Engl. J. Med. **297:**1437, 1977.

Feigan, R.D., and Cherry, J.D.: Textbook of pediatric infectious diseases, Philadelphia, 1981, W.B. Saunders Co.

Gellis, S.S., and Kegan, B.M.: Current pediatric therapy 10, Philadelphia, 1982, W.B. Saunders Co.

Katz, M.: Parasitic infections, J. Pediatr. **87:**165, 1975.

Krogstad, D.J., et al.: Amebiasis, N. Engl. J. Med. **298:**262, 1978.

Shantz, P.M., and Glickman, L.T.: Toxocaral visceral larva migrans, N. Engl. J. Med. **298:**436, 1978.

29 Diseases of the Nervous System

NEUROLOGIC EVALUATION

Growth and differentiation of the nervous system proceed rapidly during gestation and the first year of life. As a result, the head circumference increases approximately 1 cm/month during the first 6 months, and more slowly over the succeeding months. By 1 year, the head circumference has attained about 80% of its adult size as a result of growth and differentiation of the brain. A number of active processes are involved in this, including an increasing number of cells, proliferation of axons and dendrites, myelination, and neovascularization. Clinical correlates of this include development of more sophisticated motor and sensory functions, behavioral maturation, personality development, and gradual loss of the developmental primitive reflexes.

Evaluation of nervous function in the neonate, infant, or child is based on an understanding of what is normal for age. This may be difficult at times, because the typical process of brain maturation may be only delayed, rather than reversed, by an active disease process. In these situations, it is particularly important not only to compare the patient's performance with the norms for age, but also to assess the rate of acquisition or loss of skills to determine the tempo of the disease process. By the time previously acquired skills are lost, the disease is usually advanced and early therapeutic intervention is no longer an option.

Sometimes a static insult to the developing nervous system results in what seems to be a progressive disease. An example of this is the static encephalopathy resulting from hypoxia during the prenatal or perinatal period. Over the ensuing months, spasticity and pathologic reflexes gradually develop; movement disorders may also occur. Because of this changing neurologic picture, the patient may appear to have a progressive rather than a static nervous system disease. A similar impression is sometimes gained when neurologic signs appear months or years following a static central nervous system insult. This is sometimes referred to as unmasking of neurologic signs and does not necessarily imply new or active disease.

There are other unique features of the neurologic evaluation of infants and children that should be emphasized. Localizing the lesion is frequently more difficult than in older patients. The patient's cooperation is often difficult to enlist, particularly for sensory testing, assessment of muscle strength, optic fundi examination, and mental status evaluations. This does not mean that precise localization of the lesion is impossible, but it does place a greater reliance on the history and careful clinical observations. Disorders of the developing nervous system may also have clinical features suggesting a systemic disease rather than one localized to the brain. The reason for this is that the disease process may not be confined to the nervous system in the very young. In degenerative, infectious, and genetic diseases particularly, multiple organs may be involved as part of the primary disease.

History

The history is particularly important in neurologic diagnosis. It is often stated that accurate diagnosis is more dependent on history than on physical examination; this is particularly true in pediatrics.

The age of the patient in hours, weeks, or months is important to document accurately, because nervous system function is changing constantly during this time and certain diseases are specific for age. For the neurologic examination to be meaningful, it has to be interpreted in terms of precise chronologic age. The significance of historical details varies greatly with the nature of clinical problems, but some are important to obtain in every case. Chief among these are the details of pregnancy, labor, delivery, and the specifics of the perinatal period. This should be verified when possible by obtaining the patient's newborn record from the hospital. Important motor and mental milestones leading to the onset of the present illness should be recorded accurately. Obtaining the history in chronologic sequence helps to ensure that important details are not overlooked.

History taking requires effort and patience. Repetitive questioning about all the possible factors or circumstances surrounding the present illness is essential to identify the most likely diagnosis and to be able to logically eliminate other possibilities. If the diagnosis is not suspected at the completion of the history taking, it usually means the correct questions were not asked, not answered, or not properly interpreted. Under these circumstances additional history should be taken before beginning the physical examination and laboratory studies.

Physical examination

A complete general examination is essential because it often provides insights into the nature of the underlying neurologic problem. In general, it is best to proceed with the least threatening parts of the neurologic examination first, leaving procedures such as ophthalmoscopy, sensory testing, and cranial nerve examination until the end. It is important to systematically record the abnormal findings from the entire examination before making a diagnosis. It is also important to reexamine the patient on other occasions to verify questionable findings and define other abnormalities not clarified on the initial examination. In neonates and young infants the signs may fluctuate markedly, depending on time of day and particularly relationship to feeding.

Evaluation of the premature and term infant

Advances in neonatal medicine now make it possible for very small premature infants (less than 1500 g) to survive, even though they frequently require prolonged hospitalization and ventilatory support. The box on p. 778 depicts the neurologic function in the premature infant based on gestational age. Despite the difficulty in precisely assessing neurologic function in the very small infant, every effort should be made to perform a carefully detailed examination. It should include evaluation of the cranium, including head size and contour, as well as the status of the fontanels and sutures. The head circumference should be plotted on a percentile chart and recorded every day or two during the patient's hospital stay. Transillumination should always be done; when increased it may be an early clue indicating hydrocephalus or other developmental defects such as porencephaly, hydranencephaly, or focal cerebral atrophy. Transillumination may also be reduced, particularly in acute intracranial hemorrhage. Cranial bruits in the newborn are usually benign, but auscultation of the head is an important examination in developmental neurology and occasionally will detect aneurysms or arteriovenous malformations that were not suspected. Pupillary responses, conjugate eye movement, and visual fixation and following should be evaluated carefully. The optic fundi require careful examination in all newborns, because intracranial hemorrhage and infection are sometimes associated with retinal changes. The optic disc and macula also provide important information about visual function; changes in the macula are classically seen in a number of the degenerative disorders primarily involving gray matter.

Careful neurologic examination in the newborn establishes a baseline on which to evaluate subsequent findings. The full-term infant has a number of protective reflexes that are sometimes referred to as developmental or primitive reflexes. Some of these are present at birth, others appear during the early months of life, but most disappear during the first year (Table 29-1). These are important markers of nervous system maturation. Absence of these reflexes in the

Table 29-1. Reflexes of infancy

Reflex	Appears	Disappears
Placing	Birth	6 weeks
Sleeping	Birth	6 weeks
Moro reflex	Birth	4 months
Rooting reflex	Birth	3-4 months (awake)
Palmar grasp	Birth	6 months
Plantar grasp	Birth	9-10 months
Tonic neck reflex	2 months	5 months
Landau	3 months	24 months
Neck righting	6 months	24 months
Parachute reflex	8-9 months	Persists

NEUROLOGIC EVALUATION FOR ESTIMATION OF GESTATIONAL AGE

Tone	
Undisturbed posture (characteristic position when infant is supine)	
Flexed upper extremities	34 weeks or more
Flexed lower extremities	32 weeks or more
Recoil (rapid return to flexion after fullest extension maintained for 30 seconds)	
Full	38 weeks or more
Inhibited	37 weeks or less
Dorsiflexed foot (flex foot onto leg)	
Full	39 weeks
Partial	38 weeks or less
Popliteal angle (largest angle achievable when leg flexed on knee)	
90 degrees	37 weeks or more
110 degrees	32 weeks or more
180 degrees	28 weeks or more
Scarf sign (draw hand as far as possible around neck over the opposite shoulder)	
Elbow not to midline	40 weeks
Elbow past midline	34 weeks or less
Heel to ear (with pelvis flat on table, left heel to homolateral ear or temporal region)	
Accomplished with difficulty	32 to 35 weeks
Not accomplished	36 weeks or more
Reflexes	
Moro	
Feeble, not constant	31 weeks or less
Complete, reproducible	32 weeks or more
Sucking	
Weak, unsustained	33 weeks or less
Strong, synchronized with swallow	34 weeks or more
Rooting	
Brisk, reproducible	34 weeks or more
Grasping	
Strong, lifts body	36 weeks or more
Crossed extension (rub sole while leg held in extension; on opposite side the leg flexes then extends, foot adducts, toes fan)	
Complete reaction	36 weeks or more
Stepping or automatic walk (hold trunk with baby leaning forward; soles of feet contact mattress)	
Tiptoe only, feeble	32 weeks or more
Step heel to toe	38 weeks or more
Glabellar tap (unilateral or bialteral blink in response to finger tap on glabella)	
Present	33 weeks or more
Traction (pull by wrists to sitting position, elbows flex, shoulders brace, neck flexes to raise head)	
Full response	38 weeks or more

newborn usually means marked suppression of central nervous system function as a result of injury or defective nervous system development. Their persistence is also indicative of significant brain dysfunction. These reflexes are mediated at the brain stem level and provide very little information about the functional integrity of the cerebral cortex. The earliest clinical indication of cortical activity is provided by examination of visual fixation and following. This is an important milestone to record on all examinations of newborn infants.

Evaluation of the infant and older child

As the nervous system matures, the neurologic examination becomes more detailed. In the older child mental status, cranial nerve function, and muscle strength can be accurately assessed and reliable sensory testing becomes possible. This gradually evolves over the years. A de-

Table 29-2. Developmental assessment

Age (months)	Motor skill	Social-adaptive skill	Language skill
1	Prone: lifts head; follows to midline	Regards face	Responds to bell
2		Smiles responsively	Vocalizes (not crying)
3	Follows past midline		Laughs
4	Sits with head steady		Squeals
6	Reaches for object	Smiles spontaneously	
7	Transfers 1-inch cube		
8	Sits without support	Feeds self cracker	Turns to voice
10	Pulls self to stand	Plays peek-a-boo	
11	Thumb-finger grasp		Imitates speech sound
13	Cruises	Plays pat-a-cake	"Dada" or "Mama" specific
14	Walks alone well		
16		Plays ball with examiner	
20	Builds tower of two cubes	Imitates housework	
21			Three words other than "Mama" "Dada"
	Kicks ball forward	Uses spoon	
25	Scribbles spontaneously		
28			Combines two words
36	Jumps in place	Pulls on shoes (untied)	Follows two of three simple directions
	Balances on one foot	Dresses with supervision	Gives first and last name
	Hops on one foot	Dresses without supervision	Recognizes three colors

velopmental assessment, as depicted in Table 29-2, should be done on every infant and child. Major delays in the acquisition of these skills are an important clue to the presence of neurologic disease.

As the child acquires language, accurate mental status testing becomes possible for the first time. The normal 2 year old child will use two- or three-word phrases, and over the next 4 years the vocabulary rapidly increases, as does the sophistication of language production. Some otherwise normal children develop language very slowly. If they phonate properly, hear normally, and appear to have normal intelligence, the outlook for normal expressive language is good even if speech has not developed by 3 years of age. Beyond that time evaluation by a language specialist is probably in order.

As the child develops more sophisticated motor skills, subtle but significant neurologic dysfunction may be discovered. This may be mild motor incoordination, gait abnormalities, or movement disorders such as tremor or athetosis. Assuming an active disease process has been excluded, these usually represent the unmasking of signs following an earlier static injury to the brain. The same is true of mild mental subnormality, which may only be detected when the child enters school and fails to learn at the expected rate.

Summary

Proper neurologic evaluation of infants and children requires a good history, careful observation of the patient, and a thorough examination using normative data available for the various age groups. Accurate diagnosis requires that the examiner understand whether the process is progressive or static, focal or diffuse, and ultimately whether it is inflammatory, neoplastic, dysgenetic, or metabolic. Laboratory investigation is usually necessary to define the nature of the process, but even this is dependent on an accurate history and physical examination to choose the correct studies in the proper sequence.

CONGENITAL DEFECTS OF THE NERVOUS SYSTEM

Congenital malformations involving the nervous system are common. They are sometimes found in, and presumably are factors contributing to, fetal death and spontaneous abortion. They frequently occur in association with other anomalies, particularly ones involving midline structures (e.g., heart and palate) and the integument (e.g., skin, ears, and digits). Certain of these syndromes are caused by a chromosomal defect (Chapter 7), but the majority have no known etiology. An injury to the developing nervous system resulting from an infection, toxin, or metabolic defect during a critical stage of differentiation is likely, but proof is usually lacking. A smaller number of anomalies are traceable to a primary genetic defect involving other family members over several generations. Many of the anomalies are a result of errors in neural tube differentiation affecting either closure, flexion, or neural migration.

Midline spinal defects

Spina bifida results from a defect in closure of the caudal posterior neuropore. It is usually occult and not clinically significant, or it may be associated with a dermoid cyst, lipoma, meningocele, or myelomeningocele. The latter is a defect in the lower cord and its surface coverings. It is evident at birth and usually associated with paralysis of the lower limbs and bowel and bladder dysfunction. It is almost always associated with defects at the base of the brain (Arnold-Chiari malformation). An autosomal recessive pattern of inheritance accounts for some of these cases; therefore a careful family history is required to provide proper genetic counseling. Spinal dysraphism is an extreme expression of a closure defect in which all or part of the deformed cord is uncovered; this leaves an open midline groove containing tangled neural and tissue elements. *Diastematomyelia* refers to a congenital malformation involving the midline spine in which a fibrous band or bony spicule divides the cord and causes progressive neurologic signs as the patient grows. The diagnosis is usually apparent on plain radiographs of the spine. Myelography is always indicated in any child with progressive signs of spinal cord dysfunction, because diatematomyelia is a correctable lesion if operated on before irreparable cord injury occurs.

Transillumination of midline masses is a helpful way to differentiate between clear cystic lesions (meningoceles) and those that contain neural elements (myelomeningoceles and encephaloceles). It is also important to examine the midline spine and cranium carefully for dimples, hairs, or hyperpigmentation; these are frequently associated with an underlying lesion, such as dermoid cyst, which may communicate to the exterior by a sinus tract. This is an important consideration when meningitis is recurrent or is caused by unusual organisms or when therapy is ineffective. Careful examination of the midline should be a routine part of the newborn examination because sinus tracts should be closed surgically before complications ensue.

Cerebral defects

Anencephaly results from a fundamental defect in rostral neural tube development. It is incompatible with life, although some infants will survive for months if the cranial vault is intact.

Arrhinencephaly (holoprosencephaly) is a severe malformation involving the rhinencephalon. It occurs most characteristically in patients with Trisomy 13-15 syndrome. The craniofacial anomaly known as cebocephaly is a common accompaniment of this condition. It includes hypotelorism, microphthalmia, and frequently cleft lip and palate. The component features of arrhinencephaly are agenesis or hypogenesis of the olfactory pathway as well as other anomalies, including agenesis of the corpus callosum, single ventricle, and microcephaly.

Cranium bifidum is a defect involving the midline cranium similar to the spina bifida, which occurs more caudally. It may be associated with a dermoid cyst, or the brain may prolapse through the bony defect (encephalocele). The commonest location for this to occur is the suboccipital region, although it can occur frontally and may be overlooked, particularly if it involves the midline nares.

Hydrocephalus, hydranencephaly, and porencephaly

Hydrocephalus is a condition resulting from excessive fluid accumulation within the cerebrum. As a result the cerebral ventricles enlarge, leading to progressive head enlargement when the cranial sutures are open. If it develops quickly despite open sutures or occurs after the cranial sutures have fused, raised intracranial pressure results. This is characterized by lethargy, headache, nausea, vomiting, ataxia, confusion, and a combination of signs including progressive head enlargement, papilledema, hypertonia, hyperreflexia, and sometimes convulsions.

Hydrocephalus may result from obstruction

to the flow of spinal fluid within the ventricular system (obstructive hydrocephalus) or from impaired absorption of fluid by the arachnoid villi, which project into the dural sinuses over the convexity of the brain (communicating hydrocephalus). Studies such as computerized tomography (CT) scan, ventriculography, or isotope scanning are usually required to make this determination. Meningitis or subarachnoid hemorrhage may result in communicating hydrocephalus because the subarachnoid space is constricted or obliterated during the repair process. Aqueductal stenosis is frequently the explanation for hydrocephalus present at birth, although congenital infections may produce a similar clinical picture. When all the ventricular chambers are symmetrically enlarged and the cerebral subarachnoid space is narrowed or obliterated, communicating hydrocephalus is the diagnosis. When the ventricles are asymmetrically enlarged, or the enlargement involves only the lateral or third ventricles and not the fourth, it usually means an obstructive process impeding the flow of fluid at some point along the ventricular pathway distal to the site of maximum ventricular dilation. Obliteration of the outlet foramina of the fourth ventricle is referred to as Dandy-Walker syndrome. This results in dilation of all ventricles and compression and eventual thinning of the overlying cerebellum. Enlargement of the posterior skull below the inion is a valuable clue suggesting this anomaly; increased transillumination over the posterior inferior skull is practically diagnostic of the condition.

Hydrocephalus requires early and accurate diagnosis before irreversible compressive injury to the overlying brain occurs. Treatment consists of removing the obstructive lesion (e.g., tumor, aneurysm, cyst, or abscess) when possible, and diverting the ventricular fluid by means of a variety of shunting procedures.

Hydranencephaly is a major anomaly of the cerebrum resulting from a lytic injury to the hemispheres, usually during prenatal life. This is thought to be a result of symmetric infarction of the brain supplied by the major tributaries of the internal carotid arteries. The precise etiology, however, is unknown; presumably a number of mechanisms could be involved, including infection, toxins, trauma, or possibly hematopoietic factors. These infants can look remarkably normal at birth. The head may appear normal in size and contour but usually begins to enlarge in the early weeks of life as a result of impaired fluid absorption. Prominence of transillumination is so characteristic that other diagnostic procedures are usually unnecessary. There is no satisfactory treatment. Death usually results within a few months because of infection or cardiopulmonary complications.

A porencephalic cyst is a brain cavity that connects with the ventricular system. It probably results from infarction to a portion of the hemisphere during late gestation. The patient may be asymptomatic or have a variety of symptoms and signs, including raised intracranial pressure, seizures, hemiparesis, visual field defects, and hemisensory deficits. Transillumination usually shows a focal area of increased illumination if the cavity is large. Diagnosis is confirmed by CT. Occasionally these patients require a shunting procedure to control intracranial pressure. The usual treatment is directed at minimizing the problems associated with hemiparesis and controlling seizures.

Cranial anomalies

A large head is termed *macrocephaly* and a large brain *megalencephaly*. Large heads may be familial and have no pathologic significance. Excluding this group, most children with large heads have hydrocephalus. Large brains may occur sporadically or be associated with neurofibromatosis, tuberous sclerosis, or cerebral gigantism. Megalencephaly may also be familial and associated with mental retardation, impaired motor function, and sometimes seizures. The brain is poorly organized and, although large, is simplified in structure. Microcephaly, or small head (less than the third percentile), is usually the result of a congenital infection or an hypoxic-ischemic insult to the developing brain with subsequent retardation of brain growth. Occasionally microcephaly occurs in families and is associated with normal intelligence; however, most familial cases have subnormal intelligence. The head may also be small at birth as a result of premature closure of all cranial sutures, i.e., craniosynostosis. This is a medical emergency that must be recognized immediately and treated promptly before increased intracranial pressure develops. Usually sutural stenosis is incomplete, resulting in abnormalities of cranial contour but not raised intracranial pressure.

STATIC ENCEPHALOPATHIES (CEREBRAL PALSY)

Static encephalopathies result from injuries to the developing brain during pregnancy, labor, delivery, or early childhood. The resultant neurologic dysfunction usually appears gradually as the child grows and brain function matures. The injury can affect any part of the nervous system, but the cerebral hemispheres, including the cortex, white matter, and basal ganglia, as well as the cerebellum, are most often affected.

One feature of this disorder is an abnormality of muscle tone. This is best demonstrated by a change in resistance to passive movement of the limbs. Hypertonia or increased muscle tone is usual, although hypotonia or diminished muscle tone may be present, especially during the early period following acute cerebral insults. Hypotonia is also a sign of cerebellar and spinal cord dysfunction. Movement disorders are also seen, often in association with hypertonicity. Because of imbalance of muscle activity about joints and poor control of motor movements, unusual postural features and marked deformities are common.

The incidence of this problem is not known because reporting is variable, especially when the disability is minor. With the advent of modern techniques to support life in the very small neonate, one might expect an increase in this problem since intracranial hemorrhage, hypoxic-ischemic insults, and metabolic derangements are all more common in the premature baby. It has been estimated that about 40% of cases of cerebral palsy can be traced to insults occurring prenatally and the remainder to injuries occurring in the immediate postnatal period and the early months of life. Only a small percentage are caused by trauma, meningitis, or encephalitis occurring later in childhood.

Classification. The classification of these disorders is not as neatly defined as Table 29-3 might indicate. It is difficult to localize the lesion or precisely define the type of movement disorder when the muscle tone is significantly increased. The commonest type of altered muscle tone is spasticity. This may involve a single extremity (monoparesis), one side of the body (hemiparesis), or all the extremities (quadriparesis). It is characterized by increased resistance to passive movement, weakness, hyperreflexia, deformity, and, if the lower extremity is involved, Babinski's sign. Spontaneous movement of the affected extremity is diminished, and in time muscle atrophy develops. Rigidity may be difficult to differentiate from spasticity; often elements of both are present in the same extremity. When there is uniform resistance to passive movement throughout the entire range of motion, it is referred to as *plastic rigidity;* an irregular pattern to the resistance is termed *cogwheel rigidity.* Involvement of the extrapyramidal system may also result in a movement disorder. Athetosis is a slow, writhing, twisting movement of the limbs, in contrast to the quick, jerky, purposeless movement characteristic of chorea. Dystonia refers to a postural deformity

Table 29-3. Clinical anatomic classification of neuromotor disorders

Anatomic site	Clinical manifestations	Topographic manifestations
Corticospinal tracts	Paralysis Weakness Hyperreflexia Deformity	Paraparesis, legs only; legs more than arms; quadriparesis, all four extremities; hemiparesis, half the body; monoparesis, usually one extremity
Basal ganglia	Athetosis Choreiform movements Dystonia Tremor Rigidity Mental retardation Hyperreflexia	Arms, legs, neck, trunk
Cerebellum and/or connections	Ataxia Hypotonia Tremor Incoordination	Arms, legs, trunk

of the type seen in patients with severe athetosis. Ataxia is an uncommon manifestation of an acquired or developmental encephalopathy. It may occur with injuries to the cerebellum as well as with insults to the cortex or basal ganglia. Hypotonia is an early feature following acute cerebral or spinal cord injury. By the end of the first year of life hypertonia and hyperreflexia are usually evident when the brain is prominently involved.

Associated problems. When the developing nervous system is injured by a traumatic or toxic-metabolic process, mentality is also significantly impaired. This is difficult to gauge in the young infant when motor coordination is poor, and in the older child it may be difficult to define accurately because mental status testing is interdependent on motor function involving oral and facial musculature. Lack of appropriate head growth indicates impaired cerebral growth. Seizures may develop at any time and should be anticipated in patients with significant structural injuries to the brain. Other abnormalities that may be detected in these children include visual defects, proprioceptive disturbances, cortical sensory dysfunction, and perceptual motor disabilities.

Diagnosis. The diagnosis is not difficult, assuming a progressive neurologic disorder is excluded by careful history. Investigation should include detailed evaluation of muscle strength and tone as well as an assessment of joint mobility. It is important to determine whether there are limb or spinal deformities, because these can lead to complications that may significantly impair motility. The limbs should be measured carefully and examined to exclude hip dislocations, which are a problem in infants who exhibit spasticity and are not weight bearing. The patient's intellectual function should be defined as accurately as possible, and seizures should be systematically excluded by history and electroencephalographic examination. It is seldom necessary to resort to contrast studies unless unusual features are found on examination to suggest a major cerebral anomaly such as porencephaly or hydrocephalus. Screening tests should be done to exclude an abnormality of amino acid metabolism; chromosomal studies should be considered for patients with multiple somatic abnormalities.

The child with a congenital or acquired encephalopathy should be carefully evaluated when first seen by the physician, because the parents deserve to know the extent of the disability and the prognosis. Following this, it requires a team effort involving physicians, parents, educators, and other health professionals to support and encourage the child to achieve his full mental and physical potential. Many patients have productive, purposeful lives despite major handicaps.

Management. Management begins with careful clinical assessment to define the full extent of the neurologic problem. A vigorous physiotherapy and occupational therapy program should be instituted for patients with rehabilitation potential. Special shoes and proper bracing are often indicated to minimize limb deformity and promote walking. Surgery to lengthen spastic muscles and hence reduce deformity is sometimes necessary. Speech therapy as well as special aids for children with impaired hearing may be indicated. Special educational resources are often required to help these children attain their full learning potential. When seizures are present, anticonvulsant medication should be prescribed. Medications to reduce spasticity or alter rigidity have not been particularly successful, but diazepam or related compounds seem to help some severely handicapped patients.

HEADACHE

Pain-sensitive cranial structures include blood vessels, periosteum, skin, and muscles. Within the cranial cavity these include veins, arteries, dura at the base of the brain, and the venous sinuses. Irritation of these structures, regardless of cause, can result in headache. In children this is frequently a vague, ill-defined, poorly localized symptom that requires a careful history to define the etiology.

Both local and systemic causes for headaches must be carefully considered, since headache is a common symptom with multiple causes. It can result from disorders involving the teeth, scalp, paranasal sinuses, eyes, cervical spine, and temporomandibular joints. Localized infection of the paranasal sinuses is an important treatable cause to exclude but is infrequent in the infant and young child because the sinuses are small and poorly aerated. Ocular disorders are also infrequent causes of headache, although refractive errors, astigmatism, or squints may result in extraocular muscle fatigue and headache.

Most commonly, however, headache is a nonspecific symptom in children, occurring in the course of a febrile illness. The reason for this is not well defined but presumably is related in part to vasodilation secondary to temperature elevation; there may also be toxic or metabolic factors contributing to the headache associated with febrile illnesses. Anxiety or tension is another significant cause of headaches, particularly in children whose parents have similar complaints. In these situations there is often no single situational stress or conflict that is obvious, but a combination of factors that require careful history to identify. Headache secondary to raised intracranial pressure is infrequent in children but must be considered in every patient with chronic headaches, especially if it is becoming more severe or awakening the patient at night. Vascular headaches of the migraine type are also uncommon but important to recognize, because they will usually improve with therapy. Headache may also be a presenting complaint in hypertension or a prominent feature of a seizure disorder. Headache may precede the actual seizure or be a prominent postictal symptom. It can be the sole manifestation of a seizure, but this should be considered only when all other explanations for the headache have been systemically excluded.

Headache with infections or allergy

Headache from a localized nasal infection or allergy obstructing the sinuses is usually worse in the morning and aggravated by placing the head in a dependent position. If allergy is a factor these headaches may be seasonal. Headaches occurring with meningitis or inflammatory brain disorders are usually constant and throbbing and subside only when the inflammation subsides. Mild analgesics are indicated when the headache is severe. Narcotics and depressant medication should be avoided because they can affect important markers of disease progression, such as patient responses and level of consciousness.

Tension headache

Tension headache is poorly localized. It is often described as diffuse or frontal in location, and compressing, dull, or aching in quality. It usually occurs daily and lasts for a number of hours. Frequently the cause is not obvious, yet careful questioning will eventually uncover sources of anxiety or worry that must be remedied for treatment to be successful. This type of headache occurs most commonly in school-age children whose parents are being treated for mood disorders, psychoneuroses, or even psychotic illnesses.

Investigation should exclude other causes for headache. This is usually accomplished by careful history and detailed examination, including ophthalmoscopic evaluation, blood pressure measurement, and evaluation of mental status. Occasionally, skull radiographs are indicated to help exclude raised intracranial pressure. An electroencephalogram (EEG) is helpful if seizures are a consideration. It is important to appreciate that tension headaches may be caused by anxiety as a result of unresolved conflicts that may seem trivial to the examiner and are sometimes denied by the child. Tension headaches can also occur in children with chronic diseases or recurrent pain or disability, regardless of etiology.

Migraine

Classic migraine is uncommon in young children. It is characterized by a positive family history in about 80% of cases. The headache is characteristically unilateral and throbbing. It is frequently preceded by a variety of visual symptoms, paresthesias, and occasionally by aphasia. Nausea and vomiting are common, and there may be sensitivity to sound and light during the headache.

Common migraine is more frequent in childhood. Neurologic symptoms are usually not a feature of this headache syndrome; it is a frontal headache or at least not classically hemicranial. There is usually a family history. The headache is usually severe, persists for hours, and tends to remit following sleep.

Treatment of migraine begins with explanation and reassurance. Patients and parents are usually concerned about sinister underlying brain disease. Reassurance about this will allay much of the anxiety that often precipitates attacks of migraine. Therapy rarely requires more than mild analgesic medication, fluids, rest, and quiet. This should be instituted immediately after the headache begins because it may abort the more intense discomfort that follows. When headaches are unresponsive to this regimen, and particularly when they are frequent, intense, and interfere with the child's home and school routine, more aggressive approaches are indicated. Anticonvulsant medications (phenytoin [Dilantin], mephobarbital [Mebaral], and primidone [Mysoline]) are occasionally helpful, particularly in patients with paroxysmal EEG abnormalities. Such medication should be used infrequently and with the understanding that it is a therapeutic trial to be continued only if the response is good. The ergot preparations (e.g., Cafergot) are rarely indicated in childhood migraine because the classic prodromal symptoms are unusual, and administering the drug after the headache has begun is usually ineffective. It can be tried in the older child with severe intractable headache but should not be given repeatedly if symptoms are not improved dramatically. In practice, one rarely has to resort to this type of therapy if conservative measures outlined above are instituted promptly. Migraine headaches often disappear or improve as the child matures; occasionally they may persist or worsen, but the child and the parent should be reassured about the probability of improvement with age.

Headache as manifestation of raised intracranial pressure

Headache associated with raised intracranial pressure may be caused by tumor, hydrocephalus, infections, or any lesion that obstructs the flow of cerebrospinal fluid or significantly increases the volume within the cranial cavity. The typical headache is throbbing, although this is variable. It may be dull, constant, and aggravated by lying down. It may also awaken the child from sleep or be particularly severe in the morning. Vomiting may cause temporary improvement, but the severe headache usually recurs a short time later.

Children with severe headaches, regardless of character or localization, deserve careful and repeated ophthalmoscopic evaluations to detect signs of raised intracranial pressure. Papilledema may not develop for a number of days despite significant pressure elevation. Early in the course, mild venous engorgement or retinal sheen may be the only fundal changes, even when the pressure is significantly increased. This underscores the importance of careful clinical evaluation before considering invasive diagnostic procedures such as lumbar puncture.

Skull radiographs are helpful in the evaluation of raised intracranial pressure. Long-standing pressure elevation may cause demineralization of the sella turcica, erosion of the posterior clinoids, and separation of the cranial sutures; acute pressure increases may not produce any changes on the skull radiographs in the older child once the cranial sutures are fused. CT is the most helpful diagnostic procedure to exclude a mass lesion in patients with suspected intracranial hypertension.

Treatment varies with the underlying cause for pressure elevation. Mass lesions require complete resection when possible, followed by irradiation and sometimes chemotherapy if a malignant tumor is found. Hydrocephalus usually requires a shunting procedure to reduce intraventricular pressure and relieve the headache.

CENTRAL NERVOUS SYSTEM INFECTIONS

Infections involving the nervous system are common in childhood. Any unexplained febrile illness in a child should alert the clinician to this possibility, particularly if there is alteration of consciousness, convulsions, or signs of meningeal irritation. Early recognition and prompt treatment are imperative to minimize the serious morbidity and mortality associated with these infections. Despite the best effort of the medical profession, this diagnosis is often delayed, particularly in babies and young infants in whom the classic signs of infection are not always present. Whenever this diagnosis is considered, lumbar puncture should be done.

Acute bacterial meningitis

The clinical and microbiologic features of meningitis are outlined in Chapter 27, in which the importance of an orderly approach to diagnosis, proper selection of antimicrobial agents, and general principles of management are emphasized. However, complications may occur either during the period of active inflammation while the patient is under treatment in hospital or much later after all signs of infection have subsided.

Acute complications of bacterial infection

Raised intracranial pressure is usually a feature of acute bacterial meningitis, although it may not be obvious, particularly if the patient is dehydrated as a result of vomiting or reduced fluid intake. An infant with meningitis may have a flat or sunken fontanel as a result of dehydration. As this is corrected, increased intracranial pressure may appear abruptly and result in serious complications, including brain stem compression, seizures, and altered consciousness. Papilledema or other signs of raised intracranial pressure may not be obvious early in the course of meningitis or in infants with open cranial sutures. Even when papilledema, exudates, hemorrhages, and venous engorgement are present, the intracranial pressure may not be excessive because the inflammatory process may be subsiding. For these reasons it is important not to delay lumbar puncture when meningitis is a serious consideration. This is done using a small-gauge needle, and enough fluid is removed to establish the diagnosis. If the pressure increase is excessive (greater than 400 ml of water), mannitol (1 to 2 g/kg) or other dehydrating agents can be administered to reduce the risk of transtentorial or foraminal herniation. However, this is a rare complication and hyperosmolar solutions such as urea or mannitol are seldom indicated in the management of childhood meningitis.

Subdural effusion and hydrocephalus. Subdural effusion is a common complication of meningitis in infants with *Haemophilus influenzae* infection. Usually the patient develops recurrent or persistent fever, headache, neck stiffness, irritability, or vomiting during the course of an otherwise good clinical response to therapy. As the intracranial pressure increases, seizures and depressed consciousness may also occur. There is usually a cerebrospinal fluid pleocytosis, with increased protein but no organisms, and a sterile culture. There may be signs of raised intracranial pressure, including increasing head circumference, papilledema, and sixth nerve paresis. The diagnosis is confirmed by demonstration of unilateral or bilateral cranial transillumination and recovery of proteinaceous, clear, sterile fluid following subdural taps. Hydrocephalus is another complication of meningitis that may include similar signs and symptoms, although usually there is symmetric transillumination. The diagnosis of ventricular dilation is easily confirmed by CT. Hydrocephalus may develop during the acute phase of meningitis, particularly when ventriculitis is a complicating feature. Usually, however, it evolves slowly and is not appreciated until weeks or months later when the child is at home and fully recovered from the infection.

Seizures. Convulsions are frequent complications of bacterial meningitis in infants and children. Anticipating this is important to prevent aspiration pneumonia, airway obstruction, or injury in an already seriously ill patient. Patients with altered consciousness during the course of meningitis, or who have any indication of paroxysmal motor activity suggesting seizures, should be treated promptly with an anticonvulsant drug (phenytoin [Dilantin], 5 mg/kg/24 hr). Cerebritis, cortical vein thrombosis, subdural effusion, or empyema are all potential explanations for seizures, or they may be caused by water intoxication resulting from injudicious fluid administration or inappropriate antidiuretic hormone (ADH) secretion. Regardless of etiology, seizures are a serious complication, occurring in 25% to 40% of patients with meningitis, and require prompt evaluation and therapy.

Brain abscess and subdural empyema. Brain abscess is a rare complication of bacterial meningitis if one excludes the microsuppurative foci that occur with cerebritis. The large encapsulated hemispheral abscess arises by direct extension from infection involving the sinuses or middle ear or as a complication of septic embolism. Subdural empyema is a rare complication of bacterial meningitis, yet should be considered in any patient who has raised intracranial pressure, depressed consciousness, and seizures. The cerebrospinal fluid usually contains a modest pleocytosis with an elevated protein content, and normal to slightly depressed glucose concentration. The diagnosis is confirmed by removing pus from the subdural space either by needle aspiration or surgical drainage. Treatment consists of continuous drainage and massive antibiotic therapy.

Late complications

A number of complications of meningitis may not be apparent for months or years after the acute illness. Hydrocephalus may begin during the acute phase of the illness, yet not be apparent clinically until weeks or months later when the child returns with a progressively enlarging head or other signs and symptoms of intracranial hypertension. Another complication that may not be appreciated initially is deafness. This problem is easily overlooked, particularly in a young child or when the hearing loss is incomplete; it is often initially detected when hearing is assessed as a screening procedure at school. In these situations the cause-and-effect relationship to an earlier episode of meningitis may not be appreciated. Mild mental subnormality, hyperkinesis, behavioral disorders, and motor incoordination are also recognized sequelae of meningitis that may not be apparent or problematic until much later. Seizures can occur months or years after meningitis, although this is infrequent if the child is well and seizure free for 6 to 12 months following recovery from meningitis.

Chronic meningitis

Clinical features of tuberculous meningitis or fungal infections of the central nervous system (coccidioidomycosis, cryptococcosis, blastomycosis, and actinomycosis) are extremely variable in children. Early in the course of meningitis signs of nervous system involvement are frequently minimal. However, these infections progress rapidly to cause raised intracranial pressure and signs of meningeal irritation. Fungal infections of the central nervous system are unusual in children except in the malnourished, chronically ill, or immunodeficient patient. Tuberculous meningitis is infrequently seen in childhood yet should be considered in any patient with a predominantly mononuclear cerebrospinal fluid pleocytosis and hypoglycorrhachia, regardless of the reactivity of the tuberculin test (see p. 731).

Aseptic meningitis (virus meningoencephalitis)

Almost any virus that infects humans can involve the central nervous system, although some are highly selective for neural tissue and for this reason have been referred to as neurotropic agents. On clinical grounds alone it is usually not possible to know which virus is producing the infection, but there are seasonal patterns of infection that provide important clues. During the warm months when enteric infections are prevalent enterovirus meningitis is more common; in the colder season the respiratory pathogens predominate, and viruses of this class would be expected when viral meningitis occurs. Herpes simplex virus is probably the commonest viral pathogen accounting for sporadic cases of severe meningoencephalitis in children. Meningoencephalitis may also be caused by arboviruses, but these are uncommon infections in children. Meningoencephalitis is still a serious complication of a number of common virus infections, including mumps, measles, and varicella. However, these have a different pathogenesis than the usual nervous system infection secondary to virus replication in central nervous system tissue. They are discussed separately under the parainfectious encephalitides.

Virus infections of the nervous system usually cause clinical features similar to those occurring with bacterial meningitis. The primary inflammatory reaction may involve the meninges (meningitis), or the brain (encephalitis), but usually both are affected and the term *meningoencephalitis* is applied. Cardinal symptoms are headache, confusion, fever, nuchal rigidity, and sometimes convulsions, ataxia, photophobia, and weakness. The intracranial pressure may be significantly elevated. Focal neurologic signs such as hemiparesis or dysphasia may be present. Meningoencephalitis may follow a respiratory or enteric infection or occur without any obvious antecedent illness.

The spinal fluid pressure is usually increased, and the fluid contains a moderate number of cells (10 to 500/ml^3) and an increased protein content. The cerebrospinal fluid glucose is usually normal, although occasionally it is depressed. The cells are typically mononuclear, with a preponderance of polymorphonuclear leukocytes early in the course of infection.

The clinical course and outcome are variable, depending on both virus and host factors. Usually symptoms evolve slowly over the course of 7 to 10 days and then gradually subside. Major problems in management are control of raised intracranial pressure, airway maintenance if coma develops, and effective treatment of seizures.

Since virus rarely is cultured from the spinal fluid or brain, an etiologic diagnosis is usually based on the de novo appearance of antiviral antibodies in the serum or a fourfold or greater rise in titer. Unfortunately, this is not known until later in the disease course. As a result, even though the diagnosis may be suspected on clinical grounds, cultures of the blood and cerebrospinal fluid for bacteria should be done routinely to exclude infections responsive to antibiotic therapy. Even in situations where cultures are negative, confusion may arise because patients are often given one or two doses of antibiotic before hospitalization. In general, appropriate antibiotic therapy is recommended until bacterial infection has been excluded with certainty.

Neurologic sequelae of viral infections include psychomotor retardation, behavioral disorders, seizures, and occasionally focal dysfunction such as blindness, hemiparesis, or language impairment. Residual findings like these occur in 20% to 25% of children following meningoencephalitis yet are often not apparent until several years later when the child enters school. Treatment is primarily supportive and aimed at minimizing risk of serious complications. These include raised intracranial pressure, seizures, and coma. Vidarabine is an antiviral agent that is now commercially available for treatment of virologically-proven herpes simplex virus encephalitis. Another agent, acyclovir, is undergoing treatment trials at present with promising results.

Parainfectious encephalomyelitis

Encephalitis may occur a few days to 2 weeks after a number of viral infections such as measles, mumps, and varicella. This type of infection is referred to as *parainfectious encephalomyelitis*. The clinical course varies little from that seen with the usual lytic virus infections of the nervous system. Since the virus has not been recovered from either the brain or spinal fluid obtained from patients with parainfectious encephalomyelitis, it is generally concluded that the mechanism of disease must be different from direct virus replication in nervous system tissue. At this time it is thought to be a hypersensitivity reaction to viral antigen, although the precise mechanism is unclear.

Slow virus infection

Slow virus infections are rare in childhood. They are subacute or chronic infections of the brain that occur following an extremely long incubation period during which the patient is well. The best example in childhood is subacute sclerosing panencephalitis (SSPE), a slow measles encephalitis that usually develops months to years after primary exposure to the virus. The SSPE virus, in contrast to measles, has recently been shown to lack M protein, a surface antigen responsible for virus assembly. This is presumed to be the reason for the accumulation of incomplete virus nucleocapsids in brain. The reason for the defective M protein function is not understood but presumed to be secondary to host cell factors. Clinical features of this condition include male preponderance (3:1), onset usually between 5 and 9 years, progressive dementia, myoclonus, focal motor dysfunction, and eventually stupor, coma, and death. The diagnosis is established by the demonstration of markedly elevated measles antibody levels in the serum and the demonstration of similar antibodies in the cerebrospinal fluid.

There is no treatment at present that significantly alters the inevitably fatal course of this disease. The condition has attracted great interest and attention because the virus-cell interaction is unique, and its understanding may possibly provide important new insights into the pathogenesis of other human diseases of the nervous system.

Differential diagnosis of central nervous system infection

Patients with headache, fever, nuchal rigidity, and altered consciousness should be evaluated for conditions other than infection. A patient with leukemia involving the leptomeninges may show all the signs of bacterial meningitis; the diagnosis should be apparent from history, physical examination, and the demonstration of malignant cells in the cerebrospinal fluid. Tumor involving the posterior fossa may lead to early obstruction of cerebrospinal fluid flow, with resultant signs of raised intracranial pressure, vomiting, and sometimes fever and stiff neck. A similar picture can occur with chronic lead encephalopathy or as a late sequel to trauma, complicated by the formation of a chronic subdural hematoma. Subarachnoid hemorrhage is rare but should be considered in children or infants who have headache, fever, stiff neck, and signs of raised intracranial pressure. Reye syndrome (p. 746) is an acquired hepatoencephalopathy of obscure etiology. Symptoms include rapidly deteriorating consciousness and seizures, often with fever, acidosis, and hyperpnea.

Differentiation of all these conditions from pyogenic, fungal, or viral infections of the central nervous system is based on a careful history, physical examination, and particularly critical analysis of the cerebrospinal fluid. If an intracranial tumor or abscess is considered, skull radiographs and computerized tomography should be done before lumbar puncture. The EEG is helpful in the evaluation of central nervous system infection, but is not diagnostic of any one type.

Guillain-Barré syndrome (see also p. 818)

Guillain-Barré syndrome, or infectious polyneuritis, classically includes signs of ascending paralysis in a previously well child. There may be a history of an antecedent mild respiratory or enteric infection, although this is not always obtained. Typical presenting features are paresthesias in the distal lower extremities, followed in hours or days by symmetric weakness of the proximal lower limbs, progressing to involve the trunk and sometimes the upper limbs as well as the bulbar musculature. Occasionally the weakness begins in the upper limbs or the orofacial musculature, but this is unusual. The etiology is not understood, although the temporal association with viral, bacterial, and mycoplasmic infections suggests an autoimmune or hypersensitivity response, possibly to a number of different antigens. The pathologic lesion is an inflammatory demyelinating process, affecting primarily the proximal motor roots, but any nerve may be affected. The diagnosis is suggested by the findings of weakness, areflexia, and an elevated cerebrospinal fluid protein. The latter may not be present until later in the disease course. Careful evaluation of pulmonary function is essential; assisted ventilation is often required and should be anticipated by repeated measurement of vital capacity and blood gases, rather than delayed until respiratory failure develops. Occasionally, raised intracranial pressure occurs. Bladder and bowel dysfunction are common, and autonomic imbalance may result in severe postural hypotension and cardiac arrhythmias.

Treatment consists of optimal supportive care. If complications are prevented, complete recovery can be expected despite the severity of the paralysis.

INTRACRANIAL TUMORS

Brain tumors in children are important to recognize early and treat promptly, because a significant percentage of these children recover completely and others may survive for years with minimal problems. About 60% to 70% of tumors in the childhood years are located in the posterior fossa, and the majority are in the midline. There are localizing and nonlocalizing signs that suggest the presence of an intracranial mass lesion. The most important nonlocalizing sign is raised intracranial pressure, either secondary to obstruction of the ventricular pathway or displacement of tissue by the mass.

Raised intracranial pressure

Headache. The headache caused by a brain tumor fluctuates in severity. It tends to worsen after a period of recumbency or with straining or coughing. It may spontaneously remit for a period, but eventually recurs and progressively worsens. It is often accompanied by nausea and eventually vomiting. Irritability and lethargy usually accompany significant pressure increases.

Papilledema. Papilledema, or choked discs, may not be present in infants and young children with open cranial sutures, despite significantly elevated intracranial pressure. However, pressure that rises acutely may produce venous engorgement, retinal edema, hemorrhages, and papilledema, regardless of the status of the cranial sutures. Since papilledema is not a sensitive indicator of the status of intracranial pressure, skull radiographs, EEG, and CT should be obtained whenever an intracranial mass lesion is suspected. Lumbar puncture should be avoided under these circumstances, even if the optic fundi appear normal.

Diplopia and strabismus. The sudden onset of double vision or the appearance of a squint as a result of lateral rectus weakness (sixth nerve palsy) is an important sign of raised intracranial pressure. A child may tilt the head to minimize the effects of diplopia or to lessen the traction on the basal meninges.

Macrocephaly. An intracranial mass lesion may produce obstructive hydrocephalus, separation of sutures, and increasing head circumference. This underscores the importance of sequential measurements of head circumference from birth through the first 2 years of life. Unexplained acceleration of head growth may be an early sign of an intracranial mass lesion in an infant before other symptoms develop. Transillumination also provides valuable information to help differentiate the nature of the intracranial mass in an infant with an enlarging head.

Nausea and vomiting. Nausea and vomiting also may occur as a result of the intense headache or encroachment of the tumor directly on the emetic center in the brain stem. This is important to recognize because it is a valuable localizing sign for the surgeon and radiotherapist.

Posterior fossa neoplasms

The presenting features of brain tumors involving the posterior fossa are variable. Most result from raised intracranial pressure associated with signs of cerebellar dysfunction. The most important localizing sign is ataxia, usually primarily truncal as a result of midline cerebellar involvement; or the lateral portions of the cerebellum may be affected, resulting in appendicular ataxia. The cerebellar signs are ipsilateral, in contrast to pyramidal tract signs that are contralateral to the side of the lesion.

Whenever a mass compresses the limited space within the posterior fossa, the pressure effects are directed toward the foramen magnum. Occasionally, upward herniation may occur through the tentorium cerebelli. Compression at the level of the foramen magnum may result in a head tilt, severe suboccipital tenderness, or neck spasms. Tumors involving the cerebellum may also lead to hypotonia and decreased deep tendon reflexes, at least early in the clinical course. With brain stem compression, or with tumors involving other brain stem structures, hypertonicity, hyperreflexia, clonus, and extensor plantar responses are usually found.

It is difficult to distinguish between a medulloblastoma and an astrocytoma using clinical criteria alone. In general, medulloblastomas grow more rapidly and are usually associated with midline truncal ataxia and early appearance of increased intracranial pressure. Cerebellar astrocytomas, on the other hand, are more benign histologically, grow more slowly, and usually involve the cerebellar hemisphere primarily. However, it is always important to make a tissue diagnosis, because the prognosis for a cerebellar astrocytoma is extremely good. The cure rate following surgery is 80% to 90%, provided the tumor is excised before secondary pressure effects result in irreversible brain injury.

Other tumors involving the posterior fossa are less common. Brain stem glioma deserves special consideration. This tumor, which primarily involves the pons, results in early signs of cranial nerve dysfunction and usually does not produce increased intracranial pressure until late in the course of disease. It may also be associated with nystagmus, ataxia, and pyramidal tract signs. The course is one of progressive deterioration, leading to death within a few months to 1 or 2 years, despite irradiation and chemotherapy.

Cerebral tumors

Supratentorial tumors. Supratentorial tumors in childhood are usually malignant gliomas. Ependymomas may also occur, within either the hemisphere or ventricles, and are histologically benign. Calcification on skull radiographs is a clue to the presence of an ependymoma. The meningioma is a tumor occasionally seen in patients with multiple neurofibromatosis (von Recklinghausen disease), but rarely in otherwise well children. Choroid plexus papilloma is another rare tumor. It produces hydrocephalus secondary to excessive cerebrospinal fluid production. Calcifications are sometimes seen within these tumors.

Suprasellar tumors. Suprasellar tumors include a number of different tumors that produce a variety of signs and symptoms because of their proximity to the optic pathway, hypothalamus, and pituitary gland. The commonest variety is the craniopharyngioma, although optic nerve gliomas are also important tumors to consider in children. Less common tumors in this region include hypothalamic gliomas, epidermoids, and teratoid tumors.

Craniopharyngioma. The craniopharyngioma is the most common nonglial tumor of childhood. It classically produces a deformity of the sella turcica and in children almost always shows calcification on plain skull radiographs. These patients usually display growth failure or delayed sexual maturation, but raised intracranial pressure may be an early presenting feature with the hormonal dysfunction only a secondary discovery. Encroachment on the optic pathway by this tumor is common, yet many children, particularly very young patients, do not complain of a visual difficulty. It is important to examine the patient for visual field defects; these are classically bitemporal but may be extremely variable. Unfortunately, when compression by the tumor has gone unrecognized, papilledema or even optic atrophy may be present by the time the patient is first seen. Remarkable improvement in surgical treatment in recent years has made it possible to eradicate the tumor, particularly if it is recognized early. Replacement hormone therapy is now available to help these children lead a near-normal life.

Optic nerve glioma. It is important to recognize optic nerve glioma early before it extends intracranially to involve the optic chiasm. Presenting clinical features include unexplained strabismus, optic atrophy, or nystagmus; it may also involve the orbital portion of the optic nerve and produce displacement of the globe. Radiographic examination of the orbit frequently reveals enlargement of the optic foramen when the tumor involves the retro-orbital portion of the optic nerve.

Evaluation of intracranial tumors

Radiographs of the skull may show changes indicative of chronic raised intracranial pressure or calcifications. They may also show abnormalities of the clinoid processes, changes in the optic foramina, or alterations in the size and shape of the sella turcica.

Slowing of the EEG occurs with raised intracranial pressure. When this is asymmetric, it suggests the presence of a hemispheric mass lesion that must be confirmed by other studies. Whenever brain tumor is a serious diagnostic consideration lumbar puncture should be avoided, because the sudden pressure change following the removal of cerebrospinal fluid can result in transtentorial or transforaminal herniation. Occasionally, a diagnosis of tumor may be made on the basis of cells shed into the cerebrospinal or ventricular fluids. Studies of this type should be done carefully and in collaboration with neurosurgery.

CT is a noninvasive, highly sensitive technique now available to define not only the presence of an intracranial mass lesion but also its relationship to the ventricles and midline structures. Its availability has made most other diagnostic studies practically obsolete in the investigation of an intracranial mass lesion. Once a mass is detected, additional contrast studies may be necessary to define the relationship of the tumor to other structures in the region, particularly blood vessels. Selective cerebral angiography before surgery is valuable for this purpose.

Benign intracranial hypertension (pseudotumor cerebri)

Raised intracranial pressure associated with normal cerebrospinal fluid findings and small or normal-sized ventricles is referred to as *benign intracranial hypertension* or *pseudotumor cerebri*. Presenting symptoms are usually headache and vomiting unrelated to the usual causes of raised intracranial pressure, such as trauma, tumor, or infection. Examination may be normal or indicate a sixth nerve paresis and papilledema; other focal neurologic signs are unusual. If pressure increase is excessive and duration prolonged, blindness can result. The illness usually lasts several weeks and is followed by complete recovery.

Precise explanation for this pressure increase is unknown, although venous congestion resulting from sinus thrombosis is a popular explanation. This has been documented by arteriography in some cases. The condition has been attributed to hormonal imbalance, such as adrenal insufficiency after corticosteroid therapy. Ear infections, mastoiditis, thrombosis of the lateral sinus, vitamin A intoxication and deficiency, tetracycline administration, and viral infections have all been implicated in the pathogenesis of this condition. Fortunately the prognosis is excellent, despite absence of specific therapy. Corticosteroids may result in temporary improvement, but the pressure usually recurs when they are discontinued. Repeated lumbar punctures have been used effectively to control the pressure in hospitalized patients. Surgical decompression of the optic nerve has been advocated by some when progressive visual loss develops.

SPINAL CORD TUMORS

Spinal cord tumors are uncommon in children but merit careful consideration because their early recognition and treatment are necessary to prevent permanent cord injury. The commonest complaints are weakness and pain. The patient's only complaint may be a limp or some change in ability to run or climb. The pain is variable, depending on the site of cord or root compression. Persistent or intermittent pain in the back or extremities always deserves careful evaluation to exclude the possibility of an intraspinal tumor. Changes in bladder or bowel function, unexplained scoliosis, or gait disturbances are also important clues. Sensory disturbances including dysesthesias and patchy sensory loss may occur, but a discrete sensory level is unusual.

Tumors may be intramedullary or extramedullary. The commonest intramedullary tumors are gliomas. These are not approachable surgically, and the prognosis is poor despite irradiation and chemotherapy. The extramedullary tumors, on the other hand, are often curable. Intradural extramedullary tumors are primarily meningiomas or neurofibromas. Extradural tumors include metastatic tumors, lymphomas, and the primary tumors involving the vertebrae, nerves, and blood vessels in that region.

Signs and symptoms. Extramedullary neoplasms may produce continuous pain as a result of stretching or compression of nerves. Weakness in the distribution of the compressed nerve roots may develop, and, if severe, muscle fasciculations and focal atrophy can ensue.

When tumors involve the cord directly, unilateral or bilateral spastic paralysis and sensory dysfunction are usually demonstrable below the level of the lesion. Disturbances of bladder function may develop, depending on the level of cord compression. When the lesion is above the sacral segment, a constricted, small, spastic bladder develops; with involvement at the level of the sacral outflow pathways the bladder wall tends to become flaccid, resulting in overfilling and overflow dribbling of urine. Constipation or fecal incontinence may occur. Intramedullary cord tumors often produce dissociated sensory changes such as loss of temperature sensation with intact pain and touch.

Diagnostic evaluation. Radiographs of the spine are abnormal in a high percentage of spinal cord tumors. There may be widening of the spinal canal or erosion of the posterior surfaces of the vertebral bodies at the level of the tumor. Scoliosis may develop, and thinning or absence of one of the pedicles and lamina may be seen radiographically. Vertebral tumors can produce erosion of the bodies of the involved vertebrae and destruction of the intervertebral discs. A spinal tap should not be done when a spinal cord tumor is suspected, except as a preoperative study in which manometrics and isophendylate (Pantopaque) myelography are done to localize the tumor. Examination of spinal fluid obtained under these circumstances usually reveals xanthochromia, mononuclear pleocytosis, and significantly elevated levels of protein, particularly when there is obstruction to the flow of the cerebrospinal fluid.

Management. Treatment of spinal cord tumors depends on location and type of tumor. Any tumor progressively impairing spinal cord function requires surgery. If the tumor is an intramedullary inoperable glioma, decompressive laminectomy will help preserve the remaining cord function for a time; in cases in which the tumor is resectable, recovery may be complete and lasting. Chemotherapy and irradiation are potentially beneficial, depending on the tumor type.

CRANIOCEREBRAL TRAUMA

Head trauma is common in childhood, particularly among boys from 2 to 10 years of age. There are many causes, but most are deceleration injuries from falls or automobile accidents. Head injuries can also occur when a moving object (e.g., a ball or stone) strikes the head, but this is less common and usually better tolerated. It is important to consider all the intracranial structures when diagnosing head trauma, since the primary brain injury usually results from compression of the relatively soft brain against the tough dura (falx or tentorium) or the skull table and bony protuberances that characterize the intracranial compartment. This accounts for contusion to the surface of the brain at the site of injury or on the opposite side (contrecoup). Movement of the brain against these structures may also cause laceration and sometimes hematoma formation.

Cerebral concussion

Cerebral concussion occurs commonly in children following blunt trauma to the head. It is characterized by transient alteration of consciousness followed by a period of amnesia that may be difficult to define accurately in children. When seen later, the diagnosis is frequently uncertain, especially if the patient is asymptomatic. When there are signs of scalp laceration, swelling or contusion, confusion, and gross memory impairment, the diagnosis of amnesia is more certain. The child may appear pale, flushed, or diaphoretic and complain of headache, nausea, or vomiting. Recovery is spontaneous, usually within a few hours, although headache and mild confusion may persist for several days.

A careful neurologic examination should be performed to exclude signs of focal neurologic dysfunction or raised intracranial pressure. The optic fundi, pupils, pulse, blood pressure, and level of consciousness should be carefully evaluated. A complete blood count including hematocrit is important to rule out significant intracranial bleeding. Skull radiographs are indicated whenever there is a history of significant head trauma, focal neurologic dysfunction, or altered consciousness. This should include cervical spine films if the trauma was severe, or whenever there is pain or limitation of movement about the neck. Lumbar puncture should not be done unless there is clinical suspicion of meningitis. A history of head trauma is obtained quite commonly in patients with bacterial meningitis, but its role in the pathogenesis of the infection is probably unrelated in most instances.

Management of cerebral concussion consists of careful evaluation and observation until symptoms subside. This can be done at home, although significant concussive injuries usually require observation in the hospital for 24 to 48 hours. Mild analgesics can be given for headache, but sedatives should be avoided. During the period of observation the patient should be roused periodically for evaluation of level of consciousness, pupillary reactions, and gross motor function.

Skull fractures

A skull fracture is an important sign of recent head trauma. However, a simple linear fracture does not correlate with the severity of the trauma or the presence of underlying brain injury. In fact, a major cerebral injury can occur without any detectable skull fracture or external evidence of injury to the face or scalp. Compound fractures, on the other hand, are usually suspected clinically because of swelling, scalp laceration, and bony depression at the site of trauma.

Whenever a skull fracture is discovered, complications such as cervical spine injury or leakage of cerebrospinal fluid should be searched for carefully. The latter is a sign of basilar skull fracture that may not be demonstrable on radiographs. It requires prompt diagnosis and therapy to prevent meningitis. Both rhinorrhea and otorrhea require proper positioning and prophylactic antibiotics; surgery is sometimes indicated, especially for rhinorrhea that does not subside under conservative management.

Patients with linear skull fractures or significant blunt head trauma without fracture should be observed for a few days, either at home or in hospital, for complications secondary to intracranial bleeding. Depressed or compound fractures require immediate surgical treatment. Whenever fractures are unusually severe for the type of injury described, the examiner should consider child abuse and initiate appropriate investigation.

Major cerebral trauma (contusion, laceration, edema, and intracerebral hematoma)

Cerebral contusion is a bruise to the brain surface that occurs either directly below the site of trauma or on the surface of the opposite hemisphere (contrecoup). Laceration of the brain surface may occur as a result of compound skull fracture in which the bony fragments penetrate the dura and injure the surface of the brain. Compression of the brain against the falx or tentorium may also cause a laceration. This type of injury may be difficult to distinguish from other forms of major cerebral trauma, including severe concussion, edema, or intracerebral hematoma. Such severe brain injuries are frequently accompanied by shock, pallor, and sweating. Lethargy, stupor, convulsions, paresis, and signs of raised intracranial pressure also occur.

Investigation should include radiographs of the skull and spine and CT scan when focal neurologic signs are discovered or significant intracranial pressure elevation develops. Invasive diagnostic studies (arteriography, ventriculography) are rarely indicated. Lumbar puncture should not be done when intracranial pressure is elevated because of the risk of herniation. Significant intracranial bleeding can be detected early by serial hematocrit determination.

Treatment is directed at preventing complications from raised intracranial pressure, coma, or bleeding. Antipyretics should be given and cooling blankets used when hyperpyrexia develops, because this contributes to brain swelling. Corticosteroids (prednisone, 2 mg/kg/24 hr) are sometimes used to combat brain swelling, although their effectiveness is unproven. Mannitol (1 or 2 g/kg) will temporarily reduce life-threatening intracranial pressure, but under these circumstances the prognosis is grim and not significantly affected by this form of therapy. Some patients are now being treated with barbiturate anesthesia and hypothermia during the period of maximal brain swelling following head trauma. This requires continued intensive care by a team trained to manage critically ill patients in coma for several days to a few weeks.

Extracerebral (subdural and epidural) hematoma

Differentiation between a subdural and epidural hematoma is frequently difficult in children. Both may develop rapidly or gradually over days following an apparently incidental minor head injury. The reason for this is that subdural hematomas following a laceration to the dural sinuses will form rapidly, whereas those resulting from seepage from small bridging veins will evolve more slowly. An epidural hematoma following rupture to the middle meningeal artery is usually acute, whereas one resulting from injury to smaller vessels may present more gradually.

Signs and symptoms of an extracerebral hematoma are secondary to raised intracranial pressure and, to a lesser extent, the focal mass effect. Headache, irritability, lethargy, vomiting, and ataxia are often mild initially, but as pressure increases these symptoms worsen. In a smaller infant, a bulging fontanel, retinal hemorrhages, and separation of the sutures are obvious signs of raised intracranial pressure. Seizures and anemia are other signs of an extracerebral hematoma, particularly in a small infant.

Diagnosis is based on careful history and examination. In young infants an increasing cranial circumference and diminished transillumination may be seen with extracerebral bleeding. Skull radiographs may show a fracture or suture separation indicative of increased intracranial pressure. Fracture of the temporal bone overlying the middle meningeal artery or presence of a compound fracture should alert the examiner to the possibility of an extracerebral hematoma. Radioisotope scanning and CT are both valuable procedures to investigate the possibility of a subdural or epidural hematoma. Neurosurgical consultation should be requested early in the evaluation of any child with raised intracranial pressure following trauma. Subdural taps are done in infants with open sutures and increased transillumination, but these should be done only after consultation with a surgeon because proper drainage may require burr holes or craniotomy.

Although an extracerebral hematoma is a curable lesion if the diagnosis is made early, it still accounts for significant morbidity and mortality in pediatric medicine. Patients who arrive at the hospital with signs of herniation represent a failure of medical management. It is important to emphasize that head trauma is a problem for the pediatrician to understand and manage intelligently. Only a small percentage of cases have a complication requiring surgical therapy. A significant percentage of children (10% to 20%) who have had serious head injuries are left with major neurologic sequelae, including seizures, motor disabilities, and especially learning and behavioral problems. For this reason pediatricians must become child advocates by advising parents as well as local pediatricians how to prevent head injury (helmets, seat belts, proper sports attire, etc.). Pediatricians must also learn

incoordination are associated features. Without treatment patients are often totally incapacitated within 5 to 7 years, although there are exceptional patients who remain stable for a number of years. Neurosurgical intervention has been beneficial in some cases and deserves serious consideration for any patient with rapidly progressive disease, particularly if it is primarily unilateral.

Jewell C. Ward
John F. Griffith

SEIZURE DISORDERS

Epilepsy is the word used to describe a state of chronic, recurrent seizures. *Convulsive disorder, seizure disorder,* and *recurrent cerebral seizures* are synonymous terms in common usage.

A seizure is a sign of disordered brain function. At the cellular level a seizure begins with depolarization of the neuronal membrane. When this spreads to involve adjacent nerve cells, an excessive discharge results that either stimulates or inhibits a number of body functions controlled by these neurons. There are many disease states that are associated with seizure. Some of these are progressive disorders; others are static yet result in repetitive seizures that are often difficult to control.

It is estimated that 3% of children experience at least one seizure during their early years. The majority are benign, self-limited convulsions associated with fever. Regardless of the suspected cause, the first seizure should be carefully evaluated in the hospital to exclude a serious and potentially remedial underlying brain disease.

Classification of these disorders is difficult. The International Classification of Seizures (box, p. 806) is a help because it defines seizure types based primarily on clinical expression and presumed site of origin.

Partial seizures

Partial seizures with elementary symptomatology. The classic jacksonian seizure begins with a discharging focus in a discrete area of the motor cortex that spreads to involve contiguous neurons. It often begins with twitching of the mouth or eyes, followed by involvement of the face, arm, trunk, or leg muscles. The other side of the body may be affected as the seizure becomes more generalized. Todd's postictal paralysis sometimes follows the seizure.

Focal sensory seizures are characterized by paresthesias, numbness, tingling, prickling, or pain sensations originating in the extremities or the face and spreading to other parts of the body. This is similar to the jacksonian march, originating in the parietal sensory cortex. A compound form involving motor components can also occur. Frequently in young children the full description of the sensation during seizures is not appreciated. Instead the child will express fear or anxiety by running to a parent. The sensory symptoms may be visual, auditory, olfactory, vertiginous, or abdominal. Visual sensations, such as flashing colored lights in a kaleidoscope array, usually arise from the occipital cortex and may remain localized to the contralateral visual field. Formed images usually indicate discharges from the posterior-temporal region.

Many focal seizures are accompanied by disturbances of the autonomic nervous system. The patient may manifest pallor or flushing, changes in heart rate, and alterations in gastric motility with occasional nausea and vomiting. These seizures are most often associated with electrical discharges in the frontotemporal cortex or in the insula.

Partial seizures with complex symptomatology (complex partial seizures). Partial seizures with complex symptomatology were formerly called *temporal lobe* or *psychomotor* seizures. During the seizure, automatisms or automatic activity may be evident. The majority of automatisms consist of confused, repetitive, purposeless behavior during which the patient has limited awareness and no memory of the activity following the seizure. It has been estimated that 10% to 20% of children in most pediatric seizure clinics have complex partial seizures. These seizures may be caused by focal lesions, but most occur as a result of diffuse cerebral disease. Space-occupying lesions, including neoplasms, vascular formations, porencephalic cysts, and abscesses, occasionally account for this type of seizure. Since the diseased tissue is not necessarily confined to the temporal lobe, the term *temporal lobe seizures* should be avoided.

The child rarely describes the unusual distorted sensory perceptions, such as macropsia or micropsia, that adults report with this type of seizure. Neither olfactory nor gustatory hallucinations are usually reported by children.

INTERNATIONAL CLASSIFICATION OF SEIZURES

The International Classification of Epileptic Seizures is now accepted, even though the old nomenclature continues to be used. The new terms describe the clinical phenomena better than old terms such as *grand mal, petit mal, Jacksonian,* and *temporal lobe epilepsies*. The following outline of the new classification is a useful and simple method to diagnose and manage convulsive disorders based on clinical and electroencephalographic features.

- A. Partial seizures (seizures beginning locally)
  1. Partial seizures with elementary symptomatology (generally without impairment of consciousness)
     - a. With motor symptoms (includes jacksonian seizures)
     - b. With special sensory or somatosensory symptoms
     - c. With autonomic symptoms
     - d. Compound forms
  2. Partial seizures with complex symptomatology (temporal lobe or psychomotor seizures) (generally with impairment of consciousness)
     - a. With impairment of consciousness only
     - b. With cognitive symptomatology
     - c. With affective symptomatology
     - d. With psychosensory symptomatology
     - e. With psychomotor symptomatology (automatisms)
     - f. Compound forms
  3. Partial seizures secondarily generalized.
- B. Generalized seizures (bilaterally symmetric and without local onset)
  1. Absences (petit mal)
  2. Bilateral massive epileptic myoclonus
  3. Infantile spasms
  4. Clonic seizures
  5. Tonic seizures
  6. Tonic-clonic seizures (grand mal)
  7. Atonic seizures
  8. Akinetic seizures
- C. Unilateral seizures (or predominantly)
- D. Unclassified epileptic seizures (because of incomplete data)

There are two main types of seizures, partial and generalized. Partial or focal seizures arise from a circumscribed area of the cerebral cortex. They are divided into two main groups, one with elementary symptomatology without impairment of consciousness, and the other with complex symptomatology, usually with altered consciousness. Generalized seizures result from a widespread, diffuse discharge, originating in the central portions of the brain and projecting to the cortex and brain stem structures.

From Gastaut, H.: Clinical and electroencephalographic classification of epileptic seizures, Epilepsia (Amsterdam) **11:**102-113, 1970.

Complex motor movements or automatisms such as lip smacking, body rubbing, sucking, swallowing, chewing, walking, or running in circles are occasionally seen. The speech is often unintelligible mumbling. Autonomic vasomotor disturbances including salivation, vomiting, flushing, or pallor may also occur. Postictal phenomena include headache, lethargy, vomiting, hunger, thirst, or impaired speech, and focal or generalized paresis may be fleeting or may last for hours.

Generalized seizures

Absence (petit mal) seizures. Absence seizures are brief episodes characterized by staring or repetitive blinking for 5 to 30 seconds. They usually are seen in children between 5 and 12 years.

Absence attacks may also be associated with motor manifestations such as eye blinking, lip smacking, and mouth twitching. Postural tone may be increased or diminished, resulting in a sudden loss of balance and fall. Sudden pallor or changes in pupillary size are additional clinical features that sometimes make it difficult to distinguish absence attacks from complex partial seizures.

When absence attacks last for prolonged periods, the term *petit mal status* or *absence continuing* is used. An absence attack can be precipitated by hyperventilation. The attack is associated with paroxysmal generalized 3-second spike-and-wave discharges on the EEG. When the lapses are frequent, the child may appear to be daydreaming and perform poorly at school. These seizures may be completely controlled with anticonvulsant medication, although occasionally they are refractive to all therapy. Absence status does not appear to have any prognostic implication and can usually be treated effectively by intravenous diazepam followed by oral administration of ethosuximide, valproic acid, or both.

The two most effective drugs for the prevention of absence attacks are ethosuximide and valproic (Table 29-5). The latter is indicated when the child also has generalized tonic-clonic seizures. Clonazepam may be effective in controlling absence seizures, particularly those associated with myoclonus.

Prognosis for remission is favorable when onset of absence is between 5 and 9 years of age and not associated with intellectual dysfunction or other seizure types.

Generalized tonic-clonic (grand mal) seizures. The attack begins with a violent tonic contraction of all the body muscles and upward rolling of the eyes. There may be a cry caused by forced expiration of air from the lungs. The tongue is frequently bitten, and fecal and urinary incontinence may occur. The heart rate and blood pressure increase, and there is often excessive salivation with foaming. The tonic phase is followed by a clonic state, during which the trunk and limbs jerk violently. This is followed by gradual relaxation, during which the patient slowly regains consciousness. The patient may be confused and somnolent for a few hours. Mental retardation, behavioral disorders, learning difficulties, or motor deficits are less frequent in children whose generalized convulsions begin after 4 years of age.

The interictal EEG pattern may be completely normal or slightly slow for age. In some children there is a frontal or temporal cortical spike focus from which secondary centrencephalic discharges arise and spread to produce a generalized discharge.

Infantile spasms (infantile myoclonus). Infantile spasms are a type of convulsion that usually begins between 6 months and 3 years of age. It consists of sudden, brief, symmetric flexion of the head or trunk along with mild clonus of arms and legs. The eyes may roll upward or inward. In some patients there is sudden extension of the head and trunk, while the limbs are flexed or extended. These single, shocklike contractions also may occur in clusters many times daily without postictal drowsiness or sleep.

Anoxic and mechanical brain injury during the perinatal period are the commonest causes of infantile spasms. Perinatal infections and metabolic disorders, including hypoglycemia, cerebral lipodoses, or aminoacidurias, may also result in this type of seizure. Frequently there is no obvious underlying disease. The idiopathic variety occurs in infants who are developing normally; despite early diagnosis and treatment a high percentage of these patients are left with permanent psychomotor retardation.

The EEG abnormality seen in many of these patients is termed *hypsarrhythmia*. It consists of irregular, high-voltage, slow waves and spikes from both cerebral hemispheres.

Cranial computerized tomography will usually not define the underlying cerebral disorder. It should be done, however, whenever the etiology is obscure, because cerebral atrophy, agenesis of the corpus callosum, calcified nodules characteristic of tuberous sclerosis, and porencephaly have been associated with infantile spasms.

Drug treatment with adrenocorticosteroids (prednisone) or adrenocorticotropic hormone (corticotropin) frequently results in partial or complete seizure control and improvement in the EEG abnormalities. However, delayed psychomotor development is present in the majority of patients, despite steroid therapy.

Myoclonic epilepsy of older children. Myoclonic epilepsy generally consists of sudden forward jerking of the head with an associated outward movement of both arms. When the child is standing, the seizure consists of sudden head nodding with simultaneous extension of the up-

Table 29-5. Anticonvulsant drug therapy

Drug	Indications	Dosage (mg/kg/ day)	Therapeutic blood level (mg/ml)	Time to reach steady state (days)	Side-effects*
Phenobarbital	†Neonatal seizures †Febrile seizures Tonic-clonic seizures Simple and complex partial seizures	3-5	15-40	10-18	A, D, H, R
Primidone (mysoline)	†Complex partial seizures Tonic-clonic seizures	15-25	8-15	2-3	A, D, L, R
Phenytoin (Dilantin)	†Tonic-clonic seizures †Simple and complex partial seizures	5-8	10-20	5-7	A, D, R Gum hyperplasia, lupus, nystagmus, hepatitis, megaloblastic anemia, and hirsutism
Ethotoin (Peganone)	Same as phenytoin	50-60	—	—	Same as phenytoin but does not cause gum hypertrophy
Valproic acid (Depakene)	†Absence seizures Myoclonic seizures Atonic seizures Akinetic seizures Infantile spasms	30-60	50-100	2-3	A, D, N & V Hepatotoxicity and thrombocytopenia
Ethosuximide (Zarontin)	†Absence seizures Atonic seizures Akinetic seizures	20-25	40-100	2-5	A, D, N & V, R
Carbamazepine (Tegretol)	†Complex partial seizures Tonic-clonic seizures Simple partial seizures	15-25	6-12	4	A, D, L, N & V, R Bone marrow suppression and hepatotoxicity
Clonazepam (Clonopin)	Absence seizures Akinetic seizures Myoclonic seizures Infantile spasms	0.02-0.2	0.02-0.05	4	A, D, L, N & V, R Hepatitis
Mephobarbital (Mebaral)	Substitute for phenobarbital in child with hyperactivity (?)	8-10	—	—	Same as phenobarbital
Acetazolamide (Diamox)	Myoclonic seizures Absence seizures †Catamenial seizures	15-30	10-75	—	Dehydration, acidosis, agranulocytosis, and thrombocytopenia
Corticotropin	†Infantile spasms	40-80 units intramuscularly	—	—	Complications associated with all steroid preparations, e.g., Cushingoid state, growth suppression, peptic ulcer, and fluid retention.
Prednisone	†Infantile spasms	2	—	—	

*A, Ataxia; D, drowsiness; H, hyperactivity; L, leukopenia, N & V, nausea and vomiting; R, rash.
†Drugs of choice.

per extremities. This may cause a forward fall, resulting in facial injury if the child is not wearing a protective helmet. The attacks last only a few seconds, but may be associated with more prolonged generalized seizure activity. The EEG of patients with myoclonic epilepsy reveals bursts of irregular spikes and high voltage slow waves, often superimposed on a disorganized background.

Neonatal seizures. Seizures in neonates differ significantly from those occurring in older infants and children. The expression of seizure originating in the immature nervous system is often fragmentary and poorly organized. Clinical varieties include subtle, multifocal clonic seizures, myoclonic jerks, focal clonic seizures, or tonic seizures. Subtle seizures may consist only of brief apneic episodes with circumoral cyanosis, or the seizure may be more obvious and result in deviation of the eyes, posturing or tremor of a limb, chewing, sucking, or excessive drooling. Subtle seizures may also be suggested by a history of choking spells during feedings, a changing respiratory pattern, or any unexplained change in behavior that is repetitious.

Focal clonic seizures in this age group usually begin with either twitching of the facial muscles or one of the limbs, with subsequent spread to involve other ipsilateral structures. The baby usually remains conscious. Hemiconvulsions with accompanying adversive movements of the head and eyes are rare in the newborn period. A more common seizure in early infancy is the multifocal clonic type in which the clonic movements migrate from one limb to another in an irregular manner. Generalized tonic seizures with opisthotonic posturing and focal tonic spasms may also be seen in newborns.

Myoclonic jerks consist of sudden involuntary contraction of the muscles of the trunk or extremities. These must be differentiated from jitteriness that occurs normally in newborn infants and in drug withdrawal states. Jitteriness is not associated with abnormal eye movements.

Following is an outline of possible etiologic factors responsible for neonatal seizures.

A. Mechanical and hypoxic birth injury
B. Metabolic disturbances
   1. Hypocalcemia
   2. Hypoglycemia
   3. Hypomagnesemia
   4. Hypernatremia
   5. Pyridoxine dependency or deficiency
C. Central nervous system infection
D. Congenital cerebral malformation
E. Drug withdrawal
F. Miscellaneous

Febrile seizures. A critical effort should be made to differentiate the simple form of febrile seizure from epileptic seizures that may occur with fever. Some consider febrile seizures to be all seizures occurring during the first few years of life associated with fever, except those secondary to central nervous system infection. This would include patients with an underlying seizure disorder who will later develop recurrent afebrile seizures (i.e., epilepsy). Some of these patients may have structural brain lesions with associated neurologic dysfunction to account for their seizures; others may have unusually severe, prolonged, recurrent, or focal seizures associated with interictal EEG abnormalities.

There is now a practical schema for classifying and managing this problem. A febrile seizure is currently defined as one occurring between the ages of 3 months and 5 years, associated with fever but without evidence of intracranial infection or other defined cause. Risk of recurrence following the first seizure in children who are untreated is 30% to 40%. The risk of developing subsequent nonfebrile seizures is insignificant, unless at least 2 of 3 high-risk factors are present. These are (1) family history of nonfebrile seizures, (2) abnormal neurologic or developmental status before the first seizure, and (3) an atypical febrile seizure that is exceptionally prolonged or has focal features. If none of these are present, the risk of developing nonfebrile seizures is only 2% to 3%, which is not significantly more than the risk in the population at large. The latter group requires no therapy unless the seizures recur because therapy does not change the prognosis, although it does reduce the number of seizures during the period of treatment. When high-risk factors are identified, treatment with phenobarbital is indicated for at least 2 years in dosages adequate to maintain a minimum therapeutic blood level of 15 μg/ml. There is no place for sporadic anticonvulsant administration at time of fever because a therapeutic drug level cannot be achieved by episodic oral administration.

Other age-related seizures. In addition to febrile seizures, neonatal seizures, infantile spasm, and absence attacks, there are other age-

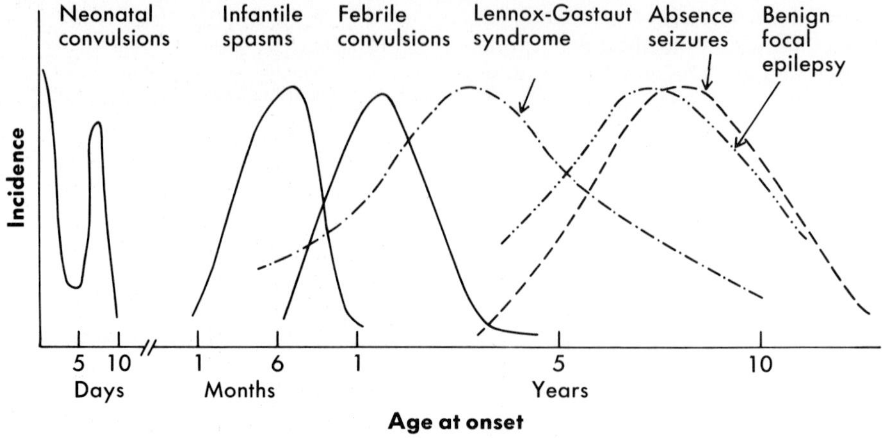

Fig. 29-1. Age-related seizures.

related seizures. Some are associated with well known clinical syndromes (Fig. 29-1).

Lennox-Gastaut syndrome. Lennox-Gastaut syndrome usually begins in infancy or early childhood with myoclonic, generalized tonic-clonic, akinetic, or atonic seizures that are poorly responsive to anticonvulsant treatment. Some of these children have a history of previous infantile spasms. There are a number of predisposing causes, including perinatal hypoxia, intrauterine infections, developmental brain anomalies, aminoacidopathies, and head trauma; often an etiology is not defined. The EEG characteristically shows multifocal or generalized slow spike and waves (2 to 12.5 complexes/second). The majority of patients have impaired intellectual development.

Benign focal seizures (sylvian seizures). Sylvian seizures are a benign form of epilepsy occurring between 4 and 10 years of age. Seizures are usually infrequent and consist of orofacial numbness, jerky facial movements, speech arrest, drooling, and mild tonic or clonic movements of one of the upper limbs. The typical EEG shows repetitive midtemporal central spikes, often activated by sleep. Most children with sylvian seizures are neurologically normal. In 75% of patients these attacks spontaneously subside within 5 years. There appears to be a tendency toward remission of seizures with or without anticonvulsant therapy.

Diagnostic evaluation of seizure disorders

A careful history is essential to determine the type of seizure, as well as possible precipitating factors. Fever, infection, falls, injuries to the head, anxiety, fatigue, and puberty may all be precipitating factors in onset of seizures. It is also important to define duration of the seizure, its pattern of progression, and all postictal phenomena such as confusion, hemiparesis, aphasia, amnesia, headache, or sleep. Clinical response to anticonvulsant medication and degree of compliance to the drug regimen should also be determined by history.

Laboratory studies should include a complete blood count and urinalysis. Aminoacid screening of urine and blood should be done whenever a metabolic disorder is suspected, particularly in infants who have seizures and lethargy.

Serum calcium, glucose, blood urea nitrogen, phosphorus, sodium, potassium, and magnesium should be determined for any patient after the first seizure if the etiology is not obvious. Similarly, the cerebrospinal fluid should be examined, primarily to exclude infection, although hypoglycemia and degenerative nervous system disease may also be associated with abnormal spinal fluid findings.

Radiographs of the skull are an essential part of the investigation of any patient with epilepsy of recent onset. Skull asymmetry, separation of sutures, calcification, or changes in thickness of the calvarium suggest an underlying brain disorder. Intracranial calcifications are seen with intrauterine infection, arteriovenous malformations, cerebral tumors, tuberous sclerosis, or Sturge-Weber disease. Occasionally, an old calcified tuberculoma may be found on skull radiographs.

The EEG is a safe, noninvasive procedure that can be used to confirm the clinical diagnosis of a seizure disorder and to classify the seizure type. An abnormal interictal EEG usually implies a serious prognosis, although normal interictal tracings can occur in patients with seizures that are poorly controlled. EEGs obtained during sleep have proved useful and are now a standard part of the investigation of any patient suspected of having seizures.

CT has revolutionized the approach to the evaluation of patients suspected of having an intracranial mass or cerebral anomaly. It has been estimated that one third of patients with chronic epilepsies will demonstrate a definite abnormality on CT scan. Generalized atrophy, hydrocephalus, porencephaly, focal atrophy, mass lesions, and calcium deposits may be detected by this procedure. This noninvasive technique has replaced angiography and pneumography as the procedure of choice for the workup of a child with a complicated seizure disorder.

Management of seizure disorders in children

Comprehensive management of a child with a convulsive disorder includes careful selection of appropriate anticonvulsant medication, evaluation of educational potential, and management of the psychologic problems that frequently complicate chronic nervous system disorders. Family members should be knowledgeable about the problem, including the side effects of drugs and the long-term treatment plan. This helps achieve better patient cooperation and understanding.

Anticonvulsant drug therapy. Treatment should be started as soon as it is clear that the seizures are recurrent. This will vary with the patient's age, type of seizure, and certainty of the diagnosis. A single drug is begun initially and increased to a maximum tolerated dosage before a second anticonvulsant is added (Table 29-5). In most children a single anticonvulsant is usually sufficient to control the seizures. Initial dosage is based on a milligram per kilogram per 24 hour formula, and is given one or more times per day, depending on the drug being administered. Drugs that are rapidly absorbed may cause toxic side effects related to intermittent peak serum concentrations. This effect is most troublesome when using drugs that require frequent administration because of a short half-life. As shown in the table, this problem may be encountered in patients receiving diphenylhydantoin, valproate, or carbamazepine. Smaller and more frequent drug doses are suggested for these anticonvulsants. Liquid medication is usually preferred for children less than 2 years of age, with tablets or capsules available for older children. Choice of drug to initiate therapy is determined by type of clinical seizure and EEG pattern. Phenobarbital is preferred over phenytoin (Dilantin) in young girls, since the latter may cause hirsutism and gingival hypertrophy.

Anticonvulsants are usually ineffective unless therapeutic blood concentrations are attained. If the seizures are not controlled by one drug, a second is usually added. The combination chosen is often empiric, but the type of seizure influences the selection in some instances. In patients who respond poorly to treatment it is usually necessary to try a number of drugs, using serum anticonvulsant levels as a guide to determine the most effective drug combination.

Ketogenic diet. A ketogenic diet is effective therapy for certain seizures that are not controlled by conventional anticonvulsant therapy. The mechanism of its action is unclear, although sustained ketosis appears to correlate with seizure control.

Children under 5 years of age are given a 3:1 ketogenic diet; those over 5 years are placed on a 4:1 ketogenic diet. The ratio refers to the fat-to-nonfat proportions by weight. While the child is on the diet, concentrations of ketones in the afternoon urine should remain in the moderate-to-high range. This can be checked routinely in the home. Substituting fatty foods with the more palatable medium-chain triglycerides may be necessary in some children.

On this diet the patient should receive 10,000 IU of vitamin D each week. Transient gastrointestinal disturbances such as nausea and vomiting may occur. A small amount of orange juice may help the gastrointestinal upset. During intercurrent febrile illnesses the child may require hospitalization and treatment with intravenous fluids. Acetazolamide (Diamox) should be discontinued while the patient is on a ketogenic diet to prevent the occurrence of severe metabolic acidosis. Hypoglycemia develops in most patients during the first few days after initiation of the ketogenic diet, but it is usually asymptomatic.

Surgical treatment. Various surgical procedures have been tried for the treatment of intractable epilepsy.

Cortical resection of the epileptic focus is the usual procedure. The operation should be carried out by an experienced neurosurgeon using electrocorticography to map the boundaries of the epileptic focus. In the immediate postoperative period there may be increased seizure frequency, but after 1 or 2 weeks the patient usually begins to improve and the requirement for anticonvulsants is reduced.

Use of serum anticonvulsant level. One of the recent major advances in management of seizure disorders is availability of methods for rapid determination of anticonvulsant blood levels. The enzyme-multiplied immunoassay technique (EMIT) provides an affordable and simple method for this, although gas-liquid chromatography and radioimmunoassay are also excellent methods. Dosage schedule of anticonvulsants can now be adjusted to maintain serum drug levels within the therapeutic range. This provides a means of checking patient compliance and provides insights into drug metabolism. Marked variability occurs in the metabolism of these compounds in normal individuals, particularly in young infants who may have variable absorption and excretion of the drug. Blood levels of a particular anticonvulsant should be determined whenever seizures are uncontrolled on therapy, drug toxicity is suspected, or changes in drug treatment are planned.

Status epilepticus

Status epilepticus is a state of continuous seizure activity. Clinically, this includes either a very prolonged single seizure (greater than 20 minutes) or repetitive seizures between which the patient fails to regain consciousness. Convulsive status epilepticus is a serious problem because it is associated with major morbidity and mortality if it persists longer than 1 hour. This is a medical emergency requiring prompt therapy. A proper airway must be ensured, oxygen administered, blood pressure supported, and intracranial pressure controlled regardless of the underlying cause of the seizures. Choice of anticonvulsants to control status epilepticus is not as important as knowing how much to administer and the potential complications of therapy. Phenobarbital and phenytoin (Dilantin) are given in combination in many centers, since these are reliable agents to control seizures when prescribed correctly. The following is a treatment regimen that has been used successfully to treat status epilepticus for a number of years.

1. Support blood pressure, respirations, and cardiac function
2. Reduce significant raised intracranial pressure
3. a. Phenobarbital: 5 to 10 mg/kg intravenously initially; repeated every 2 to 6 hours; maximum total dose 20 to 30 mg/kg/24 hr.
   b. Phenytoin (Dilantin): 5 to 10 mg/kg intravenously slowly; repeated every 2 to 6 hours; maximum total dose 20 to 30 mg/kg/24 hr
   c. Diazepam (Valium): 0.25 mg/kg intravenously in 2 minutes initially (not in combination with phenobarbital)
   d. Paraldehyde: 0.3 to 0.4 ml/kg/rectally; useful as supplemental therapy when seizures recur despite above drug regimens

Diazepam (Valium) is a good agent to arrest status epilepticus, but should not be used in combination with phenobarbital because of the risk of hypotension and respiratory depression. If it is used, phenytoin should be added to minimize the risk of subsequent seizures following the period of status epilepticus.

Paraldehyde mixed with vegetable or mineral oil and given rectally is both safe and rapid. However, it is a sclerosing solution that can cause mucosal irritation in young infants. Because it is excreted by the lungs, paraldehyde should not be administered in patients with pulmonary disease.

Occasionally general anesthesia is required to arrest status epilepticus refractive to the preceding measures.

John F. Griffith
Lawrence T. Ch'ien

NEUROMUSCULAR DISEASES

This section concerns diseases affecting (1) the anterior horn cell, (2) the peripheral nerve (neuropathies), (3) the neuromuscular junction (myasthenia gravis), and (4) the muscle (myopathies). To localize these processes and establish an accurate diagnosis, it is essential to know the symptoms, signs, and laboratory findings that accompany these diseases.

Symptoms and signs in neuromuscular disease

Weakness and atrophy. The most important and frequent symptom among patients suffering from neuromuscular diseases is weakness and subsequent wasting or atrophy of muscles. Characteristically, weakness is more proximal in the myopathies and is usually symmetrical, whereas in peripheral neuropathies, it is usually distal and symmetrical, with muscle wasting in distal arms and legs. In some neuropathies, however, multiple nerves are affected individually and in a somewhat random manner (mononeuritis multiplex). In the infantile form of spinal muscular atrophy (Werdnig-Hoffmann disease) weakness is typically generalized. In the juvenile form (Kugelberg-Welander disease) weakness is predominantly proximal.

Fasciculations. A fasciculation results from spontaneous activation of one motor unit and contraction of its muscle fibers (a motor unit is formed by one anterior horn neuron, its axon, and all the muscle fibers innervated by that neuron). Fasciculations are observable through the skin as a small muscle twitch. These can occasionally be seen in normal people, especially those under stress, but, when fasciculations are accompanied by weakness and atrophy, motor neuron disease is likely. Fasciculations can also be seen in peripheral neuropathies and radiculopathies. Tongue fasciculations are typically seen in Werdnig-Hoffmann disease.

Cramps. A cramp is a muscle contraction produced by firing of many motor units spontaneously. It is often referred to as a "charley horse" and is seen most often in patients with disease of the anterior horn cell or peripheral nerve. In muscle phosphorylase deficiency (McArdle disease), contraction of the muscle without electrical activity is seen after exercise, and therefore is not a real cramp.

Hyporeflexia. Deep tendon reflexes are decreased or absent early in peripheral neuropathies, especially distal reflexes. In myopathies, reflexes are affected later. Distribution of hyporeflexia in anterior horn cell diseases corresponds to distribution of weakness. In Werdnig-Hoffmann disease, reflexes are usually depressed.

Hypotonia. Hypotonia or lack of normal resistance to passive movements of the muscle is frequently seen, accompanied by weakness, in many of the diseases affecting the motor unit. When present in the newborn, hypotonia gives rise to the floppy infant syndrome. Hypotonia is also a prominent clinical feature of other diseases that do not affect motor units, such as Down syndrome and congenital abnormalities of the brain. Neuromuscular diseases that may manifest as the floppy infant syndrome include infantile spinal muscular atrophy (Werdnig-Hoffmann disease); congenital neuropathies; neonatal and congenital myasthenia gravis; infantile botulism; Pompe disease (acid maltase deficiency); and the so-called congenital myopathies, including central core disease, rod (nemaline) disease, myotubular myopathy (type I hypotrophy with central nuclei), and others.

Myotonia. Myotonia refers to a clinical phenomenon characterized by slow relaxation of muscle after a contraction. Myotonia is usually worse in cold environments. The patient refers to it as muscle stiffness, rigidity, and even sometimes weakness that improved after warming up. It is characteristically found in some myopathies such as myotonic dystrophy, myotonia congenita, and hyperkalemic periodic paralysis.

Sensory deficit. Symmetrically decreased distal sensation is present in most neuropathies. In some the presentation can be asymmetric. Sensory loss is seldom a complaint in children, but may be detected during physical examination. Sensory deficits may be accompanied by ulcer formation and inadvertent burning resulting from lack of sensitivity to pain or temperature. In the rare condition of familial dysautonomia, it is accompanied by lack of lacrimation and salivation.

Myoglobinuria. Myoglobinuria, or presence of myoglobin in the urine, may appear after muscle destruction, producing a characteristic dark red urine that should be differentiated from hemoglobin. Causes of myoglobinuria include trauma, toxins, and some myopathies such as McArdle disease, muscle phosphofructokinase deficiency, carnitine-palmityl transferase deficiency, malignant hyperthermia, and, in children, influenza myositis.

Neuromuscular diseases, particularly those that are hereditary, may be associated with skeletal deformities such as high arched feet (pes cavus), hammer toes, scoliosis, and kyphoscoliosis. Cardiac anomalies may occur in some neuromuscular diseases, as in Friedreich ataxia, myotonic dystrophy, and Duchenne muscular dystrophy.

Diagnostic tools in neuromuscular diseases

A variety of diagnostic tests and procedures are useful in the differential diagnosis of neuromuscular disorders.

Measurement of serum enzymes. Creatine kinase (CK), aldolase, SGOT, and SGPT are elevated in some myopathies, especially in dystrophies, polymyositis, and metabolic myopathies.

Nerve conduction studies. Measurement of the time it takes an electrical impulse to travel a segment of a nerve is used to calculate conduction velocity. Nerve conduction velocities are often slowed in peripheral neuropathies, particularly in demyelinating neuropathies; they are usually normal in myopathies and in anterior horn cell diseases. In compression or entrapment neuropathies (e.g. carpal tunnel syndrome of the median nerve) conduction will be slow only across the area of compression. Sometimes, measurement of nerve conduction velocity in proximal segments of nerve are useful in detecting slowing that occurs in some neuropathies or radiculopathies, such as in Guillain-Barré syndrome, in which measurement of the latency of the H reflex and F responses are very useful in diagnosis.

Electromyography. Electromyography (EMG) is a useful tool for detecting abnormalities of motor units and can differentiate myopathies from neuropathies or anterior horn diseases, especially neuropathies in which reinnervation has occurred. It is also useful in localizing the territory of involvement of one nerve or nerve root. The EMG recording should show no activity (electrical potentials) at rest. When denervation of muscle fibers has occurred, fibrillation potentials are frequently seen. Fasciculations are frequently found in anterior horn cell disease.

Motor units potentials have characteristic amplitudes and durations. In myopathies these potentials are reduced in amplitude, brief, and polyphasic, but normal in number on maximal contraction. The potentials will be large in disease of the anterior horn cell or the peripheral nerve, due to reinnervation; of course, the number of motor units on maximal contraction will be decreased in these diseases.

Repetitive nerve stimulation. Normally, the amplitude of the compound muscle action potential (summation of all motor units of the muscle during electrical stimulation) will not decrease when the nerve is stimulated at slow frequencies (2 or 3 Hz), but a significant decrement is seen in myasthenia gravis and in botulism, a disease in which the initial response is small.

Ischemic exercise test. The ischemic exercise test consists of exercise of an arm under ischemic conditions to see if there is a rise in serum lactate, as normally occurs. This test is most useful in diagnosis of some of the glycogen storage diseases in which serum lactate does not increase during ischemic exercise (muscle phosphorylase and phosphofructokinase deficiencies).

Muscle biopsy. Muscle biopsy will usually detect abnormalities in different neuromuscular diseases and is useful in arriving at a definitive diagnosis. Normally, muscle fibers are polygonal in transverse sections, and types I and II muscle fibers are distributed in a typical checkerboard pattern. These different types of muscle fibers are determined by their staining characteristics when histochemical techniques are used. For example, type I fibers stain dark when oxidative stains like NADH-TR are used because these fibers are rich in oxidative enzymes, whereas type II fibers stain lightly; the reverse occurs when a phosphorylase stain is used. The histochemical and physiologic characteristics of muscle fibers of one motor unit are identical, and its characteristics are determined by their motor neuron.

In neuropathies or anterior horn cell diseases, denervated fibers become angular or atrophic; if reinnervation is established, groups of fibers of the same type are seen clustering together, forming type grouping because of collateral sprouting. If the unit innervating a group of fibers becomes damaged, the entire group becomes atrophic (group atrophy).

Among the myopathies, muscle biopsy may reveal structural abnormality in muscle fibers, as in congenital myopathies; necrosis and increase in connective tissue, as in dystrophies; inflammation in inflammatory myopathies; or vacuolization in some of the metabolic myopathies in which biochemical studies on biopsied tissue will detect enzymatic abnormalities.

Nerve biopsy. Nerve biopsy is reserved for special problem cases. In a peripheral neuropathy, the nerve may show evidence of demyelination or axonal degeneration. In chronic neuropathies, the so-called onion bulb formation of Schwann cell processes around axons may be observed. In some diseases, detection of abnormally deposited material in the biopsied nerve, as in metachromatic leukodystrophy and particularly amyloid neuropathy, is the best means of establishing a diagnosis.

Cerebrospinal fluid examination. A slight-to-moderate increase in total protein is frequently observed in chronic neuropathies and is greatly increased in the acute inflammatory radiculoneuropathy (Guillain-Barré syndrome).

Major categories of neuromuscular diseases

Table 29-6 lists the clinical findings of neuromuscular disease categories. The laboratory findings are listed below.

- Anterior horn cell disease
  - Nerve conduction velocity: normal
  - Fibrillations (EMG): + + +
  - Motor units: giant polyphasic
  - Repetitive stimulation: normal
  - Muscle biopsy: angular and atrophic fibers; fiber grouping
  - Nerve biopsy: axonal degeneration in motor nerves
  - Blood chemistry: normal; CK slightly elevated occasionally
  - Spinal fluid protein: normal
- Peripheral neuropathy
  - Nerve conduction velocity: slow
  - Fibrillations (EMG): + +
  - Motor units: giant polyphasic
  - Repetitive stimulation: normal
  - Muscle biopsy: Atrophic angular fibers; fiber grouping
  - Nerve biopsy: axonal degeneration segmental demyelination; wallerian degeneration
  - Blood chemistry: diabetes, uremia, etc.
  - Spinal fluid protein: normal
- Diseases of the neuromuscular junction (myasthenia gravis)
  - Nerve conduction velocity: normal
  - Fibrillations (EMG): 0
  - Motor units: normal or small polyphasic
  - Repetitive stimulation: decrement of the muscle action potential
  - Muscle biopsy: rarely atrophic angular fibers
  - Nerve biopsy: normal
  - Blood chemistry: normal
  - Spinal fluid protein: normal
- Myopathies
  - Nerve conduction velocity: normal
  - Fibrillations (EMG): ±
  - Motor units: small polyphasic
  - Repetitive stimulation: normal
  - Muscle biopsy: according to the type; fiber degeneration, phagocytosis, increased connective tissue, storage material, inflammation
  - Nerve biopsy: normal
  - Blood chemistry: high CK, increased sedimentation rate (polymyositis)
  - Spinal fluid protein: normal

Disease of the anterior horn (spinal muscle atrophies)

Infantile spinal muscular atrophy (Werdnig-Hoffmann disease). Infantile spinal muscular atrophy is an autosomal recessive disease with an incidence of one in 25,000 live births. The disease starts early in life (the mother may notice decreased fetal movements during pregnancy). The newborn appears floppy and adopts a classic frog-leg position. The child may be anoxic at birth and have abdominal respirations and poor sucking reflex. The babies are usually intelligent and look cheerful. In about 50% of cases, fasciculations may be seen in the tongue,

Table 29-6. Major categories of neuromuscular diseases: clinical findings

Disorder	Distribution of weakness	Reflexes	Tone	Sensory deficit	Fasciculations
Anterior horn cell disease	Proximal or distal; may be asymmetric; involvement of motor cranial nerves, but ptosis and/or opthalmoplegia not found	Decreased*	Decreased* or increased	None	+ + +
Peripheral neuropathy	Distal	Decreased early	Decreased	Distal	+
Diseases of the neuromuscular junction (myasthenia gravis)	More proximal, ocular muscle movement involvement and ptosis common	Normal	Normal	None	0
Myopathies	Proximal	Normal early; then decreased mostly proximally	Decreased	None	0

*Hyperreflexia and increased tone are seen in some diseases of the anterior horn cell with involvement of the pyramidal tract; this is very rare in children.

which can also be atrophic. The disease is often progressive. Death from respiratory insufficiency or secondary infections usually occurs within the first 2 years of life. More benign forms of the disease are not unusual, and some authors have subclassified this disease in various subtypes, according to severity.

Muscle enzymes are usually normal or very mildly elevated. The EMG shows denervation, fasciculations, and decreased number of motor units. Nerve conduction velocities are normal. The muscle biopsy typically shows groups of atrophic fibers, some hypertrophic type I muscle fibers, and increased endomysial connective tissue.

Differential diagnosis includes the congenital myopathies and acid maltase deficiency as well as the rare congenital neuropathies. There is no effective treatment for Werdnig-Hofmann disease, and for this reason the diagnosis must be clearly established and distinguished from diseases with a more benign course.

Juvenile spinal muscular atrophy (Kugelberg-Welander disease). Kugelberg-Welander disease is first noticed between the ages of 5 and 15 years. It begins gradually with proximal wasting and weakness, waddling gait, and difficulty climbing stairs. The condition closely mimics a myopathy, and patients may even exhibit hypertrophy of calf muscles. Facial weakness is rare, but fasciculations are frequently present. The disease is inherited in an autosomal recessive manner, and progression is very slow.

Serum CK may be mildly elevated. The EMG shows giant motor units that are decreased in number; mild denervation and fasciculations are also seen. Muscle biopsy shows fiber-type grouping and angular fibers.

Differential diagnosis includes congenital myopathies, especially central core disease, limb-girdle dystrophies, Becker muscular dystrophy, and metabolic myopathies.

Peripheral neuropathies. Neuropathies have been classified in a variety of ways, including (1) symmetric (as with most polyneuropathies) versus asymmetric (as with most entrapment neuropathies); and (2) axonal (caused by nerve cell damage and dying back of the axon as in most toxic neuropathies) versus demyelinating (as found in neuropathies associated with lesions of the Schwann cell such as Charcot-Marie-Tooth disease and diphtheria).

The following is an etiologic classification of the neuropathies:

A. Metabolic
   1. Diabetes
   2. Uremia
   3 Vitamin deficiency
   4. Porphyria
   5. Amyloidosis
   6. Ataxia telangiectasia
   7. Abetalipoproteinemia
   8. Metachromatic leukodystrophy
   9. Globoid leukodystrophy
   10. L-Lipoproteinemia
B. Congenital, hereditary without demonstrable metabolic deficit
   1. Peroneal muscular atrophy (hereditary motor sensory neuropathy [HMSN] types I and II; or Charcot-Marie-Tooth disease)
   2. Hypertrophic interstitial neuropathy (Déjérine-Sottas disease HMSN III), hypomyelinating neuropathy
   3. Friedreich ataxia
   4. Progressive sensory neuropathy
   5. Hereditary sensory radicular neuropathy
   6. Congenital sensory neuropathy
   7. Congenital indifference to pain
   8. Familial dysautonomia
C. Idiopathic, infectious, and postinfectious
   1. Guillain-Barré syndrome
   2. Bell's palsy, brachial neuritis
   3. Chronic relapsing polyneuropathy
   4. Diphtheria, herpes zoster
   5. Leprosy
D. Toxic
   1. Antibiotics
   2. Antimetabolites
   3. Glue sniffing
   4. Heavy metals
E. Neoplastic
F. Traumatic, mechanical and entrapment
G. Vascular

Peroneal muscular atrophy (Charcot-Marie-Tooth disease). Peroneal muscular atrophy is a disease inherited in an autosomal dominant form that becomes evident during the first 20 years of life. There is distal wasting and weakness, especially of muscles innervated by the peroneal nerves, producing bilateral foot drop. Patients usually have high arches and hammer toes, and the legs have the appearance of inverted champagne bottles. The sensory deficit may be mild. Disease progression is slow but variable. The hereditary neuropathies have been divided into various categories; the peroneal muscular atrophies are classified as hereditary motorsensory neuropathy (HMSN types I and II). HMSN I is the demyelinating type in which patients have enlarged nerves and slow nerve conduction velocities. Pathologically there is severe demyelination and onion bulb formation caused by fibrosis and reduplication of Schwann cells, producing remyelination of nerve. In the HMSN type II, or neuronal type of peroneal muscular atrophy, nerves are not enlarged, onset of symptoms appears later, weakness of small hand muscles is not very severe, and muscles of the posterior compartment of the legs are weaker than in type I. Nerve conduction velocities are not as slow.

There is no specific treatment for this disease. Braces are most useful for foot drop.

Déjérine-Sottas disease (hereditary interstitial hypertrophic neuropathy or HMSN type III). Déjérine-Sottas disease has an autosomal recessive mode of inheritance, although this is variable. It may present clinically early in life in the form of the floppy infant syndrome, or a milder form may appear later in childhood. There is symmetric distal limb weakness, hyperreflexia, and sensory loss, especially position and vibration sense. The nerves are usually enlarged, and spinal fluid protein is elevated. Pathologically there is demyelination of nerves and onion bulb formation. A severe hypomyelinating neuropathy in children is believed to be a variant of this condition.

Hereditary sensory neuropathy. Hereditary sensory neuropathy is an autosomal recessive disease that starts in early childhood. It is characterized by progressive sensory deficit in a stocking and glove distribution, painless ulcers, dysesthesias, and unsteadiness of gait. Pathologically there is degeneration of the posterior root ganglia, spinal nerve roots, and sensory nerves. There is no specific treatment. According to the classification of Dyck and Lambert, this disease is called hereditary sensory neuropathy type II (HSN II). The HSN type I is an autosomal dominant disease with onset in the second decade or later.

Familial dysautonomia (Riley-Day syndrome). Familial dysautonomia is an autosomal recessive disease that affects children of Jewish extraction. It is characterized by early feeding difficulties and delayed development, hyperhidrosis, blotchy skin, absence of tears, labile blood pressure, hypotonia, and hyporeflexia. There is also absence of the fungiform papillae of the tongue, as well as absence of the normal wheal and flare formation after intradermal injection of 1:1000 histamine. Prevention of corneal ulcerations and respiratory tract infection is indicated. There is no specific therapy.

Refsum disease, (heredopathia atactica polyneuritiformis). Refsum disease is a rare hereditary disease characterized by peripheral neuropathy, deafness, ataxia, retinitis pigmentosa, and ichthyosis. It is caused by a metabolic block in the oxidative degradation of phytanic acid. Clinical improvement can be obtained by administration of a diet low in phytols and plasmapheresis (see also p. 799).

Friedreich ataxia. Friedreich ataxia is an autosomal recessive disease characterized by progressive ataxia, dysarthria, scoliosis, pes cavus, and hammer toes. Physical examination reveals presence of nystagmus, broad-based ataxic gait, and mild-to-moderate muscle weakness with hyporeflexia but present Babinski's sign. There is evidence of marked vibratory and position sense deficit with intact or only slight reduction of pain and temperature sensations.

Cardiac complications of the disease are frequent, characterized by conduction abnormalities and, frequently, ventricular septal hypertrophy.

Pathologically the disease is characterized by demyelination and gliosis of posterior columns, spinocerebellar and pyramidal tracts, loss of Purkinje cells in the cerebellum, and decreased number of large myelinated fibers in the peripheral nerves.

Friedreich ataxia should be differentiated from other spinocerebellar degenerations, multiple sclerosis, and, in adults, from subacute combined degeneration of the spinal cord.

Abetalipoproteinemia may resemble Friedreich ataxia because of hyporeflexia, Babinski's sign, evidence of ataxia, and posterior column involvement. These patients, however, also have retinitis pigmentosa, evidence of malabsorption, acanthocytes in the peripheral blood smear, and absence of betalipoproteins.

Ataxia with myoclonic jerks is seen in dentate cerebellar ataxia (Ramsay Hunt syndrome), but there is no evidence of spinal cord or peripheral nerve involvement in this disease.

The cause of Friedreich ataxia is unknown, yet several studies suggest a deficiency in the activity of the pyruvate dehydrogenase complex. No specific therapy is available. Conservative therapy should be directed at preventing complications. Surgery for scoliosis is beneficial to prevent respiratory complications.

Amyloidosis. Familial amyloidosis is characterized by a predominantly sensory neuropathy with severe involvement of the autonomic nervous system. Deposition of amyloid substance in the pulmonary valve may cause a heart murmur. The diagnosis may be established by the demonstration of deposits of amyloid substance in nerve and muscle. As the disease progresses, the patient exhibits marked orthostatic hypotension, urinary retention, and recurrent infections.

Ataxia telangiectasia (Louis-Bar syndrome). Ataxia telangiectasia is an autosomal recessive disease of children characterized by ataxia and peripheral neuropathy, with telangiectatic lesions visible in the conjunctivae and ears. Patients may develop choreiform movements. Abnormal laboratory tests include decreased serum gamma globulins, IgA, IgE, lymphopenia, and neutropenia. The disease is progressive, and patients usually die from intercurrent infections or tumors of the reticuloendothelial system.

Acute intermittent porphyria. Patients with acute intermittent porphyria frequently experience a seizure disorder, changes in mental status, and/or neuropathy. A history of abdominal pain, thought to be caused by autonomic involvement, may be elicited. Occasionally the neuropathy may have an acute onset resembling Guillain-Barré syndrome. Electrocardiographic changes, arrhythmias, and hypertension may occur secondary to autonomic involvement. Diagnosis is established by demonstrating elevated porphobilinogen and uroporphyrins in the urine, although false positives and negatives can occur. Deficiency of uroporphyrinogen I synthetase in erythrocytes is found in acute intermittent hepatic porphyria. Therapy includes a high-carbohydrate diet and use of intravenous hematin, both of which suppress porphyrin precursor production. A number of medications such as barbiturates, sulfonamides, methyldopa, chlordiazepoxide, hydantoins, alcohol, and others are contraindicated in patients with porphyria because they might precipitate an acute attack.

Guillain-Barré syndrome. Guillain-Barré syndrome is believed to be produced by an autoimmune mechanism and is frequently seen 1 or 2 weeks after an upper respiratory tract infection and other viral infections, particularly infectious mononucleosis or a stressful event such as surgery. Weakness usually develops in the legs first, followed by upper extremity involvement in both proximal and distal muscles. The patient may complain of tingling sensations, muscle aches, or numbness of hands and feet. Facial muscles are frequently involved. There is another variant in which the extraocular muscles are involved in patients with ataxia. The disease usually progresses rapidly and, although this is variable, respiratory paralysis may occur in a matter of hours. For this reason the patient in whom the diagnosis is suspected should be hospitalized and carefully monitored, especially when respiratory involvement becomes evident.

On examination there is usually proximal and distal weakness, hypotonia, and hyporeflexia, but minimal sensory findings despite sensory complaints. Classically, spinal fluid protein is elevated with no increase in cells, although mild pleocytosis may be present. Normal cerebrospinal fluid protein concentration early in the course of disease does not exclude the diagnosis. Nerve conduction velocities can be slow or normal; but, since the damage may be in the proximal segments of the nerve, measurement of the latency of the F wave and H reflex may detect proximal slowing. The EMG shows reduction of the number of motor units recruited in maximal effort. Denervation potentials are absent initially but appear approximately 2 weeks after the onset of the disease.

Pathologically, there is primary demyelination and lymphocytic infiltration, which occurs primarily in nerve roots, but patchy lesions are seen in peripheral nerves.

There is similarity between Guillain-Barré syndrome and experimental allergic neuritis in animals; the disease can be transmitted to experimental animals by inoculation of patients' sera and lymphocytes.

Treatment of Guillain-Barré syndrome is supportive and particularly aimed at preventing complications. Careful monitoring should be done to provide respiratory assistance when necessary. Corticosteroids and immunosuppressants have not proved useful. Early reports of successful therapy with plasmapheresis have not been confirmed, and in a randomized trial plasmapheresis did not prove to be beneficial. Good physical and respiratory therapy remains the best available therapy.

Prognosis for complete recovery is excellent.

Differential diagnosis includes porphyria,

diphtheria, poliomyelitis, and transverse myelitis; milder cases may resemble a myopathy because of proximal weakness. The so-called brachial neuritis may be a forme fruste of the disease. A chronic autoimmune peripheral neuropathy, or chronic relapsing polyneuropathy, or chronic Guillain-Barré syndrome, is characterized by slowly progressive muscle weakness with glove and stocking sensory deficit, arreflexia, markedly slow nerve conduction velocities, and high spinal fluid proteins. This disease responds to corticosteroids or immunosuppresant therapy as well as to plasmapheresis.

Toxic neuropathies. A number of toxins have been associated with diffuse peripheral neuropathies. One of the better known is arsenic poisoning. This substance is present in insecticides and rodenticides. Chronic intoxication is characterized by skin rashes, hyperkeratosis, and sensorimotor neuropathy. Transverse white lines (Mee's lines) in the nails are a diagnostic clue. Diagnosis is facilitated by finding arsenic in the urine (more than 0.1 mg/dl in a 24 hour specimen) and in the hair (more than 0.1 mg/dl).

Chronic lead intoxication in children usually produces encephalopathy, whereas in adults a predominantly motor neuropathy is seen affecting especially the radial nerve. Neuropathies can be seen in intoxication with insecticides, such as DDT or pentachlorophenol, or from administration of isoniazid or phenytoin. Glue sniffing may also produce a neuropathy.

Other common causes of neuropathy include uremia, diabetes, hypothyroidism, and vitamin B_1 deficiency, as well as the collagen-vascular diseases. Trauma is an important cause of neuropathy in children, and plexus injuries are well known in the newborn, particularly lesions affecting muscles innervated by C5 and C6 roots (Erb palsy). Lesions of the lower brachial plexus (Klumpke paralysis) are rarer, producing weakness of the hand muscles, sometimes accompanied by ipsilateral Horner syndrome.

Diseases of the neuromuscular junction

Myasthenia gravis. Myasthenia gravis is a disease characterized by fluctuating weakness and fatigability. The muscles most frequently involved are those supplied by the cranial nerves and those involved in respiration. The juvenile form of the disease has the same presentation and responds to the same therapy as the adult form.

This disease is believed to result from blockage of acetylcholine receptors at the myoneural junction by an immunoglobulin (IgG), which not only blocks neuromuscular transmission but also degrades acetylcholine receptor with activation of complement. It is an autoimmune disease in which the thymus gland plays an important role and usually is hypertrophic. Myasthenia gravis is sometimes associated with other autoimmune diseases and thyroid disorders.

Neonatal myasthenia. About 20% of children born to myasthenic mothers develop a transient weakness that may last a few hours or days but usually requires only temporary treatment. This condition results from the ability of myasthenic blocking globulin to cross the placenta. It may be treated with anticholinesterase medications and in severe cases with plasma exchange.

Congenital myasthenic syndromes. Congenital myasthenic syndromes usually have a familial incidence. They start early in life with a characteristic fluctuating muscle weakness and extraocular muscle involvement. Acetylcholine receptor antibodies are not increased, and patients do not respond well to anticholinesterase medication, corticosteroids, or thymectomy. Recently, patients have been described as having abnormalities of neuromuscular function attributable to acetylcholinesterase deficiency with small nerve terminals, and others have increased opening time of the ionic channels. In these syndromes repetitive nerve stimulation characteristically shows a decremental response, but single nerve stimuli shows double responses as if the patients are being overtreated with anticholinesterase drugs. No treatment is available for this condition.

Diagnosis of myasthenia gravis. The differential diagnosis of myasthenia gravis includes other diseases that produce ptosis and weakness, such as ocular myopathy lesions involving the third (oculomotor) nerve. Oculomotor involvement may erroneously suggest a brain tumor, and patients may unnecessarily undergo painful and costly tests. The diagnosis can usually be established at the bedside using the edrophonium (Tensilon) test: 0.15 to 0.2 mg/kg edrophonium given intravenously will promptly reverse the muscular weakness in 30 to 45 seconds. Repetitive supramaximal motor nerve stimulation usually reveals a decremental response in the compound muscle action potential when the nerve is stimulated at two or three stimuli per second. Increased jitter and blocking is found during single fiber electromyography. Measurement of acetylcholine receptor antibodies is very useful; titers are elevated in over 80% of patients.

Overmedication with anticholinesterase agents used in treatment of myasthenia may aggravate the weakness, resulting in a cholinergic crisis. The presence of muscarinic side effects such as increased lacrimation, salivation, abdominal cramps, and diarrhea should suggest this possibility. The use of the edrophonium test is helpful to differentiate these two conditions. If the patient's symptoms worsen rather than improve, it is an indication of overmedication.

Certain medicines make myasthenia gravis worse. Some (neomycin and kanamycin) block neuromuscular transmission, and others, such as diuretics, have an adverse effect by lowering serum potassium. Other dangerous drugs include streptomycin, bacitracin, lincomycin, colistin, procainamide, quinine, chlorpromazine, curare, succinylcholine, excessive sedatives, trimethadione, and propranolol. Penicillamine may induce a fairly classical picture of myasthenia gravis in some patients.

Treatment. Symptomatic treatment includes anticholinesterase drugs such as neostigmine (Prostigmin) and pyridostigmine (Mestinon). Thymectomy has a beneficial effect in over 50% of myasthenic patients, and remission of the disease may be induced in some cases. The use of steroids (prednisone) in high dosage on alternate days is now the most effective way of controlling the disease. Dosages of steroid are reduced as the disease remits. Plasmapheresis is an effective therapy for refractory cases. Immunosuppressants are also useful in those patients who do not respond to corticosteroids.

Myopathies

Muscular dystrophies. Four types of muscular dystrophies are classically recognized: pseudohypertrophic (Duchenne); limb-girdle; fascioscapulohumeral; and myotonic dystrophy.

Pseudohypertrophic (Duchenne) muscular dystrophy. Duchenne is the commonest type of muscular dystrophy. It is a sex-linked recessive disease that occurs in early childhood. Symptoms include a waddling gait and proximal muscular weakness. Affected children have difficulty going up stairs and arising from a chair or floor, and when rising from the floor they "climb over their legs," producing the Gowers' sign (Fig. 29-2). The calf muscles are frequently hypertrophic. Obvious proximal muscle weakness is detected early. Patients walk on their tiptoes with marked lordosis. They have winging of the scapula and later develop a fixed scoliosis and tendon contractures. The IQ, although variable, is usually somewhat lower than in the normal population. Serum CK is markedly increased. The EMG shows brief polyphasic motor unit action potentials. Muscle biopsy reveals necrosis and phagocytosis of muscle cells, fiber atrophy, and increased endomysial fat and connective tissue. Calcium accumulation in muscle fibers and large dark fibers ("overcontracted") are seen.

The disease has a progressive course, and most children are unable to walk by the age of 10 to 12 years. Death usually occurs during the teen years as a result of respiratory infections. A cardiomyopathy associated with cardiac arrhythmias is frequently seen, and the ECG is abnormal and has characteristic features that correspond to the pathologic findings of fibrosis and fat accumulation in basilar and lateral aspects of the ventricles.

There is no known specific treatment for the disease at this time, as the exact cause of muscle destruction is unknown; however, there is evidence of muscle calcium accumulation that is thought to be caused by abnormal muscle membranes. This is believed by some to trigger the mechanism of muscle necrosis.

Intensive therapy aimed at preventing contractures, scoliosis, and other complications is important. Children should remain active and ambulatory as much as possible, even with braces. Some female carriers of the disease have elevated CPKs, abnormal EMGs, and muscle biopsies, but others have completely normal studies.

There is a more benign form of muscular dystrophy, also inherited as sex-linked recessive (Becker variant), with similar distribution of weakness and EMG and muscle biopsy abnormalities. Differential diagnosis of Duchenne muscular dystrophy includes juvenile spinal muscular atrophy, childhood polymyositis, limb-girdle dystrophy, late infantile acid maltase deficiency, and other metabolic myopathies.

Limb-girdle dystrophy. Limb-girdle dystro-

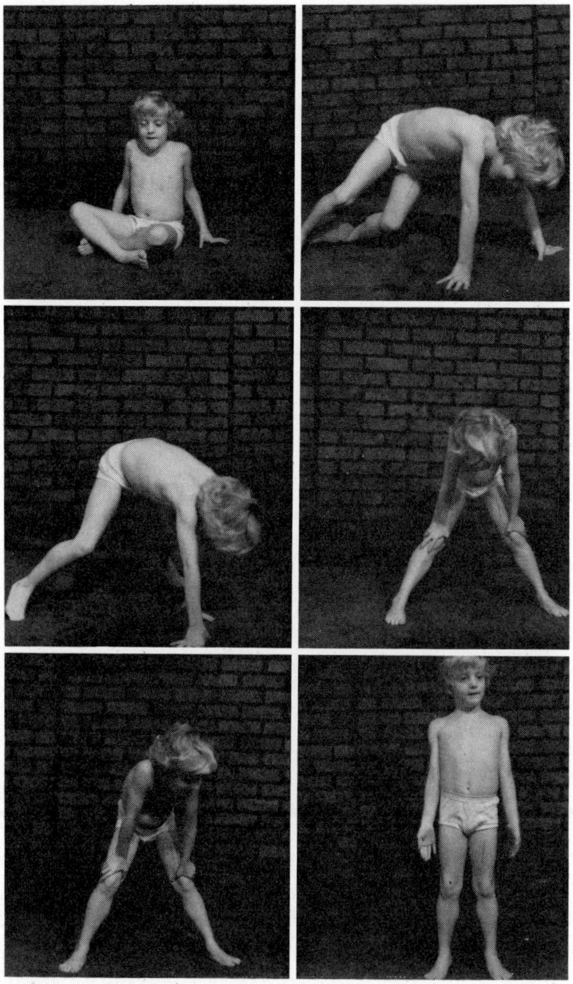

Fig. 29-2. Positive Gowers' maneuver in a patient with Duchenne muscular dystrophy. Notice the difficulty in standing up and the patient's need to "climb up his legs."

phy is usually an autosomal recessive disease. Patients have weakness in proximal muscles of the upper and lower extremities. The course is characteristically slowly progressive and may be compatible with an almost normal life span. It is believed that the "disease" is really a mixture of different syndromes.

Fascioscapulohumeral (Landouzy-Dejerine) muscular dystrophy. Fascioscapulohumeral dystrophy is an autosomal dominant disease characterized by facial muscle involvement, ptosis, and horizontal smile. Neck and shoulder girdle weakness are also prominent. The prognosis is variable, but generally the course is more benign than that of the Duchenne form. An infantile form of the disease is usually more severe and rapidly progressive.

Myotonic dystrophy. Myotonic dystrophy is an autosomal dominant disease characterized by weakness, ptosis, myotonia, early cataracts, testicular atrophy, baldness, and diabetes. The symptoms usually appear later in life but may become obvious much earlier in the neonatal period, producing a weak sucking reflex and facial diplegia with minimal or no myotonia. The weakness may be more distal than proximal in this type of dystrophy. Other features include mental deficiency, heart block, and decreased serum IgG. The EMG reveals typical spontaneous myotonic discharges known as the dive-bomber pattern. Muscle biopsy shows hypotrophy of type I muscle fibers, internalized nuclei, and frequent ring fibers. The disease is slowly progressive.

Myotonia congenita. Myotonia congenita is a benign disease in which weakness is not evident. The main symptom is myotonia that is aggravated by cold. The children have a herculean appearance with very well-developed muscles. Myotonia can be treated symptomatically with phenytoin (Dilantin) or procainamide, and recently the use of acetazolamide has been recommended.

Congenital neuromuscular diseases. Weakness appearing in early infancy may be a manifestation of a number of diseases that are best differentiated by muscle biopsy.

Central core disease. Central core disease is the most benign of these conditions. It is inherited as an autosomal dominant disease. Weakness improves as the patient ages. As in most of these diseases, type I muscle fiber predominance is seen in the muscle biopsy. A core area devoid of oxidative enzymes is demonstrable with histochemical staining. An increased incidence of hip subluxation is seen, and there is a predisposition to the malignant hyperthermia syndrome during anesthesia.

Nemaline myopathy (rod disease). Nemaline myopathy is characterized by more marked muscle weakness. A high arched palate and kyphoscoliosis are associated clinical features. Rod bodies are seen in myofibers in the muscle biopsy. These are formed by Z band material in muscle fibers.

Myotubular myopathy (type I hypotrophy with central nuclei). Myotubular myopathy is characterized by generalized weakness and ptosis. On biopsy the muscle fibers have the appearance of myotubules and are small in caliber with centrally located nuclei.

Other congenital myopathies. Other congenital myopathies include congenital fiber type disproportion, sarcotubular myopathy, reducing body myopathy, and other less known syndromes.

Childhood oculocraniosomatic neuromuscular disease with ragged red fibers. Childhood oculocraniosomatic neuromuscular disease is not truly congenital but has its onset in childhood. Clinical features include ophthalmoplegia, proximal weakness, ataxia, retinitis, deafness, heart block, and endocrine abnormalities. Usually the patients have high spinal fluid protein; spongiform changes in the cerebral white matter have been demonstrated in some. Muscle fibers have abundant and abnormal mitochondria, giving the ragged red characteristics of muscle fibers when studied with the modified Gomori trichome stain.

Inflammatory myopathies

Polymyositis and dermatomyositis (see also p. 484). Polymyositis and dermatomyositis are inflammatory myopathies that may present at any age with subacute onset of muscle weakness. An erythematous skin rash with heliotrope formation is present in dermatomyositis.

The childhood form of this disease is almost always accompanied by a rash, and subcutaneous calcifications may also be present. The disease may be associated with a diffuse vasculitis and multiple organ involvement. Evidence of other collagen vascular processes may be present. The association with neoplasms seen in adults is not present in children with this disease.

Patients may complain of generalized muscle aches and malaise. Difficulty in swallowing is not unusual. If untreated, the disease may progress to involve the muscles of respiration and deglutition.

The sedimentation rate is frequently elevated. CK is usually elevated but can be normal. The EMG reveals fibrillation potentials and brief polyphasic motor unit action potentials.

Muscle biopsy may show muscle necrosis and perivascular lymphocytic infiltration. In some cases, signs of inflammation are minimal and the biopsy shows only characteristic perifascicular muscle fiber atrophy.

The disease is believed to be an autoimmune disorder, although the exact mechanism is still obscure. The response to steroids and immunosuppressants is excellent. In refractory cases plasmapheresis may be beneficial.

Differential diagnosis includes Duchenne muscular dystrophy, limb-girdle dystrophy, carnitine deficiency, and acid maltase deficiency. Rarely the Guillain-Barré syndrome may resemble polymyositis.

Metabolic myopathies

A number of myopathies that have a metabolic basis have been defined in recent years.

Hypokalemic periodic paralysis. Hypokalemic periodic paralysis is usually transmitted as an autosomal dominant disease. It is characterized by intermittent weakness associated with hypokalemia. This may develop after heavy meals, late at night, or early mornings. Some cases are associated with hyperthyroidism, particularly in orientals. Muscle biopsy shows centrally located vacuoles. Treatment includes potassium supplements and acetazolamide. Occasionally, periodic paralysis also develops in secondary hypokalemia caused by gastrointestinal, renal, or endocrinologic problems. Diagnostically, an attack of paralysis may be induced by glucose and insulin.

Hyperkalemic periodic paralysis. Hyperkalemic periodic paralysis is also a genetic disorder of the autosomal dominant type. It is characterized by intermittent weakness associated with hyperkalemia, frequently precipitated by cold or rest after exercise. Myotonia is frequently present. It is treated with thiazides or acetazolamide.

Glycogen storage disease. As in most metabolic myopathies glycogen storage disorders have an autosomal recessive inheritance. Deficiencies of muscle phosphorylase and phosphofructokinase are characterized by muscle cramps and myoglobinuria with exercise. This is the result of inadequate glycogen breakdown to provide energy. The diagnosis is facilitated by demonstrating the failure of serum lactate to increase during ischemic exercise. Muscle biopsies may show subsarcolemmal accumulation of glycogen and absent phosphorylase and phosphofructokinase activity in specific histochemical stains. Biochemical determinations are diagnostic.

Acid maltase deficiency (1,4- and 1,6-alphaglycosidase deficiency). Acid maltase deficiency is caused by a deficiency of the enzyme that breaks down glycogen in the lysosomes. Infants may develop hepatosplenomegaly, muscle weakness, and cardiac insufficiency (Pompe's disease). It may also present during childhood with only muscle weakness (late infantile acid maltase deficiency) or occur in adulthood. Serum CK is elevated. The EMG shows myotonic discharges, although no clinical myotonia is evident. Muscle biopsy is characterized by multiple PAS-positive vacuoles and increased acid phosphatase activity on histochemistry. No treatment is available for this disorder.

Muscle weakness may also be seen in patients with branching and debranching enzyme deficiencies although the main problems are related to liver enlargement, and in debranching enzyme deficiency there is also hypoglycemia.

Disorders of lipid metabolism

Muscle carnitine deficiency. Muscle carnitine deficiency is characterized by progressive weakness in the limb-girdle distribution as a result of deficient carnitine, a substance necessary for the transport of fatty acids into the mitochondria. Muscle biopsy shows characteristic neutral lipid accumulation in muscle fibers, particularly in type I fibers. Carnitine is deficient in muscle and in serum of some patients. A systemic carnitine deficiency is characterized by muscle weakness, encephalopathy, and liver failure. Improvement in this condition has been obtained by the use of corticosteroids and by the administration of exogenous carnitine.

Carnitine-palmityl-transferase deficiency. Carnitine-palmityl-transferase deficiency is caused by a deficiency of the enzymes necessary for the incorporation of fatty acids into the mitochondria. Patients usually have muscle aches, and myoglobinuria occurs after heavy exercise or fasting. Patients are unable to produce ketone bodies during fasting because of a liver deficiency of the enzymes.

Disorders of mitochondrial function

A variety of metabolic disorders caused by abnormal mitochondrial function has been described in deficiency of NADH-coenzyme Q reductase and a deficiency of cytochrome *b*. Patients have muscle weakness that increases with exercise. A deficiency of cytochrome *c* oxidase has been described as associated with lactic acidosis, features of the De Toni-Fanconi syndrome, muscle weakness, dementia, and death in infancy.

Malignant hyperthermia syndrome. The cause of malignant hyperthermia syndrome is unknown. It is characterized by the development of high fever, muscle contractures, necrosis, and myoglobinuria during halothane and succinylcholine anesthesia, although other anesthetics and even stress have been implicated. The syndrome has an autosomal dominant pattern of transmission. Susceptible individuals can sometimes be detected by the presence of an elevated serum CPK. The myopathy seen in this condition is nonspecific, but it has been associated with conditions such as central core disease, myotonic dystrophy, myotonia congenita, and recently with Duchenne muscular dystrophy. The treatment should be preventive, although promising results have been obtained with the use of dantrolene sodium (Dantrium). Some susceptible individuals have increased serum CK. Screening of persons at risk also includes the in vitro muscle contracture test.

Tulio E. Bertorini

SELECTED READINGS

History and examination

Amiel-Tison, C.: Neurologic evaluation of the maturity of newborn infants, Arch. Dis. Child. **43:**89, 1968.

Dodge, P.R.: Neurologic history and examination. In Farmer, T.W., editor: Pediatric neurology, New York, 1964, Paul C. Hoeber.

Gesell, A., and Amatruda, C.S.: Developmental diagnosis, New York, 1956, Paul C. Hoeber.

Illingsworth, R.S.: The development of the infant and young child, ed. 5, Baltimore, 1972, The Williams & Wilkins Co.

Paine, R.S., and Oppé, T.E.: Neurological examination of children. Clinics in developmental medicine, vol. 20/21, London, 1966, National Spastica Society.

Congenital defects

Alter, M.: Anencephalus, hydrocephalus, and spina bifida, Arch. Neurol. **7:**411, 1962.

Ames, M.D., and Schut, L.: Results of treatment of 171 consecutive myelomeningoceles, 1963-1968, Pediatrics **50:**466, 1972.

DeMyer, W., et al.: The face predicts the brain: diagnostic significance of median facial anomalies for holoprosencephaly (arhinencephaly), Pediatrics **34:**256, 1964.

Fishman, M.A.: Recent clinical advances in the treatment of dysraphic states, Pediatr. Clin. North Am. **23:**517, 1976.

Fishman, M.A.: Hydrocephalus. In Eliasson, S.G., et al., editors: Neurological pathophysiology, New York, 1978, Oxford University Press.

Griffith, J.F., et al.: Hydrocephalus: medical and surgical considerations, Clin. Pediatr. **6:**494, 1967.

Keucher, T.R., and Mealey, J., Jr.: Long-term results after ventriculoatrial and ventriculoperitoneal shunting for infantile hydrocephalus, J. Neurosurg. **50:**179, 1979.

Russell, D.S.: Observations on the pathology of hydrocephalus, London, 1966, Her Majesty's Stationery Office.

Static encephalopathies

Ellis, E.: The physical management of developmental disorders. Clinics in Developmental Disorders, vol. 26, London, 1967, National Spastics Society.

Kurland, L.T.: Definitions of cerebral palsy and their role in epidermiologic research, Neurology **7:**641, 1957.

Low, N.L., and Downey, J.A.: Cerebral palsy. In Downey, J.A., and Low, N.L., editors: The child with disabling illness, Philadelphia, 1974, W.B. Saunders Co.

Malamud, N., et al.: An etiologic and diagnostic study of cerebral palsy, J. Pediatr. **65:**270, 1964.

Towbin, A.: The pathology of cerebral palsy, Springfield, Ill., 1960, Charles C Thomas, Publisher.

Headache

Ad Hoc Committee on Classification of Headache: Classification of headache, JAMA **179:**717, 1962.

Friedman, A.P.: Headache. In Baker, A.B., and Baker, L.H., editors: Clinical neurology, New York, 1971, Harper & Row, Publishers, Inc.

Haywood, T.J., et al.: Headache in children. III. Headache due to systemic disease, Headache **2:**41, 1962.

Holquin, J., and Fenichel, G.: Migraine, J. Pediatr. **70:**290, 1967.

Rothner, A.D.: Headaches in children: a review, Headache **19:**156, 1979.

Rushton, J.G., and Rooke, E.D.: Brain tumor headache, Headache **2:**147, 1962.

Central nervous system infections

Bell, W.E., and McCormick, W.F.: Major problems in clinical pediatrics, vol. 12, Neurologic infections in children, Philadelphia, 1975, W.B. Saunders Co.

Butler, I.J., and Johnson, R.T.: Central nervous system infections, Pediatr. Clin. North Am. **21:**649, 1974.

Gibbs, C.J., and Gajdusek, D.C.: Atypical viruses as the cause of sporadic epidemic and familial chronic diseases in man: slow viruses and human diseases, Perspect. Virol. **10:**161, 1978.

Hall, W.W., et al.: Measles and subacute sclerosing encephalitis virus proteins: lack of antibodies to the M protein in patients with subacute sclerosing panencephalitis, Proc. Natl. Acad. Sci. USA **76:**2047, 1979.

Smith, D.H.: The challenge of bacterial meningitis, Hosp. Pract. **11:**71, 1976.

Intracranial tumors

Bell, W.E., and McCormick, W.F.: Major problems in clinical pediatrics, vol. 8, Increased intracranial pressure in children, Philadelphia, 1972, W.B. Saunders Co.

Farwell, J.R., et al.: Central nervous system tumors in childhood, Cancer **40:**3123, 1977.

Gold, E.B., and Gordis, L.: Determinants of survival in children with brain tumors, Ann. Neurol. **5:**569, 1979.

Van Eys, J., and Cangir, A.: Chemotherapy for childhood brain tumors, J. Pediatr. **93:**554, 1978.

Walker, M.D.: Diagnosis and treatment of brain tumors, Pediatr. Clin. North Am. **23:**131, 1976.

Craniocerebral trauma

Gil, D.G.: Physical abuse of children; findings and implications of a nationwide survey, Pediatrics **44:**857, 1969.

Griffith, J.F., and Dodge, P.R.: Transient blindness following head injury in children, N. Engl. J. Med. **278:**648, 1968.

Jennett, B.: Head injuries in children, Dev. Med. Child Neurol. **14:**137, 1972.

Manucher, J.: Head injuries, N. Engl. J. Med. **890:**892, 1974.

Mealey, J., Jr.: Pediatric head injuries, Springfield, Ill., 1968, Charles C Thomas, Publisher.

Shulman, K., and Ransohoff, Jr.: Subdural hematoma in children: the fate of children with retained membranes, J. Neurosurg. **18:**175, 1961.

Wilson, C.B.: Complication of head injuries in children, Postgrad. Med. **51:**130, 1972.

Cerebral vascular diseases

Banker, B.Q.: Cerebral vascular disease in infancy and childhood. I. Occlusive vascular diseases, J. Neuropathol. Exp. Neurol. **20:**127, 1967.

Gold, A.P.: Cerebral arteriovenous malformations, Dev. Med. Child Neurol. **15:**84, 1973.

Golden, G.S.: Strokes in children and adolescents, Stroke **9:**169, 1978.

Neurocutaneous syndromes

Alexander, G.L., and Norman, R.M.: The Sturge-Weber syndrome, Bristol, England, 1960, John Wright & Sons, Ltd.

Chao, D.H.C.: Congenital neurocutaneous syndromes in childhood. I. Neurofibromatosis, J. Pediatr. **55:**189, 1959.

Gold, A.P., and Freeman, J.M.: Depigmented nevi: the earliest sign of tuberous sclerosis, Pediatrics **35:**1003, 1965.

Gomez, M.R., editor: Tuberous sclerosis, New York, 1979, Raven Press.

Sedgwick, R.P., and Boder, E.: Progressive ataxia in children with particular reference to ataxia telangiectasia, Neurology **10:**705, 1960.

Neurodegenerative diseases

Adams, R.D., and Lyon, G.: Neurology of hereditary metabolic diseases of children, New York, 1982, McGraw-Hill Book Co.

Brady, R.: Sphingomyeline lipidoses: Niemann-Pick disease. In Stanbury, J.B., et al., editors: The metabolic basis of inherited disease, New York, 1983, McGraw-Hill Book Co.

Freeman, J.M., and McKhann, G.M.: Degenerative disease of the central nervous system, Adv. Pediatr. **16:**131, 1969.

Johnson, W.G., and Rapin, I.: Progressive genetic metabolic diseases. In Rudolph, A.M., Hoffman, J.I.E., and Epstien, C.J., editors: Pediatrics, New York, 1982, Appleton-Century-Crofts.

Kolodny, E.H., and Moser, H.W.: Sulfatide lipidoses: metachromatic leukodystrophy. In Stanbury, J.B., et al., editors: The metabolic basis of inherited disease, New York, McGraw-Hill Book Co.

Menkes, J.H.: Child neurology, ed. 2, Philadelphia, 1980, Lea & Febiger.

O'Brien, J.S.: The gangliosidoses. In Stanbury, J.B., et al., editors: The metabolic basis of inherited disease, New York, 1983, McGraw-Hill Book Co.

O'Neill, B.P., et al.: Andrenaleukodystrophy: elevated C-26 fatty acids in cultured skin fibroblasts and correlation with disease expression in three generations of a kindred, Neurology **32:**540, 1982.

Robinson, F., et al.: Necrotizing encephalomyelopathy of childhood, Neurology **17:**472, 1967.

Stanbury, J.B., et al., editors: The metabolic basis of inherited disease, New York, 1983, McGraw-Hill Book Co.

Convulsive disorders

Dodson, W.E.: Pharmacology and therapeutics of epilepsy in childhood, Clin. Neuropharmacol. **4:**1, 1979.

Dodson, W.E., et al.: Management of seizure disorders: selected aspects, I., Pediatrics **89:**527, 1976.

Dodson, W.E., et al.: Management of seizure disorders: selected aspects, II., Pediatrics **89:**695, 1976.

Emerson, R., et al.: Stopping medication in children with epilepsy, N. Engl. J. Med. **314:**1125-1129, 1981.

Johnston, M.V., et al.: Pharmacologic advances in seizure control, Pediatr. Clin. North Am. **28:**179, 1981.

Kendig, E.L., Jr., et al.: Febrile seizures: long-term management of children with fever-associated seizures, Pediatrics **66:**1009, 1980.

Lombroso, C.T.: The treatment of status epilepticus, Pediatrics **53:**536, 1974.

Nelson, K.B., and Ellenberg, J.: Prognosis in children with febrile seizures, Pediatrics **61:**720, 1978.

Thurston, J.H., et al.: Prognosis in childhood epilepsy, N. Engl. J. Med. **306:**831, 1982.

Neuromuscular diseases

Bender, A.N.: Congenital myopathies, in Vinken, P.J., et al., editors: Handbook of clinical neurology, vols. 40 and 41, Diseases of muscle, New York, 1979, Elsevier North-Holland, Inc.

Bertorini, T.E., et al.: Muscle calcium and magnesium content in Duchenne muscular dystrophy, Neurology **32:**1088, 1982.

Bradley, W.G.: Disorder of peripheral nerves, Edinburgh, 1975, Churchill Livingstone.

Brooke, M.: A clinician's view of neuromuscular diseases, Baltimore, 1977, The Williams & Wilkins Co.

Byers, R.K., and Banker, B.Q.: Infantile muscular atrophy. Arch. Neurol. **5:**140, 1961.

Drachmann, D.B.: Myasthenia gravis, N. Engl. J. Med. **298:**138, 1978.

Dubowitz, V.: The floppy infant. In Clinics in Developmental Medicine, London, 1969, Heinemann Ltd.

Dyck, P.J., et al.: Peripheral neuropathy, Philadelphia, 1975, W.B. Saunders Co.

Engel, A.G., et al.: A newly recognized congenital myasthenic syndrome attributed to a prolonged open time of the acetylcholine-induced ion channel, Ann. Neurol. **11:**553, 1982.

Fenichel, G.: Clinical syndromes of myasthenia in infancy and childhood, Arch. Neurol. **35:**97, 1978.

Griggs, R.C., and Moxley, R.T., editors: Treatment of neuromuscular diseases, Adv. Neurol. **17:**1, 1977.

Moosa, A., and Dubowitz, V.: Spinal muscular atrophy in childhood: two clues to clinical diagnosis, Arch. Dis. Child. **48:**386, 1973.

Niakan, E., et al.: The use of immunosuppressive agents in corticosteroid-refractory childhood dermatomyositis, Neurology **30:**286, 1980.

Schotland, D., editor: Disorders of the motor unit, New York, 1982, John Wiley & Sons, Inc.

Swaiman, K.F., et al.: Late infantile acid maltase deficiency, Arch. Neurol. **18:**642, 1968.

Walton, J., and Gardner-Medwin, D.: Progressive muscular dystrophy and the myotonic disorders. In Walton, J., editor: Disorder of Voluntary Muscle, Edinburgh, 1981, Churchill Livingstone.

30 Pediatric Dermatology

This chapter emphasizes three aspects of pediatric dermatology: skin disease in the newborn and small infant; a few of the commonest skin problems of children and adolescents such as acne, warts, and eczema; and a few skin diseases of potentially serious medical importance such as erythema multiforme and the staphylococcal scalded skin syndrome. Also included in this chapter is a brief outline of the principles of therapy of skin diseases.

NEONATAL DERMATOLOGY

The majority of cutaneous eruptions in the neonatal period are benign and several are transient in duration.

Milia. Milia are 1 to 2 millimeter white to yellow papules usually occurring in clusters on the nose, chin, cheeks, and forehead and occasionally on the trunk (Fig. 30-1). They form when the tiny follicular ducts become plugged with keratin. This results in retention of sebaceous gland secretions and keratin, forming pinhead-sized epidermal cysts. The papules are transient and will rupture spontaneously, expressing their contents by the end of 2 months. They are present in 40% of neonates. Treatment is unnecessary.

Epstein's Pearl is an ectopic milia lesion located on the hard palate, usually near the midline.

Miliaria. Miliaria are skin eruptions caused by sweat retention. When eccrine sweat gland ducts become plugged at the level of the superficial stratum corneum, tiny (1 to 2 mm) delicate, thin-walled clear vesicles (miliaria crystallina) appear anywhere on the body (Fig. 30-2). Clear sweat fluid can be expressed when the vesicle roof is opened.

When the level of obstruction is lower in the epidermis, pressure in the duct is greater and sweat leaks out, causing a local inflammatory reaction. A clear vesicle appearing on an erythematous base is termed *miliaria rubra* (prickly heat).

Miliaria rubra is not uncommon in babies kept in incubators. There is no effective topical therapy. The rash disappears when the sweat glands are allowed to rest; this occurs at temperatures less than 29° C (84° F).

Sebaceous gland hyperplasia. Hyperplasia of the sebaceous glands manifests pinhead-sized, flesh-colored to yellow papules that may appear in clusters on the nose, cheeks, and upper lip. This hyperplasia results from maternal androgens in the fetal circulation, stimulating gland development. Histologically, these are enlarged sebaceous glands, not plugged cysts as in milia or in acne. They resolve spontaneously.

Acne neonatorum. Acne neonatorum is a mixed papular and pustular dermatitis localized on the face, with inflammation of involved sebaceous glands. This is believed to occur from transplacental transfer of maternal androgens that stimulate an increase in sebaceous gland activity. This is a self-limited and transient condition usually requiring no treatment.

Transient neonatal pustular melanosis. Pustular melanosis in the neonate consists of thin-walled, easily ruptured blisters usually located on the trunk and extremities. Removal of the blister roof reveals a hyperpigmented macule. Because most blisters rupture during birth, the common lesion seen is a hyperpigmented macule with a collarette of fine scale. This is a benign dermatosis that clears spontaneously and requires no treatment. The etiology is obscure.

Erythema toxicum neonatorum. Erythema toxicum neonatorum is a two-component lesion consisting of either a pale, flesh-colored papule or a pustule on an erythematous macule. The lesions may be present anywhere on the body except the palms and soles, and may be present at birth. Histologically, one sees a clustering of eosinophils around sebaceous glands and hair

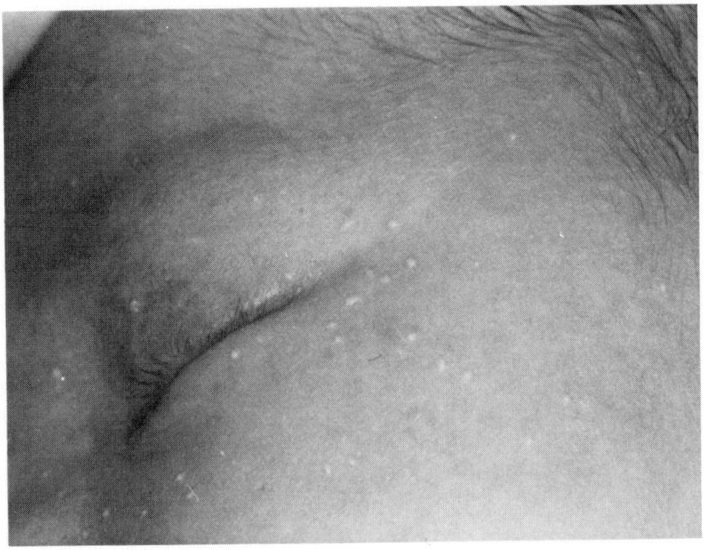

Fig. 30-1. Milia.

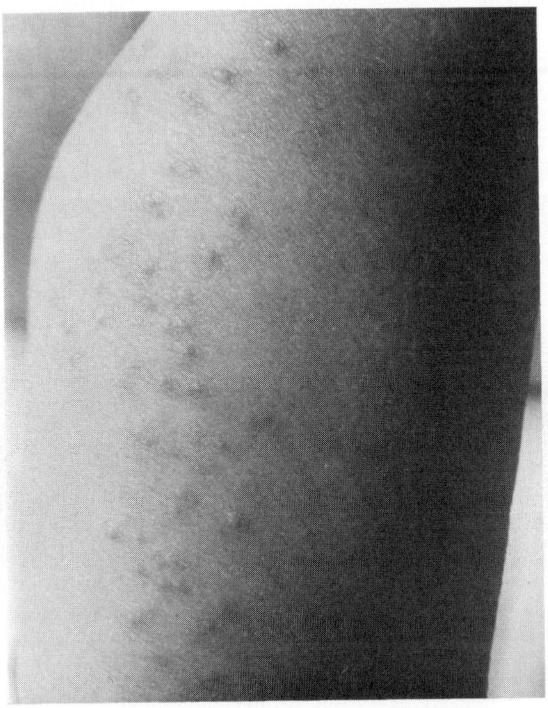

Fig. 30-2. Miliaria crystallina; miliaria rubra are those lesions with erythematous base.

follicles. Pustules result when eosinophils aggregate intradermally. The etiology is unknown, but this eruption resolves spontaneously shortly after the first week of life.

Impetigo neonatorum. Impetigo is an important bacterial infection of the newborn. The appearance is of superficial vesicles, pustules, or blisters on an erythematous base. These may evolve into denuded areas with crusting. A gram stain and culture will help identify the infectious agent, usually staphylococcus or streptococcus. This pyoderma responds well to antibiotic therapy. It is contagious and requires appropriate precautions in the nursery.

Congenital candidiasis. Candidiasis in the newborn manifests at birth as a widespread, intense erythema with small white pustules that increase in number. The eruption appears moist and usually progresses to maceration. The head, face, and neck are major sites of involvement, with the trunk and limbs also often affected. The diaper area is usually spared. Congenital candidiasis represents an intrauterine infection with *Candida albicans*. This differs from neonatal candidiasis, which is acquired when a neonate traversing the birth canal is infected with vaginal yeast organisms. Cutaneous lesions are not present at birth but will develop within the first week of life. A gram stain and fungal culture of pustule material will establish the diagnosis. Topical clotrimazole, miconazole, and nystatin are effective and recommended.

Congenital herpes. Congenital herpes may appear as solitary or grouped vesicles associated with surrounding erythema. The vesicles become pustules and may crust or become hemorrhagic. Lesions are located mainly on the presenting part at birth (i.e., face or scalp). More than half of neonates with congenital herpes will have cutaneous lesions. This can be a devastating illness, approximately half of all patients affected die or have severe neurologic or ocular sequelae. Diagnosis can be made rapidly by unroofing a vesicle and scraping its base with a small blade. A smear of the scrapings stained with Giemsa or Wright stain will demonstrate multinucleated giant cells with intranuclear inclusion bodies diagnostic of a herpes infection (Tzank test). These neonates require systemic evaluation and systemic antiviral therapy.

Early congenital syphilis (see also pp. 736-740). The earliest syphilitic lesions in newborns may have a bright reddish-pink color, evolving later into the more familiar coppery-brown lesions of cutaneous syphilis. Lesions occur mostly on the face and dorsal surface of the trunk and legs, as well as on palms and soles. Hemorrhagic blisters on the palms and soles are rare but when seen are almost always diagnostic of early congenital syphilis. These neonates are frequently premature and many will have an osteochrondritis that may present as a painful limb. Asymptomatic neonates may show lytic bone lesions on radiologic studies. Serum FTA and spinal fluid VDRL determinations are necessary to establish the diagnosis of congenital syphilis and rule out neurosyphilis. In late congenital syphilis (i.e., infection occurring in third trimester), neonates appear normal at birth but later manifest interstitial keratitis, Hutchinson incisors, mulberry molars, or eighth nerve deafness.

Treatment of congenital syphilis is discussed in Chapter 27.

Blueberry muffin syndrome. A combination of petechiae, ecchymosis, purpura, and pale red to blue dermal papules, gives the clinical picture of a blueberry muffin. This neonatal condition is seen in patients with congenital TORCH (*t*oxoplasmosis, *o*ther, *r*ubella, *c*ytomegalovirus, and *h*erpes) infections (see pp. 319 and 322), especially rubella, toxoplasmosis, and cytomegalovirus. The petechiae and purpura are secondary to thrombocytopenia and vasculitis. The red-blue papules represent extramedullary hematopoiesis. These neonates may also have hepatitis, splenomegaly, encephalitis, osteomyelitis, and congenital heart disease, especially patent ductus arteriosus or ventricular septal defects. Retinopathy consisting of deposition of black pigment in the retina is a common feature.

Blistering diseases of the neonatal period

Neonatal skin is especially subject to blistering, and many skin diseases that do not blister in older children or adults may manifest as bullous disorders in the newborn.

Incontentia pigmenti. Incontentia pigmenti starts with inflammatory vesicles or bullae in crops over the trunk and extremities. Ninety percent of afflicted neonates will develop lesions within the first 2 weeks of life. Microscopic examination reveals intraepidermal vesicles filled with eosinophils. This is the first of four stages. The next consists of diffuse warty lesions located on an extremity. Later, development of the characteristic whorled hyperpigmentation over the trunk and extremities occurs. The last stage consists of streaked, hypopigmented lesions, often limited to the calves and seen in late childhood. Incontentia pigmenti is found almost exclusively in girls (97%) and is believed to be either an X-linked dominant or an autosomal dominant trait that is lethal to boys.

Sucking blister. Bullae or an erosion without an inflammatory border usually present on the forearms, wrists, thumbs, or upper lip. These probably occur from vigorous sucking by the fetus. This lesion resolves spontaneously without treatment.

Epidermolysis bullosa. The term *epidermolysis bullosa* encompasses a group of similar disorders that present as small or large, clear, noninflammatory bullae or erosions that develop after trivial trauma (Fig. 30-3). Epidermolysis bullosa is categorized by mode of inheritance, type of healing, and histologic level of cleavage where the blister forms. The central problem is an exaggerated response of the skin to insignificant friction or trauma. Two types of these disorders, junctional epidermolysis bullosa and recessive dystrophic epidermolysis bullosa (Fig. 30-4), carry a high mortality rate during infancy from associated complications such as sepsis and fluid and protein loss (Table 30-1). The chronic blistering, infection, and scarring may lead to development of mittenlike deformities of the hands and feet. Involvement of esophagus, rectum, urethra, conjunctivae, and teeth can be severely debilitating. Phenytoin (Dilantin), which inhibits the enzyme collagenase thought responsible for blistering in the recessive dystrophic form, has been successful in the treatment of this specific form of epidermolysis bullosa.

Ichthyosis. The term *ichthyosis* means thickened, scaly, fishlike skin (Fig. 30-5). Ichthyosis encompasses a group of disorders of hyperkeratosis (thickened stratum corneum) categorized by mode of inheritance, type of scale, and pathogenesis (see Table 30-2). Histologically these disorders show a marked increase in thickness of the stratum corneum. There are thought to be four main types; all have been reported at birth. The "collodion baby," a neonate born encased in a parchmentlike membrane, is a severe presentation of the lamellar ichthyosis variety. This membrane is believed to be the remnant of the fetal outer membrane, the periderm, which protects the underlying developing epidermis during gestation. This is normally shed during the twentieth week of gestation. Lamellar ichthyosis may be associated with severe medical and psychologic disability. Some degree of symptomatic relief can be obtained with topical agents such as lactic acid (Lacticare), salicylic acid (Keralyt), and 13-Cis-retinoic acid (Accutane) may help some cases of lamellar ichthyosis.

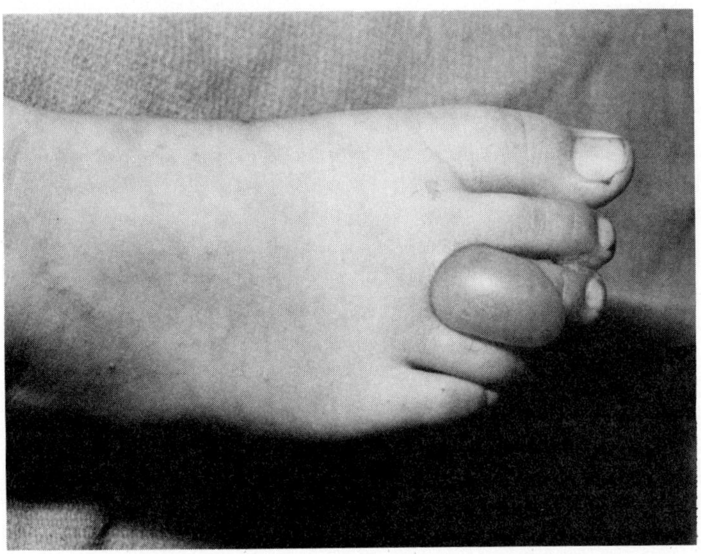

Fig. 30-3. Epidermolysis bullosa simplex.

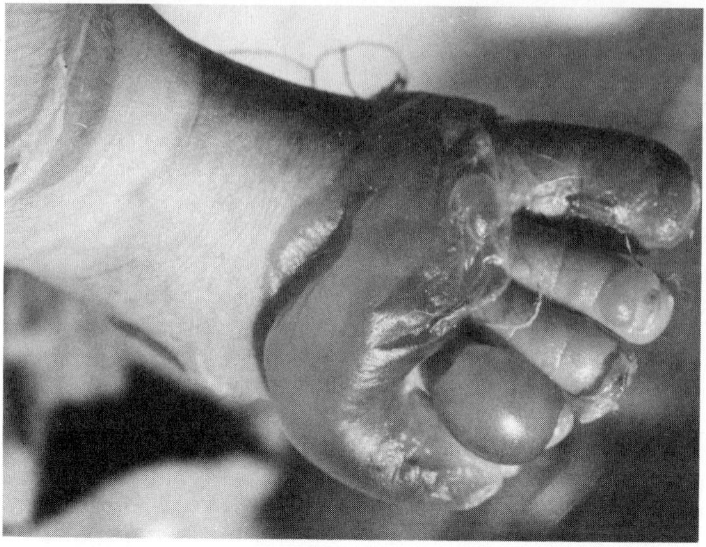

Fig. 30-4. Recessive dystrophic epidermolysis bullosa.

Table 30-1. Classification of different forms of epidermolysis bullosa

Autosomal dominant	Autosomal recessive
Nonscarring	
Generalized (Koebner)	Junctional (Letalis/Herlitz)
Weber-Cockayne (hands and feet)	
Norwegian	
Scarring	
Cockayne-Touraine	Dystrophic Localized Generalized
Pasini (albopapuloid)	

Lymphangioma circumscriptum. Lymphangioma circumscriptum appears as a group of thick-walled, firm, small vesicles that give the appearance of a cluster of frog eggs (Fig. 30-6). They are usually found on the proximal extremities, neck, axilla, chest, or perineum. They have also been noted inside the oral cavity, especially on the tongue. Bleeding into these lymphatic channels is common. The lesions penetrate deep into subcutaneous tissues, making surgical excision difficult. These are benign lesions, and no treatment is required.

Herpes gestationis. Herpes gestationis may appear on the newborn as thick-walled vesicles or bullae that may be located anywhere on the body. The eruption may be present at birth or have its onset within the first week of life. Herpes gestationis appears to be an autoimmune disease in the mother manifested as a severe pruritic vesicular eruption, often with urticarial papules and placques. It occurs in women only during pregnancy or the immediate postpartum period. Flare-ups have occurred with menses and use of oral contraceptives. Histologic features are the same for both mother and neonate and show subepidermal vesiculation with deposition of C3 at the basement membrane zone. A circulating IgG known as herpes gestationis factor has also been identified. In the neonate the eruption is usually asymptomatic, benign, and self-limited, with full resolution occurring within 2 weeks. This is not a serious disease of the neonate and there is no increased fetal risk with this maternal condition.

Pigmentary lesions in the neonate

The melanocyte is the cell responsible for all melanin pigmentation. It has its origin in the neural crest cells and migrates during embryogenesis with the mesenchymal somites. This migration distributes melanocytes to all parts of the skin. By the sixth month of gestation the melanocytes align at the dermal-epidermal junction and shortly thereafter invade the lower epidermis.

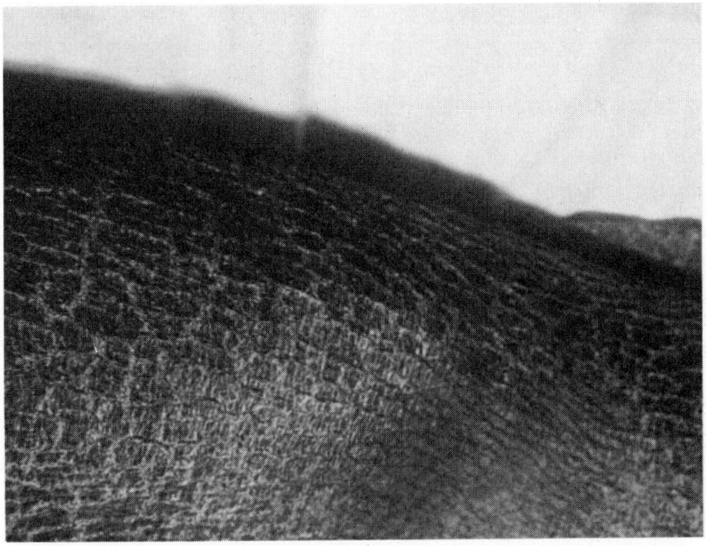

Fig. 30-5. Ichthyosis vulgaris. Notice small fishlike scales.

Table 30-2. Classification of ichthyosis

Type	Onset	Clinical features	Mode of inheritance
Ichthyosis vulgaris	3-12 mo	Mildest form—scales are platelike and on extensor surface of extremities Spares flexures Tendency for atopy	Autosomal dominant
X-Linked ichthyosis	Birth to 3 mo	Seen mainly in males—associated with deep corneal opacities involving Descemet's membrane Sparing of palms and soles Associated with deficiency of steroid sulfatase	X-linked
Lamellar ichthyosis	Birth	Collodion membrane Face all flexures involved Dense, platelike scales, yellow to brown Associated with ectropion	Autosomal recessive
Epidermolytic hyperkeratosis	Birth	Greasy brown with eythroderma Spiny ridges formed, blisters present Face spared Nitlike encasement of scalp hair	Autosomal dominant

Hyperpigmented lesions

Mongolian spot. The mongolian spot is a small or large diffusely bordered, blue-black macule usually overlying the sacrum and posterior trunk. Lesions may be solitary or numerous and are located on the extremities and trunk. These are benign lesions, seen in 90% of black and American Indian neonates and 80% of Oriental neonates. The lesion occurs when melanocyte migration in affected areas is arrested at the dermal-epidermal junction. Location of melanocytes under the basement membrane zone gives this lesion its blue-black color and diffuse border. Resolution of these lesions occurs gradually during childhood as the melanocytes slowly enter the epidermis.

Café au lait spots. Café au lait spots are sharp-bordered round or oval light-brown ma-

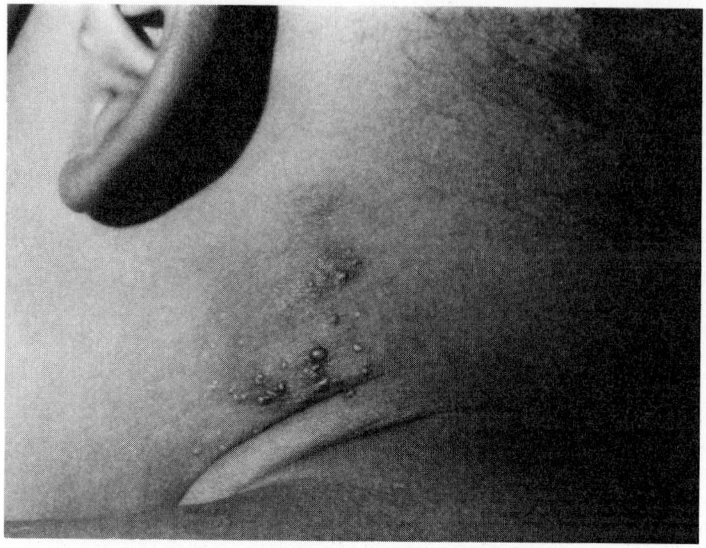

Fig. 30-6. Lymphangioma circumscriptum. Notice resemblance to cluster of frog eggs.

cules located anywhere on the body. Histologically, one sees an evenly distributed but increased amount of pigment within the epidermis. These are benign lesions, present in 10% to 20% of the general population. However, three significant medical disorders are associated with café au lait spots. Six or more lesions greater than 1.5 cm in size suggest neurofibromatosis. Freckling in the axilla (Crow's sign) occurs in about 20% of these patients and is considered pathognomonic of neurofibromatosis. Approximately 25% of patients with tuberous sclerosis will also have café au lait spots. One must always look for ash leaf spots (see under hypopigmented lesions) as well. A specific type of irregularly bordered, elongated unilateral café au lait spot known as the Coast-of-Maine spot is associated with Albright syndrome of polyostotic fibrous dysplasia and precocious puberty in females. Radiographic evaluation will often reveal pseudocystic bone lesions in early childhood.

Congenital pigmented nevi. Congenital pigmented nevi are pigmented papules or placques that vary in size, shape, and texture (Figs. 30-7 and 30-8). Their color may range from light brown to almost black, and their size from a few millimeters to as much as 35% of the total skin surface. Some lesions are uniformly brown, as in café au lait spots, but others may be mottled, rough, or thickened, with coarse hairs. In contradistinction to café au lait spots, however, all congenital nevi are elevated and palpable. They may be located anywhere on the body. Histologically, there are nests of nevus cells in the epidermis, dermis, or both. Some lesions are very extensive and may invade subcutaneous fat, fascia, and even skeletal muscle, making surgical excision very difficult. The major medical concern regarding congenital nevi is that approximately 4% to 10% of these lesions give rise to malignant tumors that carry a greater than 40% mortality rate.

It has been shown that dermabrasion in the first few weeks of life removes many of the pigmented cells from the skin and gives an improved cosmetic result. Other studies, however, suggest that the majority of malignancies arising in congenital nevi originate deep in the dermis, in areas unlikely to be extirpated by dermabrasion. For that reason, total surgical excision deep to the fascia has been recommended as the only sure treatment for these lesions. This subject has become one of great interest at this time.

Urticaria pigmentosa. Urticaria pigmentosa presents as multiple, reddish-brown or yellow-brown lesions that can range from macules to papules or nodules. When these lesions are stroked they will urticate (Darier's sign). Lesion size varies from a few millimeters to several centimeters. Lesions tend to be larger in children. Histologically, large numbers of mast cells

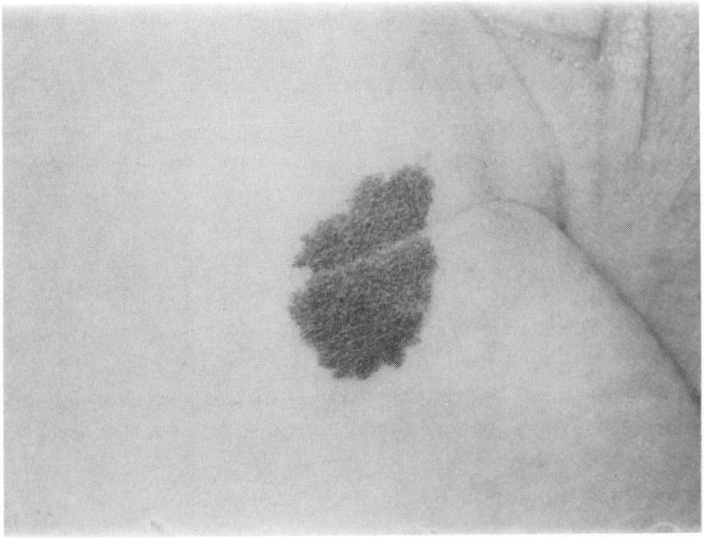

Fig. 30-7. Congenital pigmented nevus, junctional type. As a result of superficial involvement, skin furrows are preserved.

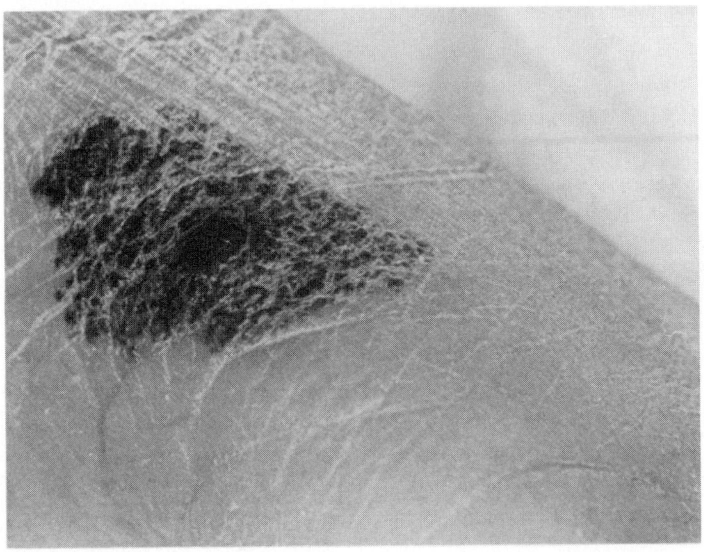

Fig. 30-8. Congenital pigmented nevus, compound type. Notice central nodule.

with intracytoplasmic granules can be demonstrated in the upper dermis using Giemsa or toluidine blue stains.

Patients developing urticaria pigmentosa at an early age (less than 10 years) have an excellent prognosis because the incidence of systemic involvement increases with age of onset. Any organ system may be involved, resulting in a wide variety of potential symptoms including intense pruritus, headaches, tachycardia, flushing, syncope, and various gastrointestinal complaints.

Sebaceous nevus of Jadassohn. The sebaceous nevus of Jadassohn is a yellow-brown or orange-pink pebbly, solitary lesion usually found in the scalp or face (Fig. 30-9). These tend to be small but may be several centimeters

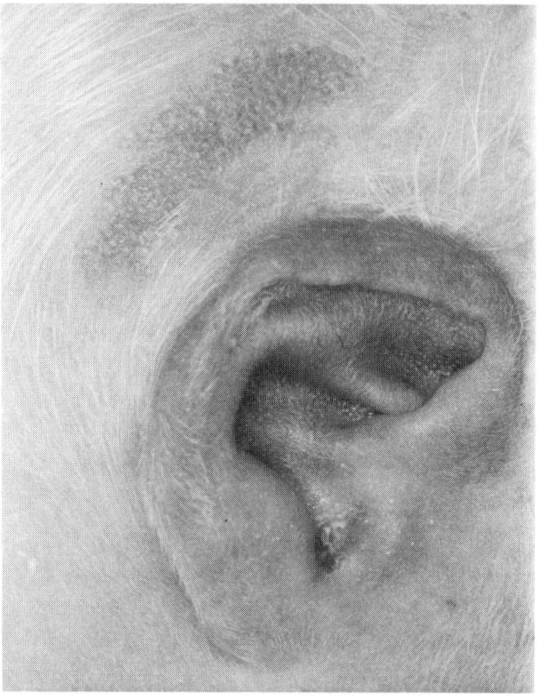

Fig. 30-9. Sebaceous nevus of Jadassohn. Notice pebbly surface.

in diameter. During infancy and childhood the histologic features include clusters of immature but benign sebaceous glands. At puberty these lesions enlarge, and the ducts dilate and penetrate deep into the dermis. Two forms of skin cancer, basal cell carcinoma and synringocystadenoma papilliferum, may arise in up to 15% of these nevi. Most dermatologists recommend total excision of these lesions before puberty.

Hypopigmented lesions

Ash leaf spots. Ash leaf spots are white or hypopigmented oblong lesions averaging 1 cm to 3 cm in size. They have an irregular outline resembling an ash leaf. This is the characteristic skin sign of tuberous sclerosis and can best be seen in a dark room using a Woods lamp. Ash leaf spots are usually located on the abdomen, back, and anterior surfaces of the extremities. Whenever such a lesion is seen, evaluation for tuberous sclerosis is mandatory. Interestingly, there is an increased incidence of partial albinism in patients with tuberous sclerosis. Any child with seizures and a white tuft of hair should also be evaluated for tuberous sclerosis.

Table 30-3. Syndromes associated with oculocutaneous albinism

Syndrome	Associated manifestations
Hermansky-Pudlak	Oculocutaneous albinism and Von Willibrand disease
Cross-McKusick-Breen	Oculocutaneous albinism, Von Willibrand disease, spasticity, mental retardation, murophthalmus
Chediak-Higashi	Oculocutaneous albinism, abnormality of polymorphonuclear phagocytosis
Tietz	Oculocutaneous albinism, deaf-mutism, hypoplasia or absence of eyebrows, normal eye color

Vitiligo. Vitiligo appears as ivory-white, sharply marginated macules with hyperpigmentation of surrounding skin. These lesions usually have a symmetric distribution and occur anywhere on the body but with a higher predilection for the face, neck, and dorsum of the hands and forearms. The size may vary from pinhead-size macules to almost total body involvement. Lesions may enlarge or may repigment. Vitiligo appears to be an autosomal dominant trait, but its onset in infancy is rare. The etiology may include an autoimmune component that results in destruction of the melanocytes in the lesions, and there appears to be a higher incidence of other autoimmune diseases in patients with vitiligo. Histologic examination of vitiliginous areas reveals absence of melanocytes, with large melanocytes at the border of the lesion. Lesions rarely repigment fully or permanently, and progression to total body involvement is possible. Treatment with 8-methoxypsoralen taken before sun exposure sometimes provides limited benefit. In general, treatment should be reserved for blacks; most whites, if prevented from tanning with sunscreens, find the spots of vitiligo not very different in color from their natural state. The condition may be emotionally disabling in blacks and deserves serious attention.

Albinism

Albinism describes a group of genetic disorders of enzyme deficiencies or aberrations in the metabolic pathway of melanin synthesis. A localized variant, ocular albinism, is loss of ret-

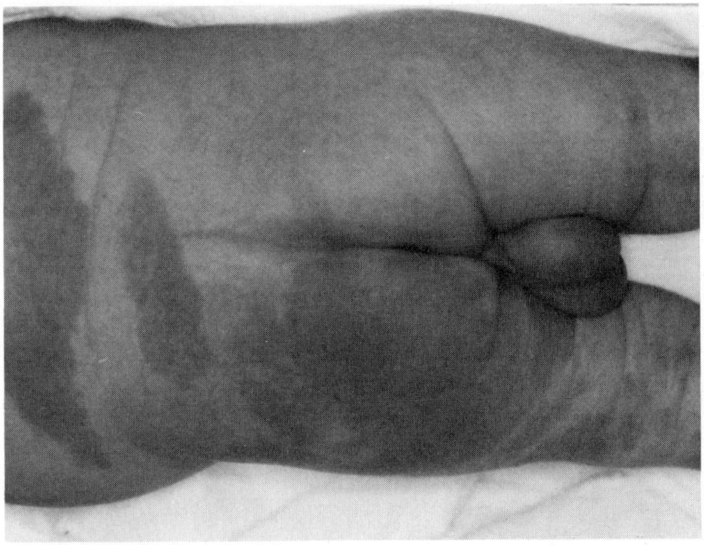

Fig. 30-10. Port wine stain. These are flat and nonpalpable.

inal pigment. Skin and hair are normal. Five other varieties are of the oculocutaneous category (see Table 30-3). Clinical features are present at birth and include white hair, pink skin, and blue or gray irides. Examination of the red reflex with an ophthalmoscope will demonstrate that it extends beyond the borders of the pupil out to the margins of the iris.

Vascular lesions

Salmon patch. The salmon patch (nevus simplex) is a faint pink macule most frequently located on the glabella (angel's kiss), nape of the neck (stork bite), or upper eyelid. It is present in approximately 40% of all newborns. Histologically, this lesion represents dermal vessels of the residual fetal circulation of the skin. These are benign lesions. Lesions on the glabella and eyelid usually fade and disappear; stork bites persist.

Port wine stain. The port wine stain (nevus flammeus) is a pink to bright red or bluish purple macule located anywhere on the body (Fig. 30-10). These grow in proportion to the growth of the child. They may also thicken to become palpable, and assume a deeper purple color as they age, signifying increased blood flow through this vascular network. Histologically, these are mature capillaries. Port wine stains are benign, but they may be associated with other syndromes such as Trisomy 13, Rubinstein-Taybi, Beckwith-Wiedeman and Sturge-Weber syndromes.

Sturge-Weber syndrome. Sturge-Weber syndrome (encephalotrigeminal angiomatosis) includes a port wine stain involving the first branch or more of the trigeminal nerve, along with vascular malformations of the ipsilateral meninges and cerebral cortex. The angioma is seen on the forehead and upper eyelid. Other features of this disorder include seizures (80%), mental retardation (60%), and contralateral hemipareses. Port wine lesions involving the first and second branches of the trigeminal nerve are associated with glaucoma (45%).

Hemangiomas. Strawberry hemangiomas are mixtures of capillaries and venules. These appear at birth as well-demarcated pale areas with telangiectasia. During the first 6 months these tend to grow rapidly but usually do not double in size. They then appear bright red. These lesions almost always involute spontaneously. No treatment is necessary unless the hemangioma overlies an eye, obstructs its vision, or interferes with some vital structure.

Cavernous hemangiomas contain larger vascular elements than are present in the strawberry hemangioma and do not involute as completely as the smaller lesions (Fig. 30-11). They grow in proportion to the growth of the child. His-

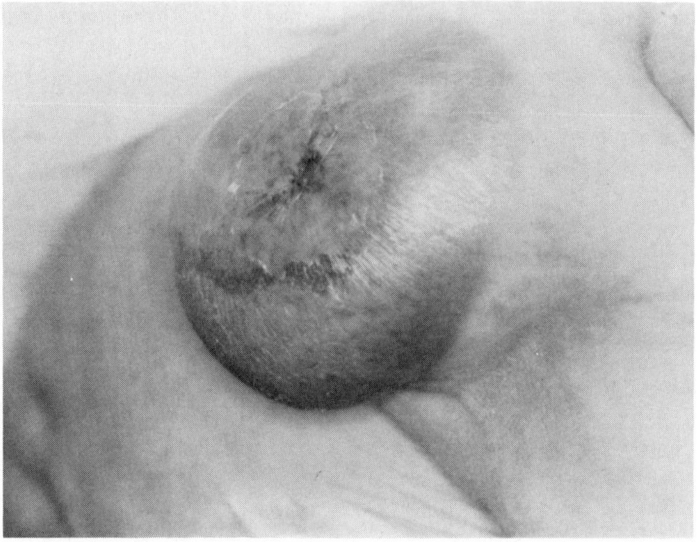

Fig. 30-11. Cavernous hemangioma. Notice central ulceration.

Table 30-4. Syndromes associated with cavernous hemangioma

Syndrome	Associated manifestations
Kasabach-Merritt	Thrombocytopenia that may result in hemorrhage
Klippel-Trenaunay-Parkes-Weber	Local overgrowth of bone and soft tissue by vascular elements resulting in hypertrophy of involved limb in both length and circumference
Maffucci	Dyschondroplasia associated with vascular hamartomas; patients clinically normal at birth develop multiple hemangiomata and dyschondroplasias seen as hard nodules on fingers and toes and then on remainder of extremities; 30% of patients develop chondrosarcoma or angiosarcoma

tologically, the vessels are lined by a single layer of endothelial cells. These lesions will undergo some degree of spontaneous involution in 90% of cases. Rarely, lesions may become extremely invasive, causing death from hemorrhage, infection, or high output congestive heart failure (see Table 30-4).

Dermatoses in the diaper area

Diaper dermatitis. Diaper dermatitis is a generalized term used to describe a cutaneous eruption in the pelvic girdle area. Usually, this eruption is characterized by erythema, inflammation, and maceration. This description, however, may apply to many cutaneous disorders, including candidiasis, irritant dermatitis, seborrheic dermatitis, and psoriasis. *Candida* infection will usually produce pustules and satellite lesions. A gram stain of a scraping from a pustule will reveal pseudohyphae and spores. Irritant dermatitis is localized to contact surfaces and spares the inguinal folds and skin creases. Seborrheic dermatitis tends to be more generalized and frequently is associated with cradle cap.

Psoriasis usually presents as localized placques that are resistant to conventional therapy for diaper dermatitis. Skin biopsy may be required to confirm the diagnosis.

Letterer-Siwe disease. Letterer-Siwe disease is a systemic histiocytic infiltrative disease that carries a grave prognosis. Clinically, these patients manifest scaly papules or vesicles usually involving the trunk or scalp. The eruption may be mild or severe and may be associated with secondary bacterial overgrowth and marked inflammation. This severe seborrheic–dermatitis-like condition is usually refractory to therapy and may be associated with petechiae. Biopsy of a petechial lesion will reveal the intense histiocytic perivascular infiltrate. Recent advances in systemic chemotherapy have improved the outlook for some of these patients.

Leiner disease. Leiner disease presents as greasy scaling of the skin, with underlying erythroderma and draining erosions and edema. This rare condition appears between the second and sixth months of age and is associated with a defect in the fifth component of complement. These infants are susceptible to gram-negative and *Candida* infections. They generally do well, but some may require blood transfusion therapy for C5 replacement.

Acrodermatitis enteropathica. Acrodermatitis enteropathica consists of the triad of periorificial dermatitis, diarrhea, and alopecia. The dermatitis consists of moist, erythematous lesions varying from papules and excoriations to vesiculobullae located characteristically at the orifices and acral areas. Infants may be listless and anorexic with growth retardation and foul-smelling stools. Systemic zinc replacement results in full resolution (see also pp. 166 and 167).

Juvenile xanthogranuloma. Xanthogranuloma in the infant appears as small red papules that evolve into discrete orange, golden, or brown nodules ranging in size from 2 to 8 mm. These lesions have a classical distribution involving the scalp, face, trunk, and proximal extremities, thus differentiating them from the lesions of infantile xanthoma associated with hypercholesteremia, which are distributed over the ankles, knees, and buttocks.

In the localized cutaneous form, juvenile xanthogranuloma is a self-limited benign disease that involutes spontaneously by age 5 years. If a child has juvenile xanthogranuloma associated with café au lait spots, or relatives with café au lait spots or neurofibromatosis, the child is at risk for the following disorders:

1. Subcutaneous orolaryngeal tumors.
2. Slight hepatomegaly, pulmonary infiltration of histiocytes, anemia, or leukocytosis.
3. Severe myeloproliferative disorders, including monomyeloid leukemia, hepatosplenomegaly, and pulmonary infiltration. The monomyeloid leukemia variant has a significant associated mortality.

Disorders of skin texture

The following cutaneous disorders appear as abnormalities in texture of the skin and not necessarily as discrete individual lesions.

Shagreen patch. Shagreen patch is a localized area of thickened collagen that on the surface appears as a firm diffuse patch with a papular-pebbly surface. Histologic examination reveals excessive collagen in the dermis. This nevus is a common feature of tuberous sclerosis.

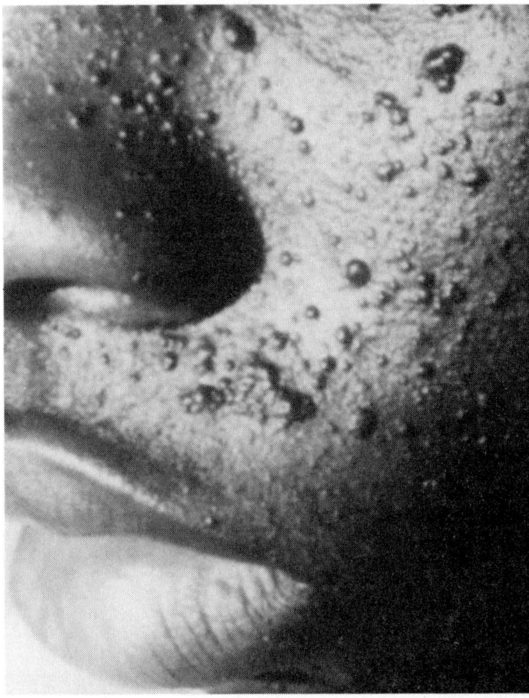

Fig. 30-12. Adenoma sebaceum in patient with tuberous sclerosis.

Neonatal fat necrosis. Fat necrosis in the neonate appears as reddish, firm, subcutaneous nodules and placques of various size, usually located over the cheeks, back, arms, and thighs. These areas appear indurated but are nonpitting. They are usually present shortly after birth but are not associated with trauma or ill health. During the next several weeks these lesions tend to soften and resolve spontaneously without atrophy.

Scleroderma neonatorum. The neonatal form of scleroderma is an infiltration of the skin in a symmetric distribution in which the dermis loses elasticity and becomes hard and cold. Progression to involve the entire integument is rapid and carries a grave prognosis. This is most common in critically ill premature neonates.

Adenoma sebaceum. Adenoma sebaceum are 1 to 3 mm size reddish-brown or flesh-colored smooth papules appearing over the sides of the nose and anterior cheeks (Fig. 30-12). Microscopic examination reveals that this lesion is an angiofibroma and not a sebaceous adenoma. When these are seen in clusters on the nose and cheeks, the diagnosis of tuberous sclerosis must be suspected. The presence of ash leaf spots, café au lait spots, a shagreen patch, and the history of seizures or mental ratardation will aid in the diagnosis. Intracerebral calcifications seen on computed tomography scan or skull radiographs can be helpful in diagnosis.

COMMON SKIN DISORDERS IN INFANTS AND CHILDREN

Acne

The treatment of acne has improved dramatically in recent years. Most patients with acne should achieve a satisfactory clinical result with straightforward office management.

Neonatal acne. Newborns may exhibit acne. It results when maternal hormones stimulate sebaceous glands of the face to make more oil than the small openings can easily empty. It goes away without treatment by the third or fourth month of age and ordinarily requires no management. When treatment is desired, very light application of 0.05% retinoic acid cream is safe and reasonably effective over a period of several weeks.

Adolescent acne. In Western societies acne is so common as to be almost expected in young people between the ages of 12 and 22. The reason for this great frequency is not at all understood. It has been suggested that Western diet may trigger acne by promoting earlier than desirable sexual maturation in 12-year-olds while the skin is still unready to cope with the demands placed on it.

Whether this is true or not, acne once developed is managed best by external therapy rather than by drastic changes in diet. The basis of topical therapy must be an understanding of the pathogenesis of the disease, and success in treating acne depends to a large degree on the patient's understanding of precisely the same factors of pathogenesis so he can manage the skin problems with minimal direction from the physician.

Ordinarily, acne begins about the nose and over the ensuing months and years spreads to the center portion of the cheeks, the forehead, the lateral portion of the cheeks, and the neck, back, and shoulders. At the same time that acne lesions are appearing on new portions of the face and upper trunk they are ordinarily disappearing from older ones. Thus a 13-year-old patient often has mild acne just on the center of his cheeks, whereas a 17-year-old patient with extensive acne on the lateral portion of his cheeks ordinarily has no lesions at all in the center.

Acne occurs when sebum is produced in quantities in excess of what the small, immature follicular openings can empty without plugging. Small children do not have acne because they make no sebum, even though their follicular openings are minute, and thus their skin has the characteristic smooth look of childhood. Most adults do not have acne, even though they make substantial quantities of sebum, because their facial follicular openings have achieved the characteristic large adult size. Adolescents are caught in the middle of this, making some sebum but having openings not yet large enough.

Patients with acne must understand that they will outgrow the disease when their skin develops the typical adult-size openings. In the meantime, it is necessary to take steps to try to prevent the openings from plugging. Once this happens, oil is trapped and the complicating bacterial invasion leads ultimately to the fully developed acne lesion.

Principles of treatment are listed below.

1. Avoid the application of anything to affected areas that will increase the tendency to plugging. This includes oily or lubricating soaps, oil-containing make-up, most suntan lotions, and rubbing by overlying hair.

2. Apply a preparation that will cause a mild peeling of follicular plugs. Benzoyl peroxide seems to be the most useful agent for this, and many patients can be managed with nothing more than nightly applications of benzoyl peroxide products. These are available both over-the-counter and in prescription brands in 2.5% to 10% strength. The right way to use benzoyl peroxide is to apply a little bit every night to the affected area whether there are pimples in that area or not. The treatment is designed to produce a mild erythema that looks more or less like that produced by a half-hour of sunshine. Over a period of weeks the production of new pimples decreases. The treatment must be continued until the disease is outgrown.

3. Treatment with topical antibiotics. The difference between a small plugged follicular opening and the inflamed red pustule seems in

most cases to be due to bacterial invasion. Topical antibiotics are then helpful and can be applied 2 or 3 times a day. Clindamycin is the most frequently prescribed topical antibiotic. Other useful ones are erythromycin and tetracycline. The advantage of a topical antibiotic is that, unlike topical benzoyl peroxide and topical retinoic acid, it does not cause appreciable skin irritation or erythema. It is an excellent agent to be used in conjunction with either benzoyl peroxide or retinoic acid.

4. Treatment with retinoic acid. This derivative of vitamin A makes the superficial layers of stratum corneum thinner. The follicular walls become thinner and the affected opening becomes slightly wider. There is thus less tendency for follicular plugging. There is a possibility that by virtue of its tendency to thin the stratum corneum it also increases the penetration of topical antibiotic. The side effect of topical retinoic acid is redness and chapping, quite similar to that caused by benzoyl peroxide. Some patients can use and need both retinoic acid and benzoyl peroxide, but the two agents should not be started simultaneously. Once a patient is comfortable with one he can usually add the second.

5. Treatment with tetracycline by mouth. This is also an effective agent in control of acne. However, recent studies have shown that topical antibiotics are as good as, or almost as good as, oral tetracycline. In general, it seems wiser to stay with them and to reserve the use of systemic antibiotics for patients who do not respond to topical ones.

6. The newest agent for the treatment of acne is 13-Cis retinoic acid (isotretinoin, Accutane). It is a synthetic retinoid analogue of vitamin A, similar to the topical product retinoic acid. Taken by mouth, it is profoundly effective in diminishing sebaceous flow and in reversing the course of acne. Because of the number of side effects, Accutane is indicated in the less than 5% of acne patients who do not respond to the full panoply of conventional treatment with benzoyl peroxide, topical retinoic acid, and topical and systemic antibiotics. When used in the resistant cases for which it is indicated, isotretinoin seems to be effective in some 90% of treated patients.

Dermatitis

Seborrheic dermatitis. Seborrheic dermatitis is the name given to a characteristic scaly erythema occurring on the scalp, eyebrows, mid-chest, groin, umbilicus, and axillae (Fig. 30-13). It is seen commonly in newborns, where it is associated with thick, greasy scales (''cradle cap'') and a nonpruritic erythema most evident deep in the folds and crevices of the baby's limbs. By age 3 or 4 months this infantile seb-

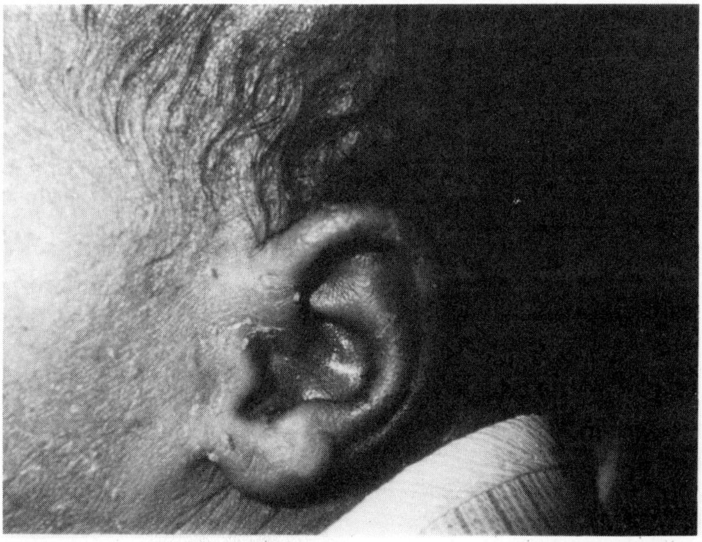

Fig. 30-13. Seborrheic dermatitis of infancy. Notice scaling of scalp, cheek, and ears.

orrheic eczema has cleared; the condition is rare in little children. (Scaly conditions of the scalp should not be attributed to seborrheic dermatitis when seen in small children. Most such scalp diseases in children have microbial causes, usually an inapparent fungus infection or a bacterial folliculitis.)

Seborrheic dermatitis recurs as dandruff and as an erythema in the characteristic sites at puberty and is common through adult life.

The present consensus is to consider seborrheic dermatitis a disease of unknown cause and to manage it empirically. In the past, seborrheic dermatitis was thought to be caused by the yeast *Malassezia ovalis (Pityrosporum ovale),* which is an important part of the normal flora in the so-called seborrheic areas. The occurrence of the disease in infancy and again in adolescence and beyond is thought to be related to a hormonal effect on sebaceous gland function in those areas at those ages. The *Malassezia ovalis* is a lipophilic yeast that increases in number in areas of abundant sebaceous flow. An important distinction from atopic dermatitis is that seborrheic dermatitis ordinarily does not induce scratching. Also, the infant with seborrheic dermatitis is ordinarily younger than the one with atopic eczema, the latter disease being rare before the fourth of fifth month.

Whatever the cause, seborrheic dermatitis does best when treated with topical corticosteroid and with agents that kill the yeast. Combinations of miconazole or clotrimazole cream along with hydrocortisone are useful in treating seborrheic dermatitis of the glabrous skin. Cradle cap is effectively treated with sulfur and salicylic acid creams (Pragmatar), as well as the usual dandruff shampoos such as Selsun or Fostex.

Hard-to-treat cases of seborrheic dermatitis must be suspected of being psoriasis, a disease that shares both clinical and histologic features with seborrheic dermatitis. Although relatively rare in children, psoriasis is far from unknown and should be considered in otherwise hard to understand cases of seborrheic dermatitis.

Atopic dermatitis (see also Chapter 26). Some 10% of the general population apparently inherit a tendency to either asthma, eczema, or hay fever. The term *atopic dermatitis* or *infantile eczema* is used for skin manifestation of the atopic state.

The condition ordinarily manifests itself at age 4 to 6 months and frequently appears as redness on the cheeks or a patchy, somewhat irritated erythema. An important differentiating point from seborrheic dermatitis and other forms of eczema is the intense itching that characterizes atopic dermatitis. Severely affected infants are fretful, fussy, and very uncomfortable because of itching. In small children the diagnosis is best made by the combination of intense itching and family history. The characteristic distribution of atopic dermatitis is an unreliable guide to diagnosis in infants.

Most infants with eczema experience some degree of relief as they reach age 3 or 4 years. The disease worsens at puberty, this time in the characteristic distribution of the sides of the neck, elbow and knee creases, flexor surfaces of the wrists, and to a lesser degree on other parts of the trunk. Distribution of the disease in older children is more helpful in diagnosis than specific appearance of individual areas. Depending on stage and severity of the disease, affected areas of skin may look red, oozing, crusted, or thick and lichenified. Sometimes all phases are seen at once, and not infrequently the dermatitis is complicated by secondary bacterial infection, with further redness and purulence present. There is no general agreement about the mechanism of atopic dermatitis. In most cases the kinds of allergic management that depend on scratch testing and desensitization do not appear to work nearly so well as they do for hay fever or asthma.

Treatment of atopic dermatitis is strictly palliative. A tendency to dry skin can be managed by the use of lubricating soap (Dove) and the addition of oil to the bath tub. An inexpensive homemade bath oil may be made by mixing 1½ caps full of Joy dishwashing solution in a pint of mineral oil. This is shaken up, and an ounce or so is added to the tub when bathing. A bland lubricating cream such as Eucerin may also be useful.

Topical corticosteroids are the mainstay of management. If possible, control should be attempted with use of 1% hydrocortisone cream. This will avoid possible complications of the more potent substituted corticosteroid products. When indicated, the stronger creams can be used in limited amounts for short periods. Tars are presently enjoying a comeback in the management of atopic dermatitis. These are available in somewhat weak forms as Chester Baker's P&S Plus Cream, or as an old-fashioned 5% crude coal tar in zinc oxide ointment that must be mixed by the pharmacist. Oral antipruritics such as diphenhydramine or hydroxyzine may be used with caution.

The use of systemic corticosteroids in atopic dermatitis is almost always a mistake and should be resisted strongly.

Most patients with eczema do fairly well most of the time. Although severe flares of eczema may sometimes be caused by the natural course of the disease, in most cases they represent one of two complicating factors. These are either secondary infection, usually with *Staphylococcus aureus,* or an acquired intolerance to one of the topical products that is being applied. A useful strategy to follow in case of severely flaring eczema is to obtain a bacterial culture and sensitivity of the organisms from the skin, treat with an appropriate systemic antibiotic, and discontinue the previous topical therapy. When topical therapy is thought to be causing irritation, a nonsensitizing and nonirritating product can be made with 5 g of 0.5% Aristocort cream in Crisco shortening to make 240 g. This gives a 0.01% triamcinolone acetonide cream that is roughly as potent as 1% hydrocortisone. The ordinary cream base of the triamcinolone is highly diluted in the Crisco and can be tolerated by most patients, including those who have a sensitivity to the preservatives and other ingredients of ordinary dermatologic vehicles.

In other instances in which patients find themselves unable to tolerate conventional therapy an alternative treatment program consists of having the patient first apply a few drops of .01% Synalar solution to the skin and then cover the skin with Cetaphil lotion. This is repeated twice a day, and these two agents are the only ones to touch the skin. No ointments or creams are ever used in this program. The applications of Cetaphil replace the ordinary use of baths for cleansing (Scholtz regimen).

Warts

Warts are a common affliction of children. They are caused by the wart virus and are considered mildly contagious from one child to another but are not an indication for any kind of protective isolation; their contagiousness is not an indication for immediate treatment. (This is in contradistinction to lesions of *Molluscum contagiosum,* which are highly contagious both by autoinnoculation of the affected child and by transmission to other children. Any lesion of *M. contagiosum* once diagnosed should be treated with as little delay as possible, and repeat visits should be scheduled in a timely enough fashion to ensure eradication of the infection.)

The main difference between the experienced and inexperienced physician in the management of warts is that the former knows his limitations, makes no promises, and knows that there are really no experts. Based on a large experiment in Edinburgh, Bunney and her collaborators showed that the best treatment for most warts is the careful application of minute quantities of a salicylic acid–lactic acid in collodion mixture such as Duofilm. This treatment should be continued daily for 12 weeks before any decision about further treatment is made. It can be expected to cure some 60% to 80% of all warts, including hand warts, plantar warts, and even some periungual warts.

Another useful treatment of warts is the application of 40% salicylic acid plaster. A small piece of this plaster is cut precisely to the size of the wart and held in place with an additional piece of adhesive tape. The wart underneath becomes soft and macerated and can be wiped off in stages over a period of several weeks. This is a particularly useful treatment for plantar warts.

Genital and perianal warts are not ordinarily a problem in small children. When they need to be treated the application of a very small amount of 15% to 25% podophyllum in alcohol, or compound benzoin tincture, repeated once or twice a week for several weeks is the classic treatment. Presence of such lesions in small children should raise suspicions of aberrant sexual practice in the household.

Dermatologists will sometimes treat warts with repeated applications of liquid nitrogen or with the electrodesiccating needle.

Flat warts or juvenile warts are sometimes hard to diagnose. They appear as small, round, only slightly elevated, tan to red spots on children's cheeks. Similar lesions may be seen on legs, particularly in young women who are shaving their legs. These very superficial warts will sometimes respond to the kind of peeling medicines that are ordinarily used to treat acne. These include retinoic acid cream and sulfur-containing products such as Fostex. A traditional acne treatment sometimes useful in treating flat warts is the nightly application of Vleminckx's solution in the form of hot compresses. Bunney's book on the treatment of warts is recommended highly and deserves a place in most pediatric libraries.

INFECTIONS OF THE SKIN

Superficial fungal infections

Superficial fungal infections occur on the skin, nails, and hair.

Superficial fungal infections of the skin classically present as red, scaly patches with a heaped-up advancing border and a clearing center. However, dermatitic, pustular, vesicular, hyperkeratotic, and granulomatous lesions may be caused by a fungus. Diagnosis is accomplished by microscopic examination of potassium hydroxide (KOH) preparation of skin scrapings and culture of skin scrapings on Sabouraud's agar. Topical antifungal agents usually clear most fungal infections of skin, but oral griseofulvin is sometimes needed in extensive infections. Commonly isolated organisms are *Microsporum canis, Microsporum audouini, Trichophyton mentagrophytes,* and *Trichophyton rubrum*.

Onychomycosis. Onychomycosis (fungus infection of the nail) is uncommonly seen in children. Usually only one or several nails are involved; seldom are all affected. Nails appear opaque white, yellow, or brown and are thickened, deformed, and lifted off the nail plate by subungual debris. The diagnosis is made by microscopic examination of KOH preparations of subungual debris. Treatment is with oral griseofulvin for 6 months for fingernail infections and up to 18 months for toenail infections. Commonly isolated organisms are *Trichophyton rubrum* and *Trichophyton mentagrophytes*.

Tinea capitis. Fungal infection of the scalp *(tinea capitis)* occurs frequently in pediatric patients. The two organisms most commonly responsible are *Trichophyton tonsurans* and *Microsporum audouini. T. tonsurans,* the most common organism, produces the "black dot" type of infection. Clinically, this infection appears as alopecia studded with numerous black dots (Fig. 30-14). The black dots are actually

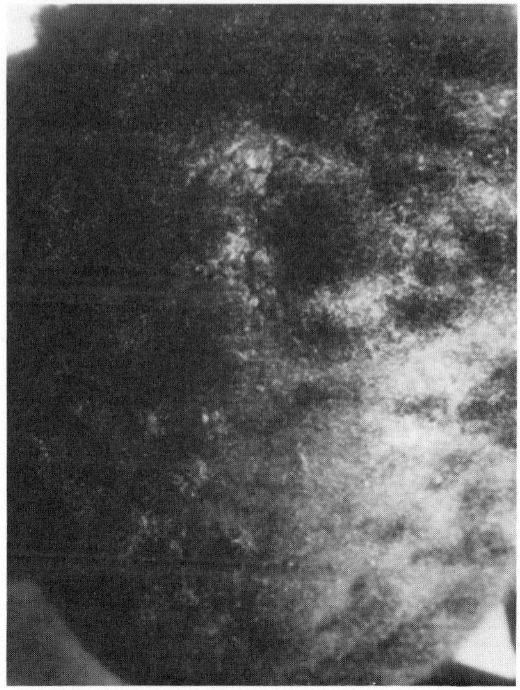

Fig. 30-14. Tinea capitis. Notice thick scale and diffuse alopecia.

short hairs that are broken off near the skin surface. When these black dots are extracted with a needle and examined microscopically, the dots reveal short hairs filled with endospores.

M. audouini produces the so-called gray patch ringworm type of tinea capitis. This infection appears as circular areas of alopecia with scaly erythematous centers and heaped-up borders. Broken hairs are also apparent but are several millimeters long. An accelerated inflammatory response consisting of a well-demarcated boggy tumefaction is called a kerion. This type of response is not specific and is seen in tinea capitis caused by most of the common dermatophytes. Diagnosis of tinea capitis is accomplished by microscopic examination of scales or black dots and culture on Sabouraud agar. The Wood's light (blacklight) examination for fluorescent broken hairs is useful only in *Microsporum* infections and is negative in Trichophyton-induced ringworm. Because the latter is now the overwhelmingly more common of the two kinds of infection, Wood's light examination is of much less importance than a microscopic search for spores in broken hairs or a positive culture. Oral griseofulvin is required to cure tinea capitis.

Tinea versicolor. Tinea versicolor is a common superficial fungal infection caused by *Pityrosporum orbiculare*. The lesions are circular macules that may be either hypopigmented or hyperpigmented. The upper trunk, front and back, is most commonly affected, but any area may be involved. Diagnosis is made by microscopic examination of skin scrapings revealing the characteristic short filaments and clusters of spores (''spaghetti and meat ball'' appearance). Treatment consists of topical imidazole antifungals, Tinver lotion, or any dandruff shampoo such as Selsun, Head and Shoulders, or Sebulex. Recurrence is common.

Impetigo. Streptococci and staphylococci both produce the superficial skin infection called impetigo, although the clinical presentations differ in appearance. Streptococci produce vesicopustular lesions that rupture and exude a yellow, serous fluid. This fluid dries, producing the thick honey-colored crusts characteristic of group A beta-hemolytic streptococcal infections. Staphylococci produce bullous lesions initially containing a clear yellow fluid that subsequently becomes cloudy and dark yellow. When these bullous lesions rupture, a thin brown crust is produced characteristic of phage group II staphylococci. Soap and water and topical antibiotics may be effective treatment for impetigo, but oral antibiotics produce a more rapid clinical response. Oral erythromycin is the drug of choice and is usually effective for both staphylococcal and streptococcal impetigo. Cases resistant to erythromycin (usually of mixed staphylococcal and streptococcal origin) and severe bullous infections should be treated with oral dicloxacillin. Glomerulonephritis is an uncommon complication of streptococcal impetigo, but it should be observed for if a nephritogenic strain of streptococcus has been reported in the community.

Folliculitis (Bockhart impetigo). Superficial folliculitis is usually caused by *Staphylococcus aureus* infection of the hair follicle opening. The lesions are small pustules with a central hair and surrounding erythema. Common locations include the scalp, buttocks, arms, and legs, but any hair-bearing area may be affected. Soap and water and topical antibiotics usually are effective for treatment, but oral antibiotics are needed for severe or resistant infections.

Ecthyma. Ecthyma is a deep pyoderma caused by group A beta-hemolytic streptococcus. Ecthyma begins as a vesiculopustular eruption with surrounding erythema-like impetigo, but quickly penetrates through the epidermis to produce a shallow ulcer. The ulcer has a punched-out appearance when the thick, dirty, gray crust is removed. These lesions occur most commonly on the lower extremities of children and are painful and slow growing. Treatment consists of gentle debridement and systemic antibiotics. *Pseudomonas* sepsis may also produce a clinically similar lesion.

Cellulitis. Cellulitis is a rapidly spreading inflammation of the skin extending to the subcutaneous tissue. The affected area is tender, erythematous, edematous, and warm, but the borders are not well circumscribed or elevated. The two most common organisms producing cellulitis are group A beta-hemolytic streptococci and *Staphylococcus aureus*. In children under 2 years of age, *Haemophilus influenzae* commonly produces a characteristic dusky red to purple cellulitis. Treatment is with systemic antibiotics based on clinical evaluation and Gram stain, culture, and sensitivity pattern of organisms recovered by needle aspiration.

Erysipelas. Erysipelas is a superficial type of skin cellulitis with intense lymphatic involvement. The involved area is hot, tender, edematous, brawny, and bright red, with an advancing border that is raised and well demarcated. Erysipelas is usually produced by group A beta-hemolytic streptococci infection, but staphylococci can coexist. Penicillin is the treatment of choice, but a penicillinase-resistant penicillin is necessary if penicillin does not produce the usual rapid response.

Staphylococcal scalded skin syndrome (see also p. 725). The staphylococcal scalded skin syndrome is clinically similar to the usually drug-induced toxic epidermal necrolysis seen in adults. The syndrome is preceded by a staphylococcal infection. Clinical manifestations are produced by an exfoliative toxin (exfoliation) elaborated by group II staphylococci. The staphylococcal infection is usually of the conjunctivae, middle ear, nose, or pharynx. Tender patches of erythema develop after a prodrome of fever, malaise, and irritability. Large flaccid bullae follow the erythema. These lead to desquamation of large sheets of stratum corneum. Nikolsky's sign (shearing of skin with pressure) is positive in noninvolved areas, and mucous membranes are spared. Patients are treated with a penicillinase-resistant penicillin. The prognosis is good.

Erythema multiforme. Clinical manifestations of erythema multiforme vary from a mild cutaneous disorder to a life-threatening multisystem disorder. Erythema multiforme presents a polymorphous appearance because of the waxing and waning of new crops of macular, urticarial, and vesicobullous lesions. The characteristic lesion of erythema multiforme is the iris or target lesion, which is an urticarial plaque with a dusky or vesicular center. This lesion is considered diagnostic of erythema multiforme and should be sought on the palms, soles, and extensor surfaces.

Erythema multiforme has many causes, the commonest of which are infections and drug reactions. Frequently reported infectious agents include *Mycoplasma* and herpes simplex, as well as other viruses. *Mycoplasma* infection responds to treatment with tetracycline or erythromycin. Viral agents are treated symptomatically.

Drugs reported to cause erythema multiforme include penicillin, phenolpthalein, sulfonamides, barbiturates, salicylates, hydantoins, halogens, phenylbutazone, and tetracycline. If a drug is the suspected etiologic agent it must be discontinued.

Other less common causes of erythema multiforme include malignancies, connective tissue diseases, and numerous bacterial, fungal, and protozoan infections.

Wet compresses may be used for erosive lesions. Analgesics are indicated for pain. Antihistamines are sometimes effective for relief of pruritus.

The severe form of erythema multiforme is called Stevens-Johnson syndrome. This may be preceded by a prodrome of flulike symptoms. It is a multisystem disorder and necessitates hospitalization. The same factors that produce erythema multiforme also produce Stevens-Johnson syndrome, but drug causes predominate. Severe mucous membrane ulceration produces the most disabling problem, as patients have difficulty eating. Most patients respond to viscous lidocaine and liquid diet. However, with severe oral involvement intravenous nutrition is required. Ocular, pulmonary, and renal complications may occur. Systemic steroid treatment for Stevens-Johnson syndrome is controversial. The most recent studies suggest that oral steroid therapy leads to more complications and affords no benefit.

Erythema nodosum. Lesions of erythema nodosum are characteristically red, tender nodules that last from 2 to 6 weeks and resolve, leaving ecchymotic areas. The most common location is the anterior tibial region, but lesions can occur anywhere on the body. The most common causes of erythema nodosum in children are streptococcal infections, upper respiratory infections, and primary tuberculosis. Other less common causes are sarcoidosis, histoplasmosis, ulcerative colitis, regional enteritis, lymphogranuloma venereum, psittacosis, coccidiodomycosis, and yersiniosis. Drugs such as iodides, sulfonamides, and oral contraceptives have been reported to cause erythema nodosum. Treatment of erythema nodosum is with bedrest and nonsteroidal antiinflammatory agents.

DISEASES OF HAIR AND SCALP

Alopecia

Alopecia areata. The usual clinical presentation of alopecia areata is a well-circumscribed, circular patch of alopecia, with smooth normal scalp completely devoid of hair. On the periphery of the alopecic area, short stubby hairs (''exclamation point'' hairs) can sometimes be found. Fine stippling of nails is occasionally associated with alopecia areata. Multiple patches may arise and coalesce, leading to alopecia totalis (complete loss of scalp hair) in less than 10% of cases. Loss of hair beginning in the occipital area and advancing anteriorally along the hair margin is called ophiasis, and portends a poor prognosis. The cause of alopecia areata is unknown. Recent opinion is that it may be caused by an immune disorder.

A variety of treatments have been advanced for alopecia areata in children, including applications of topical steroids, injection of intralesional steroids, contact sensitization, and irritant provocation with anthralin. Their multiplicity suggests their questionable efficacy. Topical Minoxidil is currently being evaluated as a possible treatment. Because approximately 95% of children with alopecia areata completely regrow hair within 1 year, reassurance and a wait-and-see attitude are indicated as the initial management.

Telogen effluvium. A number of factors including febrile illness, surgery, starvation diets, severe emotional stress, accidents, certain drugs, discontinuation of birth control pills, and childbirth can alter the hair cycle by placing a greater than normal percentage of hairs (greater than 15%) in the telogen phase of growth. When these hairs begin a new anagen phase, a shedding of hair occurs. Thus about 2 to 4 months after a stressful event a diffuse thinning and excess daily loss of hair occurs. Unless there is a recurrence of the stressful event, complete regrowth of hair is the usual result.

Trichotillomania. Angular and odd-shaped areas of alopecia are the usual presentation of trichotillomania. The area of alopecia is never completely bald, and short, broken hairs of varying lengths remain. The hair is removed either consciously or unconsciously. One should look for an underlying psychologic disorder. Ointments or oils that make hair slippery aid in the treatment of this difficult-to-treat disorder.

Traction alopecia. Plaiting, or braiding, of hair may lead to alopecia in areas in which the hair is subjected to pulling stress. These areas usually occur in the frontal and temporal areas but may occur anywhere on the scalp, depending on hair style. If the braiding is continued over a long period of time, hair may not regrow in the alopecic area. Sudden patchy loss of hair in children with broken hairs in the alopecic area suggests the possibility of child abuse. Such lesions are caused by abusive parents yanking on the child's hair.

Scarring alopecia. Scarring alopecia can be the end result of many disorders, including traction alopecia of long duration, severe viral, bacterial, and fungal infections, trichotillomania of long duration, burns, lichen planus, lupus erythematosus, and scleroderma. Once scarring alopecia has developed, hair will not regrow in the affected area.

PRINCIPLES OF DERMATOLOGIC TREATMENT

Wet compresses. The basic principle in topical therapy of skin disease is to use bland, soothing treatment on severely and acutely inflamed skin and stronger forms of therapy on older or more indolent eruptions. Translated into actual practice, this means that the best single treatment for the most severely inflamed skin is immersion in a tub of tepid tap water. Lesser degrees of inflammation can be treated with continuous or intermittent compresses of cool to tepid tap water soaked into soft cotton cloth, such as old torn-up pillow cases or sheeting.

Topical corticosteroids. The mainstay of treating most inflammatory skin disease is the application of a topical corticosteroid. There are some special precautions to be used in children in whom adrenal suppression from absorption of the more potent substituted corticosteroid molecules may be a problem. In general it is best to go no higher in strength than 1% hydrocortisone as the initial treatment for inflammatory skin disease in infants and children. Complications induced by the more potent substituted products include not only adrenal suppression but also the development of local atrophy and striae at sites of prolonged application. However, there will be instances in which 1% hydrocortisone is not strong enough to produce the desired effect; in those cases stronger products may be used. This must be done, however, with a clear understanding that their use is to be limited as much as possible and for a temporary period only. Hydrocortisone is a safe and effective product for nonprescription use at 0.5%. A 1% strength is a reasonable prescription that can be written without hesitation by the pediatrician for children of any age. Stronger corticosteroid products should be prescribed in 15 g amounts only, with a strict control over refills.

Tar. Tar ointments have been a traditional bulwark of dermatologic therapy. With the recognition that strong corticosteroid creams may induce unwanted side effects, tars are now enjoying somewhat of a revival. There are several proprietary products available in strengths of 1% to 3%. The classic tar ointment (which patients may find difficult to have mixed) is 5% crude coal tar in zinc oxide ointment. Tars are most useful in indolent and chronic forms of inflammation to be used in place of, or as an adjunct to, the stronger corticosteroid products.

Antimicrobial therapy. In general, it seems best to treat bacterial infections of the skin with systemic antibiotics, reserving antibiotic ointments for very minor problems of bacterial infection. Conversely, most fungal and yeast infections of the skin should respond to topical antifungals of the imidazole class, with systemic griseofulvin therapy reserved for fungus infections of the scalp or nails and for unusually severe forms of fungus infections of the skin.

Michael J. Bond
Robert B. Skinner, Jr.
E. William Rosenberg

REFERENCES

Abramson, J.S., et al.: Antistaphylococcal IgE in patients with atopic dermatitis, J. Am. Acad. Dermatol. **7**(1):105-110, 1982.

Albright, F.: Syndrome characterized by osteitis fibrosa disseminata, areas of pigmentation and a gonadal dysfunction, Endocrinology **22:**411-426, 1938.

Argyle, J.C., and Zone, J.: Dermal erythropoieses in neonates, Arch. Dermatol. **117:**492-494, 1981.

Bauer, E.A., and Cooper, T.W.: Therapeutic consideration in recessive dystrophic epidermolysis bullosa, Arch. Dermatol. **117:**529-530, 1981.

Bauer, E.A., et al.: Phenytoin therapy of recessive dystrophic epidermolysis bullosa, N. Engl. J. Med. **303**(14):776-781, 1980.

Brough, A.J., et al.: Dermal erythropoiesis in neonatal infants: a manifestation of intrauterine viral disease, Pediatrics **40:**627-635, 1967.

Bunney, M.H.: Viral warts: their biology and treatment, New York, 1982, Oxford University Press.

Carney, R.G.: Incontentia pigmenti: a world statistical analysis, Arch. Dermatol. **112:**535-542, 1976.

Carr, J.A., et al.: Relationship between toxic erythema and infant maturity, Am. J. Dis. Child **112:**129-134, 1966.

Chi'en, L.T., et al.: Antiviral chemotherapy and neonatal herpes simplex virus infections: a pilot study–experience with adenine arabinoside (ARA-A), Pediatrics **55:**678-685, 1975.

Cooper, L.Z., et al.: Neonatal thrombocytopenic purpura and other manifestations of rubella contracted in utero, Arch. J. Dis. Child **110:**416-427, 1965.

Crowe, F.W.: Axillary freckling as a diagnostic aid in neurofibromatosis, Ann. Intern. Med. **61:**1142-1143, 1962.

Crowe, F.W., and Schull, W.J.: Diagnostic importance of the Café au lait spot in neurofibromatosis, Arch. Intern. Med. **91:**758-786, 1963.

Fitzpatrick T., et al.: Dermatology in general medicine, New York, 1979, McGraw-Hill Book Co.

DesGrosciliers, J.P., and Brisson, P.: Localized epidermolysis bullosa, Arch. Dermatol. **109:**70-72, 1974.

Eisenberg, M., et al.: Epidermolysis bullosa—new therapeutic approaches, Aust. J. Dermatol. **19**(1):1-8, 1978.

Farber, E.M., et al.: Recent advances in the treatment of psoriasis, J. Am. Acad. Dermatol. **8**(3):311-321, 1983.

Fitzpatrick, T.B., et al.: White leaf shaped macules: earliest visible sign of tuberous sclerosis, Arch. Dermatol. **98:**1-6, 1968.

Frost, P., and Vanscott, E.J.: Ichthyosiform dermatoses, Arch. Dermatol. **94:**113-126, 1966.

Gerson, A.A.: Herpes simplex infections. In Gelles, S.S., and Kagan, B.M., editors: Current pediatric therapy, ed. 8, Philadelphia, 1978, W.B. Saunders Co.

Hanifin, J.M.: Diet, nutrition and allergy in atopic dermatitis, J. Am. Acad. Dermatol. **8**(5):729-731, 1983.

Harter, C.A., and Benerscke, K.: Fetal syphilis in the first trimester, Am. J. Obstet. Gynecol. **124:**705-711, 1976.

Harper, V.A., and Rutter, N.: Sweating in preterm babies, J. Pediatr. **100**(4):614-618, 1982.

Hendrickson, M.R., and Ross, J.C.: Neoplasma arising in congenital giant nevi: morphological study of seven cases and a review of the literature, Am. J. Surg. Pathol. **5:**109-135, 1981.

Hurwitz, S.: Clinical pediatric dermatology, Philadelphia, 1981, W.B. Saunders Co.

Jacobs, A.H.: Pediatric dermatology, Pediatr. Clin. North Am. **25:**189, 1978.

Kaplan, E.: The risk of malignancy in large congenital nevi, Plast. Reconstr. Surg. **53**(4):421-428, 1974.

Kaplan, J.M., and McCrackin, G.H.: Clinical pharmacology of benzathine penicillin G in neonates with regard to its recommended use in congenital syphilis, J. Pediatr. **82:**1069-1072, 1973.

Kietel, H.G., and Yadav, V.: Etiology of toxic erythema, Am. J. Dis. Child **106:**306-309, 1963.

Komorous, J.M., et al.: Intrauterine herpes simplex infections, Arch. Dermatol. **113:**918-922, 1977.

Leyden, J.J., and Kligman, A.M.: The role of microorganisms in diaper dermatitis, Arch. Dermatol. **114:**56-59, 1978.

Lentz, C.L., and Altman, J.: Lamellar ichthyosis: the natural course of collodion baby, Arch. Dermatol. **97:**3-13, 1968.

Mansour, A., and Gelfand, E.W.: New approach to the use of antifungal agents in infants with persistent oral candidiasis, J. Pediatr. **98**(1):161-162, 1981.

Manues, P., et al.: Early diagnosis of neonatal syphilis: evaluation of a gamma M fluorescent treponemal antibody test, Am. J. Dis. Child **120:**17-21, 1970.

Marino, L.J.: Toxic erythema present at birth, Arch. Derm. **92:**402-403, 1965.

Mark, G.J., et al.: Congenital melanocytic nevi of the small and garment type clinical, histologic and ultrastructural studies, Hum. Pathol. **4**(3):395-418, 1973.

Mulliken, J.B., and Glowacki, J.: Hemangiomas and vascular malformations in infants and children: a classification based on endothelial characteristics, Plast. Reconstr. Surg. **69**(3):412-420, 1982.

Nahmias, A.J., et al.: Significance of herpes simplex viral infections during pregnancy, Clin. Obstet. Gynecol. **15:**929-938, 1972.

Pearson, R.W., et al.: Epidermolysis bullosa hereditaria letalis, Arch. Dermatol. **109:**349-355, 1974.

Ramamurthy, R.S., et al.: Transient neonatal pustular melanosis, J. Pediatr. **88:**831-835, 1976.

Rhodes, A.R., et al.: Nonepidermal origin of malignant melanoma associated with a giant congenital nevocellular nevus, Plast. Reconstr. Surg. **67**(6):782-790, 1981.

Robinson, R.C.V.: Congenital syphilis—review article, Arch. Dermatol. **99:**599-610, 1979.

Rosenberg, B.S., and Krib, B.S.: Acne diet reconsidered, Arch. Dermatol. **117:**193-195, 1981.

Silvers, D.N., and Helwig, E.B.: Melanocytic nevi in neonates, J. Am. Acad. Dermatol. **4:**166-175, 1981.

Solomon, L.M.: The management of congenital melanocytic nevi, Arch. Dermatol. **116:**1017, 1980.

Solomon, L.M., and Esterly, N.B.: Transient cutaneous lesions. In neonatal dermatology, Philadelphia, 1973, W.B. Saunders Co.

Stein, H.: Diaper rash with cloth versus disposable diapers, J. Pediatr. **107**(5):721-723, 1982.

Szentivanyi, A.: The beta adrenergic theory of the atopic abnormality in bronchial asthma, Allergy **42:**203, 1968.

Turner, R., et al.: Shedding and survival of herpes simplex virus from "fever blisters," Pediatrics **70**(4):547-549, 1982.

Wells, R.S., and Kerr, C.B.: Genetic classification of ichthyosis, Arch. Dermatol. **92:**1-6, 1965.

31 Cancer in Childhood

Cancer is the leading cause of death from disease in children between the ages of 1 and 15. Types of cancer seen in children are different from those seen in adults. Although treatment principles for cancer at any age are similar, programs designed for the specific tumors of children vary considerably from those used for treatment of adult cancers. Furthermore, treatment of the child with cancer must take into account other important features such as growth and development.

There are about 6000 newly diagnosed children with cancer in this country annually. Because of these limited numbers, it has become customary to refer a child with cancer to a center where sufficient facilities and experience are available to provide the best treatment. Most of these centers work in close cooperation with the referring physician to provide the kind of continuous care and support needed for the child and the family. In spite of the fact that at diagnosis most children with cancer have dissemination of their tumor beyond the site of origin, more than half the affected children can achieve cure with proper treatment. This improved outlook has developed during the past 20 years, and one can anticipate continued advances in the future.

After some general remarks concerning cancer in childhood, this chapter discusses the specific tumors seen most frequently in this age group. Leukemia is the most common form of childhood cancer, accounting for about one third of the total cases. Next in line are a group of tumors with a similar incidence. Brain tumors, the second most frequent form of cancer in children, are discussed on pp. 789 to 791. The other solid tumors in children account for a remaining one half and are made up of uncommon tumor types.

ETIOLOGY

In adults most cancers occur on such exposed surfaces as skin, lung, gut, and bladder. It is believed that most adult cancers are caused by exposure of these surfaces to a variety of environmental agents. In contrast, in children most cancers occur in deep tissues such as blood and bone marrow, brain, kidney, neural crest tissue, and skeletal tissues. The number of environmental agents implicated in the cause of childhood cancer is very few. It is important to realize that in utero exposure to carcinogens has been related to subsequent development of cancer during childhood. For example, diethylstilbestrol was given to mothers to prevent miscarriages, causing vaginal cancer in female offspring during the second decade of life. Presumably, other carcinogens taken by mothers during pregnancy could similarly affect offspring, but no other specific instances have been identified.

Irradiation to the head and neck area during infancy and childhood has been related to subsequent development of thyroid cancer. Other physical and chemical agents have been only rarely implicated as a cause of cancer in children.

At this time there has been no definitive demonstration that oncogenic viruses are implicated in cancer of childhood. Some children with cancer, however, had predisposing conditions that increased their risk of specific forms of cancer in some as yet unknown manner. Such conditions are the immunodeficiency states, which predispose primarily to lymphoid malignancies; renal dysplasia associated with the development of Wilms tumor; repair defects for DNA, such as ataxia-telangiectasia and xeroderma pigmentosum (with increased susceptibility to ionizing irradiation); and chromosomal abnormalities such as Down syndrome, which increase the risk of leukemia. In other children there appear to be single-gene disorders, unassociated with specific phenotypic markers, that enhance the susceptibility to developing specific cancers. One such heritable form of cancer is retinoblastoma, which will be discussed specifically later in this chapter. It appears that in most common childhood cancers a specific proportion of patients inherited the predisposition as a single-gene disorder. As yet there are no specific ways of identifying these patients, except through the demonstrated familial pattern of the specific form of cancer.

GENERAL PRINCIPLES OF TREATMENT

Prevention. The pediatrician is primarily concerned with preventing rather than treating disease. Unfortunately for childhood cancers, as previously mentioned, we currently know very little about the cause. Therefore no effective ways of preventing cancer are available, except for avoiding those specific agents such as ionizing irradiation that are known to increase the frequency of malignancy. This area remains an important one for research.

Initial studies. It is important that at the time of diagnosis the child have the complete range of necessary studies to guide therapy and assign prognosis. It is possible at this time to identify many factors that can be associated with prognosis and response to therapy, including age, tumor type, histologic pattern, extent of disease at diagnosis, and specific biologic tumor cell characteristics. The importance of each of these factors varies with the specific tumor. Age is important, for example, in neuroblastoma. Histology is important in Wilms tumor and Hodgkin disease. The anatomic extent of disease at diagnosis is important for most tumors and is described by assigning a specific stage, usually indicated by a Roman numeral. The most limited extent of disease, in which the tumor can be completely excised, is indicated by stage I, with progressively greater extent as higher stage numbers are assigned. Stage IV disease generally designates widespread, hematogenous, metastatic dissemination.

In recent years it has been possible to demonstrate specific biologic markers that are important in relationship to clinical behavior. In non-Hodgkin lymphoma, for example, the characteristics of the tumor cells may be related to their normal T-lymphocyte and B-lymphocyte counterparts. Each type has a specific clinical behavior, as is discussed later. Because of the importance of defining all these features, the initial studies should be done in an institution capable of providing a broad range of necessary diagnostic tools.

Treatment programs. At diagnosis of most children with cancer, their disease has disseminated beyond a point at which it could be completely excised surgically. Therefore treatment for childhood cancer almost always involves a combination of operative procedures, irradiation therapy, and chemotherapy. The specific treatment program must be designed according to the type of tumor and the other initial features (as already described) found at diagnosis. Proper treatment necessitates the coordinated effort of a group of skilled and experienced physicians of the appropriate different disciplines. Today, most treatment for children with cancer in this country is by a research protocol that is designed not only to provide the best treatment but also to collect information in such a way as to learn more about therapy for this disease. Because of this research approach, treatment programs are in constant change, and therefore the general outlines of therapy for the specific cancers do not involve recommendations of specific treatment regimens that might shortly be out of date.

Supportive care. It is important to realize that as a consequence of the disease and its treatment, certain complications may arise. Frequently bone marrow is suppressed either by disease or the chemotherapy regimen, and there will be a need for transfusion of blood products. Infections are frequent consequences of treatment not only because of marrow suppression leading to neutropenia but also because of generalized immunosuppression leading to predisposition to viral and fungal infections. Anorexia is a frequent feature of the clinical course of childhood cancer, and much attention must be paid to proper nutrition. Of greatest importance is the realization of the emotional impact of childhood cancer on the child and the family: there must be facilities for providing good psychosocial support, and the physician must be constantly alert to emotional problems, both potential and immediate.

ACUTE LEUKEMIA

A classification of childhood leukemia follows:

A. Lymphoid cell line
   1. Acute lymphocytic leukemia (ALL)
      a. Standard, or common, form (ALL antigen, Ia like antigen)—about one third have cytoplasmic immunoglobulins in chains
      b. T cell form (rosette formation sheep erythrocytes and/or T cell antigen)
      c. B cell form (surface immunoglobulins)
      d. Null cell (no characteristic surface markers)
   2. Chronic lymphocytic leukemia (exceedingly rare in children)

B. Myeloid cell line
   1. Acute myeloblastic leukemia (AML)
   2. Erythroleukemia
   3. Eosinophilic leukemia
   4. Promyelocytic leukemia
   5. Monoblastic leukemia
   6. Chronic myelocytic leukemia (CML)
      a. Adult form (Ph^1 chromosome positive)
      b. Juvenile form (no specific chromosome abnormality)

Leukemia is the most common form of cancer in childhood, with about 2000 newly diagnosed cases in this country annually. Acute lymphocytic leukemia (ALL) accounts for most of these cases and represents 80% of all leukemias of childhood. ALL is itself subdivided into specific types, as indicated in the outline. The standard ALL represents two thirds of this type and has a median age of onset of 4 years. T cell leukemia is the second most frequent form and has a slightly older median age of about 10 years. The other forms are infrequently encountered. Acute myeloblastic leukemia (AML) is less frequent in children and represents the remaining 20%. It can be subdivided, as indicated, into specific groups according to the morphologic appearance of the cells, representing specific differentiation features. In children chronic myelocytic leukemia is an uncommon form of this disease.

Clinical manifestations. The principal findings at diagnosis are similar for all the acute leukemias. In general, the period of symptoms before diagnosis is brief, frequently being only 2 to 4 weeks. The usual complaints are progressive fatigue, irritability, and anorexia. At times there may be complaints of bone pain. As replacement of the bone marrow by leukemic cells progresses, production of normal cells fails. The child will develop anemia, neutropenia, and thrombocytopenia. The associated physical features are the development of pallor, fever, and bleeding manifestations. The fever may be associated with the findings of a specific site of infection, or may have no evident cause. The physical findings at diagnosis, in addition to the features mentioned, may include some degree of hepatosplenomegaly and lymphadenopathy. This finding is usually most notable in those patients with T cell leukemias, in which a greater degree of organomegaly is characteristic.

Laboratory findings. Confirmation of diagnosis is easily achieved in almost all instances. On blood counts, the patient will be found to be anemic and thrombopenic. The white blood count may be in a low or normal range, with the presence of leukemic blast cells on the blood smear. In some patients with low initial white blood counts, there may be too few leukemic blast cells to be seen easily on the blood smear. In other patients the white blood count may be considerably increased. This increase is particularly noticeable in those with the T cell leukemias, in which the median white count is $100{,}000/mm^3$ at diagnosis. On inspection of the blood smear it is important to determine carefully the cytologic features so that lymphocytic and myeloblastic leukemias can be differentiated. There are no blood smear features of the lymphocytic leukemias that are helpful in defining the specific type. Bone marrow examination is the next step in diagnosis. Usually, complete replacement of normal bone marrow elements with leukemic blast cells will be found. In a few patients, initial attempts to obtain marrow samples by aspiration will yield scanty specimens inadequate for diagnosis. In these a needle biopsy should be done, primarily to differentiate acute leukemia with pancytopenia from aplastic anemia. The findings of the marrow biopsy are almost always definitive. For patients with ALL, specific surface markers should be determined to define the subtypes. These markers and the specific cell types they define are indicated in the preceding list. A chest radiograph should be obtained to determine if there is a mediastinal mass, which is characteristic of the T cell leukemias. It is most important at diagnosis to determine the level of uric acid in the blood. Some patients with leukemia may have hyperuricemia, which can, in turn, lead to renal damage and failure. A lumbar puncture should be done at diagnosis to determine whether leukemic cells are present in the cerebrospinal fluid.

Treatment. Treatment for acute leukemias is undergoing continual change. Only general principles will be defined here. Following is a general description of an effective treatment regimen for childhood ALL, the most common form of leukemia in children.

There are three phases of treatment for leukemia. The important first phase is *remission induction*. A combination of agents is given to reduce the number of leukemic cells as rapidly as possible and to allow for return of normal marrow cell production. In standard ALL this remission is usually achieved within 4 weeks. It has been recognized that there are sanctuary areas, particularly in the central nervous system, in which the leukemic cells are spared the effects of chemotherapy. The second phase of treatment is the destruction of blast cells in these sanctuary areas, or *preventive central nervous system therapy*. Finally, it has been recognized that for complete disease control, it is necessary to continue therapy with another group of drugs for an appropriate period of time. This third phase is *continuation therapy,* or *remission maintenance*. The duration of this period has not been definitely established for maximal results. In general, however, after 2½ to 3 years it does not appear that additional maintenance therapy provides any advantage for the patient in disease control and increases risk of both short- and long-term side effects from treatment. After cessation of therapy for the patient who has been in remission from initiation of therapy, 80% will subsequently continue in remission and appear to be cured.

Drugs that have proven useful for remission induction include prednisone, vincrinstine, daunomycin, l-asparaginase, and a combination of epipodophyllotoxin, teniposide (VM-26), and cytosine arabinoside. Preventive central nervous system therapy has been accomplished by cranial irradiation in doses of 1800 or 2400 rads with intrathecal methotrexate. In another approach, higher doses of methotrexate given intravenously are combined with intrathecal methotrexate to achieve spinal fluid levels cytotoxic to leukemic cells. Continuation therapy or remission maintenance usually includes the combination of 6-mercaptopurine and methotrexate, to which may be added pulses of reinduction therapy or cycles with such non–cross-reactive agents as teniposide and cytosine arabinoside, or adriamycin and cyclophosphamide. For those patients with initially high-risk features the chemotherapy regimens are generally designed to be more intensive, especially in the earlier phases of treatment.

Treatment of acute myeloblastic leukemia (AML) is somewhat different with respect to the drugs used, but the general principles remain the same. The most important aspect of therapy is a rapid induction of remission. Most treatment regimens include the use of daunomycin and cytosine arabinoside during this period. The complications of remission induction for AML are severe, and about one fourth of patients die from bleeding or infection during this time. Central nervous system prophylaxis is of less benefit to these patients because the subsequent duration of remission tends to be too brief for the benefits to be recognized. There is even some question as to whether continuation therapy is of value, although most regimens incorporate some form of continuing drug treatment.

Patients with T cell leukemias are treated generally in the same way as are those with standard ALL. Responses to the initial phase of induction and central nervous system prophylaxis are similar to those of patients with standard ALL. The major complication of treatment is the rapidity with which these patients relapse during therapy in the continuation phase. The median time of this relapse, after remission induction, is 1 year.

There are various induction regimens for patients who have failed initial induction therapy or who have relapsed during subsequent maintenance periods. For most patients who fail primary therapy, subsequent remissions, if they can be induced, tend to be brief.

During the time of treatment, meticulous care must be given to the side effects of bone marrow suppression and immunosuppression. The patients are susceptible to the wide range of bacterial, viral, and fungal infections. During treatment, fever must be viewed as caused by infection until proved otherwise. Careful studies must be done to determine the etiology of the fever, and appropriate therapy should be instituted when the diagnosis is established. For patients in whom the clinical findings suggest bacterial sepsis, treatment must be instituted to cover both gram-negative and gram-positive organisms until the specific cause can be defined. Bleeding as a complication occurs mostly during the period of remission induction and is related to thrombocytopenia. Most episodes of bleeding can be effectively treated by the administration of platelets. Patients with acute promyelocytic leukemia have a predisposition to the development of disseminated intravascular coagulation because of the release of the cytoplasmic procoagulant from the leukemic cells. For patients with this rare form of AML, heparin is usually given during the remission induction period.

An alternative form of treatment for acute leukemia is bone marrow transplantation. Current guidelines when HLA–identical siblings are available are to perform transplants on AML patients in first remission and on ALL patients in second or subsequent remissions. Some studies with autologous marrow infusions have been done, but results are still too preliminary to know the eventual role of this approach.

Prognosis. The prognosis for children with ALL has improved considerably during the past 2 decades. At the present time, more than half the children with ALL can be expected to be alive, well, and in remission 5 years after diagnosis. In fact, during the past 20 years fully one third of the children with ALL have probably been cured of their disease by modern treatment methods.

Several clinical features have been associated with a less favorable response to treatment. These clinical features are white blood counts greater than 100,000, central nervous system involvement at diagnosis, presence of a mediastinal mass, failure to achieve remission within the first 4 weeks of treatment, and presence of this disease in children who are black. More recently, it has been possible to identify the specific subtypes of ALL. The finding of T cell or B cell leukemia is definitely an unfavorable prognostic indicator. With the possibility of being able to identify the specific subpopulations of ALL, it will now be important to determine if the clinical features just mentioned have independent prognostic significance for children with this disease. The best prognosis with treatment is for those patients with standard, or common, ALL. Many of these children are probably going to be cured of their disease. On the other hand, the prognosis for T and B cell leukemia at this time is quite poor. The leukemic cells of the T cell variety of ALL seem to have the ability of rapidly acquiring drug resistance. New treatment approaches must be developed for this form of ALL. The B cell leukemias, on the other hand, are characterized by an initial resistance to achieving disease control. It may very well be that the T cell and B cell leukemias, in fact, represent early leukemic transformation of the T cell and B cell non-Hodgkin lymphoma, which will be discussed later in this chapter.

CHRONIC MYELOCYTIC LEUKEMIA

Chronic myelocytic leukemia (CML) accounts for less than 3% of all childhood leukemia. It may be divided into adult and juvenile forms. The adult form in children is characterized by the presence of the Philadelphia[1] (Ph[1]) chromosome and has the usual clinical features and typical response to treatment seen in adults with this form of CML. The juvenile form, on the other hand, is not characterized by a specific chromosomal abnormality in the leukemic cell populations, generally occurs earlier in life, and runs an unremitting and generally treatment-unresponsive course. The distinguishing features of these two forms of CML in children are shown in Table 31-1. Treatment for the Philadelphia chromosome–positive adult form of CML is similar to that used for the disease in adults and depends mostly on the administration of busulfan (Myleran) to reduce the white blood count and the degree of hepatosplenomegaly characteristic of this form of leukemia.

Table 31-1. Features at diagnosis of adult and juvenile types of chronic myelocytic leukemia in children

Feature	Adult type	Juvenile type
Age of maximal incidence (yr)	10-12	1-2
Philadelphia chromosome	Present	Absent
Fetal hemoglobin values	2%-7%	30%-70%
Splenomegaly	Marked	Moderate
White blood count (100,000/mm^3)	Frequent	Rare
Thrombocytopenia	Uncommon	Usual

NEUROBLASTOMA (see also pp. 898-899)

Neuroblastoma is derived from the primitive sympathetic neuroblasts of neural crest origin; therefore it can develop in a primary site in many places in the body. Characteristically it develops in the adrenal gland or in the parasympathetic ganglia along the vertebral column, either in the abdomen or in the thorax. Histologically the tumor consists of undifferentiated small round cells, or it may be a mixture of these undifferentiated neuroblasts and mature ganglion cells. A characteristic feature is the presence of rosettes, which consist of neuroblasts surrounding an area filled with fibrillar material.

In most patients with neuroblastoma the onset of disease occurs within the first 5 years of life. However, the tumor can develop at any time during childhood. It is uncommon during the second decade of life. The usual presenting feature is a mass, most commonly in the abdomen. At times a thoracic primary lesion may be found on routine chest radiograph or one obtained because of pulmonary symptoms suggesting an acute inflammatory process. In about two thirds of children with this tumor, there is widespread dissemination at diagnosis. Therefore the initial finding may relate to metastatic disease with such clinical features as lymph node enlargement, bone pain, scalp nodules, and proptosis or with clinical features of the pancytopenia associated with diffuse marrow involvement. In these patients with disseminated disease, fever is common, and there is the associated fatigability, irritability, and anorexia.

Initial diagnostic studies include radiographs of the skeleton and chest. If the primary tumor appears to be in the abdomen, an intravenous pyelogram may define the site of origin by the presence of downward or lateral displacement of the kidney. Sometimes calcification can be demonstrated in the tumor mass. Skeletal films may demonstrate the osteolytic metastatic lesions. Blood counts may indicate pancytopenia, suggesting marrow infiltration. A bone marrow examination should be done to determine if marrow infiltration has occurred. In most children with neuroblastoma the urinary excretion of catecholamines will be found to be increased. This finding is useful in defining the specific nature of the tumor. The final diagnosis, however, must rest with histologic demonstration of the tumor, either by complete excision of a localized primary lesion or biopsy of a tumor in which dissemination has taken place.

For patients with localized tumor, complete excision may be effective in achieving cure. Most patients, however, have dissemination beyond the point that a complete excision can be achieved. For those with residual regional disease, radiation therapy may be effective in killing the remaining tumor cells. For most patients, chemotherapy is an essential part of the treatment regimen because the tumor has spread beyond the point of which either surgery or irradiation therapy can be completely effective.

There are two drug combinations that have proved most useful for the treatment of neuroblastoma. They are cyclophosphamide and doxorubicin (adriamycin), and teniposide and cisplatin. Less effective drugs are vincrinstine and dacarbazine (Dtic-Dome).

The prognosis for children with this tumor depends in large part on the age at diagnosis and the degree of dissemination. About 50% of all children under the age of 1 year will survive their disease, irrespective of the tumor stage at diagnosis. Above the age of 1, the prognosis is primarily dependent on the stage. For patients with tumors that can be completely excised or in whom only microscopic residual disease amenable to irradiation exists, cure may be achieved and almost all such patients can be cured. On the other hand, for patients over the age of 1 in whom either regional or distant metastasis has occurred, complete clinical response to chemotherapy can be achieved for the majority, but cure is rare.

WILMS TUMOR (see also p. 898 and pp. 941-942)

Wilms tumor (nephroblastoma) is the most common malignant abdominal tumor of childhood. It occurs most frequently during the first five years of life, with rare occurrence after the age of 8. In the newborn period the usual cause of a renal tumor is nephroblastomatosis, a benign condition requiring no specific treatment other than removal when indicated. There should be careful review of the histology of any tumor of the kidney appearing during the first weeks of life. Wilms tumor consists of mixed histologic elements, abortive tubules and glomeruli appearing in combination with undifferentiated cellular elements. In about one tenth of patients a sarcomatous appearance predominates, which carries a poor prognosis.

The usual initial finding is the presence of an abdominal mass. At times this mass can be appreciated by the parents, or it may be discovered by the physician as an incidental finding on routine physical examination. At this stage the tumor is usually asymptomatic. With further tumor growth the patient may develop abdominal symptoms such as pain, pressure, and anorexia. Later on fever may be present, as well as hypertension and hematuria. The usual site of metastasis is to the lungs. Therefore, with progressive metastatic growth, pulmonary insufficiency with dyspnea and tachypnea may be found.

At the time of finding an abdominal mass the physician should give the patient a careful complete physical examination to look for other evidence of tumor, as well as features indicating an underlying predisposing condition. These features are hemihypertrophy, aniridia, and other evidence of genitourinary anomalies. In the usual patient, only the presence of a smooth, firm, nontender flank mass in the abdomen will be found. A chest radiograph should be done to determine if pulmonary metastasis is present. An intravenous pyelogram will indicate the presence of an intrarenal mass distorting the caliceal system. The most important point in differentiation is to distinguish this abdominal tumor from the benign tumor of hydronephrosis and from the other abdominal malignant tumor, neuroblastoma. In Table 31-2 the characteristic features of these three abdominal tumors are shown as an aid to differential diagnosis. The blood counts are usually normal, and in a patient with Wilms tumor a bone marrow examination is not indicated.

The urinalysis usually is normal, but hematuria or proteinuria may be found in a few patients. The final diagnosis must rest on histologic examination of the tumor. It is important to determine at that time whether the sarcomatous elements carrying a poor prognostic outlook are present in the tumor. It is also important to establish the extent of tumor in the renal bed. Therefore the pathologic examination should be done with great care. A tumor should be established as being completely within the renal capsule (stage I), extending through the capsule but completely removed (stage II), or extending into or beyond the renal bed (stage III). If tumor is demonstrated in the lungs by radiograph, the patient is assigned a stage IV classification.

Fortunately this tumor is quite responsive to chemotherapy. Most patients have tumor completely removed at diagnosis and are classified as stage I or II disease. Of these, stage I patients require vincristine and dactinomycin, but stage II patients require both chemotherapeutic agents and irradiation to the renal bed. For patients in stages III and IV, doxorubicin is generally added to the two drugs already mentioned, with irradiation being given to residual areas of tumor.

The prognosis depends greatly on the histology of the tumor and stage at diagnosis. For patients with the unfavorable sarcomatous histology, regardless of stage, only 40% can be expected to achieve long-term, disease-free control. More than 90% of stage I patients with favorable histology can be cured. Patients in stages II and III also can expect a good chance of cure—60% or more. In about 10% of patients the tumor will be present in both kidneys at diagnosis. Even these patients, with removal of the most affected kidney and irradiation and che-

Table 31-2. Differential diagnosis of abdominal tumors

Feature	Hydronephrosis	Wilms tumor	Neuroblastoma
Physical examination	Smooth, cystic	Smooth, firm	Nodular, firm
Intravenous pyelogram	Delayed or absent filling, dilated pelvis and calices	Intrarenal distortion of calices	Downward or lateral displacement of kidney, frequent calcification of tumor
Urine	Normal, or hematuria or proteinuria	Normal or hematuria	Increased catecholamines
Metastasis	None	Lung	Bone, bone marrow, liver, lymph nodes

motherapy to the residual kidney, can achieve long-term, disease-free control in more than one half of instances. In addition, partial nephrectomy of the least affected kidney can sometimes remove all gross evidence of tumor.

RHABDOMYOSARCOMA

Rhabdomyosarcoma may occur at any age during childhood. Because it arises from striated muscle, it can also occur at almost any location throughout the body. Histologically it is a small round cell sarcoma, most commonly appearing as an embryonal form. The cells are somewhat pleomorphic, with evident pinkish cytoplasm, which in some cases is elongated so that it tends to form the appearance of a tail on a cell, resembling a tadpole. In some of these cells the cross striations characteristic of muscle can be seen. Other histologic forms are the alveolar rhabdomyosarcoma and sarcoma botryoides, which is the characteristic appearance when this tumor extrudes from a surface such as in the vagina. The mass may appear similar to a bunch of grapes, and histologically the cells are separated by an edematous stroma.

The initial clinical features depend on the site of origin and the rapidity of tumor growth. In the head and neck area the tumor may initially resemble more common childhood problems such as chronic otitis media or an infection of the nasopharynx. A persistent painful middle ear condition or an unexplained mass of the nasopharynx or face should raise the possibility of rhabdomyosarcoma. Frequently there is delay in diagnosis (with a median of about 2 months) because of the initial resemblance to other conditions. Rhabdomyosarcoma can also arise on the trunk or an extremity. Tumors in these sites present initially as painless, unexplained swellings that are firm and usually fixed to underlying tissue. The tumor may arise along the genitourinary tract and present as a vaginal mass in girls or a paratesticular tumor in boys. There also may be an intra-abdominal origin for this tumor, usually in the retroperitoneal area.

About two thirds of these patients have extension of their disease beyond the opportunity for primary excision at diagnosis. There may be extension to regional tissues and lymph nodes or hematogenous dissemination to lungs, bone, and bone marrow.

Initial studies of a patient suspected of having rhabdomyosarcoma should include the appropriate radiographic studies, depending on the region of origin. There also should be a complete blood count, a skeletal survey, chest radiograph, and bone marrow examination. The definitive diagnosis must be made by histologic examination. In some patients it may be necessary to await the findings of electron microscopy examination before the diagnosis can be established. The major problems in differentiation are similarities to other small round cell tumors such as neuroblastoma, Ewing sarcoma, and in some cases non-Hodgkin lymphoma.

Treatment should be excision, if possible, followed by irradiation therapy, when appropriate, and combination chemotherapy. The usual drugs employed for treatment of this disease are vincristine, cyclophosphamide, dactinomycin, and doxorubicin. For patients having nonresectable regional disease, irradiation therapy is advised in addition to chemotherapy. For patients with widespread dissemination, chemotherapy is the mainstay of treatment, with radiation therapy being used for local disease control.

The prognosis for children with rhabdomyosarcoma depends most on the extent of disease at diagnosis. If the tumor can be completely excised and chemotherapy is given to suppress growth of disseminated micrometastasis, the majority of children with this tumor can be cured. With increasing extent of disease, likelihood of cure decreases, and for patients with disseminated disease at diagnosis long-term, disease-free survival is unusual with current therapy.

RETINOBLASTOMA

Retinoblastoma is a relatively rare tumor of children, but it is important for the physician to recognize it as soon as possible. This tumor arises in the retina and is usually evident within the first years of life. The initial finding may be the observation by a family member that the usual red reflex of the affected eye is missing, having been replaced by a white or gray appearance behind the pupil. The child may have strabismus on that side. On physical examination, the eye may have a whitish reflex in response to light. On ophthalmoscopic examination the whitish or gray retinal tumor is evident.

In some cases it may be necessary to sedate the child for the examination so that the full extent of the tumor can be defined. In some infants this tumor is heritable. All bilateral retinoblastomas are inherited, and about 15% of unilateral retinoblastomas represent a heritable single-gene defect. The offspring of survivors of retinoblastoma in its heritable form have a 50% chance of developing the tumor. Patients who survive retinoblastoma in infancy have about a 1% risk of subsequently developing osteosarcoma.

The recommended treatment for this tumor is undergoing change. Increasingly, in appropriate patients there is an effort to preserve sight in the affected eye by irradiation or cauterization of the tumor. It is important that the child with retinoblastoma be referred to an appropriate center so that the facilities necessary for effective treatment with minimal residual damage may be made available. For patients who have had dissemination of the retinoblastoma beyond the orbit, chemotherapy is necessary.

HODGKIN DISEASE

Hodgkin disease, a form of lymphoma, is uncommon during childhood but may occur in children during the second half of the first decade. The malignancy begins in lymphoid tissue and is characterized by the Reed-Sternberg cell, which is the malignant cell of this tumor. This cell is thought to be derived from a B-lymphocyte or T-lymphocyte, but definitive proof for this derivation has not yet been offered. The tumor spreads initially to contiguous lymphoid areas and later in its course can involve extranodal tissues such as the liver, lung, bone marrow, and central nervous system. There are four histologic types, each with its characteristic clinical features and prognosis. The most favorable is that associated with lymphocyte predominance in which there are few Reed-Sternberg cells but many normal-appearing lymphocytes. The second most favorable is the nodular sclerosing variety in which islands of Reed-Sternberg cells with associated lymphocytes, eosinophils, and histiocytes are surrounded by areas of fibrosis. Less favorable is the variety with mixed cellularity, in which increased numbers of Reed-Sternberg cells are found and there is a greater predisposition to early extranodal involvement. The least favorable prognosis is the variety associated with lymphocyte depletion, in which the Reed-Sternberg cell predominates and few normal-appearing lymphocytes are present.

At diagnosis the only finding in some patients may be the development of painless, unexplained lymphadenopathy. The cervical region is the most frequent area involved, but any lymph node area can be the site of origin. The nodular sclerosing variety frequently has associated mediastinal involvement of thoracic lymph nodes. When symptoms are present, they include weight loss, easy fatigability, fever, night sweats, and pruritus. The physical examination must be carefully done to identify all involved lymph node areas. Examination of the abdomen should include an attempt to determine if the retroperitoneal nodes are enlarged and whether there is involvement of liver and spleen, as indicated by hepatosplenomegaly.

On the initial studies the blood counts may be found to be in the normal range, or there may be a leukocytosis with a neutrophilia, eosinophilia, and monocytosis. If anemia or thrombocytopenia is present at diagnosis, it indicates an unfavorable outcome. A chest radiograph should be obtained to identify mediastinal and pulmonary parenchymal involvement. A radiologic bone survey should be done to determine if bone involvement is present. An intravenous pyelogram will be useful if lateral displacement of the kidneys and ureters indicates retroperitoneal node enlargement. A liver and spleen scan likewise may be useful in demonstrating involvement of those organs. At times, lymphangiography of both lower extremities is indicated to attempt demonstration of iliac and lower periaortic node involvement.

The definitive diagnosis must come from histologic examination of one of the involved lymph nodes. For most patients a staging laparotomy is needed to determine conclusively if there are areas of disease within the abdomen. At that time, lymph nodes and liver are biopsied and the spleen is removed. Also, bone biopsies can be obtained to determine if bone marrow involvement is present. At the conclusion of these studies a stage is assigned the patient. Stage I disease involves only one lymph node area. Stage II disease indicates involvement of two contiguous lymph node areas. In stage III disease there is involvement of lymphoid tissue above and below the diaphragm. In stage IV disease extranodal involvement is present.

The treatment depends on the stage of disease at diagnosis. For stages I and II, radiation therapy is used primarily to treat the involved areas. In most treatment regimens, stage II patients also receive combination chemotherapy. For stages III and IV, chemotherapy is the primary treatment modality, but in some treatment regimens irradiation of axial node areas of the trunk and cervical region is also given. Effective agents for treatment of Hodgkin disease are prednisone, cyclophosphamide, or nitrogen mustard, procarbazine, and vincristine. Standard chemotherapy includes a combination program of four of these agents. Another effective four-drug combination includes adriamycin, bleomycin, vinblastine, and DIC.

The prognosis depends largely on the stage of disease at diagnosis and the histologic type. Patients in stages I and II with favorable histology have an excellent prognosis; more than 90% of them achieve long-term, disease-free control. Patients with more disseminated disease at diagnosis, but having favorable histology, may expect long-term, disease-free control in at least half the instances.

NON-HODGKIN LYMPHOMA

Non-Hodgkin lymphomas of children can occur at any age. Although they initially arise in an area of lymphoid tissue, there is a great predisposition to early dissemination to extranodal sites. With newer methods of identifying specific features of T-lymphocytes and B-lymphocytes, as well as the various degrees of differentiation of these cells, the classification of lymphomas is undergoing revision. As for childhood ALL patients, it is important that complete studies be done at diagnosis for patients with lymphoma. The clinical course and prognosis depend greatly on the specific cell type involved. At this time it is possible to identify lymphomas as belonging to either the T-lymphocyte or B-lymphocyte line according to their surface marker expressions. Histology is also useful in further classifying the cell type as to degree of differentiation.

The initial findings may be the development of enlarging lymph nodes that are painless but firm. The rate of enlargement tends to be greater than for Hodgkin disease. The tumor may arise in lymphoid tissue of the nasopharynx, the mediastinum, or the gastrointestinal tract. The initial signs and symptoms of these patients depend primarily on the effect of the growing mass in the area. Patients with mediastinal lymph node enlargement may rapidly develop respiratory distress from tracheal compression. Involvement of the gastrointestinal tract may produce symptoms of obstruction, and in some cases intussusception may occur with the lymphoma serving as the lead point. Because of the tendency to early dissemination, the initial finding might include involvement of the central nervous system, bone marrow, liver, or spleen. At times the lymphoma may develop in the epidural space in the spinal cord, producing cord compression. The generalized symptoms of weakness, fatigue, irritability, and anorexia may be present.

The definitive diagnosis must depend on biopsy, with histologic examination and appropriate studies of biologic markers. The extent of disease is determined from physical examination and specific diagnostic studies. A chest radiograph and bone survey should be done. The liver and spleen scan may indicate involvement of those organs. An intravenous pyelogram is useful to demonstrate abdominal node involvement. Blood counts and examination of bone marrow and spinal fluid are necessary to determine if extension to those areas is present. A uric acid level should be obtained because there may be hyperuricemia, especially with treatment, which can lead to renal failure.

The treatment program depends to some degree on the initial extent of disease. Irradiation therapy is used for those few patients with only one lymphoid area involved. For more extensive disease, chemotherapy is used; the effectiveness of additional radiation therapy is yet to be proved. The chemotherapy involves a combination of agents, including prednisone, vincristine, cyclophosphamide, L-asparaginase, and doxorubicin during the remission induction period. Methotrexate and 6-mercaptopurine can be effective agents for maintenance of remission, as for childhood ALL. Particular care must be taken during the induction phase to avoid the hazards of hyperuricemia, by administering allopurinol and by achieving fluid loading and alkalinization.

The prognosis depends in large part on the

initial staging. For stage I the prognosis is excellent for long-term, disease-free control. For stages III and IV the prognosis tends to be poor. The lymphomas of the B cell variety, arising primarily in the abdomen, have a particularly unfavorable outcome.

BONE TUMORS

Bone tumors in children usually occur during the second decade of life. The most common of the primary bone tumors are osteogenic sarcoma and Ewing sarcoma.

Osteogenic sarcoma

Osteogenic sarcoma arises most frequently in the metaphysis of one of the long bones, such as the femur or tibia. Less common would be development of the primary tumor in one of the flat bones of the trunk. This tumor has followed exposure to irradiation, and may also be seen in patients who have survived retinoblastoma. Histologically the tumor contains primitive cells that are forming osteoid. In the tumor there may also be areas of malignant cartilage formation and areas resembling fibrosarcoma. The tumor metastasizes to the lung and other bones.

The usual complaint at onset is localized pain in the affected bone. Sometimes this pain appears to follow trauma, and in some patients there may be a delay in diagnosis because the pain is thought to be caused by the injury. In any patient having prolonged, and especially unexplained, bone pain a radiograph should be obtained. With progression of the tumor there may be local swelling, tenderness, and heat.

On radiographic examination there is evidence of bone destruction and periosteal new bone formation. Frequently a soft tissue mass containing calcification can be demonstrated. A chest radiograph and bone survey should be done to determine if metastases have occurred. Definitive diagnosis is established by biopsy.

The treatment is by amputation of the affected extremity, with a sufficient margin of normal bone to ensure complete removal of the tumor. Whenever possible, the amputation should be transmedullary to provide for fitting of an effective prosthesis. Subsequently, adjuvant chemotherapy is given for a period of 1 year. Effective agents have been cyclophosphamide, doxorubicin, and high-dose methotrexate with a Leucovorin rescue. These drugs must be given by an experienced physician with sufficient facilities for careful monitoring of this treatment regimen.

Ewing sarcoma

Ewing sarcoma may occur in any bone but more frequently involves long bones such as the femur and tibia. Flat bones of the trunk may be involved more frequently than is the case with osteosarcoma. The tumor consists of an undifferentiated small cell sarcoma that grossly is soft and friable. At times it has been considered by the surgeon at biopsy to be an abscess because of this feature. The tumor metastasizes to lung and other bones.

Initial findings are localized pain in the affected bone, with subsequent development of localized swelling, tenderness, and heat. These findings are indistinguishable from those of osteosarcoma. Later in the course, fever may develop, as may symptoms of lung and bone metastasis.

The radiographic appearance may resemble a bone abscess and is characterized by bone destruction and a soft tissue mass. In some tumors a sunburst appearance of calcification can be seen in this soft tissue mass. Initial studies should include a radiograph of the lungs and a bone survey to determine if metastases are present. The definitive diagnosis is established by biopsy.

Treatment of Ewing sarcoma includes radiation therapy to the involved bone and chemotherapy with combinations of vincristine, dactinomycin, and cyclophosphamide. Doxorubicin has also been found to be an effective agent for patients with advanced disease. A recently described approach begins with chemotherapy (cyclophosphamide and doxorubicin) to reduce tumor bulk before irradiation therapy. Radiation can then be delivered through a smaller port, sparing normal tissue and in some cases in a smaller dose.

RETICULOENDOTHELIOSIS (HISTIOCYTOSIS X)

The poorly defined group of conditions known as reticuloendotheliosis (histiocytosis X) is rare in children. They are assumed to represent malignancies of the monocyte-macrophage system, but definitive proof has not yet been established. Initially three conditions were described that subsequently have been considered to be clinical representations of the same primary disease, differences depending primarily on the age of onset.

Letterer-Siwe disease

The Letterer-Siwe form usually has its onset during the first 2 or 3 years of life. There tends to be widespread organ involvement, with infiltration by typically undifferentiated cells of the monocyte-macrophage line (histiocytes). Characteristically lymphadenopathy and hepatosplenomegaly are present. The skin may be involved with a seborrheic-like lesion, most prominent over the scalp and upper trunk. In some patients there may be lung and bone marrow involvement, with clinical manifestations of pulmonary insufficiency and marrow failure, respectively. Treatment, especially for the patient in whom the onset is during infancy, is difficult. Combinations of prednisone with other chemotherapeutic agents such as vincristine, cyclophosphamide, and methotrexate have been used.

Hand-Schüller-Christian syndrome

As initially described, the Hand-Schüller-Christian syndrome included a triad of exophthalmos, diabetes insipidus, and membranous bone defects. This triad is actually rarely seen together, and the eponym is reserved for this disease when it occurs later in childhood and is characterized primarily by punched-out lesions in the bones, most characteristically of the skull. These patients may have chronic draining ear lesions and may also have the skin lesions described for Letterer-Siwe disease. Fever and other systemic manifestations are less frequent. The course tends to be more prolonged and more responsive to therapy. Organ involvement such as lungs, liver, and bone marrow may occur but is less frequent than when the disease occurs during infancy. The diagnosis is established by biopsy of an involved site. Treatment includes the combinations of chemotherapeutic agents mentioned for Letterer-Siwe disease. At times local irradiation is effective in treating symptomatic bone lesions.

Eosinophilic granuloma

Eosinophilic granuloma occurs in older children and in adolescents. It primarily affects bones and may be solitary or multiple. The histologic features resemble those of a granuloma, with the presence of macrophages and eosinophils. The involved bone may be painful and tender or may be entirely asymptomatic. There may be a spontaneous fracture through the lesion. Surgical curettage may be curative, but in some recurring lesions, radiation therapy may be needed.

Alvin M. Mauer

SELECTED READINGS

General review

Mauer, A.M., et al.: Current progress in the treatment of the child with cancer, J. Pediatr. **91:**523, 1977.

Acute leukemia and chronic myelocytic leukemia

Mauer, A.M.: Leukemias of childhood. In Hickey, R.C., editor: Current problems in cancer, vol. II, Chicago, 1977, Year Book Medical Publishers, Inc.

Neuroblastoma

Evans, A.E., et al.: A proposed staging for children with neuroblastoma, Cancer **27:**374, 1971.

Wilson, L.M.K., and Draper, G.J.: Neuroblastoma, its natural history and prognosis: a study of 487 cases, Br. Med. J. **507:**301, 1974.

Wilms' tumor

Beckwith, J.B., and Palmer, N.F.: Histopathology and prognosis of Wilms' tumor, Cancer **41:**1937, 1978.

D'Angio, G.J., et al.: The treatment of Wilms' tumor, Cancer **38:**633, 1976.

Lemerle, J., et al.: Wilms' tumor: natural history and prognostic factors, Cancer **37:**2557, 1976.

Pendergrass, T.W.: Congenital anomalies in children with Wilms' tumor, Cancer **37:**403, 1976.

Rhabdomyosarcoma

Lennox, E.L., et al.: Retinoblastoma: a study of natural history and prognosis of 268 cases, Br. Med. J. **282:**731, 1975.

Maurer, H.M., et al.: The intergroup rhabdomyosarcoma study, Cancer **40:**2015, 1977.

Retinoblastoma

Shidnia, H., et al: Treatment results of retinoblastoma at Indiana University Hospitals, Cancer **40:**2917, 1977.

Hodgkin's disease and non-Hodgkin's lymphoma

Murphy, S.B., and Davis, L.W.: Hodgkin's disease and the non-Hodgkin's lymphomas in childhood, Semin. Oncol. **1:**17, 1974.

Murphy, S.B., et al.: A study of childhood non-Hodgkin's lymphoma, Cancer **36:**2121, 1975.

Reticuloendotheliosis (Histiocytosis X)

Lahey, M.E.: Histiocytosis X—comparison of three treatment regimens, J. Pediatr. **87:**179, 1975.

Lahey, M.E.: Histiocytosis X—an analysis of prognostic factors, J. Pediatr. **87:**184, 1975.

Lucaya, J.: Histiocytosis X, Am. J. Dis. Child. **121:**289, 1971.

32 Pediatric Intensive Care

In the last 15 years pediatric intensive care has developed as a bona fide subspecialty of pediatrics. The increasing sophistication and cost of life support systems have necessitated a reorganization of services for critically ill children, including specialized training for pediatricians, nurses, and auxilliary personnel; concentration of equipment and other resources into specified units; and regionalization of services. Furthermore, the critically ill child frequently has derangements of several organ systems. This requires an interdisciplinary approach coordinated by a pediatrician trained in the practice of intensive care medicine.

The inclusion in *Synopsis of Pediatrics* of a chapter dealing exclusively with intensive care medicine is an acknowledgement of the rapidly evolving and highly specialized nature of this type of pediatric medicine. This chapter discusses four general categories of critical pediatric illness in terms of pathophysiology and general principles of management: low cardiac output states; acute respiratory failure; central nervous system disorders, especially increased intracranial pressure; and nutritional support. Cardiac arrest and brain death are also discussed. They are topics that have become important as a direct result of the rapidly changing practice of intensive care medicine, cardiac arrest, and brain death.

LOW CARDIAC OUTPUT STATES

The topic of shock in the pediatric patient has been recently reviewed by Perkin and Levin (see Selected references). *Shock* is defined as insufficient delivery of oxygen and energy substrates to meet the metabolic demands of cells in peripheral tissues and organs. Low cardiac output states are the most common cause of shock. However, not all shock states are necessarily associated with low cardiac output, and mildly reduced cardiac output may not necessarily produce shock.

Cardiac output is the product of heart rate and stroke volume, expressed in liters per minute or milliliters per minute. Cardiac output, standardized for surface area, is called cardiac index. Cardiac index is expressed in liters per minute per square meter and standardizes normal values independent of age.

Cardiac stroke volume is directly proportional to preload and myocardial contractile state and inversely proportional to afterload.

Cardiac output, then, is determined by only four factors: heart rate, preload, contractility, and afterload. Any reduction in cardiac output reflects a derangement in one or more of these determinants. Recognition of the specific deranged variable or variables in a patient with low cardiac output will indicate the most appropriate specific therapy for correction.

Preload. *Preload* is defined as the length of the ventricular sarcomere immediately before contraction. The relationship between stroke volume and preload is represented by the Frank-Starling curve as shown in Fig. 32-1. Because of the circumferential arrangement of sarcomere fibers, end-diastolic sarcomere length corresponds very closely to end-diastolic volume. Thus any decrease in end-diastolic volume is likely to produce a low cardiac output state as a result of decreased preload. On p. 861 is a list of some causes of decreased preload. Hypovolemia is the most common cause of decreased preload in pediatric patients. Absolute hypovolemia occurs with severe dehydration or severe hemorrhage. Relative hypovolemia, from extensive vasodilation, is seen in early septic shock, severe hypothermia, as a complication of spinal or general anesthesia, and in autonomic nervous system dysfunction.

Less frequently, cardiac tamponade impairs

CAUSES OF DECREASED PRELOAD

Hypovolemia
Tamponade
Arrhythmias
  Atrial (loss of atrial augmentation)
  Tachyarrhythmias
Decreased ventricular compliance
  Myocarditis
  Infarction
  Ventriculotomy
  Mechanical trauma
  Fibrillation

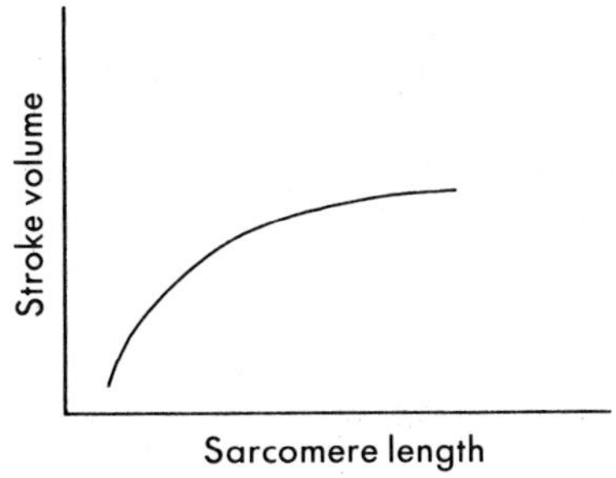

Fig. 32-1. Relationship between stroke volume and preload as represented by Frank-Starling curve.

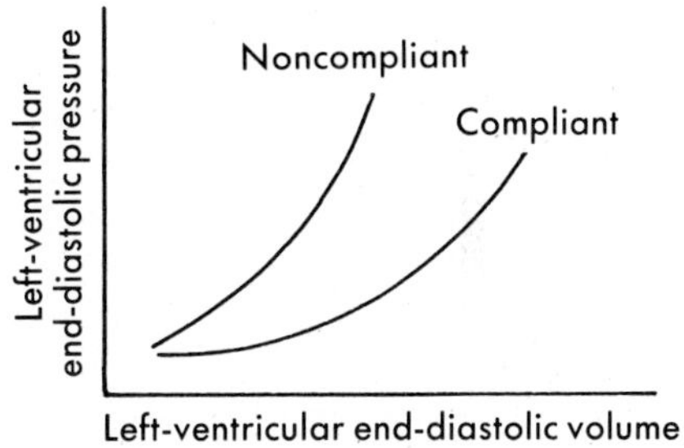

Fig. 32-2. Ventricular compliance as described by volume-pressure relationship.

preload in pediatric patients. This may occur as a result of hemorrhagic complications of cardiac surgery, as a complication of pericarditis, or rarely as the result of a pneumopericardium complicating mechanical ventilation. The presence of blood, fluid, or air in the pericardium, or the constriction of an inflamed pericardium, effectively restricts the distensibility of the ventricle, preventing optimal stretch of the sarcomeres before contraction.

Loss of atrial augmentation as a result of an atrial arrhythmia or complete heart block is an uncommon cause of decreased preload. In children with normal contractility, loss of atrial augmentation results in a less than 10% decrease in cardiac output. However, if contractility or other cardiac output determinants are deranged, loss of atrial augmentation may be responsible for as much as 50% reduction in cardiac output.

Cardiac output increases linearly with heart rate to a maximal rate of 180 beats/min in adults and 200 to 210 beats/min in children. Heart rates above this maximal rate critically shorten diastolic filling time, reducing end-diastolic volume. The decreased preload results in low cardiac output despite increased heart rate.

Many factors may influence the distensibility of the myocardium. This property of the myocardium is termed *ventricular compliance* and is described by the volume-pressure relationship in Fig. 32-2. Optimal sarcomere stretch is more easily achieved in the compliant ventricle. Reduced ventricular compliance limits optimal sarcomere stretch, and a reduced preload results. For example, myocarditis and infarction with inflammatory changes or fibrosis, contusion from mechanical trauma, and the tetanic contraction of ventricular fibrillation cause decreased ventricular compliance. Ventricular compliance is also altered by sympathetic tone, administration of exogenous catecholamines, or marked increases in intrathoracic pressure associated with positive-pressure mechanical ventilation.

Contractility. Myocardial contractility is defined as the force generated by a contracting sarcomere when preload and afterload are held constant. The contractile state of the myocardium is influenced by sympathetic nervous system stimulation, circulating catecholamines, heart rate (Bowditch "staircase" effect), and plasma concentrations of certain cations (particularly sodium, potassium, and calcium). Alterations in myocardial contractility may be detected as changes in stroke volume. These relationships can be illustrated as a family of Frank-Starling curves, each depicting a different state of contractility as in Fig. 32-3. Causes of impaired contractility are listed below.

Metabolic derangements are the most common cause of acute depressions of contractility in pediatric patients. Hypoxia, acidosis, hypoglycemia, and hypocalcemia are common derangements that may impair contractility in critically ill pediatric patients.

Many drugs commonly used in a pediatric intensive care unit may adversely affect myocardial contractility, including anticonvulsants, sedatives, anesthetic agents, and even antibiotics. A physician selecting any pharmacologic agent for a patient with or at risk for low cardiac output must consider the possible effects on myocardial contractility.

Afterload. *Afterload* is defined as the impedance to sarcomere shortening, and corresponds to the resistance against which the ventricle must eject its volume. The relationship between stroke volume and afterload can be described as a family of curves, each representing a different contractile state of the myocardium. This is illustrated in Fig. 32-4.

Increased afterload as a primary factor causing decreased cardiac output can be on an anatomic or functional basis, as listed below. Anatomic outflow obstruction can occur in the right or left ventricle. Functionally, the most common cause of increased afterload is vasoconstriction in response to absolute hypovolemia. In absolute hypovolemia, vasoconstriction is a physiologic and life-saving mechanism conserving central blood pressure. This must be differen-

CAUSES OF IMPAIRED CONTRACTILITY

Metabolic derangements
Myocardial fibrosis
Coronary insufficiency
Congestive heart failure
Myocarditis
Drugs
Mechanical trauma
Depressed catecholamine secretion

CAUSES OF INCREASED AFTERLOAD

Anatomic

Aortic valvular stenosis
Idiopathic hypertrophic subaortic stenosis
Coarctation of the aorta
Infundibular pulmonic stenosis
Pulmonary valvular stenosis
Hypoplastic pulmonary artery
Peripheral pulmonic stenosis
Severe pulmonary embolus

Functional

Systemic hypertensive disease
Peripheral vasoconstriction (e.g., secondary to sepsis or drugs)
Pulmonary vascular hypertension

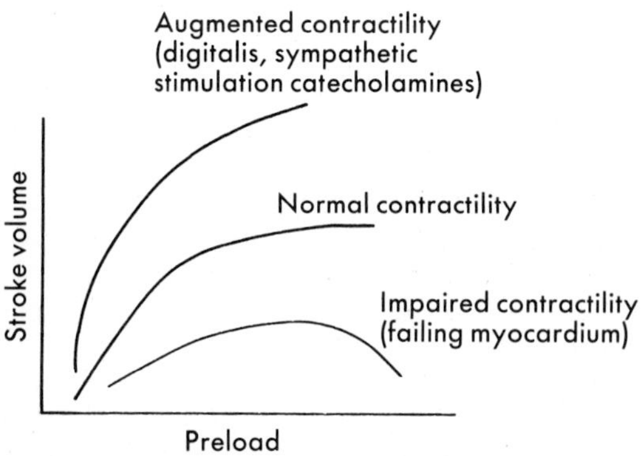

Fig. 32-3. Frank-Starling curves depicting different states of contractility.

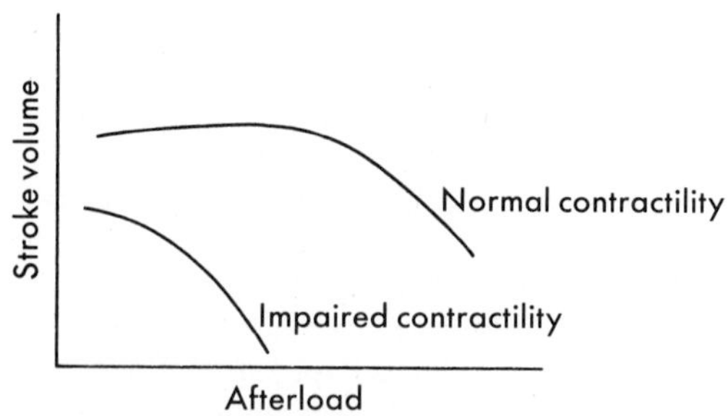

Fig. 32-4. Curves representing different contractile states of the myocardium.

tiated from vasoconstriction occurring with normal or elevated preload, in which the increased afterload is a *primary* determinant of low cardiac output. The latter situation occurs most commonly in the vasoconstrictive stages of septic shock. In the former situation, vasoconstriction may persist after preload correction, and then the increased afterload may contribute to the low cardiac output state.

Several drugs commonly used in a pediatric intensive care unit can alter peripheral vascular resistance and cause decreased cardiac output. This is particularly true of norepinephrine, epinephrine, and, in high doses, dopamine.

Finally, pulmonary vascular hypertension may cause increased afterload to the right ventricle, producing a low cardiac output state. This is the pathophysiologic hallmark of "persistent fetal circulation" of the neonate. It is also commonly seen in patients with long-standing left-to-right intracardiac shunts, and in patients with severe parenchymal pulmonary disease.

Heart rate. As mentioned earlier, cardiac output will increase linearly with increasing heart rate to a maximal 200 beats/min after which cardiac output fails. With decreases in heart rate, stroke volume is augmented by sympathetically mediated increases in contractility and by mobilization of additional venous return from venous capacitance vessels, allowing maintenance of normal cardiac output. Heart rates of 50 beats/min may be tolerated by the healthy school-age child but lower rates can impair cardiac output. Neonatal compensatory capabilities are less well developed, and the neonate in particular is more dependent on normal heart rates for maintenance of cardiac output.

Below is a list of causes of bradycardia that may produce decreased cardiac output. Neonates may present with low cardiac output because of congenital heart block. Acquired abnormalities of conduction pathways resulting in bradycardia may occur as a complication of cardiac surgery or may be associated with myocarditis and other cardiomyopathies. Metabolic abnormalities are a common cause of bradycardia in a child under intensive care. Hypoxia, acidosis, hypothermia, hypoglycemia, and electrolyte imbalance (sodium, potassium, calcium, magnesium) all can produce bradyarrhythmias that may result in low cardiac output states. Many drugs frequently used in the intensive care unit may produce bradycardia: digitalis, intravenous calcium, barbiturates, and cholinesterase inhibitors. Finally, reflex-mediated bradycardias, particularly those associated with severe central nervous system injury, may produce bradycardias severe enough to impair cardiac output.

CAUSES OF SLOWING OF HEART RATE

Conduction block
Anatomic or acquired abnormality of conduction pathways
Metabolic abnormalities
Drugs
Reflexes

Assessment and monitoring of low cardiac output states. The low cardiac output state is suggested to the clinician by a number of nonspecific symptoms and signs. Older patients may have an altered level of consciousness, manifested by lethargy, agitation, delirium, or stupor. Muscle weakness and pain, reflecting the decreased perfusion to muscles, are sometimes noted. Peripheral perfusion will be poor, with acrocyanosis, delayed capillary refill, pallor, and mottling. Tachycardia is common. Hypotension, in contrast to the common misconception, is a late development and reflects a particularly severe low cardiac output state. Reduced urine output is a sensitive clinical parameter of low cardiac output, and hourly urine output must be monitored by an indwelling catheter. Oliguria less than 0.75 to 1.0 ml/kg/hr, in the absence of intrinsic renal disease, probably reflects decreased renal perfusion secondary to low cardiac output.

Certain laboratory values may be altered by the low cardiac output state but are not diagnostic. Serum sodium and hemoglobin may be elevated, normal, or decreased, depending on the hemodilution or hemoconcentration effects of changes in extracellular water. Metabolic acidosis is common; serum lactate and lactate/pyruvate ratios will be increased, reflecting a shift to anaerobic metabolism. The acidosis may, in fact, be more prominent after improvement in the low cardiac output state, as improved perfusion "washes out" peripherally pooled metabolic acids.

Assessment and monitoring begin with frequent, serial measurement of the above parameters. However, in the patient with severely impaired cardiac output, the clinician must rely on invasive monitoring to refine his assessment and to guide specific therapy.

The first task is quantification of preload. The ideal assessment of left ventricular preload is quantification of left ventricular end-diastolic volume. This is possible to a limited degree with two-dimensional echocardiography, and more precisely by radionucleotide imaging techniques. However, these techniques are not routinely available at the bedside or applicable to the minute-by-minute monitoring necessary in the intensive care unit.

Left ventricular end-diastolic (LVED) pressure is related to left ventricular end-diastolic volume. However, LVED pressure cannot be monitored clinically, and left atrial pressure can be used. The left atrial pressure (LAP) correlates with LVED pressure only in the presence of a normally functioning mitral valve. Unfortunately this measurement is possible only in the postoperative cardiac surgery patient after placement of a left atrial catheter. For the patient who has not undergone cardiac surgery, one must rely on remotely related indicators of left ventricular preload. Central venous pressure (CVP), measured by a superior vena caval or right atrial catheter, actually reflects right ventricular end-diastolic pressure (assuming normalcy of tricuspid valve). The right ventricular filling pressure approximates the left ventricular filling pressure in normal states. Below is a list of conditions in which the CVP become unreliable as an indicator of left ventricular preload.

The relative unreliability of CVP measurement as an indicator of left ventricular preload led to the development in the late 1960s of the Swan-Ganz catheter. This is a quadrilumen catheter that may be inserted percutaneously into the central venous circulation and easily passed into the main pulmonary artery without the need for fluoroscopy. In this position, pulmonary artery pressures, pulmonary capillary wedge pressures (PCWP), and cardiac output can be measured.

Catheters are now available for use in the pediatric patient, including the neonate. Through the use of this catheter, it is possible to quantify changes in each of the parameters that influence cardiac output.

The pulmonary capillary wedge pressure correlates well with left atrial pressure, allowing a reliable assessment of left ventricular preload.

The thermistor contained in the catheter allows determination of cardiac output by a thermodilution technique, which correlates well with widely accepted dye dilution measurements. Afterload, or vascular resistance, can be separately determined for the systemic or pulmonary circuits using measured pressures and cardiac output. Measurement of specific cardiac output determinants allows specific identification of the deranged parameter, allowing specific therapeutic manipulation. In addition, pulmonary arterial blood may be sampled to mea-

CAUSES OF UNRELIABILITY OF CVP MEASUREMENT

Rapid changes in blood volume
Myocardial depression or stimulation
Administration of vasoactive agents
Pulmonary hypertension and right ventricular dysfunction
Tricuspid valve abnormalities
Severe pulmonary disease
High levels of intrathoracic pressure

CIRCULATORY PARAMETERS ACCESSIBLE WITH SWAN-GANZ CATHETER

Measured variables

Pulmonary artery pressures
Separate right and left ventricular filling pressures
Cardiac output
Mixed venous oxygen saturation

Derived variables

Right and left ventricular work
Pulmonary and systemic vascular resistances
Oxygen availability and consumption

sure a true mixed venous oxygen saturation. This variable then allows calculation of intrapulmonary shunt, oxygen consumption, and oxygen availability. Parameters accessible by use of the Swan-Ganz catheter are found on the opposite page.

Accurate and continuous measurement of arterial blood pressure is performed by cannulation of a peripheral artery. Percutaneous insertion is accomplished with relative ease, even in the neonate, although a cutdown is occasionally necessary. The preferred locations are the radial, dorsalis pedis, or posterior tibial arteries. In selected situations, the brachial or femoral arteries are used. Umbilical and temporal artery catheters, popular in neonates, should be avoided, as the complications are more frequent and serious.

Treatment of low cardiac output states. After determining derangement of one or more of the determinants of cardiac output, specific therapy is undertaken. Ongoing monitoring of the above discussed methods allows quantification of response to therapy.

When decreased heart rate is the primary factor responsible for the low cardiac output state, treatment involves accelerating the heart rate to appropriate values for age. Any metabolic abnormalities responsible for the bradyarrhythmia must of course be corrected. Atropine then may be effective, particularly when the bradycardia is sinus in origin. More frequently, catecholamine agents with significant chronotropic properties must be used, such as isoproterenol or epinephrine. If the cause of the bradycardia is an anatomic or traumatic abnormality of the conduction pathways and is expected to be persistent, insertion of a temporary pacemaker is indicated.

When decreased preload is the primary factor responsible for the low cardiac output state, the cause of the impaired preload must be corrected. Cardioversion or antiarrhythmics may be indicated to correct an arrhythmia causing loss of atrial augmentation. In selected cases of myocarditis, antiinflammatory agents may be useful. Correction of decreased preload usually involves intravascular volume expansion. The choice of volume expander—crystalloid, colloid, whole blood, packed cells, or Dextran—is based on factors such as the cause of the intravascular volume depletion and the patient's baseline hemoglobin and serum protein. The crystalloid versus colloid controversy remains to be settled, but a conservative approach involves the use of colloid only when serum protein and oncotic pressure are less than normal.

The goal of intravascular volume expansion is achievement of an optimal filling pressure, rather than some arbitrary "normal" value for CVP or PCWP. The shape of the Frank-Starling curve for the normal myocardium demonstrates that a PCWP greater than 7 to 10 mmHg produces minimal further increase in cardiac output. In the sick myocardium, the Frank-Starling curve is shifted downward and to the right, with a flatter slope (see Fig. 32-3). With such a curve, "normal" PCWP will not maximize cardiac output, and optimization of preload may not occur until a PCWP of 18 to 22 mmHg is reached. Optimization of cardiac output might not occur until even higher filling pressures in the failing and noncompliant myocardium. However, further increases are limited by effects on the pulmonary capillary bed. Even with normal pulmonary vascular permeability, interstitial pulmonary edema will develop with LAP or PCWP in excess of 22 to 24 mmHg. This occurs at lower pressures if there is increased capillary permeability such as with septic shock, longstanding shock of other types, or primary lung injury.

Treatment of impaired contractility involves (1) correction of metabolic derangement, such as hypoxia, hypocalcemia, hypoglycemia, electrolyte abnormalities, and acidosis; (2) digitalization when long-term inotropic support is necessary; or (3) use of catecholamine inotropic agents.

The use of catecholamine agents requires a basic understanding of adrenergic receptor physiology. Table 32-1 describes the important adrenergic receptors, their location, and the physiologic effects of their stimulation.

Each of the clinically available catecholamine agents has different relative effects on each of the receptor sites. These relative effects are summarized in Table 32-2.

Selection of a catecholamine agent should consider the effects on each of the four determinants of cardiac output. For example, if increase in heart rate is required for correction of low cardiac output, an agent with greater chronotropic effect is indicated; if increase in heart rate might be detrimental, another agent is in-

Table 32-1. Important adrenergic receptors

Adrenergic receptor	Site	Action
$Beta_1$	Myocardium	Increased atrial and ventricular contractility
	Sinoatrial node	Increased heart rate
	Atrioventricular conduction	Increased rate of conduction
$Beta_2$	Arterioles	Vasodilation
	Lungs	Bronchodilation
Alpha	Peripheral arterioles	Vasoconstriction
Dopaminergic	Mesenteric, renal arterioles	Vasodilation

Table 32-2. Relative effects of catecholamine agents on receptor sites

	Alpha peripheral	$Beta_1$ cardiac	$Beta_2$ peripheral	Dopaminergic—renal, mesenteric
Norepinephrine	++++	++++	0	0
Epinephrine	++++	++++	++	0
Dopamine	++++	++++	++	++
Isoproterenol	0	++++	++++	0
Dobutamine	+	++++	++	0
Methoxamine	++++	0	0	0

dicated. Similarly, afterload may be increased or decreased, depending on the vascular properties of a particular agent. Another consideration is the effect on myocardial oxygen consumption. This is a more important consideration in the adult patient, and perhaps the adolescent, whose coronary perfusion may not be sufficient to meet the increased oxygen demand created by the use of inotropic agents. Although this is less of a concern in pediatric patients, it does remain a consideration.

The most commonly used catecholamine agents are epinephrine, isoproterenol, dopamine, and dobutamine. For detailed discussion of these agents, see Goodman and Gilman's *The Pharmacological Basis of Therapeutics*.

Epinephrine was one of the earliest catecholamine agents to be used in clinical situations. It possesses approximately equal alpha and beta stimulating properties. It is a powerful inotropic and chronotropic agent and produces large increases in myocardial oxygen demand. In very high doses alpha vasoconstriction predominates, and epinephrine may in fact cause an increased afterload and impaired peripheral perfusion; this is a limitation on its use as a continuous infusion.

Isoproterenol is the most potent beta stimulant of all the catecholamine agents and possesses virtually no alpha effects. It also has greater chronotropic properties than other catecholamine agents. $Beta_1$ stimulation with isoproterenol produces a marked increase in cardiac output, whereas $beta_2$ receptor stimulation produces peripheral vasodilation and reduction in total peripheral resistance.

Dopamine was developed in the late 1960s as an agent to provide inotropic effects without chronotropic effects, which were detrimental in many adult patients. In addition, dopamine has unique effects on "dopaminergic" receptors located in the renal and mesenteric vascular beds, producing there a vasodilation. Thus dopamine possesses dose-dependent effects on dopaminergic, alpha, and beta receptors. In low doses, total renal blood flow and cortical nephron flow increase. In middle-dose ranges, $beta_1$ and $beta_2$ stimulation occurs, with improved contractility and small increase in heart rate and vasodilation in skeletal muscle vascular beds. In higher doses, alpha effects predominate and widespread, significant vasoconstriction occurs. In doses greater than 20 μg/kg/min the increase in total peripheral resistance may actually decrease cardiac output by increasing afterload. Table 32-3 lists the dose ranges over which clinically significant effects occur with dopamine.

Dobutamine is a recently released catechol-

Table 32-3. Dose-related effects of dopamine

Dosage	Type	Effect
2-4 μg/kg/min	Dopaminergic receptor	Renal and mesenteric dilation, natriuresis, diuresis
5-15 μg/kg/min	Beta receptors	Increased contractility, mild increased heart rate, mild vasodilation
15-20 μg/kg/min	Further beta receptor, early alpha receptor	Further increase in contractility, variable early vasoconstriction
Greater than 20 μg/kg/min	Alpha receptor	Increasing predominance of vasoconstriction, increased peripheral resistance and afterload, possible decreased cardiac output

amine agent similar in many ways to dopamine. It has similar inotropic ($beta_1$) properties with minimal chronotropic effects. Unlike dopamine, however, alpha-mediated vasoconstriction does not occur to a clinically significant degree until doses are increased to nearly 40 μg/kg/min. Dobutamine also lacks the dopaminergic-stimulating properties of dopamine.

The use of vasodilator therapy to decrease afterload has been a major development in the treatment of low cardiac output states. Occasional situations exist in which cardiac output is reduced primarily by increased afterload secondary to pathologic vasoconstriction. As mentioned earlier, such is the case in some stages of septic shock and occasionally after correction of previously existing preload and contractility problems. Specific treatment of the increased afterload with vasodilators can produce a normal cardiac output. Afterload reduction therapy has become much more widespread than in these specific applications. As discussed earlier, a family of afterload curves can be described (see Fig. 32-4). In the severely dysfunctional myocardium, small amounts of afterload can reduce cardiac output. Even "normal" values for total peripheral resistance may represent a substantial afterload. In such a patient, small amounts of afterload reduction will significantly increase cardiac output.

The newer vasodilators, nitroprusside and nitroglycerin, have replaced the older chlorpromazine, trimethaphan, and phentolamine. Nitroprusside, given by continuous intravenous infusion, is a nearly ideal drug for afterload reduction therapy. Its onset of action is rapid, and it is extremely potent. Its dose-response relationship is essentially linear over the dose range clinically used, and its effects are extremely short-lived when the drug is discontinued. The major complication with nitroprusside, other than potential excessive vasodilation and hypotension, is related to cyanide and thiocyanate toxicity. The drug is converted to cyanide, which is responsible for its vascular smooth muscle–relaxing effects, and the cyanide is converted to thiocyanate. Both metabolites may be toxic. The toxic effects are seen generally with high doses for prolonged periods of time and are more prevalent in adult patients than pediatric patients. Within the last year, nitroglycerin has become available for intravenous infusion. It has the same advantages as nitroprusside and apparently lacks toxicity. Additionally, nitroglycerin has specific coronary vasodilating properties. This offers the advantage of increased myocardial perfusion. The major difficulty with nitroglycerin is its tendency to adhere to intravenous tubing, making its delivery less predictable and less easily controlled.

VASOCONSTRICTING PRESSORS

Norepinephrine
Mephentermine
Ephedrine
Metaraminol
Phenylephrine
Methoxamine

A discussion of vasoactive agents must include mention of vasoconstricting agents, if only to condemn their use in most clinical situations. These agents, listed above, are primarily alpha agonists and act by producing widespread vasoconstriction. Thus blood pressure is temporarily increased by a marked increase in total peripheral resistance, but the substantial increase in afterload ultimately reduces cardiac output. These agents have been advocated in the past to temporize hypovolemic shock. It is our feeling that this need virtually never exists, and clearly the treatment of hypovolemia is volume expansion. Their use is limited to two situations: hypotension associated with spinal or general anesthesia, and right-to-left shunt emergencies, such as a life-threatening "tetralogy" spell that has not been relieved by the usual interventions. The initiation of a vasoconstricting agent may reduce the extent of right-to-left shunting long enough to allow the infant to be taken to the operating room.

ACUTE RESPIRATORY FAILURE

Respiratory failure signifies the inability of the lungs to maintain adequate arterial tensions of oxygen or carbon dioxide. Acute respiratory failure may be of two types, hypoxemia with or without associated hypercapnia. (See also pp. 410-413.) The pathophysiologic derangement most often accounting for hypoxemia is ventilation/perfusion mismatching on the basis of airway obstruction (such as bronchospasm or luminal debris) and less commonly by intrapulmonary shunt on the basis of alveolar filling (such as consolidation or alveolar edema). Hypercarbia occurs when hypoventilation ensues, most often from muscular fatigue secondary to increased respiratory effort and increased work of breathing associated with most respiratory disorders. Occasionally, a central or peripheral neuromuscular disturbance reduces ventilatory effort. A list of causes of acute respiratory failure in children has been reviewed elsewhere in this volume (see p. 411 for a more detailed examination of physiology and causes).

The diagnosis of acute respiratory failure can be strongly suspected by clinical presentation of severe respiratory distress. Objective respiratory tract findings include any of the following: tachypnea, retractions, cyanosis, rales, rhonchi, wheezes, decreased inspiratory breath sounds, and apnea. Nonrespiratory symptomatology may include tachycardia, bradycardia, fatigue, agitation, diaphoresis, stupor, or coma. If time permits, the diagnosis may be confirmed by arterial blood gas determination documenting hypoxemia or hypercarbia. Numerical criteria of oxygen and carbon dioxide tensions, although helpful in confirmation, should not be the sole criteria to judge whether a child is in acute respiratory failure. Serial clinical observations coupled with serial arterial blood gas measurements allow a dynamic assessment of improvement or deterioration of respiratory status, as well as response to management.

There is usually ample time to diagnose acute respiratory failure and to institute specific therapy. Nevertheless, occasional patients are seen in respiratory arrest or with imminent cardiopulmonary arrest. In these cases, therapy is directed at immediate restoration of respiratory gas exchange and adequate circulation. Cardiopulmonary resuscitative measures in pediatrics have recently been reviewed and are discussed on pp. 412-413 and 878-880.

It must be remembered that adequate ventilation and oxygenation can follow therapy other than establishment of an artificial airway with subsequent mechanical ventilation. For example, respiratory insufficiency in fully treated status asthmaticus may be significantly reversed with intravenous infusion of isoproterenol; nebulized racemic epinephrine administered intermittently can reduce the need for intubation in acute laryngotracheobronchitis. In any case, various types of adjunctive therapy may alleviate the need for intubation and assisted ventilation. These include administration of oxygen, humidification and inhalation therapy, chest physical therapy, and judicious attention to fluid therapy.

Unless a steady, adequate improvement is seen clinically and by blood gas measurement, mechanical ventilation must be undertaken. In this situation, intubation must be considered an urgent procedure but not an emergency procedure. Ventilation can be maintained by bag-and-mask technique while preparations for intubation are made. Necessary equipment should be at hand and functional before any intubation attempt. The proper orotracheal tube size for children older than 2 years of age may be estimated according to the formula that the tube internal diameter is equal to 4 plus one fourth of the child's age. For most preterm infants, a 3.0 mm tube is used; from birth to 6 months, 3.5 mm; and from 6 to 18 months, 4.0 mm. A quick and easy guide is that the diameter of the tube should be the same as that of the patient's little finger. Preparations before any attempt at intubation include (1) ensuring the availability of suction and a working laryngoscope blade of correct size, (2) prior oxygenation for several minutes, (3) administering atropine 0.02 mg/kg intravenously, and (4) placing the patient's head in the "sniffing" position. After these preparations, the endotracheal tube is inserted just past the vocal cords. The patient's lungs are then ventilated by bag-to-endotracheal tube technique and the patient is checked for synchronous chest wall movement during inhalation, absence of breath sounds over the stomach, and presence of bilaterally equal breath sounds.

Once intubation has been successfully accomplished and the endotracheal tube properly secured, assisted ventilation can be instituted. The purpose of any mechanical ventilator is to replace the bellows function of the diaphragm and chest wall musculature. The goal of assisted ventilation is achievement of proper alveolar ventilation. As an initial guide to institution of ventilation, the following guidelines have been developed. For all patients weighing more than 5 kg, a volume-cycled, constant-flow generator is used. The initial respiratory frequency should be that which is normal for the child's age: from birth to 1 year, 30 breaths/min; from 1 to 5 years, 25 breaths/min; from 5 to 10 years, 20 breaths/min; for adolescents, 15 breaths/min. Tidal volume requirements are difficult to predict for any given clinical situation, but the initial tidal volume used is 10 to 15 ml/kg of body weight/breath. The initial concentration of oxygen required is variable, but generally a high rate of forced inspiratory oxygen (FIO_2) will ensure adequate arterial oxygen saturation. A 100% concentration of oxygen has been shown to increase intrapulmonary shunt, and therefore an initial FIO_2 of 80% to 90% is preferable. The mode chosen for ventilatory support is that of intermittent mandatory ventilation (IMV), which allows the patient not only to breathe on his own but also to receive a mandatory tidal volume from the respirator at the preset frequency. The mandatory breath is independent of the patient's ventilatory pattern. Because of continuous flow of gas through the ventilator circuit, the patient breathing spontaneously will receive fresh gas at his own tidal volume. The IMV mode is more physiologic than the control mode, in which a spontaneously breathing patient cannot receive a self-initiated breath, or the assist mode, in which the initiation of a breath may not occur because of inadequate patient effort or machine insensitivity. The initial setting for the inspiratory to expiratory ratio should be 1:2, which is that of a spontaneously breathing patient. The application of small amounts of positive-end expiratory pressure (PEEP) may be beneficial to patients who have evidence of diffuse alveolar collapse or persistent severe hypoxemia in the face of high oxygen concentrations. Once the initial settings are determined and the child is placed "on the ventilator," he must be examined for adequacy of breath sounds, chest wall motion, skin color, and peripheral perfusion. Arterial blood gases are checked no later than 20 minutes after ventilation is instituted if there are no signs of clinical deterioration. Achievement of proper alveolar ventilation is the major goal of assisted ventilation and must be assessed by serial determination of P_aCO_2. Readjustment of the respiratory frequency and tidal volume must be made according to the serial P_aCO_2 determinations. Reduction of P_aCO_2 can be accomplished by increasing respiratory rate or tidal volume, or both. Oxygenation should improve as alveolar ventilation improves. If this is not the case, gradual increases of PEEP or reversal of the inspiratory-to-expiratory ratio may improve oxygenation and reduce the FIO_2 requirement. Tissue oxygenation must be assessed by clinical observations of heart rate, blood pressure, skin color, capillary refill, level of consciousness, pH, electrolyte balance, and urine output. Appropriate monitoring and supportive measures are integral parts of the approach to the management of acute respiratory failure.

Weaning from mechanical ventilation requires resolution or adequate improvement of the underlying cause of acute respiratory failure. Blood gases must be improved as much as can be reasonably expected on the basis of the clinical course. For withdrawal of support, ventilator settings discussed above are slowly reduced, while clinical evaluation of respiratory effort and serial arterial blood gases demonstrate continued adequacy of ventilation and oxygenation. Once the patient demonstrates that he can ventilate adequately with no ventilator mandatory breaths and that physiologic levels of constant positive airway pressure (CPAP) are being tolerated, extubation is undertaken. This trial-and-error approach may be replaced by measurement of physiologic parameters of "readiness" of extubation in older, more cooperative patients.

CENTRAL NERVOUS SYSTEM INJURY

The increasingly sophisticated care available to children with respiratory, cardiovascular, and other catastrophic disorders has improved survival in critically ill children. Advances in the intensive care of the central nervous system have come more slowly, and this improved survival has been achieved at the expense of increased neurologic morbidity. Recent advances, however, in the monitoring and therapeutic modalities available for the management of patients with central nervous system injuries have begun to reverse this trend and to give cause for greater optimism for improved quality of survival in these children.

Central nervous system insults severe enough to be threatening to life or to the quality of life may be divided into four general categories:

1. Trauma
2. Anoxia/ischemia (such as drowning, smoke inhalation, and cardiac arrest)
3. Infectious (such as meningitis and encephalitis)
4. Metabolic (uremia, hepatic encephalopathy, Reye syndrome, and diabetic ketoacidosis)

The first step in the management of patients with these types of central nervous system injuries involves the scrupulous and continuous monitoring of neurologic function.

Monitoring

Monitoring of the central nervous system has taken many forms over the years. Below is a list of modalities that have found varying degrees of usefulness in the intensive care unit monitoring of a patient with central nervous system dysfunction.

CENTRAL NERVOUS SYSTEM MONITORING

- Neurologic examination
- X-ray examination
- Cerebral electrical activity
- Intracranial pressure
- Cerebral metabolic function
- Cerebral blood flow

Clinical evaluation of the patient in the intensive care unit with craniocerebral injury should be a complete neurologic examination, but it should emphasize especially two areas: level of responsiveness and brain stem function. The level of responsiveness should be described in more detail than simply using terms such as coma, semicoma, etc. The Glasgow Coma Scale provides a format for the quantification of the level of responsiveness. This 15-point scale has been shown to correlate with long-term outcome and is used by many centers as one criterion for the institution of different levels of intervention.

Evaluating the patient by using the Glasgow Coma Scale yields a score range of 3 to 15. This scoring system, though correlating with eventual outcome, is not particularly sensitive and therefore not well suited for the hour-by-hour monitoring necessary in the intensive care unit. For this purpose, several other scales and scoring systems have been developed. These usually include all of the parameters used in the Glasgow Coma Scale, in addition to other parameters such as specific tests of brain stem function.

Evaluation of brain stem function should in-

GLASGOW COMA SCALE

Eye-opening	
Spontaneous	4
To speech	3
To pain	2
None	1
Best motor response	
Obeys commands	6
Localizes pain	5
Nonpurposeful withdrawal to pain	4
Abnormal flexor response	3
Extensor response to pain	2
No response	1
Verbal response	
Oriented	5
Confused conversation	4
Inappropriate words	3
Incomprehensible sounds	2
None	1

clude a detailed examination of all important brain stem reflexes:

- Respiratory pattern
- Oculocephalic and oculovestibular reflexes
- Pupillary and corneal reflexes
- Pharyngeal, laryngeal, and tracheal reflexes
- Supracervical motor responses
- Autonomic function
- Peripheral tone and posture

The frequent performance of a detailed neurologic examination is important for several reasons. It allows some crude prediction of eventual outcome. It allows for some degree of localization of injury to the brain. Finally, it allows for the detection of changes in the patient's condition.

It is not uncommon in the intensive care unit that patients with neurologic injury will require therapies such as continuous sedative or anesthetic agents, neuromuscular blocking agents, and so forth, which render the neurologic examination useless. In these patients, particularly, we must resort to intensive care technology for the monitoring of the patient's condition.

Recent advances in x-ray technology have made radiographic examination of the patient with central nervous system injury extremely important. Skull films, echoencephalography, angiography, and various types of radioisotopic brain scans are useful in selected patients in intensive care units.

The most important radiologic advance for patients with central nervous system injury is the computerized tomography (CT) scanner. Obviously, all patients with significant head trauma should have a CT scan as part of their initial evaluation, and as indicated during the subsequent course, because of the high risk of hematomas, contusions, and late-developing hydrocephalus. Many patients with central nervous system injury other than traumatic injury will also require CT scan examination to define the nature and extent of injury.

All radiographic evaluations of patients with central nervous system injury suffer the limitation of being only sporadically performed. Although it is possible to perform most of these examinations on a daily basis, sometimes even more frequently than daily, they still do not lend themselves to the continuous monitoring of the patient's neurologic status that is required in the intensive care unit. For these purposes, the clinician must turn to other modalities.

One such modality is electroencephalography (EEG), in which recent technologic advances have improved its suitability for continuous monitoring purposes. Initial attempts at monitoring cerebral electrical function came with the use of the conventional EEG in the intensive care unit. This obviously presented some difficulties. The EEG machine is cumbersome, requires a trained technician for its operation, and, if run continuously, involves the consumption of prohibitive quantities of paper. Furthermore, the interpretation of the conventional EEG requires a physician specifically trained in the field. For these reasons, efforts were directed toward the development of electroencephalographic techniques that condense and simplify the information generated by the conventional EEG.

One example of such a modification of the conventional EEG makes use of a minicomputer and techniques called fourrier analysis and spectral display. With these techniques, information can be generated from the EEG and displayed in a form that lends itself to ready interpretation by physicians relatively unfamiliar with conventional EEGs. These displays give discrete information about overall amplitude and frequency of cortical electrical activity, and can do so globally over the entire cortex, over each hemisphere separately, or over quadrants or even more discrete segments of cortex. This information can be generated as frequently as the programer desires, even as often as every few seconds. The disadvantage of the technique is the prohibitive cost of the necessary equipment, although the use of microprocessors is likely to reduce the costs of such equipment substantially over the next few years.

A cruder but simpler and less expensive modification of the conventional EEG is the Cerebral Function Monitor (Critikon, Incorporated). This instrument uses a single bipolar EEG lead, with one electrode placed over each parietal area of the cortex. The trace generated by this device is a composite of amplitude and frequency and thus does not give discrete information about either parameter separately. However, the recent addition to this device of a channel that records the average frequency over 14-second epochs allows the instrument to give more information than earlier prototypes. The cerebral function monitor provides an easily interpreted monitor of generalized cortical electrical activity and may therefore be used to reflect functional changes resulting from decreased perfusion pressure, acute metabolic derangements, and centrally active drugs. It is also useful for the detection of seizure activity, an important monitoring capability for patients who are at risk for seizures but are receiving neuromuscular blocking agents, in whom no other indication of ongoing seizure activity is available.

The final electroencephalographic technique to be mentioned is that of evoked potentials. The majority of work done thus far with the use of evoked potentials in the intensive care unit has used auditory evoked brain stem responses. These have been shown to be somewhat predictive of long-term outcome in head injury patients, as well as relatively sensitive indicators of some forms of neurologic deterioration. Extensive work has not yet been done with the use of auditory evoked potentials in pediatric patients in the intensive care setting, but it is likely that auditory evoked potentials and somatosensory evoked potentials will prove to have a role in the intensive care unit.

Intracranial pressure

Monitoring. The most significant advance in the monitoring of neurologically injured patients has come in the form of intracranial pressure (ICP) monitoring technology. The first report of clinical monitoring of intracranial pressure in patients did not appear until 1951. Subsequent reports did not appear until the early 1960s, and reports of extensive use of intracranial pressure monitoring in patients did not appear until the early 1970s. The first description of intracranial pressure monitoring in a small but exclusively pediatric population appeared in 1975, and the technique was not widely accepted as a routine standard of care for indicated patients until the late 1970s.

Techniques available for monitoring of intracranial pressure include the intraventricular catheter, the subarachnoid bolt, the epidural transducer, and the noninvasive "fontanometer." The last two techniques have fairly limited applicability. Epidural transducers are expensive and are subject to considerable electronic vagaries. The fontanometer, although it has the advantage of being noninvasive, is less accurate than other methods and is applicable only to the young infant with an open fontanelle.

In general, intracranial pressure monitoring is accomplished in older patients by one of two methods: the intraventricular catheter or the subarachnoid bolt. Both methods yield accurate measurements of intracranial pressure, and both are associated with acceptably low complication rates. Each has its own particular advantages and disadvantages, and some patients may be more suitable for monitoring by one technique as opposed to the other. Complications of intracranial pressure monitoring include infection (less than 2% in experienced centers), bleeding (less than 0.5%), and subdural cerebrospinal fluid (CSF) "leaks" after removal of the instrument (less than 3%).

Indications for invasive monitoring of intracranial pressure are simple. Patients who have a disorder known to be associated with increased intracranial pressure, and whose level of responsiveness is impaired to the extent that elevated pressure cannot be ruled out on clinical grounds, must be invasively monitored. To rule out clinically the presence of elevated pressure requires that the patient be able to respond to stimuli in ways that require fairly complex cortical function. For example, the ability to follow verbal commands or a brisk, purposeful, and localizing response to a painful stimulus have been used in many centers as clinical indicators of the absence of threatening intracranial pressure. In addition, the patient must not be displaying intermittent abnormal or posturing responses to pain.

Using these liberal criteria for the institution of invasive monitoring has yielded interesting information in recent years. These criteria undoubtedly will include for invasive monitoring some patients who do not have elevated intracranial pressure at the time the monitoring device is placed. However, prior placement of the monitoring device allows for protection from potentially life-threatening increases in intracranial pressure that have now been shown to occur in advance of any change in the patient's clinical status. In other words, aggressive and early use of intracranial pressure monitoring in indicated patients allows for early detection of increased intracranial pressure before such pressure causes irreversible secondary brain injury and before it causes clinically detectable changes in the patient's condition.

Valid questions may be raised about the role

of intracranial pressure in eventual outcome and about the efficacy of controlling intracranial pressure in improving mortality and morbidity. The importance of intracranial pressure and its control with aggressive management has been clearly demonstrated in both adult and pediatric patients with head trauma. Most experienced clinicians who care for patients with Reye syndrome also recognize the importance of intracranial pressure and its control in the outcome of patients with this condition, although the data have been less convincingly compiled than those for head trauma. Intracranial pressure is also believed to play a role in the outcome of some patients with meningitis and encephalitis; with some metabolic encephalopathies, such as hepatic encephalopathy and diabetic ketoacidosis; and possibly also in patients with anoxic encephalopathy. However, patients with these disorders have not been able to be studied in any prospective fashion in sufficiently large numbers to generate definitive data. It is also unlikely, for ethical reasons, that any such prospective studies will ever be carried out. In any case the use of intracranial pressure monitoring in patients with these disorders, known to be associated with life-threatening intracranial pressure, is considered the state-of-the-art in pediatric intensive care.

Pathophysiology. Intracranial pressure is determined by the total volume of intracranial components relative to the total volume of the intracranial vault. In general, the intracranial vault, with its relatively fixed volume, contains four components:

1. Cerebrospinal fluid—CSF accounts for approximately 10% of the intracranial volume, is produced at a rate of 0.35 ml/min, and its synthesis and reabsorption are somewhat influenced by the intracranial pressure.
2. Blood—The cerebral blood volume is roughly proportional to the cerebral blood flow. Cerebral blood flow is governed by local tissue and CSF pH, arterial (and CSF) P_{CO_2}, arterial P_{O_2}, cerebral metabolic rate, and numerous other less important factors. A certain quantity of cerebral blood volume may be displaced from the venous sinuses, independent of cerebral blood flow, with no adverse effects.
3. Brain—The major portion of the intracranial vault is occupied by brain. This includes brain tissue and brain water. Brain water is contained both in the intracellular compartment of the brain as well as in the interstitium or extracellular compartment of the brain. A certain amount of brain water can be removed from the brain with no adverse effects.
4. Other—Other components may take up intracranial volume, such as tumors, hematomas, abcesses, and effusions.

The volume of any one of the components that occupy a portion of the volume of the intracranial vault can increase only at the expense of the displacement of an equal volume from one or the other components. As mentioned above, substantial amounts of cerebrospinal fluid, cerebral venous blood volume, and brain water, as well as any extraneous intracranial masses, can be removed from the intracranial vault with no adverse effects. When the displacement of an equal volume of a nonessential component from the intracranial vault is no longer possible, further expansion of the volume of one of the other components occurs with the production of sudden and marked increases in intracranial pressure. This relationship between intracranial pressure and intracranial volume is described in Fig. 32-5.

As can be seen in Fig. 32-5, the intracranial vault can accomodate significant increases in volume. Ultimately, however, after the accomodation of a large increase in volume, a very small addition in volume produces a significant increase in the intracranial pressure. It is at this point that the compensatory mechanisms—displacement of CSF, cerebral venous blood, and excess brain water from the intracranial vault—have been exhausted.

Intracranial pressure is important to the survival of patients with central nervous system injuries because it is an important determinant of cerebral perfusion pressure:

$$\text{cerebral perfusion pressure} = \text{mean arterial pressure} - \text{ICP}$$

Cerebral perfusion pressure, in turn, is important because it is a determinant of cerebral blood flow as defined by Poiseuille's law:

$$\text{cerebral blood flow} = \text{cerebral perfusion pressure} \div \text{resistance}$$

Thus as intracranial pressure increases one might expect a proportional decrease in cerebral blood flow. However, this does not occur strictly according to Poiseuille's law because of the exquisite autoregulatory capabilities of the cerebrovascular bed. In this vascular bed, as perfusion pressure increases or decreases, the diameter of the blood vessels changes in response

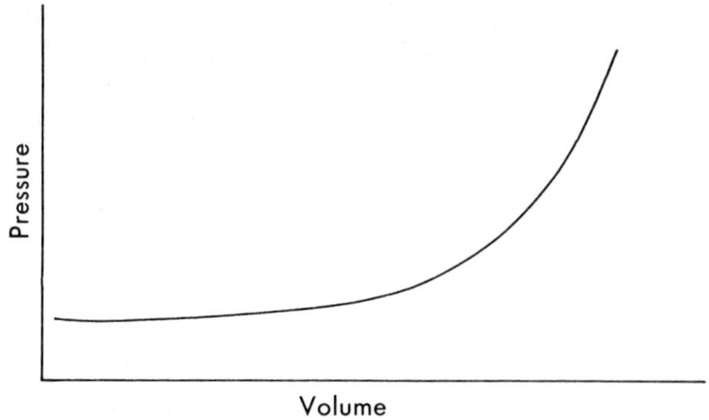

Fig. 32-5. Relationship between intracranial pressure and intracranial volume.

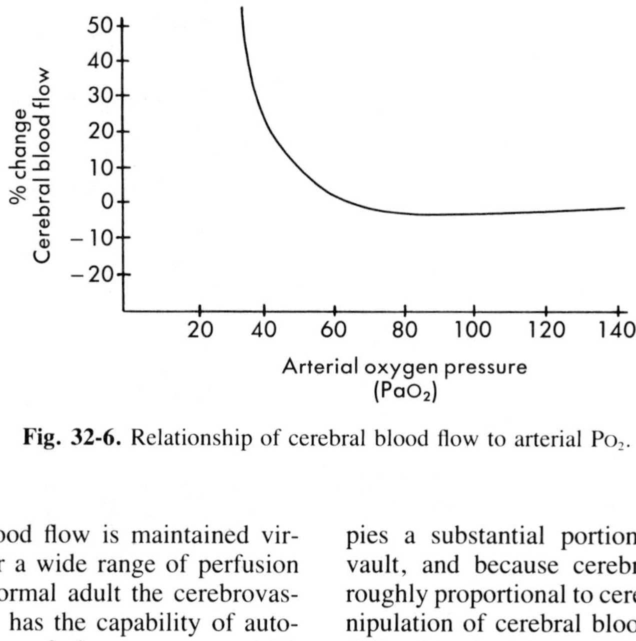

Fig. 32-6. Relationship of cerebral blood flow to arterial Po_2.

so that cerebral blood flow is maintained virtually constant over a wide range of perfusion pressures. In the normal adult the cerebrovascular bed generally has the capability of autoregulation between perfusion pressures of 50 mmHg up to 130 to 150 mmHg. However, when perfusion pressure varies as a result of changes in intracranial pressure, the cerebrovascular bed begins to lose its ability to autoregulate, and cerebral blood flow becomes much more pressure dependent and much more likely to follow Poiseuille's law.

Cerebral blood flow is important from a clinical point of view for two obvious reasons. First, the goal of most therapy is to preserve cerebral blood flow adequate to guarantee brain cell viability and preservation of brain cell function. Secondly, because cerebral blood volume (particularly cerebral venous blood volume) occupies a substantial portion of the intracranial vault, and because cerebral blood volume is roughly proportional to cerebral blood flow, manipulation of cerebral blood flow will substantially alter the blood volume. Thus controlling the factors that regulate cerebral blood flow provides a means of controlling the intracranial pressure.

The two major and easily controlled factors that influence cerebral blood flow, and therefore cerebral blood volume, are the arterial Po_2 and Pco_2. Cerebral blood flow is related to arterial Po_2 as in Fig. 32-6. As can be seen in Fig. 32-6, cerebral blood flow remains constant over a wide range of Po_2. However, when the arterial Po_2 falls below 60 torr, one sees an exponential increase in cerebral blood flow. This increased flow, which is homeostatic and preserves oxygen delivery to the brain in the normal situation, is achieved by a cerebral vasodilation. This can be lethal to the patient with an injured brain and altered cerebral hemodynamics. The vasodilation in these situations produces a sudden and acute increase in cerebral blood volume, thus producing a potentially life-threatening increase in intracranial pressure. For this reason, efforts must be made to guarantee adequate oxygenation at all times in patients with central nervous system injury.

Cerebral blood flow is linearly related to arterial P_{CO_2}. Between P_{CO_2} of 20 and 80 torr, cerebral blood flow changes about 2 ml/100 g/torr. The vasodilation responsible for this increased blood flow with increasing P_{CO_2} produces an increased cerebral blood volume at a rate of 0.04 ml/100 g/torr change in P_{CO_2}. In the adult brain weighing approximately 1400 g this represents an increase of between 10 and 15 ml of blood volume for a 10 torr increase in P_{CO_2}. This increased volume, trivial in a patient with normal cerebral hemodynamics, may produce a life-threatening increase in intracranial pressure in the patient with an injured brain.

Treatment. A basic understanding of the pathophysiology of increased intracranial pressure leads to the development of some fairly routine measures for the care of the patient at risk for increased intracranial pressure. The following list of guidelines should be considered routine for these patients because of their efficacy and low risk.

1. Maintain head elevated at 30° to 45° and in midline position to facilitate cerebral venous drainage.
2. Avoid the use of internal jugular catheters to facilitate cerebral venous return.
3. Minimize positive airway pressure as much as possible to facilitate cerebral venous drainage.
4. Use fluid restriction and diuresis to achieve a euvolemic hyperosmolar dehydration (sodium 145 to 150, osmolarity 300 to 310, CVP and PCWP 2-5 cm/H_2O).
5. Oxygenate to maintain P_{O_2} greater than 100 torr.
6. If baseline intracranial pressure is elevated, or acute increases of intracranial pressure are documented, hyperventilate to maintain baseline P_{CO_2} of 24 to 27 torr.
7. Maintain "normal" blood pressure.
8. Use sedation and neuromuscular paralysis and avoid noxious stimulation to reduce afferent stimulation and muscle movement.
9. Use antipyretic therapy to maintain afebrile state.
10. Control gastric pH.

The first three steps described above are all designed to help facilitate cerebral venous drainage. The fourth step attempts to reduce intracellular and extracellular brain water to a minimal amount.

Maintenance of a P_{O_2} greater than 100 torr provides some margin of error to prevent the potentially life-threatening vasodilation that occurs when the P_{O_2} drops to below 60 torr. Hyperventilation to the range described in step 6 reduces cerebral blood flow to the point that cerebral blood volume is optimally minimized, but with little likelihood of more detrimental reduction in cerebral blood flow.

Avoidance of febrile states will prevent the marked increase in cerebral metabolic rate, accompanied by proportional increases in cerebral blood flow and blood volume, that are associated with increased temperature. Finally, with the incidence of hemorrhagic gastrointestinal complications in patients with central nervous system injury exceeding 80%, the routine control of gastric pH should be considered mandatory.

The immediate management of acute, life-threatening intracranial hypertension, documented by monitoring or strongly suspected on clinical grounds, should include the following triad: (1) manual hyperventilation, (2) intravenous mannitol, and (3) intravenous thiopental.

Manual hyperventilation, even if the baseline P_{CO_2} is already in the 25 to 27 torr range, usually produces an immediate and potentially life-saving reduction in the intracranial pressure. This occurs as a result of the hypocarbia-induced reduction in cerebral blood flow, which in turn produces a reduction in cerebral blood volume. This maneuver is particularly effective early in the course of the development of increased intracranial pressure and usually produces a relatively sustained reduction in intracranial pressure even after the arterial P_{CO_2} has returned to its baseline value.

If manual hyperventilation fails to reduce the intracranial pressure within 30 to 60 seconds, or if manual hyperventilation is occurring more frequently than four to five times per hour, preparation should be made for the administration of an intravenous dose of mannitol (0.25 to 0.5 gm/kg). This dose of mannitol will produce within 5 to 10 minutes a sustained reduction in the intracranial pressure. It tends to be less effective if the patient is already extremely hyperosmolar, and its use in patients who are known to have subdural or epidural hematomas is controversial.

If hyperventilation and mannitol have failed to produce reduction in the intracranial pressure, or if the intracranial pressure is elevated to extremely critical levels that must be reduced within minutes, an intravenous dose of thiopental should be given (2 to 5 mg/kg). This drug must be given extremely carefully because of its potential to produce severe hypotension, especially in a severely dehydrated or hypovolemic patient. For this reason it is best to give a test dose of approximately 15% to 20% of the total dose, slowly. If this is tolerated, it is generally safe to give the remainder of the dose over several minutes.

The exact mechanism whereby thiopental produces a reduction in the intracranial pressure, usually over a period of 60 to 90 seconds, is unclear. The effects on intracranial pressure occur too rapidly to be related to effects on cerebral metabolic rate, and they occur in the absence of changes in blood pressure. Whatever the mechanism, the effects of the drug are usually sustained for several hours, particularly early in the course of the development of elevated intracranial pressure, and the onset of action is so rapid as to make the drug indispensable in management.

Patients who have increased intracranial pressure refractory to the therapies outlined above will require more complicated forms of intervention. Modalities available to these patients include the use of high-dose barbiturates to produce "barbiturate coma." This modality has been shown to produce good survival in up to 40% of patients whose intracranial pressure was of such severity as to be associated with 100% mortality or vegetative survival only. It has also been used with success in patients with Reye syndrome with similarly refractory intracranial pressure.

Several actions of barbiturates probably play a role in their mechanism for the reduction of intracranial pressure when used in high doses. Clearly, they markedly reduce cerebral metabolic rate and thereby produce proportional and well tolerated decreases in cerebral blood flow and cerebral blood volume. In addition, they are known to be free radical scavengers and lipid membrane stabilizers, and thereby may interrupt the processes that produce ongoing cell damage in the central nervous system. The administration of high dose barbiturates, however, is associated with a high incidence of complications, the most important of which are peripheral vascular instability and myocardial depression. These combined effects are likely to produce a low cardiac output state, and cardiac output, cardiac filling pressures, and other hemodynamic parameters must be monitored closely when barbiturate coma is induced.

Total body hypothermia is also known to produce sustained reductions in refractory intracranial pressure. Mechanisms for the efficacy of hypothermia are probably related to the reduction in cerebral metabolism, with proportional decreases in cerebral blood flow and blood volume. The production of hypothermia to 32° to 33° C (90° to 92° F) can usually be achieved safely in the intensive care unit setting. Reduction to less than 32° C (90° F) is associated with a very high incidence of cardiac arrhythmias and with the production of widespread peripheral vascular instability. Hypothermia has been used in conjunction with barbiturate coma; however, additional benefits from the two therapies in combination have not been demonstrated, whereas complications with the two therapies combined are more frequent than with either therapy used alone.

The final intervention available for patients with refractory intracranial pressure is that of a decompressive craniectomy. Several neurosurgical procedures have been used in the past to effectively decompress the swollen brain. Enthusiasm for these procedures has been scant because of the high incidence of complications, particulary infectious, and the low rate of improved survival. Some centers are currently renewing interest in decompressive craniectomy, believing that the intervention in the past has been reserved for patients so far progressed in their disease state as to be nonsalvageable at the time of the procedure. In addition, with the advent of good intensive care and the use of good sterile technique, the infectious complication rate may be substantially less than previously described.

Future outlook for neurologic intensive care

At the current rate at which understanding of neurologic injury is increasing, there are likely to be major advances in the field of neurologic intensive care in the next 10 to 20 years. New monitoring capabilities that will improve our ability to care for such patients include the increased availability of techniques allowing measurements of both total and regional cerebral blood flow. Techniques allowing for improved monitoring of cerebral metabolism as an indicator of brain cell function and viability are already being explored in some centers. Information being generated by positron emission tomography (PET) scanners, available in some selected centers, is already changing notions of cerebral blood flow and metabolism in man, both in the normal and in the diseased state. Finally, new therapeutic modalities, particularly those that afford "brain protection" (such as membrane stabilizers, prostaglandin inhibitors, and calcium channel blockers) are likely to increase the armamentarium with which physicians work to improve survival rate and the quality of survival in the neurologically injured child.

NUTRITIONAL CARE OF THE CRITICALLY ILL CHILD

The critically ill child has the potential for multiple system involvement. More often than is recognized, metabolic failure is present along with circulatory, ventilatory, renal, hepatic, or gastrointestinal failure. The nutritional aspect of multiple system failure in critically ill children is beginning to be appreciated and approached with various management techniques. Acute protein-energy malnutrition occurs in 20% to 30% of children in intensive care units.

The majority of patients admitted to the intensive care unit should have nutritional screening performed. Those patients with history of 5% weight loss, a decreased weight-for-height ratio, a decreased serum albumin, or diagnoses associated with development of protein-calorie malnutrition must be further evaluated. Complete evaluation can be used to classify patients into levels of nutritional need. Patients in the high priority group include: (1) those with anergy, severe hypoproteinemia, or severe lymphopenia with weight-for-height and arm muscle circumference in the abnormal range; (2) those whose skeletal or visceral protein status is marginal and who have marked stress; and (3) those with extensive burn injury. Patients who are initially normal but have marked stress, such as sepsis, major surgery, iatrogenic starvation, or multiple system failure demand repeat evaluation within the first week of admission, if not early institution of nutritional support.

Nutritional needs are drastically altered in critically ill patients. The initial metabolic response to critical illness is a hormone-mediated mobilization of endogenous substrate in support of preservation of homeostasis. A generalized increase 30% to 40% greater than resting metabolic rate occurs. Labile protein reserves are mobilized. The net catabolism in skeletal muscle results in maintenance of circulating amino acid levels in support of protein biosynthesis. Increased rates of glucose oxidation and gluconeogenesis result in hyperglycemia. A "hypercaloremic" state results as circulating levels of major building blocks and energy substrates are increased, even in the absence of nutritional support. This hypermetabolism occurs in support of sustained organ function, tissue repair, and host defense. Endogenous protein and energy stores in well-nourished patients can withstand a short period of severe stress. However, if malnutrition was present at admission or critical illness persists, serious losses of lean body mass occur, setting the stage for sepsis, sequential organ failure, and increased mortality. These metabolic alterations impair both use of dietary nutrients and attempts at restoration of nutritional losses. Nutritional support in such critically ill children must be instituted early to limit depletion of amino acid pools and body mass before serious depletion of reserves occurs. Preservation of body cell mass is easier than replacement of lost stores.

There are various routes of nutritional support, and the method used depends on the state of the individual child. Enteral feedings by means of a functional gastrointestinal tract are physiologic. Very few critically ill children will be able to maintain adequate nutrition by mouth, but small amounts of solid food or liquids may supplement other intake. Inability to chew may be bypassed with blenderized diets or one of the many commercially prepared complete liquid formulas. For patients with intolerance to certain components, "modular diets" can be mixed using commercially available separate sources for protein, carbohydrate, and fat mixed with electrolytes, water, minerals, and vitamins. If digestive ability is limited, elemental diets made up of amino acids, simple sugars, and medium-chain triglycerides can replace these "modules" to allow complete absorption.

Most patients will be unwilling or unable to maintain adequate nutritional support by mouth, and for them feeding by a nasogastric, or better yet, a nasojejunal tube, is safe and efficient. All of the above blenderized, liquid, or defined formulas can be used in this manner. Constant infusion by pump is preferable, although intermittent bolus infusion may be used, depending on tolerance and needs. Small volumes of dilute formula are initiated, followed by increasing volume and strength until projected protein and energy requirements are achieved. Potential complications of the above oral or tube feedings include osmotic diarrhea, electrolyte imbalance, gastric retention, fluid overload, vomiting, and risk of aspiration.

In the critically ill child whose gastrointestinal tract is dysfunctional because of injury, gastrointestinal disease, or surgery, total parenteral nutrition (TPN) is mandatory. Children who may benefit from TPN include burn patients, patients with congenital gastrointestinal anomalies, patients requiring prolonged respiratory support, patients with hepatic failure, and malnourished oncology patients. Ideally, the TPN solution should be delivered by means of a silicone rubber, Teflon, or polyvinyl chloride catheter aseptically placed in the superior vena cava by way of the internal or external jugular or subclavian vein. Peripheral hyperalimentation can utilize any peripheral vein. Central TPN solutions consist of glucose for calories, a protein hydrolysate or crystalline amino acid mixture for nitrogen, and fat emulsions. Electrolytes, minerals, trace elements, and vitamins are also added to the solution. The usual central solution contains 20% to 30% glucose and 3% to 4% protein equivalent. With peripheral hyperalimentation, fat becomes the major calorie source and the usual solution contains 10% glucose, 1% to 2% protein equivalent, and 10% Intralipid. The most serious complications of total parenteral feedings are infectious and metabolic. Catheter sepsis, usually heralded by fever, leukocytosis, and intolerance to glucose, may be fungal or bacterial. Prompt removal of the catheter may be adequate treatment. More commonly, metabolic complications are encountered that include electrolyte imbalance, hypoglycemia or hyperglycemia, liver enzyme elevations, trace mineral deficiencies, or essential fatty acid deficiency.

The most important consideration in nutritional support during the hypermetabolic state is to supply sufficient energy and protein to limit depletion of body stores. Daily intake should contain 100 to 125 calories/kg/day for critically ill infants, 75 to 100 calories/kg/day for older children, and 50 to 75 calories/kg/day for adolescents. The corresponding nitrogen requirements are 0.75/kg/day for infants, 0.5 g/kg/day for older children, and 0.3 g/kg/day for adolescents; 150 to 250 nonprotein calories per gram of nitrogen are required for nitrogen accumulation in ill infants and children. These values must be used as guidelines regardless of type of feeding and adjusted as surveillance of response indicates. Surveillance must include serial nutritional assessment as mentioned earlier, attention to glucose tolerance, and measurement of nitrogen balance. Fine tuning of feeding regimens is beyond the scope of this chapter.

Early use of nutritional support in critically ill children, by fulfilling hypermetabolic energy and protein requirements, will maintain host defense and preserve organ function and allow time for stabilization of clinical status.

CARDIAC ARREST

Cardiopulmonary arrest may be defined as cessation of effective ventilation and circulation. Knowledge of predisposing situations can alert the pediatrician to this untoward possibility. Cardiorespiratory arrest is more likely to occur in the following conditions: hypoxia; acidosis; shock caused by, for example, sepsis, trauma, or postoperative low cardiac output; congenital heart disease; severe respiratory distress; central nervous system disorders such as increased intracranial pressure, trauma, or ingestion; metabolic abnormalities; and near drowning. The mechanism of cardiac arrest is either ventricular standstill or, much less frequently, ventricular fibrillation. Hypoxemia, hypercarbia, and marked acidosis ensue rapidly. Increased vagal tone can lead to further asystole and bradycardia.

The cardinal signs of cardiorespiratory arrest are: (1) apnea or gasping, (2) impalpable major arterial pulses, (3) cyanosis or pallor, (4) absent or faint heart sounds, (5) loss of consciousness, and (6) dilated pupils. Presence of dilated pupils indicates at least 3 to 4 minutes of absent cerebral blood flow but does not contraindicate full attempts at resuscitation. Cardiopulmonary resuscitation (CPR) should be started immediately on diagnosis of arrest, without electrocardiographic confirmation.

Resuscitation should be carried out in a thoughtful, organized manner. Ideally, resuscitation is a team effort under the direction of the most experienced resuscitator who uses a rational approach and clears the scene of all extraneous persons. Resuscitation as developed by the American Heart Association involves basic and advanced life support techniques and concepts. Basic resuscitation is *A*irway management, *B*reathing, and *C*ardiac massage. The patient should be supine on a firm surface, with the head and thorax readily accessible. Any foreign material in the mouth is cleared by suctioning or finger sweep. The airway is straightened and opened by extending and lifting the neck (with one hand or by towels uner the shoulders), while tilting the forehead slightly backward. Overzealous extension can occlude the infant airway. Better airway opening may be achieved by drawing or pushing the mandible forward to bring the tongue anterior; if available, this position can be maintained by insertion of an oropharyngeal airway. Mouth-to-mouth, mouth-to-nose, or bag-and-mask ventilation is undertaken after airway patency is assured. The adequacy of each breath is confirmed by synchronous rise of the thorax with inspiration and audible air escape during expiration. Because a resuscitator's exhaled air contains only 17% oxygen, supplemental oxygen should be used if available, preferably above 50% concentration. External cardiac compression is started simultaneously with ventilation. Effective circulation is achieved by downward displacement of the sternum and ventricular compression against the thoracic vertabrae. The lower one third of the sternum should be displaced ½ to ¾ inch in young children and ¾ to 1 ½ inch in older children. In infants, encircle the chest with both hands and compress with both thumbs; in older children, support the spine with a firm board and compress with two or three fingers, the heel of one hand, or the two-hand adult method, depending on the child's size. Compressions should be smooth and regular, not sudden or jerky. Compressions are interspersed with ventilation at a ratio of one breath for five compressions. The appropriate rates per minute for age are as follows for heart rate to respiratory rate: infant, 120:24; young child, 100:20; older child, 80:16.

Once reasonably effective circulation and ventilation are achieved, as documented by palpable major arterial pulse, reduction of cyanosis, and reduction in pupil size, advanced life support techniques are undertaken. This includes *D*rugs, *E*lectrocardiography, *E*ndotracheal intubation, *F*luids, and *F*ibrillation treatment. More simply this means *D*efinitive therapy.

Establishment of an adequate intravenous line (for drug administration) is crucial to advanced life support. In the event of intense vasoconstriction, a scalp vein needle may be inserted in a peripheral vein until a larger vein can be cannulated. A 20 or 22 gauge over-the-needle catheter can be inserted into the brachial, cephalic, external jugular, femoral, saphenous, or dorsal hand vein. The femoral vein is often chosen because of its accessibility without the need to interrupt CPR. Central venous cannulation offers the advantages of fast delivery of the infusate and measurement of central venous pressure. We prefer superior vena caval or right atrial lines introduced through the internal jugular or subclavian vein by a wire-through-the-needle technique. An infusion of 5% dextrose in 0.9% NaCl should be started. The patient's weight or a reasonable estimate must be used to select proper fluid infusion rates as well as drug dosages.

The fundamental drug used is oxygen in the highest concentration available. Tracheal intubation should be performed as soon as basic resuscitation has become effective, or earlier if the previously described basic techniques cannot maintain airway patency. Details of tracheal intubation have been described in the section on acute respiratory failure. A 100% concentration of oxygen should be used once endotracheal intubation and controlled ventilation are established. Reversal of hypoxemia is the first aim of drug therapy. The second is correction of acidosis, which has developed because of carbon dioxide accumulation as well as lactic acidosis from a shift to anaerobic metabolism. Sodium bicarbonate is used to improve cardiac contractility and to improve response to circulating or exogenous catecholamines. The initial dose is 1 to 2 mEq/kg with subsequent doses based on arterial blood gas results, or 1 mEq/kg for every 10 minutes of continuing cardiac arrest. The final aims of drug therapy are to accelerate cardiac rate and reverse hypotension. Atropine, calcium, and sympathomimetic inotropic agents are all useful in this regard. Atropine, by virtue of its vagolytic action, may be used in an initial dose of 0.02 mg/kg (minimal dose 0.15 mg). This dosage can be repeated as necessary to a maximal total dose of 2.0 mg. Sympathomimetic agents are useful because of their stimulation of adrenergic receptors. Beta receptor stimulation increases heart rate and augments cardiac contraction, resulting in improved cardiac output; alpha receptor stimulation increases systemic vascular resistance, resulting in higher systemic blood pressure. Epinephrine, having much beta and some alpha activity, has been shown to stimulate spontaneous cardiac contractions, to improve myocardial contractility and tone, and to elevate perfusion pressure during cardiac compression. The dose is 0.1 ml/kg of a 1:10,000 solution initially and every 5 to 10 minutes as necessary. In the event of delay in intravenous placement, this dose can be administered by means of the endotracheal tube. Intracardiac injection is not to be used. In addition, calcium may be useful to increase myocardial contractile force. The dosage of 10% calcium chloride is 0.3 ml (30 mg)/kg initially and every 10 minutes. Once spontaneous cardiac activity is restored, cardiac output may continue to be reduced. Cardiac massage must continue and constant inotropic infusion should be considered. Epinephrine is effective even with reduced circulating blood volume; if volume is adequate, isoproterenol increases stroke volume and heart rate with a decrease in systemic vascular resistance; dopamine, which increases stroke volume with little effect on systemic vascular resistance or heart rate, is useful in patients with tachycardia.

In contrast to adults, cardiac asystole, not fibrillation, is common in children, and defibrillation is rarely necessary. If needed, a direct current defibrillator should be used with appropriately sized paddles. The initial energy dose is 2 watt seconds/kg, which may be gradually increased to 10 watt seconds/kg (maximal dose 400 watt seconds) if not successful.

Immediately after successful resuscitation, treatment is directed at the underlying cause of arrest as well as its sequelae. Sequelae include metabolic acidosis, hyperkalemia, vasomotor nephropathy, anoxic encephalopathy, and a low cardiac output state.

Decision to terminate an unsuccessful resuscitation is based on one or more of the following criteria: (1) no restoration of cardiac activity, (2) presence of other factors such as brain trauma or massive hemorrhage that make recovery impossible, or (3) presence of a known fatal disease in its terminal state.

High success rates in cardiopulmonary resuscitation, especially in infants and children, indicate that in most instances an all-out effort must be made to restore effective ventilation and circulation.

BRAIN DEATH

The increasing sophistication of life support technology in the last 20 years has created a complication, by now familiar to most practicing physicians, that presents the critical care practitioner with a medical, legal, and ethical dilemma—the diagnosis of brain death. Philosophic questions regarding the actual definition of death, medical questions about clinical and nonclinical criteria for diagnosis of patients who fit the definition, and ethical questions such as those surrounding termination of life support in such patients and procurement of donor organs for potential transplant recipients continue to haunt the physician, despite the substantial body of literature on the topic that has accumulated over the last two decades.

Not only has survival improved because of increasingly sophisticated care of critically ill children but also the number of children with irreversibly damaged brains has increased.

Cessation of cerebral function is a medical and legal criterion of death. Simply, brain death is "a state when the brain no longer functions and has no possibility of return of function, despite the possible continuation of cardiac activity." However, considerable discussion of medical criteria for the diagnosis of brain death persists. Several sets of criteria are currently in use, each with its own subtleties.

The demonstration of absent brain function presents little difficulty. However, the question of irreversibility poses some problems. There are two ways of predicting irreversibility of loss of brain function. The first has been to categorize patients who die in spite of maximal support by sets of clinical criteria. Such criteria indicate irreversibility. A second approach is to demonstrate that such criteria predict widespread neuronal necrosis at autopsy. The generally accepted criteria employed in most centers are based on clinical studies using the former approach.

The criteria listed in the following box are those established as having 100% accuracy in predicting somatic death in adults.

A number of additional studies have been advocated for use in the diagnosis of brain death. The most commonly used, and currently most controversial, is the electroencephalogram. A few extensive and prospective studies have established the effectiveness of a single isoelectric EEG as a predictor of failure of survival when it accompanies a clinical examination compatible with brain death. However, isolated reports of recovery after an isoelectric EEG are frequent. Most of these are cases of drug intoxication, especially barbiturates, diazepam, meprobamate, methaqualone, and trichlorethylene.

A higher incidence of false negative and false positive results occurs in pediatric patients. In one study, five children met clinical criteria for brain death and had absent cerebral blood flow by angiography. Despite such unequivocal evidence of brain death, EEG activity was present in the delta and theta ranges. All five patients died in spite of maximal support; postmortem examination of each brain revealed liquefaction necrosis. The same author has also reported patients with isoelectric EEGs despite the clinical presence of brain stem function. We have confirmed this experience in three nonanesthetized patients with isoelectric EEGs who retained brain stem reflexes, including spontaneous respirations. We view an isoelectric EEG as supportive of the diagnosis of brain death, but neither mandatory nor routine.

Recently, cerebral circulation studies have been used to support the diagnosis of brain death. Their utility arises from two facts: (1) absent cerebral circulation for greater than 30 minutes is incompatible with brain survival; and (2) cerebral circulation ceases shortly after cessation of brain cell function. The cessation of

CRITERIA FOR CEREBRAL DEATH (BRAIN DEATH) PROPOSED BY THE COLLABORATIVE STUDY OF CEREBRAL DEATH

I. Prerequisite: all appropriate diagnostic and therapeutic procedures have been performed

II. Criteria (to be present for 30 minutes at least six hours after the onset of coma and apnea):
   - A. Coma with cerebral unresponsivity (see definition 1)
   - B. Apnea (see definition 2)
   - C. Dilated pupils
   - D. Absent cephalic reflexes (see definition 3)
   - E. Electrocerebral silence (see definition 4)

III. Confirmatory tests: absence of cerebral blood flow

Definitions

1. Cerebral unresponsivity: a state in which the patient does not respond purposefully to externally applied stimuli, obeys no commands, and does not phonate spontaneously or in response to a painful stimulus.
2. Apnea: the absence of spontaneous respiration, manifested by the need for controlled ventilation (that is, the patient makes no effort to override the respirator) for at least 15 minutes.
3. Cephalic reflexes: pupillary, corneal, oculoauditory, oculovestibular, oculocephalic, ciliospinal, snout, cough, pharyngeal, swallowing.
4. Electrocerebral silence: an electroencephalogram with an absence of electrical potentials of cerebral origin for over two microvolts from symmetrically placed electrode pairs over 10 centimeters apart with interelectrode resistance between 100 and 10,000 ohms.

From J.A.M.A. **237:**982-986, 1976. Copyright 1976, American Medical Association.

flow after cell death occurs because of: (1) widespread cerebral edema raising intracranial pressure above arterial pressure, thus stopping cerebral flow, or (2) intravascular obstruction because of vasospasm and thrombus formation, which occur shortly after neuronal death. Two methods are currently available to demonstrate cessation of cerebral blood flow. Contrast angiography, performed by the injection of radiopaque dye into both carotid arteries and the vertebral artery, will show no flow above the circle of Willis. Using this technique, no false positive indications are encountered, and false negative indications are rare. Disadvantages include inability to perform the procedure at the bedside and the risk of further injury to abnormal cerebral vascular bed by hyperosmolar dyes. Radioisotope bolus angiography has recently been used in children. Increasing use in this country, combined with the extensive Scandinavian experience, suggests that the technique may be among the more reliable ancillary studies supporting the diagnosis of brain death. Some have suggested that demonstration of absent cerebral blood flow is necessary for diagnosis of brain death.

Other ancillary tests include measurement of midline cerebral structure pulsatility by echo, contrast-enhanced CT scans, and doppler demonstration of retrograde carotid flow. All examine cerebral blood flow but must be considered supportive to the diagnosis because experience with their use is limited currently.

Based on the current understanding of reliability of criteria for the diagnosis of brain death, guidelines have been established at Le Bonheur Children's Medical Center. These are summarized below.

BRAIN DEATH DIAGNOSIS GUIDELINES AT LE BONHEUR CHILDREN'S MEDICAL CENTER

Requisite

1. Absent brain stem reflexes
2. Absent spontaneous movement
3. Absent response to pain above foramen magnum
4. Apnea test (90 seconds, initial P_{CO_2} of 40 torr)
5. Hypothermia, sedation, intoxication, metabolic derangement ruled out
6. All above criteria present on two examinations no less than 12 hours apart
7. One examination as above by pediatric neurologist

Supportive

1. Isoelectric EEG
2. Atropine test
3. Contrast or isotope angiography

Presenting the diagnosis of brain death to family members of the child is one of the most difficult tasks ever faced by a physician. Ambiguity and misunderstanding created by much imprecise reporting have further complicated this task.

The most crucial factors in the presentation of the diagnosis to family members are the development of trust and early introduction of, and ongoing communication about, severe brain injury and possible brain death. Time for the parents to grasp the meaning of these terms and concepts is essential. Of equal importance is the creation of adequate family support within the hospital environment, using chaplains, social workers, and mature nurses. The objectives of family support are threefold: (1) to assure understanding of the diagnosis and its meaning, (2) to facilitate accelerated movement through the stages of grief, and (3) to set the stage for normal grief and coping mechanisms later.

The following are keys to family support that we have found useful in our experience:

1. *Establish rapport with one primary physician.* Care of the critically ill child usually involves input from several specialists. However, the family of a brain-dead child must be able to identify one physician as the care taker, decision maker, and spokesman. Inconsistencies introduced by multiple discussants, who may be providing the same information, but doing so in different manners, can cause misunderstanding.
2. *Introduce the concept of brain death early.* We introduce the concept to the family when the severity of the brain injury is appreciated. This is often at a time when prognosis is speculative, but the entire spectrum of possibilities is presented, from the remote possibility of full neurologic recovery to the possibility of brain death.

3. *Provide repeated "updates."* Frequent interaction with the parents is crucial to their understanding and facilitates their movement through the stages of grief. When the neurologic examination becomes consistent with brain death, we share this information with the parents, explaining that if there is no change within the next 12 to 24 hours, the diagnosis of brain death is confirmed. In the intervening time, regular meetings are used to advise of any changes, provide further explanation if needed, and answer all questions.
4. *Do not imply that parents are being asked to make decisions about termination of support.* The decision to terminate life support of a child who is no longer living is the physician's decision, not the parents'. However, it is important that the physician's decision take into consideration the parents' feelings, needs, and progress through the stages of grief.
5. *Use auxiliary personnel.* It is important to include social workers, primary nurses, and chaplains in most of the conversations with parents. They may more easily spend the time to fully ascertain the parents' understanding.
6. *Use medical colleagues.* We use a pediatric neurologist to confirm our neurologic examination and diagnosis.
7. *Do not prescribe sedatives for the family.* The primary physician is frequently requested by concerned family members to provide sedatives for the parents. Parents without predisposing emotional disorders need no sedation. Evidence suggests that sedation may prolong and complicate the normal grief process.
8. *Provide follow-up.* Parents are contacted by a social worker or physician 3 to 4 weeks after the death of the child. Especially in the case of the child with brain death, significant questions may arise days or weeks after the death. Establishing this contact to provide medical information and emotional support significantly facilitates resolution of the grief process.
9. *Take time.* There is simply no way to provide successful family support without an extensive time commitment by the primary physician, social work staff, and nursing staff.

Gregory L. Stidham
David F. Westenkirchner

SELECTED REFERENCES

Low cardiac output states

Perkin, R.M., and Levin, D.L.: Shock in the pediatric patient. Part I, J. Pediatr. **101**(2):163-169, 1982.

Perkin, R.M., and Levin, D.L.: Shock in the pediatric patient. Part II, Therapy, J. Pediatr. **101**(3):319-332, 1982.

Respiratory failure

Newth C.J.: Recognition and management of respiratory failure, Pediatr. Clin. North Am. **926**(3):617-643, 1979.

Central nervous system injury

Shapiro, H.M.: Intracranial hypertension: therapeutic and anesthetic consideration, Anesthesiology **43:**445, 1975.

Bruce, D.A.: Cerebrospinal fluid pressure monitoring in children: physiology, pathology and clinical usefulness, Adv. Pediatr. **24:**233-290, 1977.

Cardiac arrest

Galvis, A.G.: CPR in Children. In Averbach, P.S., and Bodassi, S.A., editors: Cardiac Arrest and CPR, Rockville, Md., 1983, Aspen Systems Corp.

Nutrition

Reimer, S.L., et al.: Nutritional support of the critically ill child, Pediatr. Clin. North Am. **24**(3):647-660, 1980.

Brain death

Black, R.M.L.: Brain death, N. Engl. J. Med. **299:**338, 1978.

33 Pediatric Surgery

In the surgical management of infants and children it is important to be familiar not only with the specific disease processes but also with the physiologic and psychologic peculiarities that make these small patients different from adult patients.

Many of the conditions necessitating surgical treatment are the result of congenital abnormalities. Interference with proper development in one organ system may have been associated with changes in another organ system in a different phase of its development. The result is the occurrence of multiple apparently unrelated abnormalities in a single child and it is important for the physician to suspect such additional problems when treating these patients.

The small size of the patient may itself lead to special problems of management. The trachea and bronchi in tiny infants are only a few millimeters in diameter, greatly increasing the risk of respiratory complications, especially those caused by aspiration. The circulating blood volume, although proportionately about the same as that of an adult, is so small as to be greatly affected by loss of amounts of blood that appear insignificant. Loss of 35 ml blood in a 5-pound infant is roughly equivalent to 1 liter of blood loss in an adult. Body fluid compartment differences are of special importance in newborn infants, in whom the extracellular fluid volume is relatively increased. Renal function in the very young lacks certain efficiencies present in older patients and must be considered in preoperative and postoperative fluid therapy. It is important to know that infants undergoing operation tolerate mild underhydration far better than overhydration.

Anesthesia for children has been perfected to a fine degree so that it is possible to manage successfully even small premature infants. Skillful choice of anesthetic agent, use of endotracheal techniques when necessary, controlled body temperature during anesthesia, and maintenance of circulating blood volume based on respect for the special problems of the small patient can make pediatric anesthesia safe and reliable.

CLEFT LIP AND CLEFT PALATE

The most common facial anomaly is cleft lip or cleft palate, resulting from failure of fusion of the maxillary and premaxillary processes at about the fifth week of intrauterine life. When the maxillary and premaxillary processes fail to fuse, the resulting defect runs from the vermilion border of the lip to the inferior surface of the nostril. Cleft lip may be unilateral or bilateral and complete or incomplete. When the cleft is bilateral and complete, it is almost always associated with a complete cleft palate and a complete absence of the gingiva bilaterally in the region of the lateral incisor teeth. The premaxillary process is displaced anteriorly, and the columella of the nose is almost absent. This is the most severe form of the defect, and good cosmetic results are difficult to obtain.

Cleft palate may be complete or incomplete; the smaller clefts involve only the uvula or soft palate, whereas large clefts affect the entire palate and gingiva. These defects may or may not be associated with cleft lips.

Treatment. Immediately after birth the problem is primarily the severe emotional disturbance of the parents, requiring sympathetic and careful orientation by the physician, who should emphasize the improvement that can be achieved by proper surgical treatment. The infant is sent home from the hospital with the parents for approximately 1 month, during which time they learn to feed the child with a special cleft lip feeder. The parents usually adjust reasonably well to the cosmetic deformity and more fully appreciate surgical correction when it is carried out at a later date. It seems unwise, as is sometimes done, to correct the deformity without letting the parents see the infant because they may then be unhappy with the surgical cosmetic result. A 1-month delay also allows the surgeon to be sure there are no severe associated congenital anomalies that might be unrecognized in the neonatal period.

At 1 month, surgical correction of the cleft lip is performed. The incomplete or complete unilateral cleft lip can be repaired with little residual cosmetic deformity. The bilateral cleft lip is always associated with a mild degree of residual deformity because of the considerable anterior displacement of the premaxillary process and the absence or marked shortening of the columella of the nose. In the postoperative period the child is fed with a cleft lip feeder and is converted to a cup and spoon at about 3 months of age.

Repair of the cleft palate is delayed until the child is approximately 14 months of age, weighs 9 kg (20 pounds), and has two front teeth. Using bilateral relaxing incisions, repair of the palate and gingival margin can be carried out satisfactorily.

It is most important in children with cleft palates that proper speech therapy be carried out over the next 4 to 5 years. If the gingival margin is involved, deformed or supernumerary teeth must be removed, and a bridge or braces are frequently necessary when the child is about 5 years of age.

Proper surgical treatment of unilateral cleft lips and complete cleft palates results in good cosmetic appearance and essentially normal speech. Although after operation for bilateral cleft lip cosmetic results are not as good, the appearance of the child is greatly improved, despite the fact that the nose is somewhat flattened and the nostrils are widened.

THYROGLOSSAL CYSTS AND SINUSES

In the embryo the thyroid anlage is a midline structure attached to the foramen cecum of the tongue, subsequently descending into the neck. Defective development may produce a fistula from the foramen cecum to the midline of the neck or a cystic structure in the midline of the neck, usually attached to the foramen cecum by a sinus tract. The cyst may be anywhere in the midline of the neck down to the suprasternal notch. It is ordinarily in the region of the hyoid bone and is generally 1 to 2 cm in diameter. The most common complication of these cysts is infection.

A thyroglossal cyst must be differentiated from (1) a dermoid cyst, (2) submental lymphadenitis, and (3) ectopic thyroid tissue. Dermoid cysts are frequently in the midline of the neck but usually lie closer to the suprasternal notch and are often attached to the overlying skin. In submental lymphadenitis the enlarged node is more anterior, lying just beneath the symphysis of the mandible. Rarely, the midline mass is a solid piece of ectopic thyroid gland, which is often the only thyroid tissue present. In such a case, this small piece of gland is seldom large enough to maintain the patient in the euthyroid state and is also more likely to undergo malignant degeneration than the normally placed thyroid. Its removal must be followed by thyroid replacement.

Treatment. All thyroglossal duct cysts should be removed because they are likely to become infected, and it is more difficult to remove these lesions after infection. It is important that the entire cyst, as well as the sinus that attaches to the foramen cecum, be completely removed. This necessitates a fairly large transverse incision over the mass and dissection down to the hyoid bone. The center portion of this bone is excised, along with an additional block of tissue up to the base of the tongue.

BRANCHIAL CYSTS AND FISTULAS

Defects in the development of the branchial arch system may result in fistula or cyst formation in the lateral portion of the neck. The most common is a remnant of the second branchial cleft, resulting in a fistula extending from the tonsillar fossa through the bifurcation of the carotid artery and opening on the neck just anterior to the sternocleidomastoid muscle about 2.5 cm above the sternoclavicular joint. Occasional fistulas are seen just anterior to the lobule of the ear, the tract running posteriorly, hooking around the facial nerve, and then emptying into the external auditory canal. Sometimes cystic formations occur in association with these fistulas, but in children fistulas without cysts are more common.

Treatment. Branchial fistulas drain mucus from the pharynx onto the neck and frequently become infected. For this reason surgical excision is advised. It is important that the entire tract from the skin to its opening in the pharynx be completely removed; otherwise recurrent infection and fistula formation will result.

CYSTIC HYGROMA

A cystic hygroma is a multicystic lesion of lymphatic origin seen almost exclusively in infancy and childhood. It is more frequently found in the axilla and the neck but may be in the abdominal cavity, the chest, or elsewhere. The lesion may be extensive, involving the entire lateral portion of the neck, the floor of the mouth, and the tongue. Such hygromas frequently extend along the axillary vessels to form a dumbbell second lesion filling the entire axilla. The cysts are soft, have indefinite edges, and in infancy may enlarge at an alarming rate. The major concern in large hygromas of the neck is their interference with respiration and deglutition, which may cause death.

Treatment. *Radiation therapy has no effect on cystic hygromas;* partial removal is the most satisfactory treatment. Surgical aspiration and injection of sclerosing agents have little or no effect. On the other hand, excision of a massive cystic hygroma in the neck is tedious because hygromas have indefinite borders. Indeed, these cysts are found lying within muscle tissue, within the tongue, and within the floor of the mouth. Also, important blood vessels and nerves course directly through the tumor. The operation is thus essentially a nerve-vessel-tumor dissection, removing as much tumor as possible and at the same time preserving all vital structures in the neck. Small recurrent masses can usually be removed with ease at a later date if necessary.

When the operation is planned carefully, when blood replacement is adequate, when anesthesia is good, and when all vital structures are preserved, the surgical result is excellent.

ESOPHAGEAL ATRESIA; TRACHEOESOPHAGEAL FISTULA

(see also p. 296)

Congenital atresia of the esophagus and congenital tracheoesophageal fistula may occur as separate entities or in combination. The various types are illustrated in Fig. 33-1. It should be noted that type *C* is the most common form, occurring in 90% of patients. In this type the esophagus ends in a blind pouch just inside the thoracic inlet, and the upper end of the lower esophageal segment forms a fistula with the trachea, usually in the region of the carina. The next most common forms, each occurring in about 4% of the patients, are type *A*, consisting of esophageal atresia without tracheoesophageal fistula, and type *E*, tracheoesophageal fistula without esophageal atresia. Types *B* and *D* are extremely rare.

Clinical manifestations. Excessive salivation and drooling during the first day of life should always suggest esophageal atresia. If fed, the child reacts in a hungry manner but soon gags, coughs, regurgitates, and often becomes cyanotic.

An attempt to insert a nasogastric tube reveals obstruction in the upper esophagus. The physician must be careful that the tube does not curl upon itself in the upper esophageal pouch, deceiving the examiner into thinking it has passed into the stomach.

Diagnostic proof may be obtained by inserting a tube into the upper esophagus, instilling 1 ml of a contrast medium, and obtaining an upright radiograph of the chest and abdomen. The blind upper esophageal pouch is revealed. The presence of any gas in the intestinal tract then indicates that a tracheoesophageal fistula is also present because air could not otherwise have reached the bowel. If there is no air in the intestines, the physician can surmise that the lesion consists of esophageal atresia without fistula.

Diagnosis of simple fistula without atresia is more difficult. The infant may have little or no trouble in the neonatal period unless the fistula is so large that strangling occurs with each feeding. Findings leading to diagnosis are occasional strangulation with eating; recurrent pneumonia, particularly in the right upper lobe; and excessive abdominal distention from the large amount of air crossing the fistula and entering the intestinal tract when the infant cries. X-ray confirmation is best accomplished with cinefluoroscopy while feeding the child a barium meal in the prone position. A negative radiograph does not rule out the possibility of a fistula, and if the physician is still highly suspicious, we advise bronchoscopy. The physician can often identify the fistulous opening in the trachea just above the carina and pass a ureteral catheter

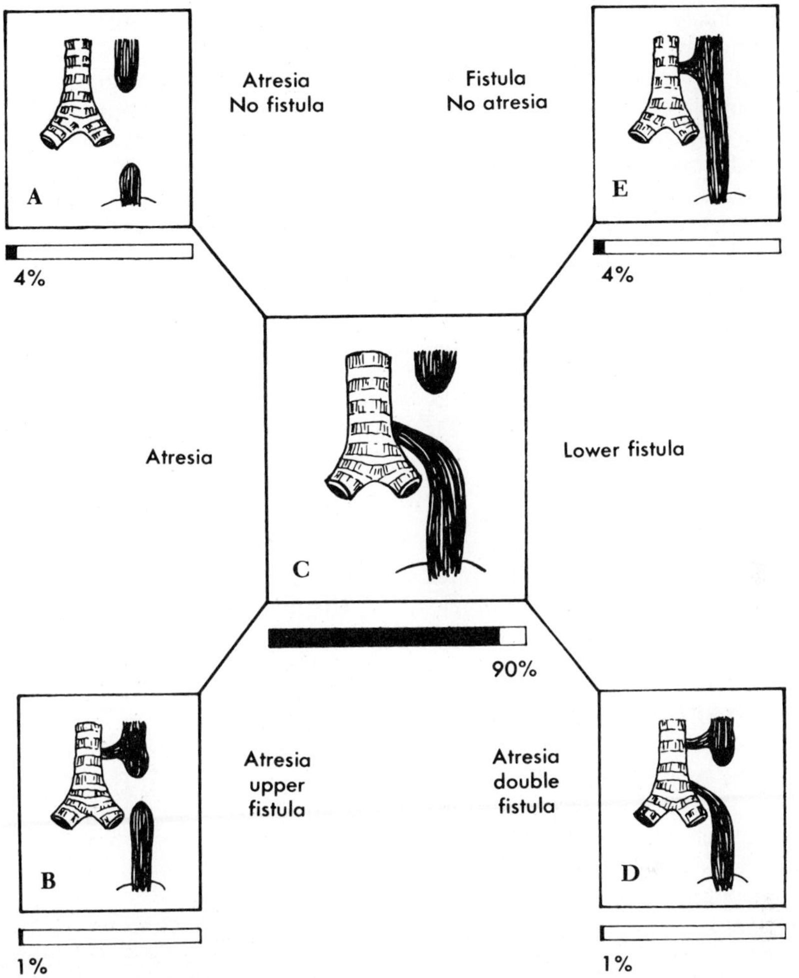

Fig. 33-1. Various types and frequencies of congenital atresia of the esophagus and tracheoesophageal fistulas. The most frequent form by far (90%) is type **C,** in which the upper segment of the esophagus ends as a blind pouch and the lower segment forms a fistula with the trachea. Types **A** and **E** each contribute about 4% of the cases, whereas types **B** and **D** contribute only 1% each. (Illustration prepared by Dr. R.N. Paul, Le Bonheur Children's Medical Center, Memphis.)

through this opening from the trachea into the esophagus. The bronchoscope can be removed from the trachea and inserted into the esophagus, and the ureteral catheter can be identified coming through the esophageal side of the fistula.

If the tracheal opening cannot be identified at bronchoscopy, a rather snug-fitting endotracheal tube is inserted into the trachea and an esophagoscope is inserted into the upper esophagus. Methylene blue, 0.5 ml, is instilled into the trachea, and in a high percentage of cases the dye can be seen entering the esophagus through the esophageal end of the fistula.

Treatment. Surgical procedures indicated depend on the type of anomaly present. Discussion will be limited to the type *C* anomaly, with upper esophageal atresia and lower tracheoesophageal fistula. Primary repair is carried out shortly after birth unless the infant is in poor condition because of aspiration pneumonia, prematurity, congenital heart disease, or other severe associated anomaly. First, a tube gastrostomy is done with either local or general anesthesia. Division of the tracheoesophageal fistula and anastomosis of the esophagus may then be delayed for several hours or even several days, during which time intermittent endotracheal suctioning and antibiotic therapy are used to correct pneumonitis and atelectasis, which are usually present when the diagnosis is established. Extrapleural exposure of the esophagus is preferred. In tiny premature infants, staged repair of the defect may be done, dividing the fistula first and then, weeks or months later, anastomosing the esophagus. This technique is also useful if the esophageal ends are too far apart for anastomosis at the first attempt, but might become close enough after a period of growth. If the esophagus cannot be repaired, esophageal replacement with a colon segment or gastric tube can be done later. With careful preoperative management, about 90% of patients with this malformation can be expected to survive.

CONGENITAL DIAPHRAGMATIC HERNIA (see also pp. 296-297)

Congenital hernia of the diaphragm usually represents an acute surgical emergency. If untreated, 75% of patients die by 1 month of age. Those who survive longer have smaller hernias without the severe pulmonary compression seen in more serious cases.

The diaphragmatic defect is generally in the posterior lateral portion, more commonly on the left; rarely, it is retrosternal. There is seldom a hernial sac, but sometimes a thin pleuroperitoneal sac separates the abdominal viscera from the lung. If there is no sac, almost all the abdominal viscera may be displaced into the thoracic cavity. On the left it is not uncommon to find the stomach, small intestine, spleen, left lobe of the liver, left kidney, and the entire colon, with exception of the descending colon, lying in the thorax. On the right, one is likely to find part of the liver, the transverse colon, and a large amount of small intestine.

Complete collapse of the lung occurs on the involved side, and marked mediastinal shift and partial collapse of the lung occurs on the opposite side. The compressed lungs are often dysplastic and incapable of normal function. The abdominal cavity is underdeveloped and so much smaller than normal that it may be difficult to return the abdominal viscera to the abdominal cavity once the diaphragm is repaired.

Clinical manifestations. Symptoms are primarily related to degree of thoracic encroachment by abdominal viscera and the degree of pulmonary dysplasia. Tachypnea, cyanosis, dyspnea, and severe acidosis often occur within a few hours after birth. The infant often vomits when fed. If an operation is not performed promptly, respiratory and circulatory collapse ensue. Occasionally infants with large hernias are relatively asymptomatic in the newborn period, the hernia not being recognized until months or years later.

Retrosternal hernias cause vague symptoms consisting of substernal pain and indigestion from pressure on the intestines involved in the hernia. Such hernias usually produce no problems in the newborn period.

Diagnosis. The presence of a lateral diaphragmatic hernia is suggested when a child has respiratory difficulty and cyanosis in the newborn period, associated with absence of breath sounds and dullness to percussion on the involved side, with significant shift of the heart to the opposite side. The physician may hear intestinal gurgles in the chest. The abdomen is usually scaphoid and appears small because most of the abdominal viscera lie within the chest.

Radiographic findings vary, depending on location of the hernia and which viscera have entered the chest. On the right the liver may produce a homogeneous shadow. On the left circular gas shadows similar to those of cystic disease of the lungs may be seen. The mediastinum is shifted to the opposite side.

Recurrent lower respiratory tract infection occurs often in older children with diaphragmatic hernia caused by compression of the lower lobe of the lung. This may be confused with resolving staphylococcal pneumonia because the circular gas shadows seen on the chest film resemble pneumatoceles. If plain radiographs are not diagnostic, a barium enema may reveal part of the colon to be intrathoracic, thus confirming the diagnosis.

Treatment. Immediate operative repair is indicated and may be lifesaving.

Because the lungs have been compressed during their entire development, they are hypoplastic. Even moderate anesthetic positive pressure may rupture alveolar sacs, producing bilateral pneumothorax. An endotracheal tube is indicated, but respiratory exchange should be extremely gentle to avoid pneumothorax.

Most diaphragmatic hernias are best repaired from an abdominal approach. Usually enough diaphragm is present to permit primary closure of the defect. In rare instances of almost complete absence of one leaf or the diaphragm, a woven Teflon prosthesis is employed. A chest tube is placed into the thoracic cavity on the side of the defect and is attached to a water seal or minimal suction.

Children with diaphragmatic hernia have malrotation of the midgut, and the Ladd procedure may be performed to avoid subsequent duodenal obstruction (pp. 892 and 894). The abdominal viscera are then returned to the abdominal cavity. In most instances the abdomen can be closed primarily, but sometimes the abdominal cavity is so small that it is necessary to leave the peritoneum and muscle layers of the abdominal wall open, merely covering the intestines with skin or with an externally exposed Silastic sheet.

Postoperatively the lungs usually expand gradually over a period of 12 to 48 hours. Then the chest tube can be removed.

The operation is successful in about one half of newborn infants with diaphragmatic hernia. In the total group the overall survival rate is higher than 80%. The frequent association of congenital heart defects adversely affects the prognosis.

OMPHALOCELE

Arrest of development of the abdominal wall during the sixth to tenth week of embryonic life leaves part of the abdominal viscera out in the base of the umbilical cord and a defect in the abdominal wall. This may be small or may involve most of the ventral aspect of the abdomen. The viscera are covered by a thin transparent membrane. This membrane may rupture in utero or at birth. The abdominal cavity may be too small to contain all the viscera.

Treatment. Surgical and nonsurgical methods of management are available. Small defects can be closed readily immediately after birth. When the defect is large and the viscera cannot be completely replaced within the small abdominal cavity, the skin may be widely mobilized and brought over the omphalocele sac. Secondary closure of the resulting ventral hernia may be difficult and hazardous. To avoid this, primary treatment of the large omphalocele may be by the use of a Silastic membrane to form a temporary covering. The size of this sac is reduced every few days to achieve complete repair of the abdominal wall in 2 weeks or less. A nonoperative method of repair consists of repeated applications of 2% mercurochrome to the sac. A tough eschar forms, and gradual closure of the defect occurs in a period of weeks or months. This method is slow and not infrequently associated with late rupture of the sac. Mercury poisoning can occur with too frequent application of the medication. This method is seldom used at the present time.

UMBILICAL HERNIA

The umbilical ring may fail to close completely in the newborn period, leaving a circular fascial defect beneath the umbilicus. This is usually small, but in older children it may reach several centimeters in size. A hernia sac develops, covered by skin and lined by peritoneum. The sac may become large in the early months of life. Most small umbilical defects will close spontaneously within the first year or two; however, some of the larger ones will persist.

The protruding umbilicus is generally the only symptom of this defect. Incarceration, with associated pain and signs of intestinal obstruction, is rare.

Treatment. Traditionally, adhesive strapping has been advised for umbilical hernias, but there is no real evidence that this is beneficial. Because most of these hernias disappear within a year or two, no specific treatment is indicated except in extremely large or symptomatic hernias or in those that persist beyond the age of 5 years. Operative repair is performed through a curved incision in the umbilical skin. After the sac is excised and its neck closed, the edges of the rectus fascia are approximated in the midline over the defect. The umbilicus should not be excised. Recurrence is rare.

INGUINAL HERNIA

Indirect inguinal hernias occur commonly in young children; about 90% occur in males. The right side is involved more frequently than the left. The hernias are frequently bilateral. In children under 2 years of age with one clinically apparent hernia, 60% or more will be found at operation to have bilateral hernias. In many cases there is an associated hydrocele. Intestine and omentum are the common contents of the hernia sac. In female infants it is not unusual for an ovary or fallopian tube to descend into the hernia.

Inguinal and scrotal swelling of varying degree is generally noted. This may disappear spontaneously, especially when the child lies down. There may be no associated complaint; however, in some cases a varying amount of discomfort, and possibly intense pain, is present. Pain is usually severe when the hernia becomes incarcerated. Incarceration occurs frequently, most often in the first 6 months of life. If the incarceration is not promptly treated, strangulation of the involved intestine, with signs of intestinal obstruction and eventually gangrene, may develop.

If the inguinal swelling is present during examination, the hernia contents may be palpated and usually may be reduced with little effort. Often the hernia fails to protrude during examination but can be detected by palpating the increased thickness of the inguinal cord structures. This increased thickness is the most constant finding. Attempting to palpate the size of the external inguinal ring and the presence of an impulse in that area yields little information in small children. If the hernia is incarcerated, the mass in the inguinal canal may be moderately or extremely tender, and it may be impossible to reduce completely the swelling.

Treatment. Surgical repair can be performed safely in tiny infants. Because of this, it is best to repair hernias when they appear rather than to defer treatment until later, unless the general condition of the infant precludes operation. Trusses are unsatisfactory in young children. The increased likelihood of incarceration in the younger age group increases the necessity for early operation. Spontaneous cure of inguinal hernias in infants probably does not occur with any significant frequency. The operation for inguinal hernia in infants and children consists mainly of high ligation of the neck of the hernia sac. Skin line incisions are closed with subcuticular sutures and are sealed with liquid collodion to avoid irritation or infection by wet diapers.

HYDROCELE

Hydroceles of the tunica vaginalis occur frequently and may be bilateral. Fluid accumulates within the tunica vaginalis, forming a soft translucent swelling. Usually there is no communication with the peritoneal cavity. However, the condition may be associated with an inguinal hernia or with a small patent processus vaginalis, creating a communicating hydrocele. If there is no communication, hydroceles of infancy usually disappear spontaneously within the first 6 months.

Hydroceles of the spermatic cord (or of the canal of Nuck) may occur without an associated hydrocele of the tunica vaginalis. Again, there may be a communication with the peritoneum through a patent processus vaginalis or an inguinal hernia sac. In some cases it may not be possible to distinguish these lesions from inguinal hernias.

Presence of the swelling is generally the only symptom of a hydrocele. If there is great variation in size, an indirect inguinal hernia or a communicating hydrocele must be suspected. An acute hydrocele or one that is associated with local pain and tenderness must be considered possibly to be an incarcerated hernia, torsion of the testis or appendix testis, or testicular inflammation.

Treatment. Aspiration of hydroceles, either for diagnosis or for treatment, is inadvisable in children. If the hydrocele is of significant size and persists after 1 year of age, it may be removed surgically. Recurrence is extremely rare.

UNDESCENDED TESTICLE (see also pp. 933-934)

During fetal development the testicle descends from its point of origin in the retroperitoneal space through the inguinal canal into the scrotum. Descent may be arrested at any point, or the testicle may follow an abnormal path, coming to lie in an ectopic position. In most instances there is an associated indirect inguinal hernia. Complete absence of one or both testicles is exceedingly rare. Thus it can be assumed that if the testicle is not in the scrotum, it is in an abnormal position.

Normal spermatogenesis seldom occurs in a testicle that fails to descend into the scrotum. Therefore sterility can be anticipated in patients with persistent bilateral undescended testicles. The testicle lying in the inguinal canal is more subject to trauma than is a scrotal testicle. Torsion of the undescended testicle is somewhat more common than of the normal testicle. Development of malignant tumors is slightly more common in undescended than in normally descended testicles. The defect may lead to significant psychologic problems.

Examination reveals that the testicle is absent from its normal scrotal position. A testicle that has actually descended into the upper scrotum may, under the stimulus of examination, be retracted into the inguinal canal by a strong, short cremaster muscle. This must not be confused with a truly undescended testicle. The retracted testis may be palpated in the inguinal canal and by gentle manipulation can usually be forced into the scrotum. Such a testis will descend spontaneously with growth and without specific treatment. Truly undescended testicles are also frequently palpated in the inguinal canal or in the lower abdomen in thin individuals. These cannot be manipulated into the scrotum. Ectopic testicles are found in several typical locations, such as in a subcutaneous pocket in the lower abdominal wall, the medial aspect of the thigh, or the perineum. Examination generally shows no evidence of hormonal disturbance, and the penis is usually of normal size.

Treatment. It is usually possible to determine by the time the child is 5 years of age whether a testicle is likely to descend spontaneously or not. Spontaneous descent is unlikely if no testicle can be palpated or if a testicle felt in the inguinal canal cannot be manipulated into the scrotum. Hormonal treatment has been recommended; however, testicles that descend during hormonal therapy would probably have descended spontaneously without treatment. The necessity of repeated injections and the expense of this treatment, without definite permanent benefit, contraindicate its routine use.

Operation is the treatment of choice. To permit development of normal spermatogenesis early operation is indicated, preferably at 2 to 4 years of age or earlier. Almost all undescended testicles can be brought into satisfactory position in the scrotum by an extensive freeing of vas and vessels through an inguinal incision. The testicle should not be sutured to the thigh, as in the former methods of treatment, but should be held in the scrotum, using a rubber band for elastic traction, or placed into a dartos pouch and anchored in it with a suture.

Results of treatment are usually good. The likelihood of future malignancy is not decreased by bringing the testicle into the scrotum operatively, but it is possible to discover such change much earlier with the testicle in its normal position.

HYPERTROPHIC PYLORIC STENOSIS

Obstruction at the pylorus caused by hypertrophy of the circular pyloric musculature is one of the most common surgical conditions in infants. It occurs four times more frequently in males than in females. In a significant number of instances another sibling or a parent will have had the disorder. Its etiology is unknown.

Generally, at about 10 to 14 days of age there is an onset of vomiting, which becomes progressively greater and projectile in nature. The vomitus does not contain bile. Vomiting occurs during or shortly after a feeding. The child is usually hungry and will nurse the breast or take another bottle immediately after vomiting. The stools become smaller in size than normal and are passed less frequently than usual.

Dehydration and weight loss become increasingly pronounced. The distended gastric outline with visible left to right peristaltic waves may be seen. In almost every case it is possible to palpate a 1.5 to 2 cm firm, movable, olive-shaped mass in the epigastrium. This is called the pyloric tumor. It can be felt more easily when the abdominal muscles are relaxed during a feeding or immediately after vomiting has occurred. The examination requires patience and persistence.

Diagnostic studies. If the pyloric tumor is not palpable, barium study of the stomach is performed. This reveals delayed gastric emptying and elongation and narrowing of the pyloric canal (Fig. 33-2). As the disease progresses, dehydration and hypochloremic alkalosis occur, as well as a total body deficit of potassium (Chapter 10).

Treatment. Surgical relief of the obstruction

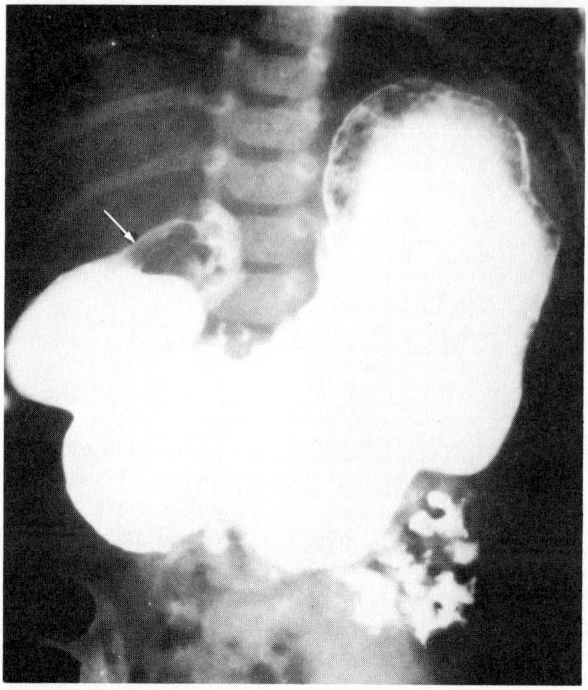

Fig. 33-2. Pyloric stenosis in a 2-month-old infant. Note large, hyperperistaltic stomach (''caterpillar sign'') and elongated pyloric canal (''string sign'') (*arrow*). (Courtesy Dr. W. Webster Riggs, Le Bonheur Children's Medical Center, Memphis.)

is advisable, although some authors have reported success with medical management. Good results depend on careful preoperative preparation. Blood chemical determinations are necessary guides to preoperative preparation. Dehydration and alkalosis should be corrected by appropriate fluid therapy, as discussed in Chapter 10. Transfusion is indicated if the hemoglobin is less than 10 g/dl.

The operation for hypertrophic pyloric stenosis is the Ramstedt pyloromyotomy, consisting of longitudinal splitting of the pyloric muscle.

Postoperative care consists of small frequent feedings beginning 4 to 6 hours postoperatively. One ounce of glucose water may be given every 2 hours, followed by formula in similar amounts, gradually increasing the volume and decreasing the frequency of feedings over the next several days. The prognosis is excellent, and the mortality rate is low.

CHALASIA (see pp. 333-335)

NEONATAL INTESTINAL OBSTRUCTION

Vomiting occurs frequently in newborn infants, but normal infants do not vomit bile. Bile-stained vomitus is evidence of intestinal obstruction distal to the ampulla of Vater until confirmed or disproved by investigation. Usually the more distal the point of obstruction, the greater is the degree of associated abdominal distention. At times severe distention may precede significant vomiting. Many conditions may cause neonatal intestinal obstruction, but only the more frequently encountered are discussed here. Differential diagnosis is chiefly by x-ray examination, preferably an upright film of the abdomen. Early diagnosis is essential.

Intestinal atresia

Complete intestinal obstruction may result from a mucosal diaphragm, or there may be complete interruption of continuity of the bowel, sometimes at several points, resulting in multiple blind segments. The duodenum and lower ileum are the most common sites. The colon is rarely involved. Duodenal atresia is often associated with Down syndrome.

Upright plain radiographs reveal distended intestinal loops with fluid levels and no air distal to the obstruction. If the duodenum is the site of blockage, the film will show gastric and duodenal air-fluid levels, the so-called double-bubble sign. When many distended loops are present, barium enema is indicated to distinguish small from large bowel. *Microcolon* is typically observed in the presence of atresia proximal to the colon.

Treatment. For duodenal atresia, duodenoduodenostomy or duodenojejunostomy is preferred to gastrojejunostomy. Distal to the duodenum, end-to-end anastomosis or anastomosis combined with several varieties of temporary enterostomy is done.

Intestinal stenosis

Stenosis is similar to atresia, but obstruction is incomplete. Milder degrees of blockage may not become clinically apparent for weeks or months, but more often the picture is acute, resembling atresia. Radiographic findings are the same as for atresia, except that varying amounts of air are present in the bowel below the obstruction.

Treatment. The treatment is the same as that for atresia.

Annular pancreas

The duodenum may be encircled by an unyielding ring of pancreatic tissue resulting from failure of proper rotation and development of the ventral pancreatic anlage. Obstructive vomiting is the characteristic feature. The radiograph resembles that of duodenal stenosis.

Treatment. A side-to-side duodenojejunostomy is performed. The ring of pancreatic tissue is not disturbed.

Malrotation of the midgut

Under normal circumstances the midgut, that part of the intestinal tract supplied by the superior mesenteric artery, returns to the intraabdominal position during the tenth or eleventh week of embryonic life, and the root of the mesentery rotates in a counterclockwise direction. This causes the colon to cross ventrally, the cecum moving from the left lower quadrant to the right lower quadrant and the duodenum crossing dorsally to become partly retroperitoneal. If this rotation is incomplete, the posterior fixation of the mesentery is inadequate, leaving a narrow pedicle-like mesentery, which permits volvulus of the bowel from the ligament of Treitz to the midtransverse colon. The volvulus may be mild or severe, with clinical findings varying from vague digestive disorders to complete intestinal obstruction leading to gangrene. A second type of obstruction may be produced by peritoneal folds attaching the abnormally placed cecum to the right peritoneal gutter, crossing and obstructing the duodenum.

Barium enema reveals the abnormal position of the cecum. Upper gastrointestinal x-ray studies, done only when obstruction is not acute, show partial obstruction of the duodenum, or the upper small bowel may lie in the right instead of the left side of the abdomen.

Treatment. The Ladd procedure for malrotation consists of rotating the midgut counterclockwise to reduce the volvulus. Peritoneal bands crossing the duodenum are then divided, and the entire colon is placed to the left and the duodenum to the right. Symptoms seldom recur.

Meconium ileus

Patients with cystic fibrosis may have obstruction at birth caused by incompletely digested meconium, which has become thick and inspissated, completely blocking the intestinal lumen. The level of obstruction varies but is usually in the ileum. The abdomen is distended, with dilated loops of intestine. These tend not to shift much in position with changes of body position. Portions of the intestinal contents give a granular or mottled x-ray shadow resembling small soap bubbles.

Treatment. Some patients may be managed by rectal irrigations with acetylcysteine or diatrizoate methyl glucamine (Gastrografin), the latter under fluoroscopic guidance. Acetylcysteine may also be administered by nasogastric tube. If conservative measures fail or if perforation of the intestine is suspected, surgery is necessary. The abnormal meconium may be liquefied by instillation of acetylcysteine, then it may be aspirated or milked into the colon. Enterostomy may be needed temporarily if other procedures fail. If pancreatin powder is added to the feedings postoperatively, a normal diet may be taken.

Hirschsprung disease (p. 350)

Congenital megacolon may cause acute obstruction in newborn infants, with severe abdominal distention. The abdomen is filled with dilated bowel. In the infant the large and small bowels are not readily distinguishable on plain radiographs. Barium enema will show that the colon is dilated as well as the small bowel. Characteristically there is a prolonged delay in expulsion of the barium. In the newborn infant the barium enema may reveal little contrast in caliber of the narrowed rectosigmoid area and the descending colon.

Treatment. If enemas and rectal irrigations do not relieve the obstruction, a temporary colostomy is necessary. At a later date, resection of the constricted segment is performed by an abdominoperineal pull-through procedure.

Meconium plug syndrome

Rarely an infant will have obstruction due to a plug of inspissated mucus in the rectosigmoid area. The x-ray findings may resemble those of Hirschsprung disease or other low bowel obstruction. The mucous plug may be outlined by barium enema.

Treatment. The plug is usually expelled after enemas. The possibility of this condition makes barium enema a necessary part of the workup in newborn infants who have obstruction and in whom plain abdominal films show many dilated loops that cannot be differentiated into small or large intestine.

Imperforate anus

The normal anal opening is absent. The colon may end as a blind pouch. More often there is a rectoperineal or rectovaginal fistula in the female or a rectoperineal, rectovesical, or rectourethral fistula in the male. Abdominal distention and vomiting occur if a fistula is absent or small. Meconium is passed in the urine in some cases with fistulas into the urinary tract. An anal dimple may be present. Meconium may be noted passing from the vagina or urethra.

Treatment. Perineal anoplasty is performed when there is a rectoperineal or rectovaginal fistula or when a blind pouch ends at the anus. Abdominoperineal or sacroperineal pull-through anoplasty is necessary for higher blind pouches or fistulas into the urinary tract. Better results are achieved if anoplasty is deferred for several months. External fistulas are dilated, or colostomy is done to permit adequate bowel movements during the interval.

INTUSSUSCEPTION

Telescoping of a proximal segment of intestine into a distal segment may lead to gangrene by obstructing the blood supply of the involved bowel. Although there may be a lead point, such as a polyp or an invaginated Meckel diverticulum, the great majority of cases in children are idiopathic. The disease occurs more often in infants between 3 and 12 months of age. Ileocolic intussusception is the most frequent type.

Sudden onset of severe intermittent cramping abdominal pain in a previously healthy child is characteristic. Vomiting may accompany the pain. Passage of bloody mucoid stools resembling currant jelly occurs in about 85% of the cases. There may be pallor, sweating, and drawing up of legs with the pain. However, early in the disease, infants may appear well between paroxysms. Fever is absent in the early stages. A sausage-shaped mass is often palpable in the right upper abdomen or epigastrium, with emptiness to palpation in the right lower quadrant. The mass may be slightly tender and somewhat movable. Rectal examination may reveal the bloody mucoid material (currant jelly stool). Signs of shock and advancing intestinal obstruction develop as the disease progresses.

If the typical mass is not felt, x-ray studies may be required for diagnosis (Fig. 33-3).

Treatment. Early diagnosis is of extreme importance. Suspecting the disease on the basis of the history should be emphasized. It may be necessary to correct shock and fluid imbalance before carrying out definitive treatment. This must be done as rapidly as possible because any significant delay increases the likelihood of gangrene of the bowel. Surgical treatment is by direct manipulative reduction of the intussusception. If it cannot be reduced or if gangrene of the intestine has already occurred, primary resection or exteriorization of the damaged intestine may be necessary. About 60% of the early intussusceptions can be reduced by barium enema under fluoroscopic control. This should be attempted only by persons well versed in the hazards and safeguards of this technique.

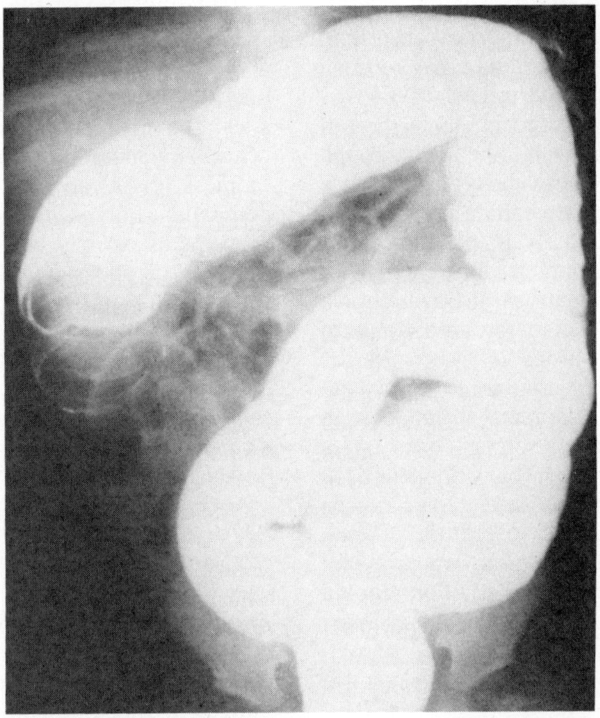

Fig. 33-3. Ileocolic intussusception in a 4-month-old infant. Retrograde flow of barium enema was stopped by ileal loops in ascending colon and was subsequently reduced by sustained hydrostatic pressure from the enema. (Courtesy Dr. W. Webster Riggs, Le Bonheur Children's Medical Center, Memphis.)

HIRSCHSPRUNG DISEASE (CONGENITAL MEGACOLON) (p. 350)

Absence or deficiency of the ganglion cells of the myenteric plexuses of the rectum and distal colon results in lack of propulsive peristalsis in the involved bowel, producing chronic functional obstruction. The aganglionic segment tends to maintain a fairly normal caliber, whereas the bowel above this obstruction becomes greatly dilated and hypertrophied. In the vast majority of cases the involvement extends from the anus for varying distances proximally into the distal colon.

Chronic constipation is the chief complaint. In the newborn infant, obstruction may occur within the first few days. This may require colostomy or may be relieved spontaneously or by enema. For the next several weeks, stools may be passed fairly normally. Thereafter a chronic state develops in which the patient may pass few spontaneous stools without the benefit of laxatives or enemas. Stools that are passed tend to be soft or liquid. The patient does not have intermittent passage of very large, firm stools, as noted in some other forms of chronic constipation. The abdomen becomes greatly enlarged. The disease may be complicated by acute or protracted episodes of enterocolitis, with vomiting and diarrhea, which may prove fatal.

There is marked soft distention of the abdomen. At times evidence of a dilated colon may be seen or palpated on examination of the abdomen. Chronic distention may cause flaring of the costal margins. On rectal examination the ampulla is empty and is not dilated. A rectal tube inserted high enough to reach above the point of obstruction may yield an explosive flow of gas and fecal material. Malnutrition is the rule in severe cases.

Barium enema reveals a typical picture of a rather normal-appearing narrow rectosigmoid leading upward to a greatly dilated colon above the obstruction. It is important to avoid filling the dilated colon with barium; this may form an impaction that is difficult to relieve.

Examination of biopsy specimens of the full thickness of the rectal wall, obtained through the anal approach, will show the typical absence of ganglion cells in the myenteric plexus.

Treatment. In extremely ill patients or infants temporary colostomy is the treatment of choice. For definitive treatment the aganglionic segment of bowel is excised by an abdominoperineal pull-through procedure such as the Swenson operation or by the more recently developed retrorectal or endorectal techniques. In caring for the child before surgery, enemas are necessary. The fluid must be siphoned back through the rectal tube because it may not be evacuated spontaneously. Absorption of enema fluid from the dilated colon is a problem; therefore physiologic saline solution should be used rather than tap water, which may produce severe, or even fatal, water intoxication.

GASTROINTESTINAL BLEEDING

(see also p. 331)

Bleeding into the upper gastrointestinal tract may result in vomiting of blood or passage of black tarry stools, whereas bleeding into the lower tract results in passage of red blood. Differential diagnosis is often difficult because of the large number of possible causes of bleeding. In the following sections, surgical causes of such bleeding will be included, but it should be remembered that there are also nonsurgical causes (blood dyscrasias, etc.).

Swallowed blood

The newborn infant may have swallowed sufficient amounts of maternal blood during delivery to produce vomiting of blood and melena. This condition is suggested by failure of the patient's hematocrit or hemoglobin levels to decrease and absence of signs of shock. Laboratory studies can identify the hemoglobin in the stool as being maternal in origin rather than fetal. No treatment is necessary. Other sources of swallowed blood are nosebleed, injuries to the mouth and pharynx, and blood coughed up from the lungs.

Polyps

Benign polyps develop frequently in children and may cause melena. There is usually only one polyp, but there may be several in various sites. The rectum and sigmoid are involved more often than more proximal areas of the colon. Painless bright red rectal bleeding is the usual complaint. Polyps may prolapse during bowel movements or may be felt on rectal examination. Rectal and sigmoid polyps can be visualized during sigmoidoscopy. Air contrast barium enema will demonstrate polyps that cannot be reached by the sigmoidoscope.

Treatment. Most polyps may be removed or fulgurated through the colonoscope. For those located higher, laparotomy and colotomy may be necessary.

Familial multiple polyposis

The entire lining of the colon and occasionally varying lengths of small intestine may undergo diffuse progressive polypoid change. This condition is hereditary. Almost all such individuals develop carcinoma of the colon in early life if untreated. Bleeding is the earliest sign.

Treatment. Treatment is total colectomy. In young children a portion of rectosigmoid is sometimes left in to maintain normal rectal function, this portion being inspected regularly by sigmoidoscopy. By election in adolescence the remaining rectosigmoid is removed or the mucosa is stripped from the rectum, and an ileoanal anastomosis is performed.

Peutz-Jeghers syndrome

Peutz-Jeghers syndrome is another familial disorder manifested by multiple intestinal polyps, usually of the small intestine. It is characterized by the associated presence of melanin spots on the lips and buccal mucosa. Intussusception or bleeding frequently ensues. Treatment is excision of the larger polyps when symptoms are noted.

Meckel diverticulum

In approximately 1.5% to 2% of the general population a diverticulum persists on the antemesenteric aspect of the terminal ileum 45 to 90 cm above the ileocecal junction. Its diameter may approach that of the ileum. It varies in length from less than 2.5 cm to several centimeters. The lining contains ectopic gastric mucosa and pancreatic tissue in most instances. This results in peptic ulceration in the diverticulum or in the adjacent ileum.

Painless bleeding is the most common complaint. Bleeding is often acute and massive but may be chronic. Blood passed in the stools tends to be brick red in color. Meckel diverticulitis may produce a symptom complex indistinguishable from appendicitis. Chronic abdominal pain may also result from the ulceration. An invaginated Meckel diverticulum may precipitate intussusception of the ileum, with typical cramping pain and vomiting. Perforation may occur. Blood in the rectum, pallor, and signs of shock may be the only physical findings in bleeding Meckel diverticulum. Physical findings in acute diverticulitis may mimic those of appendicitis. In intussusception caused by Meckel diverticulum the palpable mass is likely to be in the lower abdomen rather than in the upper abdomen, as in idiopathic ileocolic intussusception. Meckel diverticula are rarely seen on x-ray examinations but are sometimes visualized with radioisotope scans for ectopic gastric mucosa.

Treatment. Exploratory laparotomy should be performed if no other explanation for bleeding is apparent. The diverticulum is resected obliquely to avoid narrowing the lumen of the ileum.

Esophageal varices

Portal hypertension caused by extrahepatic or intrahepatic block in the portal venous drainage may result in bleeding from esophageal varices. This may be massive and life threatening. More cases in children are of the extrahepatic type, with associated splenomegaly and neutropenia secondary to hypersplenism. The portal vein in these patients is obstructed and has frequently undergone cavernous transformation. Intrahepatic block occurs in cirrhosis, which may follow neonatal hepatitis and other liver diseases.

Melena occurs with or without vomiting of blood. There is no pain. Shock may develop. In some patients an abnormal venous pattern over the abdominal and chest walls is present. If the umbilical vein has remained patent, a caput medusae of dilated veins may radiate from the umbilicus. The liver may or may not be enlarged if there is intrahepatic disease. The spleen is usually enlarged.

Barium swallow outlines varices in the esophagus. Percutaneous or operative portal venography visualizes the abnormal venous flow.

Anemia from blood loss and probably leukopenia or pancytopenia secondary to hypersplenism will be present. Liver function studies remain normal in extrahepatic portal block but indicate varying degrees of liver impairment if the block is intrahepatic.

Treatment. Acute bleeding can be controlled with the triple-lumen, double-balloon esophageal tube or by injection of sclerosing agents through the esophagoscope. Creating a portal systemic venous shunt is the definitive surgical treatment. In the more common extrahepatic blocks, splenorenal shunt is the procedure of choice. Less often a patent portal vein is present, permitting direct portacaval anastomosis. Splenectomy alone should not be done. Splenorenal anastomosis in patients under the age of 6 years is unlikely to remain patent. Therefore, in this age group, bleeding must often be controlled temporarily by direct ligation of the esophageal varices or esophagoscopic sclerosis. Aspirin must be avoided by these patients.

Peptic ulceration (see also pp. 335-336)

Peptic ulceration occurs in the esophagus, stomach, or duodenum but is uncommon in children except after stress, such as a central nervous system injury or operation (Cushing ulcer) or a major burn (Curling ulcer). The diagnosis is established by x-ray demonstration of the ulcer or endoscopy, and treatment is chiefly medical.

Duplication of the intestine

Duplications are either closed cysts or elongated tubular structures, the latter communicating at one or both ends with the intestine. They are composed of the same serosal, muscular, and mucosal layers that make up normal intestine. The size varies from cysts a few millimeters in diameter to long duplications. Their location varies from the base of the tongue to the anus, with the greatest incidence being in the small bowel. Intestinal duplications usually lie in the mesentery of the adjacent normal bowel, sharing a common seromuscular coat. The mucosal lining may resemble that of any part of the intestinal tract. Tubular duplications tend to be lined at least in part by gastric mucosa.

Some cystic duplications form asymptomatic palpable abdominal masses that may be movable and nontender. Cystic duplications may give rise to intestinal obstruction by pressure on the adjacent bowel, may cause a volvulus, or if small, may lead to intussusception. Tubular duplications are likely to be complicated by peptic ulceration with bleeding or perforation. Shock can follow bleeding from a tubular duplication.

X-ray studies tend to be negative unless the duplication is large or unless obstruction is present. Vertebral anomalies are often found in patients with duplications.

Treatment. Resection of the duplication necessitates resection of the adjacent small or large bowel sharing the common blood supply. In long tubular duplications the normal bowel may be preserved by stripping out only the mucosal lining of the duplication. Duodenal duplications may be marsupialized into adjacent duodenum because resection may be too hazardous.

RETROPERITONEAL TUMORS

Wilms tumor is the most common abdominal tumor in childhood and must be suspected whenever there is a retroperitoneal mass. Neuroblastoma (pp. 942-943), retroperitoneal teratomas, hydronephrosis, and cystic kidneys may present a similar clinical picture. Pancreatic pseudocysts, choledochal cysts, and liver lesions are rare causes of large masses in the same area.

WILMS TUMOR (see also pp. 853 and 941)

Nephroblastoma is a highly malignant neoplasm that may grow to extremely large size. It arises in the parenchyma of the kidney and grows by expansion within the renal capsule but may eventually invade perirenal structures. Vascular invasion occurs early, and the tumor may extend into the renal vein and vena cava. There is also lymphatic invasion with spread to the local lymph nodes. Distant metastasis is usually first seen in the lungs. The tumor occurs most often in children between 2 and 3 years of age but may be present at birth. Often it is bilateral.

Abdominal enlargement or the incidental discovery of an abdominal mass is usually the first indication that a Wilms tumor is present. Rarely, there may be pain associated with rapid enlargement related to hemorrhage into necrotic areas. Hematuria is unusual, and when present, is indicative of a poor prognosis.

A mass in the flank is generally present. It is ovoid, firm, smooth, and nontender. The tumor is only slightly movable. It is not as likely to cross the midline as is a neuroblastoma. A low-grade fever is often present, and hypertension is not uncommon. Urinalysis is usually normal. In the plain radiograph a soft tissue mass may be noted, displacing intestinal gas shadows. Intravenous pyelograms show distortion and displacement of the renal pelvis (Fig. 33-4). The displacement is almost always medial and may be upward or downward. Failure of dye excretion by the involved kidney occurs rarely, such a finding being more suggestive of hydronephrosis or multicystic kidney. It is seldom necessary to perform retrograde pyelograms. One of the more important findings on the intravenous pyelogram is the presence of a normally functioning opposite kidney, the presence of which must be proved before the involved kidney is removed. A chest radiograph should be made to detect evidence of metastases.

Neuroblastoma (see also pp. 853 and 942-944)

Neuroblastoma is a highly malignant lesion that develops most commonly in the abdomen but is also seen in the central nervous system, pelvis, thorax, neck, and elsewhere. The greatest number develop in the region of the adrenal glands and attain extremely large size. Metastasis is mainly by local invasion and through the bloodstream but also by way of the lymphatics. The liver or the skeletal system may be the only apparent sites of metastases. Massive metastases limited to the liver and skin metastases occur chiefly in very young infants.

Enlargement of the abdomen is frequently the first change noted by the parents. General malaise, weight loss, and loss of appetite are also noted. Skeletal metastases may result in bone pain or even pathologic fractures. A protrusion of one or both eyes from orbital metastases may be the primary complaint.

A large mass in the flank is commonly found. This is fixed, firm, and nontender. Its surface is irregular and nodular. It frequently crosses the midline. The liver may be greatly enlarged with a nodular surface. Bone metastases frequently

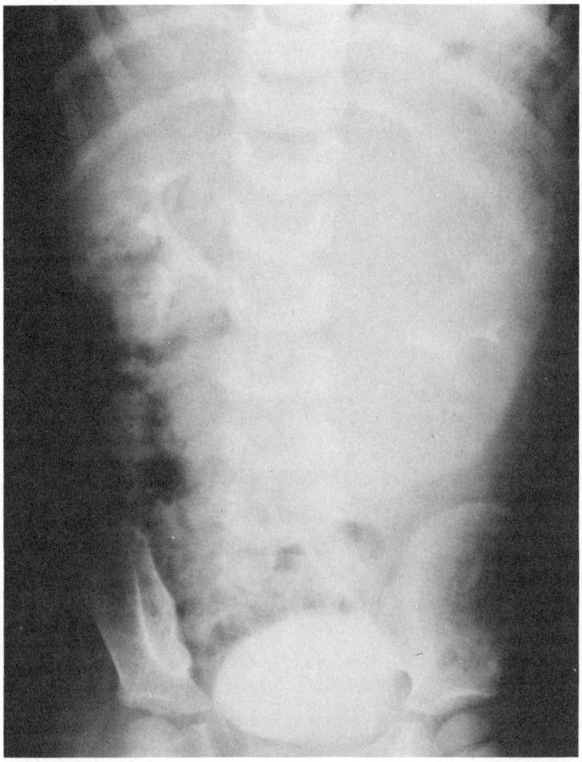

Fig. 33-4. Wilms tumor (nephroblastoma) of left kidney. Intravenous urogram shows soft tissue mass filling left abdomen and distortion of left pelvocalyceal system. (Courtesy Dr. W. Webster Riggs, Le Bonheur Children's Medical Center, Memphis.)

involve the skull, giving raised areas beneath the scalp or unilateral exophthalmos.

The plain radiograph may reveal a large soft tissue mass. A few scattered calcifications are occasionally seen in the mass. An intravenous pyelogram will show displacement of the kidney, depending on the site of origin of the tumor. Displacement is usually lateralward, as opposed to medial displacement by Wilms tumor. Function in the involved kidney is almost always preserved. Ultrasound and computerized axial tomography (CT) scans may be useful. Chest radiographs seldom reveal lung involvement, but a skeletal survey may show punched-out-lesions characteristic of metastases. Urinalysis is generally normal but urinary catecholamine levels are frequently elevated. Typical abnormal cells are sometimes seen in the peripheral blood and in the bone marrow.

Treatment. For treatment of neuroblastoma see the discussion on pp. 854-855 and 943.

Retroperitoneal teratoma

Large teratomas not specifically related to any of the normal retroperitoneal viscera may develop in the flank. These unattached teratomas may be cystic or solid and contain various types of well-differentiated tissues. Many such tumors have malignant components, varying from fairly well-differentiated sarcomas and carcinomas to highly undifferentiated anaplastic tumors.

The lesion is usually detected in the first year or two of life by the onset of painless swelling of the abdomen or by the discovery of an abdominal mass located in the flank or lateral aspect. It is nontender and may be ovoid and smooth or somewhat irregular.

Plain radiographs of the abdomen reveal a soft tissue mass in which there are usually irregular calcifications. Well-formed teeth or bones may sometimes be identified. Intravenous pyelograms may show displacement of a normally functioning kidney unless pressure on the ureter has caused hydronephrosis.

Treatment. Surgical excision of the intact tumor should be performed promptly. If examination shows malignant changes in the tumor, postoperative irradiation of the tumor area may be useful. If the tumor is inoperable, irradiation and chemotherapeutic agents should be employed. The prognosis for benign lesions is excellent. If malignant lesions are totally extirpated before metastasis is apparent, cure is sometimes achieved. However, inoperable lesions or those that have metastasized usually respond poorly to treatment.

ACUTE APPENDICITIS

The diagnosis of acute appendicitis may be a most perplexing problem. Abdominal pain is one of the commonest complaints of childhood, occurring in many diseases, primarily intraabdominal or elsewhere in the body. Although appendicitis is rare before 1 year of age, it has caused the death of newborn infants. Confusion in diagnosis results in delays, permitting appendiceal rupture before treatment in more than one half the patients under 6 years of age. The course of the disease in young patients tends to be rapid. The likelihood of generalized peritonitis in the very young is great, apparently because of inability to wall off the inflamed area.

Clinical manifestations. Almost invariably pain is the first complaint. It is usually periumbilical or generalized but subsequently becomes localized in the right lower quadrant. Nausea, vomiting, and anorexia follow. Although constipation is more common, diarrhea may occur early when the appendix lies in the pelvis against the rectum. The patient is generally most comfortable lying still, with the knees drawn up, and it may become painfully difficult to walk upright. Low fever develops early. There may be a history of recent upper respiratory tract infection or intestinal upset.

Early in the disease the general condition may appear good. Later, evidence of toxicity supervenes, with dehydration and an increase in pulse and respiratory rates. Temperature is seldom as high as 39.4° C (103° F), unless dehydration is great or peritonitis is present. In the apprehensive child it may be difficult to define localized muscle spasm, tenderness, and rebound tenderness. However, by gentle, patient palpation the physician can usually detect these findings, most obvious in the right lower quadrant. Light percussion of the abdomen may elicit tenderness over the inflamed appendix. Auscultation usually reveals peristaltic sounds unless generalized peritonitis is present. Abdominal distention occurs as the disease progresses. When walling-off has occurred, the mass of an abscess may become palpable. Definite rectal tenderness on digital examination is highly significant.

Laboratory findings. The white blood cell count cannot be relied on completely in the diagnosis but is useful to confirm clinical impressions. The total white blood cell count is usually elevated above 10,000/mm^3, with a definite shift to the left. The total count seldom exceeds 20,000 to 25,000/mm^3. Urinalysis is negative, although occasionally an inflamed appendix lying against the ureter may cause pyuria. Acetonuria is not unusual when dehydration or fever is present.

X-ray examinations are seldom helpful in the diagnosis. Sometimes a fecalith may be visualized. Even in the absence of acute symptoms, appendectomy should be performed for known appendiceal fecaliths because such patients will almost invariably have a ruptured appendix if they subsequently develop acute appendicitis.

Differential diagnosis. It is frequently impossible to differentiate acute mesenteric lymphadenitis from acute appendicitis. Mesenteric lymphadenitis is more likely to be accompanied by pharyngeal inflammation, with enlargement and tenderness of the cervical lymph glands. Certain viral infections or bacterial infections such as yersinia enterocolitica tend to produce intense abdominal pain, with tenderness and muscle rigidity. High temperature is usually a manifestation of these diseases. When the fever subsides, abdominal complaints may also subside. Acute gastroenteritis of bacterial, viral, or toxic origin may mimic acute appendicitis. Right lower abdominal pain may be the initial complaint in patients with such diseases as measles, poliomyelitis, encephalitis, rheumatic fever, and many others. Urinary tract infections, especially those limited to the right kidney, are frequently suspected of being acute appendicitis, as are lesions of the ovary. Pneumonia, particularly when involvement is in the lower lobes, may give symptoms and signs that appear to arise in the abdomen.

To avoid confusion with these various diseases, a carefully taken history and complete physical examination are essential. Observation with repeated examinations over several hours may be necessary. Fatal or disabling complications have resulted from appendectomy during the acute course of some other illness. A low enema and an appropriate dose of aspirin or acetaminophen will relieve many of the patients with acute abdominal pain not due to appendicitis.

Treatment. Appendectomy should be performed as soon as the patient's condition permits. The temperature should be brought below 38.9° C (102° F). The pulse rate should have dropped below 120 beats/min. Dehydration and electrolyte deficiency require intravenous fluid replacement, given as rapidly as is safe to permit early operation. If peritonitis is obvious, antibiotic therapy may be started preoperatively. After uncomplicated unruptured appendicitis, chemotherapy is not indicated. Drains should be left in the wound if the appendix has ruptured. The prognosis in appendicitis, even when rupture has occurred, is excellent if treatment is prompt and proper.

OBSTRUCTIVE UROPATHY (see also pp. 921-926)

The occurrence of urinary tract infection or difficulty in voiding in young males should lead the physician to suspect an abnormality of the urinary tract, producing partial obstruction. The same is true of female children but less consistently. Partial obstruction results in progressive dilation of the urinary tract with stasis of urine proximal to the point of blockage, which predisposes to infection. The obstruction may be at any level of the upper or lower urinary tract. The consequence of partial obstruction is progressive loss of renal function. When infection is present, loss of function is far more rapid.

Bladder outlet obstruction

Female children who have repeated bouts of urinary infection are frequently found to have significant amounts of residual urine in the bladder after voiding. Passage of urethral dilators may demonstrate distal urethral stenosis. Cystograms with voiding urethrograms may show a dilated urethra or a flat base to the bladder and may reveal vesicoureteral reflux. Cystoscopy may show the thickened muscular ridge of the hypertrophied bladder neck. This is occasionally encountered in male children and is frequently seen in neurogenic defects of the bladder. When the obstruction is of mild degree, urethral dilation may correct the problem. In greater degrees of hypertrophy, transurethral resection or open resection of a wedge of bladder neck by the suprapubic approach may be necessary.

Posterior urethral valves (see also p. 924)

In the male urethra at the level of the verumontanum, two semilunar valve cusps may occur. These produce a considerable degree of obstruction, resulting in dilation and hypertrophy of the bladder, ureterectasis, and hydronephrosis. A catheter passes readily into the bladder past the obstructing valves, revealing significant postvoiding bladder residual. Cystograms and voiding urethrograms reveal the dilated trabeculated bladder. Distal to the bladder neck a greatly dilated posterior urethra is seen. There is usually marked bilateral vesicoureteral reflux. Diminished renal function manifested by an elevated BUN concentration and by poor visualization of the kidneys on intravenous pyelograms is frequently encountered. It is possible in most patients to remove the valves by transurethral resection.

Ureterocele (see also p. 923)

Constriction of the mucosal orifice of the ureter may result in dilation of the distal ureter inside the bladder wall. A cystic mass protruding into the bladder at the site of the stenotic orifice develops. Proximal to this obstruction the ureter and kidney pelvis are dilated, at times severely. This abnormality occurs more frequently in females. It may be unilateral or bilateral. Its greatest incidence accompanies complete doubling of the kidney pelvis and ureter. The ureterocele typically involves the orifice of the ureter draining the upper pole of the kidney. This orifice enters the bladder caudad to the ureter from the lower pole of the kidney. The dilated ureter produces secondary blockage of the accompanying lower pole ureter, resulting in the hydronephrosis of both the upper and lower portions of the double kidney. Large ureteroceles may block the bladder neck, causing damage to the opposite kidney.

Diagnosis of ureterocele is made by observing a filling defect in the bladder on the cystogram. Intravenous pyelograms demonstrate the presence of hydronephrosis and hydroureter, with delayed emptying. During cystoscopy the ureterocele, bulging into the bladder lumen, may be visualized. The stenotic ureteral orifice may be difficult to demonstrate.

Treatment of ureteroceles by transurethral enlargement of the orifice is sometimes attempted, but the suprapubic approach is probably best. If the orifice is enlarged too much, reflux from the bladder into the ureter will cause persistence of the hydronephrosis and hydroureter after surgery. Ureteroneocystostomy may be required to overcome this reflux. If ureterocele accompanies double ureter, the involved ureter, the portion of kidney that it drains, and the intravesical portion of the ureterocele may be resected. It is usually the upper pole that is involved, and this may comprise only a small segment of the entire kidney. If the upper pole is in good condition, the two pelves or ureters may be joined and only the distal ureter excised.

Ureteropelvic obstruction

One of the most common causes of hydronephrosis is obstruction at the ureteropelvic junction, usually unilateral but sometimes bilateral. Several conditions may cause this. Blockage may result from an aberrant or accessory renal vessel, which crosses the ureter enroute to the lower pole of the kidney. Intrinsic stenosis may be present, with a short stricture or a long area having a narrow, irregular lumen. An obstructing valve mechanism may result from a mucosal flap or from origin of the ureter high on the wall of the kidney pelvis. There may also be kinks in the upper ureter that are maintained by fibrous bands.

Obstruction may be of mild degree, repeated examinations showing little progression of the hydronephrosis over a period of years. At the other extreme, obstruction may be almost complete, with considerable impairment of the kidney's function.

Abdominal pain, nausea, or vomiting may occur without infection; however, in many cases no symptoms develop until there is secondary infection. Frequency, burning during voiding, chills, and fever accompany the infection. The hydronephrotic kidney may be palpable. If acute infection is present, tenderness may be noted in the kidney area. Hypertension is only rarely encountered.

Intravenous pyelograms may be adequate to show the hydronephrosis and obstruction. If renal function is greatly diminished, retrograde pyelograms are necessary. In the uncomplicated case the urine is usually normal. However, often there is chronic pyuria and occasionally gross hematuria. The BUN concentration is normal unless bilateral involvement is present.

Treatment. In the asymptomatic patient with minimal dilation of the renal pelvis and no evidence of urinary infection, no specific treatment may be necessary. However, if significant dilation or persistent infection is present, surgical relief is necessary to avoid loss of kidney function. Aberrant vessels should usually be bypassed by dismembered pyeloplasty. At times intrinsic stenosis of the ureter will be present, in addition to the abnormal vessel. Strictures and valvelike obstruction at the ureteropelvic junction are treated by plastic enlargement of the ureteropelvic orifice by such techniques as the Foley Y-V plasty. At times it is necessary to reimplant the ureter into the kidney pelvis, and it may be necessary to reduce the size of a greatly dilated kidney pelvis by partial excision of its wall. The results are good in a large percentage of those patients in whom preexisting kidney damage and infection are not of great degree.

Double kidneys

Duplication of the kidney and ureter is not rare. The two halves of a double kidney are not completely separated, although there may be a constriction between them. However, the drainage system is completely separate. The ureters may remain doubled throughout their length, opening into the bladder through different orifices. In many cases doubling will be only partial, the two ureters joining as a Y somewhere between the pelvis and the bladder. When the ureters open through separate ureterovesical orifices, the more distal orifice is that of the ureter from the upper pole.

This anomaly has no clinical significance unless complicated by ureteral obstruction or ectopic placement of the ureteral orifice. Obstruction is usually the result of some additional defect, most commonly a ureterocele. The ureterocele is ordinarily at the orifice of the ureter from the upper pole of the kidney.

Symptoms of urinary infection are usually the

first complaints in patients with obstruction. Even in the absence of infection, hydronephrosis and hydroureter may become so severe as to cause abdominal enlargement. Urinary incontinence results when an ectopic ureteral orifice lies beyond the urinary sphincters. Because the ureter from the upper pole of the kidney enters the bladder more distally, it is this ureter that may drain into the urethra or the vagina. Such a situation leads to constant dribbling of urine, even though the patient may also void normally.

When dilated, the ureter may be large enough to be felt on abdominal or rectal palpation. There may be tenderness if acute infection is present. Sometimes the abnormally placed orifice can be seen on endoscopic examination of the vagina, urethra, or bladder.

Intravenous pyelograms are generally adequate for accurate diagnosis of these abnormalities. Each portion of the double kidney will contain only part of the usual number of major and minor calyces so that visualization of one half the collecting system can lead the physician to suspect the presence of the other half.

Treatment. No treatment is necessary unless obstruction or incontinence is present. Upper pole heminephrectomy is most commonly required, but anastomosis of the two pelves or ureters may occasionally be done.

EXSTROPHY OF THE BLADDER
(see also p. 935)

Exstrophy of the bladder is a defect of the lower abdominal wall and bladder in which the interior of the bladder lies completely exposed. Ordinarily, there is also total epispadias. The umbilicus lies unusually low, and the exposed bladder membrane extends from the umbilicus to the tip of the phallus. The pubic bones, with attached rectus sheaths, are widely separated. The bladder wall makes up the full thickness of the abdominal wall in its area. Indirect inguinal hernias and occasionally undescended testicles may be present as associated defects. Total urinary incontinence is the most distressing problem of these patients. There may be some discomfort from irritation of the exposed bladder mucosa. The epispadic penis does not permit normal sexual function. Separation of the pubic bones lead to an abnormality of gait.

Treatment. In recent years there has been increasing interest in reconstruction of the bladder to restore its normal function. In a reasonable percentage of patients total surgical correction of the abnormality may be successful. To facilitate reconstruction of the bladder and abdominal wall, bilateral pelvic osteotomy may be done. When primary reconstruction is not feasible or fails, the ureters may be transplanted. Transplantation into the rectosigmoid is feasible if there is good anal continence. Other techniques are available that reduce the likelihood of hyperchloremic acidosis from mucosal reabsorption of urine, such as implanting ureters into an isolated segment of ileum or colon, which drains into an ostomy bag. The rectum may be isolated from the fecal stream and may serve as a substitute bladder, the colon terminating as an abdominal colostomy or as a perineal colostomy brought out behind the rectum but through the rectal sphincter to attain continence. After the ureters have been transplanted, the excess bladder membrane is excised, and the penis and urethra are reconstructed for reproductive function and a satisfactory cosmetic appearance.

HYPOSPADIAS

The urethra may terminate proximal to the tip of the penis. Its orifice may lie at any point on the shaft of the penis or in the perineum. Especially with the more proximal orifices, there is a ventral chordee, or bowing of the penis so that the tip of the glans lies near the abnormal orifice despite the essentially normal length of the corpora cavernosa.

Treatment consists of correction of the chordee at about 4 years of age and subsequent reconstruction of the urethra by various plastic techniques, performed before the patient enters school.

BILIARY ATRESIA (see also pp. 354-356)

Congenital obstruction of the bile ducts is more often caused by intrinsic obstruction than by extrinsic pressure. Blockage may result from occlusion of the lumen by inspissated bile and mucus. This may occur in such hemolytic disorders as erythroblastosis fetalis. Anatomically patent bile ducts may be functionally obstructed in neonatal hepatitis, obstruction in this case being in the finer radicals of the biliary tree. The most common cause of obstruction is biliary atresia in which there is complete blockage of the lumen of part or all of the biliary tree.

Atresias may be separated into the intrahepatic group, in which no major bile passages are identifiable within the liver substance, and the extrahepatic group, in which the intrahepatic biliary tree is patent, but obstruction is present in the main biliary passages outside the liver. Biliary cirrhosis is the eventual result of complete obstructive jaundice. Ascites, portal hypertension with esophageal varices, and vitamin deficiencies complicate the disease, leading to death in most patients before 1 year of age.

Clinical manifestations. Progressive jaundice with dark urine and acholic stools persist from the newborn period. Jaundice in the first week or two may be minimal or not noted. Stool color is somewhat dependent on the diet, and it is not unusual for the stools to be described as intermittently dark or yellow. Parents often state that the degree of jaundice varies from day to day because the apparent skin coloration varies when viewed under different conditions of light and skin temperature.

Severe jaundice is eventually the most pronounced feature. The liver is usually somewhat enlarged and becomes increasingly firm after 1 to 2 months of age. The spleen may be enlarged.

Laboratory findings. The serum bilirubin level is elevated in a range from 8 to 15 mg/dl. Stools are free of bile or urobilinogen. The prothrombin time may be somewhat prolonged. Other liver function studies have not proved of consistent value in distinguishing biliary atresia from other causes of obstructive jaundice. When the history suggests a previous hemolytic disease and when the Coombs test is positive, inspissated bile may be strongly suspected as the cause of obstruction. However, true atresia has been observed in patients who also had hemolytic problems. The radioactive isotope excretion tests have shown promise in the differentiation of complete from incomplete obstruction. Needle biopsy of the liver may be helpful.

Treatment. In past years few patients with a lesion easily correctable by surgery have been found at the time of laparotomy. Occasionally a patient will be found to have extrahepatic ducts that end blindly, which can be anastomosed to the intestinal tract. This is best accomplished by establishing a Roux-en-Y type of intestinal anastomosis, bringing a defunctionalized loop of intestine up to the ducts, which avoids reflux of intestinal contents into the biliary tree in the postoperative period. In recent years this same type of procedure has been performed even though no visible ducts have been seen in the hilum of the liver. At the present time it is believed that exploration should be carried out as soon as the diagnosis of biliary atresia seems reasonably certain, preferably between 3 and 6 weeks of age. At that time the gallbladder is explored and a cholangiogram performed if there is a lumen available. If no ducts are found at the time of cholangiogram, complete exploration of the hilum of the liver is performed. Even if no ductal system is seen in the hilum of the liver, a Roux-en-Y type of intestinal anastomosis is performed, and the defunctionalized jejunal end is brought up to the hilum of the liver and simply sutured around this area in the hope that bile will escape from the liver into the intestinal tract. Long-term results for this type of procedure are unclear, but currently the procedure appears encouraging. Liver transplants can now be offered to patients who fail to impove following such procedures.

CONGENITAL HEART DISEASE

Surgical aspects

At present, certain congenital malformations of the heart and great vessels can be corrected completely without the use of the heart-lung machine. Another large group of malformations can be corrected with the use of the heart-lung machine and total cardiopulmonary bypass. Certain other cardiac anomalies can be corrected only partially, with or without the use of bypass. Finally, many such malformations are still uncorrectable surgically but will probably be curable within the next decade.

Heart-lung machine

Open heart surgery was made possible by the development of successful pump oxygenators that permit temporary total cardiopulmonary bypass. Several types of heart-lung machines, which provide satisfactory bypass for about 3 hours, have been developed.

Despite the multiplicity of machines, they all must perform certain functions satisfactorily. Blood must be taken from the patient and pumped back into the circulation at a satisfactory rate. The ideal flow rate should be about equal to the patient's own cardiac output at rest.

A normal oxygen–carbon dioxide exchange

is accomplished in the oxygenator so that the blood returned to the systemic circulation will be fully saturated with oxygen. Blood temperature must be controlled, preferably by a suitable heat exchanger. The blood temperature can be kept normal, or induced hypothermia can be used when necessary.

It is important that different components of the blood not be destroyed by the mechanical heart-lung machine. Specifically, there should not be excessive hemolysis, destruction of platelets or fibrinogen, or any degree of coagulation during the bypass procedure.

The institution of cardiopulmonary bypass is a fairly simple procedure. All blood returning to the heart through the superior and inferior vena cavae is diverted to the heart-lung machine through plastic tubes inserted into these veins. These plastic cannulas are usually inserted through the right atrial appendage, one being threaded into the superior vena cava and one into the inferior vena cava. Blood flows to the heart-lung machine by gravity and passes through the oxygenator, where oxygen–carbon dioxide exchange takes place. It is then propelled back to the systemic circulation by the pump at a flow rate equal to the patient's cardiac output. The blood is returned to the systemic circulation by a cannula placed into the aortic arch.

The following is our method of managing infants and children at the present time. In most cases we use moderate to profound hypothermia in conjunction with cardiopulmonary bypass. Cardiac arrest is accomplished by placing a clamp across the ascending aorta just proximal to the aortic cannula. Through a separate small cannula the aortic root is perfused with a cardioplegia solution made up of potassium, calcium, glucose, and steroids. This solution stops cardiac action and at the same time keeps the myocardium at a temperature of less than 18° C, allowing excellent visualization during intracardiac repair.

In some infants complete circulatory arrest is used. In these cases the core temperature of the infant is taken down to between 15° and 18° C, at which time the heart is arrested with a cardioplegia solution, the pump completely turned off, and the patient's total blood volume drained into the pump. At this point the patient's heart is decannulated so that excellent visualization can be obtained in any chamber. This affords an absolutely quiet, dry, unobstructed field so that complex anomalies can be fixed rapidly and accurately. Complete circulatory arrest is safe for approximately 45 minutes as long as the patient's body temperature is maintained between 15° and 18° C. During circulatory arrest temperatures are monitored in the rectum, esophagus, nasopharynx, tympanic membrane, and myocardium. It is mandatory that the temperature be kept below 18° during circulatory arrest.

When the repair is complete, the patient is recannulated, the pump is turned back on, and the body temperature is warmed to normal.

Results of surgery

Little risk is associated with cardiopulmonary bypass alone. For patients having a simple atrial septal defect, ventricular septal defect, pulmonary stenosis, or aortic stenosis, there is almost no mortality associated with surgery. Patients with total anomalous pulmonary venous return or complete atrioventricular canal defects and infants with complex multiple cardiac anomalies carry a higher mortality, depending on the degree of heart failure, cardiac size, pulmonary resistance, and the number of defects that must be corrected at the time of surgery.

In the following discussions brief descriptions are given of some surgical procedures currently available for various types of congenital heart disease. Each of the entities described from the surgical viewpoint is discussed more fully in its clinical and diagnostic aspects in Chapter 18.

Coarctation of the aorta

(see also pp. 438-440)

Constrictions in the aorta may occur at any site from just above the aortic valve down to its bifurcation, but 98% are located immediately distal to the arch in the vicinity of the ductus arteriosus. The constriction may be proximal to, immediately adjacent to, or just distal to the ductus arteriosus, and in a certain percentage of cases there is persistent patency of the ductus.

Coarctation results in hypertension proximal to the constriction and hypotension distal to the constriction. In some cases there is little or no opening in the aorta. Collateral circulation develops between the subclavian arteries, the vessels around the shoulder girdle, and the intercostal arteries, just distal to the coarctation. This collateral circulation is usually not evident in infants but is frequently evident by 8 years of age. By this time these large intercostal arteries often produce notching on the lower borders of the fourth, fifth, and sixth ribs.

Approximately one half of all patients with coarctation have symptoms in the first year of life, consisting of dyspnea, congestive heart failure, and poor weight gain. The other one half of these patients have no symptoms in infancy and early childhood, the diagnosis being suggested by detection of hypertension in the arms. Hypertension in the arms should always alert the physician to check the blood pressure and pulses in the lower extremities; if they are diminished or absent, the diagnosis of coarctation is evident.

Treatment. In the past, surgical treatment of coarctation consisted of excising the narrowed segment of the aorta and reestablishing continuity of this vessel either by end-to-end anastomosis or by insertion of an arterial graft when necessary. We have recently discarded this technique in small infants because end-to-end anastomosis was associated with recoarctation in approximately 35% of the cases when performed in the first few weeks of life.

Currently we incise across the coarcted segment anteriorly and patch the surface of the aorta with either the subclavian artery, which is opened and hinged down across the coarcted segment, or with a free diamond-shaped patch of pericardium. Patch angioplasty across the coarcted segment has essentially prevented the problem of recoarctation in small infants. In older children end-to-end anastomosis or patch angioplasty gives good results.

In infants under 1 year of age with severe symptoms, a short trial of digitalis therapy is indicated, but if the infant does not show immediate and significant improvement, operation should be performed. If the child improves temporarily with digitalis administration and then relapses into cardiac failure, operation should likewise be performed promptly. If with digitalis therapy the child improves and has no trouble through the first year or two of life, digitalis can frequently be discontinued, since by this time the child will have developed enough collateral circulation to relieve the severe hypertension in the upper extremities, and normal growth and development will take place.

In patients without symptoms in infancy and in those who have been treated successfully through infancy with digitalis, the ideal time for operation is between 5 and 7 years of age.

Results of surgical treatment. In older children the mortality rate associated with surgery is less than 2%; in 90% of these children the blood pressure returns to normal. In infants requiring operation during the first year of life the mortality rate is between 10% and 30%. This high mortality rate results from associated left ventricular failure, lack of collateral circulation, and at times coexisting cardiac defects such as a ventricular septal defect and patent ductus arteriosus.

Patent ductus arteriosus
(see also pp. 431 and 433)

At the present time it is believed that all patients with patent ductus arteriosus without cyanosis should have surgical division. Cyanosis implies pulmonary arteriolar disease with increased resistance and reversal of the shunt; operation is contraindicated in these patients. Infants under 1 year of age who show signs of heart failure should have division of the ductus at that time. If the child is asymptomatic, operation is advised between 1 and 2 years of age. The mortality rate in all surgical cases of patent ductus arteriosus should be less than 1%, and the recurrence rate is nil if these lesions are divided and not simply ligated. For this reason all ductuses should be divided, and the ends should be oversewn with nonabsorbable suture.

Atrial septal defects (see also pp. 426-428)

Atrial septal defects are of three types: (1) ostium secundum defects, by far the most common, in which the opening lies centrally in the septum; (2) high atrial septal sinus venosus defects, in which the opening is just beneath the superior vena cava and is usually associated with pulmonary veins from the right lung draining directly into the superior vena cava; and (3) ostium primum defects, in which the opening lies above or adjacent to the atrioventricular junction. The latter is commonly associated with a cleft in the mitral and tricuspid leaflets, permitting free regurgitation.

At present, closure of the high atrial septal defect and the ostium secundum defect with the aid of the heart-lung machine and total cardiopulmonary bypass carries such a low mortality that the mere presence of these defects warrants surgical closure. Operation is usually performed between 2 and 5 years of age.

The ostium primum defects produce symptoms in infancy: congestive heart failure and frequent lower respiratory tract infections. These children require operation, and it is preferable that the disorder be corrected by 6 years of age if possible. There is about a 2% mortality rate associated with correction of ostium primum defects, but the outlook without operation is poor.

Patent atrioventricular canal (endocardial cushion defects)

(see also pp. 430-431)

A patent atrioventricular canal is one of the most severe congenital anomalies of the heart. There is absence of the lower atrial septum and upper ventricular septum so that a large common hole exists, partly above the atrioventricular junction and partly below. There is also a great deficiency of valve substance in the septal leaflets of both the tricuspid and mitral valves. Seventy percent of these children die in the first year, and 95% die within 5 years if not treated. Surgical correction is difficult because these infants develop cardiac enlargement and pulmonary vascular disease, resulting in poor cardiac reserve. The lesion is difficult to repair because of severe defects of both the ventricular septum and the tricuspid and mitral valves.

Ventricular septal defects

(see also pp. 428-430)

Results of operation for ventricular septal defects are directly related to degree of pulmonary hypertension. In patients in whom the pulmonary artery pressure is below 50 mmHg, correction carries a 0.5% mortality rate. These defects can be closed by direct suture or with a Dacron or Teflon patch when the opening is too large for simple closure. If the pulmonary artery pressure is between 50 mmHg and the patient's own systemic pressure, the mortality rate is about 5% to 10% and is directly related to the secondary lung disease. Again, if the patient has reversal of the shunt because of increased pulmonary pressure exceeding the systemic pressure, surgical intervention is contraindicated.

An unpleasant complication with ventricular septal defects is dehiscence of the ventricular septum after closure. This occurs in about 5% of the patients because the ventricular septum is more difficult to close than the atrial septum for several reasons. The atrioventricular node and bundle of His are immediately adjacent to the ventricular defect. Deep stitches in this area will result in complete heart block, necessitating the insertion of a pacemaker. The aortic valve leaflets are adjacent to the upper border of the defect. Deep sutures in this area will result in aortic regurgitation and death. Finally, the septum is thick immobile muscle, and sutures placed in the rim of the defect are likely to tear because of the high pressure and forceful activity of the ventricles when the patient is disconnected from the heart-lung machine. Newer operative techniques for repair of these defects have gradually led to more secure closures without heart block or aortic regurgitation, and most of these patients have a normal outlook after surgical correction.

Currently, with profound hypothermia and circulatory arrest, ventricular septal defects can be closed in infants under 1 year of age with very low mortality. This is the procedure of choice at this time rather than banding the pulmonary artery, which was a palliative procedure used in the past in these very sick small patients.

Valvular pulmonary stenosis

(see also pp. 436-437)

Pulmonic stenosis consists of a fusion of the semilunar cusps, resulting in a small opening in the pulmonary valve. This opening may be as small as 1 mm in some patients. Rare cases of pure infundibular stenosis have been reported in which localized muscular and fibrous thickening project as a circular ridge into the body of the right ventricle 1 to 2 cm beneath the pulmonic valve. In any case there is partial obstruction to blood flow from the right ventricle into the pulmonary artery. A right ventricular pressure of more than 80 mmHg at rest, with a corresponding normal or decreased pulmonary artery pressure, indicates the need for surgical correction.

Two surgical procedures are available. A closed Brock valvulotomy, which can be done quickly and with little risk, will partially open the valve, but usually stenosis of some degree will be persistent. This procedure is still occasionally done in infants under 1 month of age. With the heart-lung machine, valvulotomy under direct vision can be accomplished with a low mortality rate and excellent long-term results. In all patients over 1 month of age who require valvulotomy, an open procedure is performed.

Aortic stenosis (see also pp. 433-436)

Congenital stenosis of the aortic valve usually results from simple fusion of the semilunar cusps, resulting in a narrowed valve outlet. Infundibular stenosis is occasionally seen. Rarely, supravalvular stenosis occurs in which there is essentially coarctation of the aorta approximately 1 cm distal to the valve attachment.

Aortic valvuloplasty is performed, employing total cardiopulmonary bypass in association with hypothermic cardiac arrest. It is important not to create aortic insufficiency by overzealous valvulotomy. The operative mortality rate with congenital aortic stenosis is less that 1%.

Tetralogy of Fallot (see also pp. 442-445)

The choice of surgical procedures for the tetralogy of Fallot is judged by the degree of cyanosis. The basic procedures in use today are (1) a systemic pulmonary artery shunt and (2) total correction using the heart-lung machine.

In 1945 Taussig and Blalock introduced the systemic pulmonary artery shunt procedure. Anastomosis of either the right or left subclavian artery to the corresponding pulmonary artery acts as a bypass around the severe pulmonary stenosis, allowing for increased blood flow to the lungs. Potts later devised a technique whereby the descending aorta could be anastomosed directly to the left pulmonary artery, and, more recently, Waterston devised a method to anastomose the ascending aorta to the right pulmonary artery, both procedures being useful in tiny infants in whom the subclavian artery is very small. However, these anastomoses are easily made too large and are often associated with overflow of blood into the lungs. In recent years we have instituted a tubular shunt created from a rectangular patch of pericardium, which is sutured between the stump of the subclavian artery and the side of the corresponding pulmonary artery. This provides an adequate-sized shunt and at the same time avoids the danger of overflow through the shunt because the stump of the subclavian artery governs the amount of blood entering the pulmonary circuit.

Total correction. With the advent of open heart surgery, Lillehei was the first to correct completely the cardiac defects of this disease. With the use of the heart-lung machine, the ventricular septal defect was closed, and the infundibular or valvular stenosis was completely relieved by resection and reconstruction of the outflow tract to make it of adequate size.

Present approach to tetralogy. In recent years the trend in all cardiac surgery is to attempt a total correction in one procedure rather than multiple operations. At the present time we would rather totally correct all patients with tetralogy of Fallot at one operation when possible. The limiting factor at this time is the size of the pulmonary valve and the pulmonary vascular bed. At the time of cineangiography, if the left ventricle is found to be of adequate size and the pulmonary vascular tree is not severely hypoplastic, we would prefer to perform total correction for tetralogy even in the infant who is less than 1 year of age. However, in those cases of severe tetralogy where the pulmonary outflow tract, pulmonary valve ring, and main pulmonary arteries are severely hypoplastic, a two-stage operation still seems to be indicated. First, a shunting procedure is performed, usually a Blalock procedure or a modified Blalock procedure using a pericardial extension graft. The shunt procedure increases the blood flow to the lungs and left ventricle and in a sense primes these two areas for the full cardiac load they must accept with total correction. Approximately 2 years after the shunt is created, it is obliterated, and correction of the tetralogy is performed, using the heart-lung machine. With this approach approximately 90% of the patients with the tetralogy of Fallot can be cured at the present time.

Tricuspid atresia (see also pp. 450-452)

Several surgical procedures are employed to aid these children.

Shunt procedure (Blalock or modified Blalock with a pericardial graft). With tricuspid atresia the only blood flow to the lung is through the bronchial arteries or through a small ventricular septal defect into a vestigial right ventricle, present in a small percentage of patients. The shunt procedure is merely a method of increasing blood flow to the lungs so that more blood can be oxygenated per minute. This has proved to be very helpful in some children with tricuspid atresia.

Enlargement of the atrial septal defect. A small number of children with tricuspid atresia have a very small atrial septal defect so that there is essentially no way for blood to get out of the right atrium. The atrial septal defect can be enlarged by several methods not involving use of the heart-lung machine, thus permitting a satisfactory right-to-left shunt to take place. After the atrial defect is enlarged, the patient should still have a Potts or Blalock shunt to increase the blood flow to the lungs.

Glenn procedure. In recent years, efforts have been made to bypass completely the right side of the heart by anastomosing the superior vena cava directly to the right pulmonary artery. Blood then runs from the superior vena cava to the pulmonary artery without traversing the right side of the heart. This operation has been successful, particularly in children over 6 months of age, but it is usually associated with a high mortality rate before 6 months of age.

Total correction. In some patients it is possible to perform what can be called total correction. Fontain, in France, first described the insertion of a conduit between the right atrium and the pulmonary artery with simultaneous closure of the atrial septal defect. In these cases the right atrium becomes the pump for the pulmonary circulation. This has been associated with a reasonably high mortality. The use of a valve conduit (insertion of a porcine valve inside a Dacron graft inserted between the right atrium and the pulmonary artery) has lessened the mortality accompanying this procedure.

A small percentage of patients with tricuspid atresia have a moderate-sized right ventricle that is kept open by a ventricular septal defect. This ventricle does not communicate with the right atrium. In patients who have a moderate-sized right ventricle a valve conduit can be sutured between the right atrium and the right ventricle on the outside surfaces of each chamber. This indeed does accomplish a total correction for tricuspid atresia and is associated with an extremely low mortality.

Transposition of the great vessels
(see also pp. 445 to 448)

In transposition of the great vessels the aorta arises entirely from the right ventricle, and the pulmonary artery entirely from the left ventricle. If no other defects existed, these children would die immediately after birth because no oxygenated blood would be able to reach the systemic circulation. In all patients with transposition there is an atrial septal defect, a ventricular septal defect, a patent ductus arteriosis, or any combination of these, which allows for some intracardiac mixing of blood and permits these patients to survive to an average of 3 months of age. Coexisting congenital valvular disease, particularly stenosis between the left ventricle and the pulmonary artery, is common.

The multiplicity of defects makes total correction of this disease difficult at the present time. In small infants it is most helpful to create a large interatrial septal infect. This can be performed by a cardiologist using an atrial septosomy balloon catheter, as described by Rashkind. The catheter is slipped across the foramen ovale from the right atrium to the left atrium, the balloon is inflated with 4 to 5 ml saline or radiopaque dye, and the balloon is forcibly pulled from the left atrium to the right atrium, tearing the septum open. This sometimes will allow adequate mixing for several months to a year, but in many instances the atrial septum must be excised surgically, utilizing either inflow occlusion or the Blalock-Hanlon technique. In an occasional case where there is severe stenosis between the left ventricle and the pulmonary artery, either a Blalock shunt or a Glenn shunt is used to increase the blood flow to the lungs. On the other hand, in those patients who have a large interventricular septal defect, banding of the pulmonary artery before 6 months of age is necessary to prevent irreversible pulmonary vascular disease resulting in pulmonary hypertension.

Total correction. Total correction of transposition of the great vessels is now associated with low mortality. Correction in most cases is performed by transposing normal venous inflow so that it matches the transposed cardiac outflow. Several technical methods are available for transposing the venous inflow. The most popular are the methods introduced by Sennig, some modification of that method, or the method introduced by Mustard. In both cases the original atrial septum is completely removed and a new septum made in a fashion that reverses the venous inflow.

In recent years Jatene in South America has

switched the origin of the great vessels along with the coronary arteries, which would seem to be the most ideal method for correction of transposition. However, this has been associated with high mortality because of the difficulty of moving the small coronary arteries in infancy.

Total anomalous pulmonary venous drainage (see also pp. 452-453)

A multiplicity of variations can occur in total anomalous pulmonary venous drainage. All blood returning from the pulmonary veins flows by various routes into the right atrium. There is an associated atrial defect permitting some of this blood, with the unoxygenated blood from the two venae cavae also emptying into the right atrium, to shunt across to the left atrium. This will, of course, cause some cyanosis because of the shunting of venous blood to the left side of the heart. These patients also have an enormous left-to-right shunt, since all the pulmonary venous blood returns to the right atrium. About 70% of such children die in the first month of life and 80% in the first year of life.

With the heart-lung machine, profound hypothermia, and complete circulatory arrest, all forms of total anomalous pulmonary venous return can be corrected in infancy with reasonably low mortality. Surgery should be performed as soon as the diagnosis is established, which is not infrequently during the first week of life. The mortality in even these small infants is now less than 15%.

Single ventricle

In those patients who have a single or common ventricle with two normal AV valves through which blood enters the ventricle and two great vessels carrying blood away from the ventricle, septation is possible, although the mortality with this procedure is reasonably high.

Truncus arteriosus (see also pp. 448-450)

Type I. In cases of type I truncus arteriosus there is one large trunk overriding both the right and left ventricles, with the ventricular septal defect just beneath the truncal valve. The pulmonary arteries arise from the side of the truncus just distal to the truncal valve.

In past years pulmonary artery banding was the only surgical treatment available for controlling congestive heart failure in these infants, and for the most part it yielded a reasonably poor palliation. At the present time we feel there is no place for pulmonary artery banding in type I truncal lesions. Total correction is carried out between 3 and 12 months of age, at which time the ventricular septal defect is closed and a porcine valve conduit inserted from the right ventricle to the pulmonary artery. This in itself might be considered a palliative procedure, since the conduit will obviously have to be changed to a larger size at some later date. The low mortality associated with early total correction and remarkable clinical improvement, compared with the miserable ongoing congestive heart failure and chronic pulmonary problems associated with banding, leaves little argument concerning the efficacy of early total correction.

Types II and III. Infants with types II and III may have decreased, ideal, or increased pulmonary blood flow. Most patients in this group have moderate to severe hypoplasia of the pulmonary arteries and have restricted pulmonary blood flow. Palliative shunting is indicated in the hope that the pulmonary artery system will increase in size so that eventual total correction will be possible. In those infants with pulmonary arteries just the correct size to deliver an adequate but not overwhelming amount of blood to the pulmonary vascular bed, early surgical intervention is unnecessary. In rare cases large pulmonary arteries arise from the ascending aorta so that early total correction is feasible and ideal, just as in type I truncus.

Vascular ring (see also pp. 440-441)

Several types of vascular malformations in the superior mediastinum, causing compression of the esophagus and trachea, have been grouped under the term *vascular rings*. Only a few of the more common ones will be described here. The three principal types of aortic arch anomalies producing esophageal and tracheal obstruction are (1) double aortic arch, (2) right aortic arch with left ligamentum arteriosum, and (3) aberrant subclavian artery.

Double aortic arch. Occasionally infants are born with two aortic arches. One passes in front and to the left of the trachea, and the other passes to the right and posterior to the esophagus and trachea. These limbs then join to form a common descending aorta. Usually one arch is larger than the other, more commonly the right or posterior one. The smaller of the two arches is the one that should be divided to relieve the obstruction.

Right aortic arch and left ligamentum arteriosum. In patients with a right aortic arch and left ligamentum arteriosum, the aorta ascends to the right of the trachea and esophagus rather than to the left, and the ligamentum arteriosum extends from the left pulmonary artery across the left posterior aspect of the trachea and esophagus, joining the aorta behind the esophagus. A vascular ring capable of causing symptoms is thus formed.

Aberrant subclavian artery. Of the numerous types of aberrant subclavian artery, the most common is a right subclavian artery that passes behind the esophagus to the right arm. This may cause no symptoms, or it may cause difficulty in swallowing.

Clinical manifestations. Difficulty in swallowing, dyspnea, severe retraction, and crowing type of respirations in infants are suggestive of vascular rings. The child tends to lie with his head in hyperextension to open the thoracic inlet. If the child's head is flexed, complete tracheal obstruction may occur.

Diagnosis is usually made by barium swallow, but occasionally a tracheogram and aortogram are necessary. With barium swallow a persistent distortion of the esophagus will be seen. If a tracheogram is performed, narrowing of the trachea will be found. Although aortograms delineate more accurately the type of vascular ring, they are not always necessary. Newer testing with digital subraction techniques clearly defines the defects.

Treatment. With double aortic arch the smaller of the two arches is divided. With right aortic arch and left ligament the ligamentum arteriosum is divided. Aberrant subclavian arteries can be divided with impunity. These operations tend to relieve partially or completely esophageal and tracheal obstruction. In all cases the thymus is removed, and any vascular structure anterior to the trachea is attached to the posterior surface of the sternum, further alleviating tracheal compression. Results are excellent, and morbidity and mortality are extremely low.

Robert G. Allen
Earle L. Wrenn, Jr.

SELECTED READINGS

Rickham, P.P., et al.: Neonatal surgery, ed. 2, Boston, 1978, Butterworth & Co., Inc.

Keith, J.D., Heart disease in infancy and childhood, ed. 3, New York, 1978, The Macmillan Co.

Ravitch, M.M., et al.: Pediatric surgery, ed. 3, Chicago, 1979, Year Book Publishers, Inc.

Eckstein, H.B., et al.: Surgical pediatric urology, Philadelphia, 1977, W.B. Saunders Co.

Coran, A.G., et al.: Surgery of the neonate, Boston, 1978, Little, Brown & Co.

34 Pediatric Urology

The number of congenital urologic anomalies seen in the pediatric population is significant and is a source of major morbidity and occasional mortality. In addition, urinary tract infection is one of the commonest bacterial diseases seen in childhood and is frequently the first indication of a urinary tract abnormality. The maturity of pediatric urology as a specialty and the rapid expansion of our knowledge of urologic problems in children has led to increased diagnostic capability and improved treatment methods. It is truly unfortunate when the signs or symptoms of urologic disease go unnoticed, because many of the conditions encountered can be managed or surgically corrected. The following discussion and outline is not intended to be a complete accounting of pediatric urologic knowledge as it is today but rather represents the latest thoughts on old problems and some new ideas concerning their diagnosis and treatment.

EVALUATION OF THE PEDIATRIC UROLOGIC PATIENT

Although older children can express their symptoms to some degree, the history obtained from the pediatric patient is, in many cases, secondhand from the parents and can be influenced a great deal by the parents' powers of observation and expression. Despite such possible limitations, an attempt must be made to obtain a complete history. A high index of suspicion concerning the possibility of uropathology may be necessary, especially when the clinical picture is unclear. It is important to obtain any family history of a urologic disease to recognize hereditary or genetically transmitted diseases.

Urologically, the physical examination is directed primarily to the abdominal and genital examinations in both the boy and the girl. General examination can be important, as there are well-known associations of certain urologic abnormalities with other physical abnormalities such as low-set ears and Potter's facies. Other congenital anomalies associated with urologic abnormalities include cardiac anomalies, musculoskeletal anomalies, hemihypertrophy, the absence of abdominal musculature, and the presence of a single umbilical artery in the newborn. Patience and persistence when using light palpation of the abdomen can be most rewarding in examining for flank masses, renal enlargement, evidence of a distended bladder, or the evaluation of tenderness in the abdomen. Percussion, auscultation, and transillumination can be helpful in determining the nature of an intra-abdominal or flank mass.

Inspection and examination of the external genitalia will disclose such abnormalities as hypospadias, epispadias and exstrophy, undescended testicle, imperforate hymen, and anal and sacral anomalies. A urologic evaluation is important in the patient with suspected neurogenic bladder or sacral spinal anomalies. Early detection of abnormalities of anal sphincter tone or lower limb reflexes may be key indicators of neurologic deficits predisposing to a neurogenic bladder.

Signs and symptoms of urologic disease can be varied. Irritative symptoms include dysuria, urgency, and frequency, and are usually of bladder or urethral origin, appearing acutely during an inflammatory process. Obstructive voiding symptoms such as straining, decreased caliber of urinary stream, intermittency, or dribbling associated with incontinence are important signs and should not be ignored. Enuresis is usually thought of as nocturnal, occurring during sleep, or diurnal, occurring during the waking hours. Nocturnal enuresis alone is infrequently associated with uropathology, whereas persistent diurnal incontinence or reversion to nocturnal and diurnal incontinence in an older child are associated with a higher incidence of uropathology.

Nonspecific signs or findings may be the only

clues leading to discovery of urologic disease. Failure to thrive is frequently associated with demonstrated urologic abnormalities, particularly vesicoureteral reflux. In many cases, fever of unknown origin is found to originate from infection in the urinary tract. Abdominal pain of a vague and repetitive nature in many children can be the only symptom of significant urologic disease. Back pain is infrequently a symptom of urologic disease in children, but when it is present, only the older child is able to localize and verbalize his complaints. In most cases, abdominal pain associated with urinary tract anomalies is primarily expressed as periumbilical. A high index of suspicion may be necessary to make an early diagnosis of urologic disease by obtaining appropriate x-ray studies.

Laboratory diagnostic evaluation. Urinalysis is the cornerstone of laboratory evaluation in the patient suspected of urologic disease. Urinalysis should be a routine study performed in the outpatient setting. Collection methods vary with age of the child and degree of cooperation. In the newborn or young infant or the moribund patient, suprapubic aspiration of urine is a safe and easy method of urine collection. Results of urine analysis and culture are the most accurate when this collection method is used. On a routine basis in the older infant, a bagged specimen obtained after thorough cleansing of the external genitalia with sterile saline can be reliable, especially if there is no evidence of infection. If such specimens are positive or equivocal they should be repeated using more accurate collection techniques. For the older more cooperative child, a midstream urine sample obtained after thorough cleansing of the external genitalia by sterile saline is still the safest and easiest method of urine collection. When necessary, catheterization can be safely performed in the older child when other collection techniques have failed. However, this is infrequently required, and such an invasive technique should be used only when noninvasive methods have not given the necessary information.

Urinalysis can be quickly and conveniently performed in the outpatient setting using any of the current commercially available reagent strips. These strips are impregnated with individual reagents that give information about urinary constituents such as glucose, protein, hemoglobin, nitrites, pH, and specific gravity. Microscopic examination of the urinary sediment gives additional information about the presence of red blood cells, white blood cells, or bacteria. In the centrifuged urinary sediment, greater than 3 red blood cells and greater than 5 white blood cells per high-power field is considered abnormal. Pyuria suggests urinary tract infection, but accurate diagnosis is made by means of urine culture. Previously, urine culture techniques were both difficult and expensive to perform; however, with the advent of the newer office or clinic screening systems, there is no longer any reason to deny the patient an accurate diagnosis made through urine culture.

Hematuria is described as gross or microscopic and painful or painless. Gross hematuria can be further characterized by noting whether the blood is present in the initial portion of the urinary stream, the end of the stream, or throughout the urinary stream. Microscopic hematuria refers to red blood cells noted only on examination of the urinary sediment. Most instances of hematuria in children have their origin in the kidney and, more specifically, the glomerulus. The association of inflammatory symptoms with hematuria makes one suspect urinary tract infection, and a urine culture is definitive. The presence of casts and large amounts of protein on urinalysis immediately establishes the bleeding to be of glomerular origin. Hematuria can occur in conjunction with viral, respiratory, or other febrile illnesses and usually clears with the passing of the illness and poses no threat to the child. Other more serious sources of hematuria in these cases must, of course, be excluded. A history of trauma, or a family history of renal difficulties or renal failure, can be important in determining the cause of hematuria. Blood spotting on the underclothes or diapers is noted particularly in children with urethritis or ammoniacal meatal inflammation. When the cause for hematuria cannot be determined on history, physical examination, and urinalysis, radiographic evaluation is indicated. Voiding symptoms, gross hematuria, or demonstrated urographic abnormalities usually indicate the need for cystoscopy in these patients.

Measurement of serial creatinine clearance is the most accurate way to measure and follow a child's level of renal function, though more sophisticated techniques such as inulin clearance may be necessary when special information is required or there is evidence of significantly reduced renal function. The screening measurement of renal function is reflected as serum creatinine or blood urea nitrogen (BUN). At 7 to 10 days after birth, the serum creatinine of an infant falls from the maternal level to represent true infant renal function. In the early days of life, the BUN is more informative of renal function, taking into account the state of hydration of the child.

The excretory urogram still serves as the mainstay for obtaining anatomic knowledge of the upper urinary tract. In the first week of life, the excretory urogram is of limited value because of poor concentration of the contrast medium by the kidneys and because of overlying gas and bowel shadows, which can obscure anatomic detail. In the newborn, renal scanning techniques can be more informative. Perhaps the most helpful addition to our radiographic armamentarium for investigating the urinary tract has been the voiding cystourethrogram. This study gives both anatomic and functional information about the lower urinary tract.

Renal scanning techniques provide a great deal of functional information about the kidneys. These studies can give information concerning differential renal function and also can determine when significant obstructive lesions are present. With the use of the diuretic renogram enhanced with furosemide (Lasix), one can obtain a definition of obstruction of the upper urinary tract in a noninvasive manner. Although scanning techniques lack the resolution and anatomic details obtained with the excretory urogram, these studies remain complementary. When used together they give a comprehensive assessment of anatomy and function of the upper urinary tract.

Abdominal ultrasound is becoming more helpful in children with increased use. It is particularly helpful in diagnosing abdominal masses, hydronephrosis, renal agenesis, and other similar urologic conditions. Use of ultrasound in the pregnant female may reveal urologic abnormalities in the fetus, particularly fetal hydronephrosis. The appropriate way to manage such antenatally diagnosed problems will become an increasing challenge to the pediatric urologist. CT is an effective way of evaluating intra-abdominal and retroperitoneal structures in a child, but as yet its use is not clearly defined.

The urodynamic evaluation of a child includes the cystometrogram, the measurement of urinary flow rate, and sphincter electromyography. These studies give exact functional information regarding lower urinary tract function and are chiefly applied in children with neurogenic bladder dysfunction. They can also be used to investigate severe voiding dysfunction in the absence of a demonstrated neurologic abnormality.

The role of cystoscopy in children has changed as pediatric urology has matured. In the past it was virtually a routine procedure in every form of evaluation for suspected urinary pathology. Cystoscopy is now used much more selectively. It is used primarily in the evaluation of those children with demonstrated radiographic abnormalities, gross hematuria, frequent and recurrent urinary tract infections, severe voiding dysfunction manifest by incontinence, and as an adjunct for those patients undergoing urodynamic testing.

URINARY TRACT INFECTIONS

(see also p. 562)

Urine is normally sterile. Urinary tract infection is said to exist when bacteria are actively multiplying in the urinary tract. When bacteria are confined to the bladder, cystitis occurs. When bacteria are found in the kidneys, pyelonephritis occurs, and it is this condition that poses the threat of renal damage with its long-term consequences.

Several epidemiologic studies document the incidence of urinary tract infection in children have shown that 3% of girls and 1% of boys will have a symptomatic urinary tract infection by 11 years of age. These studies have shown, however, that important differences do exist based on age and sex. Girls have a higher incidence of urinary infections than boys, and whites have a higher incidence than blacks.

In neonates with urinary tract infections, boys predominate and it is felt that these are hematogenous in origin. Congenital abnormalities associated with these neonatal infections are found in significant numbers when these children are studied and should be sought even though the origin of the infection is thought to be hematogenous rather than ascending.

There is a shift from male to female predominance in the occurrence of urinary tract infections that begins in infancy and persists through the preschool and school-age years. Structural abnormalities have been shown to occur in up to 80% of infants and preschool children investigated for bacteriuria. This is an especially important statistic when one considers that renal damage secondary to infection occurs predominantly in children under 5 years of age. Beginning with school-age children, there is a trend toward decreasing incidence of bacteriuria with advancing age. Even so, several studies have shown that covert or asymptomatic infections exist in significant numbers, and it has been estimated that 5% to 6% of all school-age girls will acquire at least one episode of bacteriuria. The search for structural abnormalities and continued surveillance are important in this group, as they are known to be at especially high risk of developing symptomatic infections associated with the onset of sexual intercourse and pregnancy.

Enteric bacteria are responsible for the majority of urinary tract infections. The most frequent causative organism is *Escherichia coli*. Also seen are strains of *Klebsiella, Proteus,* and *Pseudomonas*. In approximately 5% of urinary tract infections, gram-positive organisms such as *Enterococcus* and *Staphylococcus* are isolated. The route of entry for these infections is usually through the urethra. Hematogenous sources of urinary tract infections are infrequent and occur mainly in the neonate.

Host resistance factors play an important role in the etiology and pathogenesis of urinary tract infections. Urine is generally a suitable culture medium but does contain some bacterial inhibitory characteristics such as increased osmolality, urea concentration, and low pH. Bladder emptying is a major defense mechanism in addition to certain poorly understood mucosal properties that allow for the binding and phagocytosis of bacteria. Any lesion such as obstruction that hinders periodic bladder emptying leads to stasis and residual urine, causing increased susceptibility to infection. Increased intravesical pressure is another mechanism predisposing to infection. This can occur secondary to obstruction, neurogenic dysfunction, or functional bladder abnormalities arising from other causes. High intravesical pressures are thought to lead to submucosal ischemic changes that disrupt normal defense mechanisms of the bladder and provide fertile ground for bacterial multiplication. The role of immunoglobulins in urinary tract infections is poorly defined.

Urinary tract infections are thought of as high risk (pyelonephritis) or low risk (cystitis) as they pertain to renal damage in children. The most accurate method of localizing infection is by ureteral catheterization, bladder washout techniques, or renal biopsy. These are all invasive and are of little practical routine use. Indirect attempts at localization, using measurement of C-reactive protein, urinary enzymes, and other measurements have not been successful. It is also difficult to distinguish between upper urinary tract and lower urinary tract infections purely on a clinical basis. There is evidence, however, that the presence of fever, with or without abdominal or flank pain, is reasonably reliable to clinically distinguish pyelonephritis from simple cystitis. In the infant and younger child, nonspecific symptoms such as failure to thrive, gastrointestinal disturbances, weight loss, or malodorous urine may be the only findings leading one to suspect urinary tract infection. Frequency, urgency, and dysuria without fever or abdominal pain are generally indicative of lower urinary tract infections and are seen typically in the older child who is better able to communicate. It is stressed, however, that the severity of underlying urinary pathology does not always correlate well with the types or severity of symptoms associated with the urinary tract infection. It is therefore important to initiate an evaluation of each child with a documented urinary tract infection regardless of the accompanying symptoms or inability to localize that infection.

The diagnosis of urinary tract infection can be suspected by the patient's clinical presentation and the finding of pyuria on urinalysis, but definitive diagnosis is made only by urine culture. Care must be taken in collection of the urine specimen for culture because collection techniques, as has been mentioned, can influence the results of these cultures. It is generally believed that urinary tract infection is present when more than 100,000 colonies per milliliter of an organism in pure growth are isolated in the culture of a clean-catch specimen. Any growth seen on the culture of a specimen collected by suprapubic aspiration, and more than 10,000 colonies grown on the culture of a specimen obtained by catheterization is thought to be indicative of true bacteriuria. Multiple organisms encountered in the urine culture can indicate contamination and the culture should be repeated. It is on the basis of antibiotic sensitivities of the organism cultured that the treatment regimen is determined.

Confirmation of bacterial urinary tract infection indicates the need to obtain an excretory urogram and a voiding cystourethrogram. There is no sound basis for the widely accepted thought that radiographic studies of female children are necessary only with the second infection, or that only boys should undergo investigation following the initial urinary infection. The same incidence of renal scarring and structural abnormalities is seen in children with overt urinary tract infections as in those with covert or asymptomatic infections discovered through screening procedures. Also, an equal incidence of abnormalities has been demonstrated in studies where initial versus recurrent infections were compared. Some studies have indicated that covert infections are even more common than overt infections. This would indicate that when one sees children with symptomatic urinary tract infections this may very well not be the true first episode of bacteriuria. When one considers the above and the fact that both asymptomatic and symptomatic urinary tract infections have up to an 80% chance of recurrence, it is clear that there is no justification for waiting for a second infection before conducting a radiographic evaluation of these children.

Initial evaluation of these children is primarily a radiographic one that consists of the excretory urogram and voiding cystourethrogram. Additional studies including cystoscopy or urodynamic evaluation may be undertaken on those children with demonstrated abnormalities or certain specific recurrent symptom complexes. The accompanying figure outlines in general the steps for investigation and management of the pediatric patient with urinary tract infection (Fig. 34-1).

Treatment of urinary tract infections. Therapy for children with urinary tract infection is based on urine culture results and bacterial sensitivity to the antibiotic. The clinical condition of the patient plays an important role in deciding on a treatment schedule. The length of therapy has traditionally been a 10-day course of antibiotics, with long-term low-dose prophylaxis being reserved for those children with frequent recurrences or who have known urinary tract abnormalities. Short-course therapy consisting of a single dose, or 1 to 5 day therapy, is under evaluation, but early results are incomplete. Short-course therapy may be most appropriate in those children with known radiologically normal urinary tracts. Until more information is available, short-course therapy should be viewed with caution because of early reports indicating a higher than desired reinfection rate. An integral part in the management of the child with a urinary tract infection is a follow-up urine culture to be done in 3 to 4 days following treatment to evaluate the effect of that treatment.

Initial therapy is begun in the afebrile patient with oral medication using oral sulfonamides or nitrofurantoin. Therapy can be started after initial assessment and a urine culture have been obtained. A change of antibiotics may sometimes be necessary when the culture and sensitivity reports are obtained 24 to 48 hours later. In the child who is febrile and clinically ill but remains well hydrated and able to take fluids and medication, outpatient therapy is begun using one of the penicillin derivatives such as cephalosporin. An increased bacterial resistance to ampicillin has been noted, and it seems best that this not be used as first-line treatment in the febrile child with a urinary tract infection. For the child who is febrile, clinically septic, and unable to take oral medication, parenteral antibiotics in the hospital setting are necessary. Initial treatment of these patients includes an aminoglycoside in combination with carbenicillin or ampicillin. In a child with sepsis, a 10-day to 2-week course of parenteral therapy is recommended with follow-up outpatient oral therapy. Once treatment has begun, a urine culture should be obtained in 48 to 72 hours to document the effectiveness of that treatment. Urine culture should then be repeated 4 to 5 days after the medication has been stopped to make sure that no relapse has occurred.

Radiographic evaluation of the urinary tract has traditionally been delayed for several weeks following treatment. This has been done to reduce the incidence of inaccurate results obtained on the basis of acutely inflamed tissues, such as reflux and bladder changes secondary to edema. An excretory urogram can be performed at any

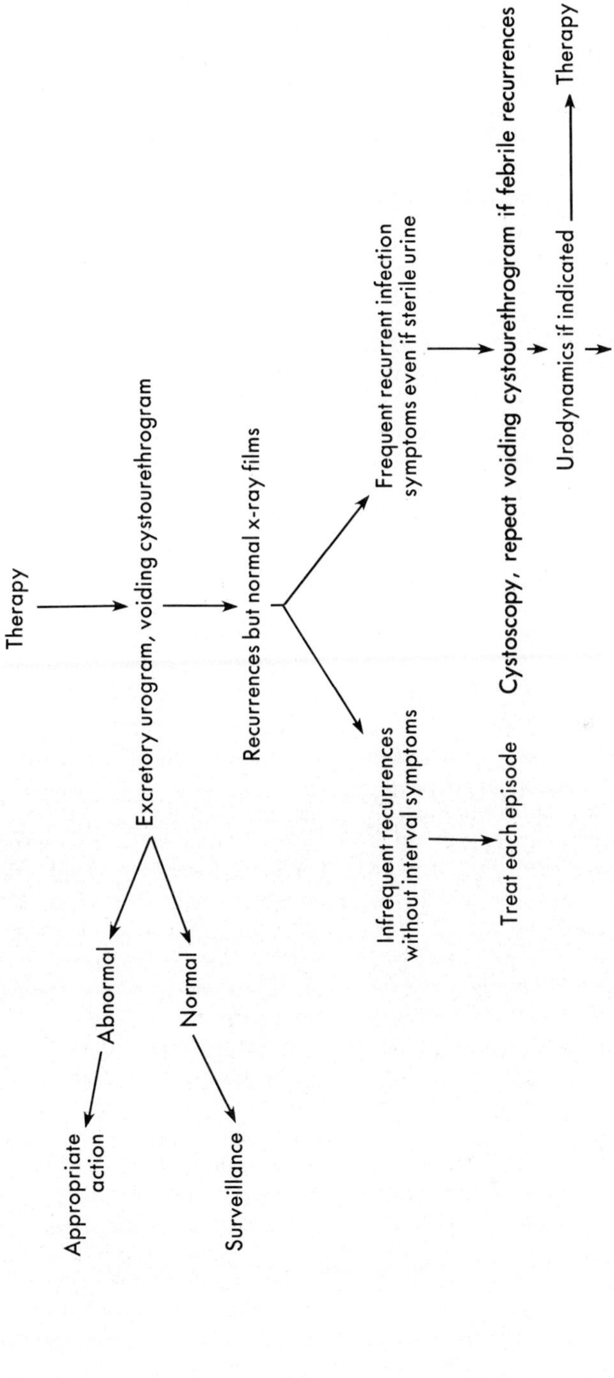

Fig. 34-1. Evaluation of patient with documented urinary tract infection.

time during therapy, particularly when one suspects an acute obstruction or a perinephric abscess or when the child is not responding clinically to initial treatment. If it is not possible to wait for several weeks to perform the voiding cystourethrogram, this can be done when a negative urine culture has been obtained and the child is near the end of the course of treatment.

In the child with recurring urinary tract infections and a normal excretory urogram and voiding cystourethrogram, prevention of further recurrences may only be possible through the use of low-dose antibacterial medications over an extended period. The etiology of these recurrent episodes in children is unknown but may center around a localized deficiency regarding bladder defense mechanisms. Of special interest in this category is a condition known as cystitis cystica. This is a disease diagnosed by typical endoscopic appearance of the bladder showing proliferative cystic changes over the entire bladder mucosa. Children with cystitis cystica particularly require long-term low-dose antibacterial prophylaxis for a minimum of 6 months and may in some cases require medication for 12 to 36 months.

Perineal hygiene is of questionable value in preventing infections, but in many cases it does give the parents a feeling of participating in the child's care and adds to the child's comfort. Labial irritations may be associated with recurring lower urinary tract infections. These are best handled by sitz baths and local application of creams, including steroids and antimicrobials. Alteration of clothing such as the use of cotton panties as well as a diligent search for abnormalities such as pinworms are of little proven benefit for the prevention of infections but can provide a measure of patient comfort. Constipation associated with an increase in urinary tract infection is best manipulated by diet and bowel training.

Nonbacterial urinary tract infections. Viral infections usually presenting as hemorrhagic cystitis do occur. These are caused primarily by adenovirus type 11 and 21 and require sophisticated culture or serum techniques for documentation.

Posterior urethritis or deep urethral inflammatory disease is seen frequently in young males. This is thought to be caused by a viral infection and presents as a sudden onset of urgency, urinary frequency, and dysuria. This can follow a respiratory or viral illness. The pain is usually referred to the tip of the penis, and, on occasion, there may be microhematuria or terminal hematuria. These children can exhibit significant voiding discomfort and in many cases will clutch at the tip of the penis in an effort to alleviate their pain. Urine cultures are negative for bacteria, and radiographic studies are normal. When this diagnosis is suspected clinically, an excretory urogram with a voiding film spotting the urethra is obtained. In the light of negative radiographic and culture results, endoscopic evaluation of these children is usually not necessary. Treatment is symptomatic and in many cases may require several days to several weeks before the symptoms regress. There is likewise a tendency for this disease to recur.

Fungal urinary tract infections usually result as an overgrowth following broad-spectrum antibiotic therapy in a child with urologic pathology, particularly in the presence of foreign bodies. Premature infants and infants and children who are immunosuppressed typically have increased susceptibility to fungal infections.

VESICOURETERAL REFLUX

Vesicoureteral reflux refers to the regurgitation of bladder urine back into the kidneys. The normal ureterovesical junction functions as a valve mechanism that prevents this reflux. Thus the antireflux mechanism normally present serves to protect the upper urinary tract from infection and increased intravesical pressures. Only in the last 3 decades has the importance of reflux been realized, particularly as it relates to renal damage in children. It is now known that reflux is the most frequent abnormality found in children investigated for urinary tract infection.

Careful studies of the normal ureterovesical junction have shown the ureter to pass obliquely through the muscular bladder wall, after which the ureter pursues a submucosal course known as the submucosal tunnel before the longitudinal muscle of the ureter then forms the base, or trigonal area, of the bladder. It is the length of the submucosal portion of the ureter that is directly related to the prevention of reflux. Normally the submucosal length is 5 times the width of the ureter. Such a submucosal tunnel produces a flap-valve mechanism that allows urine to enter the bladder but prevents its back-passage into the ureters and kidneys.

Any alteration of the configuration of the normal ureterovesical junction can cause reflux. Embryologically, the length of the submucosal ureteral tunnel is determined by the site of origin of the ureter, which arises from the wolffian duct. If this step in formation occurs abnormally, a primary ureterovesical junction abnormality exists that gives rise to what is termed *primary reflux*. This is the most common form of reflux encountered. Secondary reflux is that in which conditions exist that cause distortion or destruction of what was an otherwise normally formed ureterovesical junction. Such conditions include paraureteral diverticula, the neurogenic bladder, and distal obstruction such as with posterior urethral valves. Cystitis or acute inflammation can likewise paralyze the normal ureterovesical junction, permitting reflux, but this usually disappears when the inflammation is successfully treated medically.

Genetic factors influence reflux. There is a known decreased incidence of reflux in black children in relation to white children, and there is also a known tendency for familial reflux to occur. The inheritance of reflux is multifactorial. A study of the siblings of children known to have reflux has recently shown that 30% of such siblings exhibit reflux. The majority of the discovered siblings with reflux had no urinary tract symptoms or prior history of urinary tract infections. Several exhibited evidence of renal scarring. Whether this scarring is secondary to unrecognized infections, sterile reflux, or dysplasia acquired in utero is as yet unknown. What is clear is the need for the screening of siblings of children known to have reflux, particularly those under 5 years of age, in whom susceptibility to renal scarring is known to be greatest. Although it is often stated that girls predominate over boys with reflux, this is possibly not true. It is true that girls have a higher incidence of urinary tract infections and therefore are possibly investigated more frequently, but it has been shown in the screening study that reflux probably occurs equally in the sexes.

The mechanism of renal scarring secondary to reflux is still a subject of debate. All investigators agree that reflux with accompanying bacterial infection of the urine is damaging and cannot be tolerated. Some feel that, with the more severe degrees of reflux, even sterile urine can induce renal scarring and create changes known as reflux nephropathy. Others, countering this argument, have attributed these changes to unrecognized urinary tract infection or possibly dysplasia induced in utero. This question can perhaps be answered by screening newborn siblings of children known to have reflux and assuring urine sterility in those found to have reflux as they are followed or treated during the first 5 years of life.

The diagnosis of vesicoureteral reflux is a radiographic one and requires a voiding cystourethrogram (Fig. 34-2). The severity of reflux is of practical significance in the management of this abnormality and is classified below.

Grade I	Reflux into the ureter only
Grade II	Reflux into the ureter, pelvis, and calyces without dilation
Grade III	Mild or moderate dilation with little or no blunting of the calyces
Grade IV	Moderate dilation and/or tortuosity of the ureter and moderate dilation of the renal pelvis and calyces
Grade V	Gross dilation and tortuosity of the ureter and gross dilation of the renal pelvis and calyces

In general, the more severe the grade of reflux, the greater the likelihood that renal damage has occurred or will occur. Since the voiding cystourethrogram gives only information about reflux, it is essential that the child known to have this condition undergo an excretory urogram. This allows one to assess the degree of renal damage or renal scarring and provides a means of following this child in relation to developing changes in the kidney (Fig. 34-3).

It is known that vesicoureteral reflux ceases with advancing age. This is thought to be the result of a maturation process that increases the competency of the ureterovesical junction, thus allowing children to "outgrow" their reflux. Cystoscopy is an integral part in the evaluation of the child with known reflux, seeking to identify those who will spontaneously cease their reflux as opposed to those who will need surgical correction. The length of the ureteral tunnel is observed at cystoscopy, and, in general, the more nearly normal the ureteral orifice and the longer the submucosal tunnel the greater the likelihood the child will spontaneously cease refluxing with growth and control of urinary tract infections. Also, in general, the more severe degrees of reflux are associated with great-

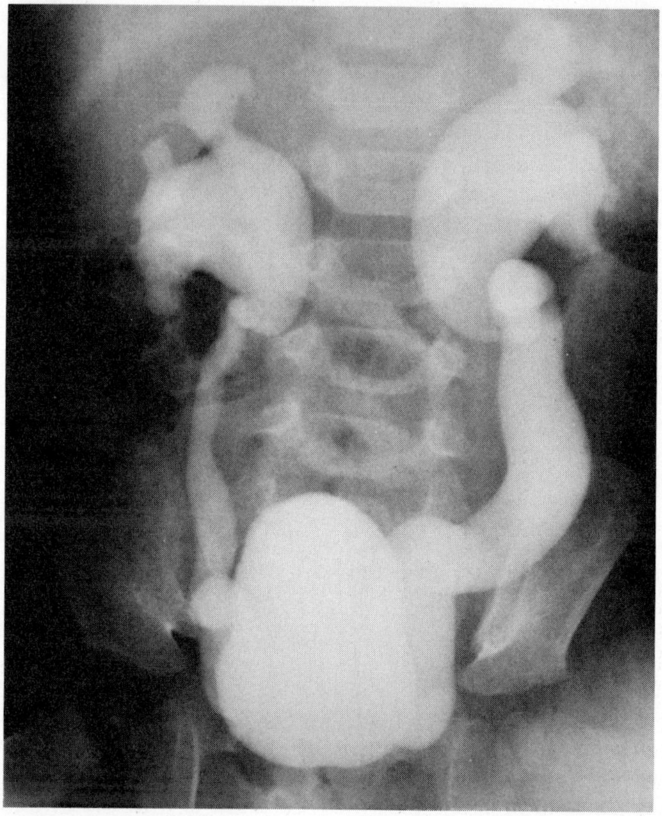

Fig. 34-2. Marked vesicoureteral reflux demonstrated on cystogram.

er ureterovesical abnormality. The child with grade I reflux is not at significant risk, and cystoscopy is withheld from these children unless other indications are present. In children with grade II reflux and higher, endoscopic assessment of the ureteral orifice anatomy can be helpful in predicting which child may spontaneously cease refluxing or which child will most likely require immediate or near-term surgical therapy. It can also help in determining the proper timing of follow-up radiographic studies should immediate surgery not be required.

If it is elected not to surgically correct reflux when first discovered, maintenance of a sterile urine by continuous low-dose antibacterial prophylaxis is essential. This is best accomplished by use of sulfa drugs, nitrofurantoin, or trimethoprim-sulfamethoxazole combination. Interval cystograms and intravenous pyelograms are indicated. Their timing is dictated by the age of the child, the severity of the reflux, and the degree of orifice abnormality seen at cystoscopy. Nuclear cystograms can be helpful in following children known to have reflux.

The indications for surgical correction (ureteral reimplantation) in children with reflux are infections that occur in spite of prophylactic antibacterial therapy, severe orifice abnormality unlikely to mature and improve with time, and the higher grades of reflux present with or without established renal damage. Other indications include the presence of a fixed anatomic deformity (paraureteral diverticulum, duplication, ureteral ectopia, etc.), and children in whom adequate follow-up and close clinical supervision and urine sterility cannot be assured. It is likewise known statistically that children beyond age 10 are unlikely to spontaneously cease refluxing. It would thus seem unwise to continue simply to follow these children into young adulthood, as most agree that a lifetime of reflux is undesirable, particularly in the female child who

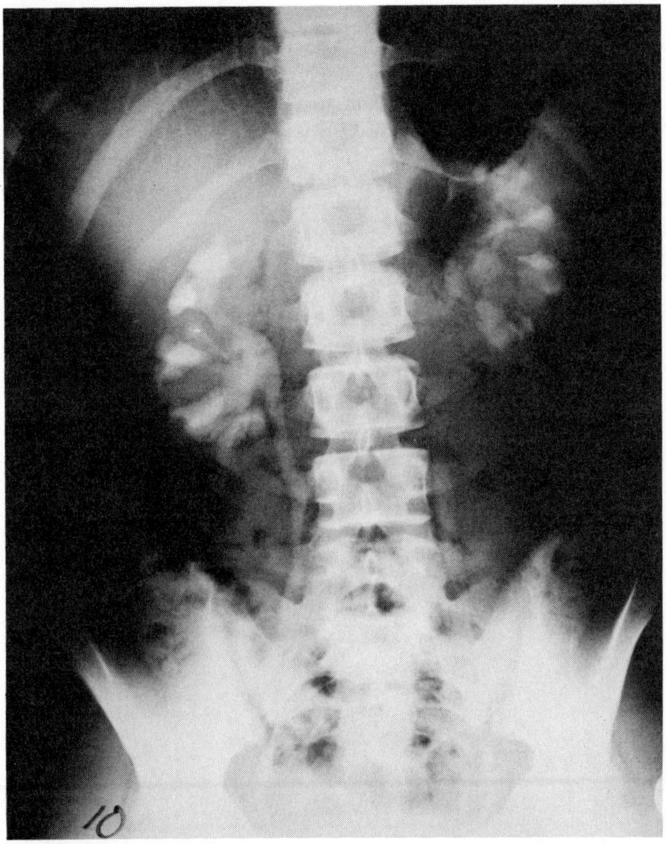

Fig. 34-3. Reflux nephropathy with parenchymal loss and calyceal clubbing.

faces the problem of urinary infections with the onset of sexual activity, and the deleterious effect that such infections might have on pregnancy.

The correction of reflux by ureteroneocystostomy has become highly successful by any one of several techniques. Successful ureteral reimplantation in the uncomplicated case is easily attained in greater than 95% of patients in the hands of those familiar with antireflux techniques. The intraoperative surgical and anesthetic management of these children makes it a safe procedure with a hospital stay that has been significantly shortened. All of these factors should be considered when deciding on the length of time to continue to follow children with reflux and whether or not continued radiation exposure, urinary instrumentation, medication, and other interventions are acceptable.

OBSTRUCTIVE UROPATHY

(see also pp. 901-902)

Obstruction is second only to reflux in frequency when an abnormality of the urinary tract is found in children. Obstructive uropathy can lead to renal damage caused by decreased renal blood flow, decreased filtration pressure, and altered renal tubular function. Additionally, the problems of infection and calculus formation can occur because of urinary stasis and create further damage superimposed on the obstruction.

The presentation of obstruction varies according to the age of the child. Older children characteristically appear with symptoms of infection, abdominal and flank pain, hematuria, obstructive voiding patterns, incontinence, or other signs of voiding dysfunction. In the neonate or younger child, nonspecific symptoms indicative of infection can be present, or an abdominal mass simply may be discovered on routine examination.

The diagnosis of obstruction is primarily radiographic. The intravenous pyelogram will usually delineate upper urinary obstruction. Other studies that include ultrasound and renal scanning can be helpful in making the diagnosis. Under certain circumstances, dilation of the urinary system can occur without true obstruction being present. When this is suspected, a diuretic renal scan or direct perfusion pressure studies can be helpful in determining whether obstruction truly exists. The voiding cystourethrogram, cystoscopy, and direct urethral calibration are methods for determining the presence of lower urinary tract obstruction. Once the level and type of obstruction have been defined, surgical correction is necessary.

Upper urinary obstruction. The renal calyx can be obstructed by congenital and intrinsic abnormalities or more often by compression of a vessel crossing the neck of the calyx. Radiographic appearance of hydrocalycosis is distinct. When such an appearance is proved to be obstructive or is accompanied by flank pain or infection, surgical correction is indicated.

The ureteropelvic junction is the most common site of obstruction in the upper urinary tract. The point of obstruction occurs where the renal pelvis narrows to form the ureter (Fig. 34-4). The obstruction is caused by either an intrinsic abnormality, obstructing bands, or an abnormally placed crossing vessel. In addition to the usual symptoms associated with urinary infection, this condition can present as hypertension, an abdominal mass, or recurrent ill-defined abdominal pain. When ureteropelvic junction obstruction is present on the excretory urogram, a voiding cystogram should be performed to rule out reflux and the possibility of a secondary ureteropelvic junction obstruction. The treat-

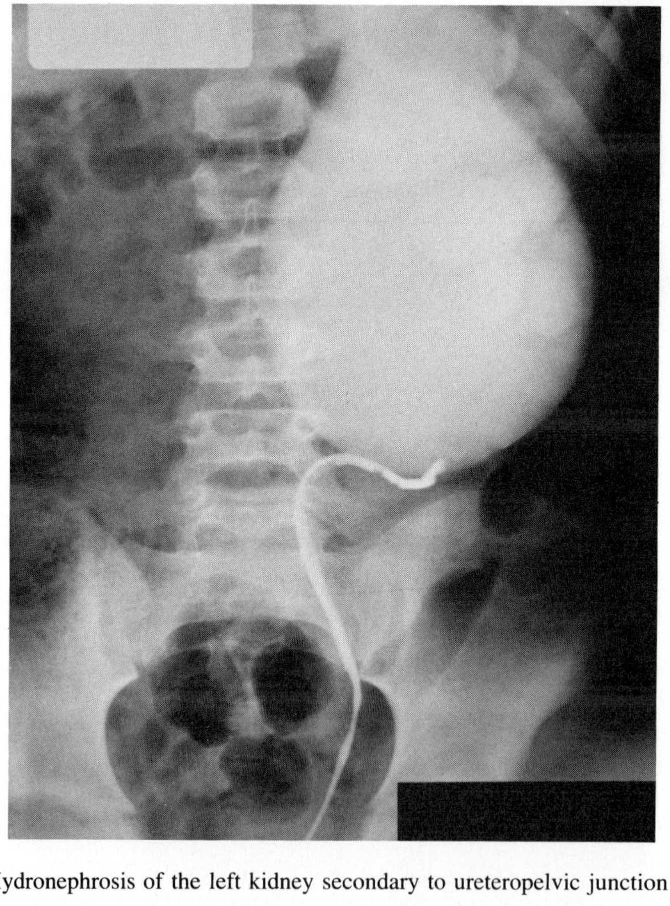

Fig. 34-4. Hydronephrosis of the left kidney secondary to ureteropelvic junction obstruction.

ment of this condition consists of excision of the obstructing segment and reanastamosis of the patent ureter to the renal pelvis. The overall success rate in older children approaches 90%. The surgical task is more complicated in the neonate, but good results are attainable. Not all kidneys with ureteropelvic junction obstruction are salvageable. Whenever possible, however, attempts are made to conserve renal parenchyma even when poor function is present initially. If necessary, secondary nephrectomy can always be performed.

Congenital ureteral obstruction distal to the ureteropelvic junction is seen infrequently but can occur secondary to ureteral valves, obstructive polyps, or retrocaval position of the ureter.

A frequent obstruction seen at the level of the ureterovesical junction is a condition known as *megaureter*. Megaureter, or large ureter, is secondary to obstruction, reflux, or a physiologic consequence known as nonrefluxing and nonobstructing. The term *primary obstructive megaureter* applies when the distal 2 to 3 cm of the ureter is found to be patent and nonstenotic but is not functionally effective in peristalsis. This leads to a functional obstruction and ureteral dilation above this level. A characteristic radiographic appearance results (Fig. 34-5). The treatment for this condition is excision of the dysfunctional ureteral segment with tailoring and reimplantation of the remaining ureter into the bladder. Other conditions causing ureteral enlargement are treated as dictated by the primary disease process.

Ureteroceles are cystic dilations of the distal ureter as they enter the bladder (Fig. 34-6). Ureteroceles vary in size and can obstruct the ipsilateral ureter or, in cases of marked enlarge-

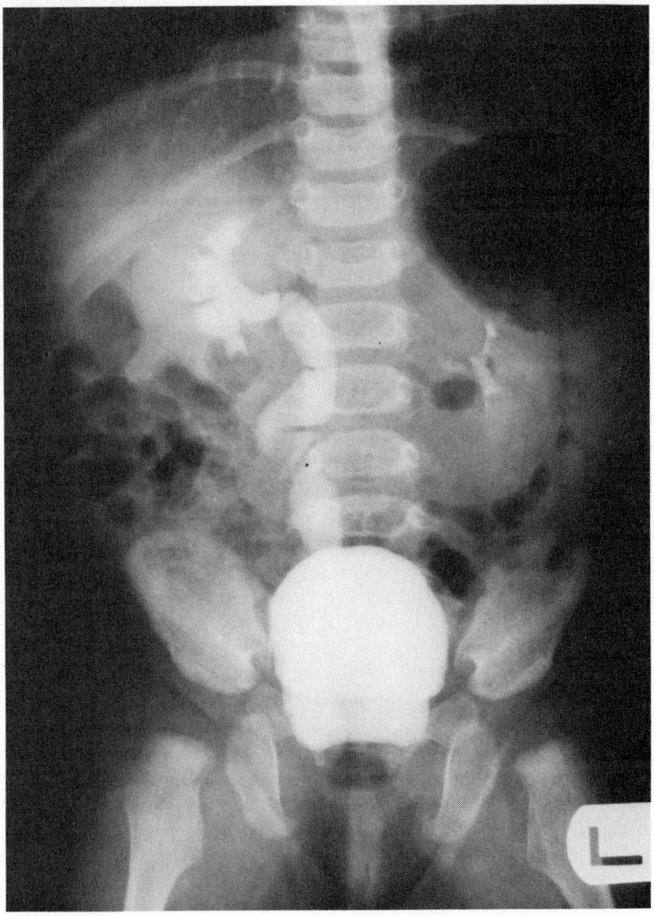

Fig. 34-5. Hydronephrosis secondary to obstructive megaureter (right kidney).

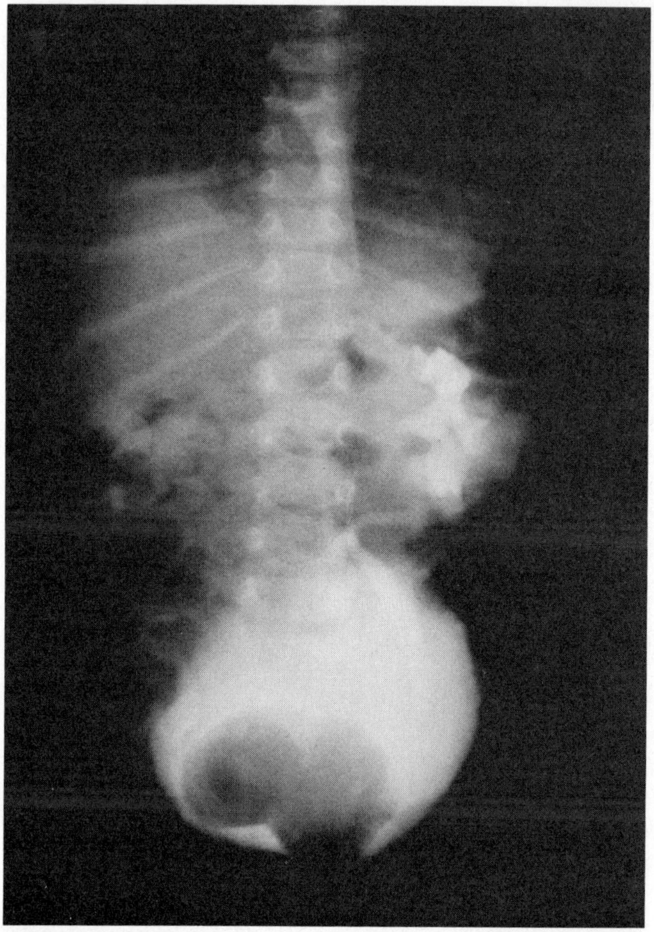

Fig. 34-6. Large filling defect in base of bladder secondary to ureterocele obstructing right kidney.

ment, the contralateral ureter as well.

A ureter can end ectopically outside the normal location of the bladder. When this occurs, it can be associated with urinary incontinence, urinary infection, and obstruction of the ectopic ureter. A ureteral duplication can be associated with either ureterocele or ectopia and usually affects the ureter draining the upper portion of the kidney.

Lower urinary obstruction. Bladder neck obstruction is mentioned only for completeness and occurs rarely, if ever, as a primary process in children. It can occur secondary to neurogenic bladder, posterior urethral valves, or previous surgical procedures on the bladder neck. Treatment should be directed toward the primary process leading to the abnormality at the bladder neck. Müllerian duct cysts are rarely seen but can cause obstruction at the bladder neck.

Posterior urethral valves are probably the best known and most spectacular form of infravesical obstruction in childhood. The classic presentation is in the male infant discovered with sepsis, a urinary tract infection, an abdominal mass, alteration of the urinary stream, or failure to thrive. Obstructive symptomatology, incontinence, and infection are usually the predominant symptoms in older children. The diagnosis is established radiographically by the voiding cystourethrogram (Fig. 34-7). Initial treatment of children with posterior urethral valves may require a period of metabolic normalization and catheter drainage before proceeding with primary transurethral fulguration of the valves. Modern instruments allow fulguration of the valves in even the youngest and

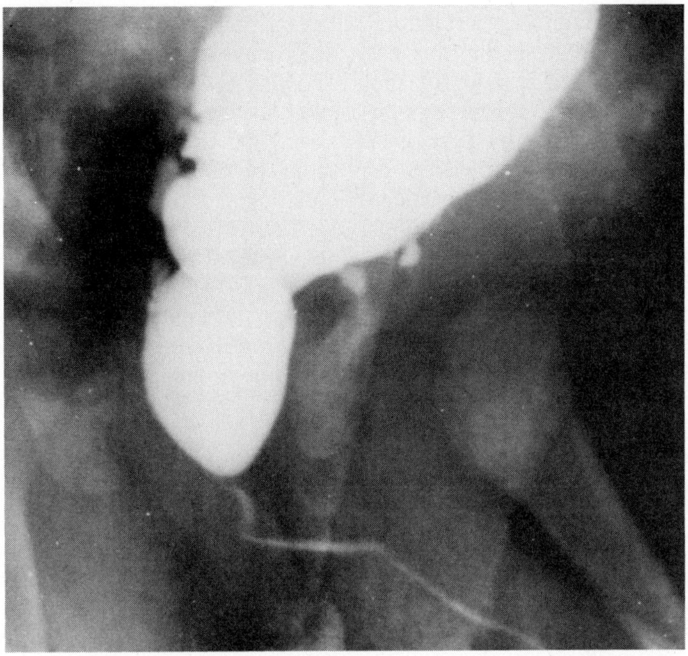

Fig. 34-7. Large dilated posterior urethra secondary to valvular obstruction. Note thin, poorly distended urethra distal to obstruction.

smallest children. Fifty percent of patients with posterior valves will have reflux noted on the initial examination. At least half of these will show spontaneous cessation of the reflux after valve removal. Residual ureteral dilation without reflux after valve fulguration has been a point of discussion in pediatric urologic circles. It was thought at one time that such dilation represented persistent obstruction, but this has been proved not to be true in most cases. Diuretic renography and pressure perfusion studies have proved such ureteral dilation to be nonobstructive and nondamaging to the upper urinary tract. Such ureteral dilation has been noted to improve with time, with improvement being documented by serial measurement of creatinine clearance and renal growth. In children with valves in whom there is ureteral obstruction or persistent reflux, tapering and reimplantation of the dilated ureter is indicated. It should be remembered that a significant degree of renal dysplasia can be present in children with posterior urethral valves at the time of the discovery of their condition. In many cases, this limits their potential for future renal function, and successful surgical management simply provides time before dialysis or renal transplantation will be necessary. Close follow-up of renal function and blood pressure measurements is indicated in all patients with posterior urethral valves.

Anterior urethral valves are encountered infrequently and have basically the same clinical presentation and mode of management as seen in those with posterior urethral valves. The renal consequences of anterior urethral valves are usually less severe.

Urethral strictures in male children are classed as congenital, traumatic, inflammatory, or iatrogenic. These patients usually have obstructive voiding patterns, hematuria, or urinary tract infection. A voiding cystourethrogram gives the characteristic appearance of a narrowed urethral lumen. Dilation of urethral strictures has generally been ineffective in children. Visual urethrotomy with injection of steroids appears to be the most efficient endoscopic method of treating these children. When such an approach is not successful, surgical correction by urethroplasty is necessary.

In the past, distal *urethral stenosis* has been a frequent diagnosis in female children with urinary tract infections or lower urinary tract symptomatology. The exact importance of this entity is still a matter of debate. Children with a clearly obstructive voiding pattern, urinary retention, and urethral voiding complaints such as dysuria undoubtedly benefit from the rupture of the dense urethral fibrous ring that constitutes the narrowing. The diagnosis is made by direct calibration of the urethra, usually performed before cystoscopy. It has been proposed that turbulent flow caused by this distal urethral narrowing leads to the backwash of bacteria from the distal urethra back into the proximal urethra and bladder, thus contributing to recurrent urinary tract infections. Arguments for and against this thesis exist, and as yet the role of the female urethra in recurrent urinary tract infection is not completely clear. Dilation or nonradical internal urethrotomy have not produced harmful effects in the hands of the experienced pediatric urologist and does play a role in the symptomatic relief of a number of children with voiding symptoms and complaints concerning lower tract voiding. It remains unclear whether this procedure will influence the incidence of urinary tract infections.

There is equal controversy regarding the importance of *meatal stenosis* in male children. This is a common finding in the population and is found primarily in circumcised boys. Removal of the foreskin apparently leaves the glans and urethral meatus unprotected, allowing recurrent episodes of meatal inflammation that eventually leads to narrowing of the urethral meatus. In the past, meatal stenosis has been blamed for a number of urinary problems. Little objective evidence has been presented that meatal stenosis, in the absence of urinary tract infections or other abnormalities, poses a serious health threat to the child. Symptoms related specifically to obstruction at the meatus are penile tip pain, a needle-like stream, a stream that is deviated upward, and one that creates irritation with flow. These symptoms form the main reasons for performing meatotomy, which can be done in the older child as either an outpatient or a day surgical patient. Radiographic procedures in these children are performed only in the presence of urinary tract infections or other symptoms.

INCONTINENCE (see also pp. 86-88)

The development of bladder control usually occurs uneventfully in the normal child. Though the act of urinary continence and controlled voiding seems simple, it is, in reality, a complex event involving coordination of multiple neural pathways and muscle groups. In some children, however, the attainment of urinary control at a reasonable age may be delayed. When this occurs, the child should be assessed for possibilities of underlying urinary tract abnormalities leading to this delay in functional development.

Enuresis simply refers to the involuntary loss of urine. Classification of this form of incontinence as to time of day can be important when looking for underlying risk factors. *Diurnal incontinence* refers to daytime wetting during waking hours. *Nocturnal incontinence* or *enuresis* refers to involuntary loss of urine during sleep.

The child with diurnal incontinence past the age of 3 years seems to be at increased risk of having urinary tract anomalies. Neurologic as well as anatomic abnormalities can be the source of incontinence. A continuous incontinence in association with normal voiding intervals can be secondary to an ectopically placed ureter in the female child that drains into the vaginal or periurethral area. Urgency or precipitous incontinence can be seen with the neurogenic bladder, and overflow incontinence is sometimes encountered with obstructive uropathy. Children with recurrent urinary infections and reflux may initially have the problem of persistent or reversion diurnal incontinence. In addition to careful history and physical examination, the child with diurnal incontinence past 3 years of age should be evaluated for structural abnormalities with an intravenous pyelogram and voiding cystourethrogram.

Though the majority of children do attain nighttime continence by the age of 5 years, there is a small percentage with normal anatomy that persist in wetting. A primary enuretic child is a child who has never experienced a dry night and who wets on the average of one night per week beyond 5 years of age. Secondary enuretic children are those who have had a period of dryness but who have reverted to a nocturnal wetting pattern. The child with solely nighttime incontinence or nocturnal enuresis infrequently is found to have underlying structural urinary abnormalities. Theories concerning the etiology of nocturnal enuresis include maturational delay of the nervous system, generalized developmental delay, and sleep disorders. Genetic factors seem to be present in many of these patients, as it is known that a strong family history of enuresis frequently is found on evaluation. Though psychologic stresses can be a cause of wetting problems, it infrequently is found with nocturnal enuretic patients. Evaluation of these children should begin with a history and physical examination and urine culture. Radiographic evaluation is not necessary unless an abnormality is found on examination, a positive urine culture or history of urinary tract infection exists, or diurnal incontinence is present.

Treatment of these types of incontinence differs depending on the etiology. In the child with diurnal incontinence, specific treatment is directed toward correction of a structural abnormality, treatment of a recurrent inflammatory process, or management of a specifically defined functional abnormality. Anticholinergics and bladder sedatives such as propantheline (Probanthine) and oxybutynin are helpful in those children with functional bladder disturbances. The treatment of the nocturnal enuretic child includes the use of tricyclic antidepressants, anticholinergics, and behavioral modification techniques.

Nonneurogenic neurogenic bladder. A special problem known as the *nonneurogenic neurogenic bladder* has been increasingly recognized in children who fail to gain normal urinary and sometimes bowel control. The etiology appears to be the occurrence of an emotional or physical insult to the lower urinary tract during the critical toilet training period. Emotional disturbances in these patients are frequent. In attempts to combat spontaneous bladder contractions, these patients try to maintain continence by increasing the tone of the external urinary sphincter. This becomes exaggerated and a functional form of obstruction develops. In advanced cases, the bladder is found to be severely hypertrophied and has a neurogenic appearance on radiographic studies. Reflux and hydronephrosis may be present, and urinary tract infections develop in many of these children. Treatment is directed toward the control of infections and retraining the child to develop proper detrusor sphincter coordination. Anticholinergics and biofeedback training have been helpful in the latter.

NEUROGENIC BLADDER

Congenital anomalies of the spinal cord are the most common causes of neurogenic bladder in children. Myelomeningocele, spinal dysraphism, and sacral agenesis are the most common of these abnormalities. Other diseases include brain and spinal cord tumors, vascular anomalies of the nervous system, and generalized neuropathies such as multiple sclerosis. Trauma to the brain and the spinal cord can also cause permanent neurologic deficits that can affect the bladder.

The physiology of micturition is a complex sequence of events involving all levels of the nervous system. Any disease process at any level can have potentially serious effects on bladder function. Urinary tract changes secondary to the neurogenic bladder are common in children with these disorders. The problems associated with neurogenic bladder dysfunction include incontinence, recurrent urinary tract infections, urinary stones, hydronephrosis, and vesicoureteral reflux.

The neurogenic bladder can be classified in a number of ways. The most useful classifications take into account the etiology of the neurogenic bladder and the functional capacities of the bladder and the urinary sphincter mechanism. Improved urodynamic testing techniques have made it easier to evaluate the pediatric patient and, in many patients, is invaluable in planning the long-term management of the child with neurogenic vesical dysfunction. Such management has improved in recent years as the result of an improved understanding of the neurologic processes involved in bladder control and the advent of clean intermittent catheterization.

Myelomeningocele. Myelomeningocele and related spinal cord abnormalities account for the majority of children with neurogenic bladder. This spinal abnormality is manifested by failure of fusion between arches of the vertebrae and associated dysplasia of the spinal cord or its membranes. This is a common abnormality, occurring in 2 in 1,000 live births in the United States. The lumbosacral spine is involved in the majority of cases, with less frequent involvement of the thoracic and cervical spine. Aggressive neurosurgical treatment has led to a higher percentage of children surviving this congenital defect. Since less than 10% of children with myelomeningocele survive past infancy without a neurogenic disability, the majority of these children probably will have some problems with neurogenic bladder dysfunction.

Early assessment of the urinary tract is mandatory in these children. A baseline intravenous pyelogram and voiding cystourethrogram are important in determining the status of the kidneys, the ability of the bladder to empty, the presence of vesicoureteral reflux, and defining, if possible, the relationship of sphincter activity to attempts at bladder emptying. Because rapid changes in the status of the urinary tract can occur during infancy, these studies should be repeated every 6 months until the child is 2 years of age. If the urinary tract appears stable at that time, repeat studies can be made on a yearly basis.

Frequent urinalysis and culture are important in these children, because they are at an increased risk for urinary tract infections. Seventy-five percent of such patients will have a urinary tract infection by 4 years of age. Nearly 25% of these patients will exhibit vesicoureteral reflux, and 30% will develop an abnormal intravenous pyelogram. The changes in the collecting system and kidneys are secondary to bladder problems associated with incomplete emptying and the high pressures generated by uninhibited bladder contractions (Fig. 34-8).

Urodynamic evaluation of these children can be helpful in assessing the functional nature of the bladder and sphincter. This includes cystometry and sphincter electromyography. Since stabilization of the bladder may not occur until 18 to 24 months of life, such urodynamic studies are postponed until that time. It is important to define the functional capacity of the bladder, the ability of the bladder to empty, and the ability of the urinary sphincter to function in coordination with attempts at bladder emptying. It should be noted that the child with a very low myelomeningocele and good lower extremity function can be the one with the more severe problems of bladder and sphincter dyscoordination. If the infant empties well without high

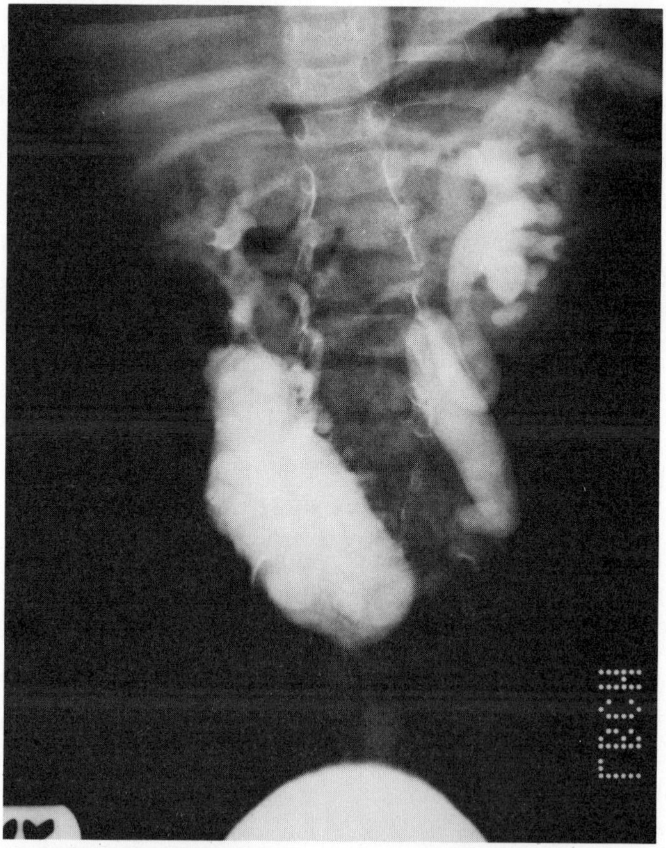

Fig. 34-8. Neurogenic bladder with associated hydronephrosis.

residuals, a combination of spontaneous voiding and Credé maneuver can be successful as bladder management. For the infant bladder that does not empty well, particularly with the presence of reflux or hydronephrosis, a temporary vesicostomy closure can be beneficial in lowering emptying pressures of the bladder and allowing decompression of the urinary tract. Later vesicostomy closure and development of alternative bladder management can be carried out.

Whereas the goals of bladder management in the younger child are to protect renal function, in the older child the additional challenge becomes how to gain social acceptance without urinary incontinence. Attainment of continence depends on the type of neurogenic bladder involved. Successful management is frequently achieved through the use of clean intermittent catheterization, or a combination of medication and intermittent catheterization. The success of managing such patients with intermittent catheterization is emphasized by the decrease in permanent urinary diversion and its accompanying upper tract damage in children with myelodysplasia. In those in whom continence cannot be achieved, the development of the artificial urinary sphincter provides a viable alternative to urinary diversion.

URINARY DIVERSION

Over the past several years, fewer indications have been found for permanent urinary diversion in children. Recent advances in reconstructive surgery, the use of clean intermittent catheterization, and the development of the artificial urinary sphincter have led to improved primary treatment of many diseases previously treated by diversion. Long-term problems with urinary diversion have been the deterioration of the upper urinary tract, recurrent urinary tract infections, urinary stones, stomal management, and psychologic distress. Because these problems were noted with increasing frequency in the long-term follow-up of these children, alternatives to diversion were developed.

When permanent urinary diversion is unavoidable, the nonrefluxing colon conduit has recently been used successfully and offers some advantages over the ileal conduit. Colon conduits provide fewer stomal complications, and at the time of surgery an antireflux anastamosis can be made between the ureter and the colon segment. Such an anastamosis seems to prevent ongoing damage to the upper tracts secondary to infection. Permanent urinary diversion may still be required in severely affected children with myelodysplasia and an unmanageable neurogenic bladder. Also, the child with exstrophy, in which the bladder is unusable as a urine reservoir, will require permanent urinary diversion.

Temporary diversion. Temporary urinary diversion continues to be a viable alternative in managing the child with poor emptying of the urinary tract. These temporary measures are usually instituted in infancy or when the child is severely ill and needs immediate drainage of the urinary tract to assist with treatment and stabilization. Types of temporary diversion include cutaneous ureterostomy, cutaneous pyelostomy, and vesicostomy. Intubated temporary diversions such as nephrostomy tubes and suprapubic catheters have a high rate of morbidity and are rarely used for extended periods.

Indications for temporary diversions include a poorly emptying urinary tract such as with posterior urethral valves, severe prune belly syndrome, and a neurogenic bladder with poor emptying and high pressures associated with reflux or hydronephrosis. The nonintubated temporary measures of diversion allow the urinary tract to drain under low pressures. Though the incidence of urinary tract infection remains low in these patients, they may require prophylactic antibiotics during the period of diversion. Such temporary measures allow for growth and development of renal tissue, and when the child is stable and can tolerate more extensive surgery definitive procedures with undiversion can be completed.

Urinary undiversion. Because of improvements in the management of neurogenic bladder and obstructive uropathy and the development of the artificial urinary sphincter, many patients that have previously undergone urinary diversion are now likely candidates for urinary undiversion. Before undiversion, these children go through extensive evaluation of the upper and lower urinary system, particularly sphincter and bladder function. Even the child with a nonfunctional bladder secondary to urinary diversion can be a good candidate for undiversion. Depending on the status of the bladder, the ability to manage original pathology, and the level of renal function, several techniques are available for regaining continuity of the urinary tract. These range from simple reanastamosis of the ureters to using bowel seqments to regain continuity and augment the bladder capacity. Fortunately, as indications for urinary diversion become fewer, the candidates for undiversion will be seen less frequently.

GENITAL ABNORMALITIES IN THE MALE

Abnormalities of the penis

Development of the indifferent gonad into a testis results in the secretion of testosterone. This hormone stimulates wolffian duct development and the formation of male external genitalia. It is thought that inadequate testosterone stimulation is responsible for virtually all forms of incomplete penile and urethral development in the male.

Hypospadias. *Hypospadias* refers to the abnormal placement of the urethral meatus on the ventral surface of the penis proximal to the tip of the glans. It is a common anomaly, occurring in approximately 1 in 250 live male births. Eighty-five percent of these cases are of mild severity, with the meatus at a glandular or coronal location. Fifteen percent represent the more severe types of hypospadias (Table 34-1). Nonelastic fibrous tissue representing the underdeveloped corpus spongiosum produces ventral curvature (chordee) of the penis, which is particularly exaggerated on erection. The foreskin fails to close ventrally, leaving a dorsal hood of skin over the glans (Fig. 34-9). The description of hypospadias as to severity should be an anatomic one and is best not expressed in degrees. Hypospadias is transmitted as a multifactorial mode of inheritance, and it has been estimated that up to a 14% chance exists for a male sibling of a hypospadiac boy to likewise exhibit the abnormality.

Initial evaluation of a child with hypospadias should include a careful search for palpable gonads. Genetic evaluation is reserved for those children whose genitalia appear truly ambigu-

Table 34-1. Site of the meatus in hypospadias

Location of hypospadias	Percentage (%)
Glandular or coronal position	85
Penile shaft position	10
Penoscrotal or perineal position	5

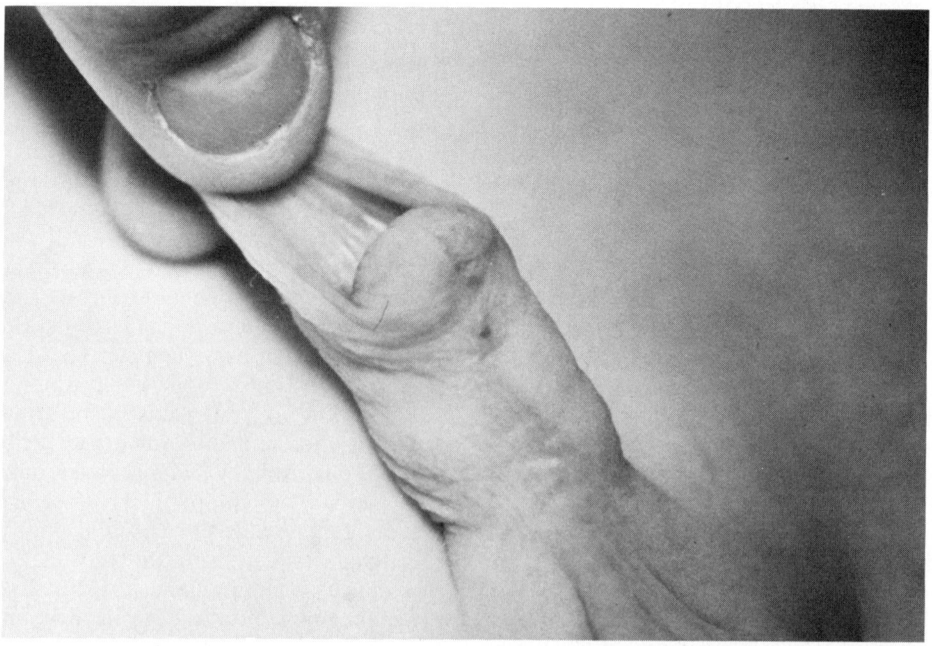

Fig. 34-9. Hypospadias. Notice dorsal hooded foreskin and proximally placed ventral meatus.

ous. Urographic evaluation is still a matter of controversy, although several reports have shown an increased incidence of reflux and other urinary anomalies likewise believed to follow a multifactorial form of inheritance. It is known that the urinary system and the genital system develop at different times embryologically, but common genetic factors could exist, and at this time we believe it is safer to screen these children with an excretory urogram and voiding cystourethrogram to uncover any associated abnormalities.

In the neonatal period, establishment of a clear diagnosis with simple observation, and avoidance of circumcision, is all that is required. Early consultation by a urologist experienced with genital reconstruction in children is desirable to counsel the family, to explain to them what the future holds for surgical reconstruction, and to allay any fears, anxieties, or guilt. The age for surgical correction, in part, depends on the severity of the defect. The more simple procedures for the less severe forms of hypospadias are done at an earlier age, approximately 12 to 18 months. The more severe or complex type of defects are usually repaired when the child is approximately 3 years of age, when he is more emotionally stable and able to cooperate.

The most important goal of surgery is to ensure correction of any chordee to produce a straight phallus, which allows for sexual intercourse. Creation of a neourethra at or near the tip of the glans penis is important to allow the child to stand to void and direct the urinary steam and subsequently to allow deposition of semen at a vaginal depth sufficient for insemination and fertilization. Achieving a pleasing cosmetic appearance is important, but ensuring adequate function is essential.

Surgical correction of hypospadias is accomplished by single or multistaged procedures. One-stage procedures have been used traditionally in the less severe forms of hypospadias, with multistaged repairs being used for the more severe defects. As techniques have improved and as surgeons become available to deal consistently with this problem, one-stage repairs have developed and produce success with even the more severe forms of hypospadias. Familiarity with the new techniques and the intraoperative use of the artificial erection and artificial urinary stream have produced excellent surgical results with one-stage repairs. Complications of surgery include persistence of chordee, urethrocutaneous fistula, and urethral or meatal stricture. The correction of each is possible with secondary surgical procedures and is usually less involved than the primary operation.

Chordee without hypospadias has become increasingly recognized. It is typified by a normally placed urethral meatus but with a dorsal hood of foreskin representing incomplete ventral fusion and abnormal skin or spongiosum development. Penile torsion without hypospadias likewise occurs, leading to an abnormal appearance of the penis and foreskin. Circumcision in these patients should be avoided until the need for surgical correction is determined.

Epispadias. Epispadias is incomplete fusion of the urethral plate on the superior surface of the penis, leaving the penis splayed dorsally and the foreskin in a ventral position (Fig. 34-10). This anomaly is much rarer than hypospadias and is classically seen in children with exstrophy of the bladder. Epispadias can occur as an isolated anomaly or can be associated with bladder neck malformation and urinary incontinence, requiring surgical procedures directed at the internal defects in addition to genital reconstruction. The repair and management of epispadias technically parallels that of hypospadias.

Microphallus. Microphallus is an abnormally small penis, which has been arbitrarily defined as one that measures less than 1 cm in stretched penile length. The resultant failure to develop normally is caused by either failure of stimulation by testosterone or failure of the tissues to respond to such testosterone stimulation. Gender reassignment in infants is based on the presence or absence of corporal bodies and whether or not the child responds to parenteral testosterone or gonadotropin administration. If it can be demonstrated that the child will be unable to function as a male at maturity, then the gender role should be assigned as female. The concealed penis should be distinguished from microphallus in that the former represents a normal size penis with normal corporal bodies simply hidden by foreskin and usually a prominent prepubic fat pad.

Foreskin. The foreskin at birth is normally not retractable. Foreskin adhesions to the glans penis loosen as the child gets older. Unless there has been difficulty with balanoposthitis or main-

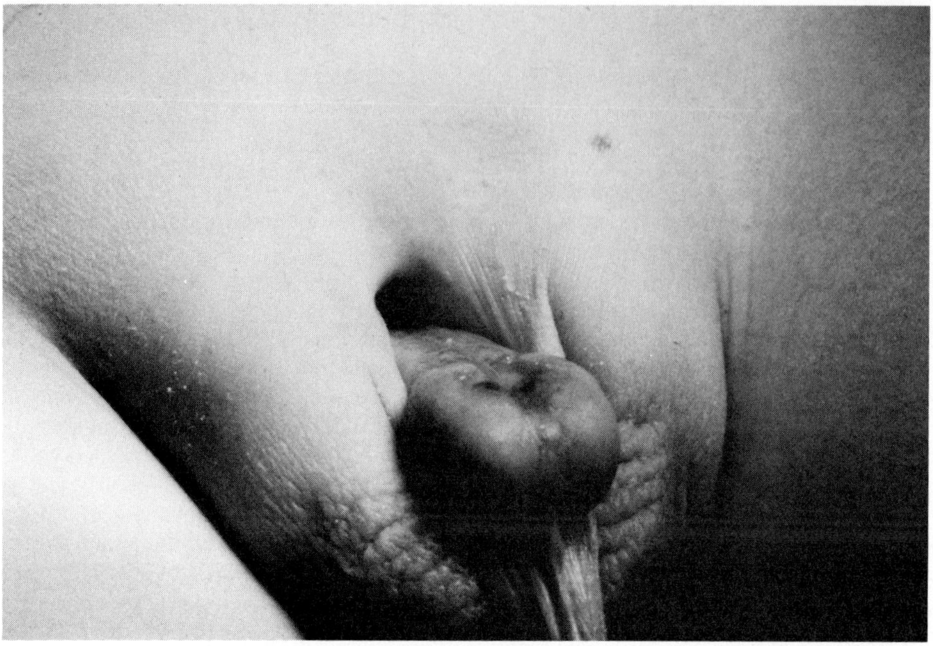

Fig. 34-10. Epispadias. Note penis splayed dorsally with ventral foreskin.

taining proper hygiene, the foreskin does not need to be routinely retracted in the infant. Phimosis is the inability to retract the foreskin beyond the glans penis secondary to circumferential scarring. Paraphimosis occurs when the foreskin has been retracted but then forms a circumferential ring proximal to the glans penis with resultant swelling and edema of the distal penis and glans. Initial management of paraphimosis is reduction of the swelling by manual pressure and replacement of the foreskin over the glans. Both conditions are clear indications for circumcision.

Circumcision. Circumcision began as a religious or social custom rather than as secondary to perceived medical needs. Modern day indications for circumcision have included the need for improved hygiene, the prevention of carcinogenesis of the penis, and treatment for phimosis and paraphimosis. In addition, circumcision is also performed for personal, cosmetic, or religious reasons. The subject of circumcision is currently one of debate and appears to lack a clear conclusion. If performed on a routine basis or for personal desires, circumcision is probably best done in the neonatal period. In older children, circumcision should be withheld except for specific medical indications.

Complications of circumcision include infection, skin adherence to the glans that can actually conceal the penis, skin bands from the penile shaft to the glans, and, rarely, urethrocutaneous fistula. Although complications of circumcision are often cited by opponents of the procedure, it must be stated that more time is spent in the operating room handling problems for noncircumcision than for handling complications of circumcision. Early unpublished observations indicate that the rate of urinary tract infections in male children is increasing as the incidence of circumcision has fallen. This issue is obviously not decided, and all factors must be kept in mind when discussing this procedure with the infant's parents.

Priapism. Priapism is persistent penile erection occurring without sexual stimulation. In children this is associated primarily with leukemia, sickle cell disease, or trauma. Priapism secondary to sickling is treated initially in a conservative fashion using analgesics and transfusion therapy. If such therapy is unsuccessful within 24 to 36 hours of its institution, surgical therapy is indicated. Surgery is performed by creating a shunt between the glans penis and the corpora cavernosa, allowing expulsion of the sludge and sickled blood cells and establishing an avenue of venous egress from the corpora cavernosa to the corpus spongiosum, which is not involved with the normal erection process. The treatment of priapism secondary to leukemia or trauma is directed at the primary disease process.

Abnormalities of the testes and scrotal contents

Cryptorchidism. Testicles form intra-abdominally in the fetus, and, in the process of differential growth and under stimuli that are incompletely understood, the testicle normally descends to its position in the scrotum. *Cryptorchidism* is the term applied to the condition in which a testicle fails to descend to a normal scrotal position. Up to 5% of male neonates will exhibit undescended testicles, but the vast majority of such testicles descend into the scrotum during the first year of life. If the testicle cannot be manipulated into the scrotum during careful examination after 1 year of life, cryptorchidism is present. The retractile testis caused by an overactive cremasteric reflex is common in children and does not represent a true abnormality. In the majority of cases of cryptorchidism, the testicle is found in the inguinal canal and is usually palpable. However, the testicle can be found anywhere along the path of normal descent (Table 34-2). Ectopic testicles are generally found in the inguinal area but are also seen at the base of the penis, the perineum, and in the thigh. The cause of cryptorchidism is probably hormonal and reflects either an intrinsic testosterone production defect of the testicle or an abnormality interfering with testicular stimulation, such as the hypothalamic-pituitary-gonadal axis.

Problems associated with maldescent are primarily those of infertility and the development of testicular malignancy. Testicular germ cells are heat sensitive and, when subjected to even a 1° C rise in temperature, as in the inguinal canal, changes rapidly occur within these reproductive cellular elements. Microscopic changes are observed in the undescended testicle as early as 2 years of age; thus it is thought that surgical therapy should be performed before the child is 2 years old if it is to be successful in increasing chances of fertility. It must be remembered that fertility is compromised in both the unilateral as well as the bilateral undescended testicle and that this could be secondary to a broader effect of hormonal understimulation such as a leuteinizing hormone (LH) deficiency.

Table 34-2. Location incidence of cryptorchidism

Location of testicle	Percentage (%)
High scrotal position	45
Inguinal canal position	45
Intra-abdominal position	10

Testicular malignancy is said to occur up to 20 to 40 times more often in the patient with an undescended testicle than in the normal population. Surgical placement of the testicle into the scrotum does not protect the individual from later development of a tumor. The primary purpose of orchiopexy is to place the testicle where palpation and examination allow early detection of any tumors that may develop and thus allow institution of appropriate therapy. It has been noted that no child who has undergone orchiopexy under 4 years of age has yet been reported to develop a testicular malignancy. This, once again, indicates that early treatment may be beneficial.

Radiographic studies of the urinary system in a child with cryptorchidism are not needed unless separate indications exist. It has been thought that in a child with impalpable testes and demonstrated renal agenesis no exploration for the testicle would be necessary. This has subsequently been found to be untrue, and in such an individual surgical exploration to determine the location of the testicle is indicated. It is important in each individual with a nonpalpable testis that the status and location of that testicle be determined.

Surgical treatment of cryptorchidism is necessary in those patients whose testicles have not descended by 1 year of age. This treatment should not be delayed and should be undertaken at any time within the second year of life. The testicle can be found anywhere along the line of descent, including intra-abdominal locations. It is most commonly found in the inguinal canal. Surgical treatment consists of locating the testicle, freeing the vas deferens and spermatic vessels from surrounding attachments, and lengthening the cord structures to allow manual placement of the testicle into the scrotum. If the testicle is found to be dysgenetic, this tissue must be removed because of the high malignancy potential. It is possible for the testicle, the vas, and the epididymis to exist separately. To truthfully say that testicular agenesis exists, both vas and spermatic vessels must be located serving a fibrous area. In general, hormonal therapy with human chorionic gonadotropin to stimulate descent has produced unsatisfactory results. An interesting new therapeutic approach in which LH releasing factor is administered by nasal spray followed by human chorionic gonadotropin stimulation has produced some early success, but the practical application of hormonal treatment remains to be clarified.

A phenotypic male with impalpable gonads, especially with any degree of hypospadias, requires at least a buccal smear to rule out congenital adrenal hyperplasia, which could be a life-threatening condition. Anorchia, although it does occur, is rare and can be diagnosed by human chorionic gonadotropin stimulation testing to determine the need for surgical exploration.

Testicular torsion. Torsion of the spermatic cord deprives the testicle of its blood supply and can lead to testicular necrosis within 6 to 8 hours of onset. Torsion in the neonatal period primarily occurs in the perinatal period with the occurrence of twisting of the entire scrotal contents and subsequent spermatic cord obstruction high in the canal. In utero torsion does occur, and if unrecognized is probably the most common cause of the atrophic testis noted later in life. Torsion in the neonate usually presents in the healthy male with an enlarged, discolored, firm hemiscrotum that is not tender. Early surgical intervention in the neonate infrequently allows salvage of the twisted testis. There is some evidence that the contralateral testicle can be preserved by prophylactic surgical fixation. In the older pubertal or prepubertal male, testicular torsion usually occurs as an acute painful scrotal swelling sometimes accompanied by abdominal pain and often with its onset at night when the child is at rest. The testis is sensitive, elevated, and swollen. This type of torsion differs from that of the neonate in that the cord is twisted inside the tunica vaginalis. Physical examination reveals a tense, tender testicle riding high in the scrotum. Elevation of the testicle can increase pain in the child with torsion. If the epididymis can be palpated, it is noted in an abnormal position rather than the normal posterolateral position.

The differential diagnosis of torsion of the spermatic cord includes torsion of the appendix testis or appendix epididymis, epididymitis, testicular tumor, orchitis, or trauma. Torsion of the appendix testis or epididymis can be diagnosed early by identifying a very localized tender swelling in the area of the head of the epididymis or upper pole of the testicle with the remainder of the testicle and epididymis being normal. Epididymitis produces a swollen, tender, enlarged epididymis usually associated with dysuria and abnormal urinalysis. Trauma can be determined by history. A tumor can cause pain because of hemorrhage into the substance of the tumor.

The diagnosis of torsion of the spermatic cord can be made by physical examination in many cases. The use of the Doppler stethoscope to determine the absence of testicular blood flow can be of some help in equivocal cases, but testicular and scrotal scanning appears to be more accurate. Scrotal scans appear to be primarily beneficial in confirming that a diagnosis other than testicular torsion exists. If a diagnosis cannot be clearly established, scrotal exploration is mandatory. At surgery, detorsion of the testicle with preservation of that organ is the primary goal of therapy if necrosis has not begun. In the majority of cases, the testicle has already perished and fixation of the contralateral testicle is the important part of the procedure. There is a high incidence of torsion occurring in the contralateral testicle, so fixation of that testicle is mandatory to preserve future reproductive and hormonal function.

Idiopathic scrotal edema is diagnosed primarily by the presentation of a swollen scrotal wall, but a palpably normal nontender testicle is noted within the scrotal compartment. Henoch-Schönlein purpura can include testicular and scrotal involvement with petechiae and some scrotal swelling but has the physical findings of a normal intrascrotal testicle, which may on occasion be tender. Testicular scans can be particularly helpful in confirming the diagnosis in these two instances.

Hydrocele hernia. A hydrocele is a collection of fluid around the testicle. A hydrocele can be considered a potential hernia in a child since it usually arises because the processus vaginalis connecting the peritoneal and scrotal cavities is patent. It is this patency that allows fluid to enter and collect around the testicle, leading to variable degrees of scrotal swelling. Hydroceles are fairly common at birth and may take up to a year to resolve totally. Hydroceles can be followed without surgery in the first year of life if there is no evidence on physical examination of inguinal swelling and hernia, or rapid change in size suggesting a widely patent processus vaginalis.

If the hydrocele fails to resolve in the newborn, or if there is evidence of herniation, surgical exploration with ligation of the patent processus and repair of the hernia is undertaken. Contralateral inguinal exploration is indicated in the younger patient because of the high statistical likelihood of an asymptomatic patent processus.

An incarcerated hernia presents as a sudden swelling in the inguinal or scrotal area and requires immediate manual reduction of intestinal contents and surgical attention within 24 to 48 hours after diagnosis. If indeed the hernia cannot be reduced, or if there are symptoms of strangulation of the bowel, immediate surgical intervention is indicated.

EXSTROPHY, CLOACAL EXSTROPHY, AND IMPERFORATE ANUS

Epispadias and exstrophy. Epispadias and exstrophy is a developmental anomaly caused by persistence of the cloacal membrane that prevents mesodermal invasion ventrally over the region of the bladder and lower abdominal wall. The abnormality includes failure of closure of the symphysis pubis, which produces an abdominal wall defect and leaves the bladder open onto the lower abdomen (Fig. 34-11). Urine is freely discharged from the ureters onto the surface of the body. The penis is epispadic. The bladder muscle in many of these cases is abnormal, with fibrosis and poor muscle orientation. The bladder mucosa develops histologic changes very early and has a potential to develop adenocarcinoma in later life. The sphincteric and pelvic muscles are abnormal and are not in a closed position. Very few renal anomalies are noted initially in association with exstrophy, but hydronephrosis will develop in a certain percentage of patients, thought to be caused by infection and fibrosis occurring at the exposed ureterovesical junction. Associated anomalies in

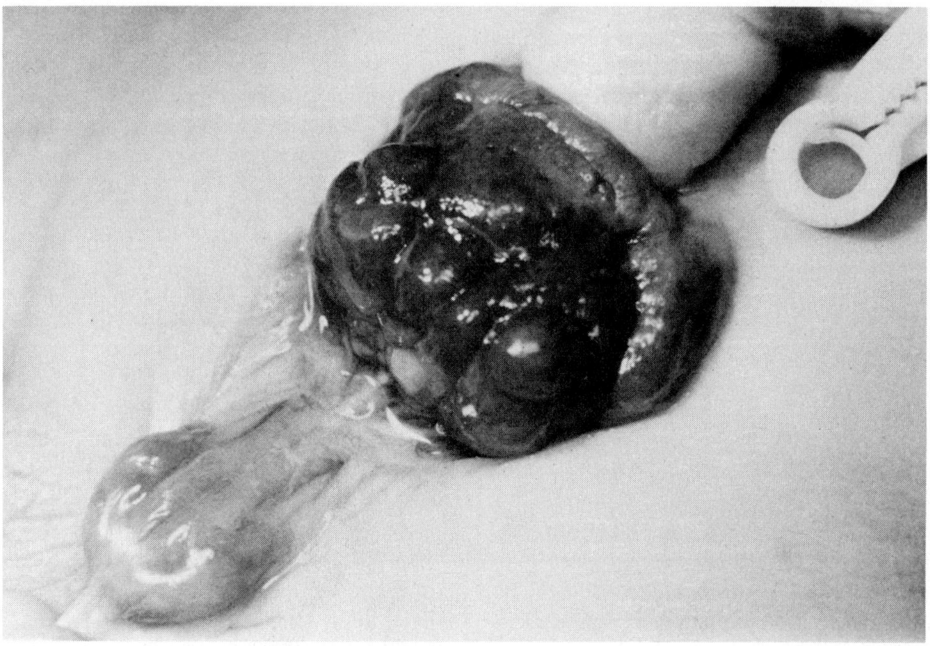

Fig. 34-11. Exstrophy of the bladder in the neonate. Note complete epispadias below and umbilicus superiorly.

addition to epispadias include the bifid clitoris in the female and an anus located more ventrally and anteriorally with a tendency for rectal prolapse. In the female, the vagina is also located more anteriorly and has a tendency to show stenosis.

Management of the child with epispadias and exstrophy complex is one of the greatest technical challenges in pediatric urology. The tendency toward development of hydronephrosis and carcinoma in the abnormal bladder does not allow the option of avoiding treatment altogether. Optimal treatment is functional closure. This is a complex, multistaged operation beginning first with closure of the bladder and usually requires iliac osteotomies for pelvic relaxation. This is best performed in a neonate or in a young infant. As a second procedure, a bladder neck and continence mechanism must be reconstructed with accompanying ureteral reimplantation. Genital reconstruction for epispadias is accomplished by additional procedures. Undescended testicles and hernias are common in the male, and hernias are sometimes seen in female patients. These, likewise, require treatment as part of the multistaged procedure.

In general, a child with greater than 5 ml established bladder capacity is a candidate for attempted closure of the exstrophy. Functional closure that produces urinary continence, preserves renal function, and leads to adequate sexual ability is usually attained in 60% of patients. Those in whom attempts at closure have failed, or who are not suitable candidates for closure, undergo urinary diversion with excision of the exstrophied bladder, repair of the abdominal wall, and reconstruction of the genitalia.

Cloacal exstrophy. Cloacal exstrophy is an even more complex set of anomalies that includes failure of the hind gut to form properly. The exstrophied mass is marked by a central bowel segment representing the cecum flanked by hemibladders with a bifid phallus or clitoris. These children represent an extreme surgical challenge if they survive. They usually have many other anomalies, many of which are incompatible with life. Bowel as well as urinary management is usually only accomplished by various forms of diversion. Female gender assignment is required because of lack of ability to construct acceptable male external genitalia.

Imperforate anus. Imperforate anus is an anomaly with a high association of genitourinary abnormalities. The initial management is directed at the bowel. The pediatric urologist is involved in these patients in management of the commonly associated genitourinary abnormalities that are primarily those of reflux, neurogenic bladder, some form of obstructive uropathy, or genital abnormality.

GENITAL ABNORMALITIES IN THE FEMALE

Abnormalities affecting the female genitalia are frequently encountered by pediatric urologists. Many conditions can be confused as being primarily urologic in nature and others may be associated with urologic abnormalities. Such genital abnormalities can also involve the urinary tract, which deserves consideration during the treatment of the primary condition.

Failure of fusion or abnormal formation involving the müllerian ducts can lead to many congenital vaginal abnormalities. Vaginal agenesis, vaginal duplication, transverse vaginal septum, and imperforate hymen are conditions that can be encountered. Vaginal agenesis can be associated with uterine malformations and is frequently associated with renal abnormalities, particularly a solitary pelvic kidney. Imperforate hymen and transverse vaginal septum can lead to obstruction of vaginal drainage and thus a collection of mucoid secretions that can become quite large and present as an abdominal mass with urinary obstruction. Most lesions are discovered as perineal abnormalities during infancy, although some are discovered in older children during menarche. Treatment of these conditions is surgical and ranges from simple incision and drainage for an imperforate hymen to complex vaginal reconstruction for vaginal agenesis. Associated urinary anomalies are managed in conjunction with the primary abnormality.

Hydrocolpos presenting as an abdominal mass is usually associated with urogenital sinus anomalies in female children. These children have a single perineal opening as opposed to separate urethral and vaginal openings. The urethral and vaginal confluence ends in a common distal sinus. In many cases, the vaginal portion is obstructed. The large size of the vagina and uterus is secondary to the build-up of vaginal and cervical secretions in the obstructed proximal vagina. A cystogram will show a bladder displaced anteriorly and a rectum displaced posteriorly, and on excretory urogram many patients will show hydronephrosis secondary to extrinsic obstruction by the enlarged vaginal and uterine cavities. Genitograms and endoscopy may be necessary for a precise anatomic definition. Prompt surgical treatment is necessary to produce vaginal decompression and establish appropriate vaginal position in the perineum to afford drainage.

Cloacal anomalies consist of those in which urethra, vagina, and rectum all drain through a distal common channel. Surgical treatment is complex and can involve urinary decompression in addition to vaginal reconstruction and management of bowel obstruction.

Introital or vaginal masses in the newborn or in infancy can be the first sign of genital abnormalities. Differential diagnosis of such a condition includes imperforate hymen with hydrocolpos, periurethral cyst, urethral prolapse, or a prolapsing ureterocele. Malignancy can occur in these children, but it is rare.

A periurethral cyst is usually noted at birth and can be quite large. The mass effect is usually greatest near the urethral meatus and may distort the position of the meatus. Aspiration, simple excision, or unroofing of the cyst is the treatment of choice. Simple observation of the smaller cysts is adequate.

A prolapsing ureterocele presenting at the introitus is almost always associated with an obstructed upper pole segment of a kidney with a duplicated collecting system. In addition to the prolapse of the ureterocele, the obstructed portion of the collecting system may be palpable as a flank mass. The ureterocele may originate from a vaginal ectopic location or can prolapse from the bladder through the urethra. An excretory urogram confirms the diagnosis of a nonfunctioning upper pole segment of a duplicated collecting system, and a voiding cystogram will usually delineate the presence of the ureterocele as a filling defect in the bladder. A vaginogram can be helpful in outlining vaginal defects. Treatment involves excision of the hydronephrotic ureter and upper pole kidney segment with subsequent decompression of the ureterocele. Occasionally enough function exists in the upper segment to warrant salvage by means of ureterocele excision and ureteral reimplantation.

Urethral prolapse usually presents as a vaginal mass (Fig. 34-12). In most cases, it is associated with necrosis of the prolapsed urethral mucosa and is the most common cause of "vaginal" bleeding seen in female children. It is more common in black female children. This must be differentiated from rhabdomyosarcoma of the vagina. Endoscopic evaluation of bladder and vagina to exclude presence of a malignancy can be performed at time of excision of the prolapsed urethral mucosa.

The neonate with apparent female genitalia but a prominent clitoris needs to be evaluated carefully for the presence of the adrenogenital syndrome or other causes of ambiguous genitalia. Diagnostic studies are discussed in the section on intersexuality. Management of the child with ambiguous genitalia is a multidisciplinary problem involving the urologist, the geneticist, and the endocrinologist.

Exstrophy of the bladder in girls is associated with abnormalities of the genitalia. Even following successful closure of the exstrophy, the vagina will usually be located more anteriorly and will lack the usual support of the urogenital diaphragm. Occasionally exstrophy will be associated with duplication or other vaginal abnormalities. Much of the reconstruction of the genitalia of these children is coordinated with closure and surgical treatment of the urinary tract abnormality.

Nonspecific vulvovaginitis is the most common abnormality seen in younger girls. The epithelial lining of this area is delicate and easily injured because of the lack of estrogen stimulation. Inflammation can be a frequent occurrence, leading to erythema and a thin vaginal discharge. Specific bacterial infections can be documented by culture. Physical examination can rule out trauma or the presence of vaginal foreign bodies. Treatment of nonspecific vulvovaginitis is by means of sitz baths and antibiotics, antibacterials, and steroid creams.

Labial adhesions can occur as a result of recurrent vulvovaginitis. Treatment is best instituted using short-course (1 to 2 weeks) estrogen cream therapy. Manual or surgical lysis is usually best reserved for those children who are not responsive to medical treatment.

Specific infections such as gonococcal vulvovaginitis should be documented by culture and treated accordingly. Condyloma accuminata

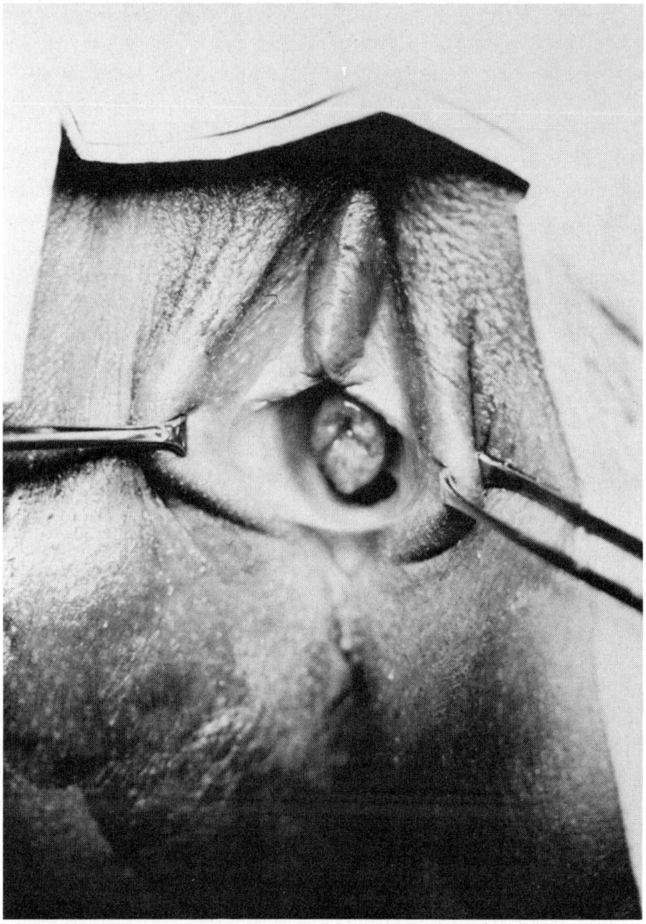

Fig. 34-12. Urethral prolapse.

are caused by a virus, preferring moist areas such as the labia and introitus. The mode of transmission in children is not known but is not always venereal. When the disease is encountered, careful examination for child abuse is mandatory. Surgical therapy for condylomata is usually curative.

INTERSEXUALITY (see also pp. 629-636)

Evaluation of the infant with ambiguous genitalia is one of the greatest challenges in pediatric urology. It requires accurate application of both practical and theoretic knowledge. Any decision as to the sex assignment should be made by a team that should include the pediatric urologist, the pediatric endocrinologist, and the geneticist.

Sexual development occurs in essentially three stages. The first stage is the differentiation of the gonad, which is directed by the chromosomal composition of the individual. Gonadal development occurs at 6 weeks gestation and differentiation is primarily dependent on the presence of a Y chromosome. The second stage is that of the development of the internal ductal systems. In the undifferentiated stage, both wolffian and müllerian ducts exist simultaneously. Gonadal development determines changes in the internal ductal structures. If a Y chromosome is present and testicular development ensues, both testosterone and müllerian-inhibiting substance is secreted in the male child. This acts to stimulate wolffian development and causes regression of the müllerian ducts ipsilaterally. In the absence of a Y chromosome, the gonad develops into an ovary, the müllerian system develops along female lines, and the wolffian duct eventually regresses. The third stage is that of development of the external genitalia, which occurs from 10 to 15 weeks of gestational age. In the absence of a testis and androgen production, normal female genitalia develop. In the male, testicular excretion of testosterone causes development of the male phenotype. For testosterone to be completely effective, the tissues of the urogenital sinus and genitalia must bind and then convert testosterone by means of the enzyme 5-alphareductase to dihydrotestosterone, which directs development of the external genitalia.

Classification of sexual disorders and syndromes is very complex. From a practical standpoint, the three most common disorders leading to abnormal sexual development are chromosomal abnormalities, excessive androgen production leading to virilization of the female, and defective androgen production or action leading to feminization of the male. The phenotypic abnormalities noted in such chromosomal syndromes as Turner and Klinefelter syndromes are readily recognizable. If one excludes these types of abnormalities, the four most common causes of intersexuality are true hermaphroditism, mixed gonadal dysgenesis, female pseudohermaphroditism, and male pseudohermaphroditism.

A true hermaphrodite is one in which both ovarian and testicular tissue occur and is an infrequent finding. Only a few hundred cases have been reported in the literature. The diagnosis is made at the time of exploratory laparotomy and gonadal biopsy or excision. The karyotype is usually XX but can be XY or mosaic.

Mixed gonadal dysgenesis is a much more common cause of ambiguous genitalia and can present with a wide variability of genital appearance. These patients have a testis on one side and a streak gonad on the other. The most common karyotype is 45X0-46XY.

Female pseudohermaphroditism occurs when there is virilization of a normal female. Exogenous androgens, such as the ingestion of progestational agents or virilizing maternal tumors, can lead to this disorder. The most common cause, however, is congenital adrenal hyperplasia in which abnormalities of steroid production lead to excessive quantities of androgen being produced by the fetus. These patients have varying degrees of masculinization that can be virtually complete except for the absence of palpable gonads. These patients are potentially fertile but are also at risk for cardiovascular collapse and death caused by salt loss and metabolic abnormalities if the diagnosis is not made early.

Male pseudohermaphroditism occurs when genetic males differentiate either partly or completely as phenotypic females. This can occur from defects in androgen synthesis, androgen action, or defective müllerian regression. Classification of this group of patients requires extensive hormonal evaluation, which includes measurement of urinary and plasma steroids, stimulated levels of plasma steroids, and the evaluation of androgen action of cultured fibroblasts.

Complete evaluation of a patient with ambiguous genitalia begins with a careful history searching for a positive family history or maternal ingestion of drugs. The physical examination is centered around the search for palpable gonads, a uterus, or midline müllerian structure on rectal examination. If gonads are palpable in the labioscrotal fold, it is almost certain they are testes, since ovaries do not descend. Increased skin pigmentation, dehydration, or failure to thrive should suggest an adrenocortical etiology for ambiguous genitalia.

A buccal smear is easy to obtain and should be the first order of laboratory evaluation. Karyotyping is helpful in assessing and defining specific chromosomal abnormalities. Hormonal evaluation should consist minimally of measurement of urinary ketosteroids, 17-ketosteroids, and pregnanetriol. Specific hormone evaluation, which includes plasma precursor hormones and hormonal stimulation studies, requires chemical measurements performed by specific research laboratories and are beyond the scope of this discussion. Genitography, uroradiography, and cystoscopy are helpful in evaluating both the urinary tract as well as the status of development of the urogenital sinus and internal ductal structures. Exploratory laparotomy is necessary in some cases to evaluate the internal ductal structures as well as to inspect and biopsy the gonads, with removal of gonadal tissue where indicated.

The sex assignment of these children should be completed in the newborn period. It should be the responsibility of a team and not a single individual. Gender reassignment should only be considered in the first few months of life and only in unusual circumstances. In each case, individualization is necessary. In general, the questions to be answered in rearing a child with ambiguous genitalia are those surrounding fertility, the possibility of future hormone production, and the ability to function sexually in the role chosen. The decision to rear an individual as a male depends on the development of the phallus and its potential for both development and adequate surgical correction of an abnormal urethral position.

Female pseudohermaphrodites are potentially fertile. Therefore attempts should be made to rear these children as females. Those with mixed gonadal dysgenesis are thought best reared as females because of inadequate masculinization, the presence of a uterus and a vagina, the almost certain sterility, and the short stature that will be achieved as adults. Likewise, as many as 25% of these patients will develop gonadal tumors if gonads are allowed to remain. Thus these patients require surgical removal of the gonads. True hermaphrodites should be reared in a gender role primarily based on the adequacy of the external genitalia.

Male pseudohermaphrodites, in many ways, pose the most difficult questions as to gender assignment. The major question is whether there will be adequate growth of the phallus for sexual function and whether the patient will be fertile. Currently there is no simple or consistently accurate way to predict the answers to these questions. Extensive hormonal and genetic studies, in conjunction with exploratory laparotomy and gonadal biopsy, may in many cases be necessary before gender can be assigned with any degree of accuracy. In most cases, the major criterion for sex assignment still basically rests on the degree of masculinization of the external genitalia.

ABDOMINAL MASSES

Approximately 55% of all children presenting with an abdominal mass have a nonsurgical cause for the enlargement. Of the 45% classified as having surgical conditions, the majority are retroperitoneal and two thirds of these have renal enlargement. It is therefore evident that urologic abnormalities are responsible for the majority of abdominal masses of surgical significance. The differential diagnosis of an abdominal mass can be an interesting and challenging problem.

After a thorough history, the physical examination may give clues and valuable information as to the etiology of the abdominal mass. Abdominal examination is best carried out using light palpation and bimanual techniques. The position, characteristics, and mobility of the mass should be noted. Transillumination of a mass can be helpful in diagnosing fluid collections such as hydronephrosis. Multiple examinations of the abdominal mass are unnecessary and may lead to rupture or spread of a malignant tumor of the kidney should one be present. Associated abnormalities noted at the time of physical examination can give a clue as to the etiology of the condition. Aniridia or hemihypertrophy would suggest Wilms tumor. Abnormalities of the ear would most likely be associated with hydronephrosis, and a webbed neck would suggest a renal anomaly such as a horseshoe kidney coincident with Turner syndrome. Imperforate hymen would lead one to suspect hydrocolpos as the cause of an abdominal mass in the female infant.

The position of the mass in the abdomen can give a clue to the tissue of origin. A pelvic mass in a male child would most likely be an enlarged bladder with obstructive uropathy. A pelvic mass in a female child highly suggests hydrocolpos. A pelvic mass could also be the result of anterior meningocele, teratoma, or ovarian cyst. Upper abdominal masses would most likely arise from the kidneys, adrenals, liver, or spleen.

Initial laboratory diagnostic evaluation of these children should include an excretory urogram and an abdominal ultrasound. In the newborn child, a renal scan can be substituted for the excretory urogram. Using these techniques, up to 95% of the abdominal masses can be diagnosed with accuracy. A voiding cystourethrogram should be ordered if the need is suggested by findings on the excretory urogram and physical examination. Further evaluation with venacavography, arteriography, or CT scanning of the abdomen would be dependent on the findings on excretory urogram and ultrasound.

Abdominal masses of urologic origin in childhood can be better understood when viewed in light of the age of the patient. The knowledge that certain conditions predominate statistically within certain age groups can help one be more accurate in diagnosing these lesions. In the neonate, the most common cause of abdominal mass is a nonfunctioning multicystic kidney followed by hydronephrosis. In infants and younger children, hydronephrosis is the most common cause of abdominal mass, with malignant lesions such as neuroblastoma or Wilms tumor increasing in incidence as the child gets older. In older children, neuroblastoma and Wilms tumor are the most common causes of abdominal masses, with hydronephrosis being third. It is thus clear that hydronephrosis and benign conditions predominate in the younger child, with malignant conditions being more common in older children.

Surgical treatment of these mass lesions, of course, should proceed without undue delay. However, it is no longer necessary to be hasty in the treatment of these children and operate on them immediately on admission. A thoughtful evaluation can help one plan the appropriate surgical approach under optimum conditions. When possible, restoration or preservation of renal function when hydronephrosis or obstructive uropathy is discovered is believed to be optimum treatment. Treatment of a malignant urologic disease is generally aimed at its complete removal and appropriate staging.

MALIGNANCIES OF THE GENITOURINARY TRACT

(see also p. 853)

Kidney. Wilms tumor, or nephroblastoma, is by far the most common renal tumor seen in childhood. The incidence of this tumor is second only to neuroblastoma as the most common solid tumor in children. The majority of cases are in children 7 years of age or younger, with the peak incidence being between 2 and 3 years of age. Symptoms and findings on presentation include gross or microscopic hematuria, abdominal pain, abdominal mass, or hypertension. A strong index of suspicion may be necessary to detect this tumor before it becomes large enough to palpate in the abdomen. Wilms tumors have been associated with other clinical findings including hemihypertrophy, aniridia, and Beckwith syndrome. However, the majority of children with Wilms tumors do not have these associated abnormalities.

Initial evaluation when Wilms tumor is suspected is the intravenous pyelogram (Fig. 34-13). This will usually show an enlarged kidney with a functioning but distorted collecting system. Other helpful studies include CT scanning of the abdomen, renal angiography, vena cavagram, and ultrasound. These studies are frequently done to determine extent of the tumor, status of the vessels as far as tumor involvement is concerned, and whether there is any evidence of metastases. Attention must also be given to the contralateral kidney because Wilms tumors are bilateral in about 5% of cases.

Once the diagnosis is made, surgical excision of the tumor is mandatory. Approximately two thirds of children with Wilms tumor have lower stages I and II.

Stage I	Tumor limited to the kidney; renal capsule intact
Stage II	Tumor extends beyond kidney or into the blood vessels but does not involve adjacent organs or regional lymph nodes
Stage III	Residual tumor in the abdomen (not involving the liver) after surgical excision of the lesion
Stage IV	Evidence of hematogenous metastases
Stage V	Bilateral tumors

Surgery is the cornerstone of therapy, and in the earlier stages excision of the tumor alone can be curative. The use of radiation therapy and chemotherapy is necessary in the higher stages of disease and has improved the prognosis in this group of children. As would be expected, prognosis depends largely on the stage of the tumor, although it has been noted that children under 2 years of age have a better prognosis than those who are older.

Mesoblastic nephroma is unusual but is the most common solid tumor of the kidney seen in infants. This usually presents as an abdominal mass. This tumor seems to be of very low-grade malignancy and may be a benign variant of Wilms' tumor. Nephrectomy is curative.

Renal cell carcinoma is predominantly seen in adulthood. There does, however, seem to be an increasing incidence of this tumor in younger age groups. The average age of presentation in childhood is 9 years. Clinical presentation and radiographic findings are similar to those in Wilms tumor, with hematuria and abdominal mass being common. Radiographic studies may not be able to differentiate between Wilms tumor and renal cell carcinoma. Frequently, the final diagnosis cannot be determined until histologic examination of the specimen is com-

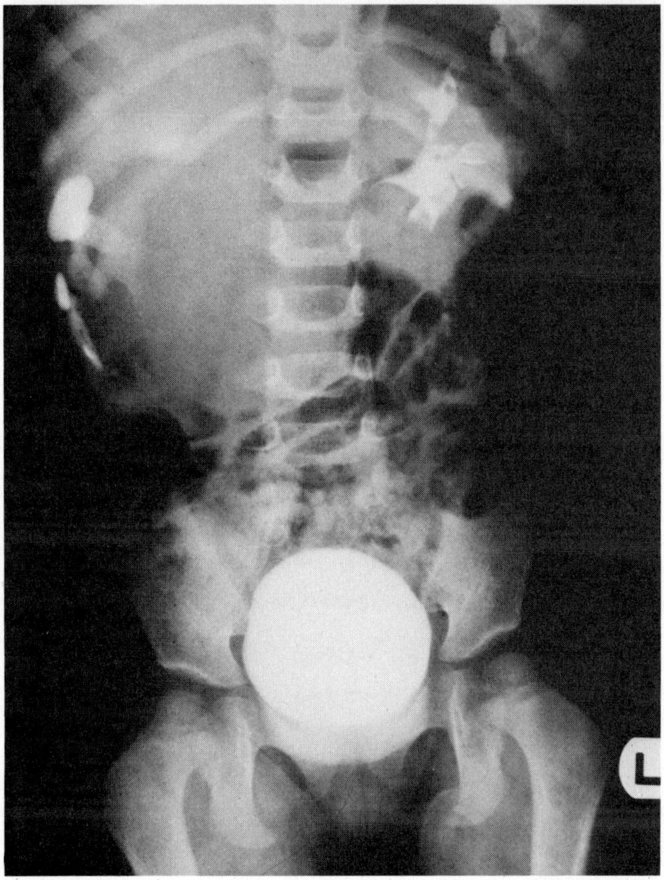

Fig. 34-13. Wilms tumor arising in right kidney showing gross distortion of collecting structures.

plete. The only effective treatment for this tumor is surgical excision. Earlier stages of the tumor have survival rates of approximately 70% at 5 years. Radiation therapy and chemotherapy have not seemed to alter the prognosis of this disease.

Metastatic malignancy to the kidney or secondary renal tumor involvement must be considered in any mass lesion of the kidney. Hodgkin disease and leukemia are the most frequent secondary renal tumors. These are usually bilateral processes, and renal failure may be associated with them. Treatment of these lesions involves attention to the primary disease process.

Adrenal malignancies. Neuroblastoma is the most common malignant solid tumor in childhood. The primary site of origin is the adrenal glands, although it can occur elsewhere. The overall incidence is higher than that of Wilms tumor. Most neuroblastomas are diagnosed in children under 5 years of age with the peak incidence at about 18 months. Fifty percent or more of these tumors are discovered because of an abdominal mass, while about 30% will present with fever, weight loss, and anemia. Unfortunately, metastatic disease is noted in approximately 70% of the children at the time of diagnosis. Findings on excretory urogram include displacement of the kidney without alteration of the collecting system, calcification in the area of the adrenal glands, and a large mass in the abdomen displacing bowel and sometimes the kidneys across the midline. These tumors typically excrete catecholamines, so that increased urinary levels of vanillylmandelic acid (VMA) or homovanillic acid (HVA) can be found in 90% of such patients.

Treatment of early stages of neuroblastoma with surgical excision has a high survival rate. Since most tumors are discovered at later stages, the overall prognosis of this disease is approximately 30% survival at 2 years. The higher stages of the tumor are treated with surgery in combination with radiation and chemotherapy. As in Wilms tumor, younger children have a better prognosis, and specifically those under 18 months of age have shown increased survival rates with this tumor.

With the exception of neuroblastoma, tumors of the adrenal gland in children are rare. Adrenocortical tumors are usually discovered because of bleeding in the retroperitoneum or because of a mass noted in the abdomen. Secondary hormonal changes may be noted because of increased or abnormal production of hormones by the tumor. Surgical excision is the primary treatment of these tumors.

Pheochromocytoma is a tumor arising from the adrenal medulla and is rare. It is a cause of approximately 1% of hypertension in children. The average age of discovery is 12 years. About 90% of pheochromocytomas are of adrenal origin with the remainder being found in the thoracic, abdominal, and pelvic areas. Though this tumor is infrequently malignant, there is a higher incidence of malignant changes of this tumor in children. Occasionally, a family history of pheochromocytoma is noted and there appears to be some increase of incidence in children with neurofibromatosis. Surgical excision of this tumor is the most successful form of treatment.

Retroperitoneal tumors. Additional tumors seen in the retroperitoneum in children include teratomas, lipomas, and neurofibromas, the majority of which present as a palpable mass and are benign. Surgical excision is the treatment of choice for each of these conditions.

Tumors of the lower urinary tract. Tumors of the bladder are rare in children, though benign papillomas have been described. Virtually all malignant tumors of the childhood bladder are rhabdomyosarcoma. This tumor is one of the most common connective tissue tumors in childhood. Fifteen percent of them are found within the true pelvis. They may arise from the bladder, prostate, or vaginal area.

Presenting symptoms of this pelvic tumor may include hematuria, vaginal bleeding, and obstructive voiding symptoms especially in the male. Physical signs in the female include protrusion of the bleeding mass from the introitus in addition to irritative voiding complaints. In the male, bleeding from the urethra with obstructive and irritative voiding symptoms may be noted. Rectal examination in the male usually reveals a mass in the area of the bladder and the prostate. An excretory urogram in these children will frequently show displacement of the bladder by the tumor or a filling defect within the bladder caused by the tumor (Fig. 34-14). In large tumors, occasionally one or both kidneys may show signs of obstruction.

The majority of children with this tumor are discovered when they are younger than 5 years of age. Treatment of rhabdomyosarcoma includes a combination approach including surgery, chemotherapy, and radiation therapy. Over the past several years, radical surgery has been used less frequently. After tissue diagnosis is obtained, chemotherapy and sometimes radiation therapy are used initially. If these should fail, radical surgery and pelvic exenteration is then indicated.

Tumors of the testicles. A firm mass in the scrotum, either tender or nontender, must be considered a tumor until proved otherwise. Differential diagnosis of intrascrotal masses includes testicular torsion, torsion of the testicular appendages, epididymitis, hydroceles, hernia, hematoceles, and tumor. Tumors within the scrotum are usually of testicular origin, but paratesticular tumors of connective tissue are also seen.

When physical examination, clinical history, and appropriate laboratory and x-ray studies fail to establish a conclusive diagnosis, scrotal exploration is necessary. When tumor is suspected, the testicle is best approached through an inguinal incision, which allows for early control of the vessels and radical orchiectomy if necessary.

Testicular tumors are of 2 types, germinal cell and nongerminal cell. Germinal cell tumors make up 75% of testicular tumors in prepubertal boys, with the remaining 25% arising from nongerminal tissues. The latter includes Sertoli cell, Leydig cell, and connective tissue cell tumors or metastatic tumors to the testis.

The most common germ cell tumors in children are embryonal cell carcinoma and teratoma. Embryonal cell tumor is less malignant than the adult counterpart, but the tumor does have the ability to metastasize. The disease also

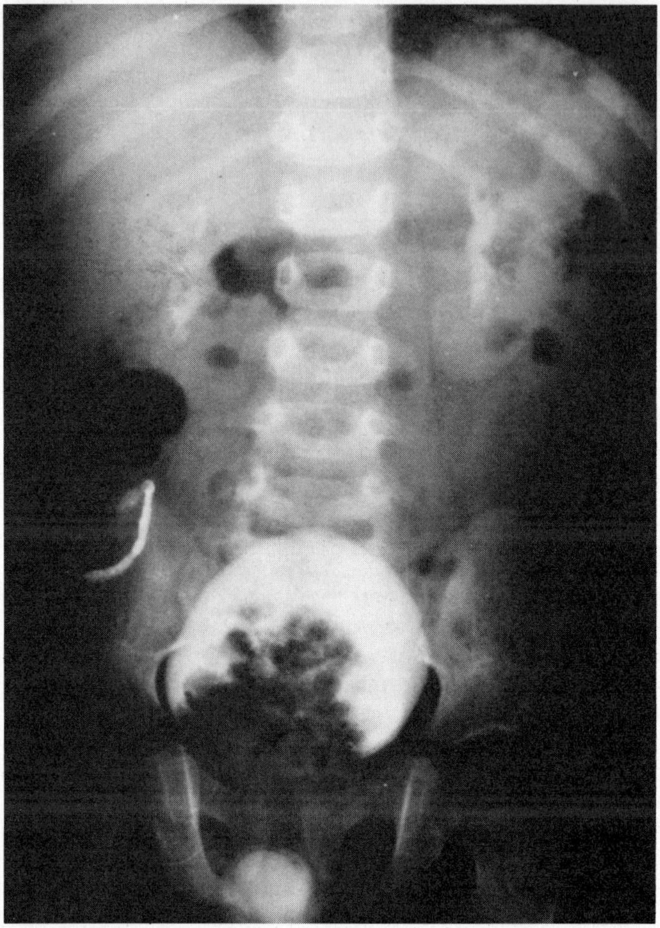

Fig. 34-14. Rhabdomyosarcoma of bladder seen as filling defect on cystogram.

seems to be more severe in older children. Treatment of the infant with embryonal cell carcinoma includes radical orchiectomy in combination with lymphadenectomy. The prognosis for treatment of children younger than 2 years of age is better than for the older child. Teratomas in children are benign and surgical excision usually results in cure.

Leydig cell tumors and Sertoli cell tumors may be first noted because of effects brought on by hormone production. Sexual precocity and changes secondary to the hormonal function of these tumors may be noted before any evidence of a testicular mass is discovered. Excision of these tumors usually results in cure and relief of symptoms.

Rhabdomyosarcomas are also seen in the scrotum and account for about 10% of intrascrotal or paratesticular malignancies in children. The average age of presentation of these tumors is 9 years. Treatment of this tumor includes excision of the spermatic cord and lymph node dissection. A combination of surgical excision with chemotherapy and radiation therapy has achieved nearly an 80% survival rate in tumors discovered in early stages.

PRUNE BELLY SYNDROME

The prune belly, or Eagle-Barrett syndrome, is characterized by absence or paucity of abdominal musculature, giving the child the characteristic "prune belly" appearance at birth.

The other classic findings include bilateral undescended testicles and a dilated urinary collecting system. Though the unique abdominal findings and urinary tract abnormalities have been described in the female, the classic syndrome affects the male. The incidence of this syndrome is about 1 per 40,000 live births. This syndrome may present with varying degrees of severity, ranging from the child with virtually no abdominal musculature and severely dysplatic kidneys to the child with the presence of abdominal muscle tissue and a dilated urinary tract with good renal function.

The etiology of the disease is unclear but it is thought that there is an arrest of mesenchymal development between the sixth and tenth week in utero. Prognosis of these children depends on the degree of renal dysplasia present. Peristalsis is usually poor in the ureters, and they appear dilated and tortuous. The distal ureter is usually affected more severely than the more proximal portion. Histologic examination of the dilated ureters reveals increased fibrous tissue and poor development of muscle fibers in the ureters. The bladder is characteristically large and usually empties incompletely. Approximately 75% of these children have vesicoureteral reflux. The urethra is generally dilated, though there are no areas of obstruction within the urethra or bladder neck. The diagnosis is confirmed when the child with the characteristic abdominal findings is noted to have an abnormal excretory urogram and undescended testicles.

The primary goal of treatment is to maintain adequate renal function and to prevent any deterioration in renal status. In those children with the milder form of the disease and good renal function, simple observation, maintenance of a sterile urine, and monitoring of the renal functional status may be all that is required. Surgical therapy is reserved for those with the more severe forms of the disease or in those who show a deterioration in renal function. One-stage reconstruction with ureteral shortening, tailoring, and reimplantation along with reduction cystoplasty is, in many cases, needed and can be performed in the neonate or infant. Temporary tubeless diversion such as ureterostomy or pyelostomy may be necessary, but one-stage reconstruction is preferable.

Fortunately, a good number of these children do not require reconstruction or diversion even though the radiographic appearance of their urinary tracts is grossly abnormal. Some will, however, develop difficulties in emptying the bladder, which can be improved by internal urethrotomy. In those who are ultimately unable to satisfactorily empty their bladder, intermittent catheterization can be used.

The testes are usually intra-abdominal in location and can be best brought into the scrotum during infancy. The results of orchiopexy in the older child are usually disappointing. To date, reports regarding fertility in these children are incomplete, although hormonal function and development of secondary sex characteristics appear to be normal.

STONE DISEASE (see also pp. 551-552)

Stone disease in children is an uncommon occurrence and accounts for less than 10% of all urinary stones seen in the United States. The incidence of urinary stone disease varies depending on geographic location. Certain areas of the United States and the world have been noted to have a high incidence of calculi, yet the reasons for this remain unclear. A combination of genetic traits and environment seems to be a plausible theory to explain the high occurrence of stone disease in certain parts of the United States. On a worldwide basis, an increased incidence of urinary calculi has been noted in the Mediterranean area, parts of India, and Southeast Asia. The highest incidence of urinary stones in the United States is in the southeastern United States.

Stones can be classified generally into four major groups: endemic stones, infection-induced stones, metabolic stones, and idiopathic stones. Endemic stones are seen today in certain underdeveloped countries such as parts of India and Asia. The stones occur mostly in males and are usually bladder stones. They are urate stones and appear to be related to dietary habits in these countries. This type of stone is seen infrequently in the United States.

Infection-induced stones account for about one third of urinary stones seen in children. They are primarily found in children having underlying congenital abnormalities that preclude normal drainage of the urinary tract. Children with a neurogenic bladder and stasis of the urine have a higher incidence of infection-induced stones, as well as children who have a long-term indwelling catheter or cutaneous urinary diversions. The stones are usually composed of magnesium-ammonium phosphate and are associated with infections caused by urea-splitting organisms.

Metabolic disease and renal tubular abnormalities are an uncommon cause of urinary calculus disease, yet proportionately there is a higher incidence of these problems in children than seen in the adult population. Below is a list of some of the causes of metabolic and renal tubular disorders causing urinary stone disease.

- Renal tubular syndromes
  - Renal tubular acidosis
    - Distal defect, type I
    - Carbonic anhydrase inhibitors
  - Cystinuria
  - Glycinuria
- Enzyme disorders
  - Xanthinuria
  - Primary hyperparathyroidism
- Hypercalcemic states
  - Primary hyperparathyroidism
  - Sarcoidosis
  - Hypervitaminosis D
  - Milk-alkali syndrome
  - Neoplasms
  - Cushing syndrome
  - Hyperthyroidism
  - Immobilization
  - Idiopathic infantile hypercalcemia
- Uric acid lithiasis
  - Idiopathic uric acid lithiasis
  - Gout
  - Idiopathic renal lithiasis
  - Myeloproliferative disorders

Idiopathic stone disease, in most clinical studies, accounts for 50% to 75% of all urinary stones seen in children. These stones are usually composed of calcium oxalate. Of all types of stone disease, this is the most poorly understood. Recent studies have determined that many of these children have hypercalciuria unassociated with hyperparathyroidism or other hypercalcemic states.

Some investigators have indicated that two major groups can be identified in those who form "idiopathic" calcium oxalate stones. One group has an intrinsic renal "leak" that is an apparent tubular defect allowing for high urine concentrations of calcium in the filtered urine. The other group has increased absorption of calcium from the intestines. This increased calcium absorption causes periods of higher than normal blood levels, which will secondarily cause an increased filtering of calcium by the kidney (hypercalciuria).

Diagnosis and treatment of stone disease. Symptoms associated with stone disease are usually noted when the stone causes obstruction, causes hematuria, or is associated with a urinary tract infection. Any child that has a sudden onset of flank or abdominal pain with associated gross or microscopic hematuria should be suspected of having a urinary calculus. Pain associated with an obstructed ureter is usually a colicky, radiating pain that extends from the renal area around to the scrotal or labial area. On occasion a stone will present as an unexplained febrile illness. This is usually because of an associated infection in the area of the urinary stasis. The urinalysis will frequently show pyuria and hematuria. The urine culture is usually positive.

Initial evaluation of the child suspected of having a urinary calculus should include a thorough physical examination and careful questioning concerning a family history of stone disease. A urinalysis is frequently suggestive of a stone, in that not only microscopic hematuria will be seen but also characteristic urinary crystals will be noted. A normal urinalysis does not exclude the possibility of calculus. A plain film of the abdomen will frequently reveal a calcification in the area of the urinary tract and will strengthen the suspicion of an obstructing calculus (Fig. 34-15). Approximately 90% of urinary stones contain calcium and, when large enough, will be radiopaque. An intravenous pyelogram confirms the presence of the calcification within the urinary tract and reveals the degree and level of obstruction.

Depending on the size, position, presence or absence of infection, and severity of symptoms, a number of initial therapeutic options are available. If the stone appears small enough to pass spontaneously, analgesics and hydration will frequently hasten the passing of the stone. However, should the stone not pass, surgical removal is necessary. A septic patient, of course, will usually require initial antibiotics before surgical intervention is undertaken. Occasionally insertion of a ureteral catheter past the obstructing stone will decompress the kidney and allow more effective use of systemic antibiotics before surgery.

An important part of the long-term management of the patient with stone disease is recov-

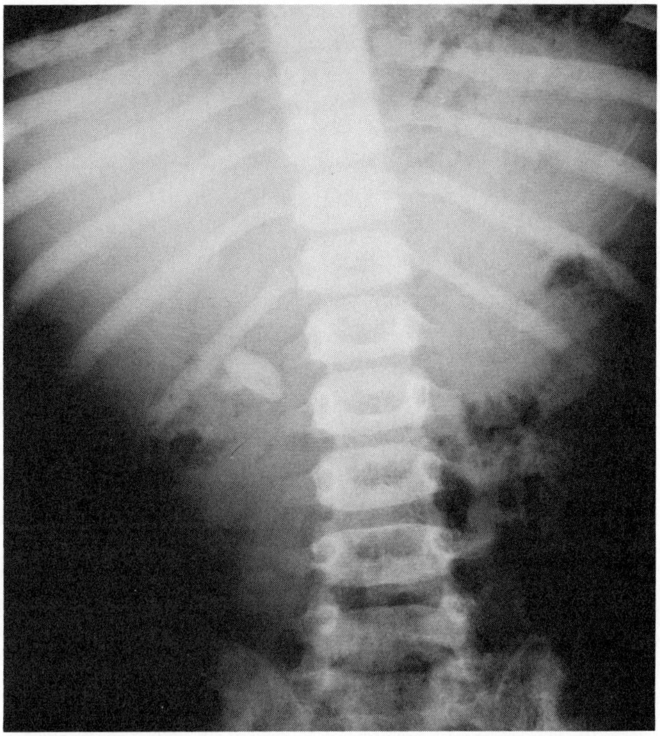

Fig. 34-15. Plain film of abdomen showing large right renal pelvic stone.

ery of the urinary calculus and analysis of its content. Once the determination is made of the type of stone present, a logical approach to the diagnosis of potential metabolic or renal abnormalities can be carried out.

The etiology of an infection-induced stone is usually obvious, and measures to prevent recurrence of such a stone are usually directed at proper management of the underlying obstruction or other abnormality. These children may even require long-term prophylactic antibiotics.

Though most of the stones seen are calcium oxalate, occasionally uric acid stones and cystine stones will be found. These will require further metabolic evaluation of the child, and treatment should be directed at decreasing the excretion of the uric acid and cystine and increasing the solubilities of these in the urine.

If a calcium oxalate stone is identified, the child should be evaluated for the presence of hypercalcemia, hypercalciuria, or hyperoxaluria. If hypercalciuria is found without evidence of underlying metabolic abnormalities, the evaluation should proceed with an oral calcium loading study to determine the type of hypercalciuria present. Results of the serum parathormone level, serum calcium and electrolyte levels, and the oral calcium loading study can frequently determine whether the hypercalciuria is secondary to an intrinsic renal leak or caused by hyperabsorption of calcium from the intestine.

Children with hyperabsorption of calcium will have normal urine calcium-creatinine ratios before the calcium loading studies but will increase this level above normal after the calcium loading study is performed. Children with the renal leak type of hypercalciuria will have an increased fasting level of their urine calcium-creatinine ratio, as well as increased urine calcium-creatinine ratio after a calcium loading study.

Treatment of these children with stone disease will be based on information gained from the calcium loading study. If the child has the hyperabsorptive type of hypercalciuria, decrease in calcium intake as well as the addition of neutral phosphates to the diet can reduce the amount of calcium excreted. The renal leak type of hypercalciuria can be treated with thiazide diuretics, which decrease the excretion of calcium in the urine by the tubules.

GENITOURINARY TRAUMA

The most common cause of death in children in the United States is accidents. Thus a significant number of children with multiple injuries will be seen initially by the pediatrician. Injuries to the genitourinary tract must be considered when evaluating these children.

Though penetrating wounds do occur in children, they are less frequently seen than in the adult population. Blunt trauma is by far the most common source of urinary tract injury to children. These injuries are usually seen following automobile accidents, motorcycle and bicycle accidents, and contact sports. Child abuse must also be suspected in the child with unexplained injuries.

Most of the injuries of the genitourinary tract are seen in boys and involve the kidneys. Children are predisposed to renal injury because the kidney is relatively large in relationship to the body size of the child. There is also less perirenal fat, and the kidney is not well protected by the ribs of the child.

Nearly 20% of renal injuries in children involve an abnormal kidney. An ectopic kidney or a kidney with tumor or congenital obstruction are more easily injured because of their intrinsic abnormality. Hematuria may be seen following relatively insignificant injury to a child with one of these renal abnormalities.

Diagnosis of injury to the kidney frequently necessitates a high index of suspicion. On physical examination, flank or upper abdominal tenderness may be seen. A mass in the flank may also be present. Serial examinations may indicate an expanding mass in the area of the kidney, indicating bleeding in the renal area. Contusions over the flank and abdomen, as well as fractured ribs, are frequently associated with renal injury. The urinalysis usually reveals either gross or microscopic hematuria when the kidney is injured. Yet, 25% of severe injuries of the kidneys will not have gross or microscopic hematuria on the initial evaluation. When a renal injury is suspected, an intravenous pyelogram should be done as early as the patient's clinical status permits.

Further evaluation and treatment will be based on the results of a carefully performed intravenous pyelogram. Minor fractures of the kidney usually do not require surgical intervention, whereas a shattered kidney with bleeding in the retroperitoneum may require surgical intervention with nephrectomy. Virtually all penetrating wounds to the abdomen will be explored, and it is of benefit to the surgeon, in determining the best treatment for the kidney, to have adequate x-ray studies of the urinary tract before surgery.

Bladder injuries account for a small portion of genitourinary trauma and are usually associated with pelvic fractures. Nearly 80% of bladder ruptures are of the extraperitoneal type. Presence of a severe bladder injury should be suspected in any crush injury to the pelvis or any injury associated with pelvic fracture. Gross hematuria is present in the majority of cases and the diagnosis is confirmed by a cystogram.

Urethral injuries are more frequently seen in the male and are associated with pelvic fractures or a straddle type of injury. Early suspicion of urethral injury in a male is important. Whenever a pelvic or perineal injury is seen and there is gross blood noted at the urethral meatus, a urethral injury should be considered. Careful evaluation of this injury should be completed before blind insertion of a catheter. Such instrumentation, before adequate assessment of the injury, can frequently convert a partial tear of the urethra to a complete tear and thus increase the severity and morbidity of the injury. Assessment of the injured urethra can be done by retrograde urethrogram in which contrast material is injected at the meatus. This radiographic study will outline the course of the urethra, presence or absence of continuity of the urethra with the bladder, and presence of extravasation of the contrast material.

Injuries of the male genitalia include blunt and penetrating trauma to the scrotum and testicles. These injuries are frequently associated with significant intrascrotal bleeding and pain. The history and physical examination usually make the diagnosis obvious. In severe injuries in which intrascrotal bleeding is persistent, surgical exploration may be necessary. It should also be kept in mind that pain in the scrotum may be attributed to an injury but may, in reality, be secondary to torsion of the testicle or torsion of a testicular appendage. Early suspicion and identification of torsion in these children will result in early surgical intervention and salvage of the testicle.

Injuries to the penis in children are infrequent and range from zipper and toilet seat injuries to the extremes of partial and complete amputation.

PRENATAL DIAGNOSIS OF GENITOURINARY ABNORMALITIES

The intrauterine diagnosis of fetal abnormalities has until recently been limited to those disorders that can be detected by either biochemical testing or chromosomal analysis of amniotic fluid obtained during the second trimester of pregnancy. Recent advances and technical improvements in the area of ultrasonic imagery have permitted identification of one or both fetal kidneys in up to 90% of 17 to 20 week old fetuses. By 22 weeks of gestation kidneys are seen in nearly 95% of fetuses examined by ultrasound. These technical advances now allow an early diagnosis of fetal urologic abnormalities, such as bilateral renal agenesis, infantile polycystic kidneys, renal cystic dysplasia, and obstructive uropathy (Fig. 34-16). Such diagnoses can be made early enough in a pregnancy so that appropriate counselling and management can be carried out.

At present it is unclear if early diagnosis and relief of urinary obstruction will improve potential of renal development and function in the fetus. Though it would seem that relief of the obstruction would benefit the kidney, some in-

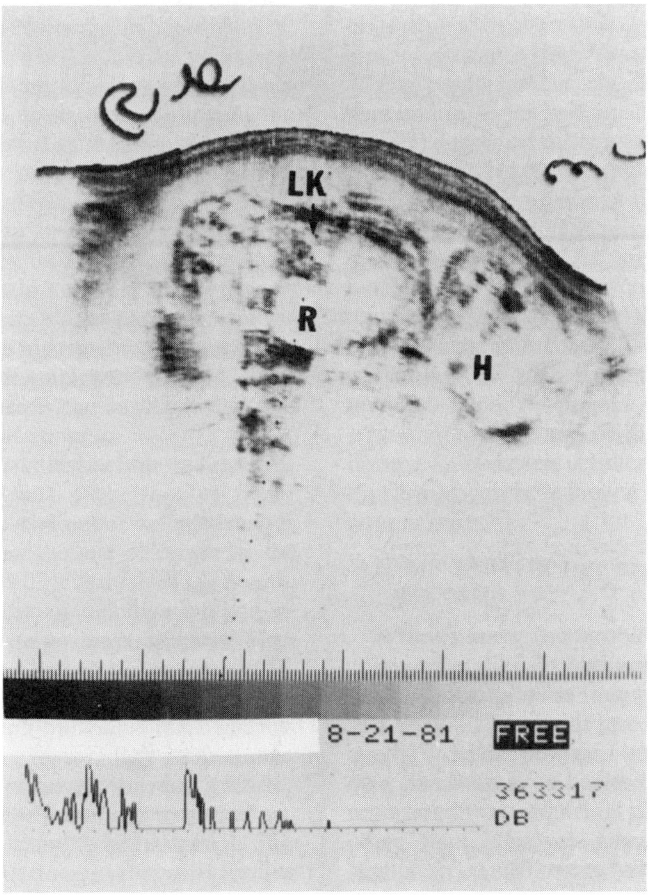

Fig. 34-16. Maternal ultrasound showing fetus with hydronephrosis *(LK)* and multicystic kidney *(R)*. *MU,* Maternal umbilicus; *H,* fetal head; *RM,* rib margin.

vestigators suspect that the major amount of damage caused by such obstruction occurs well before detection is possible by ultrasound.

The dilemma of whether to proceed with interventional therapy of the fetus mainly occurs in the fetus with obstructive uropathy. Lesions incompatible with life or those involving only one kidney will not require early intervention. The advantage of the intrauterine diagnosis of a urinary tract abnormality is twofold. The family can be counseled concerning the defect so that they can be prepared for potential problems during pregnancy or after birth of the infant. Also, it allows for referral of the mother to a center capable of handling complicated pregnancies and potentially ill neonates.

H. Norman Noe
Gerald R. Jerkins

REFERENCES

Campbell, M.F., editor: Campbell's urology, vol. 2, Philadelphia, 1979, W.B. Saunders.

Congenital anomalies of the lower genitourinary tract, Urol. Clin. North Am., February, 1978.

Jerkins, G.R., and Noe, H.N.: Familial vesicoureteric reflux: a prospective study, J. Urol. **128:**774, 1982.

Jerkins, G.R., Noe, H.N., Hollabaugh, R.S., and Allen, R.G.: Spermatic cord torsion in the neonate, J. Urol. **129:**121, 1983.

Kelalis, P.P., and King, L.R.: Clinical pediatric urology, Philadelphia, 1976, W.B. Saunders.

Noe, H.N.: Voiding dysfunction in the child with problem wetting, J. Dev. Behav. Pediatrics, vol. 1, #1, March, 1980.

Noe, H.N.: Endoscopic management of urethral strictures in children, J. Urol. **125:**712, 1981.

Noe, H.N., and Dale, G.A.: Evaluation of meatal stenosis in children, J. Urol. **114:**455, 1976.

Noe, H.N., and Patterson, T.H.: Screening urography in asymptomatic cryptorchid patients, J. Urol. **119:**669, 1978.

Noe, H.N., Stapleton, F.B., Jerkins, G.R., and Roy, S. III: Clinical experience with pediatric urolithiasis, J. Urol. **129:**1166, 1983.

Noe, H.N., Wilimas, J., and Jerkins, G.R.: Surgical management of priapism in sickle cell anemia, J. Urol. **126:**770, 1981.

Pediatric urology, Urol. Clin. North Am., June, 1980.

Report of the International Reflux Study Committee: Medical versus surgical treatment of primary vesicoureteral reflux: a prospective international reflux study in children, J. Urol. **125:**277, 1981.

Stapleton, F.B., Noe, H.N., Roy, S. III, and Jerkins, G.R.: Hypercalciuria in children with urolithiasis, Am. J. Dis. Child., vol. 136, August, 1982.

Williams, D.I., and Johnston, J.H.: Paediatric urology, second edition, London, 1982, Butterworth Scientific.

35 Pediatric Orthopedics

Because the skeletal system of the growing child may be affected by a wide variety of conditions, the physician who deals with children is frequently confronted with problems related to the bones and joints and their associated structures. Familiarity with the most common conditions is essential, particularly in view of the fact that in many instances early diagnosis and proper treatment may avert increasing abnormality. Fortunately the restorative capacities of children are great, and their growth potential is an asset toward eventual recovery.

Diseases of the bones and joints may be divided into a smaller group that is congenital in origin and a much larger group with acquired etiology. Furthermore, orthopedic problems may be localized, extensive, or generalized. Congenital abnormalities of the skeletal system may be genetically determined or may be the result of adverse prenatal circumstances. Acquired conditions include disturbances of growth and development caused by poor nutrition, local or systemic disease, metabolic defects that have skeletal repercussions (renal tubular defects leading to rickets), many forms of trauma, neoplastic processes, acute and chronic infections, and injury to the skeleton from continued intake of drugs and other toxic materials.

In this chapter the more common orthopedic problems of children are discussed briefly, and several of the rarer entities that are of special interest are reviewed.

FOOT

Pes planus. The foot of the newborn infant has no visible arch. The sole at the midfoot may even bulge with physiologic fat, and slight eversion or pronation of the heel is normal. When the child learns to stand and then to walk, a more definite pes planus may develop. The limbs are spread in a wide stance to maintain balance, and body weight stretches the ligaments of the feet, especially those on the medial side. Before the age of 2 years, if the feet are aligned satisfactorily with the legs, treatment is seldom indicated, but the parents will need reassurance. It is estimated that 97% of children under 18 months of age are flat footed by clinical examination. Only about 47% of children evaluated at 10 years of age are flat footed.

After 2 years of age a definite pes planus may require that the foot be supported. Corrective shoes with high tops and medial heel wedges 3.2 to 9.5 mm (⅛ to ⅜ inch) in height may be used, or supports may be placed inside the shoes on the posteromedial part of the soles in the form of scaphoid pads. Depending on the degree of pes planus, corrective shoes with high tops may be needed for 6 months to 6 years. Foot exercises are also prescribed. The best is simply walking on the toes to elevate and strengthen the muscles of the longitudinal arch. Lack of improvement within a few months indicates need for orthopedic referral and possibly steel arch supports (covered with soft leather padding), cast correction, or operation. The most severe type of pes planus is associated with perpendicular talus, a deformity revealed best by weight-bearing radiographs; the talus is perpendicular (its long axis parallel to the tibia). Orthopedic consultation is indicated.

Congenital malformations such as bony bridges may cause a spastic or rigid flatfoot. These bridges are not visible radiographically until the tarsal bones become sufficiently ossified, usually at about 6 or 7 years of age. When pes planus is recognized early, conservative therapy generally suffices. However, if proper conservative treatment is not given, surgical procedures may be necessary later. Examination should exclude other abnormalities such as genu valgum, femoral or tibial torsion, short Achilles tendon, and neuromuscular conditions.

Equinovarus (clubfoot). Talipes equinovarus constitutes about 25% of all congenital anomalies seen in clinics for crippled children. It occurs approximately once in each 700 to 1000 live births.

At the end of the first trimester of fetal life the feet are usually in a position of equinovarus, and during the last two trimesters they assume the normal position. However, they may remain in equinovarus for reasons of heredity, adverse prenatal influences, or abnormal intrauterine position. Investigations suggest that a disturbance in development of muscles and tendons may be a cause. The clubbed foot may be a manifestation of a neurologic problem, such as spina bifida, meningomyelocele, or diastematomyelia. Evidence for genetic factors in the etiology of clubfoot includes an increase of 300 times over the population incidence in monozygotic twin pairs and an increase of twenty-five times in relatives of affected patients. The risk of a second affected child after one affected child is about 3%.

Equinovarus may be mild, or it may be so severe that the toes point toward the medial side of the distal tibia. The Achilles tendon and anterior and posterior tibial tendons are contracted. Radiographs reveal that the long axis of the talus points medialward and plantarward and that of the calcaneus medialward; normally the talus is in line with the first metatarsal and the calcaneus with the fifth metatarsal.

When equinovarus is mild to moderate, treatment may be delayed several weeks, but when severe, earlier treatment is preferable. When mild, the parents are taught to stretch the child's feet into the corrected position. As soon as standing or walking is begun, high-top corrective tarsal pronator shoes are fitted. These may be the only measures necessary. However, if improvement is not prompt, orthopedic consultation is indicated. When the deformity is moderately severe, Denis Browne splints suffice; when severe, plaster wedging casts usually produce satisfactory correction unless the equinovarus is part of a more generalized arthrogryposis. When the deformity is severe and does not respond to conservative treatment, surgical correction is indicated. Goldner has pointed out the importance of correcting the deformity of the talotibial, subtalar, and talonavicular joints.

Calcaneovalgus. Calcaneovalgus is the next most frequent deformity of the foot. The foot is dorsiflexed and everted so that only the heel presents to the floor when standing is attempted. Correction can usually be accomplished by simple stretching—pulling the foot into the equinovarus position 12 to 15 times, 3 times a day. Furthermore, properly fitted tarsosupinator shoes with high tops are indicated. If these measures are unsuccessful, plaster casts or a Denis Browne splint in the reverse position may be necessary. Operation is seldom if ever indicated. However, because this deformity is unnecessarily alarming, the parents should be reassured.

Metatarsus varus. Metatarsus varus is a pigeon-toed or skew-foot deformity. The anterior part of the foot deviates medialward; angulation occurs at the tarsometatarsal joints. The forefoot cannot be abducted into the neutral position. Mild to moderate deformity can be corrected by repeated manipulations and a corrective shoe; both pull the forefoot from the position of adduction to that of abduction. A more severe deformity is corrected by plaster wedging casts. A severe or neglected deformity often requires operative correction.

It is important to know that a pigeon-toed gait may be the result of (1) forefoot adduction (metatarsus varus), (2) equinovarus (clubfoot), (3) internal tibial torsion, (4) internal femoral torsion, or (5) internal rotation contracture of the hip.

Cavus feet. Cavus feet are characterized by exceedingly high arches, usually associated with equinus deformity of the forefeet, mild calcaneus position of the heels, and clawing of the toes. This condition is seldom recognized before the age of 3 or 4 years; it may increase progressively. Because such conditions as a neurologic abnormality in the lower spine (Charcot-Marie-Tooth disease), poliomyelitis, or Friedreich ataxia may cause cavus deformities, a thorough neurologic evaluation is indicated.

A mild deformity is treated by gently stretching the plantar fascia; the forefoot is repeatedly dorsiflexed, thus flattening the longitudinal arch. Placing a metatarsal pad behind the metatarsal heads or a metatarsal bar in a similar position on the sole of the shoe is also helpful. A severe deformity may require operation, such as tendon transfer, capsulotomy, or triple arthrodesis, with a midtarsal dorsal wedge resection. Triple arthrodesis should be delayed until the child attains a skeletal age of at least 10 years.

Orthopaedic consultation is necessary in persistent deformity.

Trauma. Trauma is frequent in childhood. Conservative treatment results in rapid recovery from musculofascial strains, bruises, contusions, and mild ligamentous sprains. However, when acute pain in the foot is associated with hyperemia, swelling, and tenderness in the midtarsal region, a march fracture must be considered. This condition, rare in childhood, results from excessive foot strain. Diagnosis is confirmed by radiographs that reveal a transverse zone of increased density across a metatarsal bone, usually the second or third. Later a fracture line appears in the zone of condensation. Treatment consists of rest and supporting the foot in a walking boot cast. Complete recovery can be anticipated.

Freiberg disease. Osteochondrosis of the second metatarsal head occurs fairly frequently during adolescence. It is characterized by pain and swelling at the metatarsal arch and especially by tenderness over the second metatarsal head. Radiographs confirm the diagnosis. Treatment is symptomatic.

Köhler disease. Osteochondrosis of the navicular is characterized by pain, swelling, hyperemia, and tenderness along the medial side of the longitudinal arch. In the early stage the radiograph reveals increased density of the navicular; later, fragmentation becomes evident. The affection occurs chiefly between the ages of 6 and 10 years. It should not be confused with the normal multiple centers of ossification seen in the navicular before the age of 6 years. When the osteochondrosis is mild, treatment consists of using arch supports and, if necessary, crutches. When it is severe, a walking boot cast may be necessary. Proper treatment and time lead to complete regeneration and relief of symptoms within a few months.

Sever disease. Sever disease, or osteochondrosis of the apophysis of the os calcis, appears frequently in the 8- to 12-year-old age group, especially in extremely active children. It is characterized by pain in the heels occurring during activity, such as running and jumping. Examination may reveal mild swelling about the posterior aspect of the heels and moderate tenderness to palpation over the apophysis of the os calcis. Radiographs of the heel show a fragmentation and sclerosis of this epiphyseal center. The diagnosis is primarily clinical. Treatment consists of reduction in the child's activities, elevation of the heel of the shoe, removal of the heel counter or spur leather, and addition of sponge rubber inside the shoe. In the more severely involved case, plastic heel cups may be helpful. Occasionally, it may be necessary to apply a walking boot cast.

KNEE

Genu varum (bowleg). Bowlegs may be congenital in origin, may be the result of rickets, or may be caused by osteochondrosis of the proximal tibial epiphysis (Blount disease). Because an adequate amount of vitamin D is almost universally added to commercially available milks, and because this vitamin is usually added to the diets of children, rickets resulting from a deficiency of vitamin D has become rare in the United States. Congenital abnormalities of the renal tubules are now chiefly responsible for rickets. Treating the metabolic abnormalities caused by such tubular defects may decrease the severity of the associated rickets and the tendency for the legs to bow. Various anomalies of cartilage maturation (e.g., hereditary metaphyseal dysostosis) of the epiphyseal cartilages about the knee may produce bowing.

In Blount disease the bowing occurs in the region of the proximal tibial epiphysis. Radiographic changes are most evident at about the age of 2 years. Treatment usually consists of corrective splinting. Treated early, prognosis is excellent. When the deformity is severe or neglected, surgical correction by osteotomy is indicated.

Genu valgum (knock-knee). Knock-knee is not considered congenital and is seldom seen in newborn infants. Causes include rickets, poliomyelitis, debilitating diseases, and trauma or infection involving the proximal tibial epiphysis. It is more frequent in girls, probably because their pelves are wider and their ligaments and musculature are more relaxed.

When the child is standing, the knees touch each other, ankles are apart, and feet are pronated. Children with moderate or severe genu valgum should be careful while participating in body contact sports because of susceptibility to strains and fractures. Fatigability and leg pain are frequent complaints.

If the condition is caused by vitamin D–deficiency rickets, vitamin D should be administered. If it is caused by rickets secondary to renal tubular defects, treating the metabolic abnormalities may be helpful. Any other debilitating condition should be treated. Mechanical management of mild deformities consists of using knock-knee night splints and, for severe deformities, day braces also. Shoes should have high tops, elevation under the medial side of the heel, and scaphoid pads inside. Severe neglected deformities can be corrected by osteotomy.

Genu recurvatum (back-knee). Back-knee is characterized by hyperextension of the knee. It may be congenital, developmental, or the result of abnormal intrauterine position. At birth it is a striking and startling deformity. Even when severe, prognosis is good with proper treatment, which consists of repeatedly applying corrective plaster casts, wedged to flex the tibia on the femur at the knee.

Developmental genu recurvatum may be caused by trauma or infections involving the proximal tibial epiphysis. Operation may be necessary, but conservative treatment generally suffices. Shoe heels should be elevated so that the patient's weight is shifted forward on the toes at all times. Moccasins or shoes without heels should never be worn. Corrective exercises are also indicated. Any child or adolescent with 10° or more of genu recurvatum should avoid body contact sports because the ligaments of the knee are more susceptible to traumatic disruption. Further recurvature or hyperextension may cause disruption of the peroneal nerve or popliteal vessels. When a recurvatum is caused by arthrogryposis, the prognosis is extremely poor.

Internal tibial torsion. In internal tibial torsion the tibia is greatly twisted or rotated internally, usually because of an abnormal intrauterine position. The primary deformity is not, as often suspected, forefoot adduction, equinovarus, tibia vara, or internal rotation of the hips. Anteroposterior radiographs of the legs show a discrete space between the tibia and fibula at the ankle and not the overlap of these bones, as normally seen. The deformity may be self-limiting and correct spontaneously with growth, but when torsion is more than 25°, treatment is indicated. Parents are taught to derotate the tibia manually by applying corrective pressure 12 to 15 times, 3 times a day. Corrective shoes are fitted. If no improvement occurs in 3 to 6 months, corrective splinting is indicated. If active treatment is required, it should be instituted before the child is 3 years old. As the child grows older, the bone becomes harder and more resistant to the derotational forces applied by corrective splints and shoes. Faulty sitting habits of the child should be corrected.

Congenital recurrent dislocation of patella. Congenital dislocation of the patella (extremely rare) should be treated surgically by reattaching the patellar tendon more medially on the tibia. Recurrent patellar dislocation is frequent and is caused by the pull of the quadriceps mechanism in an abnormal direction. Usually there is a history of direct force applied to the patella or rotary twisting strain of the knee (common in some contortionist dancing). The dislocation generally is lateral and reduces spontaneously. The diagnosis is established by the history: "giving away" and pain, followed rapidly by transitory effusion and tenderness over the knee medial to the patella and by pain on attempting to displace the patella laterally, referred to as the apprehension test. For acute or initial dislocation, treatment consists of reducing the dislocation (if it has not reduced spontaneously) and immobilizing the limb at 0 degrees in a plaster cylinder for 4 weeks. Patients with recurrent dislocation should be referred to an orthopedist for surgical correction.

Osgood-Schlatter disease. Osgood-Schlatter disease is epiphysitis of the tibial tubercule, occurring between the ages of 9 and 15 years. It is characterized by pain at the tibial attachment of the patellar tendon and swelling and extreme tenderness over the tibial tubercle. Diagnosis is confirmed by lateral radiograph of the knee showing fragmentation of the epiphysis of the tibial tubercle. Treatment is conservative: restricting activity and applying heat locally for relief of pain. Surgery is not indicated. An uncooperative patient should be treated by immobilization in a plaster or fiberglass cylinder from groin to ankle for 3 to 4 weeks. Parents should be warned that symptoms will recur sporadically but will respond to the same treatment. Symptoms subside when epiphyseal growth is complete. If the residual deformity (a bony prominence) is cosmetically disturbing, it can be removed surgically.

Osteochondritis dissecans. In the traumatic

condition of osteochondritis dissecans an area of articular cartilage and its corresponding subchondral bone become demarcated. The area may become detached and form a loose body (joint mouse). The lesion characteristically involves the medial femoral condyle, but it is frequently seen in the ankle and may occur in any major joint. If the fragment becomes detached, it must be removed surgically. Before the fragment becomes detached, conservative treatment results in complete recovery in most children. Between the ages of 2 and 6 years irregular ossification of the femoral condyles should not be mistaken for osteochondritis dissecans.

HIP

Dysplasia of the hip. Congenital dislocation of the hip generally begins as a presubluxation or dysplasia, rather than as an actual dislocation. Before the age of 1 month physical signs are usually characteristic enough for the diagnosis to be established by a careful examination. These signs result from insecure anchorage of the femoral head within the acetabulum. Most congenitally dislocated hips can and should be diagnosed on the day of birth (see following discussion of clinical manifestations).

Etiology. Current opinion is that a variety of factors may be responsible. From early in the embryologic development of the limb bud until the end of the first trimester, chances for malformation are numerous. Delay in rotation of the limb bud or in muscle innervation during the period of rapid growth may produce changes in the acetabulum or femoral head. During the second and third trimesters, malposition in utero may predispose to dysplasia. Abnormal anteversion of the femoral neck may occur during rotation of the limb bud. Delay in development of the limbus (the fibrocartilaginous structure that forms the superior rim of the acetabulum) and inversion of the limbus may be predisposing factors. Any condition adversely affecting development and relationships of the femoral head and neck may be a cause.

Heredity plays an important role in congenital dysplasia of the hip. The condition is seven times more frequent in girls than in boys. It is twenty-five to thirty times more frequent in first-degree relatives (siblings and offspring) of affected patients than in the general population, a frequency of about 1 in 500, with a recurrence risk of 6% to 7% for sisters of affected patients. Some areas of the world, especially the continent of Europe, seem to be plagued by this malady. In the Orient the condition is extremely rare; this may be a result of the custom of carrying the baby astride the mother's hip with the legs widely abducted. Salter induced acetabular dysplasia in pigs by keeping the hips in extension for 6 weeks. The pigs were then permitted to run freely for 10 weeks, and the condition corrected itself.

Clinical manifestations. Physical findings are often more diagnostic than radiographic manifestations. On inspection of hips and thighs the most obvious abnormality involves the skinfolds anteriorly and posteriorly. This abnormality is caused by proximal displacement of the hip resulting from muscle spasm. Anteriorly, an extra fold can often be seen, as well as asymmetry of the inguinal folds. Posteriorly, an extra gluteal fold with the buttock displaced proximally on the dislocated side is common. When examined manually, hip abduction on the affected side is found to be greatly restricted. Normally abduction is possible to 90°, but in the dislocated hip it is limited to 45° or 50°. Manipulation may also reveal telescoping of the hip joint. As the dislocation increases in severity, an external rotation deformity of the limb becomes obvious. In an older child, lordosis may occur, and in bilateral dislocations the lordosis will produce a waddling gait. A positive Trendelenburg sign is found in a child old enough to stand; the opposite side of the pelvis is depressed toward the floor when the patient stands on the affected limb.

Radiographic findings. Fortunately, simple measurements on correctly taken radiographs of the hips and proper interpretation permit accurate diagnosis. The *acetabular index,* or inclination of the acetabular roof, is measured as follows: a line is drawn transversely between the triradiate (or Y) cartilages of the acetabula; a second line is drawn from the Y cartilage of the acetabulum in question proximally and laterally tangential to the ossified acetabular roof. The angle between these two lines is called the acetabular index and indicates the inclination of the roof. An angle of 30° or less is normal. A more obtuse angle means potential instability and may lead to dislocation of the femoral head.

Another useful measurement involves drawing a horizontal line between the triradiate cartilage of the hips and a line perpendicularly from the outer lip of the acetabular rim. These lines produce a cross. The head of the femur or the potential nidus of the head of the femur should lie in the medial lower quadrant of this cross. If the epiphysis lies superior or lateral to this inner lower quadrant, there is a dislocated or subluxated hip. Because the bony nidus for the capital femoral epiphysis usually does not appear until 4 to 6 weeks after birth, it may be necessary to estimate from the appearance of the femoral neck the point at which the nidus should be located and to visualize the cartilaginous femoral head by relating it to the neck.

Differential diagnosis. In differential diagnosis, coxa vara is the most important condition to consider. Coxa vara, a dysplasia of the femoral neck, may produce similar physical findings. Diagnosis is definitely established by radiographs. Differential diagnosis is concerned also with congenital absence of a part of the femur, coxa plana, slipped epiphysis, acute and chronic infections of the hip joint, neoplasms, and various metabolic diseases.

Treatment. For a mildly dysplastic hip without dislocation, simple conservative treatment is indicated; the hips are held in a position of wide abduction with several diapers or a Pavlek harness. If the results are not favorable, the patient should be referred to an orthopedist. For a definite dislocation in which the hip is not easily reduced or is unstable after reduction, manipulative reduction and plaster immobilization in the frog-legged position may be indicated. If reduction is difficult or unstable, an arthrogram is indicated. If the femoral head is riding high above the superior rim of the acetabulum, then a period of traction as recommended by Crego, or home traction used by McEwing, should be employed for several weeks before reduction is attempted.

If reduction is impossible by manipulation alone, surgical incision and repositioning of the femoral head under the limbus is usually necessary because the limbus may be folded down inside the acetabulum, preventing reduction. Early accurate reduction, either closed or open, and protection of the hip until the acetabular index is normal and ossification of the capital epiphysis is well advanced are essential. When diagnosis is prompt and reduction accurate, a good hip that will function well throughout life can be anticipated.

If, after adequate reduction and immobilization, the hip tends to subluxate or a deficient acetabulum exists, a rotational osteotomy of the femoral shaft or a Salter innominate osteotomy may be necessary. In general, the older the child when the dysplastic hip is recognized, the more likely surgical intervention will be required. The Pemberton, Colonna, or Chiari procedure may be indicated.

Coxa vara. Congenital coxa vara, a defect in the femoral neck, may be unilateral or bilateral, and although there is a hereditary tendency, it should be considered a developmental anomaly. Many etiologic factors have been implicated: rickets, debilitating diseases, fractures, osteochondrosis, chondrodysplasia, hypothyroidism, or any circulatory disturbance in the area.

Clinical manifestations. The most obvious feature is a painless waddling gait with a gluteus medius limp. The condition may be noticed from about the age of 3 years until the end of adolescence. There is considerable limitation of abduction despite normal motion in all other planes. The Trendelenburg test is positive and becomes progressively more so with increasing age. Telescoping, a prominent finding in congenital dislocation, cannot be elicited.

Radiographic findings. Diagnosis is confirmed by radiographs showing a decrease in the angle between the neck and shaft from the normal 135° to 90° or less. Typically, a triangular area of bone is demarcated in the inferior part of the neck adjacent to the head, with a band of decreased density across the neck. The femoral head is situated low in the acetabulum, which is shallow, slanting, and abnormally wide.

Treatment. Osteotomy is done to correct the abnormal angulation of the neck. Bone grafting may be necessary.

Slipping of the capital femoral epiphysis (adolescent coxa vara). Slipping of the capital femoral epiphysis is a mechanical derangement of the epiphyseal plate. It occurs in children between the ages of 10 and 16 years, most frequently in the obese child or the very tall, thin, rapidly growing child. Because girls mature earlier than boys, they are affected at an earlier age. However, the condition is five times more frequent in boys. Both hips are involved in about

40% of cases. Consequently, when slipping has occurred in one hip, the other hip must be carefully watched.

Clinical manifestations. There are three types of slipping: (1) traumatic, in which the epiphysis is actually displaced by a definite injury; (2) gradual, in which the epiphysis is gradually displaced without a definite injury (this is the most frequent type); and (3) combined gradual and traumatic slipping, in which the epiphysis is gradually displaced during several weeks or months, after which further displacement is caused by an acute injury.

The earlier a slipping is diagnosed and treated, the better will be the prognosis. The condition should always be suspected when a child between the ages of 10 and 16 years complains of acute or chronic pain in the hip or knee, especially if the child is tall and lanky or unusually obese. Because in over one half of the patients pain is referred to the knee, the physician should not be misled and fail to examine the hip. Examination of the hip reveals restriction of internal rotation and, depending on the degree of displacement, a tendency to external rotation and flexion. A common associated finding is chronic or subacute tonsillitis. Some authorities consider infection an important predisposing cause to epiphyseal involvement.

Differential diagnosis. Traumatic or infectious synovitis, tuberculosis, coxa plana, congenital coxa vara, and fracture must be considered.

Anteroposterior and lateral radiographs are essential and will show widening and rotation of the epiphyseal plate and local rarefaction of the inferior medial portion of the neck, as well as that the Shenton line is interrupted. Late callus formation appears at the superior and posterior junction of the head and neck. The bared anterosuperior portion of the femoral neck becomes humped.

Treatment. Treatment is surgical. Before actual slipping has occurred, or when displacement is less than one third of the width of the neck, the epiphysis should be pinned in situ. Fixation should be with Knowles' pins, or similar pins—never with Smith-Peterson or similar nails that are driven into the head and neck of the femur. When displacement is more than one third the width of the neck, gentle manipulative reduction or osteotomy followed by internal fixation is indicated. Obesity or any other systemic involvement should also be treated if present.

Unless adequate therapy is instituted promptly, complications such as ankylosis, pathologic dislocation at the epiphyseal plate, avascular necrosis, or sequestration of the capital epiphysis may occur.

Pathologic dislocation of the hip. Pathologic dislocation may be caused by acute or chronic infection, flaccid or spastic paralysis of surrounding muscles, or progressive central dislocation or intrapelvic protrusion of the femoral head. Orthopedic consultation is indicated.

Coxa plana (Legg-Calvé-Perthes disease). Coxa plana was first described in 1910 by Legg (United States), Calvé (France), and Perthes (Germany). This entity (flat hip) occurs in children between the ages of 5 and 10 years and progresses through three pathologic stages: condensation, fragmentation, and regeneration of the capital femoral epiphysis. Although its etiology is unknown, there is a disturbance of circulation not only in the capital epiphysis but also in the epiphyseal plate and acetabulum. Coxa plana is self-limiting and passes through its three stages in more or less than 36 months. Whether recovery is complete or a permanent deformity results is determined primarily by two factors: (1) the age of onset (the younger the patient, the more complete is the recovery) and (2) efficiency of treatment. Weight bearing must be prevented until the stage of regeneration is well advanced.

Diagnosis. Diagnosis is established by radiographic findings. Early, only the shadow of the swollen capsule and possibly a widening of the joint space are seen. The first osseous changes consist of widening of the epiphyseal plate, with a ground-glass appearance and widening of the femoral neck adjacent to the plate. The first change in the epiphysis is a "jockey cap" configuration of bone in its superior part, caused by areas of rarefaction beneath the subchondral bone plate. A little later, irregular areas of condensation are seen throughout the epiphysis. Even later, considerable fragmentation of the entire epiphysis and loss of its normal contour are seen; if weight bearing is permitted at this stage, the epiphysis will develop typical flattening and broadening (coxa plana).

In the differential diagnosis early tuberculosis, acute or chronic synovitis, rheumatoid arthritis, slipping of the proximal femoral epiphysis, congenital dysplasia of the hip, and coxa vara are to be considered.

Treatment. Weight bearing is prevented until regeneration of the epiphysis is well advanced. Bed rest, with Buck traction to the leg, and systematic exercises are ideal. When acute pain and muscle spasm have subsided, walking with crutches can be allowed and a Fort harness or nonweight-bearing brace may be used to maintain the hip in abduction and prevent weight transmission through the femoral head. Atrophy of the extremity is prevented by nonweight-bearing exercises. Osteotomies and bone grafts are of little value.

Kelly et al. reviewed 80 hips in 80 patients with Legg-Calvé-Perthes disease seen at the Campbell Clinic (Memphis), with an average follow-up of about 22½ years. They concluded the following: (1) Most of these patients can be treated by nonsurgical procedures. (2) Poor results occur in children who are beyond 6 years of age at onset of symptoms. (3) Poor results occur in Catterall types III and IV, but the Catterall classification is not adequate for determining early treatment.

Canale and Kelly have devised a dynamic abduction brace (DAB) for containment of the involved hip. When the shoe of the unaffected side is elevated 1½ to 2 inches, application of the DAB brace results in abduction of the involved hip.

Acute pyogenic arthritis of the hip. (See p. 494.)

Nonspecific synovitis of the hip. Synovitis may be acute or chronic, traumatic or infectious. Painful muscle spasms and limp are the chief clinical features. The hip is usually in a position of flexion and external rotation. Motion is severely limited, and pressure over the trochanter produces pain. It is important to realize that over 60% of all children complaining of hip pain have only synovitis that is not serious and is generally the result of trauma. Synovitis must be differentiated from affections of the hip already discussed and, in addition, bursitis about the hip or pelvis. Treatment consists of bed rest, traction, application of heat, and specific antibiotic therapy as indicated. Symptoms usually subside rapidly.

Growth of the epiphysis may be stimulated as a result of increased vascularity, resulting in a larger femoral head.

SPINE

Before abnormalities of the spine are considered, its normal physiologic curves must be mentioned. Maximal posterior curvature in kyphosis develops in the area of the fifth, sixth, and seventh thoracic vertebrae, and anterior curvature, or lordosis, develops in the lumbar spine. There is no physiologic lateral curvature.

Adolescent kyphosis (osteochondritis deformans juvenilis; Scheuermann disease). In Scheuermann disease, ossification of the vertebral body epiphyses is abnormal. The cause is unknown. Several contiguous vertebrae are involved, usually in the lower thoracic and upper lumbar areas, varying from mild irregularity of the epiphyses to severe wedging. Backache and gradually developing kyphosis generally begin between the ages of 12 and 16 years. The symptoms are self-limiting but may last for 2 or 3 years. In diagnosis, tuberculosis, brucellosis, pyogenic infection, neoplasm, or blood dyscrasia should be considered.

Treatment. Measures should be instituted to prevent deformity of the spine. Symptoms are lessened by the child's lying supine for 15 to 20 minutes several times daily. Exercises to extend the dorsal spine, obliterate the lumbar lordosis, and stretch tight hamstring muscles are extremely important. When the symptoms are severe, when there is vertebral wedging, or when deformity is shown on a standing lateral x-ray film, orthopedic consultation is indicated and a Milwaukee brace may be necessary.

Vertebra plana; Calvé disease. Vertebra plana is a rare lesion and usually develops in children between the ages of 4 and 8 years. It may be localized to a single vertebral body but occasionally involves several in different locations in the spine. Vetebral bodies may be fragmented or uniformly flattened, but the disc spaces remain normal. As healing occurs, a considerable increase in bone density is seen on the radiograph. This lesion is generally believed to result from eosinophilic granuloma, and an orthopedic surgeon should be consulted. With multiple lesions, the diagnosis of Hand-Schüller-Christian syndrome should be considered. Easy fatigability and nocturnal pain are characteristic symptoms. Muscle spasm, point tenderness, and occasionally a slight angular kyphosis are the usual physical signs.

Anomalies of the lumbosacral area

Developmental anomalies are more frequent in the lumbosacral area than elsewhere in the spine. Included are spondylolisthesis, spina bifida occulta, sacralization of the last lumbar vertebra, scoliosis, and diastematomyelia.

Spondylolisthesis. In spondylolisthesis the primary pathologic condition consists of defects in the pars interarticularis between the two vertebrae, which allows the superior vertebra to displace anteriorly. Spondylolisthesis involves the fifth lumbar and the first sacral vertebrae most often. A defect in the pars interarticularis without displacement of the vertebra is known as spondylolysis and may be unilateral or bilateral.

Clinical manifestations. Spondylolisthesis is rare in early childhood but fairly common in adolescence. Low back pain, which usually radiates into the thighs posteriorly, is the presenting symptom. Pain is accentuated by activity and relieved by rest and recumbency. Flexion is limited and painful. Straight leg raising is limited by hamstring spasm. When spondylolisthesis is severe, a tender dimple or "step-off" is present in the midline at the lumbosacral level.

Radiographic findings. Defects in the pars interarticularis are seen more easily in the lateral radiograph with the spine flexed. When the presence of a defect is questionable, oblique films are indicated and will confirm the diagnosis.

Treatment. The initial treatment should be symptomatic, with a low back brace and systematic exercises to strengthen the back and abdominal muscles. If pain persists after several months of conservative treatment or if slipping of the vertebra occurs, arthrodesis of the involved area may be necessary.

Spina bifida occulta. Spina bifida occulta is a defect of closure in the laminae of one or more vertebrae. It occurs most frequently at the fifth lumbar or first sacral level. Back pain (with or without radiation) may lead to its discovery, but more frequently the defect is noted as an incidental radiographic finding. Spina bifida occulta is ordinarily not a condition that produces symptoms requiring treatment. Involvement of more than one segment may increase one's risk for having offspring with neural tube defects. Other defects should be considered when symptoms are significant.

Sacralization of the fifth lumbar vertebra. In sacralization one or both of the transverse processes of the fifth lumbar vertebra are long and wide and are either fused to, or articulate with, the sacrum or ilium. This condition ordinarily is not a cause of symptoms in the pediatric age group. Even in adults its significance is controversial.

Scoliosis. Scoliosis is a physical sign. It is a lateral spinal curve and may be structural or nonstructural (functional). Nonstructural curves are flexible, bend equally to each side, and demonstrate no fixation or pathologic change. Structural curves do not bend equally to each side, and the curve or deformity exhibits some degree of fixation.

Structural scoliosis is characterized by pathologic changes of the spine and its supporting structures. It may be idopathic, with no apparent etiologic factor. Most idiopathic curves are believed to be familial, genetic in origin, and inherited. Poliomyelitis, nutritional factors, endocrine abnormalities, vitamin deficiencies, and stress or trauma have been considered as causes. Structural scoliosis may also be congenital and caused by hemivertebra or other congenital anomalies of the spine. Other causes are thoracoplasty, cerebral palsy, neurofibromatosis, Marfan syndrome, syringomyelia, muscular dystrophy, and amyotonia congenita.

Functional, or nonstructural, scoliosis begins without structural changes of the spine or its supporting framework.

Clinical manifestations. Deformity is the chief clinical manifestation. Unlevel shoulders or hips, a prominent scapula, an asymmetric waist, and a list of the torso are common physical findings. There is mild discomfort but seldom pain. However, pain may occasionally be a complaint. Pain, when present, demands an immediate, thorough study.

Diagnosis. Early diagnosis and prompt treatment are imperative. An attempt must be made to determine the primary cause. Neurologic consultation may be necessary. If no cause is discovered, the scoliosis is considered idiopathic.

Fixed rotation is a quality of a structural curve

that may be detected clinically by the *forward bending test*. Fixed rotation—and thus, presumably, structural scoliosis—is detected by visualizing from the head or rear a standing patient bent forward at the hips, with the head and arms down as if to dive. Asymmetric prominence of the paraspinal muscles or the ribs adjacent to the spine constitutes a presumptive positive test for structural scoliosis. The patient should be referred to an orthopedic surgeon, and no radiographs are necessary before referral. A single standing anteroposterior view at a distance of 1.8 m (6 feet) will confirm the diagnosis and is best made by the consultant who will treat or follow up the patient.

Treatment. Treatment depends on the age of the patient and the location, severity, and rapidity of increase of the curves. An orthopedist should regulate therapy.

Treatment of scoliosis is operative or nonoperative. Many types of braces or orthoses are now available to attempt to stop the progression of curves in growing patients. The basis for all such appliances is the Milwaukee brace, which has proved to be effective in halting progression but not in producing reversal of the curve or permanent improvement. Exercises and physical therapy programs are beneficial for the patient, but if used alone do not constitute appropriate therapy for a progressing curve in a growing patient.

Surgery is used most frequently for (1) congenital scoliosis; (2) deforming curves in mature patients and also in younger patients; (3) curves that progress during nonoperative or orthotic treatment; (4) collapsing spines associated with neuromuscular disorders; and (5) curves associated with neurofibromatosis. The basis for surgical treatment is a posterior spinal fusion with added bone graft—usually from the patient's iliac wings. Internal fixation, usually supplemented by plaster cast immobilization, is routinely used whenever the bones of the vertebrae are strong enough to withstand direct corrective force. When they are not, a plaster cast alone or a traction cast is used. The most widely employed type of internal fixation is Harrington instrumentation posteriorly. Dwyer instrumentation anteriorly with fusion may be indicated when posterior correction and fusion are not feasible or are inefficient. Cast immobilization for 6 to 12 months is necessary after surgical treatment.

Diastematomyelia. Diastematomyelia is a congenital anomaly in which a bony spicule protrudes posteriorly from the posterior surface of a vertebral body into the middle of the spinal canal. The spicule is attached to the posterior layer of spinal dura and divides the spinal cord or the cauda equina into lateral halves. During growth the spine normally grows faster than the spinal cord; in diastematomyelia this attachment of the dura to the bone prevents the cord from retracting normally into the thoracolumbar area. Consequently the cord is stretched. Clinically the anomaly is characterized by low back pain, limitation of flexion of the back, and severe limitation of straight leg raising. Other symptoms may relate to the bowel or bladder, motor weakness, or sensation. Neurologic examination may reveal reflex, motor, or sensory deficits. External signs include pigmented areas, hemangiomas, cutaneous growths, lipomas, and hairy patches over the involved areas of the spine. Radiographs may show congenital anomalies of the spine. The diagnosis is confirmed by a myelogram. Treatment is surgical.

CERVICAL SPINE AND NECK

The cervical spine may be affected by most of the lesions found in other parts of the spine, as well as by entities peculiar to the neck, such as torticollis, cervical rib, and other anomalies.

Spina bifida. Spina bifida of the cervicodorsal area is second in frequency to that in the lumbosacral area. Usually the dura does not protrude through the defect, and the lesion is suspected by finding a dimpling or excessive hair in the region of the seventh cervical vertebra. After the diagnosis is made by radiographs, only periodic observation is necessary. However, a meningocele may develop and protrude through the defect. When this or other neurologic defects are suspected, neurosurgical and orthopedic consultations are indicated.

Hemivertebra. Hemivertebra is a congenital spinal anomaly caused by the incomplete development of one side of a vertebra. The immediately adjacent vertebrae may grow faster than normal and produce fairly sharp and localized scoliosis. Hemivertebrae usually require no treatment, but if the scoliosis increases in severity, orthopedic consultation is indicated.

Klippel-Feil syndrome. In the Klippel-Feil syndrome one or more cervical vertebrae are usually absent, and two or more may be fused together. Often the head appears to rest on the shoulders rather than on the neck. Radiographs of the cervical spine show varying degrees of deformity. Other congenital defects of spine, chest, and limbs may occur. Treatment is indicated only when marked webbing of the skin of the neck may be improved by plastic surgery.

Sprengel deformity. Sprengel deformity is a congenital anomaly that is characterized by elevation of the scapula. Frequently an extra ossicle (the omovertebral bone) connects the scapula to the cervical spine. Mild cervicodorsal scoliosis is usual. The scapula is sometimes so greatly elevated that it appears to be attached to the mastoid process. Treatment in most instances is conservative and consists of neck and shoulder girdle exercises. When the deformity is severe, operation may be indicated.

Torticollis (wryneck). Torticollis may be congenital or acquired. When it is congenital, the pathologic change is usually located in the sternocleidomastoid muscle. There is an apparent shortening of the neck, a tilting of the head to the affected side, and rotation of the chin toward the opposite shoulder. When it is acquired, trauma, tuberculosis, osteomyelitis, acute myositis, lymphangitis, lymphadenitis, a cervical spine dislocation, or a fracture may be the cause.

Congenital torticollis. Theoretically, congenital torticollis is present at birth, but it is rarely diagnosed before the tenth to fourteenth day. It occurs more often in girls. A cylindric nontender mass is generally palpable in the sternocleidomastoid muscle. As it becomes fibrotic it shortens the muscle, and the adjacent muscles become contracted secondarily. When the condition is severe and untreated, a characteristic asymmetry of the face and neck develops. If corrected early, this asymmetry improves rapidly.

Early conservative treatment usually produces an excellent result. The neck is stretched by forcing the head away from the affected side and rotating the chin toward the shoulder of the affected side. The mass in the sternomastoid muscle is gently massaged.

When severe torticollis fails to respond to several weeks of conservative treatment and a mass is present in the sternocleidomastoid muscle, the mass should be excised. In neglected cases the sternal, clavicular, and mastoid attachments of the muscle are excised. After operation, corrective stretching and active exercises are necessary for several months.

Cervical ribs, thoracic outlet, and the scalenus muscle syndrome. After leaving the cervical plexus the seventh and eighth cervical nerves pass over the transverse process of the seventh cervical vertebra or perhaps a supernumerary rib attached to it and may be compressed against such a rib. If the compression is sufficient, symptoms are produced along the distribution of the nerve. These conditions are rare in infancy, but they may occur in adolescence. Girls are affected more often than boys.

Examination reveals considerable tenderness over the nerves in the supraclavicular area. Stretching the upper extremity, especially in a dependent position, may accentuate symptoms. When symptoms are severe, elevating the arm above the head may obliterate the radial pulse. Ischemia of the hand may occur in severe or untreated injuries and produce clawing of the fingers. In the differential diagnosis, synringomyelia, progressive muscular atrophy, ruptured cervical disc, spinal cord tumor, or localized ulnar nerve palsy must be considered.

Treatment. Conservative treatment should always be tried. Infiltrating the scalenus muscle or stellate ganglion with a local anesthetic may produce temporary relief and help confirm the diagnosis. During sleep the arm should be elevated and externally rotated at the shoulder. Corrective exercises to strengthen the muscles of the neck and shoulder girdle are extremely important. When conservative treatment fails, the cervical rib or scalenus muscle should be resected. In extreme cases when symptoms persist, it may be necessary to remove the first rib of the thoracic cage.

THORAX

Deformities of the thorax. Deformities of the thorax are infrequent and rarely disabling but may be alarming to parents.

Pectus planum. Pectus planum is characterized by flattening of the chest anteriorly, usually by moderate dorsal kyphosis and sometimes by the absence of one or more of the pectoral muscles. It seldom progresses in severity and is only important cosmetically. Treatment consists of corrective exercises to decrease the kyphosis and to strengthen the muscles of the back.

Pectus carinatum (pigeon chest). The sternum projects anteriorly in a sharp angle, like that of a pigeon. The anteroposterior diameter of the chest is increased. One side of the chest is usually more prominent than the other. It may improve spontaneously with growth. Deep breathing exercises and other exercises to strengthen the muscles of the neck and thorax may be helpful. Pectus carinatum may be a component feature of more generalized conditions such as Marfan syndrome and homocystinuria.

Pectus excavatum (funnel chest). In the congenital anomaly of funnel chest the deformity is the reverse of that seen in pectus carinatum. A funnel or deep groove is present in the midline anteriorly. The costochondral cartilages are angulated posteriorly, and the sternum is greatly depressed. Funnel chest may eventually be disabling by producing cardiorespiratory disturbances. It is disfiguring, especially in girls. When the condition is mild, deep breathing and corrective back exercises may be tried. When it is severe or symptomatic, correcting the deformity surgically is indicated and is most gratifying. Pectus excavatum may be a component feature of more generalized conditions such as Turner, Noonan, and Marfan syndromes.

SHOULDER

The shoulder's stability depends almost entirely on its ligaments, capsule, and muscles, and these are especially susceptible to trauma. Many important bursae are located about the joint and may become pathologically involved. Traumatic synovitis, bursitis, and strains of ligaments and muscles cause more than 60% of all painful shoulder conditions in children. Treatment of these traumatic conditions consists of rest with the shoulder in abduction and the use of ice packs for 24 to 36 hours, followed by heat for a similar period. When acute symptoms have subsided, active exercises are begun.

The other 40% of painful shoulder lesions in children are in the majority of instances caused by infections (acute pyogenic, tuberculous, and brucellar) and benign and malignant neoplasms.

A rare but interesting cause is traumatic pericapsulitis, unilateral or bilateral. It is caused by severe trauma, and it can be mistaken for a malignancy. The child has a swollen, painful, hyperemic shoulder that is tender to palpation and painful on manipulation. Radiographs show new periosteal bone around the entire capsule and down the humeral shaft. A carefully taken history usually reveals that a parent, maid, or another child has jerked the arm. Treatment consists of support and rest. The lesion should disappear in 2 to 3 weeks. This condition is often seen as a component of the battered child syndrome (Chapter 13).

ERB PALSY

For a discussion of Erb palsy see p. 265.

ELBOW

The elbow is a hinge joint with a normal range of motion from zero (straight) to 140° flexion. However, in the child the joint may normally hyperextend as much as 10°. Pronation and supination are also integral functions of the elbow. The joint is completely surrounded by tight capsular and ligamentous structures, which when stretched or torn may become fibrotic and limit motion. Because nerves and vessels pass so near, fractures and dislocations of the elbow may cause devastating circulatory and neurologic complications unless treated promptly and properly.

Bursitis. There are ten definite bursae about the elbow, but the important ones are the olecranon and radiohumeral bursae.

The olecranon bursa is located superficial to the olecranon, is often injured, and may become infected. Olecranon bursitis is diagnosed by obtaining a history of repeated trauma or sudden severe injury to the area, followed by pain, tenderness, and fluctuant swelling superficial to the olecranon. Traumatic or nonspecific bursitis is treated by aspirating the bursa, applying compression bandages, using heat locally, and rehabilitating the joint gradually. Infectious bursitis is treated by aspiration and then with appropriate antibiotic therapy. Chronic bursitis that fails to respond to conservative measures demands excision of the entire bursa.

Tennis elbow (epicondylitis). The term *tennis elbow* is used loosely to designate any of several painful lesions that occur on the lateral side of the elbow. The most frequent is epicondylitis, a minute tear in the origin of the common extensor muscles on the lateral humeral epicondyle. The tear causes fibrositis in a pinpoint area that becomes extremely painful and tender. Infiltrating the tender point with a local anesthetic and hydrocortisone is often curative.

Radiohumeral bursitis is one form of tennis elbow. It is diagnosed by finding a localized point of tenderness over the radial head. Treatment is the same as just outlined for epicondylitis.

Nursemaid's elbow. Nursemaid's elbow occurs in children 1 to 3 years of age. It is caused by a sudden jerk of the arm, as in picking up a child or lifting him up a step by one hand. The radius is pulled distalward, and the annular ligament is displaced proximally from its normal position around the radial neck to lock around the radial head. The extremity is maintained in a position of adduction and internal rotation, with the elbow extended. The extremity is obviously painful, and the child usually cries vigorously and constantly. Pain is accentuated by any movement of the arm. Radiographs are negative but are necessary to exclude a fracture or dislocation.

Reduction of the subluxation is relatively easy and requires no anesthesia. With the elbow flexed to 90°, the forearm is quickly and forcibly supinated and pronated while pressure is exerted over the radial head by the operator's thumb. A definite click is felt, pain is immediately and completely relieved, and the child resumes use of the arm. If the injury is recent, no immobilization is necessary. If it occurred several days previously, there may be residual soreness and local edema. In this instance the elbow is splinted at 90° for 2 or 3 days, after which complete freedom of use is allowed.

WRIST AND HAND

Tenosynovitis. Inflammation of the tendon sheaths in the hand and wrist may be acute or chronic, traumatic or infectious.

Purulent tenosynovitis requires immediate treatment with rest, elevation, local heat, antibiotics, and in the severe case early surgical drainage.

Traumatic tenosynovitis may be caused by either a sudden severe injury or repeated minor injuries to a tendon and its sheath. It usually responds favorably to immobilization, heat, and infiltration of a local anesthetic and hydrocortisone.

Congenital deformities of the hand. Supernumerary digits, syndactylism, cleft or clubbed hand, and other congenital deformities of the hand require consultation with the orthopedist before definitive treatment is undertaken.

TRAUMA

The most frequent orthopedic lesions of childhood after the first year of life are caused by trauma. Fortunately most of these injuries heal without complication or permanent disability.

Soft tissue injuries. An injured muscle, joint capsule, tendon, or soft tissue structure is best treated with rest, immobilization, and during the first 36 to 48 hours application of ice packs locally, followed then by warm packs. Gentle active exercises are begun on the third or fourth day. Activities are resumed gradually.

A muscle injury of the mildest type is caused by direct trauma and results in local muscle spasm. It responds favorably to rest. A more severe injury causes bleeding into muscle and should be treated as described in the preceding paragraph. When the injury is neglected, myositis ossificans may develop and require more prolonged immobilization and rest. An even more severe injury may rupture a muscle. When the rupture is small, conservative treatment suffices; when it is large, immediate surgical repair is indicated.

Fractures. In treating fractures, especially in children, the physician is sometimes tempted to consider the radiographic findings too seriously and to "treat the radiographs" rather than the patient. First, the patient as a whole must be carefully evaluated and treated. Next, an adequate blood supply to the injured area must be maintained. Finally, the extent of damage to the soft tissue, including nerves, and the severity of the fracture are appraised. A plan of treatment is then formulated.

Fractures in children are very different from those in adults. Injured epiphyseal plates, normal variations in bone density, congenital pseudoarthroses, birth fractures, and other conditions peculiar to children must be appraised accurately. That bones of children heal more rapidly than those of adults and that they remodel remarkably well during growth must be considered.

To evaluate a fracture properly, excellent radiographs must be available and must be interpreted correctly. Furthermore, films of the opposite normal extremity should often be made for comparison. To be of value, such films must be made in comparable planes. Failure to compare radiographs of both limbs is responsible for most errors in diagnosing fractures in children, especially those involving an epiphysis.

In a greenstick fracture the cortex on the convex side is broken, but on the concave side it is only buckled. In a torus or infraction fracture the cortex on the concave side is buckled, but the opposite cortex usually shows no injury. Multiple or repeated fractures without a history of sufficient trauma is suggestive of defective bone formation (notably osteogenesis imperfecta) and also the battered child syndrome (see Chapter 13). A single spontaneous fracture suggests a pathologic fracture through a bone cyst, a lesion of fibrous dysplasia, or a giant cell tumor. A more serious neoplasm may be present.

Fractures in children are relatively easy to treat but require mature judgment. Rotation, alignment, apposition, and length must all be considered. Rotation must be corrected early in treatment because later it becomes impossible to correct without operation. An increase in angulation of 10° to 15° in the direction of the normal curve of a bone is permissible, but never more than 5° in the opposite direction. The age of the child and the distance from the fracture to the nearest epiphysis are also important; the younger the child and the closer the fracture to an epiphyseal plate, the better angulation will correct itself with growth. Consequently the older the child and the closer the fracture to the middle of the diaphysis, the more accurate must be the reduction. When a greenstick fracture is reduced, the cortex on the concave side must be thoroughly broken before accurate alignment is possible.

Apposition and length are least important. In girls under 10 years of age or boys under 12 years a long bone may be allowed to unite with an overlap, provided rotation and alignment are satisfactory. Side-to-side apposition results in rapid union, and with growth and remodeling, normal length and contour are restored. For a fracture of the femur or humerus, overlapping is not only acceptable but is usually desirable. The acceleration in longitudinal growth after such a fracture in a child is so great that an overgrowth frequently occurs otherwise.

Fractures involving epiphyseal plates must be clearly understood by the physician and must be explained in detail to the parents. A violent longitudinal thrust that crushes the epiphyseal plate, even when deformity is minimal, invariably retards epiphyseal growth and often results in malalignment. This occurs more frequently in the lower extremity. An epiphyseal injury that does not crush the plate or disturb its blood supply rarely affects growth.

All but the simplest fractures involving joints or epiphyseal plates should be treated by an orthopedic surgeon. The parents should always be warned that there may be disturbances in growth after any epiphyseal injury.

Volkmann ischemic contracture. Failure to recognize a neurovascular complication after any fracture or dislocation about the elbow and to treat it promptly may lead to severe pathologic changes, the most disabling of which is Volkmann ischemic contracture. In this condition, contractures of the fingers and wrist are caused by ischemia of the muscles of the forearm. It usually occurs after improperly treated supracondylar fractures of the humerus. It can occur after severe trauma with or without a fracture in the forearm or hand, such as a laundry wringer injury or pressure from the tire of a vehicle passing over the arm.

Ischemic fibrosis and contracture of forearm muscles are produced by arterial insufficiency caused by spasm or rupture of the brachial artery. It is imperative after injury about the elbow or forearm that the hand be under constant observation for circulatory or neurologic impairment. Cardinal signs of vascular insufficiency indicating impending Volkmann ischemia are (1) pain disproportionate to the severity of the injury, (2) loss of pulses, (3) either pallor or cyanosis of the extremity, (4) loss of sensation, and (5) loss of motor function. If these signs are present, prompt treatment (within 3 to 4 hours) is imperative and is based primarily on reestablishment of the arterial circulation to the extremity and splitting of the fascias in the area.

Battered child syndrome. For a discussion of the battered child syndrome see Chapter 13.

CONGENITAL PSEUDARTHROSIS OF THE TIBIA

Congenital pseudarthrosis of the tibia was first described by Hatzoechor in 1708, and until 1930 amputation was the standard treatment of choice. However, since that date numerous treatment modalities have been described. However, all too often amputation has been the final treatment. Bypass and dual onlay bone grafts have proved most successful, but have of necessity been repeated every few years until the child reaches adolescence. In 1958, Boyd and Sage published a classic article. Their histologic findings noted that specimens in 13 cases showed dense cellulous fibrous connective tissue and within this matrix of fibrous tissue islands of sclerotic bone were found. Most significant, each specimen included a cartilaginous area described as fibrous cartilage, fibrohyaline cartilage, or fibrous tissue metaplastic to cartilage. Only one of 13 cases showed a true synovial-pseudarthrosis. Universally, vascularity at the nonunion site was present. In 1982, Bassett and colleagues reported on 92 patients treated by the use of Pulsing Electromagnetic Fields (PEMF). They found this the most successful and certainly the less traumatic method of treatment. However, they warn that the key to success in the treatment of infantile nonunion is the combination of PEMF treatment with good orthopedic management consisting of rigid immobilization, non-weightbearing status, and rehabilitation with impacting loading exercises. This infantile type of nonunion remains a major challenge to orthopedic surgeons, but PEMF appears to offer some important advantages for overcoming this pernicious condition.

OSSEOUS INFECTIONS

Osteomyelitis. Osteomyelitis, an important infection of infancy and childhood, is now more easily controlled than in the past but still presents problems in diagnosis and management. It occurs more commonly during infancy and in children 8 to 12 years of age. Any bone may be affected, but the most common sites are the distal end of the femur and the proximal ends of the tibia and humerus.

Etiology and predisposing factors. The most common causative organism is hemolytic *Staphylococcus aureus,* which is responsible for approximately 80% of cases. However, a wide variety of other organisms may produce osteomyelitis (especially in neonates), including various streptococci, gram-negative enteric bacteria, and *Salmonella* sp. In children with sickle cell disease, osteomyelitis is frequently caused by *Salmonellae*.

Although osteomyelitis results occasionally from a wound or compound fracture, in children it is classically blood-borne from foci of infection such as furuncles, abrasions of the skin, and impetigo. The disease is more common in children of poor socioeconomic circumstances.

In many patients there is a history of antecedent local trauma. It is thought that bacteria already in the bloodstream find in the stagnant circulation of the contused tissue an excellent opportunity to initiate growth and produce osseous infection. It begins most often in the capillary loops of the metaphyseal region of long bones adjacent to the epiphyseal plate.

Pathologic findings. The infection spreads rapidly into the spongy cancellous marrow, destroying bone and producing necrosis through thrombosis of vessels. It also extends by way of the haversian canals through the cortex to form an abscess that lifts the periosteum and spreads beneath it, thrombosing vessels in this area and adding to the bony necrosis. Thus death of bone results from a combination of septic and avascular necrosis. In infants and very young children the periosteum ruptures early, resulting in a soft tissue abscess. In older children the stronger periosteum resists rupture and contains the infection that spreads beneath it, producing intraosseous tension and bone necrosis.

Death of large portions of the cortex results in formation of sequestra—necrotic cortical fragments that cannot be absorbed and therefore become separated. The elevated periosteum begins to lay down new bone surrounding the necrotic areas—this is called involucrum. It may form in an irregular manner, leaving holes or gaps through which pus may drain to the surface or sequestra may be discharged.

As a rule, the epiphyseal plate is impervious to infection and protects the epiphysis unless the adjacent joint becomes involved. However, the hip joint is an exception to this rule because the neck of the femur is intracapsular.

In some instances osteomyelitis is not a spreading infection as just described. A walled-off, localized area of osteomyelitis 1 to 2 cm (about 3/8 to 3/4 inch) in diameter may occur (Brodie abscess). A chronic nonsuppurative sclerosing infection may produce an increased density of the cortex and is designated as osteomyelitis of Garré.

Clinical manifestations. Classically, signs and symptoms of acute osteomyelitis begin abruptly and build up to maximal intensity during the first few days of the disease. The child appears toxic, the temperature is high, the pulse is rapid, and in older children there is often a chill at onset. There may or may not be an area of localized tenderness over the involved bone. As a rule, however, there is progressively severe localized pain associated with extreme tenderness to pressure (sustained for 1 or 2 minutes) over the affected bone. Localized swelling and erythema are seldom present early but may occur later. If a subperiosteal abscess has formed, rupture of the periosteum is indicated by a sudden decrease in pain and by the appearance of local swelling and redness associated with a temporary diminution in constitutional symptoms.

Laboratory findings. Blood findings are those characteristic of severe pyogenic infection: polymorphonuclear leukocytosis with a shift to the left. Blood culture is usually positive during the early acute stage. Radiographic findings are of little value at onset or within the first 10 to 14 days, although localized soft tissue swelling may be observed. However, it is common to note after 10 to 14 days one or more small areas of rarefaction of the cortex. Soon after, radiographic evidence of new bone formation by elevated periosteum may be observed. The more chronic the process, the greater are the radiographic manifestations, often showing sequestra and involuscrum.

Diagnosis. Acute osteomyelitis may simulate acute pyogenic arthritis, cellulitis, erysipelas, rheumatic fever, and various malignant lesions, notably Ewing endothelial sarcoma. When acute osteomyelitis is a complication of another severe disease, the child may be so toxic and debilitated that bone infection may not be suspected.

Treatment. Acute osteomyelitis can be rapidly progressive and fatal. Therefore prompt vigorous comprehensive therapy is extremely important.

General supportive treatment comprises institution of strict bed rest, adequate hydration and nutrition, and symptomatic measures to relieve pain and fever. Blood transfusion may be indicated, especially in patients who develop anemia rapidly.

Local treatment comprises splinting of the affected extremity to afford complete immobilization, application of massive warm packs, and elevation of the involved member.

Specific therapy is ideally based on knowledge of the causative organism and its sensitivities to antibiotics. For this reason one or more blood cultures are obtained as soon as possible and needle aspiration is performed at the "point of maximal tenderness." However, the physician should not wait for laboratory identification of the organism and determination of its sensitivities before initiating therapy. To do so is to risk additional bone destruction and, in some cases, the patient's life. After cultures have been obtained and while awaiting results, therapy is initiated with a penicillinase-resistant, semisynthetic penicillin such as nafcillin. The patient is treated with intravenous antibiotics until there has been significant clinical improvement, at which time carefully monitored oral therapy may be considered. The total duration of antibiotic therapy generally ranges from 4 to 6 weeks.

The orthopedic surgeon should advise and help in treatment of all patients who do not respond rapidly to treatment as outlined previously. When surgical drainage is required, the insertion of polyethylene tubes will allow the administration of the appropriate antibiotic directly into the infected area. At the same time, other tubes connected to a suction apparatus maintain constant drainage of the infected area. This method often permits primary closure of some surgically drained infections.

Fortunately, modern medical management has greatly reduced the death rate as well as the incidence of chronic osteomyelitis, all too common in former days. Before the antibiotic era the mortality rate was approximately 25%, but it is now only about 2%.

GENERALIZED AFFECTIONS

Osteogenesis imperfecta. Osteogenesis imperfecta is characterized by softness and fragility of the skeleton. Multiple fractures and deformities are common.

Osteogenesis imperfecta (OI) is genetically

determined. Recent evidence indicates the existence of at least four distinct entities that conform to this term. The type constituting the largest proportion of patients (OI, type I) is inherited as an autosomal dominant, with osteoporosis that leads to fractures. Fractures are present at birth in a few cases. Associated with this are congenital blue sclerae and onset of conductive hearing loss in the third or fourth decades secondary to otosclerosis. This is a relatively mild form, and some victims have no history of fractures. This group (OI, type I) is probably further subdivisible into a form with associated dentinogenesis imperfecta and another without it. Prominent clinical variability is the rule. A second group (OI, type II), which includes most patients with neonatal manifestations, is probably inherited in an autosomal recessive manner. Affected infants have multiple congenital fractures, short and bowed limbs, characteristic broad crumpled femora, cranial osteopenia with bone islands in the skull, and beaded ribs, and all those described by Sillence et al. died before or soon after birth. Prenatal diagnosis has been successful in detecting recurrences of autosomal recessive forms.

A third group (OI, type III) also manifests fractures at birth, leading to severe progressive deformities of limbs and spine, along with ligamentous laxity. The degree of blue sclerae is much less severe than that in OI, type I, and decreases with age. Most affected patients of this third group (OI, type III) also have dentinogenesis imperfecta. According to Sillence et al., most such cases are sporadic, and this form of OI is probably genetically heterogeneous, including possibly some autosomal dominant and definitely some autosomal recessive cases. Sillence et al. currently reserve the type III label for those patients with demonstrable autosomal recessive inheritance. The fourth group (OI, type IV), inherited in an autosomal dominant manner, involves normal-colored sclerae and osteoporosis, leading to fractures and variable long bone deformity. A detailed family history, evaluation of immediate family members, and genetic counseling are recommended in all cases. OI, type I may be mistakenly diagnosed as a child abuse case; a careful history, physical examination and appropriate radiologic characteristics will help to differentiate the two.

Straightening long bones by multiple osteotomies and threading the fragments on a medullary rod that remains in place permanently may help. With growth the bone becomes longer than the rod and often fractures beyond its ends. Insertion of a longer rod is then indicated. Telescoping Bailey rods designed to lengthen automatically with bone growth may be used.

Osteopetrosis (marble bones; Albers-Schönberg disease). The chief characteristic of osteopetrosis is radiologic evidence of excessive density of most or all bones of the body. The condition is genetically determined, and two forms probably exist. The first is a more benign form, usually not recognized in infancy and inherited in an autosomal dominant manner; the second is a more severe, more rapidly progressive autosomal recessive form, generally with a fatal outcome in the first decade of life. In the autosomal recessive form particularly, anemia may develop because of bony encroachment on the blood-forming marrow. The spleen, liver, and lymph nodes may enlarge because of extramedullary hematopoiesis. Optic atrophy is frequent. Blood chemistry values are normal.

Although the bones appear intensely hard, like marble, chalky areas of softening that predispose to fracture are frequent. Such fractures are abrupt and transverse, the fragments appear chalky in the radiograph, and callus develops slowly.

Melorheostosis. A distinguishing characteristic of melorheostosis is its significant difference from osteopetrosis. Usually only one extremity is involved and only part of a single bone, which eventually becomes distorted. The radiographic appearance is suggestive of wax flowing down a candle. Often there is severe pain in the bone and limited motion in the adjacent joint. Melorheostosis generally begins in children 5 to 14 years of age. Its etiology is unknown. Scleroderma with fibrosis and thickening of muscles and other soft tissues may occasionally cause stiffness and pain in the area involved. The diagnosis is established only by radiographs. There is no specific therapy.

Multiple cartilaginous exostoses (diaphyseal aclasia; osteochondromas; hereditary deforming enchondromatosis). Multiple cartilaginous exostoses are characterized by the presence of exostoses or cancellous bone covered by a thin cortex and a layer of cartilage. It is sometimes confused with dyschondroplasia (Ollier disease). The condition is inherited in an autosomal dominant manner, about 60% of cases having a familial incidence; the other 40% of cases are sporadic, the result of a new mutation. The lesions are often present at birth but rarely cause difficulty before the age of 6 years and may not be noticed until puberty. They occur on the metaphysis and may be single or multiple. They rarely develop on the diaphysis and never on the epiphysis. The most frequent sites are the distal femoral and proximal tibial metaphyses, but they may develop on any bone of endochondral origin. Symptoms are usually pain and impairment of function because of pressure on joints, muscles, or tendons.

No treatment is indicated unless symptoms from pressure are severe enough to justify excising them. About 5% to 15% of the lesions are reported to become malignant.

Enchondromatosis (Ollier disease). Enchondromatosis is a rare developmental disorder characterized by the presence of rounded columns of displaced hyaline cartilage in the metaphyses of long bones. Although it is considered a variant of the same developmental error as diaphysial aclasia, its characteristic of remaining inside the metaphyses makes differential diagnosis relatively easy. The disorder is seen in early childhood and rarely in newborn infants; it produces a short limb. The etiology is unknown. The phalanages, the pelvis, and the ulna are frequently involved, and, as in diaphysial aclasia, the ulna is often shorter than the radius. Other long bones may be shortened as much as 2.5 cm. Characteristically the disorder is unilateral. Occasionally a lesion projects from the cortex of a metaphysis, but it usually points toward the epiphyseal plate. In contrast, osteochondromas, including those of diaphysial aclasia, always point toward the shaft.

There is little tendency for these masses of displaced cartilage to show excessive proliferation, except in the hands and feet. Here they may grow to considerable size, fungate through the cortex, and cause severe crippling. At puberty the lesions stop growing. The treatment of choice for a solitary lesion (enchondroma) is curettage and filling the defect with bone grafts. Osteotomy for correction of deformity may be done with impunity because the bones unite readily.

Enchondromatosis with hemangioma (Maffucci syndrome). Maffucci syndrome is the same disorder as Ollier disease, except for the presence of hemangiomas and phleboliths in the soft tissue.

Multiple epiphyseal dysplasia. Multiple epiphyseal dysplasia is characterized by abnormally large epiphyses and dwarfism. It is most often inherited in an autosomal dominant manner, but in a rare family a clinically indistinguishable disorder has been observed to conform to an autosomal recessive pattern. The fingers are short and thick, and their ends are blunt. The shoulders, hips, and ankles are usually affected and sometimes the knees, wrists, and elbows. The centers of ossification of the epiphyses develop slowly and mature irregularly. Peripheral stippling may be present but is never severe. Generally, many epiphyses are affected, and the joints are correspondingly deformed; the ends of the bones are small and irregular, and thus the joints tend to subluxate.

Chondrodysplasia punctata (stippled epiphyses; chondrodystrophia calcificans congenita). Chondrodysplasia punctata is a rare disorder of infancy in which discrete centers of unusual density are seen in the cartilaginous epiphyses. Both autosomal dominant (Conradi-Hünermann disease) and autosomal recessive (rhizomelic type) forms exist. The recessive form is characterized by rhizomelic dwarfism, joint contractures, scoliosis, depression of the nasal bridge, cataracts, and ichthyosiform dermatosis with alopecia. Death caused by pulmonary or renal infection is common in the first year of life; survivors are usually mentally retarded. In the presumed dominant form, findings are similar to those in the recessive form, but the prognosis for life is much better, and intelligence is unimpaired. The epiphyses appear as though many shotgun bird shot had been flung into them. The distal femur and proximal tibia and humerus are usually affected, and dwarfing with shortening of the proximal segments of the limbs is characteristic.

Osteopathia striata. Osteopathia striata is a rare condition characterized by striations in bone, especially in metaphyses of long bones and the pelvis. Vague recurrent joint pains, with or without swelling, may occur, and the gait may be abnormal. The radiographic appearance of the long bones, especially those adjacent to the knee, suggests a heavy graining similar to that seen in wood paneling. Generally the disorder is an incidental finding. Its cause is unknown.

Osteopoikilosis (osteopathia condensans disseminata). Osteopoikilosis is characterized by the presence of multiple dense spots in many bones throughout the body. It causes no symptoms. The etiology is unknown, and laboratory tests are normal.

Achondroplasia. Achondroplasia is the most common chondrodystrophy. It is inherited as an autosomal dominant disorder, but 80% to 90% of cases represent new mutations. At birth, short-limbed dwarfism of the rhizomelic type, increased skin folds on limbs, a depressed nasal bridge, and a trident hand deformity are noted. With time the head is relatively larger than the body and dorsal kyphosis and lumbar lordosis occur. Because of thorocolumbar vertebral narrowing, neurologic deficits in the lower limbs may develop with age.

Myositis (fibrodysplasia) ossificans progressiva. In myositis ossificans progressiva, columns of bone develop in the soft tissues and progressively limit motion. It is inherited in an autosomal dominant manner with nearly complete penetrance. The metabolism of calcium is normal. During infancy and childhood, localized masses of calcium develop, ordinarily painless and usually noted first in the neck. Later these deposits of calcium involve the trunk. They look like bone grafts and characteristically progress throughout the muscles and soft tissues of the back. They often bridge from the dorsal spine to the occiput. This is the disease that produces the "stone man" of the circus.

Other. More than 80 types of heritable chondrodystrophies are known. Autosomal recessive, autosomal dominant, and X-linked forms are known. Congenital forms, in addition to achondroplasia, include thanatophoric dwarfism, asphyxiating thoracic types, spondyloepiphyseal dysplasia congenita, and achondrogenesis. Hypochondroplasia, pseudoachondroplasia, spondyloepiphyseal dysplasia, and Ellis-Van Creveld syndrome may be detected shortly after birth or in infancy. Most forms may be differentiated by their radiologic, clinical, and inheritance patterns. A complete skeletal survey, including skull, AP and lateral spine, chest, pelvis, long bone, and hand-and-feet films are frequently necessary for accurate diagnosis. Types may vary as to whether a patient is short-limbed, which segment of the limb is involved (rhisomelic, mesomelic, acromelic), or whether the trunk is affected, or any combination of these factors. Epiphyseal, metaphyseal, and diaphyseal involvement varies. Correct diagnosis is extremely important as prognosis for height, neurologic complications (such as cervical spine instability), and recurrence risks differ.

Marfan syndrome. Marfan syndrome is inherited as an autosomal dominant condition and represents the most common heritable disorder of connective tissue. Ocular, cardiac, and skeletal systems are involved. Classically, ectopic lenses are detected in early childhood, but less commonly, severe myopia may be the ocular finding. Cardiovascular involvement may include dilated aortic root or mitral valve prolapse. Arachnodactyly, flatfeet, scoliosis, camptodactyly, joint instability, increased arm span related to height, and decreased upper to lower segment ratio are main skeletal manifestations. Cardiac complications may result in sudden death. All such patients should have complete cardiac, ophthalmologic, and orthopedic evaluations yearly.

NEUROMUSCULAR AFFECTIONS

(See Chapter 29.)

Poliomyelitis. For a discussion of poliomyelitis see pp. 753-756.

Dermatomyositis. For a discussion of dermatomyositis see pp. 484-488.

Arthrogryposis multiplex congenita. Arthrogryposis multiplex congenita is characterized by multiple contractures and other abnormalities of the extremities. It has been mistakenly diagnosed in cases of other conditions, including the trisomy 18 syndrome. It is not a single entity but is a clinical syndrome that may have any one of a number of etiologic-pathogenetic bases. Some cases have been familial; an autosomal dominant mode of inheritance has been suggested for these. The spine is rarely involved. Dislocations of the hips and clubbing of the feet and hands are frequent. The disorder is the result of developmental disturbances that seem to begin in the primitive myoblast. Various muscles may be completely absent or may be represented only by strands of small pink fibers. Joints are relatively normal except for being distorted by contractions of muscle and soft tissue. The number of anterior horn cells in the spinal cord is greatly reduced. Mentality is usually normal.

Treatment consists of bracing, splinting, corrective surgery, and a well-planned program of rehabilitation. Results, however, are discouraging.

MALIGNANT TUMORS OF BONE

For a discussion of malignant tumors of bone see p. 858.

BENIGN TUMORS OF BONE

Of the many benign tumors of bone in children, the most frequent are osteochondroma and unicameral bone cyst. However, other lesions may be simulated. These include such entities as acute and chronic infections, traumatic lesions, nonossifying fibromas, eosinophilic granulomas, and lesions of Hand-Schüller-Christian, Niemann-Pick, Gaucher, and Letterer-Siwe diseases.

Unicameral bone cyst. Unicameral bone cyst, according to Stewart and Hamel, is "a circumscribed area of bone destruction isolated by a zone of fibrosing osteitis with insufficient reparative properties to heal the cyst." It usually occurs in the metaphysis of a long bone. When adjacent to the epiphyseal plate, it is designated active, and when it is away from the plate, it is called latent. Clinically a bone cyst is characterized by pain and by expansion of the bone. A pathologic fracture through the cyst occurs in about half the patients. Most cysts develop in the proximal humerus, the distal femur, or the proximal tibia. They occur most often in the first and second decades of life. Diagnosis is suggested by radiographs but confirmed only by biopsy. Treatment consists of thoroughly curetting the lesion and packing it with cortical bone grafts, or resection of nonessential parts of bone. After establishing the diagnosis, injection of the cavity with cortisone has been reported effective in a number of cases. Roentgenographic therapy is contraindicated.

Giant cell tumor of bone. Giant cell tumor appears more commonly in the second and third decades of life. It is a rare tumor that begins in the epiphysis of a long bone. The usual presenting symptoms are pain and swelling in an epiphyseal region, but pain from a pathologic fracture may be the initial symptom. Giant cell tumors have been graded by Jaffe and Lichtenstein as follows: grade I, typical benign giant cell tumors; grade II, tumors not definitely malignant but occasionally showing a miotic figure in which the cells are atypical; and grade III, tumors definitely malignant. Immediate biopsy is indicated for any type. Treatment of a grade I tumor consists of thorough curettage and filling the cavity with bone grafts. Grade II and III tumors should be treated as primary malignancies. Occasionally, local resection may be adequate.

Chondroblastoma (Codman tumor). Codman tumor is predominantly cartilaginous in origin and in cellular structure. It occurs most frequently in the second decade of life. Symptoms begin with pain near the end of a long bone, often the proximal humerus. Radiographically the tumor is sharply circumscribed and is distinctly mottled by deposits of calcium in its tissue. Often bone is condensed around the periphery of the tumor, which may then simulate an osteogenic sarcoma. Diagnosis is confirmed only by biopsy. Treatment consists of resection or thorough curettage and packing with bone chips.

Osteoid osteoma. Osteoid osteoma is a localized benign lesion occurring usually in the second decade of life. It consists of a highly vascular deposit of osteoid located typically in the cortex of a long bone. The lesion is only a few millimeters in diameter but is surrounded by an area of sclerotic bone that may extend 2 or 3 cm in all directions. Radiographically it suggests low-grade sclerosing osteitis (Garré). An osteoid osteoma is cured by surgical extirpation.

Marcus J. Stewart

SELECTED READINGS

Banks, H.H., editor: Birth defects and the orthopedic surgeon, Orthop. Clin. North Am. **7**(2):259, 1976.

Bassett, C.A.L., et al.: Treatment of therapeutically resistant non-unions with bone grafts and pulsed electromagnetic fields, J. Bone Joint Surg. **64A:**1214-1220, October 1982.

Bleck, E.E.: Congenital clubfoot: pathomechanics, radiographic analysis and results of surgical treatment, Clin. Orthop. **125:**119, 1977.

Blockey, N.J.: Children's orthopaedics: practical problems, Woburn, Mass., 1976, Butterworth (Publishers) Inc.

Boyd, H.B., and Sage, F.P.: Congenital pseudarthrosis of the tibia, J. Bone Joint Surg. **40A**(6):1245-1270, 1958.

Campos. O.P.: Treatment of bone cysts by intracavity injection of methylprednisolone acetate: a message to orthopedic surgeons, Clin. Orthop. **165:**43-48, 1982.

Coleman, S.S.: Congenital dysplasia and dislocation of the hip, St. Louis, 1978, The C.V. Mosby Co.

Harris, N.H., et al.: Acetabular development in congenital hip dislocation, J. Bone Joint Surg. **57B:**46, 1975.

Hohl, J.C., editor: Fractures and other injuries in children, Orthop. Clin. North Am. **7**(3):525, 1976.

Lovell, W.W., and Winter, R.B.: Pediatric orthopaedics, Philadelphia, 1978, J.B. Lippincott Co.

Mollan, R.A.B., and Piggot, J.: Acute osteomyelitis in children, J. Bone Joint Surg. **59B:**2, 1977.

Rang, M.: Children's fractures, Philadelphia, 1974, J.B. Lippincott Co.

Reed, M.H.: Fractures and dislocations of the extremities in children, J. Trauma **17:**351, 1977.

Rombouts, J.J., and Rombouts-Lindemans, C.: Scoliosis in juvenile rheumatoid arthritis, J. Bone Joint Surg. **56B:**478, 1974.

Scaglietti, O.: Nuove prospettive nell' impiego dei corticosteroidi nella malattia neoplastica, Atti Accad. Med. Lomb. **29:**1, 1974.

Scaglietti, O., et al.: The effects of methylprednisolone acetate in the treatment of bone cysts. Results of three years follow-up. J. Bone Joint Surg. **61B**(2):200-204, 1979.

Scaglietti, O., et al.: Final results obtained in the treatment of bone cysts with methylprednisolone acetate (Depo-Medrol) and a discussion of results achieved in other bone lesions. Clin. Orthop. **165:**33-42, 1982.

Tachdjian, M.O.: Pediatric orthopaedics, Philadelphia, 1972, W.B. Saunders Co.

Tachdjian, M.O., editor: Pediatric orthopedics, Orthop. Clin. North Am. **9**(1):1, 1978.

36 Pediatric Ophthalmology

This chapter will concern those ocular conditions that are recognized and treated by the child's physician and those that are suspected by him but are referred to an ophthalmologist for diagnosis and treatment.

There are certain common conditions of the eye that the general practitioner or pediatrician will ordinarily diagnose and treat, such as foreign bodies in the eye, mild acute conjunctivitis (pink eye), styes, mild trauma, and so on; however, a pediatrician or general practitioner will probably leave most eye problems to the ophthalmologist. But even in these cases, as a family counselor, he will need to have a basic knowledge of the condition, its treatment, and its prognosis to be of help. Furthermore, in the smaller community the family physician is called on to treat certain conditions that ordinarily he would rather not manage. To know when to treat patients and when to refer them to the specialist is part of the art of the practicing physician and is also a mark of the expert and conscientious physician.

GENERAL CONSIDERATIONS

At birth the eye is well developed anatomically and measures about three fourths of its adult size. The pupil is small with a blue iris because of the lack of deposition of pigment. The anterior chamber is shallow, and the cornea does not appear to be as shiny clear as it does later on.

Within a few months the cornea becomes clear, the anterior chamber deepens, and the pupil becomes larger. In some children the pupils normally become large. The iris remains blue or becomes hazel, green, or brown, depending on the degree of pigmentation that develops. The eyeball reaches its adult size by about the eighth year of life.

The eyes remain closed during the early postnatal days and are somewhat sensitive to light. Vision is not very acute at birth, but by 6 weeks the infant will usually follow light, and by 8 to 10 weeks he will follow objects and may even reach out to grasp them. From this time onward there is a gradual increase in visual acuity until about school age (6 years), when the normal child has 20/20 vision like the normal adult. At birth the visual acuity is only in the 200/400 range.

The eyes may "wander" during the early weeks of life, but by the age of 3 months the eyes should have settled down to a binocular pattern; therefore a child with any gross and apparent deviation of the eyes from each other still present at the age of *3 months* should be seen by an ophthalmologist.

No tears appear when the baby cries until about 2 to 4 weeks after birth, when tearing becomes obvious.

Examination. Because it is important to gain the child's confidence if a satisfactory examination is to be carried out, evaluation of the eyes may well be left to follow the rest of the examination before any injections or other painful procedures are performed. Force is to be employed as a last resort because the examination cannot be completely satisfactory when the child squeezes and rolls his eyes upward. Desmarres lid retractors are helpful when the child closes his eyes very tightly. If the eyegrounds must be seen, a well-dilated pupil and the use of the indirect ophthalmoscope are easiest for the ophthalmologist. The pediatrician, however, may have to use direct ophthalmoscopy. If necessary, this examination should be carried out under general anesthesia in a young child.

Visual acuity, even in a young infant, can often be estimated by the way the child performs visually and how he follows an object such as a light. In the slightly older child, age 6 months to 3 years, observation as to how he fixates to a light and maintains that fixation when the opposite eye is covered and uncovered is of utmost value. During the fourth year of life, visual acuity of a child usually can be assessed with pictures, the "E" chart, or, later in the early school years, the Snellen chart. The intraocular pressure can be estimated by palpation, but deep sedation or general anesthesia must be used when the level of pressure is in question. The ocular rotations generally can be observed by using an attractive object, and the alternate cover test and the cover-uncover test are the "acid tests" in ruling out the presence of a strabismus. However, merely observing the light reflex on the cornea (Hirschberg test) can reveal the presence of an obvious tropia or, in contrast, a pseudostrabismus. Attractive objects in the field of vision can often be helpful to estimate the visual fields, even in the young child. The use of a loupe and good illumination to examine the external eye is usually all that is required.

The most common ocular conditions in children include vision disturbances, disturbances in the motility of the eye including strabismus, nystagmus and ptosis, associated headaches, and reading difficulties. External diseases of the eye include red eyes from conjunctivitis, blepharitis, foreign body, and trauma.

Principles of local medications. Medications in the form of drops may be the easiest to use in children, but ointments (in ophthalmic tubes) are more effective because of more prolonged contact. Ointments have the added advantage of becoming contaminated less easily from outside sources and deteriorating less rapidly.

Techniques of instillation. Proper techniques for instilling drops or ointment outside the office must be taught to the parent, who is instructed to have the child look upward so that the medication is not placed directly on the highly sensitive cornea but falls on the inner surface of the lower lid. The lower lid is held momentarily as the patient looks down, and to prolong the absorption time the patient is warned not to squeeze his eyes.

Common pitfalls to be avoided. Liquid medications used in treatment of the eye deteriorate rapidly and become contaminated easily. The physician should have only small amounts on hand and should prescribe only small amounts for home use.

Local anesthetics should never be prescribed as take-home medication because the patient may unknowingly injure an anesthetized eye. Furthermore, a local anesthetic delays wound healing.

Atropine should not be used or prescribed without definite indications because the pupil becomes widely dilated and vision becomes blurred for a period of 1 or 2 weeks.

Also, local steroids should not be prescribed without definite indications. Prolonged use of steroids may cause increased intraocular pressure and cataracts and also may give rise to secondary infection, such as fungus infections, as well as aggravate viral infections, such as herpes simplex. Steroids should never be used locally in the eyes by anyone except an ophthalmologist unless the diagnosis is certain and the indications specific.

DISORDERS OF THE EYELIDS

Blepharitis. Blepharitis is a common affection of the lid margins and conjunctiva characterized by redness and crusting. In severe cases there may also be ulceration and actual loss of eyelashes. In children it is most commonly caused by a *Staphylococcus* infection superimposed on an allergic background. The allergy is generally considered to result from the *Staphylococcus* and its toxin. The course is chronic and recurrent. Treatment consists of the local use of sulfonamide or antibiotic ointment instilled in the eye and rubbed into the base of the lashes after thorough cleansing and removal of crusts with a cotton swab. Occasionally desensitization with *Staphylococcus* toxoid is indicated. The squamosal variety may be associated with seborrheic dermatitis (and *Pityrosporum ovale*), and the child may have dandruff of the scalp or eyebrows or lashes. Treatment of the dandruff with selenium sulfide ointment, plus local treatment with an antibiotic steroid ointment, is often required.

Hordeolum. A hordeolum (stye) is an acute infection in the Zeis or Moll glands of the lid margin that results in a small abscess. Because it is superficial, it usually suppurates rapidly and ruptures spontaneously with complete healing. Application of hot packs for 20 to 30 minutes, three or four times a day, will often give comfort and hasten the pointing of the stye. The styes may come in crops and require treatment of the underlying staphylococcal blepharitis with both systemic and local antibiotics. Rarely, incision and drainage of the abscess is required.

Lid abscess and chalazion. Infections of the deep glands of the tarsal plate of the lid are uncommon in children, but occasionally a lid abscess will form that may require incision and drainage, usually from the undersurface of the lid. A low-grade chronic infection produces a granulomatous lesion, called a chalazion, which requires incision and curettage from the posterior surface of the lid. However, an occasional isolated chalazion may be left alone until the child gets older and can tolerate a local anesthetic, if it does not form a disfiguring knot on the lid.

Ptosis. In children, ptosis is usually congenital; the acquired type is caused by trauma or disease. Ptosis may be unilateral or bilateral. The upper lid generally droops to a variable degree as a result of deficient action of the levator palpebrae muscle. The child may raise his eyebrow or brows in an attempt to elevate the lid. In bilateral cases the child may extend the head to enable him to see beneath the drooping upper lids. If the pupil is covered, vision may fail to develop in the affected eye. Thus it is important that the ophthalmologist evaluate this condition early. If the vision is not threatened, surgical treatment is postponed until the age of 3 or 4 years. It consists in shortening the levator muscle, or, if this muscle is very paretic, connecting the upper lid to the frontalis muscle of the forehead with fascia lata or synthetic material. A peculiar type of ptosis, the Marcus Gunn phenomenon, or jaw-winking, consists of the elevation of the ptotic lid on chewing or shifting the jaw to the side. Most of these patients do not require surgery.

CONGENITAL OBSTRUCTION OF NASOLACRIMAL DUCT

Normally the tear duct is patent throughout its entire length at birth, but occasionally it fails to open at its nasal end or somewhere along its course. In this event, tears are stagnated in the duct, and an infection in the sac may result. This condition may be unilateral or bilateral and may become manifest by lacrimation, conjunctival redness, and a mucopurulent discharge during the second month of life. The treatment is to first massage by backward and downward pressure on the tear sac just medial to the inner angle of the eye several times a day. Sometimes this massage will force the nasal orifice of the duct to open, with rapid subsidence of all signs and symptoms. This probably should be accompanied by the instillation of a local antibiotic solution. In a large percentage of these children, even if the obstruction persists to age 3 months, it will eventually clear. It is unpredictable, however, just who will not require probing. If probing is delayed until a child is 9 to 12 months of age, simple probing may then be ineffective, and a major plastic procedure will have to be performed or polyethylene tubes inserted in the drainage system. Therefore probing should probably be done to prevent a chronic dacryocystitis if there is not significant clearing with conservative treatment by the age of 3 months.

CONJUNCTIVITIS

Conjunctivitis is the commonest of all eye diseases in the Western Hemisphere. Simple hyperemia of the conjunctiva is noninfectious in nature but is more common than the infectious variety. Zinc sulfate, 0.25% drops, and phenylephrine, 0.25% drops, are of some help. Most infectious cases are caused by bacteria. Other causes include viral infection, allergy, protozoa, and fungi.

Bacterial conjunctivitis. Bacterial conjunctivitis may be either acute or chronic. The ordinary type is often caused by *S. aureus,* pneumococcus, *Haemophilus influenzae, Moraxella lacunta,* and viridans streptococci. These organisms produce acute conjunctivitis with sudden onset, mild to moderately severe burning, redness of the conjunctival lining of the eyelids, some general injection of the bulbar conjunctiva, and mucopurulent discharge. The term *pink eye* is commonly applied to this acute condition. It may be spread from one eye to the other and may be transferred to other persons by hands, towels, etc. These infections are self-limited and last several days to 2 weeks. Treatment with local antibiotics or sulfonamides shortens the course of the disease.

Viral conjunctivitis. Viral conjunctivitis is similar to bacterial conjunctivitis except that the discharge is scanty and, of course, self-limited, but it tends to be longer in duration than bacterial conjunctivitis. Local antibiotics are not curative but may be used to avoid secondary infection.

Allergic conjunctivitis. Allergic conjunctivitis may be chronic or recurrent and may or may not be associated with other manifestations of allergy. Secondary infection is fairly common. In addition to burning, the special characteristics include itching of the eyes, which causes the child to rub them. The conjunctiva assumes a pink, skimmed-milk juiciness; there is watering of the eyes but little discharge. An allergic study sometimes is necessary, but generally the local administration of steroids for a short time, occasionally combined with local antihistamines, is all that is required in children.

Special forms of conjunctivitis

Ophthalmia neonatorum. Conjunctivitis in newborn infants can be gonococcal, staphylococcal (or other bacteria), or viral in origin.

Gonococcal ophthalmia constitutes one type of ophthalmia neonatorum that is now becoming less common but is still extremely important. Infection takes place in the birth canal and becomes manifest 2 to 5 days after delivery. There is severe edema of the lids and conjunctiva, with a copious purulent discharge. The greater danger exists because of the possibility of ulceration of the cornea, with perforation and destruction of the eyeball. Diagnosis is best made by taking a smear and culture from the conjunctiva and performing a Gram stain. Intensive treatment is then begun with parenteral antibiotics, preferably penicillin, and local irrigation with boric acid, followed by local instillation of penicillin into the eye. Treatment should also be given to the uninvolved eye. The infant must be isolated because the condition is easily transmissible.

Staphylococcal conjunctivitis and other forms of bacterial conjunctivitis usually occur between the third and fifth day after delivery, whereas viral conjunctivitis (inclusion blennorrhea) occurs around the tenth day. These conditions are less severe and cause no complications. Usually they respond readily to local sulfonamides and antibiotics.

Ophthalmia neonatorum is to be distinguished from chemical conjunctivitis produced in many newborn infants by prophylactic silver nitrate. There is an early onset of the latter (first 24 hours) and rapid subsidence without treatment.

Inclusion conjunctivitis (viral). Inclusion conjunctivitis is common during the summer months, is contracted in swimming pools, and is moderately contagious but usually not severe. Response to local sulfonamides is rapid.

Adenovirus conjunctivitis. Adenovirus conjunctivitis is associated with sore throat and fe-

Table 36-1. Differential diagnosis of red eyes

	Acute conjunctivitis	Acute iritis	Acute glaucoma	Corneal trauma and inflammation
Incidence	Common	Fairly common	Uncommon	Fairly common
Discharge	Moderate to copious	None Lacrimation	None	Watery or purulent
Visual acuity	Normal	Slightly blurred	Marked ↓	Usually blurred
Pain	None Hot gritty sensation	Moderate, worse at night	Marked, cheek and forehead	Pain or irritation
Conjunctival injection	Diffuse	Circumcorneal	Diffuse	Diffuse
Cornea	Clear	Usually clear	Steamy	Abrasion, ulcer, or foreign body
Pupil size	Normal	Small, irregular	Large, dilated oval	Normal
Pupil response	Normal	Poor	Poor	Normal
Intraocular pressure	Normal	Normal or ↓ or ↑	↑	Normal
Smear	Organisms	None	None	Organisms if ulcer
Iris	Normal	Swollen, dull, discolored	Congested, discolored, pushed forward	Normal
Anterior chamber	Normal	Exudate	Shallow, turbid	Normal unless ulcer
Ciliary tenderness	Normal	+	+	Some

ver; there may be palpable preauricular nodes. No treatment is available, but fortunately it is a self-limited disease, generally lasting a matter of days.

Vernal conjunctivitis. Vernal conjunctivitis is a peculiar allergic manifestation, the precise nature of which is still unknown. It is characterized by itching, photophobia, ropy discharge, and pale hypertrophy of the conjunctiva around the limbus or at the border of the upper tarsus. Symptoms are most severe in the spring and early summer months. Treatment is symptomatic by frequent copious boric acid irrigations and local administration of steroids. With the passage of time, children can outgrow this condition.

Phlyctenular keratoconjunctivitis. Phylctenular keratoconjunctivitis is associated with malnutrition, poor hygiene, and possibly tuberculosis. The essential lesion is a hard red elevation of the corneoscleral junction with a small depression in its apex. Treatment consists of local application of steroid ointment.

Chronic follicular conjunctivitis. Chronic follicular conjunctivitis is most commonly seen in children from orphanages and from deprived environments. It is characterized by numerous follicles along the upper and lower palpebral conjunctivae. The duration is 2 to 3 years, and treatment is usually only symptomatic.

• • •

Table 36-1 gives a differential diagnosis of the causes of "red eyes" in children.

CORNEA

The cornea has been described as the window of the eye. It is a tough, transparent, avascular membrane about 1 mm in thickness. The surface epithelium is modified conjunctiva. Many drugs pass through the cornea to gain entrance to the eye.

Lesions of the cornea are obvious because they produce opacity with consequent impairment of vision. Photophobia is also characteristic of lesions of the cornea, as well as lesions of the inner eye, such as iritis. A differential diagnosis of corneal disease is often difficult and deserves the greatest possible attention to detail.

Corneal ulcers. Corneal ulcers are common and of many varieties. They may be associated with conjunctivitis, secondary infection following trauma or presence of a foreign body, or nutritional or allergic factors, or they may be a result of endogenous infection. Severe types may cause perforation of the cornea with destruction of the eyeball. The less severe types may leave in their wake a permanent opacity with unsightly and often blind eyes. In most cases severe damage can be prevented if the ulcer is treated promptly and vigorously.

Interstitial keratitis. The commonest and most important variety of interstitial keratitis is that caused by congenital syphilis. It is usually manifested in the early teenage years but has become less common with the advent of penicillin. There may be an acute abrupt onset of inflammation of the eye(s) with severe photophobia and early clouding of the cornea. Treatment consists of local and systemic penicillin and local steroids. Fortunately the vision that is lost may be restored by corneal transplant when the disease becomes inactive.

SCLERA

Diseases of the sclera are rare in children and need not be considered here.

PUPIL, IRIS, AND CILIARY BODY

The pupillary opening is constantly being regulated to admit the proper amount of light. The iris acts as a diaphragm, and the pupil is dilated by its radial muscle fibers, innervated by the sympathetic nervous system. On the other hand, it is contracted by the circular muscle fibers, innervated by the parasympathetic supply by way of the third cranial nerve. The pupil reacts to increased light by constriction and to less light by dilation. It reacts to near objects also by constriction and to distant objects by dilation. The pupillary reactions are sensitive indicators of many neurologic disturbances affecting the child. The musculature of the ciliary body behind the iris regulates the curvature of the lens and thus is constantly changing as the eye focuses at different distances.

Inflammation of these structures, *iridocyclitis,* is not common in children but may cause serious impairment of vision should it occur. A broader term, *uveitis,* involves inflammation of not only the iris and ciliary body but also includes the choroid and surrounding layers. Inflammation may be acute, such as an allergic response to disease elsewhere in the body (exanthemas, respiratory tract diseases), or a direct infection (granulomatous diseases such as syphilis, tuberculosis, or toxoplasmosis). A severe complication of Still disease may include iritis with a band keratopathy. Symptoms may be mild or severe, with pain, pericorneal redness, cloudy cornea, muddy iris, contracted pupil, and impairment of vision.

Treatment must be instituted early to prevent permanent ocular damage. A search is first made for the possible cause before treatment is begun. Therapy consists first of treating the primary disease, should it be found, and, second, of treating the inflammation itself. This usually consists of local atropine and steroid medication, but treatment of an inflammation of the posterior segment of the eye includes either systemic steroids or retrobulbar depot steroids.

LENS

The lens, situated behind the pupil, has the function of maintaining an accurate focus of the rays of light that pass through it to the retina. The principal disease of the lens is an opacification called a cataract.

Cataracts in children are usually congenital and hereditary, evidence of the disease being present at birth or shortly after. Some cases are caused by disease in the mother, for example, rubella occurring in the first trimester of pregnancy. Other forms of cataract in children may be caused by injury or by ocular disease.

Should the vision be sufficiently affected, the only treatment is surgical removal, which should be carried out between the ages of 1 and 2 months. The younger the patient, the earlier opportunity there is for development of vision, but this must be weighed against the difficulties in operating on the eye of the young child and the problems of anesthesia. If surgery is delayed too long, there may be permanent impairment of vision, even though the cataract is removed. At present the method of removal most frequently used is to incise the cataract and then aspirate it through a large-gauge needle or aspirating-cutting machine.

CHOROID AND RETINA

Diseases of the choroid and retina are uncommon in children. In recent years much has been written on the subject of the retinopathy of prematurity *(retrolental fibroplasia)*. However, it now occurs less frequently since the discovery that the disease is associated with excessive use of oxygen, particularly in the premature infant, especially if birth weight is less than 1.3 to 1.8 kg (3 to 4 pounds). The condition is characterized by an overgrowth of newly forming blood vessels in the developing retina, caused by the stimulus of oxygen, followed by relative anoxia when deprived of oxygen. In extreme cases this leads to detachment of the retina and the formation of a white membrane behind the lens, visible by ordinary illumination.

Cases are still seen in smaller premature infants needing high concentrations of oxygen for survival. In these patients, prevention is sought by a reduction of the oxygen percentage of 30% or less if possible and as soon as possible. Because of the variability of the oxygen delivered to the incubators, the direct measurement of the arterial Po_2 should be done to follow suspected cases.

Retinoblastoma (p. 855) is an uncommon tumor of the eye seen almost exclusively in children less than 5 years of age; two thirds of the affected children are under the age of 2 years. The tumor arises in the retina and, if untreated, invades the optic nerve to destroy the eye and the brain, and then takes the life of the child. The parent usually notices a white reflex in the pupil of one eye as the first indication of an abnormality. This condition is called leukocoria and must be considered in all cases in which a white pupil appears in the child. By this time the tumor is already advancing into the eye behind the lens. The other eye is also involved in about 30% of the cases; therefore an ophthalmic examination of both eyes under general anesthesia is always indicated. The more involved eye is usually removed surgically, the optic nerve being sectioned as far posterior as possible. The opposite eye, if involved, is treated with deep x-ray therapy, diathermy, light coagulation, and antimetabolites. Rarely, both eyes must be removed to save the life of the child. The differential diagnosis of retinoblastoma includes retrolental fibroplasia, persistent hyperplasia of primary vitreous, all forms of pseudogliomas including the nematodes, retinal dysplasia, colobomas of the retina, cataracts, and so on.

The retina and choroid are affected by various malformations, abiotrophies, and intrauterine infections, which also affect other parts of the body.

NEURO-OPHTHALMOLOGY

Because of the extensive connections between the cranial nerves, the brain, and the upper spinal cord pathways, the eyes play important roles as indicators of neurologic disease. Cranial nerve VI (supplying the external rectus muscle) has a long intracranial course. Probably for this reason it participates frequently in pathologic changes. Also frequently involved is cranial nerve III and, less frequently, cranial nerve IV.

Pupil. The pupil is stimulated to contract by cranial nerve III and dilates by the cervical sympathetic nerve by way of the internal carotid plexus. The pupil constricts in response to light or near focusing and dilates in response to darkness and distant fixation. Abnormal dilation and failure to react to condensed light would mean the intentional or inadvertent instillation of a mydriatic drug into the eye, trauma to the eye with local sphincter paralysis, or pathologic changes in cranial nerve III. Failure to react to the direct light reflex would mean disease in the afferent nerve, or the retino-optic nerve pathway, such as is caused by optic atrophy. Sympathetic nerve affections involving the eye are extremely rare in children.

Extraocular muscle paralysis. Paralysis of extraocular muscles may be congenital, may result from trauma such as birth injury or accident, or may be caused by intracranial infections or tumors. Such paralysis is manifested by deviation of the eyes in a direction opposite to the action of the paralyzed muscle. In contrast to congenital strabismus, acquired strabismus results in diplopia, and this may be the presenting symptom. The prognosis depends on the cause, and attention should be directed to it first. Persistence of the muscular paralysis requires surgical correction, just as in congenital strabismus.

Nystagmus. Nystagmus is characterized by rhythmic involuntary oscillation of the eyes of varying degree. Distance vision is usually poor if the amplitude of the nystagmus is great, because the eyes are unable to fixate on an object steadily because of their wide excursions in relation to the object. Reading vision is less impaired the closer the print is held to the eyes. The child may even be able to read small print if held close enough.

Nystagmus may be congenital or acquired in early infancy as a result of poor vision or as a result of disease of the vestibular apparatus associated with middle ear infections, trauma, or tumors. Nystagmus caused by disease of the vestibular apparatus is distinguished from the congenital or ocular type by the presence of a quick jerk to one side, slow movement of recovery to the other, and its association with vertigo and deafness. Another type of acquired nystagmus may be caused by drugs, such as the vertical nystagmus produced by barbiturates or phenytoin (Dilantin). Nystagmus with head nodding that is persistent and hereditary must be distinguished from spasmus nutans, which usually disappears by the age of 3 to 4 years. The treatment of the vestibular type depends on the cause. If the nystagmus has a quiet position, that is, if it is less severe on one direction of gaze, surgery may be performed on the extraocular muscles to put this quiet phase straight ahead. This reduces the amount of nystagmus and the head turn.

Optic nerve. Optic neuritis is usually unilateral but is occasionally bilateral. It is associated with encephalitis, meningitis, or generalized infectious diseases. Frequently the cause cannot be demonstrated. It is characterized by profound loss of central vision, edema, hemorrhages and exudates of the retina surrounding the disc, and congestion of the retinal blood vessels.

Papilledema, on the other hand, is almost always indicative of a space-occupying mass such as a brain tumor. It is usually bilateral but occasionally may be unilateral. The appearance of the optic nerve and the retina is often the same as with optic neuritis (papillitis), but vision is not impaired until the increased intracranial pressure has been present for some time.

Optic atrophy. Optic atrophy, characterized by various degrees of pallor of the nerve head, may result from optic neuritis, prolonged papilledema, trauma, or pressure of a tumor, or it may be congenital with no known cause. The physician should remember, however, that the infant optic nerve head is somewhat paler than that of the adult. For this reason, diagnosis of blindness in the infant with suspected optic atrophy should not be made until the physician is sure of the findings.

Strabismus. One of the commonest ocular abnormalities in children is strabismus, or squint. It may be convergent (toward the midline) or divergent (away from the midline). Either type may be complicated by a vertical component. More than 1% of children are born with or will develop this ocular deviation. An equal number will have a significant tendency of the eyes to deviate, which is latent and is therefore called a phoria.

At birth, coordination between the two eyes is incompletely developed. There may be some deviations and wanderings of the eyes, but by the age of 3 months the eyes should be working together in following a moving object of interest and should be focusing together. If the deviation still persists at 3 months of age, the child probably has a strabismus and should be examined at this time by an ophthalmologist.

The two eyes, when developing normally, work as a unit. Images of an object focused on the retina of each eye are passed on to the brain as two sets of nervous impulses that are fused into one. This fusion faculty is deficient or absent altogether in the congenitally strabismic child who is unable to use the two eyes together. Two images are presented to the brain, and it cannot fuse them; therefore the child temporarily has double vision (diplopia).

Unconsciously the brain adopts the obvious expediency of suppressing the use of one eye and ignoring its image to avoid the confusion of diplopia. The brain has difficulty in suppressing one of these images when both are presented to it with equal intensity. But if one eye deviates so that the object visualized falls on a less sensitive area of the retina peripheral to the fovea centralis, the image passed on to the brain will be less intense and more easily suppressed. Thus permanent deviation or strabismus develops.

The strabismus may be monocular (the image of one eye is habitually suppressed) or it may be alternating (the image of each eye may be alternately suppressed). In the former the child uses or fixates with one eye habitually while the other eye is crossed; in the latter the child uses either eye indiscriminately while the opposite eye is crossed or divergent.

It is to be remembered that vision is developing at the same time that one eye is being ignored in monocular strabismus. The vision in the suppressed eye therefore fails to develop. If the condition is untreated, the result is a permanent impairment of vision, termed amblyopia. This is a major reason for early treatment in monocular strabismus.

In the alternating type of strabismus, on the other hand, both eyes are being used, even though one at a time, and vision is being developed normally.

The age of onset of strabismus varies considerably. Children who have little or no fusion faculty will show deviation at or soon after birth. Strabismus will develop later in those having less deficiency of the fusion faculty of the brain. Such a child has increasing difficulty in blending the images of the two eyes and finally gives way to suppression of one image to avoid the confusion of diplopia. This usually occurs at 1 or 2 years of age but occasionally later. The onset may be precipitated by a fall, emotional upset, or illness.

Another factor frequently entering the picture to embarrass a deficient fusion faculty is a high refractive error. High hyperopia or astigmatism may so increase the visual effort or blur the image of one or both eyes that a weak fusion faculty may give way to dilpopia and then to suppression and deviation of the eyes. It is for this reason that glasses may be needed early to correct or prevent the development of permanent strabismus.

It must be remembered that it is not known precisely whether the deficient fusion faculty, relative differences of innervation to the extraocular muscles, structural anomalies of the extraocular muscles in their relation to the globes, dysgenesis of the ocular motor nerve nuclei, or some other factor precipitates a congenital strabismus. Therefore the deficiency of fusion may be secondary rather than primary in cases of strabismus.

The diagnosis of strabismus is usually obvious, but occasionally the parents are certain their child's eyes are crossed when in fact they are not. This pseudostrabismus results from many factors, the most important being a prominent fold in the corner of the eyes in some children. This fold occasionally is a true epicanthus. On looking to one side, the opposite eye partially disappears behind the fold, thus giving the appearance of crossed eyes. True strabismus is diagnosed by the fact that the corneal reflex from a light thrown into the eyes is not centered in one of the pupils. If the light is centered in each pupil, it is easy to demonstrate to a skeptical parent that there is no strabismus. Of course, the best way to diagnose strabismus is by doing the cover-uncover test and the alternate cover test. The alternate cover test is performed by having the hand alternately cover the eyes while the child observes a fixation target such as light. This distinguishes if any deviation is present, either a phoria or a tropia, that is, a latent as opposed to a true strabismus. The cover-uncover test, on the other hand, which is performed by just covering and uncovering one eye and observing the fixation of the two eyes to a light, merely tells whether the deviation is latent or manifest, and whether it is alternating or unilateral.

Treatment of strabismus should begin early. If obvious strabismus is persistent after the age of 3 months, the child should be seen by an ophthalmologist. If it is determined that the child is using only one eye, then the eye that he habitually uses must be occluded to ensure the development of sight in the deviating eye. This occlusion is accomplished by either a patch on the face or sometimes by the use of "medical patching," consisting of instilling atropine into the better eye. In the great majority of cases, when occlusion is begun early, the child can grow up with good vision in each eye.

The eye of the strabismic child should be refracted always with maximal cycloplegia and dilation of the pupil. If there is significant refractive error, it should be corrected with glasses at this time. In accommodative strabismus the wearing of glasses alone may prevent the development of, or may correct, the ocular deviation. In extremely small children who have difficulty wearing glasses, or supplementing glasses, or occasionally in lieu of glasses even in the older child, strong miotic drops such as echothiophate iodide (Phospholine) or DFP are used to inhibit the central nervous system stimulation to the eye and thus decrease the degree of strabismus.

The great majority of patients, however, will require operation on the extraocular muscles to align the eyes. Fortunately this operation is almost always without danger to the eyesight because it is carried out entirely on the exterior of the eyeball itself. The muscles are resected, recessed, or advanced to a degree determined by several measurements with prisms in the office before the operation. When the physician is sure of the measurements and the degree of deviation, an operation is indicated, regardless of age, whether this be 3 months or 6 years, remembering that the earlier it is done the better.

It should be pointed out to the parents that more than one procedure may be necessary, particularly when the strabismus includes a vertical deviation or some other complicating factor. It is particularly important that the strabismus should be well on its way to correction before school age.

The goal of all treatment of strabismus is not only to improve and maintain good vision and to make the appearance of the eyes cosmetically satisfactory, but also to enable the functioning of two eyes together as a unit, if possible, that is, binocular vision with stereopsis. However, in most patients this goal cannot be obtained because of the inherent fusion faculty deficiency that was either the cause of the strabismus in the first place or resulted because the strabismus occurred and was not corrected before the fusion faculty was developed. Some children will develop a certain degree of binocular cooperation spontaneously after the eyes have been straightened, and in some children the deficient fusion can be strengthened further by eye exercises (orthoptic training). This requires an expert technician who knows how to elicit the active cooperation of the child and the parent. These exercises must begin sometime after the fourth year of life when the child is able to understand them.

Fortunately the lack of binocular vision is not a serious handicap to the child who has never had it. He compensates for this defect for most occupations not requiring quick and accurate judgment of distances between objects at close range; difficulty with instruments such as a binocular microscope exemplifies the problem of lack of binocular vision.

It is to be emphasized that the parents of a strabismic child can be assured that, with rare exception, when persistent treatment is given, a child can grow up with straight eyes and with eyes that see well. If the surgery is performed before the age of 1 year, there is evidence that not only will the eyes look well and see well but also the child will develop more binocular vision than if the surgery is delayed until school age.

GLAUCOMA

Glaucoma is defined as any increase in intraocular pressure incompatible with continued health of the eye. Fortunately it is rare in children, but its consequences are so devastating that everyone dealing with children should be aware of its manifestations. It is particularly important that the disease be diagnosed early in life.

It usually begins in the first few months of life, but it may be present at birth. An early symptom may be slight photophobia, which results in the infant keeping his eyes closed, turning from light, or even burying his head in the pillow. There may be slight redness and watering of the eyes. At this stage the condition may be easily passed off as a mild conjunctivitis. However, close observation reveals slight haziness of the eye caused by cloudiness of the cornea. This is the most important early sign of congenital glaucoma, and it is at this stage that treatment is most effective.

The disease often progresses rapidly with irreversible structural changes in the eye in a matter of weeks. All too frequently the diagnosis is not suspected until the eye is noted to become enlarged. Because of the distensibility of the infant's eye, the enlargement may become so great and the coats of the eye so thin that rupture of the globe may be produced by the slightest trauma. At this stage of buphthalmos, the eyes are blind, or nearly so, and no treatment is of any help. The cause of the increased intraocular pressure is failure of the drainage channels to cleave completely and open up in the embryo.

Treatment is always surgical, although medical therapy may be effective in the interim, and is highly successful if the condition is detected before enlargement of the eyes has progressed significantly. Goniotomy, the operation indicated, is accomplished by passing a pointed knife across the anterior chamber to separate the iris root from the outflow channels. Not infrequently, more than one goniotomy is necessary before a sufficient angle is opened.

Rarely, secondary glaucoma caused by developmental defects, intraocular disease, or trauma may be encountered in children. Treatment is aimed at the cause, and sometimes medical and surgical therapy are also needed.

ORBIT

Probably the most common affection of the orbit in children results from inadequately treated sinusitis. Infection from the ethmoid sinuses may extend through the thin laminar papyracea to produce a subperiosteal or retrobulbar abscess that may require external drainage. The child is quite ill, with edema being present at the nasal aspect of the orbit. The eyeball is displaced laterally and forward. Orbital cellulitis, or true abscess of the orbit, occurs within the orbital periosteum. Orbital cellulitis will cause a forward displacement of the globe with brawny edema surrounding it. (See p. 997.)

Various tumors may occur in the orbit of children, the most common of which are hemangioma and lymphoma. They usually produce a monocular exophthalmos. The lymphomas are noted in cases of leukemia. Rhabdomyosarcoma, although rare, is the most common malignant orbital tumor of childhood. Presenting in the first and second decades of life, this lesion is characterized by a rapidly developing proptosis. Early exenteration of the orbit, supplemented with radiation therapy, is the recommended treatment of choice at the present time. The prognosis is poor but not hopeless.

TRAUMA

One person goes blind in the United States every 16 minutes; one half of these cases are preventable. Trauma is the commonest cause of blindness in children after the age of 2 years. In spite of the protection afforded by the bony orbital rim, the cushioning effect of the retrobulbar mass, and the screening effect of the lids and lashes, the incidence of eye injuries in children is discouragingly high. Slingshots, bows and arrows, air rifles or BB guns, and sticks and other sharp instruments still take their toll of the eyes. Many children lose their eyes from fireworks injury, even when use of fireworks is prohibited by law.

Foreign body. The simplest form of injury is foreign body in the eye. A small particle is blown into the eye by a gust of wind or while the child is riding in an automobile or on a bicycle. The foreign body may be found caught in a shallow groove 1 mm above the upper lid margin on its posterior surface. Most foreign bodies will work themselves out of the eye in time and be washed down by the tears and be found at the inner canthus. Frequently the child rubs the eye and imbeds the foreign body in the conjunctiva of the lid or in the cornea itself. The foreign body then scratches the cornea at every blink of the lid. It is therefore important to evert the eyelid to examine for the suspected particle. It is then easily removed by a moistened cotton swab, actually without any anesthesia.

More serious is the foreign body that has struck with sufficient velocity to become embedded in the cornea. The child may have pain and photophobia and be apprehensive, making examination difficult. Local anesthesia consisting of tetracaine (Pontocaine) or proparacaine (Ophthaine) followed by fluorescein is necessary to reveal the abraded area that is otherwise not readily seen. It is preferable to use the sterile fluorescein strips moistened with sterile saline rather than fluorescein drops because of the high contamination rate of the latter. A period of 3 days is required for healing. Anesthetic ointments delay healing and give a false sense of security and therefore should not be used. A snug dressing after instillation of the sterile antibiotic drops and absolute eye rest give the most relief.

Lacerated wounds. Lacerated wounds of the eyeball require accurate suturing, and if they are deep and extensive, enucleation may be necessary. In every incidence, lacerations of the eyelids require careful suturing of the tarsal plates to prevent disfiguring cosmetic deformity. The repair should be done immediately or several days later when the acute swelling has subsided. Particular attention must be given if the canaliculi are involved.

The ordinary "black eye" is usually produced by a blow with a large blunt object, most commonly the fist. Fortunately the rim of the orbit catches most of the force of the blow, and for this reason, although swelling and bleeding under the skin may be severe, the eyeball is rarely damaged. Occasionally, however, intraocular hemorrhage and other damage are produced. A serious complication is that of blowout fracture, in which the weak orbital floor or ethmoid cells may give way to the force transmitted to the closed cavity, and a fracture occurs with herniation into the fracture site of intraorbital contents, including muscles. This may lead to the presence of diplopia and later to enophthalmos if not corrected early.

Burns. Burns of the eye may be thermal or chemical. The latter are more dangerous. No time should be lost in trying to neutralize the chemical. The eye should be irrigated immediately and copiously with water, or some water substitute, despite any fright or protest. If strong acid or alkali has been splashed into the eye, holding the eye(s) under a strong stream of water from the faucet may save sight, since the damage is done so rapidly. The role of the ophthalmologist will then be to salvage as much vision as possible.

Blood in the eye, particularly in the anterior and posterior chambers of the eye, is called *hyphema*. The commonest cause of hyphema in the child is trauma to the eyeball itself. There may be only a small amount of blood present, so little that it is difficult to see without good illumination or a loupe or even a slit lamp, or the blood may entirely fill the eyeball (an eight-ball hemorrhage). This is a serious problem, and the child should be placed at complete bed rest under deep sedation, with both eyes patched. Rebleeding or secondary hemorrhage occurs most frequently during the third to fifth day after injury and may lead to the dreaded complication of secondary glaucoma. If conservative therapy fails, surgical intervention and washing out of the clot may be needed.

SYSTEMIC DISEASES

Congenital syphilis. Congenital syphilis was formerly a common condition in the outpatient department of any large hospital. Since the advent of penicillin and early and more thorough treatment of patients, the eye manifestations of congenital syphilis, such as interstitial keratitis, chorioretinitis, and Argyll Robertson pupil are rarely seen in the clinic.

Toxoplasmosis. Toxoplasmosis has been recognized to be an important cause of ocular inflammatory disease. The organism is a protozoan parasite that affects many animals and birds. The distribution is worldwide. Most cases in children are congenital, the infection being acquired from the mother in utero. Large patches of chorioretinitis are seen that are often inactive and pigmented by the time the diagnosis is made. Manifestations of the central nervous system include cerebral calcifications and deafness (p. 322).

German measles (rubella). When rubella occurs during the first trimester of pregnancy, a high percentage of congenital anomalies may occur (pp. 319-321). The commonest ocular anomaly is congenital cataract. There are two varieties, the more severe of which almost always requires surgical removal. Prognosis is guarded because other anomalies of the eye may also be present, including microphthalmus and iris hypoplasia. Rubella retinopathy and rubella glaucoma may also occur. The latter can be transitory in nature.

Measles (rubeola). Conjunctivitis and epithelial keratitis are common early in the course of measles. Children were formerly consigned to a dark room to "protect" the eyes. This is no longer considered necessary because the ocular manifestations clear with the disease. Rarely, when encephalitis is a complication of measles, optic neuritis and other complications may occur. No treatment of the eyes is necessary. A delayed manifestation of latent rubeola may result in Dawson encephalitis (SSPE), which has visual disturbances as one of its signs.

Mumps. Involvement of the lacrimal gland beneath the upper outer border of the orbit is not uncommon with mumps. Inflammatory foci in the eye rarely occur. Mumps encephalitis may cause pupillary abnormalities and paralysis of extraocular muscles.

Vaccinia. Occasionally the vaccine virus is carried to the eye by fingers of the child from his own or another's vaccination. Typical blebs with much edema may be produced on the lids. Rarely does the cornea become involved. Treatment consists of hyperimmune gamma globulin given systemically. More recently, IDU applied locally has been found to be effective.

Chickenpox (varicella). Swollen lids and catarrhal conjunctivitis, rarely with vesicles, may be seen in chickenpox. Treatment of ocular involvement is that of the general disease.

Histoplasmosis. Histoplasmosis may be the presumptive cause in posterior chorioretinitis, in which there is usually a posterior polar lesion near the macula, with hemorrhagic borders and satellite lesions farther out in the periphery. The diagnosis is presumptive, even if histoplasmosis is confirmed elsewhere in the body. Treatment for the main part consists of local or retrobulbar cortical steroids, although histoplasmin desensitization and amphotericin B systemically have been tried. Photocoagulation of the lesion with the Zeiss photocoagulator after studying the lesion with intravenous fluorescein has been practiced. (See pp. 759-760.)

Cerebral palsy. The eye manifestations of cerebral palsy are extremely common, two out of three such children having some eye defect. The commonest eye problem is a refractive error, usually consisting of astigmatism mixed either with hyperopia or myopia. Extraocular muscle disturbances, with esotropia dominating, is the next most common anomaly. Except for the presence of other associated phenomena such as nystagmus, the ocular manifestations consist of those that one would expect with any central nervous system disease. Except for prevention of amblyopia, treatment for the associated refractive errors and strabismus is often delayed in these children, as contrasted to the treatment of the normal child. (See pp. 782 and 783.)

Leukemia. Ocular manifestations of leukemia in children are extremely common and may consist of Roth spots in the fundus. These are little red hemorrhages with white centers thought to contain leukemic cells. Retrobulbar and intraocular hemorrhage may be massive. Hemorrhage and exudation may cloud the fundus; venous engorgement, sheathing, sausage-shaped vessels, and dark-appearing vessels may also be present. Another manifestation is optic neuritis or optic nerve infiltration with leukemic cells. A sterile hypopyon appearing in a child should make the physician rule out the presence of leukemia before other conditions are considered. Leukemic cells may infiltrate other regions of the eye, such as the sclera, choroid, and conjunctiva. Actual infiltration into the orbit may occur.

Marfan syndrome. In Marfan syndrome the patient presents with bony anomalies of arachnodactyly, high arched palate, lax joints, and cardiac disease resembling aortic insufficiency or dissecting aneurysm. The most important point, however, is the presence of subluxated lenses, with the lenses usually displaced upward and outward in the presence of a tremulous iris. Associated with the condition may be glaucoma, high myopia, keratoconus, megalocornea, blue sclera, and retinal detachment. The ophthalmologist should try to refract the patient's eye both through the phakic portion and the aphakic portion with a dilated pupil before deciding on further therapy.

Homocystinuria. Homocystinuria is an inborn error of metabolism that presents with an excretion of homocystine, an amino acid seldom found in the urine. The probable deficiency of the enzyme cystathionine synthetase leads to increased levels of methionine and homocystine. The clinical manifestations include fair complexion with a mild flush, mental retardation, seizures, bone anomalies, thromboembolic phenomenon, extreme nearsightedness, and dislocated lenses. This disease should be added to the differential diagnosis of ectopia lentis, which may be its presenting sign. (See p. 650.)

Galactosemia. The deficiency of galactose-1-phosphate uridyl transferase may produce a variety of manifestations. Among the serious effects of this disease are zonular cataracts, which occur in about three fourths of the cases, are often seen in the first week of life, and are bilateral. With a high-powered lens and an ophthalmoscope they appear to be like an oil drop in the center of the pupil because of the enhancement of the refractive power around the fetal nucleus. Osmotic hydration and accumulation of galactose alcohol metabolites have been suggested as possible causes. Early diagnosis in infancy is important, since restriction of the galactose intake may cause a reversal of the cataract formation; the cataracts may sometimes regress spontaneously. (See p. 656.)

Alkaptonuria. In alkaptonuria there is a deficiency of homogentesic acid oxidate substrate, a derivate of tyrosinase that accumulates in the body tissues and is excreted in the urine. Ochronosis describes the ocher pigmentation of cartilage, especially in the ear and of the sclera, particularly on either side of the corneal limbus where the rectus muscle inserts. Conjunctival staining in the form of brown droplets and staining of Bowman's membrane of the cornea have been described. Usually pigmentation does not become striking until the second decade of life.

Cystinosis. Cystinosis is a defect in the proximal tubules of the kidney that permits the loss of phosphate, with renal rickets, glycosuria, and generalized aminoaciduria. The role of cystine throughout the body has not been carefully delineated, but cystine crystals have been found in the cornea, conjunctiva, ciliary body, choroid, iris, and sclera. Photophobia may be a complaint, but the corneal lesions may be asymptomatic. These consist of diffuse haze that may be easily overlooked. A conjunctival biopsy may be helpful. (See p. 652.)

Mucopolysaccharidoses. All of the present mucopolysaccharidoses are classified according to the by-products found in the urine. At the present time several forms are known, including Morquio, Hunter, Hurler, Sanfilippo, Scheie, and Maroteaux-Lamy syndrome, all of which (except Hunter and Sanfilippo), have eye manifestations that include corneal clouding. If congenital glaucoma is known to be absent, any child with a cloudy cornea should have a workup for mucopolysaccharidoses. (See pp. 657-660.)

Myasthenia gravis. In myasthenia gravis in children the commonest presenting sign may be ptosis, although extraocular muscle paresis can also occur. Diagnosis is confirmed with the reduction of the ptosis with edrophonium (Tensilon) and a therapeutic response to the drug when administered systemically.

Cerebromacular and macular degeneration. In this group of conditions in which there is macular degeneration, illustrated by Best's disease, and in cerebromacular degeneration with a severe central nervous system involvement with the degenerative process (illustrated by Tay-Sachs disease), there are various macular changes including degeneration, clumping of pigment, and atrophy, with subsequent decrease in visual acuity.

REFRACTION

The commonest anomaly of the eyes is refractive error. Children are profoundly affected by refractive difficulties, especially after they have reached school age, when studies demand good vision. On the other hand, children may go for a long time with undetected vision in the 20/100 range, particularly if such vision had a gradual onset. Because of visual impairment or excessive focus effort, the child may do inferior schoolwork and become nervous and irritable.

Fortunately, present-day periodic vision tests in the public and private schools uncover most errors of refraction.

A word should be said in reference to headaches and their relation to refractive errors. Although it is true that headaches can occur as a result of increased effort, particularly at the end of the day or after doing near work in the presence of refractive errors, it is often overemphasized.

There are three types of refractive errors that affect children: (1) hyperopia, (2) myopia, and (3) astigmatism. The type of error is determined by the shape of the eyeball and the relationship of the different refractive surfaces and media. The shape of the eyeball is inherited, just as any structural feature is inherited, although there is evidence that this may be modified by acquired influences. The eyeball grows as the child grows until the adult size and shape is reached. While the child grows, the refraction may change greatly in some children. Hyperopia increases until about 7 years of age and then decreases slowly until adulthood is reached. On the other hand, myopia may increase gradually from the early or teen years until adulthood is reached.

Hyperopia. In hyperopia (farsightedness) the eyeball is thought of as being too short. Rays of light passing through the cornea and the lens would, if possible, come to a focus behind the retina. The curvature of the lens must therefore be changed to bring the focus forward to the retina. This act requires effort by the ciliary muscles. If the hyperopia is great, the ciliary muscles become tired, readily producing symptoms of strain. Fortunately, children have a large amount of accommodating or focusing power. Thus in simple hyperopia, despite the strain, visual acuity is good for distance and near vision. Correction of this error is accomplished with convex lenses that reduce the excessive demand for the muscular effort of focusing.

It must be remembered that should this focusing be accompanied by a reflex stimulus to the convergence mechanism, the child may undergo an esotropia caused purely by the excessive accommodative effort. In these children, correction by medication or glasses may completely correct the strabismus. Likewise, it should be remembered that a difference between the two eyes (an anisometropia) may lead either to a small degree of strabismus or, equally important, to amblyopia caused by the difference in the retinal image sizes.

Myopia. In myopia (nearsightedness) the eyeball is too long, and the focus falls in front of the retina, producing a blurred image for distance. The nearsighted child can often read without the muscular effort of focusing. He may, however, have to hold the print close to his eyes to obtain a clear focus if myopia is of high degree. This focusing anomaly is readily corrected by concave lenses but may tend to increase gradually over a period of years until adulthood is reached.

Congenital myopia may be of high degree in the range of 10, 15, and even 20 diopters of myopia. Fortunately the vision tends to improve gradually with age and is generally in the 20/40 range by the time the teenage years are reached. Furthermore, this myopia, in contrast to the acquired variety, usually does not tend to increase. This can be consoling to the parents. Corrective lenses may not be worn by these children until they become more visually attentive, near the school-age period.

Astigmatism. In astigmatism the curvature of the cornea, instead of being the same in all meridians, is flatter in one meridian than in the meridian usually perpendicular to it. Rays of light are not focused symmetrically on the retina; objects viewed are distorted and blurred. Because the eye constantly tries to obtain a clear image, although it cannot, the muscular effort is nonrewarding and tiring. This effort is corrected by a lens that compensates for the abnormal curvature of the cornea, which is called a cylinder.

Testing for glasses (refraction) in young persons with significant refractive errors is best carried out with the accommodation or focusing power completely at rest. The state of rest or suspension of focusing permits a more accurate measurement of the refractive error, which would otherwise be constantly changing during the examination of children. Cycloplegic drugs, such as atropine, are used at the first examination. In subsequent refractions, cycloplegia may often be omitted.

The correction of refractive errors with lenses is one of the most positive therapeutic measures in medicine and brings much alleviation to the patient and gratification to the physician.

Blinking. An associated symptom with that

of refraction may be blinking. Parents of these children bring the child to the pediatrician or ophthalmologist complaining that the child blinks excessively, particularly at various times of the day. Although refractive errors and other evidences of eyestrain should be searched for, often no cause whatsoever is found. Once the presence of pathology, including local lid disease and conjunctival disease, is ruled out, these children are best left alone for a time. If blinking persists, mild sedation or use of tranquilizers is helpful.

Reading problems. The incidence of a specific reading problem (dyslexia) is much less common than reading problems in general. It has been estimated that the incidence of reading problems varies, but it may be in the range of 7% to 8% of all children in school. Only 1% are probably the result of a specific reading disability or dyslexia, with boys outnumbering girls 8:1. (See also p. 38.)

Once it has been determined that a child is reading a year or two behind his grade level, a definite reading problem can be said to exist. The actual detection that a reading problem exists will usually be initiated by the parent or teacher.

Once the children are referred for medical or other evaluation, a general physical examination, with special emphasis on the neurologic examination, should be done. If indicated, consultation in regard to hearing and sight should be sought. Special emphasis should be given to the possibility of the existence of minimal brain dysfunction (see Chapter 3). Then, in the absence of any known medical or physical disability, psychologic testing or psychiatric evaluation should be done. Reading testing and a general aptitude and specific remedial evaluation, such as those performed in a reading clinic, should of course be included.

In the absence of any known treatable condition detected during the workup, most of these children are then best helped by tutoring. It is doubtful that eye exercises or visual training to train the motor part of the visual input is worthwhile. However, in the hands of trained, effective basic reading teachers with time to spend, most of these children can be taught to read, and their reading skills and speed can be improved. Special classes for those thought to be visually perceptually handicapped should be sought out, depending on availability in the general area.

Subnormal vision. The education of children with subnormal vision uncontrolled by conventional medical, surgical, and optical treatment becomes of great concern. In general, the following facts should be kept in mind:

1. Special glasses or optical aids should be given to increase the size of the retinal image.
2. Reading aids, such as a reading stand and reading markers, can aid the child's reading.
3. The so-called "sight saving" books are reserved for children who cannot read the N-18 or 18-point type of regular books with the best optical correction.
4. Resource rooms or "sight saving" classes are helpful for the visually handicapped but are not necessary if the teacher and school system have enough special help available for children with subnormal visual problems.

Braille and schools for the blind are reserved for those blind children who must use a nonvisual method for the primary communicative skill.

Roger L. Hiatt

SELECTED READINGS

Liebman, S.D., and Gellis, S.S.: The pediatrician's ophthalmology, St. Louis, 1966, The C.V. Mosby Co.

Ophthalmology Staff of the Toronto Hospital for Sick Children: The eye in childhood, Chicago, 1967, Year Book Medical Publishers, Inc.

Parks, M.M.: Ocular motility and strabismus, New York, 1975, Harper & Row, Publishers.

Roy, F.H.: Ocular differential diagnosis, Philadelphia, 1975, Lea & Febiger.

Scheie, H.G., and Albert, D.M.: Textbook of ophthalmology, Philadelphia, 1977, W.B. Saunders Co.

37 Pediatric Otolaryngology

Pediatric otolaryngology is concerned with the diagnosis and management of diseases and anomalies of the head and neck. This includes not only the well known "ear, nose, and throat" problems but also other medically and surgically treated problems of the head and neck.

EAR AND MASTOID

Structure and function. The ear is divided anatomically into three parts, the external ear, the middle ear, and the inner ear. It is the organ of hearing and balance. Embryologically, the ear arises from the first and second branchial arches, the first branchial cleft, and the first branchial pouch. The external ear is comprised of the auricle and external auditory canal and develops around the first branchial cleft from derivatives of the first and second branchial arches. The middle ear includes the entire middle ear cleft (the tympanic cavity with ossicles), the mastoid cavity, and the eustachian tube. It arises from the first pharyngeal pouch. The mastoid cavity enlarges and becomes clinically important at about 1 or 2 years of age. The inner ear consists of the cochlea, which is the organ of hearing, and the vestibular labyrinth, which is the organ of balance. The inner ear soft tissue is neuroectodermal in origin and is fully developed at birth, although the bony inner ear capsule is not completely ossified at birth.

The auricle is composed of skin-covered cartilage. The skin is continuous down the external canal and over the tympanic membrane, becoming progressively thinner with fewer appendages as it approaches the tympanic membrane. The medial portion of the external canal is bony, and the lateral portion is cartilaginous. There are three layers found in the normal tympanic membrane: squamous epithelium is the lateral layer, mucosa of the middle ear cleft is the medial layer, and a sturdy layer of fibrous tissue lies between the two. This fibrous tissue attaches to the long process of the malleus and extends peripherally to the annulus, which attaches the tympanic membrane to the bony external canal.

The middle ear and mastoid are normally air filled and lined with pseudostratified ciliated respiratory epithelium, which is of the columnar type near the eustachian tube orifice and gradually becomes cuboidal without cilia in the mastoid cells. Development of the middle ear is largely completed by birth. The eustachian tube initially develops in a horizontal plane and in later life becomes more forward and downward, sloping into the nasopharynx. The ossicles are found in the middle ear cleft, connecting the tympanic membrane to the oval window of the inner ear. Other prominent structures in the middle ear include the round window, the facial nerve, and the promontory of the cochlea. The inner ear is embedded in the petrous bone, which is the hardest bone in the body. Inside the bony labyrinth of the inner ear is found the membranous labyrinth, which is filled with endolymph and surrounded and cushioned by perilymph. The membranous labyrinth is composed of the three semicircular canals as well as the utricle and saccule. These structures have specialized areas containing aggregates of neuroectodermal hair cells, which are the sensory end organ cells for balance. The cochlea also contains hair cells in the organ of Corti. These hair cells are the end organs for hearing. Sensory signals from the hair cells are carried along the vestibular and cochlear nerves, which eventually join to make up the eighth cranial nerve.

The external ear funnels sound to the tympanic membrane and aids in localization of sound. The tympanic membrane and ossicles have approximately a 22 to 1 mechanical advantage and transform sound energy vibrations in the air into fluid vibrations in the inner ear. The stapedius muscle and tensor tympani muscle are located in the middle ear and have a protective function to dampen middle ear vibrations when potentially damaging loud sounds occur. The cilia and secretory cells of the middle ear mucosa keep the middle ear clean, with the cilia constantly beating toward the eustachian tube to carry mucus and debris to the nasopharynx. A more important function of the eustachian tube is to equalize pressure between the middle ear and the surrounding environment. There are several theories of hearing, the most commonly accepted being the traveling wave theory, which proposes that the area of maximum displacement of the fluid waves in the inner ear determines the particular signals that are sent to the brain. This is an oversimplification but is the most generally accepted theory today. The semicircular canals monitor angular acceleration, and the utricle and saccule monitor linear acceleration.

Diagnosis. For discussion of ear examination see pp. 246-247. Pneumotoscopy is a valuable diagnostic aid in determining mobility of the tympanic membranes and the presence or absence of fluid in the middle ear cavity. In the very young child this may be difficult and often unreliable. The child will usually have to be restrained and the instrument will have to be completely sealed in the external canal. An objective and more elegant method of measuring middle ear function is available using the tympanometer. This instrument has a variety of tips to ensure a good seal in the external canal. A wide range of negative and positive pressures may be applied to the eardrum, and the compliance of the eardrum is measured using a built-in impedance bridge that bounces sound waves off the tympanic membrane and can measure the amount of sound reflected and absorbed.

The normal tympanic membrane with pressure equalized on both sides is very compliant and absorbs the highest percentage of sound. The retracted tympanic membrane or the bulging tympanic membrane are not very compliant and reflect the highest percentage of sound. The results of the test are plotted on a graph called a tympanogram. The three basic types of tympanograms are shown in Fig. 37-1. Type A tympanogram indicates normal tympanic membrane mobility and compliance. Type B tympanogram indicates poor compliance and is most commonly associated with fluid in the middle ear. Type C tympanogram indicates good compliance at a negative pressure, indicating there is negative pressure in the middle ear system, which is the result of eustachian tube dysfunction.

Additional information may be easily gathered by measuring the stapedius reflex. This is an integral part of the routine tympanogram and involves the presentation of a pure tone at various frequencies at a sound intensity of 75 to 85 dB above the hearing thresholds. At this level the stapedius muscle is activated to dampen the middle ear system and change the compliance of the tympanic membrane. The clinical application of stapedius reflex testing is that a rough estimate of hearing threshold may be obtained. There are variations of the three basic types of tympanograms that have more subtle indications. The interested student is referred to any of the modern textbooks on audiology.

Audiometry and hearing loss. Conventional audiometry is usually reliable in children age 3 and older and provides an accurate assessment of hearing. In younger children a modification of the conventional test called sound field testing may be necessary, with the disadvantage of having to test both ears simultaneously. The pure-tone audiogram is performed in a soundproof booth with headphones on the patient. Sounds are presented to one ear at a time to measure the patient's air conduction, which determines the hearing levels of the entire hearing mechanism. If this is abnormal, the patient's bone conduction is tested using a bone conduction oscillator, which is placed on the patient's skull to determine the sensitivity of the patient's sensorineural mechanism, effectively bypassing the external and middle ear.

A normal audiogram will have air conduction levels at all frequencies at a range of 0 to 10 dB of sound. A *conductive* hearing loss exists when the bone conduction level is at a lesser sound pressure than that of the air conduction level. A *sensorineural* hearing loss exists when the air conduction and bone conduction results show the same hearing loss below the 10 dB line at frequencies tested. A mixed hearing loss exists when a combination of conductive loss and sensorineural loss is present. Examples of these three basic types of hearing loss are seen in the pure-tone audiograms in Fig. 37-2. Much more

Text continued on p. 994.

NAME ______________________ DATE ____________

ADDRESS ______________________ NUMBER ____________

______________________ BIRTHDATE ____________

EQUIPMENT ______________________ EXAMINER ____________

Speech Audiometry

	SRT	% Corr.	S/N	% Corr.
R				
L				
R				
L				
Bin or FF				
Aided				

Speech Materials

SRT
Discrim.
Records:
Live Voice:

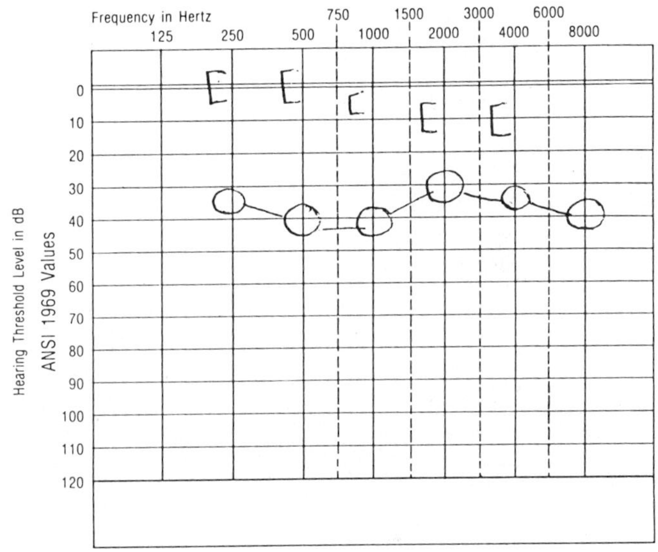

CONDUCTIVE HEARING LOSS

Masking:	Weber lateralizes to:			125	250	500	1000	2000	4000	
Complex:	Masking levels used	in right ear (testing left)	A/C							
WBTN:			B/C							
		in left ear (testing right)	A/C							
Other:			B/C							

Legend

	Right		Left
Air Conduction	O		X
A/C Masked	△		□
Bone Conduction	<		>
B/C Masked	[		]
Sound Field		*	
No Response	↙	NR	↘
	Right Ear — Red		Left Ear — Blue

Patient's Hearing Aid

Make:	
Model:	
Gain:	MPO:
Receiver:	Ear:
Other:	

Fig. 37-2, cont'd. Pure tone audiograms showing conductive hearing loss.

NAME ______________________ DATE ______________

ADDRESS ______________________ NUMBER ______________

______________________ BIRTHDATE ______________

EQUIPMENT ______________________ EXAMINER ______________

Speech Audiometry

	SRT	% Corr.	S/N	% Corr.
R				
L				
R				
L				
Bin or FF				
Aided				

Speech Materials

SRT
Discrim.
Records:
Live Voice:

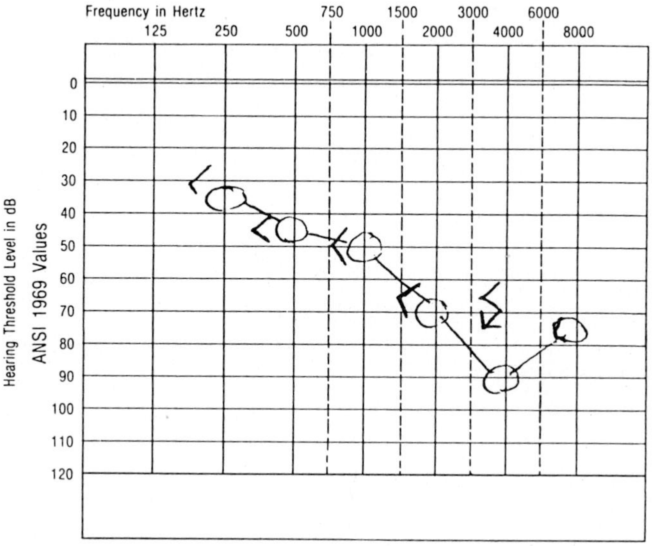

SENSORINEURAL HEARING LOSS

Masking:	Weber lateralizes to:			125	250	500	1000	2000	4000	
Complex:	Masking levels used	in right ear (testing left)	A/C							
WBTN:			B/C							
		in left ear (testing right)	A/C							
Other:			B/C							

Legend

	Right		Left
Air Conduction	○		X
A/C Masked	△		□
Bone Conduction	<		>
B/C Masked	[		]
Sound Field		*	
No Response	↙	NR	↘
	Right Ear — Red		Left Ear — Blue

Patient's Hearing Aid

Make:	
Model:	
Gain:	MPO:
Receiver:	Ear:
Other:	

Fig. 37-2, cont'd. Pure tone audiograms showing sensorineural hearing loss.

NAME ______________________ DATE __________

ADDRESS ______________________ NUMBER __________

______________________ BIRTHDATE __________

EQUIPMENT ______________________ EXAMINER __________

Speech Audiometry

	SRT	% Corr.	S/N	% Corr.
R				
L				
R				
L				
Bin or FF				
Aided				

Speech Materials

SRT
Discrim.
Records:
Live Voice:

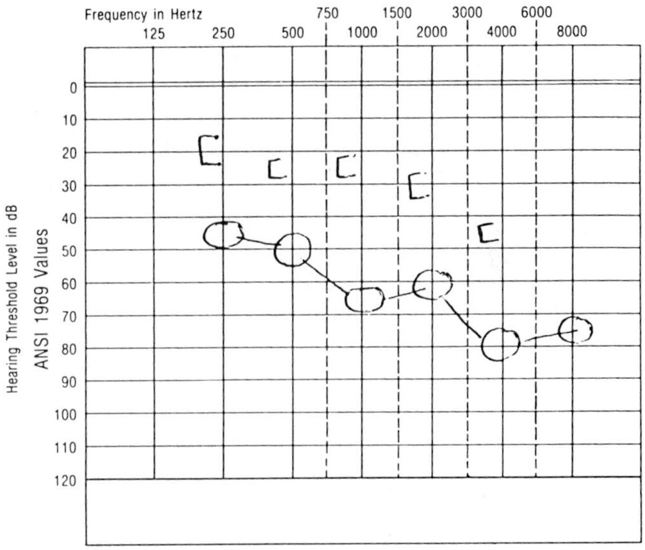

MIXED HEARING LOSS

Masking:	Weber lateralizes to:			125	250	500	1000	2000	4000	
Complex:	Masking levels used	in right ear (testing left)	A/C							
WBTN:			B/C							
		in left ear (testing right)	A/C							
Other:			B/C							

Legend

	Right	Left
Air Conduction	O	X
A/C Masked	△	□
Bone Conduction	<	>
B/C Masked	[	]
Sound Field	*	
No Response	↙ NR	↘
Right Ear — Red	Left Ear — Blue	

Patient's Hearing Aid

Make:	
Model:	
Gain:	MPO:
Receiver:	Ear:
Other:	

Fig. 37-2, cont'd. Pure tone audiograms showing mixed conductive and sensorineural hearing loss.

information is obtained in the standard audiologic evaluation, including speech audiometry, which determines the hearing level at which patients can understand speech in each ear, and speech discrimination testing, which determines the percentage of the words heard that are actually understood. For infants and uncooperative children of any age, brainstem-evoked responses, commonly known as BSER, provide objective data on the auditory pathway even when the patient is under general anesthesia.

Early identification of children with hearing loss is essential, as failure to do so leads to permanent disability in speech and language development. Children with significant hearing loss of 30 dB or more should have hearing aids and special training begun at least by 12 months of age. Neonatal screening of high-risk infants together with a high index of suspicion on the part of the pediatrician will lead to identification of children with hearing loss at an early age when they can receive the maximum benefit from available technical and therapuetic intervention.

Vestibular testing is difficult in young children but some useful information may be obtained by using the electronystagmogram in children older than 4 years of age when indicated.

A variety of congenital malformations of the ear can occur. The auricle and external canal may have aberrations varying from only very mild to extremely severe. Marked deformity of the pinna, including total absence of the pinna, may occur and is frequently accompanied by stenosis or atresia of the external auditory canal. Preauricular cysts, which develop from small sinus tracts, frequently become infected, and when this occurs they must be surgically removed. Anomalies of the middle ear may accompany external canal malformations or may occur independently. These frequently occur with Treacher Collins syndrome and Crouzon syndrome. Surgical correction of middle ear and external canal deformities is possible and is most successful in those patients with well-developed middle ear spaces. Radiologic studies are helpful in determining the best operative candidates. The presence of a tragus correlates highly with a relatively normal middle ear. Eustachian tube abnormalities with secondary otitis media can cause significant hearing loss. Inner ear deformities may result in a broad spectrum of hearing losses ranging from mild to severe. Valuable information concerning the type of inner ear deformity may be obtained by a combination of audiometric and radiologic studies.

Most of the patients with congenital deafness have no visible anatomic abnormality. Approximately 50% of congenital hearing loss is inherited, and of this approximately 90% has an autosomal recessive inheritance pattern. Many of these patients have other abnormalities, and a large number of syndromes have been defined. For example, in Usher syndrome there is an autosomal recessive hearing loss and retinitis pigmentosa. Pendred syndrome has autosomal recessive hearing loss and goiter. Alport disease is autosomal dominant sensorineural hearing loss and progressive nephritis.

This leaves another 50% of the congenital hearing loss patients who have an acquired etiology for their hearing loss. These include the TORCH group of diseases, kernicterus, and syphilis.

Another large group of sensorineural hearing loss patients are those who suffer acquired hearing loss after birth. Mumps is the most common cause of unilateral acquired sensorineural hearing loss in children. Other causes of acquired sensorineural hearing loss are measles and meningitis.

Otitis externa. Otitis externa may occur at any time but is frequently seen during swimming season and in fact is sometimes called "swimmer's ear." This diagnosis is made by eliciting pain when gently touching the auricle and by examination of the ear, revealing superficial infection of the external canal. The primary organisms associated with otitis externa are *Pseudomonas* and *Staphylococcus aureus*. Occasionally a fungal overgrowth with *Aspergillus* or *Candida* occurs. Otitis externa is treated with broad-spectrum antibiotic drops, frequently containing a steroid as an anti-inflammatory agent. These may be used directly or in more severe cases may be delivered through a wick in the external canal. If the infection does not resolve quickly, the external canal may need to be cleaned, using a small suction tip under microscopic control. Great care must be taken if any polyps are seen in the external canal, because these may be associated with a middle ear problem and may be attached to the ossicles. Tugging on the polyp may result in removal of an ossicle. Additionally, polyps may represent inflammation overlying a cholesteatoma.

Otitis media and mastoiditis. Inflammatory conditions of the middle ear are among the most common medical problems in the pediatric age group. It is important to have an understanding of their pathophysiology in approaching the patient so that rational treatment is administered. In inflammatory conditions of the middle ear an important fact to remember is that the middle ear spaces are all connected, and in acute infections all of the epithelium of the middle ear is involved to a greater or lesser degree. As discussed earlier, this includes the epithelium of the eustachian tubes, the tympanum, the aditus, and the mastoid. If the inflammatory process extends beyond the mucoperiosteal lining of the middle ear cleft, complications occur. Most common of these are mastoiditis, labyrinthitis, meningitis, and temporal or posterior lobe abscesses. Mastoiditis is often overdiagnosed; it should be remembered that mastoiditis occurs only when there is osteitis present. Otitis should not be classified as mastoiditis when there is only infection of the membranes with or without fluid in the mastoid cell system. Consequently, radiologic examination showing thickening of the epithelium and fluid in the mastoid does not indicate mastoiditis.

In almost all cases of otitis media there is *dysfunction of the eustachian tube*. This may be either primary or secondary. Treatment of recurrent inflammatory conditions of the middle ear without the realization that eustachian tube dysfunction exists leads to undue recurrent infections and complications (see Fig. 37-3). In current practice, the use of pressure-equalizing tubes through the tympanic membrane to bypass the malfunction of the eustachian tube is one of the commonest and most rewarding surgical procedures. There is not uniform agreement concerning the precise indication of pressure-equalizing tube insertion. However, it is generally accepted that, in children with frequent recurrent otitis and in children with persistent middle effusions that do not respond to medical therapy, the placement of pressure-equalizing tubes is indicated.

For discussion of *serous otitis media* and of *acute otitis media* see pp. 383 and 381-383 respectively.

Chronic otitis media results in a permanent perforation of the tympanic membrane and persistent or recurrent infection and drainage. This is probably a sequela of acute otitis media with perforation. The usual causative organisms are *Pseudomonas* and *Staphylococcus aureus*. The perforation of the tympanic membrane may be large or small and may be associated with cholesteatoma. A cholesteatoma is a growth of skin and debris in a closed area resulting in pressure necrosis of the ossicles and bony walls of the middle ear cavity. Severe complications including meningitis and brain abscess may result from

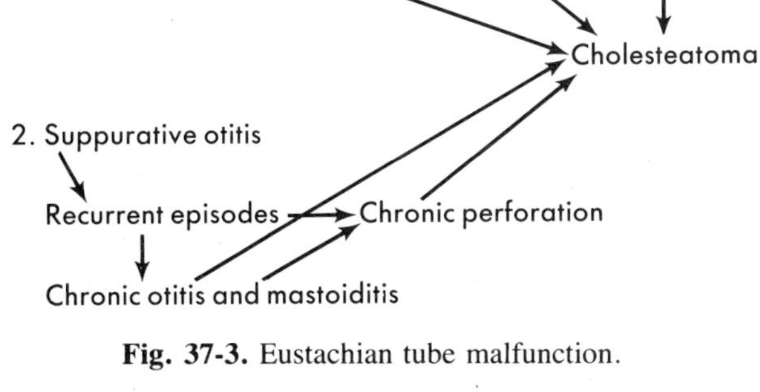

Fig. 37-3. Eustachian tube malfunction.

cholesteatoma. Chronic otitis media is usually treated with topical ear drops and systemic antibiotics. Eventually a tympanoplasty (repair of the tympanic membrane) is necessary and, in cases of persistent infection or cholesteatoma, mastoidectomy is indicated as well.

Adhesive otitis occurs as a result of repeated episodes of acute otitis, or as a complication of chronic otitis. It may also occur in cases of eustachian tube dysfunction without otitis. There is retraction of the tympanic membrane with thinning, scarring, and adhesions of the middle ear structures. Surgical reconstruction is helpful in relieving the hearing loss in many of these cases.

True *labyrinthitis* is quite rare. Authorities disagree about the existence of a viral labyrinthitis other than those previously mentioned related to mumps or measles and resulting in a hearing loss. Bacterial labyrinthitis, called *suppurative labyrinthitis,* causes permanent total hearing loss. Serous labyrinthitis is seen when nearby infection causes an inflammatory response in the labyrinth. The pathogenesis here is similar to that of sympathetic meningitis. Serous labyrinthitis is associated with hearing loss that may be either temporary or permanent.

Trauma. *Trauma to the ear* may result in perforation of the tympanic membrane. It is important to examine the patient as soon as possible to determine if any sensorineural loss has occurred in addition to the conductive loss caused by perforation of the tympanic membrane. This can usually be tested by using a tuning fork to perform the Weber test. In a patient with previously normal hearing, this test should lateralize to the injured ear if a conductive loss is the only injury. More severe injuries may involve the inner ear by rupturing the oval window or round window. These patients usually suffer significant dizziness that persists after the injury and will have associated sensorineural hearing loss. This will cause the Weber test to lateralize to the noninjured ear. A fistula test may be performed by applying gentle positive or negative pressure to the external canal, which in the presence of an inner ear injury will elicit nystagmus, vertigo, and sometimes nausea.

Significant head trauma may cause a fracture of the petrous bone, known more commonly as a temporal bone fracture or basilar skull fracture. Such fractures usually occur along the long axis of the internal auditory canal that carries the seventh and eighth nerve in the temporal bone. These are called longitudinal fractures and do not usually injure the nerves themselves. The fracture line usually runs through the middle ear and external canal, causing a hemotympanum and perforation of the tympanic membrane with subsequent bloody drainage from the ear. Audiometric studies will reveal a conductive hearing loss in the affected ear. Function of the seventh nerve is usually normal.

The less common type of fracture, called a transverse fracture, occurs at an angle other than parallel to the internal auditory canal and has a high degree of association of injury of the seventh and eighth cranial nerves. This type of fracture may or may not be associated with hemotympanum but is usually associated with severe sensorineural hearing loss and some degree of facial paresis or paralysis. It is extremely important in trauma cases to determine whether the facial nerve deficit had its onset several hours or days later. Facial paralysis of immediate onset requires surgical intervention, whereas facial paralysis of delayed onset is managed conservatively with electrical stimulation of the facial nerve and surgical intervention only if signs of degeneration of the seventh nerve develop.

Bell's palsy is an idiopathic paresis or paralysis of one side of the facial musculature caused by an abnormality of the facial nerve. It is thought to be a result of viral inflammation of the trunk of the seventh cranial nerve. It is a diagnosis of exclusion, because any treatable cause for the paralysis such as acute otitis media, cholesteatoma, or acoustic neuroma must be ruled out. Once a total paralysis is evident, facial nerve stimulation is performed regularly to monitor the condition of the nerve. Surgical decompression of the nerve is rarely necessary in children. Systemic steroids have not proved to be beneficial in studies involving children.

NOSE AND PARANASAL SINUSES

Structure and function. The nose develops from the embryonic nasal pits. The maxillary and ethmoid sinuses develop in the lateral nasal wall and are present at birth. Later in life, the frontal sinuses and the sphenoid sinuses develop as extensions of the ethmoid sinus cells. The sinuses develop in pairs, although the frontal and sphenoid sinuses are very irregular from side to side. Approximately 15% of the population have only one frontal sinus, and 5% have no frontal sinus at all.

The external nose is a cartilaginous and bony structure covered by skin. It is divided internally into two halves by the nasal septum. Forming the internal lateral wall of the nose are the three turbinates and just inferior to each turbinate is its meatus into which various sinuses and the nasal lacrimal duct drain. The anterior septum is very vascular, having a plexus of arteries and veins that is called Kiesselbach's plexus or Little's area. The maxillary sinuses gradually occupy more and more of the maxillary bone as the permanent teeth erupt and occupy their position lower in the midface. At approximately 12 years of age the floor of the maxillary sinus has descended to the same level as the floor of the nose.

The function of the nose is to clean, warm, and humidify the incoming air. This is accomplished by the tiny hairs called vibrissae located at the nostrils, by the epithelium folded over the turbinates, and by the very vascular epithelial lining of the entire nasal cavity. There is a nasal cycle that includes alternating blockage of either side of the nose as the turbinates swell and shrink. Located in the superior portion of the nasal cavity is the area of olfactory epithelium that is the end organ of the sense of smell. This is combined with the sense of taste to give the total sensation of flavor. The most significant functions of the paranasal sinuses are to warm and humidify the inspired air. The nasal cavity and paranasal sinuses do serve as a resonance chamber for the voice.

Diagnosis. The nasal cavities are fairly easy to examine, especially after the use of topical vasoconstrictors such as cocaine or phenylephrine. The sinuses are difficult to examine, although palpation is helpful to elicit tenderness indicating underlying infection. A thorough examination of the sinuses can be performed radiologically.

Congenital defects of the nose and paranasal sinuses are rare. An abnormal appearance of the nose is present in cases of complete cleft lip. Occasionally a hypoplastic maxillary sinus may be seen that is easily confused with sinusitis. Dermoid cysts develop from epithelial cell rests in the lines of embryonic fusion and must be differentiated from encephalocele or gliomas.

Choanal atresia is discussed on p. 294.

Tumors of the nose and paranasal sinuses are rare, except for *nasal polyps,* which are usually the result of allergy or infection. Nasal polyps always should alert the examiner to the possibility of cystic fibrosis.

Viral upper respiratory infections affect the entire upper airway but seem to produce the most bothersome symptoms in the nasal cavity. Symptomatic treatment is usually satisfactory. Topical vasoconstrictors may be used briefly, but their chronic use may result in rhinitis medicamentosa with thickening of the nasal mucosa and blockage of the patient's airway. This is best treated by using a brief course of oral steroids followed by a 3 to 4 week course of intranasal steroids.

Acute sinusitis is discussed on p. 385-386.

Chronic sinusitis responds poorly to medical management. Nevertheless, intensive treatment with systemic antibiotics, a brief course of topical decongestants, followed by several weeks of intranasal steroids is indicated. The usual causative organisms include a mixed flora with aerobic and anerobic organisms. Allergy is frequently associated with acute and chronic sinusitis. Cases resistant to medical therapy may need diagnostic washing of the sinuses or surgical placement of antrostomies.

Periorbital cellulitis is an important complication of sinusitis. It is usually of rapid onset and involves swelling of the periorbital area with eventual ophthalmoplegia. Once this stage is reached the morbidity is significant. Periorbital cellulitis must be treated actively with intravenous antibiotics, including staphylococcal coverage. Vigorous nasal hygiene with topical decongestants is performed simultaneously. If the patient shows no improvement in 24 to 36 hours, surgical intervention is mandatory. Untreated periorbital cellulitis may lead to meningitis, brain abscess, or cavernous sinus thrombosis.

Persistent unilateral foul-smelling purulent rhinorrhea should always suggest the presence of a foreign body in the nose.

Epistaxis occurs frequently in children, mainly in the area of Kiesselbach's plexus. The primary etiology is nose picking. Upper respiratory infections predispose the child to epistaxis. Epistaxis may be impressive to the parents, but is rarely clinically significant. Treatment consists of pressing the lateral walls of the nose together at the septum to tamponade the bleeding. Topical decongestants are occasionally helpful. Subsequent treatment involves cool-mist humidifiers and the use of topical antibiotic ointment to aid in lubricating the septum and preventing drying. Occasionally careful, light cautery to the vessels may be necessary for persistent or recurrent epistaxis.

MOUTH AND FACE

The mouth and face have begun to form by the end of the eighth week of gestation. Initially the oral cavity and foregut are separated by the buccopharyngeal membrane, which ruptures at approximately the third or fourth week of gestation. The first branchial arch gives rise to the mandible and maxillary processes, and the maxillary processes give rise to the palate. The tongue is derived from the first, second, and third branchial arches. The salivary glands develop as outpouchings of the mouth.

The mouth is divided by the dental arches into two regions, the vestibule and the oral cavity. The vestibule is that region bounded laterally by the lips and cheeks and medially by the teeth. The oral cavity is bounded laterally and anteriorly by the teeth and posteriorly by the soft palate and base of the tongue. The tongue is divided into the body, or anterior third, and the base, or posterior two thirds. Major salivary glands are paired and include the parotid, submandibular, and sublingual glands. The mouth has multiple functions. It plays a major role in the production of speech and also is important in chewing and swallowing. Additionally the taste function is performed by areas of the tongue.

The major congenital defects of the mouth and face are cleft lip and palate, which are discussed on pp. 884-885. There are many congenital syndromes that involve the mouth and face. Treacher Collins syndrome includes lateral facial hypoplasia, micrognathia and a distinctive facial morphology, as well as hearing loss. Alpert syndrome consists of craniosynostosis and midface hypoplasia. In Crouzon syndrome craniosynostosis and midface hypoplasia are present. Pierre Robin syndrome includes micrognathia, cleft palate, and glossoptosis.

Intraoral abnormalities are legion and include a number of tumors of dental origin, mucous retention cysts, ranulas, and thyroglossal duct cysts.

Open-bite deformity in children may be caused by prolonged thumb sucking or tongue-thrusting. Ankyloglossia, or tongue tie, is significant only if the tongue cannot be protruded between the teeth; if it can, the child will be able to develop normal speech patterns. Surgical clipping of the tongue is rarely indicated. It may be performed as a simple office procedure.

Viral inflammatory lesions of the mouth are discussed elsewhere in this book. Aphthous stomatitis is of unknown etiology and runs its course in 7 to 10 days. There are usually one or sometimes more than one white ulcerated lesion that is extremely painful and may originate at the sight of local trauma. Moniliasis, or thrush, is discussed on p. 758.

Ludwig's angina is a severe cellulitis of the submental and submaxillary areas. This can develop quite rapidly and cause severe respiratory obstruction if not expertly managed. Initial treatment consists of intravenous antibiotics and surgical drainage, with tracheostomy needed in many cases. There are many other types of neck infections, most of which are secondary to infectious processes in the head and neck. Treatment consists of appropriate antibiotics and surgical drainage as indicated.

Masses of the salivary glands may be divided into firm masses, of which greater than 50% are malignant in children, and soft masses, of which the majority are hemangiomas or lymphangiomas. Factors that suggest malignant salivary gland masses are rapid growth, paresis or paralysis of the facial nerve, presence of pain, and radiologic evidence of erosion of bone.

The submandibular glands are much more likely to develop *stones* than are the parotid glands because the submandibular glands are located more dependently, have more alkaline secretions, have increased levels of calcium and phosphorus in the secretions, and have tortuous ducts. Stones that do not resolve on conservative treatment of warm saline oral rinses, sialagogues, systemic antibiotics, and intraoral opening of the submandibular duct, are best handled by a submandibular gland excision or superficial parotidectomy. Although the submandibular gland more commonly has stones, the parotid gland more commonly is infected. Treatment of this parotitis should be with good hydration and intravenous antibiotics to cover *Staphylococcus aureus*.

Sjögren disease consists of keratoconjunctivitis, xerostomia, and rheumatoid arthritis. It frequently presents with bilaterally enlarged parotid glands. *Sarcoidosis* can also produce enlarged parotid glands and, when the uvea of the eye is also involved, it is called *uveoparotid fever* or Heerfordt disease.

Sialorrhea is a condition in which there is a real or apparent overproduction of saliva. This is most commonly seen in children with diseases of the central nervous system. It usually responds well to surgical division of the tympanic branch of the ninth cranial nerve, along with division of the chorda tympani nerve in the middle ear. If these simple procedures fail to slow sialorrhea, the submandibular glands can be surgically removed and the parotid duct can be reimplanted in a more posterior position to encourage swallowing of the saliva.

Facial fractures occur fairly infrequently in children, probably because of the relatively small size of the facial bones when compared to the cranial vault. Another reason for fewer facial fractures is the lack of pneumatization of the maxillary bone. Treatment of the various facial fractures is very similar to that used in adults. However, the fractures must be manipulated within several days of injury, otherwise rapid healing will prevent the fracture sites from being moved into position. With any facial fracture there is always the danger of interruption of the growth of the involved bones and the development of facial asymmetry. Children 6 to 12 years of age are in a period of mixed dentition. Therefore, the traditional wiring into intermaxillary fixation is difficult if not impossible, and innovative measures must be used.

PHARYNX

Structure and function. The pharynx is derived from the proximal portion of the foregut and is connected to the mouth after the rupture of the buccopharyngeal membrane. It may be divided into three parts, the nasopharynx, oropharynx, and hypopharynx. The nasopharynx is that region between the base of the skull and the level of the soft palate. It communicates with the nasal cavity. The oropharynx begins at the level of the soft palate and continues to the level of approximately the tip of the hyoid bone. It is continuous anteriorly with the oral cavity, and the opening between the two is known as the fauces. The palatine tonsils lie on either side of the fauces. The hypopharynx is that region from the level of the hyoid bone down to include the pyriform and the esophageal introitus. The supporting musculature of the pharynx consists of the pharyngeal constrictors that meet posteriorly in the midline raphe.

The eustachinan tubes open into the nasopharynx through the torus tubaris. Active opening of the eustachian tube is accomplished by the tensor veli palatini muscle. Also in the nasopharynx is the adenoid tissue that arises from the superior and posterior walls. The anterior boundary of the oropharynx is somewhat vague, but in general the palatine tonsils are considered to be in the oropharynx. The base of the tongue is also part of the oropharynx, including the lingual tonsils, which are found on the surface of the base of the tongue.

The pharynx serves as a conduit for air and food and plays an important role in speech production. A patent nasopharynx is essential for proper eustachian tube function and therefore proper middle ear function and hearing. As swallowing occurs, the soft palate is moved posteriorly to seal off the pharynx and prevent regurgitation of food and liquid through the nose. This movement is also essential in the production of speech. The role of the palatine tonsils, adenoids, and lingual tonsils in immunology is still unclear. It is thought that they have some role in the development of the immunologic system during the first 12 to 18 months of life. After this stage, tonsillectomy has not been proved to cause any significant deficit in human immunology.

The pharynx may be examined by direct vision, and in cooperative patients further examination may be accomplished using indirect examination with mirrors. A recent development, the flexible nasopharyngoscope, allows thorough examination of the pharynx in uncooperative children in the office.

Velopharyngeal incompetence occurs when the soft palate is unable to seal off the nasopharynx. This occurs occasionally after tonsillectomy and adenoidectomy. It is more commonly seen in patients with cleft palate both before and after cleft palate repair. Speech therapy will usually overcome most of these problems, but occasionally surgical correction may be required, such as a posterior pharyngeal flap procedure.

Acute pharyngitis and acute tonsillitis are discussed on p. 379.

Peritonsillar abscess is discussed on p. 385.

Retropharyngeal abscess is discussed on p. 385.

Juvenile nasopharyngeal angiofibroma is a benign tumor seen exclusively in pubescent males. It manifests itself initially by nasal blockage with frequent and occasionally very severe episodes of epistaxis. The most appropriate treatment is surgical removal after embolization of the blood supply. Radiation therapy may be used alone or in combination with surgery.

Other benign tumors of the pharynx are rare.

Malignant tumors of the pharynx are relatively rare in children. Nasopharyngeal carcinoma usually has its initial manifestation as a metastatic lesion to the cervical lymph nodes. This malignancy is treated primarily with radiation therapy and has a better prognosis than the same tumor in an adult. Lymphomas are also seen in the lymphatic areas of the pharynx and neck, including the tonsils and cervical nodes.

LARYNX

Structure and function. The larynx develops as an outpouching of the pharynx called the laryngotracheal groove. Further differentiation gives rise to the vocal cords, arytenoid cartilages, and epiglottis. At birth, the larynx is approximately at the level of the second cervical vertebra. Shortly thereafter, the larynx begins to descend lower in the neck to arrive at the fifth to sixth cervical vertebra in the adult.

The larynx is a complex structure of cartilages, ligaments, muscles, and membranes. The cartilages are articulated at the cricothyroid joints and cricoarytenoid joints. Numerous small muscles provide the fine movement of the vocal cords in the larynx necessary for speech. The major motor innervation of the larynx is through the recurrent laryngeal nerves bilaterally. The left recurrent laryngeal nerve loops around the aorta and is a common site for injury during surgery on nearby structures or compression by intrathoracic lesions. A minor contribution to the motor innervation is from the superior laryngeal nerve.

Developmentally, the primary function of the larynx is to protect the airway. Production of speech is a secondary development. The complex set of muscles mentioned above act to abduct the vocal cords during inhalation and adduct the vocal cords during swallowing to prevent aspiration. Much more precise positioning of the vocal cords is possible during speech to allow the wide variation of pitch and volume. A unique function of the larynx is the ability to create a cough by allowing air pressure to build in the intrathoracic area.

Diagnosis. The larynx may be examined in selected children using the dental mirror or the flexible fiberoptic nasopharyngoscope. Frequently, children will have to be placed under general anesthesia for thorough examination of the larynx. The vocal cords and epiglottis may be examined under fluoroscopy. Barium swallow will give some information regarding laryngeal anatomy and physiology.

Laryngeal stridor, including larygomalacia and congenital subglottic stenosis, is discussed on p. 389.

Juvenile papilloma is the most common neoplasm in the pediatric larynx. The onset is usually at 2 to 5 years of age. It presents with hoarseness and airway obstruction. Repeated endoscopy and removal by surgical excision or laser excision is the treatment of choice. The use of interferon in laryngeal papillomas is being investigated and shows promise. Also, vaccine made from the patient's own excised papilloma has been used with varying results. Juvenile papillomas are thought to be of viral etiology, and there is a statistical correlation between vaginal condylomas in the mother and laryngeal papillomas in the child. Tracheostomy should be avoided if at all possible, since papillomas tend to grow toward the tracheostomy site.

Subglottic hemangioma presents with symptoms of airway obstruction and stridor. The diagnosis is made by laryngoscopy. No active treatment is indicated unless serious airway obstruction occurs, in which case tracheostomy may become necessary. Steroid therapy may be helpful. Radiation therapy will reduce the size of the mass, but the carcinogenic effects of radiation therapy constitute a hazard. Endoscopic laser removal may be effective in selected cases.

Vocal cord nodules are frequent causes of persistent hoarseness in children. They occur at the junction of the anterior and middle third of the vocal cords. They usually result from vocal abuse ("screamers' nodes"). Treatment involves intensive speech therapy and surgical removal in persistent cases.

Mucus retention cysts are sometimes found on the epiglottis or surrounding areas. These respond well to surgical removal, or incision and drainage with removal of a portion of the cyst wall.

Acute epiglottitis is also called acute supraglottitis. For discussion of this topic see p. 391.

Laryngotracheobronchitis (croup) is discussed on p. 393.

Acquired *subglottic stenosis* is a significant problem and is seen as a complication of long-term endotracheal intubation in children. Since the cricoid bone is the only complete ring of bone in the upper airway, any narrowing from edema or scar tissue in this area is critical. Treatment is similar to that of congenital subglottic stenosis, except progression of the symptoms is more common in acquired subglottic stenosis.

Laryngeal trauma may occur from external blunt trauma with fracture of the thyroid and cricoid cartilages and subsequent airway obstruction. These severe injuries are treated by tracheostomy and exploration of the larynx with stenting and repair of the injury as necessary.

HEAD AND NECK MASSES

Branchial cleft cysts, thyroglossal duct cysts, and cystic hygromas are seen fairly frequently. For discussion of these topics see pp. 885-886.

FOREIGN BODIES OF THE LARYNX, TRACHEA, AND BRONCHI

The art and science of bronchoesophagology was developed by Chevalier Jackson in the early part of this century. In his cases, the mortality of foreign body aspiration decreased from 24% to 2%. Of the foreign bodies ingested by children, about one third are aspirated and become lodged in the airway. Foreign bodies lodged in the larynx are primarily problems with children younger than 1 year of age. Foreign bodies that reach the bronchi lodge more often in the right main stem bronchus.

Initial symptoms are coughing, choking, gagging, and wheezing. Following these symptoms, a significant percentage of patients will be basically asymptomatic. Once the foreign body is lodged in the main stem bronchus, it will obstruct the lung or a lobe and will produce obstructive emphysema. This will appear as hyperinflation of the involved side on the chest x-ray. Chest radiographs taken at full inspiration and full expiration are helpful in diagnosis, but fluoroscopy is more precise.

Removal of foreign bodies is best performed in the operating room where complications can be handled if they occur. Rigid instrumentation is used for exposure, and specialized instruments allow atraumatic removal of most foreign bodies. Close cooperation must be maintained between the anesthesiologist and the surgeon.

FOREIGN BODIES OF THE PHARYNX AND ESOPHAGUS

Coins in the esophagus are the commonest foreign bodies in children in the United States. Less than 50% of those who have foreign bodies will have a good history of ingestion. Therefore a high index of suspicion is necessary to reach a proper diagnosis.

Blockage of the esophagus is strongly suggested by Jackson's sign, which is the inability to swallow one's own saliva. Most foreign bodies will pass through the esophagus. Obviously, the normal esophagus is less likely to become obstructed by a foreign body than is the esophagus with pre-existing pathology. Barium esophagram may be helpful in making the original diagnosis. Endoscopy and removal can usually be done on an elective basis rather than as an emergency procedure. Once the foreign body reaches the stomach it will usually pass through the digestive tract without incident.

Charles W. Gross
Ronald H. Kirkland

GENERAL REFERENCES

Bluestone, C.D., and Stool, S.: Pediatric otolaryngology, New York, 1983, W.B. Saunders Co.

English, G.M.: Otolaryngology, New York, 1982, Harper & Row.

Paparella, M.M., Shumrick, D.A.: Otolaryngology, New York, 1983, W.B. Saunders Co.

38 Laboratory Values—the Pediatric Range

The purpose of this section is to provide the clinician with a set of "panic" values and "expected" ranges for laboratory tests in the pediatric age group. The former are concerned with certain test results that have been associated with the presence of, or the propensity to contribute to, the development of life-threatening states, including cardiac dysrhythmias, coma, convulsions, cardiorespiratory arrest, or hemorrhage. The list of "expected" ranges has been compiled from studies on our own patient population and published data in which the method and reaction conditions, when described, most nearly approximate those currently in use in the pathology department at Le Bonheur Children's Medical Center (Memphis). Ideally, each laboratory should employ a similar process in establishing expected ranges for their physicians to use as guides. Therefore, before adopting these ranges for use we strongly suggest that they be reviewed by the clinical pathologist or laboratory director for possible substitutions that would more closely reflect the method, reaction conditions, or peculiarities of the patient population in a specific institution.

Caution. It is most important that such values be regarded as expected and not as unquestionable exact limits or indicators of normality. Consequently, any panic value or result outside the expected range for age, or seemingly spurious normal value, should be investigated for "goodness of fit." That is, does the result correlate with, or is it reinforced by, the physical findings, clinical course, the potential impact of concomitant or recent drug therapy, or the results of other laboratory parameters? This is the ultimate in quality control. The clinical pathologist may be helpful in assessing the "goodness of fit" by suggesting other laboratory tests to check the result. If the result remains suspect, then the pathologist or laboratory director and medical technologist should be asked to reinvestigate the testing procedure and repeat the studies, looking to exclude any element of imprecision or the presence of interfering endogenous or exogenous agents. Obviously, a cooperative and communicative effort among the medical technologist, pathologist, and clinician is essential to ensure proper interpretation and use of laboratory results.

"PANIC" LABORATORY VALUES

Alcohol
>300 mg/dl (Coma)
>400 mg/dl (Potentially fatal)

Ammonia
>Upper expected limit for age (refer to expected ranges)

Bilirubin
Neonatal unconjugated ≥12 mg/dl (i.e., total minus direct)

Bleeding time, Ivy
>9.5 minutes

Calcium
<Lower expected limit for age, or >upper expected limit for age (refer to expected ranges)

Carbon dioxide (CO_2 content)
<Lower expected limit for age, or >upper expected limit for age (refer to expected ranges)

Carbamazipine, tegretol
>8 μg/ml

CK isoenzymes
Sudden appearance of CK_2 (MB) relative to findings in previous specimens

Digoxin
>Upper therapeutic limit
<Lower therapeutic limit (refer to expected ranges)

Dilantin
>30 μg/ml

Free thyroxine index (FT_4I)
>Upper expected limit for age (refer to expected ranges)

Free triiodothyronine index (FT_3I)
>Upper expected limit for age (refer to expected ranges)

Glucose
<Lower expected limit for age (refer to expected ranges)
>500 mg/dl

Hematocrit
<20% or >70%
Hemoglobin
<7.0 g/dl or >25 g/dl
Lactic acid
>2.4 mEq/L
Magnesium
<1.2 mg/dl
>7.3 mg/dl
Osmolality, serum
<255 mOsmol
>325 mOsmol
Partial thromboplastin time, activated
>40 seconds
Phenobarbitol
>40 μg/ml
Phosphorus
≤2 mg/dl
Platelet estimate
<2.5/oif ≥50/oif
Platelet count
<50,000/mm³ ≥ 1,000,000/mm³
Potassium
<Lower expected limit for age
>Upper expected limit for age (refer to expected ranges)
Primadone
>12 μg/ml
Prothrombin time (PT)
>14.7 seconds
Pseudocholinesterase
<Lower expected limit for age (refer to expected ranges)
PT
See **Prothrombin time**
PTT
See **Partial thromboplastin time, activated**
RBC morphology
Drepanocytosis (sickle forms) in unsuspected or undiagnosed cases
Schistocytosis present on initial peripheral smear or developing subsequent to previous smears and reinforced by diminishing platelet count
Salicylate
>29 mg/dl
Sickle cell screen
Positive
Sodium
≤120 mEq/L
≥155 mEq/L
Theophylline
>20 μg/ml
Urinalysis
Color—gross hematuria
Glucose (dipstick) 2+ or greater
WBC
<500/mm³
>50,000/mm³
Absolute calculation of leukemic blast forms
Zarontin
>100 μg/ml

NORMAL LABORATORY VALUES

ABO isohemagglutinin titer
Method: Hemagglutination
Antibodies present in patients ≥6 months of age
Acetaminophen
Method: Enzyme immunoassay (refer to Fig. 38-1)
Acetone (qualitative)
Method: Sodium nitroprusside
None detected; negative
Acid phosphatase
Method: Thymolphthalein
Adult: 0-0.8 U/L
Pediatric range under development
Activated clotting time
Method: Whole blood clot with siliceous earth
<2 minutes, 10 seconds
Activated partial thromboplastin time (APTT)
Method: Fibrin strand detection (fibrinometer)
21.6-35.8 seconds
Albumin
Method: Bromcresol dye

Age	g/dl
Newborn, cord blood (S)	3.6-4.4
1 week, premature	3.3-4.0
1 week, full-term	3.0-5.1
Newborn	2.9-4.8
Infant	2.3-3.8
1 year, premature	3.7-4.4
1 year, full-term	4.5-4.8
3-5 years	3.8-5.0
5-8 years	3.7-4.8
8-14 years	3.8-5.8
14-16 years	4.0-6.0
16 years-adult	3.5-5.5
Adult	
Man	4.2-5.5
Woman	3.7-5.3

Alanine aminotransferase (A1AT)
Method: Wroblewski (pyruvate/LDH)

Age	U/L
Birth-3 days	1-25
6 months	25-33
6 months-1 year	16-36
1-5 years	7-23
6-15 years	2-15
Adult	4-35

Alcohol (serum, ethanol)
Method: Alcohol dehydrogenase

<50 mg/dl	Nonintoxication level
50-150 mg/dl	Questionable level
>150 mg/dl	Intoxication level

Aldolase
Method: Enzymatic
1-6 U/L (Adult), serum aldolase in the neonate is four times the adult activity and in children it is twice that of adults. Adult values are attained by the time the child reaches puberty.

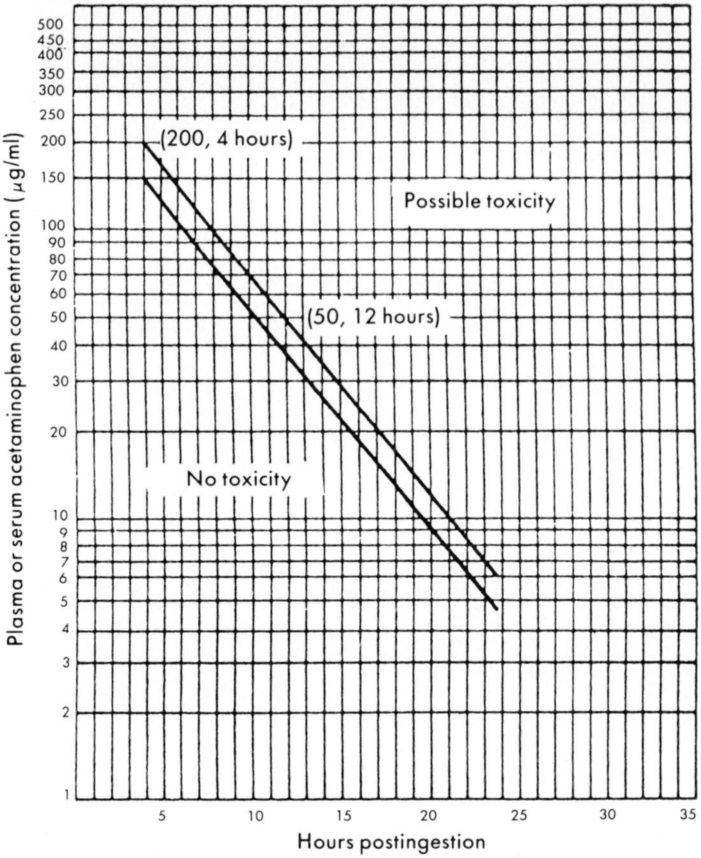

Fig. 38-1. Plasma or serum acetaminophen concentration compared to hours post ingestion.

Aldosterone

Method: RIA

Serum:

Age	Mean	2 SD*
0-1 year	43 ng/dl	5-132
1-4 years	26 ng/dl	5-60
4-8 years	19 ng/dl	4-76
8-12 years	10 ng/dl	3-28
12-16 years	9 ng/dl	1-18
Adult (supine)	2-9 ng/dl	

Urine:

0-3 weeks	6.4-37.5 μg/1.73m^2/day
Adult	2.0-11.8 μg/1.73m^2/day
Adult	
Normal salt diet	3-12 μg/1.73 m^2/day
Low-salt diet	3-5 times ad libitum salt diet

*Standard deviation.

Alkaline phosphatase

Method: Kinetic PNPP

Age		U/L
Cord blood		83-183
Newborn		62-368
6 weeks-18 months		118-354
18 months-3 years		81-339
3-10 years		108-295
10-11 years	Boys	75-347
	Girls	96-437
12-13 years	Boys	127-403
	Girls	92-336
13-14 years	Boys	100-420
	Girls	12-284
14-15 years	Boys	78-446
	Girls	78-212
15-16 years	Boys	43-267
	Girls	35-117
16-18 years	Boys	58-331
	Girls	35-124
Adult	Men	41-137
	Women	39-118

Table 38-1. Amino acid screen

AGE	TAUR	ASP	OH-PRO	THR	SER	GLU
Neonate	101-181	4-12	<80	196-238	129-197	27-77
Infant		15-23	<50	105-249		
9 months-2 years	19-91	0-9		33-128	24-172	
2-12 years	57-115	4-20		42-177	79-112	23-250
Adult	27-168	0-24	≦10	79-246	67-129	14-192
AGE	**$ASPNH_2$ + $GLUNH_2$**	**PRO**	**GLY**	**ALA**	**CIT**	**VAL**
Neonate	623-895	151-215	274-412	274-384		97-175
Infant		93-293	143-283	186-398		85-237
9 months-2 years	46-290	51-185	56-308	99-313		57-262
2-12 years	57-467	68-148	117-285	137-343		128-283
Adult	413-690	100-442	120-553	209-659	5-53	116-315
AGE	**½ CYS**	**MET**	**CYSTA**	**ILEU**	**LEU**	**TYR**
Neonate	49-75	21-37		31-47	55-89	53-87
Infant	24-60	12-24		23-55	55-119	12-96
9 months-2 years		3-29		26-94	45-155	11-112
2-12 years	30-77	10-22		28-84	56-178	31-71
Adult	48-114	6-39	10	35-97	71-175	21-87
AGE	**B-ALA**	**PHE**	**BAIB**	**HOMOCYS**	**E + $OHNH_2$**	**ORN**
Neonate		64-92				66-116
Infant		35-75				28-72
9 months-2 years		23-69				10-107
2-12 years		26-61				27-86
Adult	25-73	27-115		<50	<16	29-125
AGE	**LYS**	**HIS**	**ARG**	**TRY**		
Neonate	154-246	61-93	37-71	15-49		
Infant	79-191	50-106	44-80			
9 months-2 years	45-144	24-112	11-65			
2-12 years	71-170	24-106	23-117			
Adult	82-321	31-106	10-137	19-45		

Alkaline phosphatase isoenzyme
Method: Cellulose acetate electrophoresis
Refer to pathologist's interpretation

Alpha 1 acid glycoprotein
Method: Nephelometric
30-135 mg/dl

Alpha 1 antitrypsin
Method: Nephelometric
85-213 mg/dl

Alpha fetoprotein screen
Method: Ouchterlony
Negative

Alpha galactosidase
Method: Fluorescence enzyme assay
11-24 nmole/hr/ml plasma
0%-35% heat stability

Alpha 2 macroglobulin
Method: Nephelometric
146-369 mg/dl

Amikacin
Method: Enzyme immunoassay
Peak: 15-25 μg/ml
Trough: <6 μg/ml

Amino acid screen
Method—Ion-exchange chromatography
Plasma (quantitative): expressed in μmoles/L

Amino acid screen—cont'd
Urine (quantitative): Abnormal findings generally 3 to 1000 times normal
Pattern of increase interpreted by pathologist (see Table 38-1)

Ammonia
Method: Glutamate dehydrogenase

Age	μmole/L	
Newborn	64-107	(higher in premature and jaundiced infants)
0-2 weeks	55-90	
1 month	20-55	
Infant to child	29-57	
Adult	13-34	

Amylase
Method—Maltopentase (kinetic)
Serum: 23-85 U/L (Adult)
Pediatric: Newborns' serum shows little, if any activity. Measurable activity appears at approximately 2 months of age. Much of this activity is of salivary origin until after the first year of life.

Amylase—cont'd

Urine

Amylase/creatinine clearance ratio	1.3%-4.3%
Amylase/urine creatinine ratio	
Boys	0.06-0.20 U/mg
Girls	0.07-0.32 U/mg
Amylase/2 hours	4.00-37 U/2 hours

Anion gap

Na-(Cl + CO_2)

5-18

Anti-DNASE B

Method: Enzyme inhibition

Preschool children	60 units
School-age children	170 units
Adults	85 units

Anti-nDNA antibody

Method: Indirect fluorescence assay

<1:20

Antinuclear antibody titer (ANA)

Method: Indirect fluorescence assay

<1:20

Antistreptolysin O (ASO)

Method: Enzyme inhibition

School-age children	≦166 Todd units
Preschool children and adults	≦100 Todd units

Antithrombin III

Method: Thrombin/DTNB

Newborn, premature	20%-50% NHP
Newborn, full-term	30%-90% NHP
0-6 months	40%-90% NHP
6 months-adult	80%-120% NHP

Anti-thyroid antibody panel

Method: RIA/paper chromatography

Antithyroglobulin, adult and children: Less than 10 μ/ml

Antithyroid microsomal antibody, adult and children: less than 25 μ/ml

Ascorbic acid

Method:

Serum: Spectrophotometric

WBC: Spectrophotometric/colorimetric DNPH

Serum: 0.4-1.5 mg/dl

WBC:

Boys	4.9-14.9 μg/10^8 WBC
Girls	3.7-24.1 μg/10^8 WBC

ASO

See Antistreptolysin O titer

Aspartate aminotransferase (AspAT)

Method: Pyridoxal-5-phosphate

Age	U/L
Cord	22.0-37.8
Newborn	18-74
Infant	up to 67
18 months-5 years	16-46
5 years-8 years	20-45
8 years-12 years	15-40
12 years-14 years	15-35
14 years-16 years	15-30
Adult	
Men	8-46
Women	7-34

Autoimmune antibody test (collagen-tissue)

Method: Indirect fluorescence assay

<1:20

B-HCG

Method: RIA

Sensitivity of test: 40 mIU/ml

Bile acids (conjugated bile acids)

Method: RIA

<6 μmol/L (fasting)

Bilirubin, direct (conjugated)

Method: Diazo salt

Newborn	<1.5 mg/dl
1 month-adult	0-0.4 mg/dl

Bilirubin, total

Method: Diazo salt

Age	Premature	Full-term
	mg/dl	mg/dl
0-24 hours	1-6	2-6
24-48 hours	6-8	6-7
3-5 days	10-12	4-6
1 month-adult	up to 1.5	

Bleeding time (Ivy)

Method: Simplate method

2.0-9.5 minutes

Blood gas

Method: Electrodes (pH, P_{CO_2}, P_{O_2})

(see Table 38-2)

Bone marrow

Method: Microscopic

Myeloblasts	0.3-5	Rubriblast	0.2-8
Progran	0.5-8	Prorub	0-5.8
Myelo	5-19	Rub	5-34
Meta	5.6-34	Metarub	1.6-21.5
Band	6.1-36	Lymph	3-36
Seg	5-32	Monos	0-6
Eos	1-9	Plasmacytes	0.3-2
Basos	0-5.5		

BUN (blood urea nitrogen)

Method: Urease (conductivity rate)

Age	mg/dl
Cord	5-11
<2 months	4-15
2 months-adult	5-23
1 year-2 years	5-15
Child-adult	6-20

BUN/creatinine ratio

6-20

Calcitonin

Method: RIA

Less than 150 pg/ml (fasting)

Calcitriol

Method: Competitive protein binding

Children (6-17 yrs)	16-64 pg/ml
Adult (20-50 yrs)	26-44 pg/ml

Table 38-2. Blood gas

Parameter	Age	Source of blood	Range
pH	Newborn	Arterialized capillary; arterial	7.33-7.49
	2 months-1 year	Arterialized capillary; arterial	7.34-7.46
	Child and adult	Arterialized capillary; arterial	
		Male	7.35-7.45
		Female	7.36-7.44
		Venous	7.32-7.42
P_{CO_2}	Newborn	Arterialized capillary; arterial	26.8-40.4
	2 months-2 years	Arterialized capillary; arterial	26.4-41.2
	Child and adult	Arterialized capillary; arterial	
		Male	36.2-46.2
		Female	33.1-43.2
		Venous	40-50
P_{O_2}	Newborn	Arterial	60-76
	Child and adult	Arterial	80-105
		Venous	25-47

Calcium, total (corrected for albumin)
Method: Cresolphthalein complexone
Serum:

Age	mg/dl
Premature first week	6.0-10.0*
Full-term first week	7.0-12.0*
To 2 years	8.8-11.2
2-16 years	8.6-11.0
16 years-adult	9.0-11.0

Urine:

4-12 years	80-160 mg/24 hours
Adults	≦8.4 mg/kg body weight per 24 hours

Calcium/creatinine ratio (fasting urine): <0.21

Calcium, ionized
Method: Specific ion electrode
Children and adults 4.00-4.72 mg/dl

Carbamazepine (Tegretol)
Method: Enzyme immunoassay
4-8 μg/ml

Carbon dioxide (CO_2)
Method: Rate change of pH

Age	mEq/L
Cord blood	15.0-20.2
Child	18-27
Adult	24-35

Carcinoembryonic antigen (CEA)
Method: CEA (Abbott) RIA; CEA (Roche) EIA

CEA (Abbott)	Adults	0-3.0 ng/ml
CEA (Roche)	Adults	0-2.5 ng/ml

Carotene
Method: Spectrophotometric
50-250 μg/dl

*Due to low albumin level in newborns up to 1 week, these are not corrected for albumin.

Catecholamines (total)
Method: RIA

Age	pg/ml
0-20 years	550-2000
21-40 years	800-2900
41-60 years	1000-3800
61-80 years	1300-5300

Catecholamines (fractionated)
Method: RIA

Age	Epinephrine pg/ml	Norepinephrine pg/ml
0-20 years	<200	550-2000
21-40 years	<200	800-2900
41-60 years	<200	1000-3800
61-80 years	<200	1300-5300

Catecholamines, urine (total)
Method: Bertler Crout/fluorometric

Age	μg/24 hrs
Birth-1 year	4-20
1-5 years	5-40
6-15 years	5-80
Over 15 years	20-100
Adult	Less than 100

CBC
Method: Profile (automated laser analyzer); Differentiation (manual microscope) (see Table 38-3)

Cell count, CSF
Method: Microscopic
RBC 0
WBC

0-10 days	0-32 cells/mm^3
Under 1 year	0-10 cells/mm^3
1-4 years	0-8 cells/mm^3
Over 5 years	0-5 cells/mm^3

Ceruloplasmin
Method: Nephelometric
18-45 mg/dl

***Chlamydia* titer (FA)**
Method: Fluorometric antibody (must be correlated with clinical state)

Table 38-3. Expected CBC values

Parameter	Birth	1 month	3-12 months	13 months-2 years	3-8 years	9-14 years	15 years-adult	
							Male	Female
WBC × 10^3/mm^3	9.0-30 (18.1)	5.0-19.5 (10.8)	4.7-14.0 (9.4)	3.7-12.9 (8.3)	3.6-11.8 (7.7)	4.6-9.4 (7.0)	4.5-11.0 (7.1)	4.5-11.0 (7.1)
RBC × 10^6/mm^3	5.0-6.3 (5.6)	3.4-4.6 (4.0)	4.0-5.6 (4.8)	4.0-5.5 (4.7)	4.1-5.5 (4.8)	4.1-5.7 (4.9)	4.3-5.9 (5.1)	3.5-5.5 (4.5)
Hb g/dl	19.0-19.5 (19.2)	12.1-16.3 (14.2)	10.7-14.3 (12.5)	9.6-15.4 (12.5)	11.4-15.4 (13.4)	11.2-16.3 (13.8)	13.9-16.3 (15.1)	12.0-15.0 (13.5)
HCT %	53-65 (59)	37.3-48.7 (43)	31.4-41.8 (36.6)	31.5-42.3 (36.9)	33.4-45.1 (39.2)	32.9-48.0 (40.4)	39-55 (47)	36-48 (42)
MCV μ^3	95-115 (105)	97.5-112.5 (105)	64.7-89.3 (77)	67.1-89.2 (78.1)	74.2-88.8 (81.5)	71.5-93.2 (82.4)	80-100 (90)	79-98 (88)
MCH $\mu\mu$ g	30-42 (36)	30-42 (36)	21.6-31.5 (26.5)	22.5-30.7 (26.6)	25.2-30.2 (28.0)	24.6-32.0 (28.3)	25.4-34.6 (30)	25.4-34.6 (30)
MCHC %	32-34 (33)	31.9-35.1 (33.5)	30.3-37.6 (34.0)	31.4-36.6 (34.0)	31.8-36.7 (34.3)	32.3-36.1 (34.2)	31-37 (34)	30-36 (33)
PLATELETS × 10^3/mm^3	140-290	200-370	200-470	250-450	250-470	140-450	140-450	140-450
BANDS* %	10.1-18 (14.1)	6.5-12.5 (9.5)	0-16.1 (4.9)	0-15 (4.6)	0-19.5 (6.3)	0-27.7 (8.5)	0-13.8 (5.4)	
SEGS* %	32-62 (47)	15-35 (25)	0-44.6 (21.4)	0-48.3 (23.5)	6.2-55.8 (31.0)	9.4-66.2 (37.8)	22.6-58.2 (40.4)	
LYMPHS %	26-36 (31)	41-71 (56)	38.2-92.2 (65.2)	35.3-89.3 (62.3)	26.9-78.1 (52.5)	15.2-73.6 (44.4)	26.2-65.0 (45.6)	
MONOS %	3-11	—	0-13.8 (6.4)	0-11.4 (5.6)	0-10.6 (5.0)	0-9.5 (4.5)	0-10.0 (4.6)	
EOS %	0-6	—	0-6.7 (2.1)	0-9.7 (3.3)	0-12.4 (4.2)	0-11.6 (4.0)	0-12.3 (4.3)	
BASOS %	0-2	—	0-1.5 (0.3)	0-2.4 (0.6)	0-2.6 (0.8)	0-3.1 (1.1)	0-1.3 (0.3)	

*These ranges are based on the classification of Miale, in which the neutrophil is classified as a band as long as there is visible chromatin between nuclear membranes. The diagnostic utility of this classification is currently under review and reconsideration.

Number in parentheses is the mean for that range.

Chloramphenicol

Method: HPLC

Peak	15-25 μg/ml
Trough	5-15 μg/ml

Chloride

Method: Coulometric titration

Serum

Age	mEq/L
Newborn	96-106
Child-adult	95-105

Sweat

<8 days	23-61
"Child"	Up to 50
<17 years	7-52 (mean 23)
17-21 years	8-53 (mean 27)
>21 years	9-72 (mean 31)

Urine (24 hr volume)

	mEq/24 hr
Infant	1.7-8.5
Child	17.0-34.0
Adult	140-240

CSF

	mEq/L
Child-adult	120-128

Cholesterol

Method: Enzymatic cholesterol oxidase/cholesterol esterase

Age	mg/dl
Premature cord blood	47-98
Full-term cord blood	45-98
3 days-1 year	69-175
1-20 years	120-230
20-29 years	120-240
30-39 years	140-270
40-49 years	150-310
50 years and older	160-330

CIE

Method: Countercurrent immunoelectrophoresis

No antigen detected

Cold agglutinin titer

Method: Tube dilution

≦1:16

Complement C-3

Method: Nephelometric

80-140 mg/dl

Complement C-4

Method: Nephelometric

15-45 mg/dl

Complement CH-50 (CH^{100})
Method: Radial diffusion
25-85 CH^{100} units/ml

Complement fixation
Method: Complement fixation
Titer of <1:4 in absence of disease

Compound S, direct (following metopirone)
Method: RIA
>5 μg/dl

Compound S, specific
Method: RIA
Adult and child: Less than 120 ng/dl

Copper
Method: Atomic absorption spectrophotometry
0.4-1.4 mg/dl

Cortisol
Method: RIA
Serum:

	(μg/dl) Male		(μg/dl) Female	
Age	**Mean**	**2 SD**	**Mean**	**2 SD**
Less than 6 years	11.3	7.5-17	7.7	5-11
6-8 years	7.4	5-10.5	9.3	7-13
9-10 years	6.1	4-9	10.0	9-14
10-12 years	5.7	4-8	7.8	5.5-11
12-14 years	10.1	7.5-13.5	9.8	7-14
Over 14 years	7.6	4-16	12.6	4-19
Adult: AM	7-18			
PM	2-9			

Urine (free):

Age	μg/24 hr Mean	2 SD
Normal children	41	18-64
Obese children	24	11-67
Children under stress	99	28-170

CK (creatine kinase)
Method: Oliver (HK/G-6-PDH)

Age	U/L
Premature	0-120
Birth-3 weeks	22-267
3 weeks-3 months	15-134
3-9 months	9-97
9 months-1 year	0-47
1-3 years	0-91
3-6 years	4-88
6-15 years	4-87
Adult men	30-210
Adult women	20-128

CK isoenzymes
Method: Cellulose acetate electrophoresis
Cord blood and neonate: CK_3 and possibly CK_2 and CK_1
Adult
CK_3 (96-100%)
CK_2 (0-4%)
CK_1 (0%)
Refer to pathologist's interpretation

C-Reactive protein (CRP)
Method: Precipitation
Negative

Creatinine
Method: Alkaline picrate
Serum

Age (years)	Male (mg/dl)	Female (mg/dl)
1	≦0.6	≦0.5
2-3	≦0.7	≦0.6
4-7	≦0.8	≦0.7
8-10	≦0.9	≦0.8
11-12	≦1.0	≦0.9
13-17	≦1.2	≦1.1
18-20	≦1.3	≦1.1
Adult	0.5-1.4	

Urine (as 24-hour clearance):

Age	ml/min/standard surface area
Premature and newborn	40-65
6 months	75
12 months and over	100
18 months and over	
Boys	98-150
Girls	95-122
Adult	
Men	91-119
Women	77-113

Cryoglobulin
Method: Precipitation
Negative

Cryptococcal antigen
Method: Latex agglutination
Negative

Digoxin
Method: RIA
Newborn and infant 2-4 ng/ml
Child-adult 1-2 ng/ml

Dilantin
See **Phenytoin**

Direct antigen detection
Method: Immunofluorescence
Negative

D-Xylose absorption (1 hour)
Method: *p*-Bromaniline on whole blood
1 hour D-xylose: Less than 6 months, >15 mgm/dL; over 6 months, >20 mgm/dL

Entamobea histolytica
Method: CIE
Negative

Eosinophil count (total)
Method: Microscopic (Unopette)
Newborn-24 hours: 20-850/mm^3
1 year: 50-700/mm^3
Adults: 0-450/mm^3

Eosinophil, nasal smear
Method: Hansel stain/microscopic
0 or none seen

Epinephrine stimulation
Method: Differential (pre- and postepinephrine injection)
Total PMN count >45% over baseline values

Epstein-Barr viral capsid antigen antibody (GAM)
Method: Indirect fluorescence
<1:10 in the absence of infection or prior history of infection

Epstein-Barr viral capsid antigen antibody (IgM)
Method: Indirect fluorescence
<1:10 in the absence of infection or prior history of infection

ESR (erythrocyte sedimentation rate)
Method: Wintrobe
Children 0-13 mm/hr
Men 0-10 mm/hr
Women 0-20 mm/hr

Essential fatty acid deficiency
Method: Gas chromatography
Ratio $\begin{bmatrix} 20:3 & W9 \\ 20:4 & W6 \end{bmatrix} \leqq 0.4$

Estrogen
Method:
Serum: RIA
Urine: Chromatographic/fluorometric
Serum (total):
Adult women:

Early follicular phase:	70-400 pg/ml
Late follicular phase:	100-900 pg/ml
Luteal phase:	70-700 pg/ml
Adult men:	130 pg/mL or less

Urine (total):
Nonpregnant women:

Onset of menstruation:	4-25 μg/24 hrs
Ovulation peak:	28-99 μg/24 hrs
Luteal phase:	22-105 μg/24 hrs
Adult men:	5-18 μg/24 hrs

Ethosuximide (Zarontin)
Method: Enzyme Immunoassay
40-100 μg/ml

Factor VIII antigen
Method: Cross immunoelectrophoresis
63%-153%

FA-*Chlamydia*
Method: Fluorescent antibody
Must be correlated with clinical state

FA-pertussis
Method: Fluorescent antibody
Bordetella species: Negative

FDP (fibrin degradation products)
Method: Rapid latex agglutination
Serum: 4.9 ± 2.8 μg/ml
Urine: <0.25 μg/ml

Febrile agglutinins
Method: Latex agglutination
Febrile antigens 2+ reaction at 1:80 or higher dilution of their homologous positive control sera; negative control should be negative always

Fecal fat (72-hour quantitative)
Method: Saponification/titration
Up to 7 g/24 hr

F_ENa (excreted fraction of filtered sodium)
Less than 1 indicates prerenal azotemia
Greater than 3 indicates acute tubular necrosis

Ferric chloride
Method: Qualitative colorimetric
Negative

Ferritin
Method: RIA

Age		ng/ml
6 months-15 years		7-142
18 years-45 years	Men	36-255
	Women	10-64
45 years-older	Men	42-262
	Women	24-155

Fibrinogen
Method: Turbidimetric rate
Child-adult: 200-400 mg/dl

Folate
Method: Competitive protein binding
Serum

Children-adults:	4-25 ng/ml
Suggestive of deficiency:	3-4 ng/ml
Folate deficiency:	<3 ng/ml

RBC: 200-800 ng/ml of packed RBCs

Free erythrocyte protoporphyrin
Method: Fluorometric/extraction
0-50 μg/dl Blood or ≦160 μg/dl RBC

Free fatty acids
Method: Novak-Cobalt nitrate*
Newborns: 0-1845 μEq/L
All others: 215-875 μEq/L

Fructose tolerance
Method: Glucose (glucose oxidase); phosphorus (phosphomolylodate [UV])
Small but definite rise in plasma glucose; a small, short-lived fall in phosphorus concentration

FSH (follicle-stimulating hormone)
Method: RIA
Serum
Prepubertal children, boys and girls <5 mIU/mL
Adults
Women: 2-25 mIU/ml (except at midcycle peak)
Men: 2-20 mIU/ml
Urine
Male: 2-12 IU/24 hrs
Female
Menstrual cycle: 8-60 IU/24 hrs
Ovulatory phase: 30-60 IU/24 hrs

Fungal immunodiffusion
Method: Immunodiffusion
No bands present in absence of infection or no prior history of infection

Galactose-1-phosphate uridyl transferase
Method: NAD (UV rate)
15-33 U/g Hb (based on simultaneously assayed controls)

---

*After >10- and ≦12-hour food fast.

Gamma GT
Method: Szasz (GG-P-nitroanilide)

Age	U/L
Premature	56-233
Birth-3 weeks	0-103
1-3 days	13-198
3 weeks-6 months	4-111
6 months-5 years	0-23
6-15 years	0-23
16 years-adult	
Men	9-69
Women	3-33

Gamma GT isoenzymes
Method: Cellulose acetate electrophoresis
Fractions 2 and 3
Refer to pathologist's interpretation

Gastrin
Method: RIA

Age	(pg/mL) Mean	2 SD
Newborn	130	119-141
Prepubertal and pubertal children		
Fasting 3-4 hours	59	9-109
Fasting 5-6 hours	42	8-76
Fasting 8 hours or more	23	0-47
Adults (fasting)	Less than 100 pg/mL	

Gentamicin
Method: Enzyme immunoassay
Peak: 5-10 μg/ml
Trough: <2.0 μg/ml

Glucose
Method: Glucose oxidase
Serum

Newborn, premature	20-80 mg/dl
Newborn, full-term	20-90 mg/dl
0-2 years	60-110 mg/dl
Child-adult	60-115 mg/dl

Urine: Child-adult up to 0.5 gm/day
CSF: 50%-80% of Blood glucose

Glucose quotient: $\frac{\text{CSF glucose}}{\text{Serum glucose}} = \geqq 0.5$

Glucose tolerance: Refer to Figs. 38-2 and 38-3.

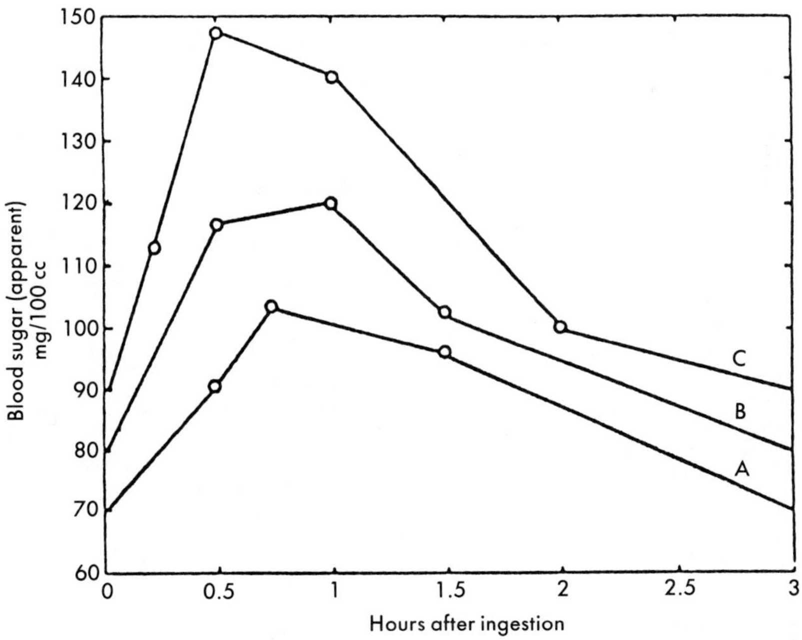

Fig. 38-2. Oral glucose tolerance test with use of capillary blood. Normal responses in children of different ages to standard test doses. *A*, Newborn; *B*, from 1 month through 5 years; *C*, more than 5 years. (From Behrendt, H.: Diagnostic tests in infants and children, ed. 2, Philadelphia, 1962, Lea & Febiger, pp. 53-55.)

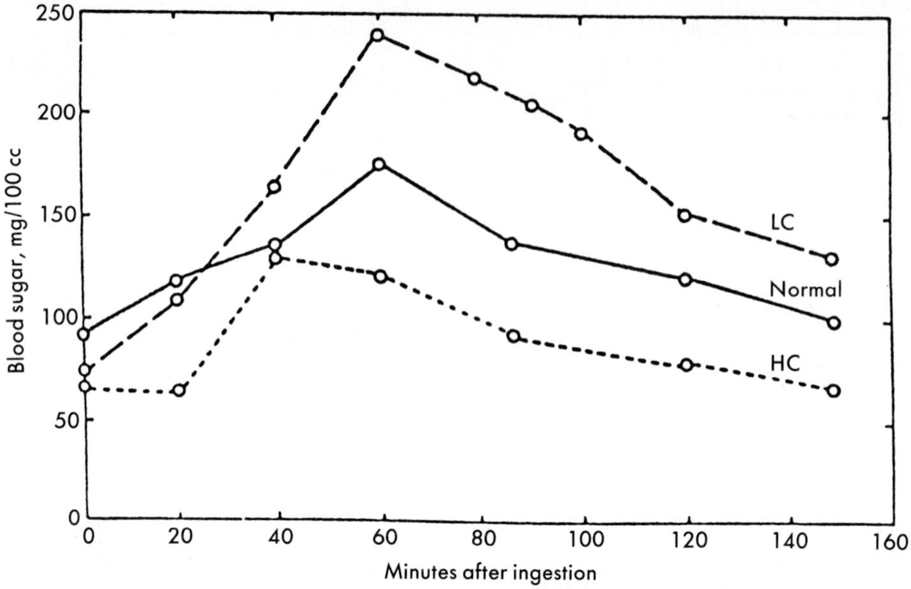

Fig. 38-3. Effect of diet on oral glucose tolerance test in normal child. Tolerance curves obtained during normal dietary regimen after low carbohydrate (LC) regimen of 3 weeks and a 5-day period of regular diet with daily addition of 150 g of glucose (HC). (From Ross, C.W.: Impaired glucose tolerance in certain alimentary disorders of children, Lancet **2**:556, 1936.)

Glucose 6-phosphate dehydrogenase (G6-PD)
Method: Fluorometric
146-376 Units/trillion RBC

Glutathione reductase
Method: GSSG (kinetic enzyme)
2.6-6.3 IU/gm Hb (no FAD added)
4.6-7.9 IU/gm Hb (FAD added)

Guaiac
Method: ColoScreen
Negative

HAA (hepatitis B surface antigen)
Method: RIA
Nonreactive

Haptoglobin
Method: Nephelometric
27-139 mg/dl

HDL cholesterol
Method: Electrophoresis
Refer to pathologist's interpretation

Hemoglobin A_1C (glycosylated Hb)
Method: Cation exchange chromatography
Child: 3.83%-7.87%
Adult: 5.85%-8.85%

Hemoglobin electrophoresis
Method: Cellulose acetate and citrate agar electrophoresis
Refer to pathologist's interpretation

Hexosaminidase, A
Method: Calculated from TOTAL-isoenzyme
51% of total hexosaminidase value

Hexosaminidase, total
Method: Fluorometric
1260-3475 nmole/ml/hr

HGPRT/APRT
Method: Radioenzymatic
Based on simultaneously assayed controls

Homocysteine screen
Method: Qualitative colorimetric
Negative

Homogentisic acid
Method: Gas chromotography
Negative

Human growth hormone
Method: RIA

Age	**Mean** (ng/mL)	**2 SD**
4 hrs after birth	32	20-44
1 day	22	18-26
3 days	16	14-18
4 days	18	15-21
5 days	12	10-14
6 days	13	11-15
7 days	13	11-15
Children	2-5	
Adults	<10	

Table 38-4 Immunoglobulins (A, M, G)

	IgA	IgM male	IgM female	IgG
Birth	0-8	0-23	0-23	800-1792
1 month	4-21	17-67	22-85	513-1182
2 months	8-55	23-89	29-114	313-827
3 months	13-71	26-106	33-136	261-687
4 months	15-84	28-117	36-150	244-661
5 months	15-88	30-123	39-157	261-713
6 months	17-95	32-128	40-164	278-766
7 months	17-105	33-134	43-171	305-809
8 months	19-109	35-140	44-178	322-879
9 months	19-120	36-145	46-185	365-948
10 months	21-126	36-150	47-192	392-1027
11 months	23-137	38-156	49-200	426-1122
1 year	25-158	39-156	50-200	452-1192
2 years	34-168	47-184	61-236	539-1401
3 years	40-235	51-201	66-257	600-1575
4 years	46-288	53-201	67-257	626-1653
5 years	59-328	54-201	68-257	661-1749
6 years	65-368	54-201	68-257	687-1879
7 years	69-393	54-201	68-257	713-1905
8 years	76-420	54-202	68-257	722-1940
9 years	84-445	54-203	68-258	740-2001
10 years	92-473	54-206	68-260	748-2001
11 years	95-498	54-209	68-264	748-2001
12 years	97-525	54-212	68-267	748-2001
13 years	99-550	54-217	70-271	748-2001
14 years	103-578	56-223	71-278	748-2001
15 years	105-603	56-233	71-285	748-2001
Adult	113-563	54-222	62-250	800-1801

17-Hydroxycorticosteroids (urine)
Method: Spectrophotometric

Age	mg/dL
0-2 weeks	0.05-0.3
2 weeks-1 year	0.10-0.5
1-3 years	0.5-1.0
3-6 years	0.6-1.8
6-9 years	0.9-3.3
9-12 years	1.2-5.2
12-16 years	
Boys	2.0-6.0
Girls	2.8-6.8
16-20 years	
Boys	3.0-10.0
Girls	2.0-7.0
Adults	
Men	5.0-10.0
Women	3.0-7.0

p-Hydroxyphenyl compounds
Method: Qualitative colorimetric
Negative

Immunoelectrophoresis
Method: Agarose electrophoresis
Refer to pathologist's interpretation

Immunoglobulins (A, M, G)
Method: Nephelometric (expressed in mg/dL) (see Table 38-4)

Immunoglobulin (IgE), prist
Method: RIA

Age	U/ml
1 year	0-58
2 years	0-61
3 years	0-61
4 years	0-70
5 years	0-221
6 years	0-221
7 years	0-221
8 years	0-337
9 years	0-337
10 years	0-337
11 years	0-187
12 years	0-187
13 years	0-187
14 years	0-187
Adult	0-150

Inborn error screen
Refer to individual components of the battery; reducing substances SC, mucopolysaccharide SC, amino acid SC, ketoacid SC, and *p*-hydroxy compounds

Indirect immunofluorescence for cytomegalovirus (CMV)

Method: Indirect immunofluorescence

<1:16 In the absence of infection or prior history of infection

Insulin

Method: RIA

Adult (fasting): Less than 20 μU/mL

Iron

Method: Bathophenan-throline

Age	μg/dl
Newborn	110-270
4-10 months	30-70
3-10 years	53-151
Adult	72-186

Iron-binding capacity (total)

Method: Bathophenan-throline/$MgCO_3$

Age	μg/dl
Newborn	59-175
3-10 years	250-400
Adult	250-400

Percent of saturation: 20%-50%

Joint aspiration

Method: Microscopic

Clarity:	Clear
Color:	Pale yellow; colorless
Mucin clot:	Compact large clot, suspended in clear supernatant, clot does not break up when tube is shaken
Viscosity:	String; 2.5 cm 4 cm long
Fibrin clot:	No clotting
WBC:	<200/mm^3
RBC:	None

Keto acid screen

Method: Qualitative colorimetric

Negative

Newborns may have moderate increase

Keto acid fractionation

Method: TLC

Small amounts of alpha-ketoglutaric and pyruvic acid (newborns exhibit excretion of pyruvic, alpha-ketoglutaric, and acetoacetic acids)

17-Ketosteroids (total), urine

Method: Zimmerman spectrophotometric

Age	mg/day (Male and female)
0-14 days	up to 1.0
2 weeks-2 years	0.0-0.5
1-3 years	<2.0
2-6 years	0-2.0
3-6 years	0.5-3.0
6-8 years	0.0-2.5
6-9 years	0.8-4.0
8-10 years	0.7-4.0
9-12 years	2.0-6.0

17-Ketosteroids (total), urine—cont'd

	Male	Female
10-12 years	0.7-6.0	0.7-5.0
12-14 years	1.3-10.0	1.3-8.5
12-16 years	3.0-12.0	3.0-14
16-20 years	5-21	4-18
Adult	7-23	5-15

Lactic acid

Method: Enzymatic (lactate-pyruvate)

Venous blood (plasma): 0.5-2.0 mEq/L

CSF: 0.9-2.8 mEq/L

Lactose tolerance

Method: Glucose-glucose oxidase

Serum: Increase of ≥20 mg/dl (as blood glucose) from fasting value

Method: Reducing substance—Clinitest pH—pH stick

Stool: Reducing substance (0-trace)

In 3-7 days old infant: 2+, 3+, 4+

pH: 7.0-7.5

LD (lactate dehydrogenase)

Method: Wacker (lactate-pyruvate)

Serum:

Age	U/L
Newborn	≥500
6 weeks-18 months	208-473
18 months-3 years	249-403
3-8 years	191-381
8-11 years	187-325
11-14 years	144-316
14-16 years	129-279
Adult	99-207

CSF:

≤1 week	22-73
>1 week	17-59

LD isoenzymes

Method: Cellulose acetate electrophoresis

LD isoenzymes 3 and 4, and in some cases 5, are higher in cord blood and infants during the first week of life (particularly days 1-3) than in older infants and children.

Refer to pathologist's interpretation.

L.E. preparation

Method: Microscopic (clot tube)

Negative

***Leptospira* antibodies**

Method: Latex agglutination

Negative

Lesch-Nyhan screen (urinary uric acid/creatinine ratio)

Method: Uric acid (uricase); creatinine (alkaline picrate)

Birth-6 months	0.2-2.9
6 months-2 years	0.5-2.5
2-4 years	0.6-1.8
6-8 years	0.3-1.5
8-10 years	0.3-1.3
12-18 years	0.4-0.7

Lipase
Method: Turbidimetric
4-24 U/dl

Lipid profile and lipoprotein electrophoresis
Method: Lipoprotein (cellulose acetate electrophoresis)

Lipoprotein	Relative %
Chrylomicrons	0%-2%
Beta	45%-56%
Prebeta	12%-21%
Alpha	28%-40%

See individual tests for cholesterol, triglyceride, and FFA.
Refer to pathologist's interpretation.

Long-acting thyroid stimulating hormone (LATS)
Method: RIA
None detected

Luteinizing hormone (LH)
Method: RIA
Serum
Prepubertal children, boys and girls: Less than 5 mIU/ml
Adult women: 2-25 mIU/ml (except at midcycle point)
Adult men: 2-20 mIU/ml
Urine
Prepubertal children (1-10 years):

Boys (IU/24 hours)	Girls (IU/24 hours)
<1.0-5.6 (Mean = 2.9)	1.4-4.9 (Mean = 2.7)

Puberty (see Table 38-5)

Magnesium
Method: Methylthymol blue
Serum:

Age	mg/dl
Birth	1.65-1.77
Newborn	2.1-2.9
Child	1.8-2.3
Adult	1.74-2.4

Urine
Infant and children: 0.9-5.2 mg/kg/day

Methyl malonic acid
Method: Qualitative colorimetric
Negative

Mono test
Method: Hemagglutination
Negative

Mucopolysaccharide, screen
Method: Dye binding
Negative (<2 mg/dl)

Mucopolysaccharide, quantitative
Method: Colorimetric/CPC precipitation

Age	mg glucuronic acid / mg creatinine
Birth-1 year	10-50
1-2 years	7-22
2-6 years	5-20
6-20 years	Upper limit declines to adult value of 4

Mysoline
See **Primidone**

Nonessential, essential amino acids
Method: Quantitative amino acid analyzer (Ninhydrin colorimetry)
≤0.5 Ratio of

$$\frac{\text{Glycine} + \text{Serine} + \text{Glutamine} + \text{Taurine}}{\text{Leucine} + \text{Isoleucine} + \text{Valine} + \text{Methionine}}$$

Nucleated red blood cells
Method: Microscopic

Age	Expressed per 100 nucleated cells
Birth-1 day	1-5
2 days	2
1 week-adult	0

5′ Nucleotidase
Method: Enzymatic
0-11 U/L (adult)

Table 38-5. Luteinizing hormone (LH)

Tanner stage	Boys		Girls	
	Age (years)	LH (IU/24 hours)	Age (years)	LH (IU/24 hours)
1	<9.8	1-5 (Mean = 2.3)	<9.2	1-5 (Mean = 3.4)
2	9.8-14.5	1.5-11 (Mean = 4.2)	9.2-13.7	3-10 (Mean = 7.0)
3	10.7-15.4	2.5-13 (Mean = 6.5)	10.0-14.4	5-18 (Mean = 10.1)
4	11.8-16.2	5-16 (Mean = 11)	10.7-15.6	6-21 (Mean = 13.5)
5	12.8-17.3	4-28 (Mean = 16)	11.8-18.6	5-24 (Mean = 14.3)
Adult:		9-23		4-30

Osmolality
Method: Vapor pressure osmometry
Serum:

Age	mOsmol
1 day	266-299
2 day	258-289
5 day-adult	270-285

Urine
Maximal (dehydration): 800-1400
Minimal (water diuresis): 40-80

Parathyroid hormone (C-terminal)
Method: RIA
Adults: 40-100 μlEq/ml
Measured as immunoreactive parathyroid hormone:

0.5-6 years	22 μlEq/ml (nondetectable-56)
6-12 years	16 μlEq/ml (nondetectable-34)
12-20 years	20 μlEq/ml (nondetectable-44)
Adult	22 μlEq/ml (nondetectable-44)

Pentobarbital
Method: HPLC
Peak: 20-40 μg/ml (Barbiturate coma)

Pertussis (FA)
Method: Fluorescent antibody
Bordetella species, negative

pH (stool)
Method: Dipstick
7.0-7.5

Phenobarbital
Method: Enzyme immunoassay
15-40 μg/ml

Phenylalanine
Method: Fluorometric
1.1-3.1 mg/dl

Phenytoin (Dilantin)
Method-Enzyme immunoassay
10-20 μgm/ml

Phosphorus
Method: Phosphomolybdate (UV)

Age	mg/dl
Cord blood	4.8-6.2
Premature	
Birth	5.6-8.0
6-10 days	6.0-11.7
20-25 days	6.6-9.4
Full term	
Birth	5.0-7.8
3 days	5.8-9.0
6-12 days	4.9-8.9
Newborn	4.2-9.0
6 weeks-18 months	3.8-6.7
18 months-3 years	2.9-5.9
3-15 years	3.6-5.6
15-16 years	2.4-5.4
Adult	2.5-5.1

Phytanic acid
Method: Gas chromatography
<0.3% Normal control

Plasminogen
Method: Streptokinase
Adult: 73%-122% NHP

Porphyrin, qualitative
Method: Fluorometric
Negative

Porphyrin, quantitative
Method: Chromatography/spectrophotometry
Coproporphyrins: <160 μg/24 hrs
Uroporphyrins: <30 μg/24 hrs

Potassium
Method: Ion specific electrode
Plasma:

Age	mEq/L
Premature	4.5-7.2
Full-term	5.0-7.5
2 days-3 months	4.0-6.2
3 months-1 year	3.7-5.6
1-16 years	3.5-5.0

Urine: 25-120 mEq/24 hrs

Pregnancy test (slide and tube)
Method: Passive hemagglutination inhibition
Men and nonpregnant women: Negative
Pregnant women: Positive

Primidone (mysoline)
Method: Enzyme immunoassay
5-12 μg/ml

Progesterone
Method: RIA
(see Table 38-6)

Prolactin
Method: RIA

Age	Mean (ng/ml)	2 SD
1 day	278	160-396
3 days	204	138-270
4 days	114	53-175
5 days	82	46-118
4 weeks	87	29-145
6 weeks	17	9-23
1 year	10	6-14
2-12 years	5	3.8-6.2
13-16 years	6	3.8-8.2
Adults	<20 ng/ml	

Protein
Method:
Serum: Biuret
CSF: Turbidimetric (trichloroacetic acid)
Urine: Turbidimetric (sulfosalicylic acid)
Serum:

Age	gm/dl
Cord blood	4.78-8.04
Birth	4.6-7.0
1 week	4.4-7.6
2 weeks-1 month	4.4-7.6
1 month-3 months	3.64-7.38
3 months-4 months	4.2-7.4
4 months-6 months	4.29-6.10
7 months-1 year	5.10-7.31
1 year-2 years	3.69-7.50
2 years-3 years	6.38-8.06
3 years-5 years	4.88-8.06
6 years-8 years	5.97-7.94
9 years-11 years	5.97-7.94
12 years-16 years	5.97-7.94
Adult	6.44-8.32

Table 38-6. Progesterone

Age	Male		Female	
	Mean (ng/dl)	**2 SD**	**Mean (ng/dl)**	**2 SD**
Cord blood	363	281-445	178	131-225
1 Day	13	10-16	12	9-15
7 Days	0.5	0.4-0.6	0.5	0.4-0.6
1 week-9 years	Less than 30		Less than 30	
9-11 years	34	29-39		
10 years			23	18-33
11 years			34	22-46
12 years	40	20-45	26	23-30
13 years	33	20-37	33	25-41
14 years	34	21-37	18	12-24
15-18 years	56	30-64		
Adults	<25 ng/dl		<100 ng/dl (Follicular phase) >400 ng/dl (Luteal phase)	

Table 38-7 Protein electrophoresis

Age	TP*	Albumin	Alpha$_1$	Alpha$_2$	Beta	Gamma
Cord blood	4.78-8.04	2.17-4.04	0.25-0.66	0.44-0.94	0.42-1.56	0.81-1.61
At birth	4.6-7.0	3.2-4.8	0.1-0.3	0.2-0.3	0.3-0.6	0.6-1.2
1 week	4.4-7.6	2.9-5.5	0.09-0.25	0.3-0.46	0.16-0.6	0.35-1.3
2 weeks-1 month	4.4-7.6	2.5-4.0	0.09-0.25	0.3-1.0	0.4-1.1	0.4-1.3
1-3 months	3.64-7.38	2.05-4.46	0.08-0.43	0.4-1.13	0.39-1.14	0.25-1.05
3-4 months	4.2-7.4	2.8-5.0	0.07-0.39	0.31-0.83	0.31-0.83	0.11-0.75
4-6 months	4.29-6.10	3.17-3.88	0.12-0.25	0.52-0.84	0.44-0.76	0.24-0.90
7 months-1 year	5.10-7.31	3.22-4.31	0.15-0.55	0.78-1.46	0.63-0.91	0.32-1.18
1-2 years	3.69-7.50	1.89-5.03	0.09-0.58	0.41-1.36	0.36-1.41	0.36-1.62
2-3 years	6.38-8.06	3.57-5.50	0.19-0.26	0.68-1.09	0.47-1.09	0.73-1.46
3-5 years	4.88-8.06	2.93-5.21	0.08-0.4	0.43-0.99	0.47-1.01	0.54-1.66
6-8 years	5.97-7.94	3.26-4.95	0.09-0.45	0.50-0.83	0.45-0.93	0.70-1.95
9-11 years	5.97-7.94	3.16-4.97	0.12-0.38	0.7-0.87	0.63-1.02	0.79-2.03
12-16 years	5.97-7.94	3.19-5.13	0.09-0.32	0.5-0.97	0.48-0.88	1.08-1.96
Adult	6.44-8.32	3.46-4.78	0.16-0.30	0.51-0.86	0.59-1.06	0.68-2.11

*All ranges are in g/dl

Protein—cont'd

CSF:

Age	mg/dl
Premature (at birth)	50-200
Full-term (at birth)	40-120
Newborn (≤1 month)	<80
>1 month	15-40
Child-adult	15-45

Urine:

Random <10 mg/dl
First AM 15-20 mg/dl
24 hours 50-100 mg/m^2 of body surface per day in patient >1 year old

Protein electrophoresis

Method: Cellulose acetate
Refer to pathologist's interpretation
(see Table 38-7)

Prothrombin time

Method: Fibrin strand detection
10.7-13.9 seconds

Pseudocholinesterase

Method: Ellman (butyrlthiocholine)
Newborn, full-term (0-5 days): 0-20.2 U/ml
Adults: 7-19 U/ml

Pyridoxine index

Method: Kinetic enzymatic

$$\text{Index of AspAT} = \frac{\text{With pyridoxal } PO_4}{\text{Without pyridoxal } PO_4} < 1.36$$

Pyruvate

Method: Photometric
0.36-0.59 mg/dl

Pyruvate kinase

Method: Kinetic enzymatic
1.9-5.2 IU/gHb

R.A. test
Method: Latex agglutination
Negative

Reducing substances, stool
Method: Clinitest, Benedict's copper reduction
3-7 Days: 2+ to 4+
>7 Days: None detected

Reducing sugar
Screen: Negative
Chromatography: Refer to the qualitative description

Renin
Method: RIA
Children*

Age	Mean ng/ml/hour	2 SD
First week	18	13-23
2-4 weeks	74	54-94
3 months-1 year	<15	
1-4 years	<10	
4-15 years	<6	
Adults (normal sodium diet):		
Supine:	1.6	0.1-3.1
Standing:	4.5	1.6-7.4

Reticulocyte count
Method: Microscopic/new methylene blue

Birth-1 week	2.0%-6.0%
2-4 weeks	0.3%-1.6%
1-6 months	0%-2.8%
6 months-6 years	0%-1.8%
7 years-adult	0.5%-1.5%

Riboflavin index
Method: Kinetic enzymatic

$$\text{Index of } \frac{\text{Glutathione reductase} + \text{FAD}}{\text{Glutathione reductase} - \text{FAD}} < 1.84$$

Rotavirus antigen detection
Method: Enzyme immunoassay
Negative

RPR
Method: Flocculation
Nonreactive

Rubindex
Method: Hemagglutination/inhibition
<1:8 In the absence of infection or with no prior history of infection

Salicylate
Method: Ferric complex
Therapeutic: 2-29 mg/dl
Lethal: >70 mg/dl

Sedimentation rate
See ESR

Selenium index
Method: Kinetic enzymatic
105-195 μg/g Hb

Sickle cell screen
Method: Tube solubility
Negative

*Samples from patients over 1 year of age are from subjects on "normal" salt intake, who were supine for a 2-hour rest between 9 AM and 11 AM.

Sodium
Method: Ion-specific electrode

	Age	mEq/L
Plasma:	Premature	132-142
	Full-term	132-142
	Child	136-142
	Adult	135-145
Urine:	Infant	0.3-3.5 mEq/24 hr
	Child	40-180 mEq/24 hr
	Adult	80-200 mEq/24 hr

Streptozyme
Method: Slide agglutination
≤200 STZ units

Sucrose tolerance
Method
Serum: Glucose oxidase
Stool: Acid/clinitest
Serum: Increase of 20 mg/dl (as glucose) over baseline
Stool: Reducing substance
Prehydrolysis (0-trace) 3-7 days: 2+ to 4+
Posthydrolysis (0-trace) 3-7 days: 2+ or greater

T_3
Method: RIA

Age	T_3RIA (ng/dl)	FT_3I
Cord	14-86	10.3-90.5
1-3 days	100-470	90.1-661.9
6 days-1 year	90-300	
1-12 months	105-245	84.0-269.2
1-5 years	105-269	84.0-295.6
5-10 years	94-241	75.2-264.8
10-15 years	83-213	66.4-234.1
>15 years	80-210	
15-20 years	80-210	64.0-230.8
Adult	70-204	59.3-234.5

T_4 (free)
Method: Dialysis
Children and adults: 1.3-3.8 ng/dl

Tegretol
See **Carbamazepine**

Testosterone
Method: RIA
Prepubertal children (boys and girls): <50 ng/dl until Tanner stage II
Adult
Women: <70 ng/dl
Men: >280 ng/dl
NOTE: Age and Tanner stage normal values for pubertal children are being developed

Theophylline
Method: Enzyme immunoassay
Apnea of newborn: 6-11 μg/ml
Asthma: 10-20 μg/ml

Thrombin clotting time
Method: Fibrinometer (fibrin strand detection)
5.7-11 seconds

Thyroglobulin
Method: RIA

Age	Mean (ng/ml)	2 SD
Term infants		
Cord blood	24	5-65
1 day	41	6-93
3 days	50	9-148
Premature infants		
27-31 weeks		
1 day	251	107-395
10 days	106	49-163
30 days	40	17-63
31-34 weeks		
1 day	212	147-277
10 days	72	32-112
30 days	35	19-51
Children		
7-12 years	35	20-50
13-18 years	18	9-27
Adults*	4.1	0-9.6

*In a study of 78 normal adults, 87% had values less than 10 ng/ml, 8% had values 11-20 ng/ml, and 5% had values 21-30 ng/ml.

Thyroid profile
Method: RIA
Cholesterol: See individual test

Age	T_4 (μg/dl)	FT_4I	T_3BI*
Cord	7.3-15.3	5.5-16.1	0.95-1.33
1-3 days	10.1-20.9	9.1-29.3	0.71-1.11
1-2 weeks	9.8-16.6	8.3-19.1	0.87-1.18
2-4 weeks	8.2-16.6	6.6-18.3	0.91-1.25
1-4 months	7.1-15.0	5.3-15.8	0.95-1.33
4 months-1 year	5.5-13.5	4.4-14.9	0.91-1.25
1-6 years	5.6-12.6	4.5-13.9	0.91-1.25
6-10 years	4.9-11.7	3.9-12.9	0.91-1.25
10-16 years	3.8-10.6	3.0-11.7	0.91-1.25
16-20 years	4.1-10.9	3.3-12.0	0.91-1.25
Adult	4.7-11.1	4.0-12.8	0.87-1.18

*T_3 Binding index.

Age	TBG* (μg/ml)
Cord	19.0-39.0
1 day-1 week	14.0-41.0
1-4 weeks	15.0-39.0
1-12 months	22.0-42.0
1-5 years	15.0-36.0
5-10 years	14.0-30.0
10 years-adult	12.0-30.0

*Thyroxine-binding globulin.

Tobramycin
Method: Enzyme immunoassay
Peak: 5-10 μg/ml
Trough: <2 μg/ml

Toxoplasma gondii
Method: Indirect fluorescence
<1:16 in the absence of infection or prior history of infection

Transferrin
Method: Nephelometric
190-290 mg/dl

Triglyceride
Method: Enzymatic

Age	mg/dl
Premature-29 years	20-150
30-39 years	20-160
40-49 years	20-170
>50 years	20-220

Trypsin, stool
Method: X-ray digestion
Activity: >1:10 (NOTE: Invalid above 4 years)

TSH (thyroid-stimulating hormone)
Method: RIA

Age	μU/ml
Cord blood	3-22
1-3 days	<40
3-7 days	<25
Over 7 days	0-10

TRP (tubular reabsorption of phosphorus)
Method: PO_4-Phosphomolybdate; creatinine-alkaline picrate
78%-97%

Tyrosinase
Method: Qualitative microscopic
May be negative or positive; refer to laboratory director's comments

Tyrosine
Method: Fluorometric
0.6-2.1 mg/dl

Uric acid
Method: Uricase

Age	mg/dl
Child	2.0-5.5
Adult man	3.0-7.0
Adult woman	2.0-6.0

Urinalysis
Method: Multi-Stix/microscopic
Color and clarity: Light yellow-amber/clear-slight hazy
Specific gravity: 1.002-1.030
pH: 5.0-8.0
Protein: Negative
Glucose: Negative
Ketone: Negative
Bilirubin: Negative
Blood: Negative
Nitrate: Negative
Urobilinogen: 0.1-1.0 Ehrlich units/dl
Reducing substance: Negative

Urinalysis—cont'd
Microscopic:
WBC: <5/HPF
RBC: <5/HPF
Cast: Occasional hyaline
Epithelial: Few
Bacteria: None

Urine drug screen (Toxi-lab)
Method: Modified thin layer chromatography
None detected

Urine output (24-hour volume)
NOTE: Test is intake dependent

Age		Volume (ml)
Newborn		19-51
1 month-1 year		25-150
1-5 years		70-300
3-6 years		100-580
3-10 years		100-600
5-10 years		175-835
10-12 years	Boys	315-1305
	Girls	325-1150
13-16 years	Boys	500-1675
	Girls	665-1305
17-20 years	Boys	1175-2000
	Girls	885-1545
Adult	Men	1385-2300
	Women	715-1615

Valproic acid
Method: Enzyme immunoassay
50-100 μg/ml

Vancomycin
Method: RIA
Peak: 15-25 μg/ml
Trough: <12 μg/ml

Vasopressin
Method: RIA
Plasma: Children and adults—random hydration
0.4-5.3 μU/ml

Vitamin A (total)
Method: Fluorometric/extraction
47-113 μg/dl

Vitamin B_{12}
Method: RIA
200-1000 pg/ml
Definite deficiency: <100 pg/ml
Probable deficiency: 100-140 pg/ml
Possible deficiency: 140-200 pg/ml

Vitamin C (ascorbate)
Method:
Serum: Colorimetric (DNPH)
Urine: Dip Stick
WBC: Colorimetric (DNPH)
Serum: 0.4-1.5 mg/dl
Urine: Negative (<0.5 mg/dl)
WBC:
Male 4.9-14.9 g/10^8 WBC
Female 3.7-24.1 g/10^8 WBC

Vitamin E (free)
Method: HPLC
Child (1-12 years): 4-7 μg/ml
Adults: 4-24 μg/ml

D-Xylose absorption (1 hour)
Method: p-Bromaniline on whole blood
1 Hour D-xylose: Less than 6 months, >15 mgm/dL; over 6 months, >20 mgm/dL

Zarontin
See Ethosuximide

Zinc
Method: Colorimetric
0.82-1.29 mg/dl

R.E. Brown
Sheon Lynch

REFERENCES

Albritton, E.C., editor: Standard values in blood, Philadelphia, 1952, W.B. Saunders Co.

Conrath, T.B., editor: Handbook of microtiter procedures, Cambridge, Mass., 1972, Dynatech Corp.

Consolidated Biomedical Laboratories: Reference ranges, 1983, Columbus, Ohio.

Davidsohn, I., and Henry, J.B.: Todd and Sanford's Clinical diagnosis by laboratory methods, eds. 15, 16, Philadelphia, 1974, 1979, W.B. Saunders Co.

Documenta Geigy: Scientific tables, ed. 6. Summit, N.J., 1962.

E.I. Dupont de Nemours & Co., Inc.: ACA III-chemistry instruction manual, Wilmington, Del., 1981.

Endocrine Sciences: Pediatric Laboratory Services, Tarzana, Calif., 1981.

Friedman, R.B., et al.: Effects of disease on clinical laboratory tests, Clin. Chem. **26**(4):1D-476D, 1980.

Fudenberg, H.H., et al., editors: Basic and clinical immunology, ed. 2, Los Altos, Calif., 1978, Lange Medical Publications.

Grist, N.R., et al.: Diagnostic methods in clinical virology, ed. 3, Oxford, 1979, Blackwell Scientific Publications.

Helgeson, N.G.P., et al.: Laboratory medicine, vol. 2, Chap. 29, New York, 1977, Harper & Row, Publishers, Inc.

Hyland: Product insert, Round Lake, Ill., 1979.

Jones, P.G., and Campbell, P.E., editors: Tumours of infancy and childhood, Oxford, 1976, Blackwell Scientific Publications.

Lancer: Acetaminophen product insert, St. Louis, 1981.

Le Bonheur Children's Medical Center: Control Population, Memphis, 1983.

Lennette, E.H., and Schmidt, N. J., editors: Diagnostic procedures for viral rickettsial and chlamydial infections, ed.5, Washington, D.C., 1979, American Public Health Association.

Meites, S., editor: Pediatric clinical chemistry: a survey of normals, methods, and instrumentation with commentary, Washington, D.C., 1977, American Association for Clinical Chemistry.

Meites, S., editor: Pediatric clinical chemistry: a survey of reference (normal) values, methods, and instrumentation with commentary, ed. 2, Washington, D.C., 1981, American Association for Clinical Chemistry.

Miale, J.B.: Laboratory medicine—Hematology, ed. 6, St. Louis, 1982, The C.V. Mosby Co.

Nichols Institute: Pediatric program catalogue, Los Angeles, 1982.

Pathologist's Service Professional Associates, Inc.: Service manual, ed. 7, Tucker, Ga., 1982.

Race, G.J., editor: Laboratory medicine, vol. 4, New York, 1977, Harper & Row, Publishers, Inc.

Rose, N.R., and Friedman, H., editors: Manual of clinical immunology, ed. 2, Washington, D.C., 1980, American Society for Microbiology.

Taylor, W.J., editor: Individualizing drug therapy, New York, 1981, Gross, Townsend, Frank, Inc.

Tietz, N., editor: Fundamentals of clinical chemistry, Philadelphia, 1976, W.B. Saunders Co.

Williams, W.J. et al., editors: Hematology, ed. 2, New York, 1977, McGraw-Hill Book Co.

Wintrobe, M.M.: Clinical hematology, ed. 5, Philadelphia, 1961, Lea & Febiger.

Young, D.S., et al.: Effects of drugs on clinical laboratory tests, Clin. Chem. **21**(5):1D-432D, 1975.

Appendix A

Nomogram for estimation of surface area

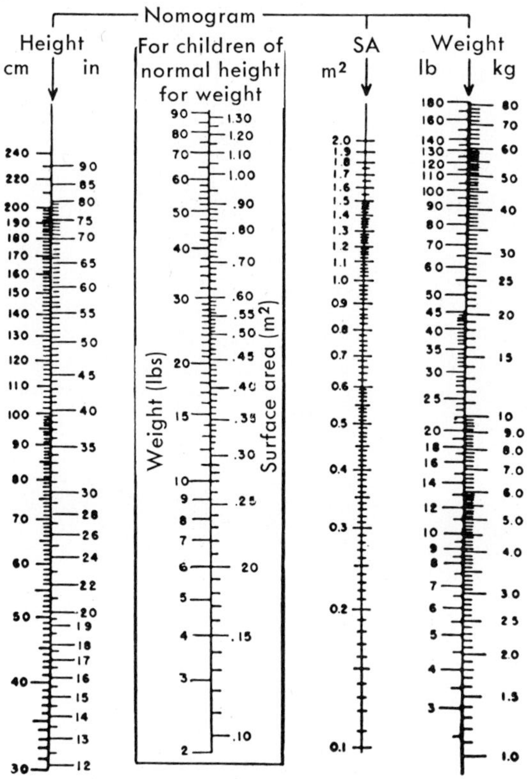

Surface area is indicated when a straight line that connects the height and weight levels intersects the surface area column, or if the patient is roughly of average size from the weight alone (enclosed area). (Modified from data of E. Boyd by C.D. West; from Shirkey, H.C.: Drug therapy. In Vaughan, V.C., III, and McKay, R.J.: Nelson textbook of pediatrics, ed. 10, Philadelphia, 1975, W. B. Saunders Co.)

Appendix B

Relations between body weight in pounds, body surface area, and adult dosage

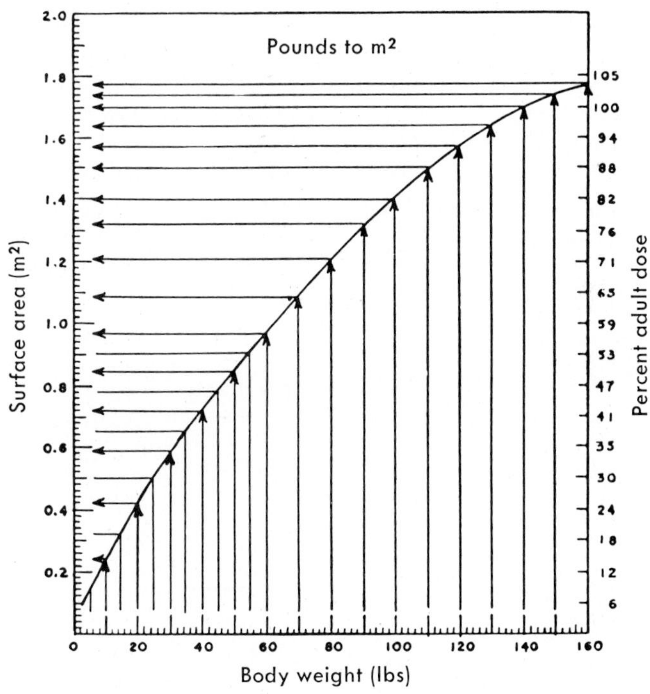

Note that the 100% adult dose is for a person weighing about 140 pounds and having a surface area of about 1.7m². (From Talbot, N.B., Richie, R.H., Crawford, J.D., and Tagrin, E.S.: Metabolic homeostasis—a syllabus for those concerned with the care of patients, Cambridge, Mass., 1959, Harvard University Press.)

Appendix C

Acid-base nomogram*

Base excess is calculated from the alignment nomogram (Sigaard-Anderson). The computation of base excess is possible when hemoglobin concentration and any two of the following parameters are known: blood pH, PCO_2 plasma bicarbonate, or total carbon dioxide content of plasma. The variables most commonly used in newborn laboratories are pH and PCO_2.

Assume that an infant in rather severe respiratory distress is admitted to your facility. Blood samples are collected soon after admission, and the following information is forwarded to you:

pH = 7.10 (normal = 7.35 to 7.44)
PCO_2 = 75 torr (normal = 30 to 37 torr)
Hemoglobin = 20 g/100 ml

The values for pH and PCO_2 are plotted on their appropriate scales at points *A* and *B*, as shown on the nomogram on p. 1025. A line is drawn through points *A* and *B* across all four scales. The base excess is read at minus 10 mEq/L at point *C*, where the drawn line intersects a grid line representing hemoglobin concentration of 20 g/100 ml. The plasma bicarbonate concentration can now also be read at 23 mEq/L. If only the pH and bicarbonate are known (as well as the hemoglobin concentration), base excess and PCO_2 can be derived by drawing a line through points corresponding to the known values.

*From Korones, S.B.: High-risk newborn infants: the basis for intensive nursing care, ed. 3, St. Louis, 1981, The C.V. Mosby Co.; illustration adapted from Winters, R.W., Engel, K., and Dell, R.B.: Acid-base physiology in medicine, Cleveland, 1967, The London Co.

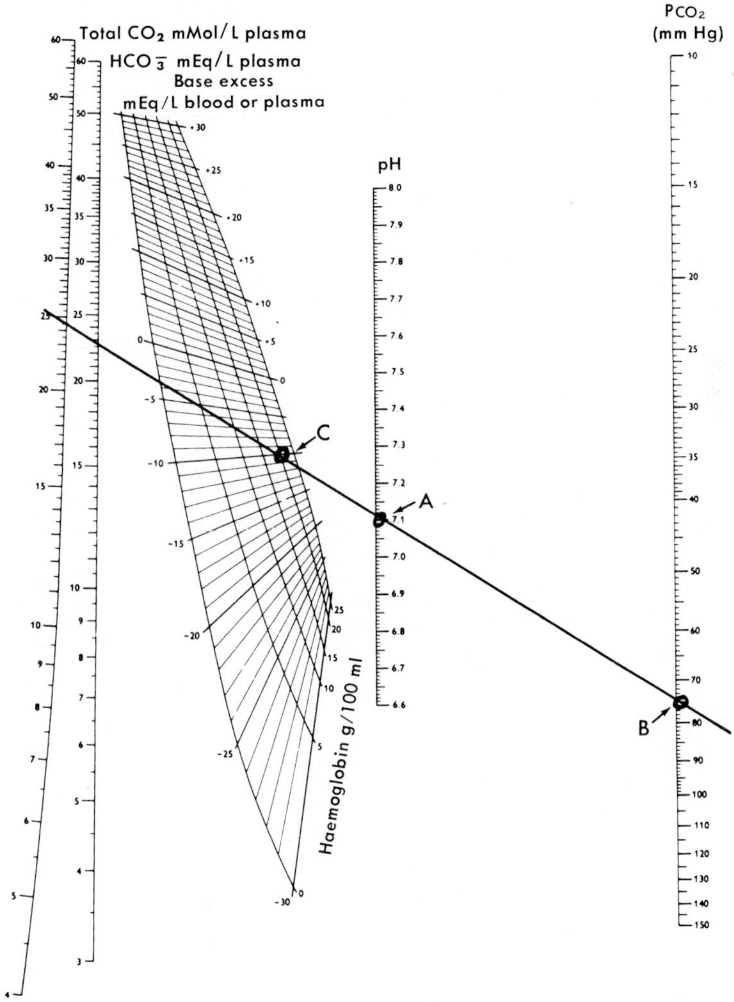
Total CO_2 mMol/L plasma
HCO_3^- mEq/L plasma
Base excess
mEq/L blood or plasma
pH
P_{CO_2}
(mm Hg)
Haemoglobin g/100 ml
A
B
C

Index

B

D

O

W